THE

NEW

GOOD

HOUSEKEEPING

FAMILY

HEALTH

AND

MEDICAL

GUIDE

THE NEW GOOD HOUSEKEEPING FAMILY HEALTH AND MEDICAL GUIDE

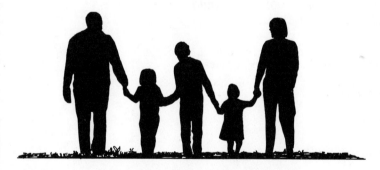

HEARST BOOKS · NEW YORK

Library of Congress Cataloging-in-Publication Data

The New Good housekeeping family health and medical
    guide.

    Rev. ed. of: Good housekeeping family health &
medical guide. c1980.
    1. Medicine, Popular.   I. Good housekeeping
(New York, N.Y.)   II. Good housekeeping family health
& medical guide.
RC81.G628   1989   613   88-11257
ISBN 0-688-06164-8

Printed in the United States of America

Revised Edition

    3 4 5 6 7 8 9 10

BOOK DESIGN BY BARBARA MARKS

CONTENTS

Good Housekeeping Staff

Editor-in-chief   John Mack Carter
Executive editor   Mina W. Mulvey
Institute director Mary E. Powers

Editorial Staff, Revised Edition

Dorsey W. Woodson, editorial manager; Millie
Poliakoff, managing editor; Pia MacDermott, Se-
nior Living editor; Adell Lubell, Wellness editor;
Sally Urang, R.N., Elise Parker, R.N., Family Medicine
and Health editors; Howard R. Goldsweig, M.D.,
Charlene Laino, Forrest V. Perrin, Beth Goldin,
R.N., Medical A to Z editors; Cynthia Pollock, First
Aid editor; Moira Duggan, copy editor; Colonel
R. M. Youngson, M.D., special medical consultant;
Amy Gash, project editor; Ann Bramson, executive
editor, Hearst Books.

The publishers are grateful to the following individuals and companies for assistance in preparation
of this book:

Richard Bonson, who drew many of the illustrations throughout the book and also produced all
the full-color artwork.

Dr. Ian Starke and Dr. Grahame Howard for help
with text for the full-color illustrations, and Sally
Walters for picture research on the full-color
illustrations.

Medtronic (U.K.), Ltd.; Technicon Instruments Co.,
Ltd.; EMI Medical, Ltd.; Philips Medical Systems; and
GEC Medical Equipment, Ltd., for technical assis-
tance in preparing certain illustrations.

Several illustrations in the full-color section on
the immune system are based on drawings in
Immunology II by Joseph A. Bellanti; this is by kind
permission of the publishers, W. B. Saunders
Company, Philadelphia, PA.

National Council of State Emergency Medical
Training Coordinators, Inc., and New York City
Emergency Medical Service Training Academy, who
served as consultants on the **First Aid** section.

Marion Laboratories for the table on "Calcium
and Caloric Content of Various Foods."

Height and Weight Tables courtesy Metropolitan
Life Insurance Company.

Contributors to First Edition

Graham H. Barker, M.B., B.S., A.K.C., M.R.C.O.G.;
Michael Hastin Bennett, M.A., M.B., F.R.C.S.; Arthur
J. Berman, M.D.; Richard J. Bing, M.D., F.A.C.P.;
John H. Bland, M.D., F.A.C.P.; Gordon Bourne,
F.R.C.S., F.R.C.O.G.; William T. Bowles, M.D.,
F.A.C.S.; Frank M. Calia, M.D., F.A.C.P.; Rachmel
Cherner, M.D., F.A.C.P.; David N. Danforth, M.D.,
Ph.D., F.A.C.S.; Joseph A. DeJulia, D.D.S.; Stephen
Engel, M.D., F.A.C.S.; Robert A. Glick, M.D.; Arlene
N. Heyman, M.D., Robert M. Hui, M.D.; Ginette
Betty Jacob, M.D.; Mark A. Jacobs, M.D.; Warren M.
Jacobs, M.D., F.A.C.S., F.A.C.O.G.; Judith K. Jones,
M.D., Ph.D.; Thomas Kalchthaler, D.O.; Lenore S.
Katkin, M.D., F.A.A.P.; Margaret M. Kilcoyne, M.D.;
Robert Lewy, M.D.; Henry O. Marsh, M.D.; Marcel-
ine Meyerriecks, R.N., B.S.N.; Lawrence G. Pape,
M.D., Ph.D.; Christopher S. Pitcher, D.M.,
F.R.C.Path.; Alexander S. Playfair, M.R.C.S., L.R.C.P.,
D.Obst.R.C.O.G.; John L. Roglieri, M.D.; Saul L.
Sanders, M.D.; Lawrence Scharer, M.D., F.A.C.P.;
Tony Smith, B.M., M.A.; Joseph E. Snyder, M.D.;
Paul S. Stein, M.D.; Richard D. Sweet, M.D.; John
Yudkin, M.D., Ph.D., F.R.C.P., F.R.I.C.; Jonathan E.
Zucker, M.D.

INTRODUCTION

Welcome to *The New Good Housekeeping Family Health and Medical Guide*. This is a totally revised edition of one of the most popular and useful health-care reference books ever published. Drawing on the expertise of scores of highly qualified professionals, the *Guide* is updated to include the latest advances in health and medical science and the most modern approaches to medical treatment. Throughout, you will find an emphasis on the *prevention* of illness, reflecting the most important trend of twentieth-century medicine.

We recognize that needs for health-care information often arise unpredictably and in different degrees of urgency. You will need some information very quickly and in small doses—the meaning of a medical term, for example. In other circumstances you will want detailed information delivered in a manner you can easily understand. With this in mind, the editors have arranged the *Guide* for ready reference.

First Aid

The **First Aid** section precedes all others. In it you will find basic, simple procedures that you can perform until professional help is available. It is a good idea to familiarize yourself with this section; note that the "Help-at-a-Glance" guide to **First Aid** is arranged alphabetically by subject for quick access.

Color Atlas of the Body

In the next section you will find 103 highly detailed, full-color anatomical drawings that show what the body looks like inside, what its component structures and organs are called, where they are located, and brief descriptions of how each system functions. The **Color Atlas** serves as a valuable reference for the entire *Guide*.

Section One: An Encyclopedia of Medicine

As with any other professional or scientific community, health care has its own language. The four chapters of the *Guide* following the anatomical plates make up, in essence, a medical encyclopedia. The *Medical A-Z* contains information about conditions, diseases, symptoms, and the function of organs, as well as definitions of technical terms. *Providers* identifies and describes the qualifications and roles of some physician specialists with whom you may have contact during diagnosis, treatment, and recovery. *Tests* familiarizes you with some of the thousands of tests used by health-care professionals to make diagnoses. And *Procedures* gives you brief explanations of some of the more commonly used treatments and surgical therapies. The **Encyclopedia of Medicine** will help you, initially, when health care professionals are not available; and it will help you ask intelligent, informed questions when they are.

Throughout these first chapters of the *Guide* you are provided with concise information written and arranged for ready access and quick comprehension. Health care, however, is more than emergencies and episodes of illness. Keeping your family and yourself healthy requires a life-style in which illness and injury are avoided. Good health care also involves an understanding of relationships and natural processes. Much of what happens to you and your family is part of the natural series of events that make up living; as such these happenings can be anticipated and managed. Helping you to do this is the purpose of the remaining sections of the *Guide*. Unlike the earlier alphabetized sections, these are designed to be read in their entirety. They provide you with points of view and rationales in addition to specific information. They also will help you understand in considerable detail the problems you and your family may encounter—including many you certainly will face—in the process of managing total health care.

Section Two: Family Medicine and Health

The chapters in this section approach health care in the context of bearing and raising children through adolescence. The physical and emotional cycles of womanhood are discussed, and in those pages you will find a wealth of detail about pregnancy, childbirth, and infancy. Special attention is paid to the care of children during preadolescence and into the teen years. The family as a group is examined in the context of family planning and therapies that can be administered to the family as a whole.

Section Three: Wellness

Since the first edition of *The Good Housekeeping Family Health and Medical Guide* was published the idea of health maintenance—the exercise of individual responsibility in keeping oneself healthy—has become an even greater factor in health care. **Wellness** is an overview of how you can best maintain the health of yourself and your family. It offers straightforward information on topics such as heart disease, cancer, drug abuse, and nutrition.

Section Four: Senior Living

The most rapidly growing segment of our society is the most health-conscious. Elderly persons are likely to have a greater and more frequent need for health care. If you do not have an elderly member in your family, remember that you yourself are a candidate for that community. If you do have an aged relative, it is essential that you be aware of the special health-care concerns of this very special group of persons. In **Senior Living** we have included important information for the families of aged persons and for the elderly themselves, who are taking an increasing role in their own health care.

Senior Living covers a wide variety of topics. Several of them, such as common disorders and diseases of aging, deal with subjects touched on elsewhere in the *Guide*, but here they focus on specific situations that accompany aging. The emotional and social elements are considered in subsections dealing with retirement, family relationships, mental health, and sources of help outside the family. Wellness for the elderly is examined as well as the physical changes that accompany the aging process.

Section Five: The Family Health Recordkeeper

The last section of the book is **The Family Health Recordkeeper**, where you can keep track of all pertinent information about the health and well-being of yourself and your family.

This edition of *The Good Housekeeping Family Health and Medical Guide* will help you to communicate better with physicians, dentists, pharmacists, and other professionals with whom you will come into contact and upon whose advice you should rely. It is not a substitute for the opinions and advice of those health-care providers. Neither is it meant to be definitive on any given subject. While we have made every effort to ensure that the information in this volume is accurate and up-to-date, we recognize the great diversity of opinion and the constant changes that mark health care in this era of greatly accelerated discovery.

How to Use This Guide

In a work this size, information is offered in many different ways and places. Be sure to refer to the index to cover all aspects of the subject you are interested in. The index is not only the quickest way to locate a subject but the best way to take advantage of the positive mine of detailed, helpful, and interesting information that is contained in this one volume.

Though related subjects are keyed to one another throughout the book (for example, in **Section One: A Medical Encyclopedia**, words set in SMALL CAPITAL LETTERS direct you to other pertinent entries within the section), this cross-referencing is no replacement for a well-used index.

THE

NEW

GOOD

HOUSEKEEPING

FAMILY

HEALTH

AND

MEDICAL

GUIDE

1
FIRST
AID

Help at a Glance

This section provides you with basic first-aid information and descriptions of treatment which you may be called upon to provide in common emergency situations. It cannot take the place of actual first-aid training such as that taught by local Red Cross chapters. But it certainly can help you and the person you are treating in an emergency. It will guide you to achieve the three important aims of first aid:

1. To keep the patient alive
2. To prevent his condition from worsening
3. To relieve anxiety, pain, and discomfort

Not all injuries are life-threatening, but they can be aggravated by improper handling. The victim may experience psychological tension as a result of the injury, and one of the goals in first aid is to provide comfort and assistance to alleviate tension as much as possible.

You must remember that first aid is *first* aid only, consisting of measures to be taken before a medically trained person provides "second aid"—that is, appropriate treatment. Your care will ensure that the patient is in the best possible condition when the professional takes over.

Throughout, you will find directions for the use of improvised materials as well as items available from a carefully prepared home first-aid kit. To prepare your own kit, follow the recommendations given in this section under FIRST-AID BOX. Experience shows that all too often such a kit is not available when the need arises.

Use this section of the book for reference and let the indexed Contents help you. It is also a good idea to read through it from beginning to end, so that when an emergency arises you will be somewhat prepared. Some parts are so important—describing urgent actions—that you should study and learn them right now. Those actions are:

Ensuring a clear airway (see UNCONSCIOUS, RE-SUSCITATION, CHOKING)
Stopping BLEEDING
Safeguarding the UNCONSCIOUS
Minimizing the risk of SHOCK

Finally, why not enroll yourself as a student in a first-aid class? You can spend productive hours deepening knowledge and experience by learning with a group under a qualified teacher. Your telephone book will give the number of the local Red Cross unit from which you can inquire.

One thing you *can* do right now is this: In the phone book, look up the number in your area for Emergency Medical Services (if 911 does not apply). Place this number, with other emergency numbers, for immediate access by your telephone.

WOUNDS

Controlling slight bleeding as a result of an accident with a razor blade or broken glass requires simple first aid. Applying a clean dressing firmly usually will control the slight bleeding in 5 to 8 minutes.

If the injury involved a blow which could have caused a fracture, *do not move the damaged part* until you have safeguarded it (see FRACTURES).

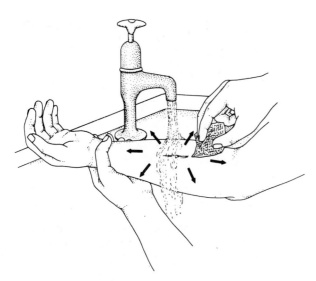

Figure 1 *For minimal bleeding, wash with clean water and wipe away from the wound.*

1. Have the person sit or lie down, particularly if he feels faint.

2. Control bleeding: as follows:

Minimal bleeding: Wash with sterile water or clean tap water (see Figure 1) and cover wound with a dressing. Stabilize the dressing with a bandage and keep the part at rest. (For example, do not attempt walking on a leg or put an arm in a sling.) Remember, it takes 5 to 8 minutes to stop bleeding—for example, a nick of the skin from a razor blade while shaving.

Severe bleeding—blood saturates the dressing completely in one minute or less:

Arterial bleeding. Critical. Blood is seen spurting from the wound with every beat of the heart. The first-aid response for spurting blood is to *immediately* apply direct pressure over the wound site. In this situation there may not be time to locate material to use as dressing. Apply firm pressure with your hand and *do not release*, because large amounts of blood can be lost from arterial bleeding.

Venous bleeding—blood flows from the wound at a rate in proportion to the size of the wound and the number of vessels damaged. Apply a clean or sterile dressing and stabilize with a bandage. If the first dressing becomes blood-soaked, apply additional dressing material without removing the initial dressing. By removing the first dressing you could disturb the clotting that has begun and delay the control of bleeding.

3. Remember, always keep at rest the part of the body where the wound is located.

4. Refer to antishock measures (see SHOCK). See also BLEEDING.

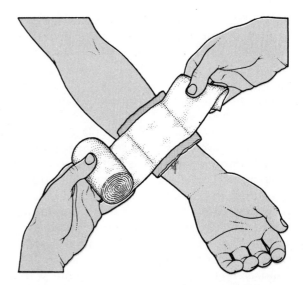

Figure 2 *Ready-prepared dressings, available in individual packages, are useful for larger wounds.*

■ *What to use as dressing*

Note that in first aid we do not use antiseptics; this is reserved for trained medical personnel.

The best cover for the wound is white gauze from a freshly opened package. A clean handkerchief or small, smooth towel will serve. But handle it carefully: Hold it by one corner, let it fall open; then, still handling only by the corners, refold it so that what was the inner aspect (unexposed to germs since it was washed and put away) becomes the outer surface that comes in contact with the wound.

For the pad you can use a thickly folded handkerchief, small towel, or even something like a clean sock. The bandage can be improvised from a stocking, necktie, small towel, or scarf; use safety pins if it is not practical to knot it.

Your first-aid kit, however, may contain more suitable items. A quite small superficial wound can be covered with a ready-prepared *self-adhesive dressing:* The protective layer is partly peeled off the front so that the gauze pad now exposed can be applied without being touched by the fingers.

For larger wounds, the prepared sterile dressing is ideal. As taken from its individual package, it consists of gauze and pad in one, already attached to its bandage (see Figure 2).

■ *When something is embedded in the wound*

Leave the object there. Loose dirt or gravel lying

on the surface certainly can be brushed away gently with a clean cloth. But anything that is *stuck in*, whether it be a sliver of glass or even a knife, should not be moved. The deep point may be lying against an important structure like a large blood vessel or nerve which may be damaged by an unplanned pull.

How then to cope? You do *not* place a dressing over an impaled object. Let your first covering layer lie loosely folded around the object. Then build around this projection a thick, firm trough of padding so that the embedded object is deeply protected within it (see Figure 3). This trough will now receive the pressure of the bandage.

The *ring pad* is a device that can be used in some cases for making this trough. Take a large handkerchief, a small towel folded into a thin band, or something like a stocking. Make a circle of the right size with one end. Now twist the long free end in and out until it is all used up. You end with a quite firm, fairly thick circle with a small hole in the center (see Figure 4).

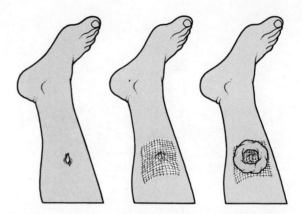

Figure 3 *Do not attempt to remove an object embedded in a wound, but surround it with a protective ring of padding before applying a bandage.*

■ The tetanus risk

Tetanus (lockjaw) can develop from many wounds, especially if they are contaminated with soil or road dust or if they come from animal bites and are deep. The germs often are found in soil or agricultural areas, and they thrive in enclosed, airless conditions in the tissues. Make sure your patient gets medical advice about protection against this risk. Following a wound, an injection of tetanus antitoxin, or the safer tetanus toxoid booster if appropriate, protects against the development of this disease.

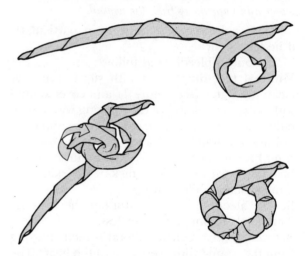

Figure 4 *A ring pad can be improvised from a hand-kerchief, stocking, or even a small towel.*

■ Eye wounds

Do not attempt any cleaning with soap and water. Bandage a smooth pad over the eye. If movement hurts the eye, it could be wise to put both eyes at rest temporarily by covering the good eye as well, since the two eyes move together.

After placing bandages over both eyes, it is important to remain in constant communication with the injured person.

See also *Chemical Burns* under BURNS. For particles in the eye, see OBJECT IN THE EYE.

■ Chest wounds

A penetrating wound of the chest wall can be extremely dangerous. As the patient breathes in,

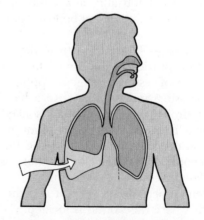

Figure 5 *In a penetrating chest wound, air may fill the space between the lung and chest wall.*

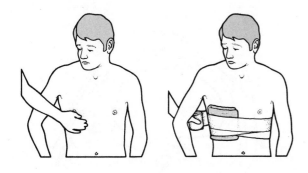

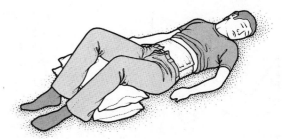

Figure 7   *Use pillows, blankets, jackets, etc., to raise the patient's legs. This relaxes the abdominal muscles and relieves pressure on the wound.*

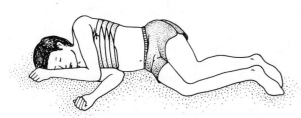

Figure 6   *First seal the chest wound with your palm. After applying a thick bandage, lay the patient on the injured side; this helps breathing.*

air may enter not only through his mouth and windpipe but also through the wound itself. From this point of entry it does not go into the lung but fills up the space between the lung and chest wall (see Figure 5). During expiration the loose tissue at the wound tends to close up like a valve flap. With each intake of breath, more and more air (which cannot get out) fills up that side of the chest. Air under tension compresses and flattens the lung and places an extra burden of work on the heart. The quicker the wound is sealed, the better.

1. Immediately close the opening in the chest wall with the palm of your hand (see Figure 6). Keep it there while:

2. You have someone prepare as quickly as possible a thick pad (towel, handkerchief) to replace your hand; if you are alone with the patient, you will have to use your free hand to accomplish this.

3. Bandage this pad firmly in position to seal off the hole. Use wide bandages, plastic wrap, aluminum foil, folded towels, stockings, or, if available, elastic adhesive strapping. The urgency to close the wound overrides the need to clean the skin around it.

4. Lay the patient on the injured side. This

helps by leaving the good side unhindered to do the breathing for both sides. It also reduces the risk that any coughed up blood will flow over into the lung. If the patient becomes short of breath, do not let him lie flat, but have him propped up (by blankets or pillows), seated half upright. Breathing becomes easier in an upright position.

■ Abdominal wounds

Muscles of the abdominal wall run lengthwise mainly from top to bottom (rib cage to pelvis). Their fibers are under some tension, much like taut rubber bands. If some of the fibers are cut, the hole will tend to widen as the cut ends pull apart. To counteract this, reduce muscular tension by "folding" the patient so as to bring pelvis and rib cage nearer to each other.

Lay the patient down on his back with his head and shoulders a little raised and knees bent; use pillows or blankets to raise up the knees and head (see Figure 7). A good alternative is to have the patient lying on his side in this "folded" position; his head will be low enough that any vomit he brings up will flow out of his mouth rather than being inspired into his windpipe.

BLEEDING

Blood at any wound tends to clot, thereby forming a "stopper" to close up the bleeding vessels. However, for this to happen bleeding must be stopped or sufficiently slowed so that the clot is not being constantly swept away as fast as it tries to form. Simple, slight bleeding will respond by clotting if the area is treated like a wound with a firmly bandaged pad over a dressing (see WOUNDS).

However, when bleeding is severe, the situation is urgent, and attempts at sterility or cleanliness may have to be sacrificed for speed.

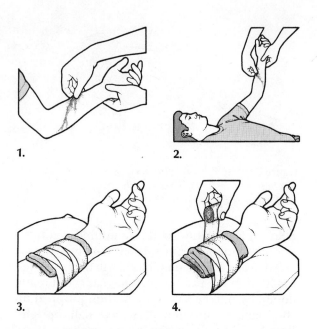

1.   **2.**

3.   **4.**

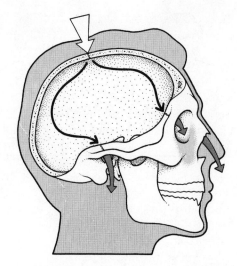

Figure 8   *Bleeding around the ear, nose, or eye can result from a blow on the head. Any sign of bleeding from such cause demands urgent medical attention.*

■ General rules

1. At once use your hand either to press hard over the bleeding area or to pinch the wound edges together with fingers and thumb. This pressure must be maintained for 10 minutes.

2. Meantime lay the patient down. Whenever possible elevate the bleeding area as this helps a little to reduce the blood flow in it. *But be careful not to move a part which may be fractured.*

3. As soon as possible replace the hand pressure with pressure from a firm pad held down by a tight bandage. If, as is likely, orthodox dressings and bandage are not immediately available use what is at hand: socks, handkerchiefs, ties, belts, stockings. *Never leave the wound without any pressure at all.* If you are alone with the patient, it may be necessary to keep one hand on him while you use the other to reach for anything suitable, including clothing.

4. Watch the bandage carefully. If it shows blood still oozing through, do not remove it but apply more pressure over it with further padding and bandage. In exceptionally difficult cases this may have to be done several times so that the dressing becomes very bulky. Control generally will be achieved.

Apply the necessary antishock measures (see SHOCK). Get medical aid or call an ambulance immediately.

■ Scalp bleeding

Elastic fibers in scalp tissue tend to pull the wound open so that bleeding is profuse. Furthermore,

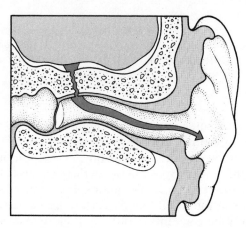

Figure 9   *Bleeding from the ear may be due to a fracture at the base of the skull.*

blood comes to any point in the scalp from a network of vessels all around it, so that local pressure may not halt the bleeding. In that case a ring pad (see Figure 4) around the wound with very firm bandaging over this may succeed.

■ Bleeding from the ear, nose, or about the eye

A blow on the head may transmit its force around the skull and cause a fracture at the base of the skull. This may show up as bleeding from the ear, bleeding from the nose (see Figure 8), or bruising around the eye.

Regard any such bleeding, however slight, with suspicion and obtain medical advice as rapidly as possible (see also HEAD INJURY).

The Ear. The amount of blood to flow out is not likely to be dangerous in itself. But if there has been a blow fracturing the base of the skull (see Figure 9), there now is an open pathway for bacteria from the ear canal to move into the skull cavity and infect the brain.

DO NOT plug the ear; this would allow blood to collect and clot in the canal, forming a nutrient medium in which bacteria could multiply rapidly. Instead, let the blood escape by laying the patient down toward the bleeding side. Lightly cover the whole ear with a dressing and bandage, which will protect against dirt but allow blood to flow out.

The Nose. If bleeding follows a blow to the top of the head, consider the possibility of a fracture at the base of the skull. If it follows a blow on the nose, then the nose may be fractured and need treatment, but the bleeding is likely to stop soon.

Most nosebleeds happen when a vessel just inside the nostril bursts because of engorgement with inflammation, because of raised blood pressure, or because of finger scratching within the nostril. Sit the patient up. Let him *pinch the whole lower soft part of the nose* between his finger and thumb *for 10 minutes without letting go.* Some blood may yet flow down the back of the throat; it will do no harm and can be spat out. The patient sits with the elbow of the pinching arm on a table, a bowl in front of him and a towel around his neck.

If this does not work, try a second bout of 10 minutes. Tell the patient not to sniff or blow his nose, which could dislodge the clot.

■ *Bleeding tooth socket*

Copious bleeding can begin a few hours after a tooth extraction. Sit the patient up in the same way as for the nosebleed victim. Have him bite hard on a thick pad of gauze or absorbent cotton bridging the area of the missing tooth but not packed into the socket, which could be injurious. The pad will tamp down to a smaller size as it gets wet, so it should start out quite big. The biting pressure is maintained for at least 10 minutes, as the patient presses his chin hard on his cupped hand, while his elbow rests on a table.

■ *Cut tongue bleeding*

The patient sits at a table with his elbow on it. He puts out his tongue and holds the bleeding area firmly within the folds of a handkerchief between thumb and forefinger for at least 10 minutes.

■ *Bleeding from cut palm*

The patient makes a tight fist over a thick pad in the palm. The whole hand is firmly bandaged in this clenched position (with the thumb *outside* the bandage).

■ *Bleeding from the lungs*

Blood may be coughed up as *a single streak* from the effort of a heavy cough. It must never be ignored, however because it could have a more serious cause.

Heavier and more alarming bleeding shows up as *bright red blood* which may be *frothy* because it is mixed with air. The matter is extremely *urgent.* Put the patient at rest and *get medical help at once.*

A patient producing copious amounts of red blood should remain in *a sitting position*—never lay him down.

BLEEDING FROM THE STOMACH

Speed of bleeding	Slow	Fast	Very Fast
FEATURES	Almost hidden; the blood passes into the bowels. It may (by action of digestive changes) color the stools black.	Blood accumulating in the stomach is digested to a black mass, like coffee grounds, which may be vomited.	Fresh-looking blood is vomited before it has time to change color.
PATIENT'S CONDITION	In time could become anemic and weak.	Feels ill and often nauseated with discomfort or pain.	Weak and shocked.
ACTION TO TAKE	Consult a doctor as soon as possible.	Put the patient to bed and get medical advice at once. Give nothing by mouth.	A severe emergency needing urgent hospital help. Apply antishock measures (see SHOCK). Give nothing by mouth.

■ *Bleeding from the stomach*

This can arise from irritation of the stomach lining by certain drugs (such as aspirin), or from an ulcer or tumor. See the table below for first-aid action.

BURNS

Injury from burns is far more than surface destruction. The greatest harm—perhaps with permanent scarring and disability—comes from heat that spreads into the deeper tissues and remains there. In particular, the liquid part of the blood, the plasma, oozes in very large amounts from the blood vessels of the area. Some of this which reaches the surface collects in blisters. But the volume lost from within the circulation is certainly more than that which fills the blister; a great deal swells up the burned tissues. A severe burn which has destroyed skin surface leaves no "roof" to contain the blister and considerable seepage may proceed from this open raw area. There is therefore a high risk of shock developing (see SHOCK).

The first-aid approach is to counteract this process by rapidly cooling the burned area with large quantities of water to stop the burning process. *Seek medical help at once.*

■ *If clothes are on fire*

Seize the first available thing to use for smothering the flames: a thick curtain or towel, a rug or even your coat which you pull off fast. Wrap it over the flames, pressing down to exclude air.

The panic-stricken child may be running around, thus fanning the flames and making things worse. Get him on the floor so that the burning surface is uppermost with the flames rising away from his body. As you apply the smothering material, do this, if you can, from his head and toward his feet so that flames are directed away from his head (see Figure 10).

Now pull away any bits of clothing which may yet be smoldering, but nothing that is adhering to the skin. Leave untouched any material that is burned but extinguished; it may be stuck to the skin.

Adults and older children should be taught that when no help is available they should STOP, DROP to the floor, and ROLL to smother the flames.

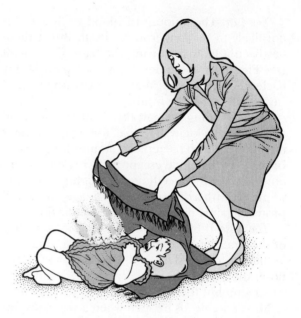

Figure 10 *Use a coat, towel, curtain, or anything handy to smother burning clothes, pressing down to exclude air. Direct the flames away from the head.*

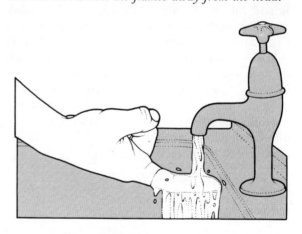

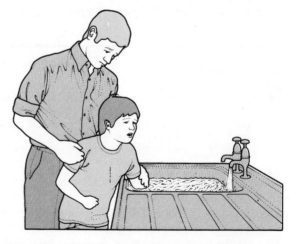

Figure 11 *Cool the burned area immediately by immersing in cold—preferably running—water.*

■ *Treating the burn*

1. Immediate cooling. Apply cold water at once and liberally (see Figure 11). A burned hand or arm is plunged into a bucket or sink of water. A simple fingertip burn can be held under running water.

A large area of the body, or a body part such as the face, cannot easily be plunged into water. Get a thick pad made by something like a folded towel; soak it in cold water and place it over the whole burned area. As this pack becomes warm, you should repeatedly remoisten and reapply it. (One thing you do NOT do is to put the patient in a cold bath, ice water, or snow pack.)

This wet cooling action gives relief of pain, and you maintain it for 10 minutes. If after this the patient still feels much pain continue for another 10 minutes.

Ordinary cold water gives best results; ice packs or ice water is less efficient.

Even if you reach the patient some 15 to 20 minutes after the burn, it is still wise to apply cooling.

2. Dress the burn. If there are any possibly constricting items in the area (rings, garters, bracelets), remove them carefully before swelling creates more problems. Pin on a dry dressing of the cleanest available material to cover the whole burned area as a protection against infection. Bandage firmly but not tightly. Where an arm or leg is involved, encasing the limb in a pillowcase is an excellent improvisation. Keep it elevated, as this reduces the swelling. DO NOT use any creams or antiseptics.

3. Antishock treatment is important (see SHOCK). When the burn is extensive and there may be delay in getting the patient to the hospital, we can break one of the rules: If he is conscious and if he is showing no signs of vomiting, get him to drink in order to compensate for the fluid and salts lost with the plasma. Prepare tepid water with half a teaspoonful of salt and a quarter of a teaspoonful of baking soda to each pint. He takes half a glass of this in slow sips every 15 minutes. Prompt medical attention is essential, however, since extensive burns are life-threatening.

■ *Blisters*

Do not rupture blisters. If blisters have formed, your first-aid measure is not to disturb them: Include them *under* the dressing.

■ *Chemical burns*

Caustic materials on the skin need to be washed away immediately with a long-continued, copious, but gentle stream of water until you are certain that none remains on the skin.

Chemicals in the eye present an extra problem in that the patient in pain tends to keep his lids tightly shut. They have to be opened gently to let the water flow over the eyeball and under the lids. Lay him down on the affected side so that the washings do not stream into the other eye or over the rest of his face. A stream of water cannot harm the eye; a 20-minute continuous wash may save a person from permanent blindness.

SPRAINS

A sprained joint has had its ligaments and fibers overstretched and partly torn by a sudden forceful movement, for example, the inward wrenching of an ankle.

A *cold compress* is helpful if applied immediately, as it helps to reduce the pain and swelling. Soak a thick pad of material (a folded small towel or a large handkerchief) in cold water; wring it out so that it is just comfortably wet; bandage it on closely with some open-weave material. Keep the joint elevated and at rest. After about 20 minutes the compress can be discarded and you move on to the next stage of support.

Firm support—absorbent cotton or thick pads applied around and interleaved with firm bandaging (an elastic bandage is useful here). Or you can closely apply firm cushioning by bandaging a cylinder of rolled-up thick material about the joint (see Figure 12).

Be careful not to make the whole so tight that it occludes the blood supply. This risk is greater

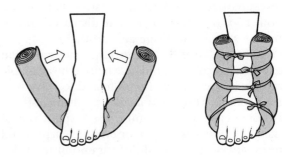

Figure 12 *A roll of thick material can be used to provide support for a sprained ankle joint.*

at the front of the elbow and back of the knee where the vessels run close to the skin. Warn your patient to ease the bandage if the body part beyond it becomes cold, numb, or puffy.

A severe sprain may be difficult to distinguish from a fracture. Whenever there is doubt, treat it *as if it were a fracture.*

FRACTURES

The important point about fractures is to suspect them *when they are likely*—that is, when the patient has received a blow or crush over an area with underlying bone (which is practically anywhere except the abdomen). Some fractures can be severe without showing much or any deformity or disability or even without causing severe pain.

Some fractures do not happen at the point that received the blow. The force of falling onto an outstretched hand may travel up the arm to jerk and break the collarbone near the shoulder. A falling person may land heavily on a heel and break, not the ankle, but the thighbone near the hip; this is especially likely in the elderly.

■ *First-aid management*

The general rules are extremely straightforward:
   1. **Warn the patient not to move.** And warn bystanders not to move him. The general tendency of solicitous but uninformed persons is to try to pick up a fallen victim.
   2. **Stop any severe bleeding** (see BLEEDING).
   3. **Dress any wound at once** (see WOUNDS), but take care not to move the fractured area. Even a hastily improvised covering is important to minimize the risk of bacteria reaching the fracture.

It may seem that so far you have done nothing specific for the fracture itself. But you have already achieved a lot. You have protected the patient against blood loss and against infection. And by his immobility you have made sure that broken bone ends do not become more displaced and do further damage to tissue around them.
   4. **Immobilize the fracture.** (If, however, you expect medical or ambulance help to be available rapidly it is wise to do no more and to leave it to the experts.) You immobilize by applying a splint. In some cases you can improvise a splint out of slabs of wood, cardboard, or even magazines and newspapers. A good splint to immobilize an injured forearm, elbow, and wrist can be made from a magazine or thick newspaper, tightly rolled and

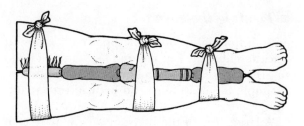

Figure 13 *A fractured leg can be immobilized by splinting it against the good one. Towels, scarves, or similar material can be used as padding.*

then padded and bandaged. However, the best and ever-present splint is the patient's own body: good leg against injured leg, or chest wall against injured arm.

■ *Principles of immobilization*

Do not move the injured part if you can avoid it. A goal in fracture immobilization is to stabilize not only the fracture site but also the joints at either end of the bone. Bring the good side (for example, the other leg) as a splint alongside the injured one. Between the two parts insert padding (wool, folded towels, scarves) to fill up hollows or prevent chafing where bumps lie against each other. Secure the injured part to the good part firmly enough to prevent movement, with real or improvised bandages. Avoid placing a bandage where you suspect the fracture to be, and tie the knots off on the good side (see Figure 13).

■ *Lower jaw fracture*

Give primary attention to the problems of the patient who may not be able to speak or swallow while his mouth is filling with blood or saliva. His tongue may have slipped back to obstruct the airway if the damage is severe. In that case keep the jaw forward with your fingers hooked over the teeth. If artificial respiration is needed, it will have to be given by someone equipped with and trained in the use of resuscitation bag and mask. The mouth-to-mouth method is not appropriate here.

Clear the patient's mouth gently. Manually support the jaw and lean the patient forward for drainage of secretions.

■ *Collarbone fracture*

The patient has pain in the shoulder and will tend to support the elbow on the injured side in order to relieve the pull of the arm on the broken bone. Maintain this support as you apply a sling.

The sling is made from a triangular bandage

(its long side about 60 inches), or it can be improvised from scarves or towels (see Figure 14).

In the absence of these, improvisation can be made by pinning up a sleeve or the turned-up lower edge of a jacket.

■ Rib fracture

In simple cases the main feature is painful breathing, not extremely severe, and the fracture tends to heal easily. No special first-aid treatment is needed, except that sometimes the patient gets relief by having the arm on the affected side in a sling. A physician should be consulted, however.

For more severe injuries of the chest wall, see WOUNDS.

■ Upper limb fracture

If the elbow can be bent without pain: Put padding in the armpit, and apply a sling, preferably using a triangular bandage as shown in Figure 15.

If the elbow cannot be bent: Keep the limb straight and secure it by three broad bandages to the side of the body. This patient should travel on a stretcher.

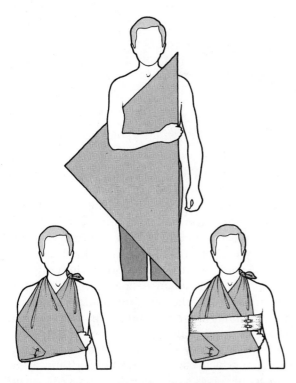

Figure 14 *Use a triangular bandage as a sling to relieve the pull of the arm on the broken collarbone. Keep the forearm sloping slightly up, and secure with a knot over the good shoulder and a safety pin near the elbow. A wide bandage to hold the upper arm against the chest completes the immobilization.*

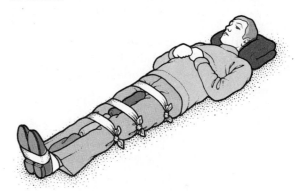

Figure 16 *The fractured leg and thigh are immobilized by bandages around the ankles, knees, and thighs, with padding between the legs.*

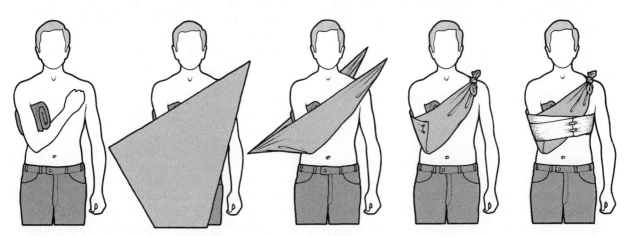

Figure 15 *To immobilize a fractured upper limb: Put thick padding (wool, rolled-up towel) in the armpit and against the chest. Carefully bring the arm to the side of the chest with the hand toward the opposite shoulder. Then apply a sling, using a triangular bandage as shown, or improvising with some other material. Give further support by firm, broad bandaging of the upper arm to the chest wall.*

■ *Pelvis fracture*

Allow the patient to lie on his back in the position he finds most comfortable. If he wishes to bend the knees (thus relaxing the pull of muscles on the broken bones), let him do so and support the bent knees with pillows or rolled blankets.

If the patient must undergo a long wait or difficult travel, then you should immobilize with two broad, overlapping bandages firmly around the pelvis, padding between the legs, a figure-of-eight bandage around the ankles and bandaging around the knees.

Take great care, since a fractured pelvis may be accompanied by severe internal damage, by a fracture of the thighbone, or by a fracture of the spine.

■ *Leg and thigh fracture*

Immobilize the leg and thigh as shown in Figure 16:
1. Bring the good leg alongside the injured one.
2. Put padding between the legs.
3. Tie a figure-of-eight bandage around the ankles.
4. Bandage the knees together.
5. Bandage just below the fracture site.
6. Bandage around the thighs.

■ *Foot fracture*

Carefully and gently remove the patient's shoe and sock; cradle the whole foot and ankle in a pillow or folded blanket firmly bandaged around it to act as splint. Keep the leg elevated (on pillows or a folded blanket), as this helps to reduce the swelling.

■ *Spine fracture*

You must take the suspected fracture of the spine *extremely seriously*. The ring-like bones of the vertebral column surround the spinal cord; if a disrupted bone fragment were to move against or into the spinal cord it could cause permanent paralysis or loss of feeling to some part of the body, sometimes very extensively. This calamity might not happen at the time of the fracture itself, but could ensue due to improper handling of the patient.

Suspect a fractured vertebra after any forceful fall or blow followed by pain in the neck or back. Immediately tell the patient not to get up, but to

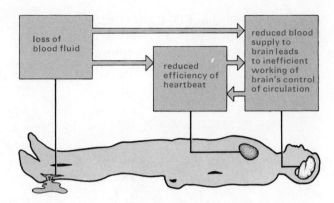

Figure 17   *The vicious cycle of developing shock is sparked off by severe blood loss.*

lie still. And make sure no bystander tries to move him—it is essential to wait for trained experts to get him on the stretcher.

While you wait, cover him with blankets or coats to keep him warm.

The mechanics of the spine are such that any "folding up" or bending forward of the vertebral column could push a piece of broken bone against the spinal cord. When it comes to getting this patient on a stretcher, the ambulance attendants may tie his legs together and go through a special lifting routine which keeps him straight and stretched. Or they may use a specially designed stretcher which can slide under him and allow him to be lifted and carried in the position in which he lies.

The head should not be hyperextended on an unconscious patient. Keep the head and neck in a straight line with the long axis of the body. Do not move the spine. Avoid flexing or rotating the head and neck. Avoid extending or twisting the spine. To establish an airway, use a maneuver known as the *jaw lift, chin lift,* or *jaw thrust.* Pull the jaw forward while keeping the neck in a stable position. Grasp the angles of the victim's lower jaw with both hands, one on each side, and move the lower jaw forward. This will pull the back of the tongue away from the pharynx and ensure an open airway.

You may find it necessary to move the patient from an urgently dangerous situation (fire, exposed mountain slope, water immersion). If time allows, get three or four helpers who will share the support of the patient evenly so that he can be lifted without folding or twisting his body or turning his head. One helper should cradle the head between his palms with outstretched fingers extending to the shoulders. Lift together at a prepared signal; carry him the minimal distance com-

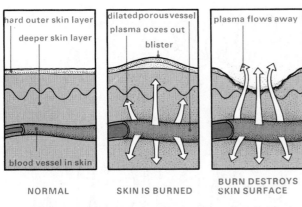

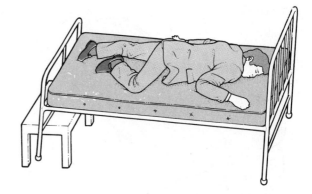

Figure 18 *By damaging surface tissue and dilating underlying blood vessels, burns can cause extensive loss of plasma and lead to shock.*

Figure 19 *Lay the patient on his side in the Recovery Position. See also Figure 23.*

patible with safety, and lower him to a firm surface still in the same position.

■ *Skull fracture*

See HEAD INJURY.

DISLOCATIONS

The features of a dislocation are very much like those of a fracture. As a first-aider you do not face the problem of making the exact diagnosis. Treat it like a fracture. In any case, many dislocations do not happen alone, but are accompanied by some bone breakage in the joint area.

SHOCK

In first aid, the term "shock" refers not to emotional upsets but to a physical condition, a failure of the heart and circulation that follows severe injury. Shock is caused by a loss of blood fluid. In *severe hemorrhage* the reduced amount of blood in the body results in a weakened heartbeat and inadequate supply of oxygen and other chemicals to all the tissues. The brain in particular is sensitive to this lack; the centers in the brain that automatically regulate respiration, blood pressure, and heart action no longer work adequately. In this way, even if the bleeding is controlled, a vicious cycle of failure may have been set in action (see Figure 17). With *large wounds and bruises* there may be extensive blood loss deep within the tissues. Although the blood is still inside the body, it has escaped from the blood vessels; it is stag-

nating and taking no part in the circulation. *Fractures* of large bones involve damage not just to the bones themselves but also to the muscles and other organs that are located around the bones, causing disruption of blood vessels and loss of blood from the circulation. *Burns* themselves can create blood loss in an extensive, if more disguised, way by dilating the blood vessels of the injured area, making them "porous" so that the plasma—the liquid component of the blood oozes out copiously (see Figure 18).

■ *The patient in shock*

One who has suffered any of the injuries described above in a severe way is therefore at risk of developing shock: a low blood volume, a failing heartbeat, a poor flow of what blood remains circulating, and inadequate nutrition to all parts of the body—specifically to brain, heart, and lungs. This steadily worsening condition could be described as a "running down of life forces."

A patient in shock is pale, cold, sweating; his pulse and breathing are fast and weak; he feels faint, nauseated, thirsty. He may become restless or irrational and eventually comatose and unconscious. In this stage, first aid is of minimal help; the patient needs the full technique of hospital treatment, including fluid transfusion.

We must realize that immediately after the injury the patient may still appear tough and resistant, but internally the machinery of shock has been set in motion. How long it will take for him to show the signs depends on such factors as his original strength and the rate and amount of blood loss. It may be a few minutes or several hours.

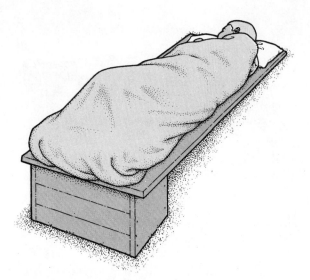

Figure 20   *Cover the patient loosely with blankets or coats to prevent undue heat loss.*

■ Preventing shock

As first-aiders we cannot treat fully developed shock. But we can prevent or minimize its development. Happily, the actions for this are very simple. Unhappily, their very simplicity often makes the first-aider overlook them. Take these measures seriously and act on them even if your patient seems in fairly good shape—do not wait for him to deteriorate.

1. **Stop bleeding at once** (see BLEEDING).

2. **Ensure rest and position.** Treat the patient where he is. Do not transport him unless you are in a danger area (fire, fumes, collapsing building). In a traffic-laden road have someone divert the cars.

Loosen tight clothing (belt, suspenders, collar, corset). Keep the patient lying down. Have him on his side to safeguard his airway (see Figures 19 and 23). However, beware of moving a patient who may have a fracture—especially if his back is involved. In some cases it is best to keep him in the position in which you have found him.

3. **Keep him warm** with loose coverings of blankets or coats (see Figure 20). See that he is protected from heat loss both above and below the body. But do *not* add electric blankets or hot-water bottles. The extra heat might improve his color by dilating the blood vessels of the skin, but that would mean drawing toward the surface a large volume of blood from the depths of the body where it is needed by the essential organs of life.

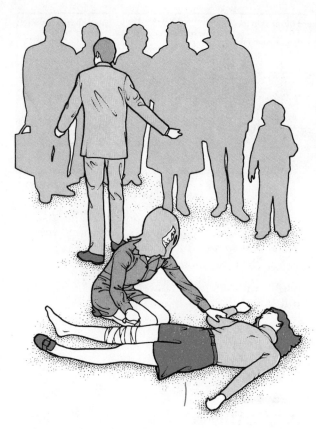

Figure 21   *Try to keep away any bystanders who could be distressing to the patient—and remember that an apparently unconscious person often can hear what is said by people nearby.*

4. **Relieve discomfort.** Reducing both pain and mental anxiety plays a great role in warding off shock. First aid does not permit giving medicine or tablets without medical authority. But the immediate dressing of wounds and the immobilization of fractures are important pain relievers. Talk to your patient with calm confidence, explaining your actions as reassuringly as possible. Answer any questions as accurately as you can, dwelling on the positive and comforting aspects only. Tactfully but firmly clear away any agitated or demoralizing bystanders (see Figure 21). Give them things to do which take them off the scene.

Never whisper to others near your patient; remember that an apparently unconscious person may be able to overhear what is said. Guard your speech.

5. **Give nothing by mouth.** Do not give hot tea or coffee. The patient may vomit. Anything he brings up may then be aspirated into his windpipe and choke him, especially if he is comatose or later under anesthesia for emergency surgery. If he is thirsty you can relieve this by giving him

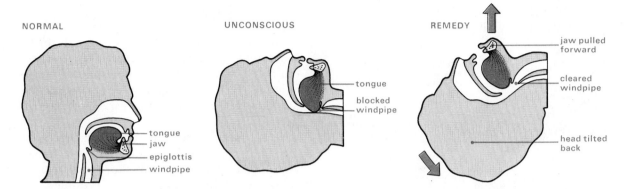

NORMAL   UNCONSCIOUS   REMEDY

jaw pulled
forward

cleared
windpipe

tongue
blocked
windpipe

tongue
jaw
epiglottis
windpipe

head tilted
back

Figure 22 *To avoid the risk of suffocation, bend the unconscious patient's head back and pull his jaw forward. This simple measure prevents the flaccid tongue from blocking air entry to the windpipe.*

a rolled-up and moistened handkerchief to suck.

Brandy or whiskey are dangerous since they can dilate skin vessels and draw blood away from the body depths.

Even a single cigarette can have a deleterious effect by reducing the oxygen capacity of the blood and by reducing the blood supply to the heart muscle.

UNCONSCIOUSNESS

■ *The risk of suffocation*

Your first-aid problem with an unconscious patient is not to find out why he is in this condition, but to protect him from the very real risk of choking. Abnormal unconsciousness allows no protective reaction from the patient if his airway gets blocked: Blood, vomit, or even saliva in the mouth may run into the windpipe of a person lying on his back. Dentures can become misplaced and cause blockage.

It is the patient's own tongue that forms the greatest threat, however. Attached by its base to the jawbone, the tongue is free to move backward and forward.

It is a muscle, and like all muscles it loses tone and becomes limp in the unconscious person. When he is lying on his back, his flaccid tongue can easily fall against the back of the throat and block the air entry to the windpipe (see Figure 22).

You can counteract these hazards by:
1. Clearing the mouth.
2. Pulling his jaw forward and bending his head back—actions that pull the tongue away from the back of the throat.

3. Positioning him with his head low to one side, so that any fluid in the mouth can flow out.

■ *Action on the unconscious person*

1. **Is he breathing?** If not, begin resuscitation at once (see RESUSCITATION).

2. **Is he trying to breathe but the airway is obstructed?** Immediately sweep a finger deeply all around his mouth to clear out any material lying there. Bend his head back and keep it thus. Generally the neck movement is enough but additional clearance achieved by pushing the jaw forward may be needed.

3. **Stop any bleeding** (see BLEEDING).

4. **Check for possible fractures** (unless the nature of the case excludes their likelihood). You want to move him into a safe position, but you must be sure that you do not first have to immobilize a broken bone (see FRACTURES). It is difficult to detect a fracture in a person who is dressed normally and unable to respond to touch or to questions. However, do your best by palpating (feeling) carefully but firmly all over without moving any part. Unless you can see a gross deformity you have to be guided by feeling for irregularities, comparing the knobs and contours of both sides.

5. **Put the patient in the Recovery Position.** In this position, the patient is lying on his side, which ensures free breathing and the outflow of any fluid coming into the mouth (see Figure 23).

Kneel at the patient's side. Put one hand protectively over his face as you pull on his hip with the other hand, rolling him toward you. This maneuver results in the patient being moved into the recovery position. It cannot be emphasized too strongly that, when a neck fracture is sus-

THE RECOVERY POSITION FOR NON-INJURED PERSONS

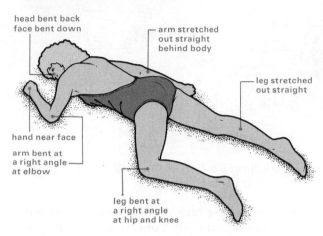

head bent back
face bent down

arm stretched
out straight
behind body

leg stretched
out straight

hand near face

arm bent at
a right angle
at elbow

leg bent at
a right angle
at hip and knee

Figure 23   *Everyone should know how to put a patient in the Recovery Position. In this position the person can breathe freely, and fluids can escape from the mouth, lessening the risk of choking. Your knowledge of this maneuver could save a patient's life.*

pected, moving the patient in this manner or extending the head can result in additional spinal injury.

6. **Dress any open wounds** (see WOUNDS).

7. **Take antishock measures** (see SHOCK).

Do not reserve the Recovery Position for the unconscious only. You will wisely use it for those who might become unconscious, the poisoned, or those who have just been afflicted with a stroke. Not only is it a safe position, it is a comfortable and relaxing one as well.

If the patient smells of alcohol this is no reason to think he is unconscious because of intoxication. The drink may have had nothing to do with his condition. Or it may be only an indirect factor, such as having made him fall and damage his skull.

Remember that a person who appears to be senseless may yet hear and understand what is said. Be very cautious with your speech.

Finally, you must *never attempt to give anything to drink to someone who is unconscious.*

DROWNING AND NEAR DROWNING

With due concern for the rescuers' own safety, the drowning victim must first be reached. If head and spinal injuries are not suspected, the first priority is to establish an airway and initiate rescue

breathing even before the victim is removed from the water.

After the victim has been removed from the water, quickly determine whether a pulse is present and begin standard cardiopulmonary resuscitation (CPR), if necessary. As soon as it is available, 100 percent oxygen should be administered to the victim.

Some complications of drowning may appear after the event, so even if a victim appears to have recovered at the scene, he or she should be transported to a hospital as quickly as possible.

Diving accidents may result in head and spinal injuries. If this type of injury is suspected and the victim is floating face down, carefully turn him over with the least amount of movement, always supporting the head and neck to keep them level with the back. Do not remove the victim from the water; instead keep him floating on his back. Wait for professional assistance if possible, because this type of victim should be immobilized with a backboard or other rigid support before being removed from the water.

The basic cardiopulmonary resuscitation rules apply for these kinds of victims (see RESUSCITATION).

FAINTING

If your patient is feeling faint and is still conscious, help him to lie down at once. Elevate his legs if you can, loosen any tight clothes, and get him covered. Ask him to relax and to take deep breaths slowly. The attack generally eases and the patient wants to struggle up. Do not let him do so until you are sure his color and strength are back to normal. Then let him change slowly from the lying to the erect position. Give him a drink of water.

Where lying down is not possible, as in the auditorium of a theater, tell the patient to bend down low, with his head between his legs.

If he has fainted, treat him as for unconsciousness (see UNCONSCIOUSNESS).

SEIZURES IN CHILDREN

Often such seizures occur as the child is developing a feverish infection. The nervous system of a small child is not as efficient in controlling body heat, and it is more sensitive to high temperatures.

The child, who may have seemed out of sorts and lacking appetite, suddenly goes unconscious and stiff with head held back and eyes rolled up.

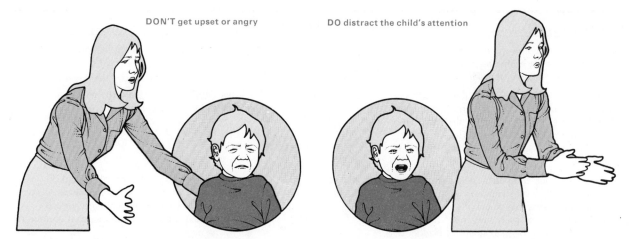

DON'T get upset or angry   DO distract the child's attention

Figure 24   *Attacks of breath-holding are best dealt with by distracting the child's attention rather than by showing signs of anger, anxiety, or concern.*

This is not the time to rush to telephone the doctor. Stay with the child; he needs your help.

Turn him into the Recovery Position (see Figure 23), and clear any fluid from his mouth. If he seems very feverish remove his clothes and reduce his temperature by cooling with an electric fan, by fanning with sheets of paper, or by gentle sponging with tap water. Your aim is not to bring the temperature back to normal but only to reduce it a degree or two—that is, to below the level which brought on the fit.

Now dry the young patient and cover him. By now he probably is conscious. This is the time to send for medical help.

BREATH-HOLDING ATTACKS

The small child over 1 year old of limited physical strength may use a psychological game presented as a physical move when he is frustrated and cannot get adults to let him have his own way. He holds his breath and consciously or unconsciously enjoys the concern caused to those in charge of him.

He interrupts crying and forceful breathing with a full expiration and gets more and more blue in the face, until he may lose consciousness and fall. This is a form of temper tantrum. Demonstrations of anxiety or punishments from the grown-up only serve to reinforce his behavior.

The attack can be interrupted if the adult both appears to be unconcerned and does something unusual which astonishes or interests the child. Not every parent can suddenly stand on his or her head and sing (which would be an excellent

move), but immediately turning your back on the child and jumping noisily, clapping your hands, or slamming a door could be effective (see Figure 24). He will stop his act just to see what is happening.

You then go to him in a friendly way and divert his attention by finding something pleasant to occupy his mind. But do not give in to the original demand.

EPILEPSY

As there are several forms of epilepsy, and attacks tend to vary with the individual, only an "average" type will be described. This is the "grand mal" form with loss of consciousness and jerking. The accompanying table outlines its various stages and the first-aid action you should take. Rarely a patient will have a succession of epileptic seizures following each other rapidly. This is a dangerous situation which needs the immediate help of a doctor.

HYSTERICAL ATTACKS

Hysteria is a physical expression of mental anguish. Society is more prone to sympathize with a bodily than with a mental disturbance. An unhappy patient may chronically or suddenly hate his frustrations, his work, his relations. The office worker may be rebelling against a mode of life from which he wants to escape, the housewife may feel imprisoned by her home tasks.

What may seem an unimportant event may trigger off the attack. A screaming and shouting ses-

Stage	Possible Duration	First-aid Action
Attacks usually come without warning. However, some sufferers get a brief premonition accompanied by hesitation and pallor.	A very few seconds	Immediately have the patient lie down.
Most lose consciousness and fall very suddenly. They are silent but a few give one brief cry as they fall. They lie still and rigid, often with limbs extended and head bent back. The mouth is clenched, the breath is held and complexion is blue.	30 to 60 seconds	Loosen tight clothing. Guard the airway by positioning the head (see Figure 22).
Still unconscious, the patient begins twitching and this passes into hard sharp jerking of muscles. These convulsions may knock the limbs against nearby furniture or walls, may make the patient bite his tongue or be incontinent of bladder and wet himself. His mouth may fill with frothy saliva.	20 to 60 seconds	Do not try to restrain the jerking but quickly push aside furniture or pack a buffer (cushions, rolled up towel or coat) between limb and surface knocked. Clear froth from the mouth. Continue to guard the airway.
The jerking ceases and the patient lies unconscious and relaxed.	2 to 5 minutes	Turn the patient into the Recovery Position (see Figure 23), but be wary lest he has sustained a fracture in his fall.
Recovering consciousness the patient is at first dazed, then fully aware of what has happened.		Do not let him rise too soon. Let him rest and sleep. Check for signs of injury from the fall. If the attack happened in the street or away from home you should send the patient to the hospital by ambulance.

sion could be apposite, but it would receive little pity. The cry for help, the advertisement of unhappiness, is disguised as a demonstration of acute or chronic illness which is likely to create sympathy.

The hysterical man or woman is not deliberately pretending. He has no true understanding of the mechanism at play and believes genuinely in the truth of his symptoms. He is frightened by them.

An acute hysterical attack can take many forms. The patient says he cannot breathe (while breathing hard all the time), that he is paralyzed (while moving), that he has uncontrollable shaking (while interrupting the movements as he speaks). He may collapse and moan but become normal as he assesses a change in the situation by the arrival of a newcomer. He may appear unconscious but be seen to follow the actions of bystanders or to have a firm muscle tone. If you lift his arm and let it go, it does not fall back flaccidly but is lowered gently by the patient.

Treatment depends on realizing that:

1. *The patient is "advertising."* The more attention he has, the more he will want to advertise. Disperse bystanders, whose presence only encourages the performance to continue.

2. *The patient is frightened.* Do not scold him, do not slap him, do not throw water over him. Speak to him very firmly but also reassuringly. Do not say that his symptoms are false. Tell him that however unpleasant they may be they are transitory and will disappear rapidly.

3. *The patient feels lost and confused.* Give him no requests or suggestions but very definite instructions. Explain that if he lies or sits down and has a drink of water (or coffee or tea) the symptoms will ease.

You may have to reassure anxious friends and relatives that your hard attitude is not a sign of cruelty but a definite attempt to help. If in any doubt, however, play safe and get medical advice.

In any case, once the attack is over, a doctor is needed to help the patient to recognize and deal with the real sources of his trouble.

STROKES

A stroke is the loss of function of some part of the brain caused by an interruption of its blood supply. The blood vessel in that area may have ruptured or it may have become blocked by a clot. The old alternative term "apoplexy" has been replaced by that of "cerebrovascular accident."

The results of a stroke depend on the part of the brain involved and the speed with which this disruption to its circulation occurred. Minor weakness of some part of the body, poor arm or leg action, altered speech, loss of bladder control, paralysis of one side of the body, difficulty in swallowing, or total unconsciousness—any one of these can happen.

If you suspect that your patient has just had a stroke, be cautious. *It may be progressive.* If the victim finds that his hand grasp has become inexplicably weak and clumsy, he may be at the beginning of a mishap which could worsen rapidly to make a leg and arm functionless.

Get him resting in bed and call for medical help. Watch him carefully to see if his state worsens. In severe cases place him in the Recovery Position (see Figure 23) until the doctor arrives.

OBJECT IN THE EYE

Tell the patient to stop rubbing his eyes—which almost certainly he has been doing, making the irritation worse.

Wash your hands. Moisten the corner of a clean handkerchief and roll it into a point. You will use this to touch and lift out the object.

Seat the patient in a good light and stand behind him, bending his head up against you. This keeps his head firm and gives you a clear vision of the eye.

The object may lie on the white part of the eye. If the attempt to pick it off fails, it is probably embedded. Do not try again. If the object is anywhere within the colored circle (see Figure 25), you should leave it alone. This area is important to vision and could be damaged by inexperienced handling. Cover the eye with a clean pad and let a doctor deal with it.

Generally the object has moved under one or the other lid, often into the corner. Look under the lower lid. The patient looks up while you evert the lid, pulling it down by the pressure of two fingers (see Figure 26).

To look under the upper lid, have the patient look down while you evert the lid over a matchstick held across the "hinge" of the lid (see Figure 27). Grasping the edge of the lid firmly is less uncomfortable for the patient than if you try a light and slippery hold.

OBJECT IN THE EAR

Do not attempt its removal since this could be dangerous without special training and instruments.

The only exception is a very fine thread or an

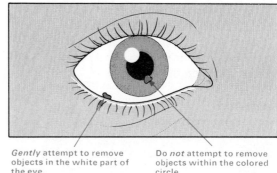

Gently attempt to remove objects in the white part of the eye.

Do *not* attempt to remove objects within the colored circle.

Figure 25   *Gently attempt to remove an object from the white part of the eye. Do not attempt to remove an object that is within the colored circle (iris).*

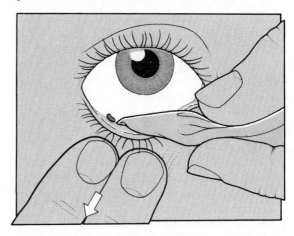

Figure 26   *Using two fingers, gently pull down the lower eyelid while the patient looks up.*

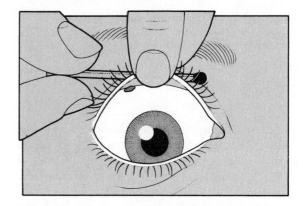

Figure 27   *Carefully pull up the upper eyelid as the patient looks down. A matchstick can help you to grip the lid as shown.*

insect, which can be intensely irritating to the patient. Lay the patient down with the ear uppermost and pour in a little tepid water or olive oil. Be very careful not to overheat the fluid. The insect will float to the top and can be wiped away.

The method is more likely to succeed if you

pull the top of the ear lobe up and back; this straightens out the external ear canal.

If there is any chance that the eardrum is perforated do not pour the fluid in; it could pass into and harm the middle ear.

OBJECT IN THE NOSE

Children in "experimental" moods often push objects up the nostril. A bean or pea tends to absorb moisture and swell and then be very difficult to dislodge.

Never try poking the object out from the depths; you will only drive it in further. Let a doctor, using special forceps, deal with it.

A small object can sometimes be expelled by blowing the nose carefully. Avoid hard blowing, however, which might cause painful air pressure inside the nose and sinuses. If there is any problem, see your physician at once.

CHOKING

Air entry into the windpipe may be blocked by:
1. An object at the back of the throat (solid food, dentures, mud).
2. The tongue in the unconscious person (see UNCONSCIOUSNESS).
3. Compression from outside (cord, strangulation, hanging).
4. An object within the windpipe itself.

The victim reacts by coughing hard in an attempt to expel the object. Muscles in the windpipe tend to tighten around it and hold it.

■ First-aid action

1. Open the patient's mouth widely; with your finger, feel deeply for anything at the back of the throat and scoop it clear.

2. The object may be too deep for you to reach. If the patient's condition is good and he is coughing well, advise him to breathe deeply and very slowly: This helps to relax the spasm of the windpipe.

3. If the obstruction does not clear and the patient is becoming blue and weak, give several hard slaps between his shoulder blades. In the case of an adult patient, this is best done when he is standing up; if he is unable to stand, roll him over onto his side. A child can be held with face bent downward over your forearm and raised

knee. A very small child can be held upside down: Grip the ankles and feet firmly with one hand, and give the slaps with the other.

4. If the patient has lost consciousness and is limp, give mouth-to-mouth resuscitation (see RESUSCITATION). In his state the windpipe spasm is relaxed and your air can pass around the object without appreciable danger of driving it further down.

■ Abdominal thrust for total obstruction: Heimlich maneuver

Sometimes trying to swallow an inadequately chewed lump of food results in total obstruction. The struggling patient is quite silent, being unable to speak or cough, and there is no whistling sound of any air moving in the windpipe.

Thrusting hard on the upper abdomen, between the navel and the lower end of the breastbone has a popgun effect, forcing air from the lungs up the windpipe to propel the object up and out. This procedure is known as the *Heimlich maneuver* (see Figure 28).

Thrust on the upper part of the abdomen hard, inward and upward. One thrust may succeed, but several may be needed. You may have to give artificial respiration after this (see RESUSCITATION).

If the patient vomits after this procedure, immediately turn him on one side and clear his mouth.

You must get medical advice after the rescue: In rare cases some internal damage occurs from the thrust. The risk of this is minimized by the correct positioning of your hands.

If you are alone and choking, the Heimlich maneuver can be self-administered. Put one fist with its thumb edge on your abdomen, slightly above the navel and beneath the ribs. Clutch your fist with your other hand; then press into the abdomen with a quick upward thrust. The movement is the same one you would use if you were attempting to save another person. An alternate method is to lean your abdomen against the back edge of a chair, porch rail, table, or sink and apply pressure against the same spot.

HANGING

As you rescue the patient, relieve the pull on his body by supporting his legs. Control his fall as the cord is cut, and ease the tight band around the neck. You may have to give artificial respiration (see RESUSCITATION).

THE HEIMLICH MANEUVER
(abdominal thrust for choking)

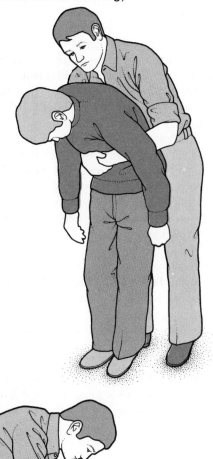

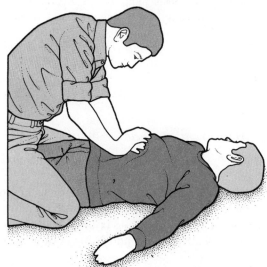

Figure 28 *This maneuver can save lives and should be learned by everyone.*

If the patient is standing or sitting: *Wrap your arms around his waist from behind. Put one fist with its thumb edge on the upper abdomen; your other hand clutches the fist. Thrust hard, inward and upward. Repeat thrusts until the food is forced out.*

If the patient is lying down: *Get him quickly on his back. Kneel astride his hips. Thrust with the heel of one hand covered by the other hand. Repeat thrusts until the food is forced out.*

ASTHMA

In an asthmatic attack, three main things happen to the tubes that form the airways of the lungs: (1) The airway tube tenses and contracts; (2) its lining becomes much thicker; and (3) this lining secretes thick mucus. All these narrow and block the tube, causing wheezing and a very difficult passage of air.

There are three likely "trigger" factors which can set this off in the asthma-prone patient: allergy, infection, and emotion. However the attack may have begun, the emotional factor plays a large part; discomfort, anxiety, and fear cannot help but build up in the victim who finds his breathing progressively more obstructed.

Your first-aid contribution will be to get the patient to relax physically and mentally and to position him to help the mechanics of breathing. A calm attitude of confidence, with advice clearly given, helps greatly.

If the patient has any tablets or inhalers prescribed for such attacks, make sure he uses them. But be certain this is done according to the doctor's instructions and do not let him take overdoses.

Let in fresh (but not cold) air and loosen tight clothing. Do not let the person crouch forward. Tell him to hold his back upright, either sitting or standing. He must relax all other parts of the body (limbs, neck, face).

Advise him to concentrate on breathing from the lower part of the chest and the abdomen. Most patients struggle to move the upper part of the chest, with poor results.

HEART ATTACK

"Heart attack" is a term that covers many types of sudden failure of the efficient beating of the heart muscle. For the first-aider there are two main forms: coronary occlusion and acute congestive failure.

■ *Coronary occlusion*

The heart muscle gets its blood supply from its own vessels, the coronary arteries, and not from the blood within its chambers. If one of these vessels suddenly becomes blocked by a clot, that part of the heart muscle which the vessel serves is deprived of blood and this is felt as pain—

although the underlying mechanisms responsible for the pain are not fully understood.

As a rule this pain is extremely severe, like a tight vice gripping the chest, and it may spread to the neck, shoulder or arm. The patient collapses, is pale or blue, breathless and sweating, with a fast, weak pulse. Sometimes he loses consciousness. Death may result.

However, please note that coronary occlusion can occur with pain of lesser severity and no marked evidence of shock. Such an attack may be mistaken for indigestion. The symptoms may be minor but the threat to the heart is nevertheless very real. For safety, in case of doubt, assume the worst.

If the patient loses consciousness, check whether the heart is beating. If it is not, proceed immediately to resuscitation (see RESUSCITATION). But never try heart compression if the heart is still beating, however weakly or irregularly.

If the patient is conscious, bear in mind that anxiety or fear produce body chemicals which can be extremely detrimental to the functioning of the heart muscle. Give sympathy with an attitude of calm confidence which can help to reassure.

Send for medical aid. Let the doctor (but not the patient) realize the degree of emergency you suspect.

Put the patient at full rest, with clothing loosened. If his breathing is difficult he should be sitting up, propped with pillows. Otherwise he should be lying down. If he is sweating, mop his face dry. Keep helpers from fussing or crowding him, which could add to his anxiety. Have the room warm but let in fresh air.

■ *Acute congestive heart failure*

In this case a fatigued or "worn" heart muscle is suddenly unable to propel blood adequately. There results congestion of blood in the lungs, whose air sacs become filled with plasma (the liquid part of blood) and some red cells that ooze from the lung vessels.

This can happen while the patient is sleeping. He wakes up very breathless, with a "bubbly" chest, each breath making a wet sound, different from the hard wheeze of asthma; he may cough up pinkish frothy fluid. He is distressed but not shocked or in pain.

Sit him supported in an upright position; be calm and reassuring, allow in fresh air, and immediately send for a doctor; this is the best you can do.

RESUSCITATION

Resuscitation consists of restoring life to someone who is near death because—

1. **his breathing has stopped** but his heart is still beating: You give artificial respiration.

2. **his breathing and his heartbeat have stopped:** You have to give both artificial respiration and heart compression.

Note that the heart can beat for a short time after breathing has ceased, but that if the heart has stopped so has breathing. Thus, in the latter case you never give heart compression alone but have to combine it with artificial respiration.

Resuscitation may be needed after:
- asphyxia
- drowning
- electrocution
- some heart attacks when the beat stops
- some forms of poisoning which affect the nervous control of heart and lungs or the ability of the blood to carry oxygen

> When resuscitation is needed you must act very fast; however, never jump to wrong conclusions. It is harmful to try it on someone who has "collapsed" but is still *conscious*, or on the unconscious person who is *breathing*. Your efforts would interfere with the still-active respiratory and cardiac functioning of the victim.

■ *Summary of method*

Airway: Position the patient so as to get his airway clear.
Breathing: Breathe the air from your lungs into his mouth; this will fill his lungs with air.
Circulation: If his color does not now improve and his pulse is absent, you add heart compression.

Airway—very rapidly:

1. If the patient is not lying flat on his back, roll him over, taking care to move the entire body at one time as a total unit.

2. Open the airway by lifting up the neck or chin gently with one hand while pushing down on the forehead with the other to tilt the head back.

3. Once the airway is open, place your ear close to the patient's mouth:

Look—at the chest and stomach for movement.

Listen—for sounds of breathing.

Feel—for breath on your cheek.

If none of these signs is present, the patient is not breathing.

4. If opening the airway does not cause the patient to begin to breathe spontaneously, you must provide rescue breathing.

Breathing

1. Take your hand that is on the patient's forehead and turn it so you can pinch the patient's nose shut while keeping the heel of the hand in place to maintain head tilt. Your other hand should remain under the patient's neck or chin, lifting up (see Figure 29).

2. Immediately give four quick, full breaths in rapid succession using the mouth-to-mouth method: Breathe in; seal your mouth over and around the patient's mouth. Then blow steadily and fully into the patient's mouth (see Figure 30). Ensure that the chest rises with each breath.

3. Check pulse. After giving the four quick breaths, locate the patient's carotid pulse to see if the heart is beating. To do this, take your hand that is under the victim's neck, or supporting the chin, and locate the victim's larynx ("voice box"). Feel for the pulse on either side.

4. If you cannot find the pulse, you must provide artificial circulation in addition to rescue breathing.

5. Send someone to call for Emergency Medical Services and medical help.

Circulation

Artificial circulation is provided by external chest compression. By applying rhythmic pressure on the lower half of the victim's breastbone, you are forcing his heart to pump blood (see Figure 31). To perform the technique properly:

1. Kneel at the patient's side near his chest. Locate the notch at the lowest portion of the sternum (breastbone).

2. Place the heel of one hand on the sternum next to the fingers that located the notch. Place your other hand on top of the one that is in position. Be sure to *keep your fingers off the chest wall* (see Figure 32). It may be easier to do this if you interlock your fingers.

3. Bring your shoulders directly over the patient's sternum as you compress downward, keeping your arms straight. Depress the sternum $1\frac{1}{2}$ to 2 inches for an adult victim.

4. Relax pressure on the sternum completely.

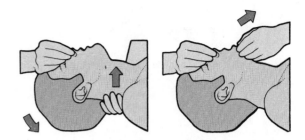

Figure 29 *With one hand under the patient's neck, tilt his head back; pinch nostrils shut.*

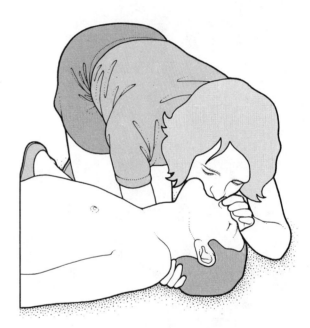

Figure 30 *Breathe in; seal your mouth over and around the patient's mouth. Then breathe out steadily and fully into the patient's mouth.*

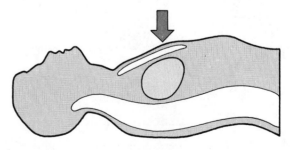

Figure 31 *In cardiac compression, depressing the breastbone squeezes the heart against the spine, forcing blood into the circulation.*

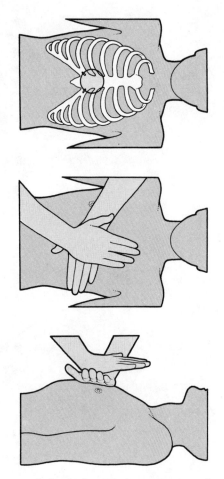

Figure 32 *It is vital to apply pressure at the correct point—the lower part of the breastbone. Press with the heel of one hand crossed by the heel of the other, keeping the fingers clear of the chest.*

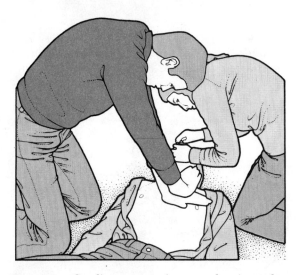

Figure 33 *Cardiac compression must be given alternately with artificial respiration. When working with a helper, always give five compressions followed by one breath.*

Do not remove your hands from the patient's sternum, but do allow the chest to return to its normal position between compressions.

5. Relaxation and compression should be of equal duration. If you do not have a helper, you must provide rescue breathing and external chest compression. The proper ratio is 15 chest compressions to 2 ventilations (breaths). You must compress at the rate of 80 to 100 times per minute when working alone since you must stop compressions when you take time to breathe.

If you have a helper, position yourselves on opposite sides of the patient if possible. One of you should be responsible for giving 1 mouth-to-mouth ventilation during the relaxation after each fifth compression. The other should compress the chest, using a rate of 80 to 100 compressions per minute with a pause after the fifth compression (see Figure 33).

■ *Resuscitating infants (birth to 1 year) and children (1 year to 8 years)*

Basic life support for infants and children is similar to that for adults. A few important differences to remember:

Airway
Be careful when handling an infant that you do not exaggerate the backward position of the head tilt. An infant's neck is so pliable that forceful backward tilting might block breathing passages instead of opening them.

Breathing
Do not try to pinch off the nose. Instead, cover both the mouth and nose of an infant who is not breathing (see Figure 34). Use small breaths with less volume to inflate the lungs. Give one small breath every 3 seconds. If the victim is a child cover the mouth and breathe every 4 seconds.

Check the *pulse in an infant* by feeling on the inside of the upper arm midway between the elbow and the shoulder. The pulse check in the *child* is the same as the adult.

Circulation
The technique for external chest compression is different for infants and small children. In both cases, use only one hand for compression. The other hand may be slipped under the infant to provide a firm support for his back.

For *infants,* use only the tips of the index and middle fingers to compress the chest at midsternum. Depress the sternum between $\frac{1}{2}$ to 1 inch

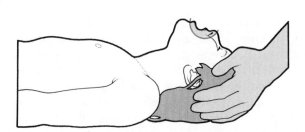

Figure 34   *When resuscitating a small child, seal your lips around the child's mouth and nose.*

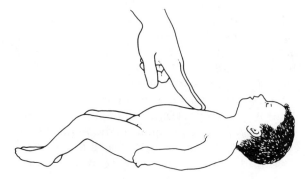

Figure 35   *For a baby, use only two fingers.*

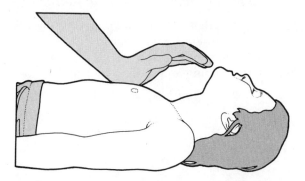

Figure 36   *Use one hand only to perform cardiac compression on a small child.*

at a rate of 100 times a minute (see Figure 35).

For *children*, use only the heel of one hand to compress the chest (see Figure 36). Depress the sternum between 1 and $1\frac{1}{2}$ inches, depending upon the size of the child. The rate should be 80 times per minute.

In the case of both infants and children, breaths should be administered during the relaxation after every fifth compression.

IMPORTANT

Resuscitation is best learned in first-aid classes under a qualified instructor. It should be practiced on a mannequin or dummy only. You must never practice on another person.

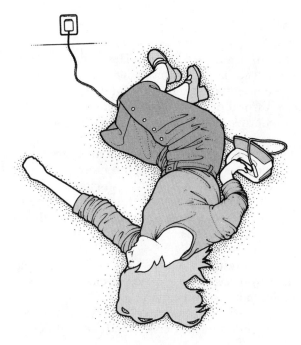

Figure 37   *Never touch a patient who is in contact with electricity; disconnect the power immediately.*

ELECTRIC SHOCK

1. When the patient is in contact with electricity
Do *not* touch him: You too may receive an electric shock or even be electrocuted. *Pull the plug at once.* If this is not possible, *wrench the plug free by the insulated cord,* or *turn off the power.* If this is not possible, *use a dry nonconducting material to push or knock the patient from this contact* (see Figure 37).

Never use a metal object. Use a wooden stick, a thick cushion, a rapidly folded coat, a chair, a wooden pole.

You may have difficulty and need to use traumatic force if the patient is holding an object that is live with alternating current (AC). This type of current puts the muscles in spasm so that the victim's hand clutches firmly.

WARNING

Where *very high voltage* is involved (some industries, power stations, high-tension towers, etc.), you must NOT attempt the rescue. This electricity can leap across gaps and hit the approaching first-aider. Keep at least 20 yards away. All you can do is to notify the authorities at once. No rescue is possible until the current has been cut off. In any case, the chance of the person's survival is extremely small.

---

2. When the patient is clear of contact

He can safely be touched. This applies also to those who have been hit by lightning.

The electric current can have—

- thrown or knocked down the victim
- burned deeply, damaging blood vessels
- caused unconsciousness
- stopped respiration and heartbeat by its action on nerves and brain center

You may have to initiate resuscitation immediately. Be on your guard for fractures and wounds from the patient's fall. Remember that a small skin burn can be a mark of extensive internal damage.

Put to rest and keep a close watch on any patient who has received a severe electric shock if he has not lost consciousness or if he appears to have recovered. He may collapse later. Call for Emergency Medical Services and medical help.

HEAD INJURY

Damage to the cranium (the upper part of the skull) can threaten the brain in several ways:

Infection. A wound of the scalp may lead to a fracture of the bone (not always exactly underneath it). The route is then open for bacteria to gain entrance to the brain.

A blow on the upper part of the head may fracture the base of the skull, on which the brain is resting. Bleeding or watery discharge (cerebrospinal fluid) from the nose or ear might result, with the risk of infection reaching the brain through the ear or nose.

Concussion. A blow on the head may give a general "shaking up" of the brain and knock out the victim. He becomes *instantly unconscious*. But if no other damage has occurred he will return to full consciousness—sometimes within seconds, sometimes within hours.

Compression. Pressure on the brain is an extremely serious matter because its soft tissues are very vulnerable and because it is tightly encased in the hard structure of the skull. Unlike other organs elsewhere (for example, the intestines in the abdomen), there is no room for displacement or an increase in size. Relatively minor changes of configuration give major pressure effects with marked consequences on the central nervous system.

Compression following injury can happen in one (or more) of three ways:

1. From depressed bone in a skull fracture.

2. From bleeding within the skull.

3. From the general swelling of brain tissue. This makes the brain fit even more tightly within the skull. It drives the brain stem downward to jam into the bony hole at the back of the base of the skull, where the medulla oblongata leaves the cranium to become the beginning of the spinal cord (see Figure 38). The brain stem contains nerve centers controlling such life functions as circulation and respiration. Subjected to pressure it may fail in its work.

Unlike concussion, which gives immediate unconsciousness, compression develops gradually. It make take minutes or hours for its effect to show, the patient gradually becoming comatose before passing into unconsciousness.

One feature which sometimes (not always) shows is enlargement of the dark pupil of the eye on one side. As a consequence, the pupils of the eyes may be unequal in size. If such a sign arises after head injury it is of grave significance.

■ *Compression following concussion*

It can happen that after a head injury the patient loses consciousness immediately from concussion and then apparently recovers ("lucid interval") before succumbing and sinking back into uncon-

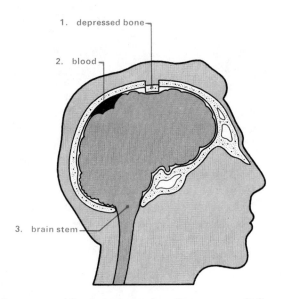

Figure 38   *After injury, compression may result from: (1) depressed bone, (2) bleeding inside the skull, or (3) pressure on the brain stem due to swelling. The effects are potentially very serious.*

sciousness due to compression which also has resulted. This is a sign of grave danger calling for urgent medical attention.

■ *First aid*

1. Treat **unconsciousness** according to the important principles outlined in the section on UN-CONSCIOUSNESS.

2. **Dress wounds** very meticulously.

3. **Beware of other injuries,** including fractures, especially fractures of the *spine* (see FRAC-TURES). Check for these as best you can before you move your patient. If in doubt, do not move him but watch his airway carefully.

4. **If you see blood or fluid from nose or ear** suspect a fracture at the base of the skull. Keep the patient on his back, or do not move because of possible spinal cord damage. Do not plug the ear but cover it with a protective dressing. If the nose is involved, warn the patient not to blow it for the act may drive contaminated fluid toward the fracture site and the brain.

5. **Get medical help as quickly as you can.**

POISONING

■ *Swallowed poisons*

Act according to this plan. The numbers refer to the notes that follow.

(1) Some poisons inhibit the respiratory control centers of the brain. Others may interfere with the blood's capacity to carry oxygen. A patient may have become asphyxiated on vomit, and the airway needs clearing. Place him in the Recovery Position (see Figure 23).

(2) *Corrosives* are chemical substances that can burn. You find them in some domestic cleaners, bleaches, rust removers, toilet bowl cleaners, and in car batteries. They include strong acids (such as sulfuric, nitric, hydrochloric) and alkalis (such as ammonia, caustic soda), which may leave marks and stains on the face and lips or where they have splashed on clothes.

On being swallowed they grossly damage the back of the throat and esophagus ("gullet"). Inside the stomach they do equal harm. Were the patient now to vomit, some of the corrosive would travel back into the mouth and aggravate the injury. Worse still, the stomach wall—weakened by the corrosive and subjected to the convulsive movements of vomiting—might perforate, letting

Swallowed poisons

Act according to this plan. The numbers refer to the notes which follow.

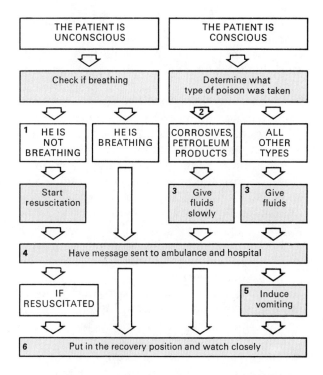

the poison leak into the abdominal cavity.

Petroleum products like gasoline or kerosene have a characteristic odor. As they are swallowed their fumes pass into the air passages and so to the lungs where they can cause great inflammation—a chemical pneumonia. A return journey by vomiting would repeat this damage.

Therefore, in both these categories—corrosives and petroleum products—*you do not want the patient to vomit.*

(3) *Give fluids* to dilute the poison. If the poison is a petroleum product, give 4 glasses of milk or water to an adult, 2 glasses to a child. But this you do to the *conscious patient only*; never give anything by mouth to an unconscious person.

The victim of a corrosive poison takes half this dose only: 2 glasses for the adult and 1 glass for the child. He must take it in slow sips; too much too fast may cause vomiting. In any case, after corrosive poisoning it will be difficult and painful to swallow.

(4) *Call for Emergency Medical Services.* It is wiser for you to remain with and attend to your patient and to delegate to someone else the message sending. He must tell the sex and age of the patient, the exact address, the poison suspected,

and the probable amount taken. Let him also explain what first aid is being given and whether or not the patient has vomited. He may be given advice on further action pending the arrival of the ambulance.

(5) *Induce vomiting only in the conscious patient who has not taken a corrosive or a petroleum product.* The best way to make him vomit is to rub against the back of his throat with your finger or with the blunt end of a spoon.

Please note that you do NOT give salt. Not only is salt an inefficient emetic, but it also can be harmful in large doses. Some premises where poisoning is a possible hazard may keep *syrup of ipecac* as an emergency emetic; the provision of this and instruction as to dosage should come through a doctor. Many doctors urge that every family should keep a supply in their medicine chest.

Keep a sample of vomit to send with the patient to the hospital if there is time.

The most important thing to do is to *get the patient to the hospital quickly.* Your attempts to induce vomiting must not delay this.

(6) The Recovery Position (see Figure 23) is necessary for any poisoned patient after you have taken other measures. The victim who has been conscious or recovered consciousness may suddenly become unconscious and start to vomit.

Always stay close by the patient in case his condition worsens. A would-be suicide, frustrated by his failure to kill himself, may make another attempt unless watched. Where you are suspicious of suicide or homicide, you should call the police; try not to handle surrounding articles.

If possible, obtain a sample of any vomit and also any containers (even if empty) from which the poison may have come; send these to the hospital with the victim.

■ Gas poisons

Carbon monoxide from incomplete burning of fuels, especially gasoline, is the most likely poison in this category. A common source is a car engine running in a closed garage or an exhaust that leaks into the inside of the car; poorly burning coal fires with inadequate ventilation can also give off poison gas. In industry, other gases, such as carbon tetrachloride, may escape in poisonous amounts. In a house fire poisonous gases may be present in a smoke-filled room.

If you have to rescue someone from an area filled with gas fumes, take a deep breath and hold it before going in. The first thing to do is to get the victim out into the fresh air; if it does not cause delay, you should also turn off the engine that is emitting the fumes and open (or break) the windows of the room or garage.

As soon as you are clear of the gas, check the victim's airway. If he is not breathing give artificial respiration. If he is breathing and conscious, advise him to take deep and slow breaths.

■ Agricultural poisons

Some pesticides can be dangerous, not only when swallowed but when invisible droplets are inhaled after the chemical has been used as a spray. Also, droplets settling or liquid splashing onto clothes and skin could be absorbed into the body.

Massive doses will produce fast and obvious poisoning. A more hidden situation is that in which the poison gradually builds up after recurrent exposure to smaller concentrations. Symptoms may develop slowly and moderately and then suddenly become severe and dangerous. The time factor may vary from minutes to days.

These symptoms are not very specific and their onset could suggest influenza. The patient has a headache, is sweating, thirsty, and nauseated. He is abnormally tired. Impaired action of nerves and muscles may lead to dimmed vision and difficulty in breathing with tightness of the chest. Eventually breathing and heartbeat could fail.

Your first-aid treatment may thus begin with suspecting the exposure in its early stages. Stop the patient from working; put him at complete rest.

Carefully remove contaminated clothing (put it in a plastic bag, working with gloves, if you can). Wash his skin very thoroughly. Irrigate his eyes with water if they could have been contaminated. He may need artificial respiration.

If he is conscious, let him drink sweetened water to which you have added a pinch of salt.

The containers of the pesticide may carry special instructions concerning emergency treatment of the poisoning. Get medical help quickly.

■ Poisonous contact plants

Poison ivy, poison sumac, and poison oak can—within a couple of hours or days after contact—cause rashes and blisters. The irritation comes from a plant resin which the patient, by scratching and manipulation, may have carried from the original exposed areas of contact (hands, wrists, face, ankles) to other parts of his body.

Take off the patient's clothes and wash his skin with copious changes of soap and water. Do not rupture blisters that form with the rash. In mild cases a simple soothing lotion (such as calamine) may be enough; but some attacks are severe—with a raised body temperature—and need medical help.

DRUG ADDICT IN CRISIS

Helping the addict who is having a severe reaction to a drug is a difficult problem. Manifestations of overdosage are so varied from drug to drug and (for each drug) from individual to individual that only the broadest outline for helping can be given. Here we consider not the basic state of addiction but the sudden crisis that can arise from self-administration.

■ *Stimulants*

Stimulants such as amphetamines ("speed") in large doses can make the taker behave very like the irresponsible, irrational alcoholic. He is energetic, loquacious, overactive. Very rarely marijuana (cannabis) can give a similar reaction.

The thing to do is to treat him like a drunken person who is behaving badly. Keep friendly with him, keep talking to him, be amenable as far as possible. Do not leave him alone at any time but keep with him and, if you can, get someone to be with you or at least close at hand and within call for help. The effect wears off with time and the addict can then be handled more easily.

■ *Hallucinogens*

Someone under the severe effect of drugs like lysergic acid (LSD, "acid") can be in danger—and so could those near him. The victim becomes psychotic, with the most bizarre ideas and behavior. He might pass through a phase of fear amounting to panic. You must constantly speak to him; be comforting and reassuring, although this may be difficult to achieve.

He might have self-destructive impulses and do almost anything, like trying to jump out of a high window. He might have delusions of being attacked or ill-treated and then suddenly could be violently hostile and attack you.

Be on your guard, seek help, and use whatever force is reasonable, but only when his safety or your self-defense makes it necessary. Calling an ambulance for his removal to the hospital is a necessary solution.

■ *Depressants*

Depressants such as barbiturates slow down a person's reactions considerably. These drugs depress and eventually induce sleep. The takers may easily be involved in traffic accidents.

Barbiturates may first put the victim briefly into a state of overactive excitement. This does not last long, and he is likely to collapse quite suddenly. At this point his life is in danger. Put him in the Recovery Position (see Figure 23) and arrange to have him sent to the hospital. If depressants have been combined with alcohol the situation is particularly perilous.

On the other hand, *withdrawal symptoms* in a drug addict can be accompanied by delirium and convulsions which need immediate medical aid. Guarding the victim's airway (see UNCONSCIOUSNESS) is your principal task.

■ *Narcotics*

Addicts often take morphine and heroin by injection into a vein, first dissolving the powder or tablet in water. One danger lies in the way these drugs depress respiration. The addict who collapsed from an overdose could cease breathing and need artificial respiration.

Another major threat is the risk the addict runs from his self-administered intravenous injection. An embolism (the blockage of a vessel) by some of the inadequately dissolved preparation can damage part of the heart, brain, or lung and cause death. First aid can help little, but you must try the general principles of resuscitation (see RESUSCITATION).

Symptoms of withdrawal from these narcotics can cause real distress. They develop gradually and can become very severe.

An addict who has accustomed himself to more or less regular doses and who, for some reason, cannot get one when it is due will soon develop a craving and will become generally anxious and restless. Some hours later symptoms like yawning, sneezing, and watering of the eyes and nose will appear. In about 24 hours these worsen. He sweats; his temperature and pulse rate are increased; his skin may itch; he is nauseated.

Though he feels very tired and hungry he can neither sleep nor eat. This may be followed by abdominal cramps, vomiting, diarrhea, and severe prostration.

Eventually he will recover but he will have been through a very high degree of mental and physical suffering. Reassure and support the patient, but do all you can to dissuade and prevent him from seeking out more of his drug for self-treatment (unfortunately, this advice usually falls on deaf ears). Medical help is needed as early as possible. Very often a dose of morphine or heroin substitute is given as effective alleviation.

INSECT STINGS

The only real dangers from insect stings are:

1. Infection at the sting site. A doctor may advise antibiotics.

2. Some insects can transmit diseases.

These two potential dangers are relatively long-term features and not factors involving first aid.

3. More immediate is the chance that the patient has acquired, from past stings, a hypersensitivity to the insect's venom. He may rapidly develop an *allergic reaction* with pallor and collapse. Some people, like beekeepers, who are exposed to this risk keep antihistamine tablets to take immediately in an emergency. The serious case needs rapid medical attention and treatment by injections, however.

The usual insect sting is only a minor matter of pain and inconvenience.

Do not use tweezers to remove insect stingers; instead, the skin where the stinger is embedded should be scraped with a knife edge. (Tweezers can further embed the stinger or pinch it into sections.) Removal of the stinger is important to stop the reaction process. Apply an antihistamine cream, smoothing it gently into the skin.

TICK BITES

The tick often remains attached to the skin. The sooner you get it off the better. Do not pull; this would leave part of it still embedded.

Either (1) "drown" the tick by covering it with a heavy oil like salad oil or machine oil. If it does not separate at once, leave the oil over it for half an hour and then slowly, carefully, remove its body with tweezers.

Or (2) light a cigarette and apply the glow-

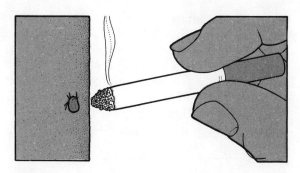

Figure 39 *One method of removing an attached tick is to apply a lighted cigarette to it, taking care not to burn the skin of the patient.*

ing end to the tick; it should now fall off (see Figure 39).

SNAKEBITES

Snakes vary so much in habitat and potential harmfulness that only general rules can be offered here. Seek expert advice about the dangerous snakes in your locality, preferably *before* any snakebite happens.

Do not lose time trying to kill the snake; try to identify it. Patient care and safety are your prime concerns.

Immediately lay the patient down; let him be at rest. Wipe away from the bite area any venom lying on the skin. Wash the area thoroughly with soap and water. Tamp it dry gently (do not rub). Put on a clean dressing.

Immobilize the bitten area as if it were fractured. This reduces the speed of flow of venom into the patient's circulation.

Pain can be very great, but do not allow the victim to take pain-relieving tablets. Fear, too, may be great; your patient may be convinced that all snakebites are fatal. They are not, and terror (not too strong a word) may be a great factor affecting the bite victim's general condition. Very strong reassurance is a great help. In the few cases where snakebite proves fatal, death generally does not happen quickly, but one or two days after the incident. Get the patient to the hospital by ambulance or car. Do not allow the victim to walk. Keep the bitten area as elevated as possible.

Send a telephone message ahead to the hospital, so that preparations can be made.

In some cases shock and respiratory difficulty occur. Watch the patient's breathing. You may even have to give artificial respiration.

YOU DO NOT

- suck the wound area
- apply chemicals to it
- cut into it
- apply a tourniquet

These maneuvers are outdated and ineffective. They may do more harm than good.

SCORPION AND SPIDER STINGS

These can give intense pain and skin damage. Some can cause general symptoms of collapse, sweating, nausea, and vomiting; it is rare for them to be fatal.

Treat as for SNAKEBITES (see above).

FROSTBITE

In severe cold the blood vessels of the skin narrow as the result of a reflex action; exposed areas blanch and may be at risk for gangrene. Parts especially threatened are extremities like fingers, toes, nose, ears, and chin. The condition worsens if partial thawing is followed by a recurrence of frosting; you must take great care to avoid this.

The affected skin is "devitalized" and must be treated gently. *It should never be rubbed.*

■ *Treatment of frostbite*

Frostbitten hands or feet should be immersed in warm water. Failing this, keep the body parts as warm as possible by bodily contact or hand covering. Do not thaw feet if the victim then has to walk. Rest after warming is important.

EXPOSURE TO COLD

Severe exposure to cold can have a devastating effect on the body, especially on the heart muscle. The general result is a progressive slowing up of the body systems; the victim may become clumsy, with poor judgment developing into mental confusion. From drowsiness he may pass into coma. He is at risk of dying of heart failure. Act as follows:

1. Give resuscitation if this is needed (see RESUS-

Treatment of Frostbite

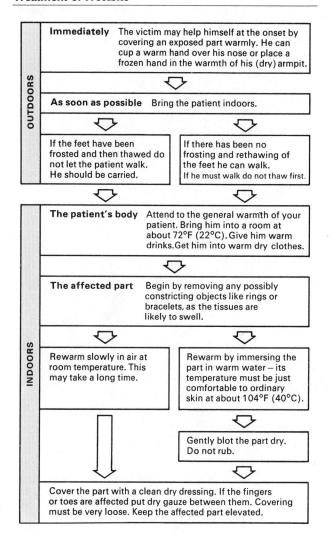

OUTDOORS	**Immediately** The victim may help himself at the onset by covering an exposed part warmly. He can cup a warm hand over his nose or place a frozen hand in the warmth of his (dry) armpit.	
	As soon as possible Bring the patient indoors.	
	If the feet have been frosted and then thawed do not let the patient walk. He should be carried.	If there has been no frosting and rethawing of the feet he can walk. If he must walk do not thaw first.
INDOORS	**The patient's body** Attend to the general warmth of your patient. Bring him into a room at about 72°F (22°C). Give him warm drinks. Get him into warm dry clothes.	
	The affected part Begin by removing any possibly constricting objects like rings or bracelets, as the tissues are likely to swell.	
	Rewarm slowly in air at room temperature. This may take a long time.	Rewarm by immersing the part in warm water – its temperature must be just comfortable to ordinary skin at about 104°F (40°C).
		Gently blot the part dry. Do not rub.
	Cover the part with a clean dry dressing. If the fingers or toes are affected put dry gauze between them. Covering must be very loose. Keep the affected part elevated.	

CITATION). Check very carefully that there is no breathing or pulse detectable. Attempts at heart massage on a heart that is still beating, however slightly, can be extremely harmful.

2. Put the patient at complete rest. Do not let him struggle on.

3. Transport him into a warm room or shelter. If there is no shelter and you have to treat him outside, shield him as best you can within a tent or by setting up a screen of poles, clothes, or blankets to protect against the wind.

4. Give him warm drinks if he is conscious. Cocoa or hot chocolate is very suitable. Let him take this slowly. NEVER give him alcohol, which would make him lose more heat by dilating the skin blood vessels.

5. Replace wet and cold clothes with warm dry covers. A plastic sheet incorporated in these would

USING TWO BLANKETS TO COVER THE COLD PATIENT

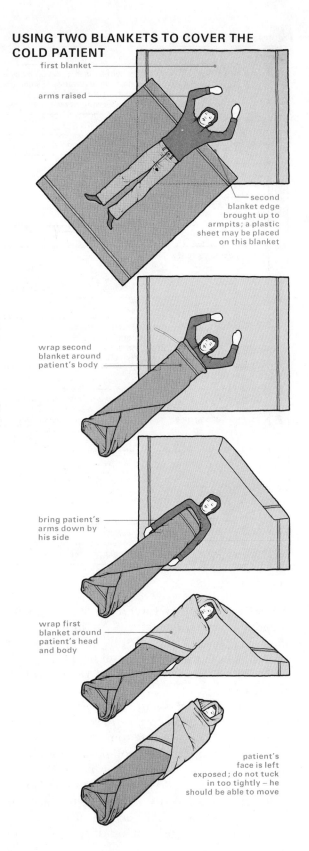

first blanket

arms raised

second blanket edge brought up to armpits; a plastic sheet may be placed on this blanket

wrap second blanket around patient's body

bring patient's arms down by his side

wrap first blanket around patient's head and body

patient's face is left exposed; do not tuck in too tightly – he should be able to move

Figure 40   *Use two blankets as shown to cover the patient who has suffered exposure to cold.*

help the body to retain heat. A great deal of heat can be lost from the head; make sure that it is within the covering, with only the face exposed. Two blankets can be used to cover the patient effectively as shown in Figure 40.

Sometimes you can use a sleeping bag; if available, a second person in the bag would be an added source of heat.

> Rapid rewarming by putting the patient in a bath of 104°F (40°C) is used sometimes, but under domestic circumstances this is best reserved for cases of sudden and relatively brief immersion, as in icy water. Where the patient has cooled slowly, the gradually altered body chemistry and heart muscle may not be able to cope with changes brought about by a sudden return to warmth.

HYPOTHERMIA

"Accidental hypothermia" is the name given to a dangerous condition of very low body temperature which can arise in the home in an almost unsuspected way. In very cold weather and where rooms are inadequately heated the occupants can gradually cool down to a body temperature of 95°F (35°C) or below. In extreme cases the body temperature can fall below 86°F (30°C).

The extremes of age are particularly prone to this mishap. The small baby, paradoxically, has a relatively large body surface from which to lose heat. He is not active and does not produce much body heat by muscle action as he lies in his crib. His temperature-regulating mechanism is not yet fully developed, and if his covers slip off he cannot pull them back.

Compared with younger people, the elderly have a slightly lower body temperature; their blood vessels are narrower; they move less in sleep; their thyroid glands (which help to produce body heat) are less active. In addition, many are taking sleeping tablets or tranquilizers which can have some temperature-lowering effect.

These patients can slip gradually into a deeply cold state, usually overnight while asleep. They are very drowsy or even in a coma, icy to the touch (even under the blankets), with pulse and respiration slow and poor in volume. The skin is puffy and pale (but sometimes rosy in babies).

You must NOT try rapid rewarming, for this might lead to circulatory collapse. Have the patient lie in bed fully (but loosely) covered, including the head. Do not warm the bed (for example, *never use an electric blanket*), but *warm the room.* If the person is conscious give him warm drinks, but *never alcohol.*

You should get immediate medical advice; some of these patients urgently need hospital admission.

HEAT EFFECTS

Perspiring as we become hot is one of our protective methods against becoming overheated. As it evaporates, sweat fluid carries heat out of the body. This effect helps to maintain normal body temperature.

Effective as it is, this mechanism has one disadvantage: The sweat carries with it a fair concentration of salts which are natural components of the body chemistry. A deficiency of these salts causes weakness and, sometimes, severe cramps.

This is the simple background to understanding the two main ways in which overheating can affect us.

ROAD ACCIDENTS

Deal with the accident by a threefold program.
1. The emergency patient
2. The urgent situation
3. The other patients

■ 1. *The emergency patient*

Just as soon as you are at the scene of a car crash, check whether or not anyone needs help for asphyxia (see CHOKING) or severe bleeding (see BLEEDING).

As far as possible, treat the patient where you find him. Tell any other injured passengers to remain where they are and that you will help them very shortly.

Always look over nearby low walls or hedges for a victim who might have been thrown there.

■ 2. *The urgent situation*

The situation could indeed be full of risk. A road that is partially obstructed as the result of an ac-

Heat Exhaustion	Heat Stroke
This can attack someone who has perspired heavily after long exertion or on a very hot day.	This can happen in a very hot region of the jungle type where the atmosphere is windless and very humid.
The body loses an excessive amount of water and salts.	There is a breakdown of the sweat-producing mechanism: Sweat is unable to evaporate into the atmosphere, which is already saturated with water vapor. The air temperature may be higher than that of the patient.
Thanks to the sweating, the patient's body temperature is normal or only slightly raised.	The body, unable to lose heat, becomes extremely hot. The body temperature may rise to 107°F (42°C) or more.
He feels faint, exhausted, and sometimes nauseated.	The patient is restless and confused and may become unconscious.
His skin is moist and may be pale.	His skin is hot, dry, and red.
His pulse is fast and feeble.	His pulse is fast and forceful.
He may develop cramps.	
First Aid	**First Aid**
Get the patient into a cool area and let him lie down.	Quickly get the patient into the coolest place, indoors if possible.
Loosen his clothing and raise his feet.	Remove his clothing.
Give him fluids with salt to drink: 1 teaspoonful of salt per glass. Fresh fruit juice is excellent for this. Let him drink slowly—half a glass every 15 minutes.	Now cool him down by sponging his body with tepid water, and by fanning him vigorously. Do not aim to bring his body temperature to normal, but only to lower it by 2 to 3 degrees F.
Recovery is likely to be good, but it is wise to get medical advice.	This condition can be mortally dangerous. You need medical help urgently.

cident and which still bears approaching traffic is full of hazards.

• *No one must smoke* because of the chance of escaping gasoline.

• If there is any *fire or smoldering* put it out at once with the fire extinguisher which you should be carrying in your car. If fire persists then you must try to get the occupants out quickly.

• *Switch off the ignition key* and turn out the lights of any car involved.

• *Put on the emergency brake.* If it does not work and the car is on a hill get something, such as a box or a rear seat, jammed up behind the wheel.

• *Get your car parked well out of the way,* off the road if you can, to leave room for police and rescue services. This is for your and your car's safety and to leave a clearing for the rescue services. At night have your headlights shining on the scene.

• *Set warnings for drivers of approaching cars.* Put a flare or a red reflector at least 200 yards on either side, or have a lookout signaling with a flashlight, a white scarf, or even a newspaper.

• *Send a message for the police and an ambulance* by one or even two messengers. Write out what is to be telephoned. Give the exact location, the number and type of casualties, and whether or not any are trapped.

It may seem as if all this is spending too much time away from the patients waiting in the car. Experience has shown that these moves avoid extra damage.

■ 3. The other patients

Now you can return to attend to patients with less urgent injuries. Carefully examine all persons involved and treat them where they are.

The person who is making a fuss or much noise is unlikely to be badly injured; he will usually respond to strong reassurance.

Beware of the unconscious victim in his seat. His neck (a possible fracture) and his airway are the most vulnerable parts. Wipe his mouth free of any fluid. Support his jaw.

You could find that the small or average-sized dressing is useless when you try to cover wounds. Wounds resulting from traffic accidents tend to be big ones, and your kit should contain some really large dressings.

It is wise not to take an accident victim to the hospital yourself; wait for the ambulance. Your

ordinary-looking car may be held up in a traffic jam. And you will be in great difficulty if the patient collapses while you travel.

In any case, you should not try to extricate patients from a smashed car. Leave this to the experts. Using special equipment they may have to remove large sections of a wrecked car to be able to get the victim out without doing him further harm.

FINALLY: If you come upon an accident scene where rescue services are already in operation, do not stop; this could impede their work. Pass very slowly and carefully.

■ Matters of priority

When facing any event with one or several accident victims, you must have a method of approach. Do not automatically tend to the nearest patient, but begin with a quick assessment of the whole situation.

There may be an immediate further risk at the scene. Walls may threaten to collapse, there may be fast-moving traffic, or there may be a fire or gas hazard. You may have to remove the patient(s) speedily and gently instead of following the rule of treating on the spot.

Survey the injured quickly. Decide which patient urgently needs your help and go to him. Call out to the others to remain still where they are, adding that you will soon attend to them. Also, warn bystanders who are not first-aiders not to try to lift up any of the victims. They may have a fracture, which could be made worse with improper movement.

Priority goes to:

• asphyxia
• resuscitation needs
• heavy bleeding

With due care, put the unconscious patient in the Recovery Position (see Figure 23).

While you work, do your best to control any gathering crowd. A voice of authority rather than of pleading works wonderfully with strangers. From the bystanders choose someone to send a message for an ambulance; this must be very definite, detailing the address, the number of casualties, and their injuries.

Get someone to clear away any dangerous debris, such as broken glass.

Your calm manner, your appearance of method and confidence can be invaluably reassuring to the patient. Establish a relationship with him. Get his name and address; give him your name. Always speak to him as you work, showing sympathy and explaining in advance anything you are about to do.

If some of his property is lying about, look after it and let him know you are doing so.

As you deal with injuries, remember to think of the hidden wound and the unsuspected fracture.

And never forget the importance of preventing shock (see SHOCK).

FIRST-AID BOX

Where do you keep it? The bathroom is not the best place for it. It should avoid steamy atmospheres; it should always be immediately accessible; it should be out of the reach of children; it should be in a zone frequently occupied by the people of the house or apartment and easily seen by guests. The upper shelf of a hall cupboard or of a dry kitchen cabinet is satisfactory.

What sort of box? It should be both roomy and portable and made of metal or plastic with a tight-fitting lid which can be opened easily by an adult. Label it very clearly.

What should it contain? Since it is for domestic use, we can presume that it will often be called upon for minor treatments which do not need a doctor. Therefore it will go beyond *first* aid and venture a little into *second* aid—that is, simple home treatments.

Instruments:
Tweezers.
Scissors (kept for this purpose only).
Thermometer.
Safety pins.

Medicines:
Acetaminophen or soluble aspirin tablets.
Simple antiseptics like cetrimide or chlorhexidine in suitable dilution ready for use, or in stronger form with the instructions on diluting carefully marked on the bottle. Ask your doctor or pharmacist.
An antiseptic cream for spreading on dressings.

Dressings:
White gauze.
Absorbent cotton.
Paper tissues.
2-inch- and 3-inch-wide plain bandages.
Ready-to-apply sterile dressings, each packed singly in its protective covering. These are obtainable in various sizes.
2-inch- and 3-inch-wide adherent dressing strips, which can be cut to size for covering simple wounds.
1-inch-wide adhesive strapping.

The above will cover most needs. It is better to keep to a few standardized items than to have a large mixed collection which can confuse. Items like absorbent cotton and gauze should be in small intact packs. Once they have been opened they should not be put back for further use later.

Anything you use from the box you should replace immediately with new items.

2
COLOR
ATLAS
OF
THE
BODY

The color illustrations on the following pages show the exact location, shape, and important details of each of the body's organs and major systems, and the brief descriptions that accompany them explain the remarkable way these systems function.

To make the descriptions as clear and comprehensive as possible, the pages have been organized so that both general as well as microscopically detailed drawings of each system appear together, on facing pages. For example, on the lefthand page of color plates IV and V, "Muscles," you can see how the muscles protect and interact with nerves, bones, inner organs, and the circulatory system. On the opposite page, the micro-anatomy of muscles is made clear in drawings that picture the incredible complexity of a single muscle fiber, the interface of muscles with the nervous system (which makes movement possible), and the detailed structure of different kinds of muscle.

The Head

The bones of the skull determine the shape of the head and also give protection to the brain and special sense organs. This view shows the intimate relationships between the various organs of the head; this compactness is one of the marvels of human evolution. The brain is by far the most complex structure in the body, and a great deal still remains to be learned about its function. With the spinal cord, it constitutes the central nervous system. The neck conveys major blood vessels, the respiratory and digestive passages and the spinal cord, and also permits extensive movement of the head around the first two cervical vertebrae.

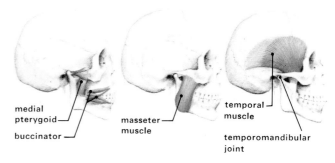

Biting and chewing muscles
Biting and chewing depend on movements at the temporomandibular joint between the lower jaw (mandible) and the rest of the skull. These movements are produced by contractions of the powerful muscles of mastication shown in the illustration above.

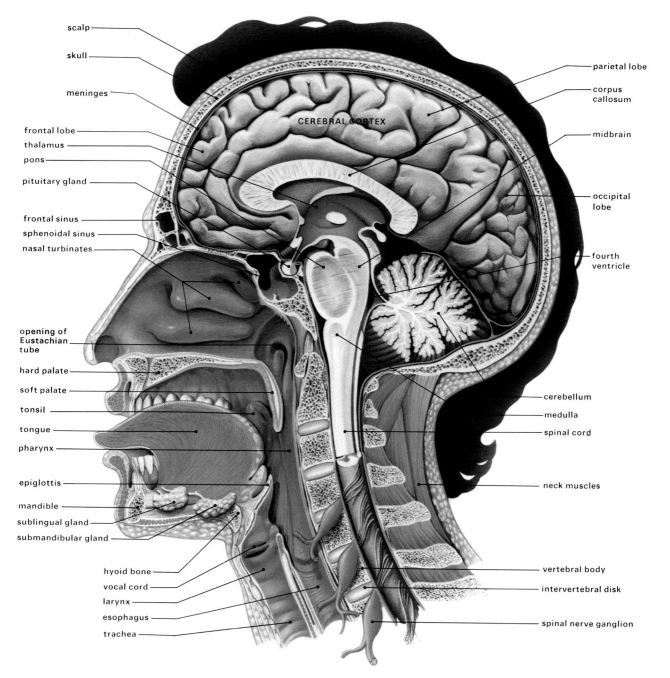

The Bones and Joints

The skeleton gives form, support and protection to the body. It consists of about 206 bones, supplemented by pieces of cartilage. The bones, especially the long bones of the limbs, act as levers operated by the muscles (connected across the joints), thus allowing movement. Some bones (e.g., the ribs and skull) also serve to protect the organs they enclose. Bones are also a reservoir of vital minerals, and some contain bone marrow, where blood cells are formed. Joints between bones are of three types: *fibrous* (allowing no movement), *cartilaginous* (limited movement) and *synovial* (freely movable).

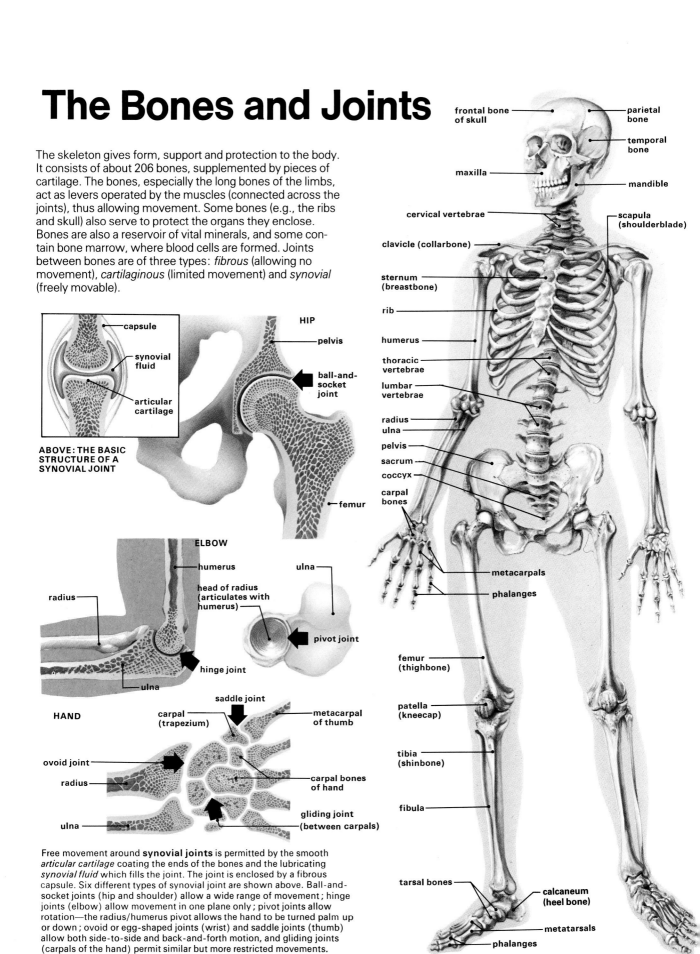

capsule

synovial fluid

articular cartilage

ABOVE: THE BASIC STRUCTURE OF A SYNOVIAL JOINT

HIP

pelvis

ball-and-socket joint

femur

ELBOW

humerus

head of radius (articulates with humerus)

radius

ulna

hinge joint

ulna

pivot joint

HAND

saddle joint

carpal (trapezium)

metacarpal of thumb

ovoid joint

radius

carpal bones of hand

ulna

gliding joint (between carpals)

Free movement around **synovial joints** is permitted by the smooth *articular cartilage* coating the ends of the bones and the lubricating *synovial fluid* which fills the joint. The joint is enclosed by a fibrous capsule. Six different types of synovial joint are shown above. Ball-and-socket joints (hip and shoulder) allow a wide range of movement; hinge joints (elbow) allow movement in one plane only; pivot joints allow rotation—the radius/humerus pivot allows the hand to be turned palm up or down; ovoid or egg-shaped joints (wrist) and saddle joints (thumb) allow both side-to-side and back-and-forth motion, and gliding joints (carpals of the hand) permit similar but more restricted movements.

frontal bone of skull

parietal bone

temporal bone

maxilla

mandible

cervical vertebrae

scapula (shoulderblade)

clavicle (collarbone)

sternum (breastbone)

rib

humerus

thoracic vertebrae

lumbar vertebrae

radius

ulna

pelvis

sacrum

coccyx

carpal bones

metacarpals

phalanges

femur (thighbone)

patella (kneecap)

tibia (shinbone)

fibula

tarsal bones

calcaneum (heel bone)

metatarsals

phalanges

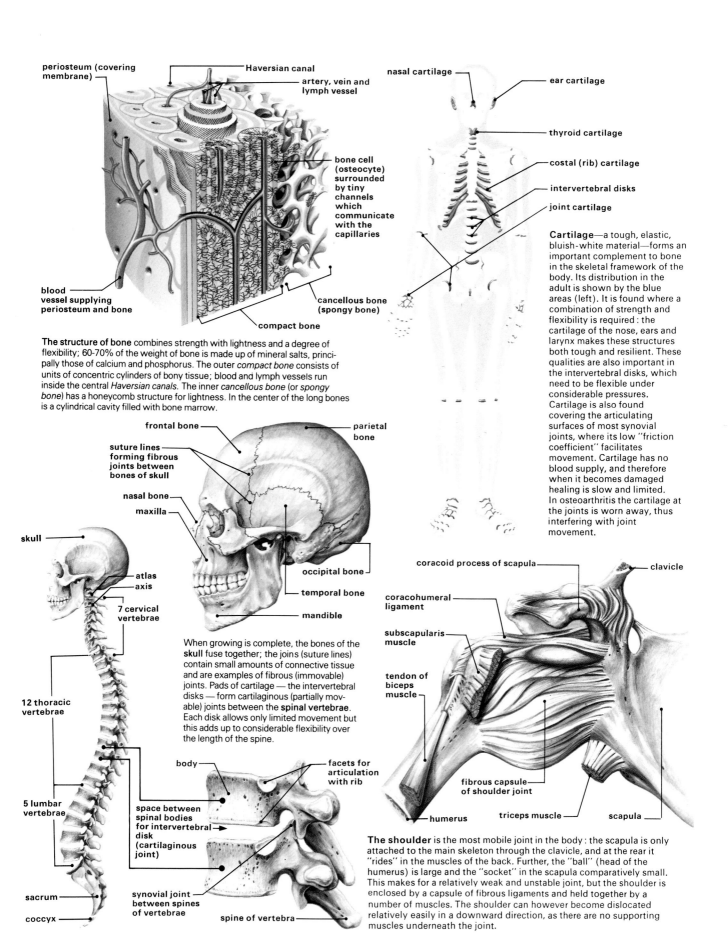

periosteum (covering membrane)

Haversian canal

artery, vein and lymph vessel

bone cell (osteocyte) surrounded by tiny channels which communicate with the capillaries

blood vessel supplying periosteum and bone

cancellous bone (spongy bone)

compact bone

The structure of bone combines strength with lightness and a degree of flexibility; 60-70% of the weight of bone is made up of mineral salts, principally those of calcium and phosphorus. The outer *compact bone* consists of units of concentric cylinders of bony tissue; blood and lymph vessels run inside the central *Haversian canals*. The inner *cancellous bone* (or *spongy bone*) has a honeycomb structure for lightness. In the center of the long bones is a cylindrical cavity filled with bone marrow.

nasal cartilage

ear cartilage

thyroid cartilage

costal (rib) cartilage

intervertebral disks

joint cartilage

Cartilage—a tough, elastic, bluish-white material—forms an important complement to bone in the skeletal framework of the body. Its distribution in the adult is shown by the blue areas (left). It is found where a combination of strength and flexibility is required : the cartilage of the nose, ears and larynx makes these structures both tough and resilient. These qualities are also important in the intervertebral disks, which need to be flexible under considerable pressures. Cartilage is also found covering the articulating surfaces of most synovial joints, where its low "friction coefficient" facilitates movement. Cartilage has no blood supply, and therefore when it becomes damaged healing is slow and limited. In osteoarthritis the cartilage at the joints is worn away, thus interfering with joint movement.

frontal bone

parietal bone

suture lines forming fibrous joints between bones of skull

nasal bone

maxilla

skull

atlas
axis

7 cervical vertebrae

occipital bone

temporal bone

mandible

12 thoracic vertebrae

When growing is complete, the bones of the **skull** fuse together; the joins (suture lines) contain small amounts of connective tissue and are examples of fibrous (immovable) joints. Pads of cartilage — the intervertebral disks — form cartilaginous (partially movable) joints between the **spinal vertebrae**. Each disk allows only limited movement but this adds up to considerable flexibility over the length of the spine.

5 lumbar vertebrae

body

facets for articulation with rib

space between spinal bodies for intervertebral disk (cartilaginous joint)

synovial joint between spines of vertebrae

sacrum

coccyx

spine of vertebra

coracoid process of scapula

clavicle

coracohumeral ligament

subscapularis muscle

tendon of biceps muscle

fibrous capsule of shoulder joint

humerus

triceps muscle

scapula

The shoulder is the most mobile joint in the body : the scapula is only attached to the main skeleton through the clavicle, and at the rear it "rides" in the muscles of the back. Further, the "ball" (head of the humerus) is large and the "socket" in the scapula comparatively small. This makes for a relatively weak and unstable joint, but the shoulder is enclosed by a capsule of fibrous ligaments and held together by a number of muscles. The shoulder can however become dislocated relatively easily in a downward direction, as there are no supporting muscles underneath the joint.

The Muscles

Muscle is a tissue with a unique property : it can shorten (contract) when stimulated by a supplying nerve. There are three types of muscle in the body : *skeletal* or *voluntary muscle* (the "meat" of the body), *smooth* or *involuntary muscle* (found in the digestive tract, blood vessels and elsewhere) and *cardiac muscle* (found only in the heart). Skeletal muscles are attached at both ends to bones, cartilage, ligaments, skin or other muscles. When a muscle contracts, one attachment will remain static, and the other will therefore move. During muscle contraction, each fiber shortens and becomes thicker, causing the muscles to swell and bulge.

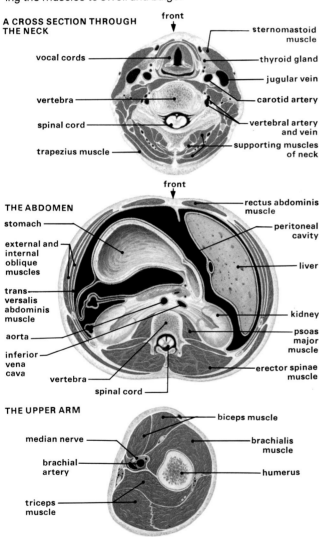

A CROSS SECTION THROUGH THE NECK

front

- sternomastoid muscle
- vocal cords
- thyroid gland
- vertebra
- jugular vein
- spinal cord
- carotid artery
- trapezius muscle
- vertebral artery and vein
- supporting muscles of neck

front

THE ABDOMEN

- stomach
- rectus abdominis muscle
- external and internal oblique muscles
- peritoneal cavity
- trans- versalis abdominis muscle
- liver
- aorta
- kidney
- inferior vena cava
- psoas major muscle
- vertebra
- erector spinae muscle
- spinal cord

THE UPPER ARM

- biceps muscle
- median nerve
- brachialis muscle
- brachial artery
- humerus
- triceps muscle

The arrangement of skeletal muscles in different parts of the body is shown by the cross sections above. The neck is crowded with important structures passing from the trunk to the head, including the windpipe, esophagus, spinal cord and major blood vessels supplying the brain. The many different muscles permit a wide range of head movements. The abdomen has three layers of superficial muscles giving support to the abdominal contents. Several important muscles support the spine and govern its movements, maintaining our upright posture. The section through the upper arm shows the arrangement of muscles around the humerus.

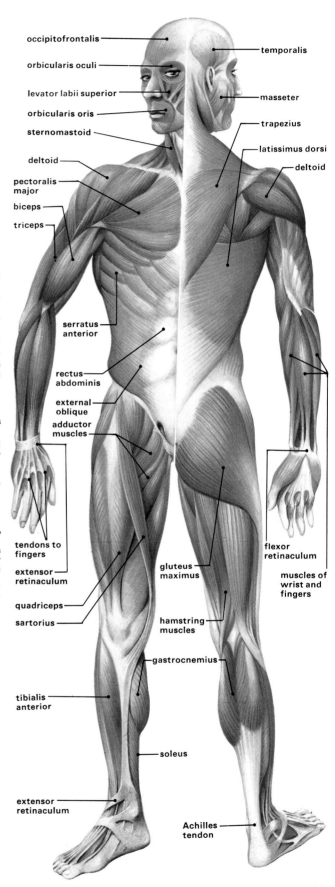

- occipitofrontalis
- temporalis
- orbicularis oculi
- levator labii superior
- masseter
- orbicularis oris
- trapezius
- sternomastoid
- latissimus dorsi
- deltoid
- deltoid
- pectoralis major
- biceps
- triceps
- serratus anterior
- rectus abdominis
- external oblique
- adductor muscles
- tendons to fingers
- flexor retinaculum
- extensor retinaculum
- gluteus maximus
- muscles of wrist and fingers
- quadriceps
- sartorius
- hamstring muscles
- gastrocnemius
- tibialis anterior
- soleus
- extensor retinaculum
- Achilles tendon

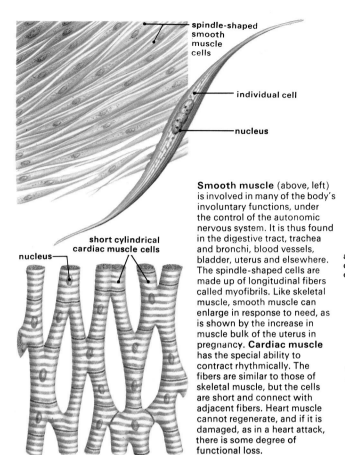

spindle-shaped smooth muscle cells

individual cell

nucleus

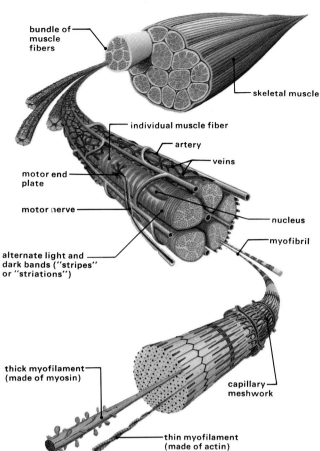

bundle of muscle fibers

skeletal muscle

individual muscle fiber

artery

veins

motor end plate

motor nerve

nucleus

myofibril

alternate light and dark bands ("stripes" or "striations")

thick myofilament (made of myosin)

capillary meshwork

thin myofilament (made of actin)

nucleus

short cylindrical cardiac muscle cells

Smooth muscle (above, left) is involved in many of the body's involuntary functions, under the control of the autonomic nervous system. It is thus found in the digestive tract, trachea and bronchi, blood vessels, bladder, uterus and elsewhere. The spindle-shaped cells are made up of longitudinal fibers called myofibrils. Like skeletal muscle, smooth muscle can enlarge in response to need, as is shown by the increase in muscle bulk of the uterus in pregnancy. **Cardiac muscle** has the special ability to contract rhythmically. The fibers are similar to those of skeletal muscle, but the cells are short and connect with adjacent fibers. Heart muscle cannot regenerate, and if it is damaged, as in a heart attack, there is some degree of functional loss.

Skeletal muscle (or striated muscle) is made up of bundles of muscle fibers grouped together. Motor nerves, which stimulate the muscle to contract, are attached to the fibers at *motor end plates*. There is a rich blood supply, able to cope with the enormous demand for blood during vigorous activity. The fibers themselves are made up of *myofibrils* which in turn contain two types of *myofilament*, thick and thin. During contraction, these interact, sliding between each other and causing the muscle fibers to shorten.

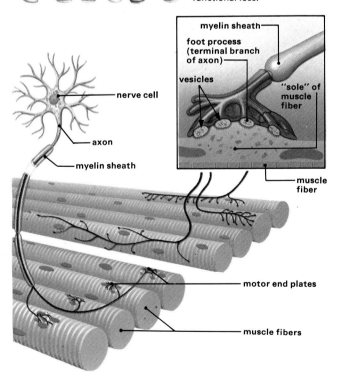

myelin sheath

foot process (terminal branch of axon)

vesicles

"sole" of muscle fiber

nerve cell

axon

myelin sheath

muscle fiber

motor end plates

muscle fibers

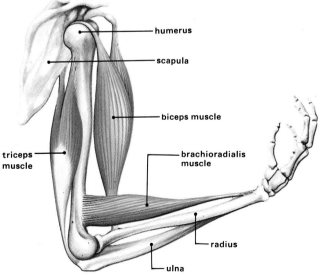

humerus

scapula

biceps muscle

triceps muscle

brachioradialis muscle

radius

ulna

A motor end plate is the junction between a motor nerve and skeletal muscle fibers. The nerve terminates in several "feet" attached to a swelling or "sole" on the muscle fiber. The nervous signal is relayed to the fibers by a biochemical "transmitter" substance stored in vesicles near the junction.

Movement of joints involves contraction of some muscles and relaxation of others (skeletal muscles are arranged in opposing groups). Thus, flexing the elbow to raise the forearm involves contraction of the biceps and brachioradialis muscles and relaxation of the triceps; to straighten the elbow, the process is reversed.

The Circulatory System

The many vital functions of the blood depend on its continuous circulation to all parts of the body. Blood is pumped by the right side of the heart through the pulmonary artery into the lungs, where it absorbs oxygen. It then returns via the pulmonary veins to the left side of the heart to be pumped through the aorta and the arterial system. It gives up oxygen – necessary for all vital bodily processes – to every tissue in the body. The deoxygenated blood returns through the veins to enter the right side of the heart once again.

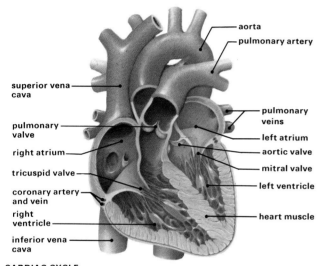

- aorta
- pulmonary artery
- superior vena cava
- pulmonary valve
- pulmonary veins
- right atrium
- left atrium
- tricuspid valve
- aortic valve
- coronary artery and vein
- mitral valve
- right ventricle
- left ventricle
- inferior vena cava
- heart muscle

CARDIAC CYCLE

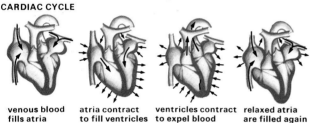

| venous blood fills atria | atria contract to fill ventricles | ventricles contract to expel blood | relaxed atria are filled again |

The heart is a double-sided pump with four chambers ; valves ensure the correct flow of blood. Venous blood enters the right atrium, passes into the right ventricle and is pumped along the pulmonary artery into the lungs. Blood returns from the lungs via the pulmonary veins into the left atrium, passes into the left ventricle and is forced out through the aorta. The sequence of these events is shown in the center diagram.

FRONT SURFACE OF HEART   **BACK SURFACE OF HEART**

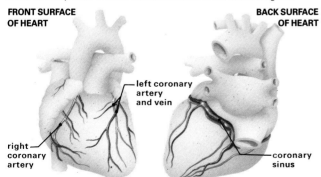

- left coronary artery and vein
- right coronary artery
- coronary sinus

The heart muscle receives its oxygen supply from the right and left **coronary arteries.** If either of these vessels becomes blocked, a "heart attack" occurs—with muscle damage, chest pain and possibly death. The **coronary veins** drain into the right atrium via the coronary sinus.

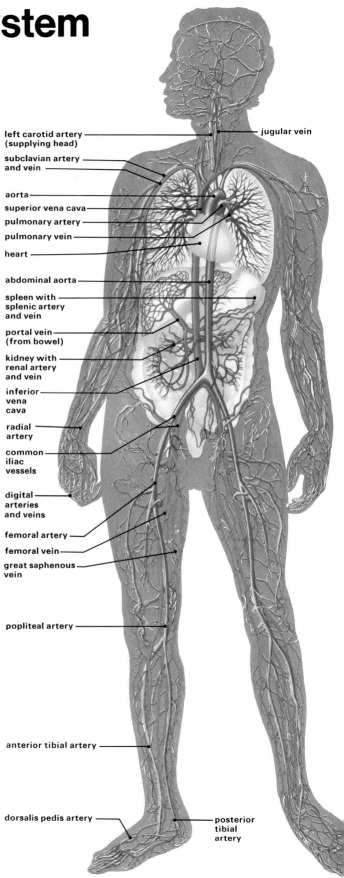

- left carotid artery (supplying head)
- subclavian artery and vein
- aorta
- superior vena cava
- pulmonary artery
- pulmonary vein
- heart
- abdominal aorta
- spleen with splenic artery and vein
- portal vein (from bowel)
- kidney with renal artery and vein
- inferior vena cava
- radial artery
- common iliac vessels
- digital arteries and veins
- femoral artery
- femoral vein
- great saphenous vein
- popliteal artery
- anterior tibial artery
- dorsalis pedis artery
- jugular vein
- posterior tibial artery

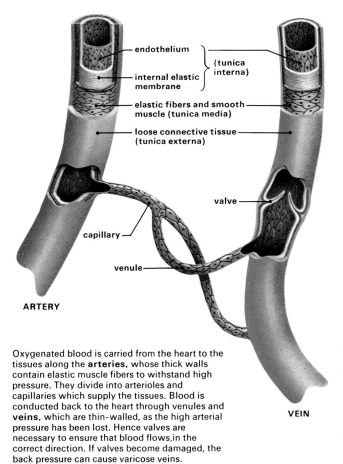

endothelium
internal elastic membrane
} (tunica interna)
elastic fibers and smooth muscle (tunica media)
loose connective tissue (tunica externa)

valve

capillary

venule

ARTERY

VEIN

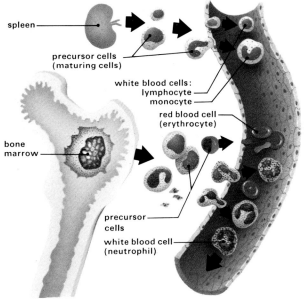

spleen
precursor cells (maturing cells)
white blood cells: lymphocyte monocyte
red blood cell (erythrocyte)
bone marrow
precursor cells
white blood cell (neutrophil)

Oxygenated blood is carried from the heart to the tissues along the **arteries,** whose thick walls contain elastic muscle fibers to withstand high pressure. They divide into arterioles and capillaries which supply the tissues. Blood is conducted back to the heart through venules and **veins,** which are thin-walled, as the high arterial pressure has been lost. Hence valves are necessary to ensure that blood flows,in the correct direction. If valves become damaged, the back pressure can cause varicose veins.

The principal blood-forming organs are the bone marrow, the lymph nodes and the spleen. The active bone marrow tissue is found at the ends of most long bones, and in the ribs, breastbone, skull and vertebrae. Red blood cells (which transport oxygen and are by far the most numerous type of blood cell) are formed in the bone marrow, passing through various stages of maturation before they are released into the bloodstream. The bone marrow also manufactures certain types of white blood cells and platelets (important in clotting). The lymphatic tissues (including the spleen) form other types of white blood cells, which similarly pass through several stages before reaching maturity. White blood cells defend the body against infection.

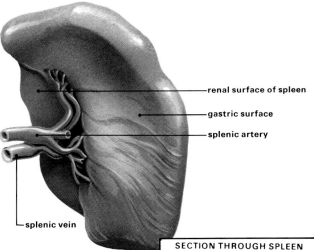

renal surface of spleen
gastric surface
splenic artery
splenic vein

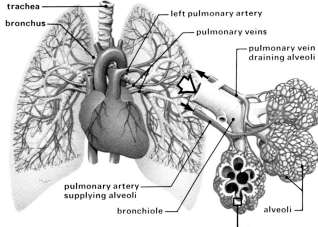

trachea
bronchus
left pulmonary artery
pulmonary veins
pulmonary vein draining alveoli
pulmonary artery supplying alveoli
bronchiole
alveoli

The spleen is a complex organ with several functions. It acts as a filter for the blood, removing old or damaged red blood cells. This takes place largely in the spaces known as the venous sinusoids. The spleen also contains lymphatic nodules which form part of the body's immune system ; they also manufacture and release white blood cells into the circulation.

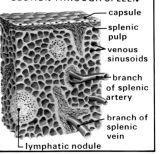

SECTION THROUGH SPLEEN
capsule
splenic pulp
venous sinusoids
branch of splenic artery
branch of splenic vein
lymphatic nodule

Gaseous interchange—the uptake by the blood of oxygen and the release of carbon dioxide—takes place in the alveoli of the lungs. There are about 300 million alveoli, each surrounded by a mesh of blood capillaries which lie very close to the air-filled space (lumen) inside the alveolus. Oxygen diffuses into the oxygen-poor blood vessels from the oxygen-rich air in the lumen, while carbon dioxide similarly diffuses from the blood into the alveolus.

lumen of alveolus
lining membrane
red blood cell in capillary absorbs oxygen from lumen
carbon dioxide in blood plasma diffuses into lumen

The Digestive System

Digestion consists of first reducing food to its constituent parts and then absorbing the essential nutrients. Food is broken down in the stomach and small intestine by the action of enzymes released from glands in the mouth, stomach, pancreas and small intestine. The absorption of nutrients into the bloodstream occurs mainly in the small intestine. In the large intestine, water is absorbed to leave semisolid waste, which is passed via the rectum as feces. The liver—the largest gland in the body—is responsible for utilizing the products of digestion absorbed into the blood.

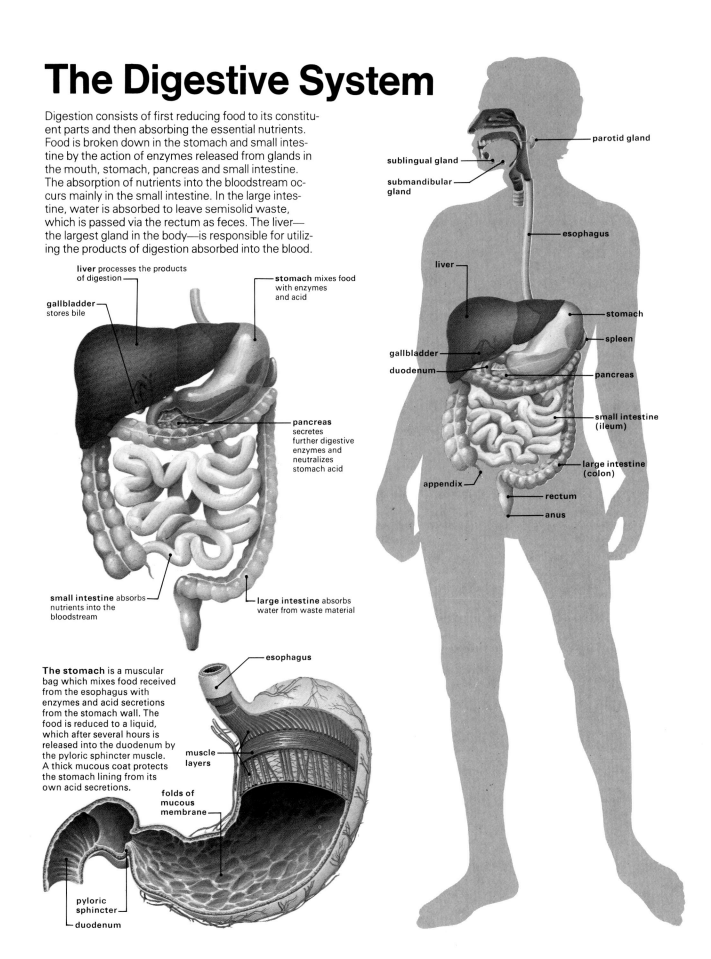

liver processes the products of digestion

gallbladder stores bile

stomach mixes food with enzymes and acid

pancreas secretes further digestive enzymes and neutralizes stomach acid

small intestine absorbs nutrients into the bloodstream

large intestine absorbs water from waste material

The stomach is a muscular bag which mixes food received from the esophagus with enzymes and acid secretions from the stomach wall. The food is reduced to a liquid, which after several hours is released into the duodenum by the pyloric sphincter muscle. A thick mucous coat protects the stomach lining from its own acid secretions.

esophagus

muscle layers

folds of mucous membrane

pyloric sphincter

duodenum

parotid gland

sublingual gland

submandibular gland

esophagus

liver

stomach

spleen

gallbladder

duodenum

pancreas

small intestine (ileum)

large intestine (colon)

appendix

rectum

anus

A CROSS SECTION THROUGH THE LIVER

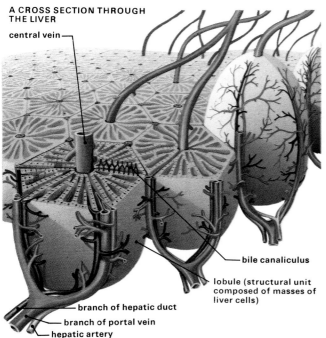

central vein

bile canaliculus

lobule (structural unit composed of masses of liver cells)

branch of hepatic duct

branch of portal vein

hepatic artery

The liver is an extremely complex gland with many vital functions. Via the portal vein it receives nutrients absorbed from the intestines. It converts poisonous ammonia compounds into nontoxic urea; it stores sugar for release into the bloodstream when necessary; it synthesizes complex proteins from simple ones absorbed from food; it makes bile which is stored in the gallbladder and is essential for fat absorption.

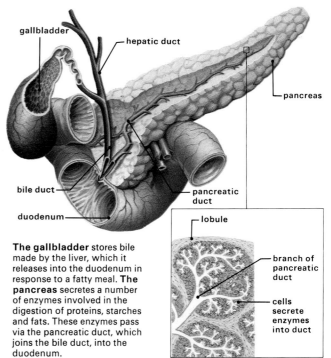

gallbladder

hepatic duct

pancreas

bile duct

pancreatic duct

duodenum

lobule

branch of pancreatic duct

cells secrete enzymes into duct

The gallbladder stores bile made by the liver, which it releases into the duodenum in response to a fatty meal. **The pancreas** secretes a number of enzymes involved in the digestion of proteins, starches and fats. These enzymes pass via the pancreatic duct, which joins the bile duct, into the duodenum.

TRANSPORTATION OF NUTRIENTS

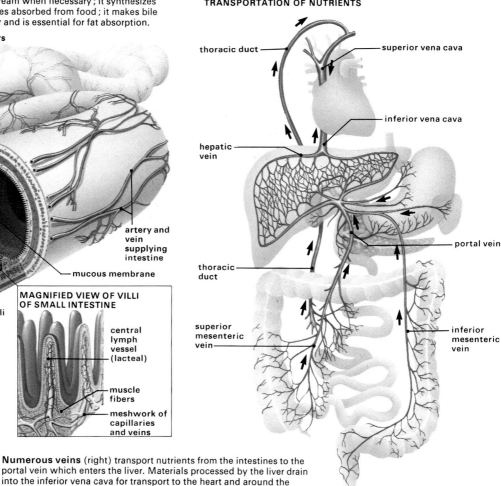

thoracic duct

superior vena cava

inferior vena cava

hepatic vein

portal vein

thoracic duct

superior mesenteric vein

inferior mesenteric vein

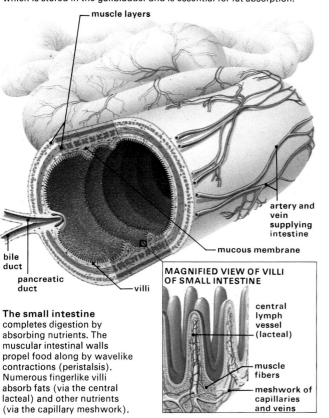

muscle layers

artery and vein supplying intestine

mucous membrane

bile duct

pancreatic duct

villi

The small intestine completes digestion by absorbing nutrients. The muscular intestinal walls propel food along by wavelike contractions (peristalsis). Numerous fingerlike villi absorb fats (via the central lacteal) and other nutrients (via the capillary meshwork).

MAGNIFIED VIEW OF VILLI OF SMALL INTESTINE

central lymph vessel (lacteal)

muscle fibers

meshwork of capillaries and veins

Numerous veins (right) transport nutrients from the intestines to the portal vein which enters the liver. Materials processed by the liver drain into the inferior vena cava for transport to the heart and around the body. Absorbed fats are carried to the heart by the thoracic duct.

The Nervous System

Nerves are complex fibers which conduct electrochemical impulses. Nerves to and from all parts of the body are grouped together within the spinal cord and conveyed to the brain, which controls and coordinates the nervous signals involved in any bodily function—innumerable in even the simplest activity. The nervous system can be divided into the *motor system* (muscular control), the *sensory system* (information from the senses to the brain) and the *autonomic nervous system* (bodily functions not under conscious control, e.g., digestion).

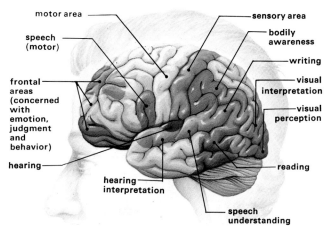

Each area of the **cerebral cortex** (outer layer of the brain) is concerned with a particular function. For example, voluntary movements are initiated in the motor area, while sensations of pain and touch are processed in the sensory area. Complex incoming signals may be collected together and processed in more than one area—for example, visual signals are perceived in one area and interpreted in another.

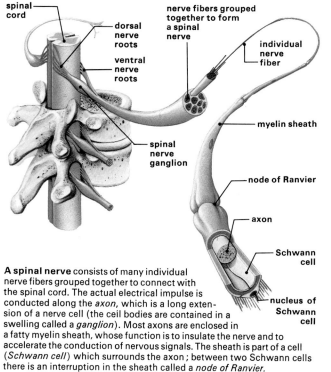

A spinal nerve consists of many individual nerve fibers grouped together to connect with the spinal cord. The actual electrical impulse is conducted along the *axon*, which is a long extension of a nerve cell (the cell bodies are contained in a swelling called a *ganglion*). Most axons are enclosed in a fatty myelin sheath, whose function is to insulate the nerve and to accelerate the conduction of nervous signals. The sheath is part of a cell (*Schwann cell*) which surrounds the axon; between two Schwann cells there is an interruption in the sheath called a *node of Ranvier*.

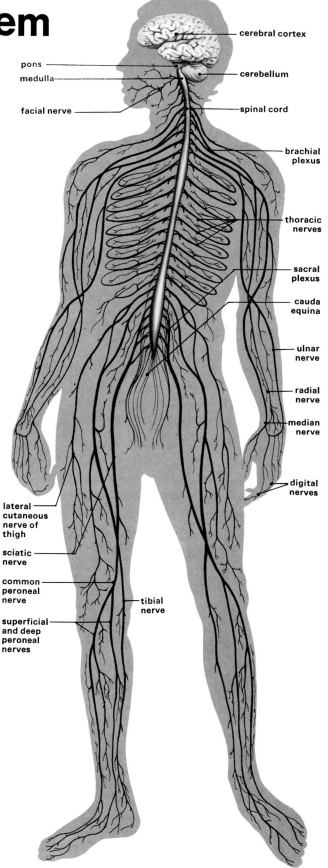

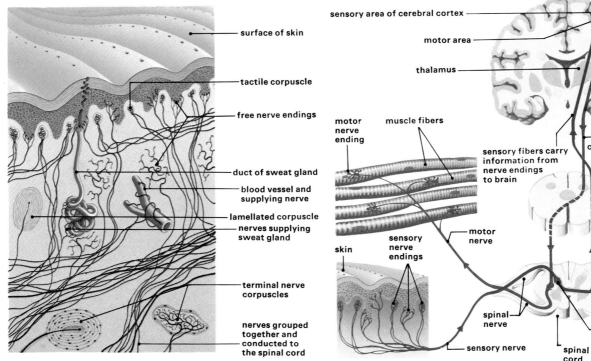

surface of skin

tactile corpuscle

free nerve endings

duct of sweat gland

blood vessel and supplying nerve

lamellated corpuscle

nerves supplying sweat gland

terminal nerve corpuscles

nerves grouped together and conducted to the spinal cord

sensory area of cerebral cortex

motor area

thalamus

motor nerve ending

muscle fibers

sensory fibers carry information from nerve endings to brain

motor fibers carry instructions from brain to muscles

medulla

motor nerve

spinothalamic tract

skin

sensory nerve endings

spinal nerve

synapse

sensory nerve

spinal cord

Nerve supply of the skin

Both motor and sensory nerves are to be found in and just below the skin. The autonomic nervous system supplies nerve fibers to the sweat glands and capillaries ; these control sweating and constriction or dilatation of the capillaries and thus heat loss from the body through the skin. Sensory nerve fibers supplying the skin may terminate in various types of structures called corpuscles. It is not certain whether a particular type is concerned with a particular sensation, though the lamellated corpuscle is thought to be sensitive to vibration and pressure. Other sensory nerves have free nerve endings, which may be concerned with the sensation of pain. Where there are hairs, the hair follicle is also supplied by nerves from the autonomic and sensory systems.

Motor and sensory nervous system

Sensory nerves carrying stimuli of pain, temperature, touch, etc., join the spinal cord via a spinal nerve. Those fibers carrying pain and temperature sensations (blue line) cross over to the other side of the cord ; this involves the transfer of the stimulus from one nerve cell to another at a *synapse.* (Other sensations, e.g. touch, are conducted along a different route.) The fibers then ascend the spinal cord in the spinothalamic tract to the thalamus, and from there to the sensory cortex. Here, with the aid of other parts of the brain, the stimulus is interpreted. Motor nerves carrying signals from the motor cortex to the voluntary muscles (red line) cross in the medulla of the brain stem before descending the spinal cord to leave via a spinal nerve.

THE PARASYMPATHETIC NERVOUS SYSTEM

THE SYMPATHETIC NERVOUS SYSTEM

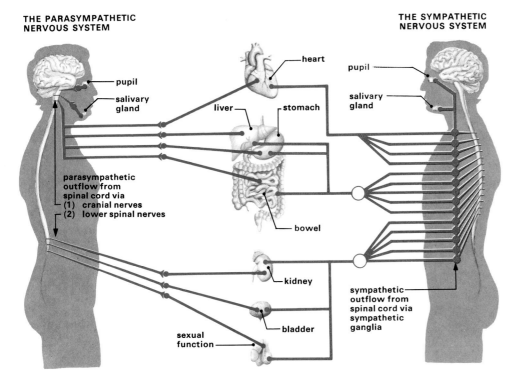

pupil

salivary gland

heart

liver

stomach

parasympathetic outflow from spinal cord via
(1) cranial nerves
(2) lower spinal nerves

bowel

kidney

sexual function

bladder

pupil

salivary gland

sympathetic outflow from spinal cord via sympathetic ganglia

The autonomic nervous system regulates the automatic functions of the body and is composed of the sympathetic and parasympathetic systems, which have opposing effects. The sympathetic system prepares the body for emergency action by reducing nonessential activities such as digestion. The sympathetic nerves are relayed from the sympathetic ganglia which form a chain along either side of the vertebral column. Stimulation of these nerves leads to increases in heart and respiration rate, blood supply to the muscles and dilatation of the pupils, while salivation, urine production and digestive activity are reduced. Ejaculation is also mediated by the sympathetic system, though penile erection is a parasympathetic function. The parasympathetic system involves the 3rd, 7th, 9th and 10th cranial nerves and the lower spinal nerves and comes into play during rest and sleep— slowing the heart and breathing, constricting the pupils and increasing digestion.

The Endocrine System

The endocrine glands (ductless glands) secrete hormones directly into the bloodstream. Hormones are complex chemical "messenger" substances; they are released in tiny amounts, yet they can produce dramatic changes in the activity of body cells. In this way they control basic body functions such as growth, metabolism and sexual development; they are also responsible for maintaining the correct levels in the blood of certain vital substances (e.g. sugar and salt).

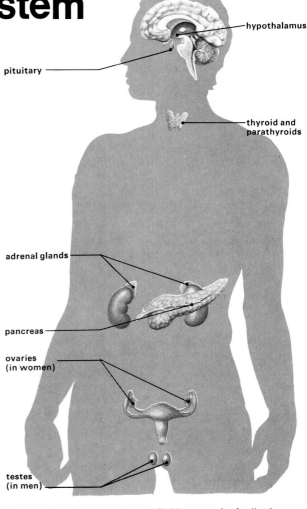

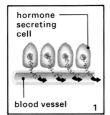
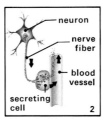
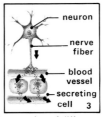

Hormones can be released into the bloodstream in a number of different ways. They may be released directly by a secreting cell (1) or when such a cell is stimulated by a nerve impulse (2). In the posterior lobe of the pituitary, nerve fibers themselves release hormones directly into the blood, which stimulate another hormone-producing cell (3).

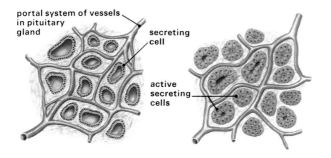

The anterior pituitary has a rich network of blood vessels connecting it to the hypothalamus. It is thought that "neurosecretions" from the hypothalamus stimulate the hormone-secreting cells.

The secretion of hormones is controlled by a complex feedback mechanism in which the nervous system is closely involved. The **hypothalamus** and **pituitary** play particularly important roles.

The pituitary gland (right) is situated at the base of the brain and is about the size of a pea; it is divided into two lobes. It is subject to the influence of the hypothalamus, to which it is connected by a slender stalk. It releases a variety of hormones which act on several "target" organs. The hormones of the anterior lobe, with the exception of somatotropin and MSH, stimulate other glands. The hypothalamus is thought to monitor the level of the hormones released by these glands and to direct the pituitary to cut off the stimulating hormone once the correct level is reached.

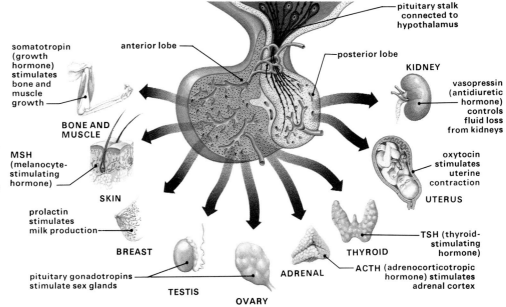

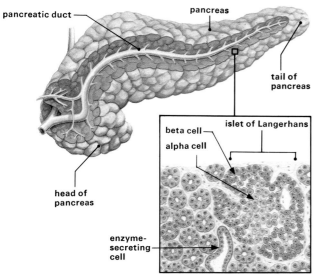

pancreatic duct — pancreas — tail of pancreas — head of pancreas

islet of Langerhans

beta cell
alpha cell

enzyme-secreting cell

The pancreas, which lies behind and under the stomach, is a mixed-function gland; as well as containing cells which secrete digestive enzymes, it has clumps of cells known as the *islets of Langerhans* which secrete hormones. These are most numerous toward the tail or pointed end of the pancreas. The islets contain two types of cells—*alpha* and *beta* cells. The alpha cells produce the hormone glucagon which raises the level of sugar in the blood; the beta cells secrete insulin which lowers blood sugar. A lack of this hormone as the result of disease or damage to the pancreas produces diabetes.

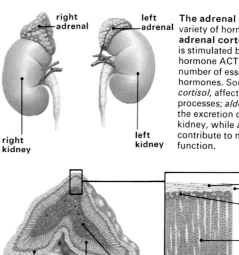

right adrenal — left adrenal — right kidney — left kidney

The adrenal glands produce a variety of hormones. The **adrenal cortex,** or outer part, is stimulated by the pituitary hormone ACTH; it secretes a number of essential "steroid" hormones. Some of these, e.g., *cortisol,* affect certain metabolic processes; *aldosterone* regulates the excretion of salts by the kidney, while *adrenal androgens* contribute to normal sexual function.

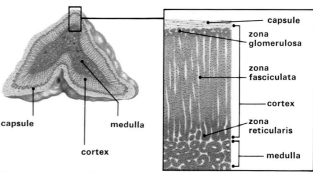

capsule — medulla — cortex

capsule
zona glomerulosa
zona fasciculata
cortex
zona reticularis
medulla

The adrenal medulla, or inner part of the adrenal glands, is entirely separate in function from the cortex and is not influenced by the pituitary gland. It secretes the hormones epinephrine and norepinephrine (adrenaline and noradrenaline) under autonomic control, in response to fear, anger or sexual desire; these prepare the body for instant action by increasing the heart rate and the blood supply to the muscles.

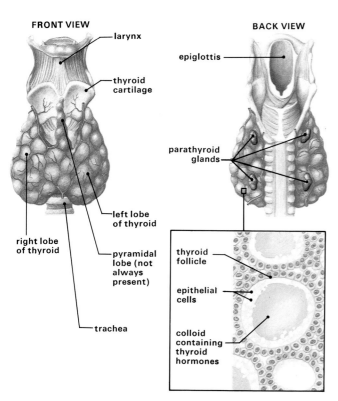

FRONT VIEW

larynx
thyroid cartilage
right lobe of thyroid
left lobe of thyroid
pyramidal lobe (not always present)
trachea

BACK VIEW

epiglottis
parathyroid glands

thyroid follicle
epithelial cells
colloid containing thyroid hormones

The thyroid gland is situated at the base of the neck on either side of the trachea, just below the larynx. It is made up of follicles containing a fluid called colloid, in which the two thyroid hormones thyroxine and tri-iodothyronine (T_4 and T_3) are stored for release into the bloodstream as necessary. These hormones control the body's metabolic rate. There are four small **parathyroid glands** situated behind the thyroid. These secrete parathyroid hormone (or parathormone), which controls the level of calcium and phosphorus in the blood.

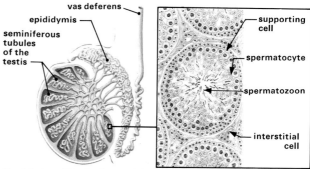

vas deferens
epididymis
seminiferous tubules of the testis

supporting cell
spermatocyte
spermatozoon
interstitial cell

The tubules of **the testes** contain cells called spermatocytes which, under the influence of gonadotropic hormones, mature into spermatozoa. These are stored in the tubules and epididymis until they are conducted to the penis at ejaculation by the vas deferens. The interstitial cells between the tubules also produce the male hormone testosterone, responsible for secondary sexual characteristics.

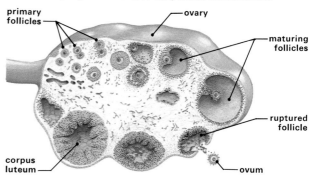

primary follicles — ovary — maturing follicles — ruptured follicle — corpus luteum — ovum

At birth, **the ovaries** contain numerous primary follicles; after puberty, these develop under complex hormonal control. At the mid-point of each menstrual cycle an ovum (egg cell) is released from a mature follicle, which then becomes a corpus luteum. If pregnancy occurs, this secretes hormones which interrupt the menstrual cycle.

COLOR PLATE XIII

The Immune System

The immune system defends the body against invasion by disease-producing organisms and against toxins they produce. It can distinguish between what belongs in the body ("self") and what does not ("non-self"), and reacts against any cells that are not recognized as "self." This reaction may be either to produce antibodies (*humoral immunity*) or to activate cells which attack the invader directly (*cell-mediated immunity*). In both cases the outcome is to make the foreign cell or invading organism subject to *phagocytosis* – destruction by certain white blood cells.

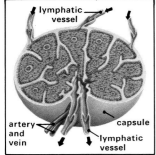

Lymph nodes (above) are pea-sized structures situated in groups at strategic points in the lymphatic vessels—the network of channels which drain the tissues and return excess fluid to the bloodstream. Foreign particles, such as bacteria, are trapped in the lymph nodes, which are inhabited by *macrophages* (white blood cells which can phagocytose, i.e. engulf and destroy, foreign particles) and *lymphocytes* (white blood cells which mount immune reactions).

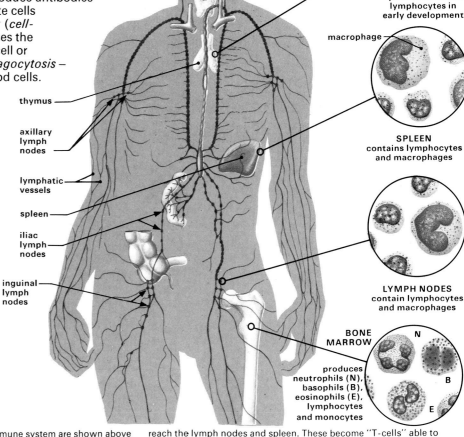

lymphocyte

THYMUS GLAND "processes" some lymphocytes in early development

macrophage

SPLEEN contains lymphocytes and macrophages

LYMPH NODES contain lymphocytes and macrophages

BONE MARROW produces neutrophils (N), basophils (B), eosinophils (E), lymphocytes and monocytes

thymus

axillary lymph nodes

lymphatic vessels

spleen

iliac lymph nodes

inguinal lymph nodes

The main components of the body's immune system are shown above (right). The lymphatic system and lymphoid tissues represent the basic structural framework. The magnified cells shown are all different types of white blood cell. Lymphocytes are concentrated in the lymph nodes and spleen: they are of two types—"T-lymphocytes" and "B-lymphocytes"—which inhabit different regions of the nodes and spleen and play different roles in the immune response. In early development, the thymus gland "processes" some circulating lymphocytes before they reach the lymph nodes and spleen. These become "T-cells" able to mount a cell-mediated immune response. Others, called "B-cells," are not processed in this way, but are capable of responding to antigens by producing antibodies. The bone marrow manufactures a variety of white blood cells: *monocytes*, which eventually become phagocytic macrophages; *neutrophils*, which are also mainly phagocytic, *basophils* (called Mast cells outside the bloodstream), which produce histamine, and *eosinophils*, which limit the effects of histamine release.

TWO METHODS OF ANTIBODY FUNCTION

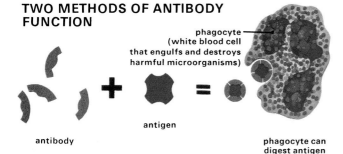

phagocyte (white blood cell that engulfs and destroys harmful microorganisms)

antigen

antibody

phagocyte can digest antigen more easily

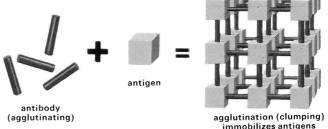

antigen

antibody (agglutinating)

agglutination (clumping) immobilizes antigens

The above diagrams illustrate two ways in which antibodies act to render the corresponding antigen harmless. **Left**: antibodies coat the surface of the antigen. As a result of this process, certain other enzymes in the blood are activated which, if the antigen is a cell or micro-organism, damage the cell wall, killing the cell. In addition, coating makes the antigen more readily destroyed by phagocytic cells: specific sites on the phagocytes attract the antibody molecules. **Right**: the antibody can combine with two molecules of antigen, thereby binding the antigen into clumps. This process of agglutination immobilizes the antigens, which can again be ingested by the phagocytes.

PHAGOCYTOSIS AND THE INFLAMMATORY RESPONSE

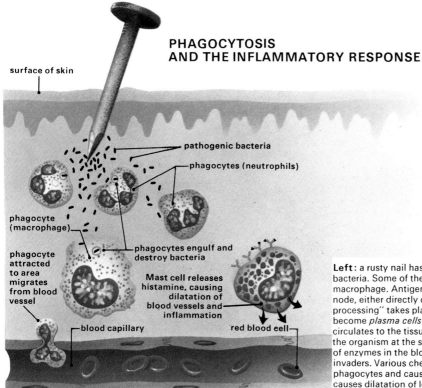

surface of skin

pathogenic bacteria

phagocytes (neutrophils)

phagocyte (macrophage)

phagocytes engulf and destroy bacteria

phagocyte attracted to area migrates from blood vessel

Mast cell releases histamine, causing dilatation of blood vessels and inflammation

blood capillary

red blood cell

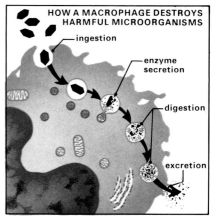

HOW A MACROPHAGE DESTROYS HARMFUL MICROORGANISMS

ingestion

enzyme secretion

digestion

excretion

Left: a rusty nail has broken the skin, carrying in with it pathogenic bacteria. Some of these are ingested by phagocytic neutrophils and by a macrophage. Antigen from the organism will reach the local lymph node, either directly or carried within the macrophage, and "antigen processing" takes place (see below). Lymphocytes are stimulated to become *plasma cells* which make the appropriate antibody; this then circulates to the tissue and combines with the antigen on the surface of the organism at the site of the wound. This reaction causes activation of enzymes in the blood, causing damage to the cell walls of the invaders. Various chemical substances are released; these attract phagocytes and cause secretion of histamine by Mast cells. Histamine causes dilatation of local blood vessels and increased migration of fluid and cells into the area, leading to the familiar features of inflammation.

DEVELOPMENT OF CELL-MEDIATED AND HUMORAL IMMUNITY

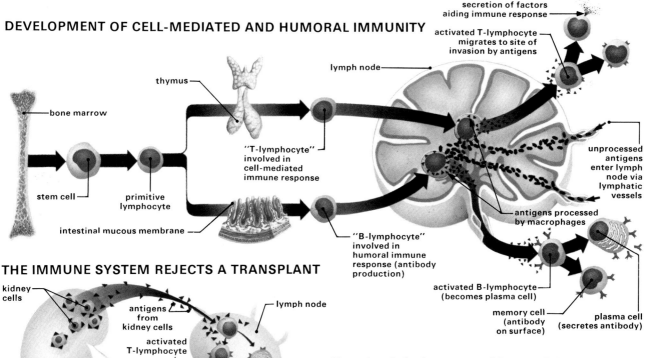

secretion of factors aiding immune response

activated T-lymphocyte migrates to site of invasion by antigens

lymph node

thymus

bone marrow

stem cell

primitive lymphocyte

intestinal mucous membrane

"T-lymphocyte" involved in cell-mediated immune response

"B-lymphocyte" involved in humoral immune response (antibody production)

unprocessed antigens enter lymph node via lymphatic vessels

antigens processed by macrophages

activated B-lymphocyte (becomes plasma cell)

memory cell (antibody on surface)

plasma cell (secretes antibody)

THE IMMUNE SYSTEM REJECTS A TRANSPLANT

kidney cells

antigens from kidney cells

activated T-lymphocyte

lymph node

donor kidney

plasma cell (secretes antibody)

antibodies

humoral attack

cell-mediated attack on donor kidney

The immune system can recognize the cells of a transplanted organ as "non-self" and attacks the organ. Both types of immune response are involved, though cell-mediated immunity plays the greater part. The rejection process can be countered by immunosuppressive drugs, or prevented by closely matching the "tissue types" of donor and recipient.

Above: in early development some of the stem cells in the bone marrow develop into primitive lymphocytes. Some pass through the thymus and become "T-lymphocytes." Others became "B-lymphocytes." (It is possible that these are processed by the intestine.) Both types of lymphocytes are stimulated by antigen: activated T-lymphocytes migrate to the point where the antigen has arisen and may destroy foreign cells themselves or activate local macrophages to do so. These lymphocytes secrete factors which "arm" macrophages and attract other white blood cells. Activated B-lymphocytes divide, and some become plasma cells. Plasma cells make large quantities of antibody; they are found in lymph nodes and bone marrow and may continue to produce low levels of antibody for many years. In addition some activated T– and B-lymphocytes become "memory cells," able to respond again if the same antigen presents itself.

The Major Sense Organs

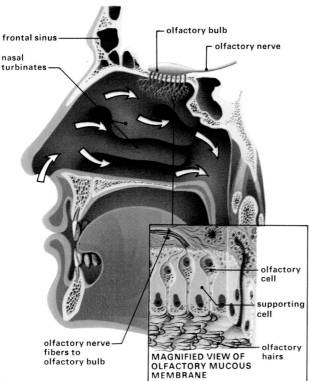

frontal sinus
nasal turbinates
olfactory bulb
olfactory nerve

olfactory cell
supporting cell
olfactory nerve fibers to olfactory bulb
olfactory hairs

MAGNIFIED VIEW OF OLFACTORY MUCOUS MEMBRANE

Smell
The olfactory mucous membrane, a small area in the nasal cavity, contains 10–20 million olfactory cells, each tipped by 10–20 tiny hairs. When air containing odorous molecules reaches the olfactory cells, certain molecules fit certain receptors on the hairs; nervous signals are then sent to the brain, where they are interpreted as odors.

Sight
Rays of light enter the eyeball through the cornea, pass through the lens and vitreous humor to the retina. The central fovea is the most sensitive area, of highest resolution. By means of a complex system of muscles and nerves, the brain ensures that the two visual axes remain parallel. The exception is when the eyes converge to read or study a close object.

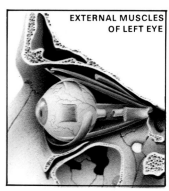

EXTERNAL MUSCLES OF LEFT EYE

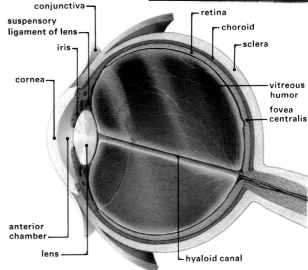

conjunctiva
suspensory ligament of lens
iris
cornea
anterior chamber
lens
retina
choroid
sclera
vitreous humor
fovea centralis
hyaloid canal

CROSS SECTION THROUGH RIGHT EYEBALL

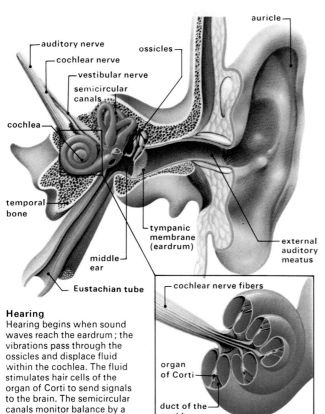

auditory nerve
cochlear nerve
vestibular nerve
semicircular canals
cochlea
temporal bone
auricle
ossicles
tympanic membrane (eardrum)
middle ear
Eustachian tube
external auditory meatus

cochlear nerve fibers
organ of Corti
duct of the cochlea

Hearing
Hearing begins when sound waves reach the eardrum; the vibrations pass through the ossicles and displace fluid within the cochlea. The fluid stimulates hair cells of the organ of Corti to send signals to the brain. The semicircular canals monitor balance by a similar mechanism.

Taste
The nervous signals responsible for our sense of taste originate in the taste buds. These microscopic structures are most numerous in the grooves around the vallate papillae of the tongue. Any substance tasted must first dissolve in saliva and then percolate through tiny pores to the hair receptors of the taste bud. There are thought to be specialized receptors for each of the basic tastes: sweet, sour, salty and bitter. All flavors are made up of combinations of these four tastes.

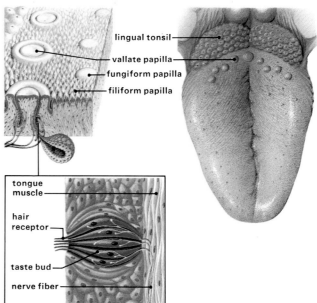

lingual tonsil
vallate papilla
fungiform papilla
filiform papilla

tongue muscle
hair receptor
taste bud
nerve fiber

AN ENCYCLOPEDIA OF MEDICINE

Section One: An Encyclopedia of Medicine

There are four chapters in this section: The *Medical A-Z* contains information about conditions, diseases, symptoms, and the function of organs, as well as definitions of technical terms. *Providers* identifies and describes the qualifications and roles of some physician specialists with whom you may have contact during diagnosis, treatment, and recovery. *Tests* familiarizes you with some of the thousands of tests used by health-care professionals to make diagnoses. And *Procedures* gives you brief explanations of some of the more commonly used treatments and surgical therapies. This section as a whole will help you, initially, when health-care professionals are not available; and it will help you ask intelligent, informed questions when they are.

3

MEDICAL A–Z

abdominal pain

Any sudden severe and continuing pain in the stomach, usually with muscle rigidity and fever. It may be due to APPENDICITIS or DIVERTICULITIS. Pain that stops and starts can indicate a blockage of the bowel, kidney stones, or GALLSTONES. The most common causes of abdominal pain are harmless conditions such as "gas" or "indigestion."

abortion

The spontaneous or contrived expulsion of the embryo or fetus. See MISCARRIAGE and also ABORTION under Procedures.

abruptio placentae

An abnormal condition of pregnancy in which the PLACENTA separates from the uterus before birth. Severe bleeding is often noted as well as pain in the lower abdomen and low blood pressure. In cases where there is only a partial separation and minimal bleeding, the mother to be

is placed on strict bed rest. In more severe cases she is hospitalized and given intravenous fluid and blood transfusions if necessary. Often the baby will be delivered by CESAREAN SECTION (see **Procedures**).

abscess

A collection of pus formed anywhere in the body.

Abscesses are caused nearly always by bacterial infection, although occasionally they result from the presence of an irritating foreign body such as a splinter.

The usual response of the body to the stimulus of local irritation or damage by bacteria is to concentrate a large number of white blood cells (leukocytes) in the affected area. While the overall effect is beneficial, the reaction has certain local disadvantages: The infected part becomes hot, swollen, red, and painful as the blood vessels dilate to carry leukocytes to the scene of action. The leukocytes pass through the walls of the blood vessels to "mop up" invading bacteria, and the area is walled off by the formation of fibrous tissue. Eventually the area of inflammation becomes localized, and the collection of dead bacteria,

An abscess is a collection of pus in a cavity. It is caused by infection with certain bacteria. Shown here are three ways in which an abscess might develop: (1) as a direct result of external infection—for example, in a cut finger; (2) by local spread from a nearby site of infection, such as an alveolar abscess in the jawbone caused by a decayed tooth; (3) as a result of bacteria being transported in the bloodstream—for example, a brain abscess may follow from a lung infection.

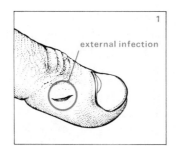

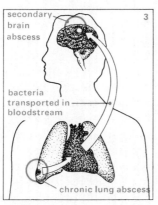

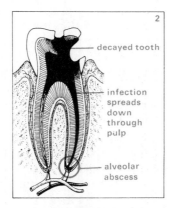

THREE ROUTES OF ABSCESS FORMATION

dead leukocytes, and exuded tissue fluid liquefies to form pus under tension.

The abscess so produced tends to find the line of least resistance in the surrounding tissues and "comes to a head" on the surface. If left to itself it bursts, but if possible the doctor hastens the process by making an incision to let out the pus and so ease the pain. It is dangerous to try to open an abscess before it is ready; an injudicious incision can only spread the infection.

achondroplasia

A congenital, frequently inherited, disorder in which the long bones of the limbs are much shorter than normal, resulting in dwarfism. The typical appearance is of disproportionately short limbs, prominent or bulging forehead, and a relatively normal body trunk size. This disorder may affect either sex and is usually obvious at birth. Adults rarely grow taller than 4 feet.

The basic problem is retarded growth of cartilage and bone in the arms and legs (the trunk is commonly unaffected). The bones of the base of the skull also fail to develop normally, and thus the forehead appears abnormally large. The bones that form the bridge of the nose fail to develop ("saddle nose"), giving a facial appearance that is virtually diagnostic of achondroplasia.

Muscular development is usually normal. Mental ability is rarely affected and achondroplastics are sexually normal and capable of parenthood. However, achondroplastic women have an abnormally small pelvis and their babies must be delivered by CESAREAN SECTION (see **Procedures**). Any person with achondroplasia should have genetic counseling before marriage.

There is no treatment. Nevertheless, the condition is compatible with a long, healthy, and fulfilled life, although it is obvious that psychological problems may have to be overcome.

acne

An extremely common inflammatory disorder of the sebaceous (oil-secreting) glands of the skin. Although several types of acne exist, described by various qualifying terms, when the term is used alone it usually refers to "common acne" (*acne vulgaris*).

Acne can affect persons at any age, but it is especially troublesome to teenagers, who may feel acute embarrassment about their personal appearance. During adolescence the sebaceous glands become particularly active and secrete large amounts of *sebum* (a fatty substance that ordinarily helps maintain the texture of the skin) owing to an increased production of *androgens* (sex hormones) in both boys and girls at the time of puberty. The sebum produced at this time is unusually thick and sticky and tends to block the sebaceous glands and their associated hair follicles. When this occurs, the follicles become dilated (stretched) with sebum and cellular debris.

If the plug of sebum extends to the skin surface, contact with the air causes its exposed surface to turn black—thus creating a *comedone* ("blackhead"). If the blockage does not extend to the surface, a "whitehead" is formed beneath the skin.

ACNE

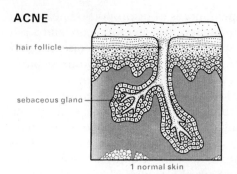

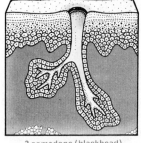

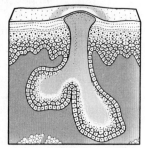

Normal skin has many microscopic hair follicles opening onto its surface (1). In acne, the mouth of the follicle is blocked by a plug of oily sebum (2). The sebaceous gland continues to secrete sebum so that the follicle becomes distended and inflamed. Bacteria then multiply in the follicle, and it becomes filled with pus (3).

Chemical changes within the blocked follicles result in the formation of irritating substances known as *free fatty acids* (FFA); retention of the secretions encourages the growth and multiplication of bacteria. As the follicles distend they form tiny cysts which eventually can rupture, releasing the free fatty acids into the immediate area and inducing an inflammatory reaction. Typically, the affected follicles (papules, or "pimples") are filled with pus which can spread the infection if the pimples are picked at or squeezed.

Acne vulgaris is further classified as *superficial* or *deep*, depending on the severity of the predominating lesions. The former is characterized by the formation of inflamed follicles, filled with pus, which "come to a head" on the skin surface. Deep acne, as the term implies, affects deeper layers of the skin; pus-filled *cysts* may form beneath the skin, some of which discharge onto the skin surface. In severe cases, as these lesions heal they may leave permanent scarring. The main site involved in acne is the face, although the neck, chest, back, and upper arms may also be involved.

At one time diet was implicated as a major cause of acne; however, modern medical opinion considers this to be unlikely in most cases. It is clear that hormonal factors during puberty are mostly responsible, although some experts believe that a hereditary influence may also contribute; this is almost impossible to document, however, since acne has a worldwide incidence and is undoubtedly the most common skin disorder of adolescence.

Treatment of acne depends largely on its severity. Often the only relief is brought by time, since the lesions tend to fade as the teenager reaches adulthood. In the meantime, it is wise to wash the affected areas gently at least daily with mild soap and water. This helps by mechanically removing some of the blackheads, scales, and bacteria. Medicated washes have proved effective in some mild cases, as has exposure to sunlight (which tends to dry up the lesions). Antibiotic ointments generally are not used, especially since they may produce further irritation of the skin in the form of a local allergic reaction. In selected cases, however, a broad-spectrum antibiotic may be prescribed to be taken orally; one of the most effective in such cases is tetracycline. Antibiotic treatment has no effect on the underlying cause of acne, but it may help reduce the number of bacteria responsible for much of the associated inflammation.

A relatively new drug, isotretinoin, has had great success in combating severe cases of acne. The drug is available by prescription only, and persons must be followed closely by a physician. It is imperative that women who are pregnant or considering pregnancy not take isotretinoin, as birth defects have been seen in children whose mothers took the drug.

Acne affects teenagers at a particularly sensitive time of life—when they are highly concerned about their personal appearance. It can be helpful to point out to them that acne is ordinarily of limited duration and that it affects large numbers of adolescents.

acromegaly

A disorder caused by the excess production of GROWTH HORMONE which occurs as a result of a tumor in the pituitary gland. This gland, which is situated in the brain, is responsible for the production of numerous hormones that affect the entire body. When a tumor develops in the part of the gland that regulates growth, two disorders can occur. If the tumor develops before puberty, while the bones still have the capacity to grow, giantism will result and the person will become excessively tall. If puberty already has occurred, the bones no longer can be affected but cartilage and soft tissues of the body will be. This disorder, known as acromegaly, occurs in both men and women.

The symptoms of acromegaly appear so slowly that a person may not even be aware of the changes in his appearance. Gradually the feet, hands, nose, lips, and tongue become larger and broader, the voice deeper. Other symptoms that often occur are an increase in body hair, joint discomfort, spinal difficulties, high blood pressure, sugar intolerance, visual problems, and headaches.

Diagnosis of acromegaly is made on the basis of the characteristic appearance and on blood

ACROMEGALY

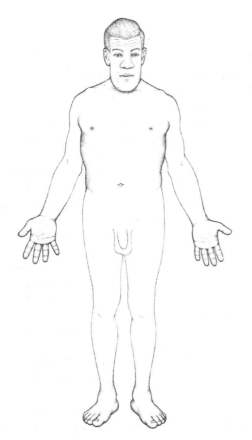

Acromegaly literally means "large extremities." This man shows the typical signs—enlarged hands and feet, massive chest, and coarse facial features with a characteristic jutting jaw. Acromegaly results from a benign tumor in the pituitary gland.

tests that measure the increased level of growth hormone. Although the physical changes cannot be reversed, they can be halted. The tumor can be treated by surgery or super voltage radiation; medications are used in some cases, though to a lesser extent. Long-term medical follow-up is essential to monitor for the possibility of the recurrence of the tumor.

acrophobia

An excessive and abnormal fear of high places. It is a natural part of human defense mechanisms to have some fear of heights because of the known danger of death or serious injury from a fall; acrophobia is merely an exaggeration of this normal fear. It has an element of unreason in it, however, since the acrophobic subject typically will exhibit fear even in a room in a high building, although the actual possibility of falling from it under these circumstances may be nil. It can be a very disabling condition since it may preclude the person from going to work or attending social functions if these involve entering a building and going above the ground floor.

As with other phobias, therapy will involve analysis in an attempt to determine the possible cause of the PHOBIA. Tranquilizing drugs may play a part in treatment, and "deconditioning" the person by teaching him to relax while in a real or imagined high place is sometimes helpful.

See also AGORAPHOBIA, CLAUSTROPHOBIA.

ACTH

Stands for *adrenocorticotropic hormone*, an essential hormone produced by the anterior (front) part of the pituitary gland, which lies at the base of the brain. It is also known as adrenocorticotropin or corticotropin. ACTH is of great importance because it provides the link between the pituitary and the cortex (outer layer) of the two tiny ADRENAL GLANDS, which lie at the back of the abdomen just above the kidneys. The cortex of the adrenal gland secretes steroid hormones such as cortisol (known as hydrocortisone when given in drug form) and aldosterone, both of which are essential for maintaining the body's biochemical balance.

It is very important that the output of steroids be carefully controlled, since too much steroid production can be very harmful. The ACTH secreted by the pituitary provides this control by means of a complex feedback mechanism: The pituitary secretes ACTH, which is carried in the bloodstream to the adrenal glands. The ACTH stimulates the adrenals to produce steroids. But when the amount of steroids in the bloodstream reaches a certain level, the production of ACTH by the pituitary is shut off automatically. This feedback mechanism produces a remarkably fine control of steroid production.

ACTH can be extracted from the pituitary glands of animals and be given by injection in the treatment of certain diseases. There are also diseases caused by the overproduction of ACTH, which can lead to severe body-wide dysfunction.

Actinomyces/actinomycosis

Actinomyces is a genus of parasitic microorganisms formerly classified as fungi but now thought to be bacteria (some experts believe them to be intermediate between fungi and bacteria).

One species, *Actinomyces israelii*, is a common inhabitant of the mouth in persons with poor oral hygiene. The parasites cling to the teeth, gums, and tonsils but rarely cause any problem— although they have been implicated in the formation of dental plaque. However, the parasites *can* cause a severe infection if they gain entrance to the tissues in some way, such as from a decayed tooth, or as a consequence of a tooth extraction or an injury to the jaw. The resulting condition is known as *actinomycosis*.

Actinomycosis is a contagious disease characterized by painful, hard swellings that progress to the formation of abscesses (localized collections of pus). The sites most commonly affected are the jaws and neck, but if the parasites enter the bloodstream they may infect the lungs, intestines, kidneys, and other organs. Early treatment with antibiotics is effective in most cases in limiting the progression of the disease.

Adams-Stokes syndrome (Stokes-Adams syndrome)

A condition, which usually affects the elderly, characterized by sudden, usually brief, episodes of unconsciousness. It can occur at any time and is not dependent on the person's bodily position. The cause is a disturbance in the conduction of the heart impulse, leading to temporary interruption of the heartbeat. Absence of the heartbeat

(*asystole*) for four to eight seconds will cause unconsciousness in the erect position; asystole of more than twelve seconds will cause unconsciousness in the recumbent position; asystole of up to five minutes leads to additional signs of CYANOSIS, fixed pupils, and neurological impairment (which may be permanent, if the person survives).

Emergency treatment usually involves the intravenous administration of isoproterenol. This may be followed by the implantation of a PACEMAKER.

See also ARRHYTHMIA, BRADYCARDIA.

addiction

Physical or mental dependence on a drug. Some experts make a distinction between *addiction* (physical dependence) and *habituation* (psychological dependence); both terms have traditionally been used to describe the adverse long-term effects of certain classes of drugs on the body and mind.

The World Health Organization, however, suggests that more meaningful diagnostic terms would be "drug dependence" and "drug abuse." The essential feature of physical dependence is the occurrence of withdrawal symptoms if regular doses are not taken.

The best-known physically addictive drugs are the opiates or "narcotics," such as morphine and heroin. Even when prescribed legally for relief of severe pain, prolonged treatment with opiates can lead to tolerance by the body of ever-increasing doses of the drug. In these circumstances sudden withdrawal of the drug will cause cramping pains, sweating, and acute mental distress. The need to relieve these symptoms by taking a further dose of the drug is the key feature of physical addiction. The fact that withdrawal symptoms occur indicates that the body itself has become dependent on the drug.

Other common drugs that may be addictive if abused include the amphetamines ("speed"), barbiturates and other types of sedatives ("sleeping pills"), and tranquilizers.

There is still a great deal of misunderstanding about the drugs that cause addiction. Many people do not realize that CANNABIS (marijuana or "pot") is not physically addictive, but that nicotine is (witness the very considerable withdrawal symptoms that occur in heavy cigarette smokers when they try to give up the habit). ALCOHOL also can be addictive, although moderate amounts do not produce addiction in the majority of people.

The treatment of addiction often is best carried out by an experienced psychiatrist working in a drug addiction program. Analysis, group therapy, and the prescription of less harmful drugs to ease the withdrawal period may all help—together with the sympathetic support of family and friends, which is essential.

See also DRUG ABUSE.

Addison's disease

A disorder in which the adrenal glands, situated just over the kidneys, cease to function adequately and thus do not produce normal quantities of the hormones called steroids. Also known as *adrenal cortical hypofunction.*

Steroids are essential to life because they enable the body to respond appropriately to stress. When there is decreased steroid production, the classic symptoms of Addison's disease will develop. These include weakness, tiredness, loss of appetite, low blood pressure, nausea, and vomiting. Changes occur in the skin as well, leading to a darker overall skin color. Discolorations also appear in the mouth.

The disease, although rare, affects both men and women at any age. In many cases, the cause is not known. In the past, tuberculosis was a frequent cause of adrenal gland destruction. Although there are still some infections that can lead to this type of damage, many cases are now thought to be caused by an autoimmune response, in which the body, for unknown reasons, begins to attack itself.

Addison's disease can be treated very successfully by giving replacement hormones. These steroids can be given by mouth or by injection, but usually must be given for life.

adenitis

Inflammation of a lymph gland (lymph node). These nodes are scattered through various parts of the body, with the main concentrations at the side of the neck, in the armpits, and in the groin. Their function is to help the body's defense against infection.

At times, however, an infection becomes sufficiently established to produce an intense inflammatory reaction in the lymph glands. These glands then become swollen and often painful.

In rare cases the inflammation proceeds to such a stage that pus is formed in the glands.

Typically, adenitis in the groin is caused by the spread of an infection in the foot or leg or in the sex organs. Adenitis in the armpits is caused by infection somewhere in the hand, arm, or in the breast. Adenitis in the neck glands (cervical adenitis) is caused by infection in the throat or ear. Chronic adenitis occurs when there is a prolonged or repeated infection. The nodes enlarge but may not be painful. Treatment depends on the cause, for example, antibiotics for repeated throat infections.

Sometimes lymphadenitis is caused by direct infection of the lymph nodes themselves, rather than by spread of infection from another site. Among the many conditions that can infect lymph nodes are TUBERCULOSIS, TYPHOID FEVER, INFECTIOUS MONONUCLEOSIS, MEASLES, and several parasitic diseases. It is also a symptom associated with AIDS.

adenocarcinoma

A type of CANCER arising in glandular tissue.

Adenocarcinomas can be distinguished under the microscope from other types of tumors, and this differentiation is of some help in assessing the likely outcome of the disease and in deciding the best method of treatment.

Adenocarcinomas can arise in the stomach, large intestine (colon), gallbladder, pancreas, uterus (womb), prostate gland, breasts, and lungs.

If they are not detected and treated early enough, these tumors may spread to other parts of the body via the blood and lymphatic systems. When such spreading occurs, the secondary tumor, which is formed at another site, has the same "glandular" appearance under the microscope as that of the "primary" adenocarcinoma (see METASTASIS). This may be a help in diagnosis if the site of the primary tumor is not yet known.

adenoids

Masses of glandlike lymphatic tissue found behind the nose on the back wall of the nasopharynx (that part of the throat located an inch or two above the area that is visible when the mouth is open). Doctors can inspect the adenoids by placing a small upward-angled mirror in the back of the mouth.

The adenoids often are referred to as the "na-

ADENOIDS

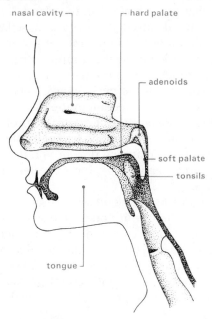

nasal cavity — ⌐ hard palate

⌐ adenoids

⌐ soft palate

⌐ tonsils

tongue ⌐

The adenoids and tonsils form part of a ring of lymphoid tissue at the entrance to the throat. Their job is to form protective antibodies against any microorganisms that attempt to enter the respiratory and digestive tracts.

sopharyngeal tonsils" because they play a role similar to that of the tonsils in helping to protect a child against inhaled germs. They sometimes become infected and grossly enlarged, making it difficult for air to pass in, through, or out of the nose. The symptoms of grossly enlarged adenoids include inability to breathe properly through the nose, a change in the quality of the voice ("adenoidal speech"), and snoring.

Adenoids usually reach their maximum size at about the age of 6 years, when the child is being exposed to a wide range of respiratory germs through contact with other children at school. From about the age of 9 or 10 they tend to shrink away. They usually disappear entirely by the time of adolescence; it is rare to find any trace of adenoids in adults. In view of their natural tendency to shrink, surgeons do not remove enlarged adenoids as readily as they once did.

adenoma

A benign tumor of glandular tissue (as opposed to ADENOCARCINOMA, which is a *malignant* tumor of the same type of tissue).

In contrast to adenocarcinomas, they do not

invade other parts of the body or destroy bodily tissues, nor do they spread to distant regions of the body to produce "secondary" tumors (metastasize). They can, however, cause harm by local pressure or by causing obstruction. Adenomas of hormone-secreting glands, such as the pituitary, can cause serious illness by excessive hormone production. Pituitary adenomas commonly cause blindness by pressure on the optic nerves.

Adenomas occur chiefly in such organs as the breast, stomach, bowel, pancreas, liver, thyroid gland, ovary, and adrenal glands. They are firm swellings formed of cells that resemble those of the tissues in which the adenoma has developed.

In the stomach and bowel an adenoma commonly develops a stalk, so that it grows into the cavity of the organ like a POLYP. In other situations (notably in the ovary), an adenoma may become cystic (filled with fluid). In the breast, an adenoma frequently contains a great deal of fibrous tissue; this type, called a FIBROADENOMA, is one of the most common of all adenomas.

Most adenomas are removed surgically. Partly this is because a *definite* diagnosis of a benign adenoma cannot be made until the lump has been removed for microscopic examination. In addition, a very small proportion of adenomas do become malignant (through changing into adenocarcinomas). Surgical excision, therefore, is not only a wise precaution, but may be essential in treating those tumors that have undergone a malignant change.

adhesion

An abnormal band of scar tissue that binds together two internal organs that normally are separate from one another. Adhesions are most commonly found in the stomach as a consequence of surgery, injury, or severe infection. Surgery may be needed to cut through the adhesions.

adipose tissue

Fat cells bound together with delicate fibrous tissue. Most lie immediately under the skin. Adipose tissue acts both as an insulator to help the body retain heat and as a source of energy for the body. This type of tissue is also found around the heart and lungs, where it acts as a cushion and provides support; around the kidneys, where it provides protection; and around the joints and muscles,

ADHESION

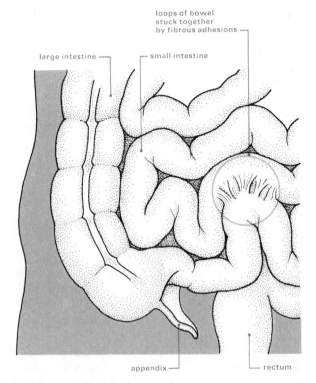

The loops of the bowel normally slide over each other freely, but occasionally they become bound together by fibrous adhesions. These may result from previous inflammation or from abdominal surgery. Adhesions may obstruct the passage of material along the bowel, in which case further surgery is necessary to divide the loops of bowel.

ADIPOSE TISSUE

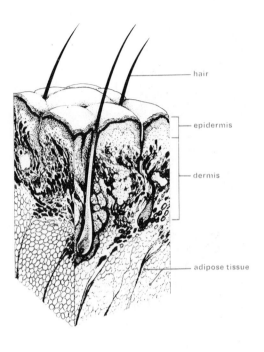

Adipose tissue is a collection of round, fat-filled cells; it is found throughout the body and acts as a reserve supply of energy. Unlike some primitive societies, Americans as a group do not have to endure periods of starvation, and thus they tend to carry excess amounts of adipose tissue. The layer (shown here beneath the skin) is also important for conserving body heat.

where it helps to prevent damage due to sudden shocks or jarring.

Excess adipose tissue anywhere in the body is known as obesity and is one of the major risk factors for CORONARY THROMBOSIS. It also greatly increases the risk of DIABETES MELLITUS and OSTEOARTHRITIS. It can be avoided by proper attention to diet and exercise.

adrenal glands

Two tiny glandular organs that lie immediately above the kidneys, at the back of the abdominal cavity. They are known also as the *suprarenal glands.*

The adrenal glands have two quite separate functions, and this is reflected by the fact that each of them is divided into two separate zones: an outer *cortex* and an inner *medulla.*

The adrenal cortex is absolutely essential to the body because it produces the cortisone-like hormones called "steroids," some of which play important roles in the metabolism of fats, carbohydrates, proteins, sodium, and potassium, and others in sexual development and the maintenance of bodily strength. If the cortex is not functioning properly because of some serious disorder (such as tuberculosis of the adrenals), then the result may be ADDISON'S DISEASE, a condition of extreme weakness and lethargy. In the past this disease proved fatal; today it is succcessfully treated with doses of adrenal steroid hormones taken in the form of tablets or injections.

The medulla of the gland is entirely separate in function. It is part of the sympathetic nervous

ADRENAL GLANDS

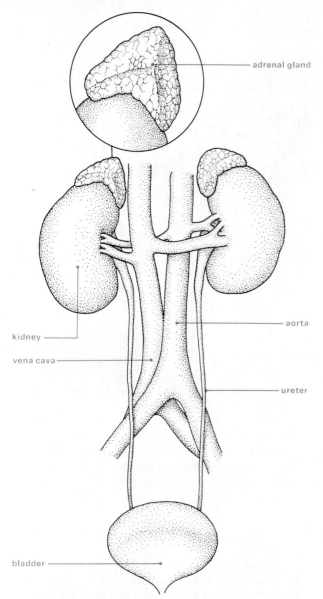

adrenal gland

kidney

vena cava

aorta

ureter

bladder

The adrenal glands sit on top of the kidneys like a pair of cocked hats. Although small, these glands are essential for life because of the hormones they produce: epinephrine and norepinephrine, which are secreted into the bloodstream when we are in stressful situations; cortisol and other stress hormones; and aldosterone, which plays an important role in regulating the blood pressure.

system, a division of the nerve communication network concerned with preparing the body for physical activity through release of epinephrine (adrenaline), the chemical that prepares muscles, heart, and blood vessels for instant action. It is often described as the hormone of "fight, flight,

or fright." The adrenal medulla is the body's primary source of this important hormone, releasing it in bursts that are triggered off by stimuli such as excitement, fear, anger, or sexual desire.

adrenaline

Another word for EPINEPHRINE (a hormone secreted by the ADRENAL GLANDS).

adrenogenital syndrome

A condition in which there is overactivity of part of the cortex of the ADRENAL GLANDS, often from tumor.

The adrenal cortex produces several steroid hormones including cortisol and androgens. The latter are male sex hormones. Overproduction of these hormones can result in the adrenogenital syndrome.

The characteristics of this condition depend on the particular "mix" of hormones being produced by the overactive adrenal gland. Chief symptoms, however, tend to be masculinization in female children and women (with excessive hairiness and enlargement of the clitoris) and precocious puberty in boys (including abnormal enlargement of the penis).

The adrenogenital syndrome is rare, and the current use of hormone therapy is usually fairly effective.

afterbirth

The PLACENTA and associated membranes expelled from the uterus (womb) after the baby has been born.

agoraphobia

An irrational fear of open places.

PHOBIAS are extremely common and agoraphobia is one of the most frequently encountered; on the most conservative estimate, there are tens of thousands of agoraphobics in the United States.

The reasons for the high incidence of agoraphobia are not known. Phobias may be linked to early childhood experiences and traumatic separations from people who are important. Agoraphobia may also be related to an underlying anxiety disorder. In this case, the person who experiences anxiety attacks when in public places eventually learns to avoid these places.

The symptoms of agoraphobia are extremely distressing for the victim. When she (the disorder is much more common in women) attempts to go out into the open, there is a terrifying feeling of panic, often with racing heart, profuse sweating, and trembling. The sufferer may be convinced that she is about to die, and this feeling cannot be alleviated until she gets back indoors again.

In variants of agoraphobia the person may fear only a particular type of open space—for instance, a park or even a supermarket with a high roof. Agoraphobics often have other phobias as well, such as a fear of cats, or insects, or of talking to other people.

Agoraphobia is difficult to treat, partly because sufferers are unable to overcome their panic in order to visit a doctor's office. The physician may be willing to make house calls, but usually what is needed is long-term therapy of the kind best given in the doctor's office. Some physicians specializing in this disorder have solved the problem by giving psychotherapy over the telephone.

Therapy may involve some form of analysis in an attempt to unravel the inner conflicts that are producing the panic. Psychiatrists and psychologists use such techniques as "deconditioning," in which the person is taught to relax while imagining herself in the feared situation. Tranquilizing drugs also have a small part to play in treatment, but they do not solve the underlying problem. In an attempt to relieve their anxiety, some persons have become physiologically and psychologically dependent on these drugs.

Research into the association between agoraphobia and panic disorders has led to new drug interventions. There are anxiety clinics that treat this disorder with increasing success.

See also ACROPHOBIA, CLAUSTROPHOBIA, PHOBIA.

agranulocytosis

A severe and prolonged decrease in the number of white blood cells (granulocytes). This condition is also known as *granulocytopenia*.

White blood cells, which are produced in the center, or marrow, of certain bones, help defend the body against many types of infection. The life span of many white blood cells in normal indi- viduals is only a few days, so they must be continuously produced in and released from the bone marrow. Agranulocytosis is caused by failure of the bone marrow to produce and release white blood cells in normal numbers.

Failure of the bone marrow may occur as a complication of malignancy. More commonly it represents a toxic reaction to drugs such as sulfonamides, gold or arsenic preparations, phenylbutazone, chloramphenicol, or certain antiepileptic and antithyroid preparations. Industrial poisons (benzol, for example) may have the same effects, as may exposure to radioactive material or X rays. Occasionally, however, the bone marrow fails to produce white blood cells for no known reason ("idiopathic" agranulocytosis).

The symptoms of agranulocytosis include those that might be expected in an individual with no real defense against infection: fever and recurrent infective ulceration of the mouth and throat, with increasing ill health and (if the condition is unchecked) eventual death.

There is no specific treatment for agranulocytosis. If the condition is a reaction to a toxic drug, the marrow will recover spontaneously (in most cases) once the drug is withdrawn. If the condition is a complication of bone-marrow tumor, this must be treated. Antibiotics are used to combat infection, and blood transfusions are given to provide a temporary source of white blood cells. Occasionally it is possible to perform a bone marrow transplant, inserting marrow taken from a donor.

AID/AIH

Terms used to indicate, respectively, *Artificial Insemination (by) Donor* and *Artificial Insemination (by) Husband*.

The term "artificial insemination" indicates the technique by means of which a man's seminal fluid is deposited in a woman's vagina or uterus under conditions other than sexual intercourse (usually with a special syringe) in the hope of achieving a pregnancy.

AIH involves taking a specimen of the husband's semen and introducing it into the wife's vagina or uterus. It is important to realize that AIH is used only in appropriate cases: when the wife has some structural or—more commonly— emotional problem that makes successful intercourse and impregnation difficult; when the husband is unable to achieve or maintain an erection long enough to have sexual intercourse; and, finally, when the concentration of sperm in the seminal fluid is abnormally low (the physician may then use special techniques to achieve a higher concentration of sperm before introducing the semen).

Much more controversial is AID, in which the seminal fluid is provided by a male donor. This method is used when the wife is fertile but the husband is not. Under current ethical guidelines, the identity of the donor should be unknown to the husband and wife, and the permission of the husband is required; in most states a legal agreement, signed by both husband and wife, is required in advance of the procedure.

AIDS (acquired immune deficiency syndrome)

First reported in the United States in mid-1981, AIDS is now regarded as a worldwide epidemic. Over 50,000 cases have been diagnosed in the United States. Though the majority of cases have occurred in homosexual or bisexual men and intravenous-drug users and their partners, anyone who is sexually active may be at risk. AIDS is characterized by a defect in the body's natural immunity against disease. People who have AIDS do not die from the disease per se, but from a number of serious, often fatal secondary or "opportunistic" infections and malignancies.

AIDS is believed to be caused by a member of the retrovirus group called HIV (human immune deficiency virus), of which there are a number of variants that also may cause AIDS. HIV attacks and destroys helper T-lymphocytes, which have a vital role in the defense against virus and fungus infections and some cancers. Once inside cells, HIV takes over the cell function and starts to reproduce, in time, producing hundreds of cloned copies of itself.

The incubation period (the period between initial infection and the development of the disease findings or symptoms) is from three to ten years or more. Even if there are no symptoms, an infected person may be carrying a live, transmittable virus—and may continue to do so for the rest of his or her life.

AIDS is spread by direct bloodstream contact with the blood or semen of an infected person. Small amounts of HIV have been identified in saliva and tears, but such body fluids are not known to be linked to the development of any AIDS cases and are not believed to be vehicles for transmission. AIDS is not transmitted by casual or household contact (touching, hugging, sneezing, etc). Deep mouth-to-mouth kissing with an infected person should be avoided, as should sharing of razors; such activities pose theoretical risks. AIDS is not transmitted by the bites of insects such as mosquitoes.

Certain behavior and practices pose high risks of HIV transmission and infection: the use of contaminated blood or blood products for transfusion or injection; the use of contaminated needles and syringes; the ingestion of an infected partner's ejaculate; unprotected (without a condom) anal or vaginal intercourse with an infected partner.

Certain measures have minimized the dangers. Condoms, properly used, greatly reduce but do not eliminate risk. All blood is now tested for HIV, so the risk in blood transfusions is practically nonexistent, though some hemophiliacs and other recipients of blood transfusions have been infected in the past. Children born to women who are HIV positive have also been affected.

The full AIDS complex may include:

• Cytomegalovirus infections, causing skin rashes, pneumonia (often fatal), hepatitis, fever, choroido-retinitis with severe loss of visual field.

• Candidiasis, the white thrush infection that starts in the mouth and genital region and spreads into the bowels and respiratory tract.

• Herpes simplex infection, which invades the interior of the body in much the same way as does candida albicans.

• Pneumocystis carinii pneumonia.

• Mycobacterium avium-intracellulare, which spreads throughout the body causing cavities filled with a cheesy material. These may occur anywhere—lungs, muscle, brain, skin, bones.

• Cryptococcus—a yeast infection that comes from pigeon droppings and mainly affects the brain and meninges (*brain linings*) causing a very slow chronic illness with memory loss, confusion, and personality changes.

• Toxoplasmosis, which causes brain abscesses and choroidoretinitis, and the main source of which is domestic cats. Cat boxes and droppings are highly infectious.

• Other conditions including aspergillosis, strongyloidiasis (a persistent worm infestation), Kaposi's sarcoma, and Burkitt's lymphoma.

The AIDS virus does not attack only the immune system. It is now known to have a definite affinity for brain tissue. Increasing numbers of cases of HIV encephalopathy (brain involvement) are now occurring in New York. This condition leads to a slow progressive dementia with eventual death.

Treatment has to be considered from two points of view—the treatment of the disorders resulting from the immune deficiency and the attack on the causal virus infection. Effective therapy exists for most of the conditions caused by immune deficiency, and, in spite of the difficulties, life can often be prolonged. Drugs such as Pentamidine for pneumocystis pneumonia, Acyclovir for herpes, Ketoconazole for candidiasis, can usually control or disperse these opportunistic infections. Recurrences are inevitably common.

The attack on AIDS itself has been mainly directed against the replication of the virus in the body, chiefly by exploiting its dependence on the enzyme reverse transcriptase. Enzyme inhibitors such as HPA-23, AL-721, Foscarnet, and, the most promising of them, Azidothymidine (AZT), are being vigorously tried. Other anti-viral drugs being investigated are Dextran sulphate, Dideoxycytidine, and Ribavirin. AZT can unquestionably prolong life, but it is a very toxic drug, and many AIDS sufferers are too weak to tolerate it.

Another approach is to try to improve the efficiency of the immune system itself. Drugs being tested for this effect include Interferon, Ampligen, GM-CSF (colony stimulating factor) Imuthiol, and the prostaglandin interleukin-2. Because there is no cure or preventive vaccine, education is the most powerful means of combating AIDS. See also IMMUNE SYSTEM.

albinism

Absence of melanin from the skin and hair, resulting in an unnaturally pale appearance. Melanin is the pigment responsible for hair and skin color and is present in persons of all races. The concentration of melanin in the skin is responsible for the production of a suntan, which is the body's way of preventing skin damage.

However, some people, owing to a genetic defect, have no melanin present. This condition has a one in 4 chance of occurring in children whose parents both carry the gene. The incidence in the United States is about one in 25,000.

Albinism causes an unnaturally white skin and hair that is white or very pale blond. Without the protective melanin, these persons are excessively sensitive to the sun and need to use extreme caution to avoid sunburn. Prolonged sun exposure puts albinos at high risk for skin cancer.

The lack of melanin also induces eye defects that cause poor vision and sun sensitivity. (There is a form of albinism that affects the eyes without affecting the skin, but this is much less common.) There is no treatment for this condition. Sunscreen lotions and sunglasses must be used to limit sun exposure.

albumin

A protein found in most animal tissues. Albumin is one of the two major proteins in human blood (the other being globulin). It is formed in the liver from protein foods in the diet. The best-known form of albumin is egg white; other types of albumin are found in milk, beans, and meat.

Albumin has an important role in metabolism. It also maintains the water-holding capacity of the blood (osmotic pressure); if it is not present in adequate concentration, excessive amounts of water pass out of the blood and into the tissues, causing EDEMA.

A low blood level of albumin is characteristic of protein malnutrition as well as certain kidney and liver disorders. Amounts and types of albumin in urine, blood, and other body tissues form the basis of many laboratory tests.

albuminuria

The presence of the serum protein *albumin* in the urine.

Albumin is one of the most important constituents of blood and is not usually found in urine. When blood passes through the kidneys, only impurities should be filtered out for excretion in the urine. When the kidney is malfunctioning, however, albumin may leak into the urine. That is why physicians make a regular practice of testing a urine specimen for albumin.

Albumin does not always indicate KIDNEY DISEASE.

alcohol/alcoholism

A type of chemical of which the most common form is *ethyl alcohol* obtained by the fermentation of sugar.

Alcohol, the main ingredient of many popular

beverages such as beer and wine, is a drug, albeit a socially acceptable one in most cultures. It is not a stimulant drug, as many people imagine, but a *selective depressant* of the central nervous system. It begins by depressing the higher functions of the brain; with increasing dosage, more basic functions are affected.

The effect of a small dose of alcohol is to depress the inhibitory or controlling centers of the brain, producing relaxation and a general loss of inhibitions. Larger quantities induce sedation and impair speech and muscular coordination. Very large quantities produce severe depression of the vital centers of the central nervous system and may be fatal.

Outside the central nervous system the physiologic effects of alcohol are less drastic. Small quantities increase the flow of gastric juices (thereby stimulating the appetite); larger amounts irritate the stomach lining, causing gastritis and even the vomiting of blood. Alcohol also increases the flow of urine.

Chronic consumption of fairly large quantities of alcohol can have highly damaging effects on body tissues, particularly those of the liver. CIRRHOSIS, a serious hardening and degeneration of liver tissue, kills many heavy drinkers. CANCER is especially likely to develop in a cirrhotic liver. Alcohol taken in excess over a long period may also cause degeneration of the heart muscle (cardiomyopathy) and serious impairment of brain function.

Alcoholism is a state of addiction to alcohol. Those who suffer from it are likely to develop the severe physical consequences of alcohol abuse that have been outlined above. Alcohol is not as addictive as heroin, morphine, or nicotine; but research indicates that most humans (and mammals generally) can be habituated to it by prolonged, constant exposure. If a person drinks enough alcohol on a regular basis, there is a strong possibility that his body will become dependent upon it. Larger and larger doses may be required, as time goes by, to keep withdrawal symptoms away.

Although stress in life plays a part in excessive drinking, alcoholism can be seen as an illness. There is evidence that genetic factors may be involved in the development of alcoholism.

Treatment of alcoholism is difficult and full of disappointments. The alcoholic must accept that he has the condition; he then needs caring support from his family, friends, and personal physician. It may also be wise for the alcoholic to consult a psychiatrist who is thoroughly experienced in dealing with the condition.

The psychiatrist might suggest psychotherapy. There are medications that are used to help the person who has difficulty refraining from drinking. One such drug, disulfiram (Antabuse), produces a severe physical reaction (including nausea and vomiting) if alcohol is taken.

Other methods employed by psychiatrists include behaviorist techniques such as conditioning the person to associate the sight and smell of alcohol with unpleasant sensations. Admission to a special alcoholic unit is often necessary so that the alcohol can be withdrawn completely ("drying out").

Alcoholics Anonymous is a leading organization whose supportive work in helping persons keep off alcohol has undoubtedly saved thousands of lives.

alkaptonuria

A rare inborn error of metabolism, which causes the excretion in the urine of a substance called homogentisic acid. This causes the urine to become dark on exposure to the air, so that urine left overnight in a pot will become almost black. (The chemical defect is the absence of an enzyme termed homogentisic oxidase, which catalyzes an important step in the metabolism of the amino acid tyrosine.)

Because of the efficiency of modern sanitation an affected individual may be unaware of the abnormality unless other symptoms develop. These include a form of arthritis and stiffness and a change in color of the cartilage in the ear and elsewhere owing to deposit of a pigment formed as a result of the chemical defect. The arthritis, which typically develops at about the age of 30, affects the larger joints, and especially the spine. There is no specific treatment, but life expectancy is normal.

This defect is hereditary and will not appear unless both parents carry the gene. If they do, then the disease will appear in approximately one in 4 of their children. Fortunately, the gene is rare; the incidence of the disease in the United States is about one in 200,000. As with other recessively inherited diseases, alkaptonuria is much more likely to appear if the parents are related to each other; thus, the disease is more common in small, inbred communities. Genetic counseling is advisable for anyone who has a relative with the disorder: The condition can be detected chemically before the symptoms develop.

allergy

The mechanism through which symptoms are caused by sensitivity to an *allergen*—an allergy-causing substance, such as pollen, feathers, fur, or dust, or a chemical such as a detergent, cosmetic, or drug. Allergy is the cause of HAY FEVER and URTICARIA (hives) and underlies many cases of ASTHMA and ECZEMA.

Allergic reactions are exaggerations of the body's normal immune responses to bacteria and viruses and their toxins. Whenever an infecting organism penetrates the skin or enters the bloodstream, the blood lymphocytes respond by forming antibodies—large protein molecules that correspond to chemical markers on the bacteria or their toxins. The allergic response is essentially similar: Antibodies are formed against pollen grains inhaled into the nose and lungs or against cosmetics coming into contact with the skin. However, whereas the normal immune response destroys bacteria and neutralizes their toxins, the allergic response causes symptoms rather than protecting against them. Characteristically, the first (sensitizing) exposure to an allergen causes no symptoms, but if the body responds by forming antibodies the stage is set for an allergic reaction on the next and subsequent exposures. Whether or not allergens such as pollen, dog hair, or strawberries provoke an allergic reaction depends on individual susceptibility. Some people are allergic to a whole range of common substances; others never develop sensitivities. Such tendencies often run in families.

The most common sites for allergic reactions are the respiratory tract and the skin. Inhaled allergens may stimulate the formation of antibodies, which become fixed to the lining of the nose or lungs. Further exposure to the same allergen will cause the antibodies and antigens to react together, with the release of chemicals such as histamine from specialized immune cells (plasma cells and mast cells) in the surface membranes. It is the histamine release that causes symptoms of hay fever such as eye-watering and sneezing from swelling and inflammation of the conjunctiva and the nasal mucous membranes. In the lungs the predominant allergic response is narrowing of the air passages, causing asthma; in the skin the response causes swelling and irritation, although the scratching this induces may lead to secondary infection. Allergy may also affect the digestive system: if certain foods are ingested to which the person is allergic, it can cause nausea, vomiting, and diarrhea.

Allergic responses may be immediate, in which exposure to the allergen causes symptoms within a few minutes, or delayed, in which there may be an interval of several days between contact with the allergen and the onset of symptoms. In delayed responses the illness may not be recognized as allergic unless careful attention is paid to the possibility.

Allergic reactions that cause troublesome symptoms can be treated with antihistamine drugs, which block the effects of histamine. Other drugs are available that suppress the formation of the antibodies. Another approach is DESENSITIZATION: Repeated injections of very small doses of the allergen responsible for symptoms are given, which over time will block the allergic response. This treatment is used most often in persons with only a few specific allergies for things such as dust or pollens. The best treatment, of course, is avoidance of the allergen but this is not always possible.

alopecia

The medical term for BALDNESS.

alphafetoprotein (AFP)

A protein normally produced by the liver and stomach tract of a human fetus.

AFP is measured in the amniotic fluid to check for fetal defects such as SPINA BIFIDA (an incomplete growth of the spine). High levels may be found in the blood of adults who have certain diseases such as liver breakdown (CIRRHOSIS), some types of HEPATITIS, and some cancers.

altitude sickness

An illness occurring in persons on high mountains or in unpressurized aircraft, as a result of the reduced quantity of oxygen in the air. Symptoms of this illness are headache, shortness of breath, and coughing. In more severe cases, the lungs may fill with fluid, a condition known as *pulmonary edema*. Usual treatment is oxygen, medication, and descent to a lower altitude.

The proportion of oxygen in the air is the same at all altitudes, but as the air gets thinner at great heights, less oxygen is available. At altitudes greater than 10,000 feet above sea level, persons generally have difficulty adapting to the reduced oxygen supply. Although one can become acclimatized to this lessened supply of oxygen over a period of weeks, it is not usually possible for people making short trips into these regions. In such cases care must be taken not to overextend oneself physically.

Alzheimer's disease

Atrophy—a shrinkage in size and weight—of the brain often occurs with advanced age but sometimes also in younger people. The age-associated condition, called *senile dementia*, is characterized by forgetfulness and slowed mental functioning. It is not a natural aging process but the result of a variety of degenerative diseases.

Alzheimer's disease is one of the most common of these diseases. Although the elderly get this disease, it is most notable for striking younger persons—some as early as in their 20s; however, it occurs most commonly in the 40-to-60 age group. The onset is very gradual but progressive. First signs may be the loss of memory of recent events, forgetfulness or repetition of routine activities, and unusual behavior.

As the disease progresses, memory loss increases, muscle coordination abilities may decrease, and irrational thinking and irritability may occur. In extreme cases, the patient loses the ability to speak, care for himself, or even think.

The cause of Alzheimer's disease is not yet known but affected brain tissue shows tangled masses of fibrillary material, most abundant in the areas most concerned with retentive memory.

There is no treatment for Alzheimer's disease, only supportive care. As the disease progresses, the person must be closely supervised and cared for, which often places great strain on the family's physical, emotional, and financial resources. In recent years, support groups have formed to offer support and counseling for families of Alzheimer's disease patients.

amaurosis

Blindness from some cause outside the eyes. Examples include the blindness sometimes associated with toxemia of pregnancy, MIGRAINE, ARTERIOSCLEROSIS, and disease of the optic nerve or brain.

In healthy persons transient amaurosis sometimes occurs when they stand up quickly from a prone position—caused simply by the draining of blood away from the head. "Amaurosis fugax" is an important symptom of brief loss of vision. It is usually due to cholesterol emboli and is a warning of high risk of STROKE.

The term "amaurotic family idiocy" refers to the inherited abnormality TAY-SACHS DISEASE (most common in people of Jewish descent) of which blindness is a feature. The blindness is due to degeneration of nerve cells, as are all the other symptoms of the disease.

amblyopia

Defective vision without any obvious diseases of the eyeball. Amblyopia may be temporary or permanent and there are several possible causes; it may be partial or it may progress to total blindness in the affected eye.

Substances that may cause it include wood alcohol, tobacco, lead, certain petroleum derivatives, and compounds that contain arsenic. *Bilateral amblyopia* may also occur as the result of poisoning with various drugs. Amblyopia can also occur as a result of damage to the region of the brain concerned with vision.

The most important preventable cause of amblyopia is STRABISMUS ("cross-eye") in infancy. In strabismus the eyes point in different directions, and the child's brain suppresses the image from one eye to prevent the confusion caused by double vision. If the squint is not treated, the eye that is not used may have permanently poor vision.

Cases of toxic amblyopia may improve if the source of poisoning is removed, but in cases due to brain damage, the blindness may be irreversible. Squint amblyopia is easily treated if found early. After age 7, little can be done.

amenorrhea

Absence of menstrual periods. Amenorrhea may be primary or secondary. In primary amenorrhea, menstruation has never occurred at all; in secondary amenorrhea, a woman who has previously been menstruating ceases to do so.

Primary amenorrhea begins to give rise to concern when a girl between 16 and 17 still has not menstruated; she should be taken to a physician for a gynecological evaluation of her condition. Primary amenorrhea at this age may be just a slight variation from normal; regular menstruation may commence shortly thereafter. But primary amenorrhea may be due to anemia, to disorders of the uterus, ovaries, or pituitary gland, or to dysfunction of the thyroid or adrenal glands. Occasionally there is *false* primary amenorrhea in which a girl is menstruating but the menstrual blood is prevented from reaching the exterior by some obstacle, such as an *imperforate hymen* ("maidenhead" without an opening). Primary amenorrhea can occur with or without the development of secondary sexual characteristics.

In a woman who has previously menstruated, the absence of the menses for a period of six months or more is called secondary amenorrhea. This is a fairly common occurrence, and there are several possible causes. In almost any woman who has secondary amenorrhea the doctor will perform a pregnancy test. Secondary amenorrhea may also be due to anemia (often provoked by heavy menstrual blood loss in the past), ovarian failure, certain pituitary diseases, or some kind of emotional disturbance or even a marked change in life-style.

Amenorrhea may also occur on use of the contraceptive pill (or after coming off it) and in AN-OREXIA NERVOSA. Treatment will depend on the underlying cause.

amnesia

Loss of MEMORY. Memories are held in the brain in short-term and long-term stores, and either or both functions may be impaired by disease, injury, or psychological stress.

Typically, the adult does not remember the events of infancy, but his recall of the rest of his lifetime is more or less continuous. In old age, however, the memory for recent events becomes impaired, while the events of childhood and early adult life are still well preserved. Loss of recent memory is also a feature of chronic alcoholism (in *Korsakoff's syndrome* the alcoholic invents stories to cover up his loss of memory) and of some other brain diseases such as DEMENTIA.

Head injuries that cause loss of consciousness—or even severe or frightening accidents that do not involve the head—may be associated with some loss of memory. Often there is a blank in the memory for some minutes or hours before the injury (*retrograde amnesia*) and for a variable period after the injury (*anterograde amnesia*). The duration of both types of amnesia tends to diminish as the person recovers from the injury, but parts of memory often never recover.

Sudden loss of memory without any injury or illness is most often due to a psychological disorder: The person who is found wandering far from home with no knowledge of his name or address usually is found to be suffering from *psychological amnesia*, a condition provoked by emotional stress.

Despite claims to the contrary, no drug has yet been found to improve failing memory.

amoeba

A microscopic, single-celled organism. Many species of amoebas are found throughout the world.

AMOEBA

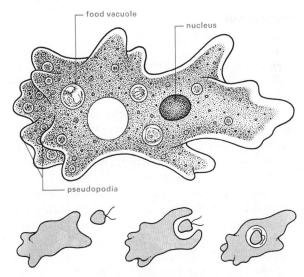

free-living amoeba ingesting a flagellate

Amoebas are single-cell microorganisms that have changeable shape. They move by putting out temporary projections called pseudopodia and flowing into them. They may be free-living or parasitic. Certain species can infect humans, causing disease—for example, one type is responsible for amoebic dysentery.

Several species live in the human body all the time; others can infect humans and cause illness.

amyloidosis

The infiltration of the liver, kidneys, heart, and other internal organs with a starch-like protein substance known as amyloid. (The exact composition of amyloid is not known, and probably varies.)

Amyloidosis is a late complication of chronic infectious diseases such as TUBERCULOSIS and OSTEOMYELITIS; it also occurs in some cancers of the lymphatic system, such as HODGKIN'S DISEASE, and in the bone-marrow cancer MULTIPLE MYELOMA. Sometimes the amyloid infiltration occurs with no predisposing cause; this *primary amyloidosis* is often a familial disorder.

The importance of amyloidosis is that the infiltration of vital organs such as the kidneys may cause their progressive failure. Vigorous treatment of the underlying infection is sometimes followed by reabsorption of the amyloid, but there is no specific treatment for the infiltration itself.

analgesia

Reduction or loss of the sensation of pain without the impairment of a person's level of consciousness.

Drugs that produce analgesia are called *analgesics*, and they can range from those used for mild pain, such as aspirin or acetaminophen, to those used for controlling more severe pain, such as codeine and morphine.

Some analgesics, such as aspirin, act by inhibiting the synthesis of pain-causing prostaglandins by damaged cells; others, such as codeine and morphine, work in the brain to alter a person's perception of pain. These latter medications can increase pain tolerance and change one's reaction to pain; the intensity of the pain remains the same but the anxiety-reducing effect of the drugs free a person from perceiving the stimulus as painful. Because of their potential for abuse, these drugs are available only by a doctor's prescription.

Analgesia can result also from diseases of the nervous system or from alcohol intoxication.

anaphylactic shock

An antigen-antibody reaction in the body which may produce a state of profound collapse. This is characterized by increasing difficulty in breathing and failure of the circulation brought about by general dilation of the small blood vessels and the escape of plasma (the fluid component of the blood) into the tissue spaces.

Anaphylactic shock may be caused by the injection of certain vaccines, antisera, or antibiotics, or by insect stings; it is a desperate emergency in which delay may prove fatal.

Treatment depends on the severity of the reaction. If the reaction is mild, steroids, antihistamines, and epinephrine can be given. In severe cases, edema of the larynx may obstruct breathing. This reaction necessitates a tracheostomy to restore breathing (the cutting of an airway into the person's windpipe—best done by experienced medical personnel). Cardiopulmonary resuscitation is necessary if the heart has stopped.

The danger of anaphylactic shock is the reason that persons who are getting injections for allergies are told to wait for half an hour before leaving the doctor's office. Persons who are allergic to bee stings should carry with them epinephrine, which they can inject into themselves in case they are stung. The epinephrine usually can ward off the anaphylactic shock for a short while so that the person has time to seek emergency medical attention.

anemia

A disease affecting the number of red blood cells (RBC) in the blood. The chief function of RBC is to carry oxygen from the lungs to all the tissues of the body. In the RBC is a substance called hemoglobin; the oxygen is attached to the hemoglobin. Anemia results in less oxygen being delivered to tissues; if severe enough, it can result in serious disease and even death.

Anemia has four basic causes. Red blood cells may be lost from the circulation through hemorrhage. There may be a deficiency of raw materials needed for the production of hemoglobin and red blood cells. The bone marrow itself may be diseased and therefore unable to produce sufficient red blood cells. Lastly, in the *hemolytic anemias*, production of red blood cells by the bone marrow is normal but the cells are destroyed unusually quickly and so do not survive for the normal period of 120 days in the circulation.

Anemia may occur also as an accompaniment of many chronic diseases such as ARTHRITIS. The reason for this type of anemia, known as the *anemia of chronic disease*, is not clearly understood and not necessarily related to any of the four basic causes.

Blood loss may be obvious, as in a person with nosebleeds or a woman with heavy menstrual periods; but when it occurs internally, the patient may be unaware of it ("occult" blood loss).

The raw materials for the production of red cells include iron for hemoglobin production and vitamin B_{12} and folic acid (another B-group vitamin). Deficiencies of these substances may be the result of dietary lack, failure to absorb them normally (though present in normal amounts in the diet), or, more rarely, an increased demand by the body (as with a need for more folic acid in pregnancy).

Diseases of the bone marrow causing a failure of red cell production include replacement of the marrow by cancer or leukemia cells and damage to the marrow caused by toxic drugs, chemicals, or radiation.

Anemia is a very common condition and in many cases goes undetected if it is not severe. For example, women, because of their menstrual blood loss, maintain their iron balance with difficulty. Surveys have revealed that 5 percent or more of women who otherwise appear healthy are in fact anemic, and up to 30 percent have no reserves of iron and are thus in danger of developing iron-deficiency anemia.

The symptoms of anemia may be minimal; but if the condition is at all severe, the patient will be pale and will complain of tiredness and shortness of breath on exertion. In addition, specific types of anemia may produce characteristic symptoms.

Blood checks for the presence of anemia and other blood abnormalities form an important part of any comprehensive medical examination.

If a patient is found to be anemic, the fundamental question for the doctor to resolve is whether the anemia is the result of a specific blood disease, such as pernicious anemia or LEUKEMIA, or whether it is a symptom of blood loss or of an underlying disease or infection.

Treatment of anemia depends on the cause. For example, in men and nonmenstruating women, iron deficiency indicates abnormal loss of blood and iron from a source such as undiagnosed tumor in the colon. Anemia is usually a sign of some other underlying condition.

anencephaly

A congenital birth defect in which the fetus has no cranium or brain, or only part of one. The baby lives only a few hours or is born dead. This defect can be detected by amniocentesis and ultrasound examination. Large amounts of ALPHAFETOPROTEIN are found in the amniotic fluid.

anesthesia

The loss of feeling, particularly the sensations of pain and touch. Anesthesia can be produced by disease or damage to the nervous system, by certain psychological states, or by the action of drugs. The term usually is applied to the deliberate induction of UNCONSCIOUSNESS (general anesthesia) so that the patient can undergo surgery. Intravenous injections of drugs such as *sodium pentothal* are used to induce general anesthesia, putting the patient quietly and agreeably to sleep. Anesthesia is then maintained with nitrous oxide gas supplemented by small doses of other anesthetic drugs.

Modern anesthesiologists have many drugs at their disposal; they can induce temporary unconsciousness, temporary paralysis, and temporary hypotension (low blood pressure) at will. Indeed, a complicated surgical operation depends for its success as much on the skill of the anesthesiologist as on the skill of the surgeon.

Anesthesia of only a part of the body (without loss of consciousness) can be produced by drugs known as local anesthetics. *Cocaine* applied to the surface of mucous membranes renders them anesthetic; but the use of cocaine has now been abandoned in favor of synthetic compounds such as *tetracaine*. Other synthetic compounds, such as *procaine* and *lidocaine*, are administered by injection; if they are injected into or under the skin they produce anesthesia of the immediate area, while if they are injected into sensory nerves they produce anesthesia of the particular region of the body supplied by the nerve.

It is possible to perform some types of major operations under local anesthesia or under *spinal anesthesia*. The latter is a technique in which the local anesthetic agent is introduced into the spinal canal under strict control to bring about temporary block of the motor and sensory nerve roots as they leave the spinal cord. The height to which the anesthetic solution is allowed to rise in the spinal canal determines the area of anesthesia (which is nearly always confined to the lower part of the trunk and the legs). An alternative technique involves injecting the anesthetic into the space just outside the membranes covering the spinal cord (*extradural anesthesia*); this method is widely used during labor and childbirth.

aneurysm

Swelling at a weak point in the wall of an artery, named according to its shape as either *fusiform, saccular, berry,* or *dissecting,* and classified as either *congenital, inflammatory, degenerative,* or *traumatic.*

Common sites for aneurysms are the aorta (the largest artery of the body), the arteries at the base of the brain (the "circle of Willis"), and the artery behind the knee. Although aneurysms can produce symptoms by pressing on neighboring structures—for example, one at the base of the brain can produce double vision by interfering with the nerves that supply the external muscles of the

ANEURYSM

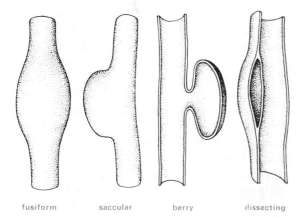

fusiform   saccular   berry   dissecting

Aneurysms form at weak points in an arterial wall. The weakness may be congenital, as with the small "berry" aneurysms in the brain, which sometimes burst, causing hemorrhage. Most aneurysms, however, are due to atherosclerosis and are fusiform or saccular in shape. A dissecting aneurysm is one where blood actually runs between the layers of the arterial wall.

eye—the chief danger is rupture, which sets up internal bleeding with possibly fatal results.

Treatment depends on the site and nature of the aneurysm. Surgery offers the only hope of cure, and an operation may or may not be possible; each case must be judged on its own merits.

angina pectoris

Sometimes just called *angina;* a type of discomfort characteristic of myocardial ISCHEMIA, in which the coronary arteries fail to supply sufficient oxygen to the heart muscle.

The discomfort usually is felt centrally in the chest but may radiate to the neck or down the left arm. It can be very severe or it may be described merely as a "tightness in the chest." The latter symptom is frequent (hence the name *angina pectoris,* "choking in the chest"), but the syndrome of myocardial ischemia may also cause discomfort in the abdomen, back, and jaw as well as breathlessness and belching.

A diagnostic feature is that the symptoms occur during activity and rapidly disappear if the person stops and rests for a few minutes. Thus, those suffering from chronic angina may come to recognize that a certain degree or duration of exercise (walking a certain distance or exceeding a certain speed) will bring on the symptoms, and they learn to avoid the symptoms by keeping within their personal exercise tolerance. Emotional factors and cold may also contribute to the onset of pain.

Angina is most often caused by the narrowing of the coronary arteries due to ATHEROSCLEROSIS with the result that the blood supply to the heart muscle is reduced. If the rate and strength of the heartbeat are increased by exercise, the blood flow required to keep the muscle adequately supplied is exceeded and the characteristic discomfort results. Reducing the requirement by reducing activity allows the blood flow to become adequate again. Less commonly the coronary arteries are normal but the heart muscle is "starved" of oxygen either because the blood is deficient in hemoglobin (ANEMIA) or the blood pressure is low from narrowing of the aortic valve (aortic STENOSIS) or other valvular abnormalities. The diagnosis depends mainly on the person's medical history, although the EKG will usually show characteristic abnormalities.

Angina is a serious disorder since its presence denotes diseased coronary arteries; all those afflicted with angina should seek early medical advice. Under good medical care, however, many live a relatively normal life for many years with the condition.

Treatment consists of easing the load on the heart by losing weight and lowering high blood pressure, giving up smoking (which aggravates the condition), and altering the diet to reduce blood levels of fat. Drugs that relieve the symptoms include glyceryl trinitrate (nitroglycerin), which dilates the coronary arteries and reduces the work load of the heart, and drugs known as "beta-adrenergic blocking agents" and "calcium channel blocking agents," which reduce the work load of the heart. In some cases, coronary angioplasty or coronary bypass surgery may be indicated.

ANKYLOSING SPONDYLITIS

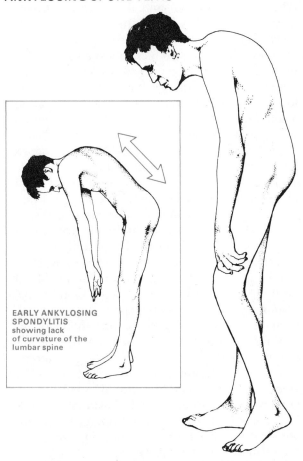

EARLY ANKYLOSING
SPONDYLITIS
showing lack
of curvature of the
lumbar spine

Ankylosing spondylitis is a progressive inflammatory disease that affects the spinal column. Movement is gradually limited, and in severe cases the backbone may become totally rigid.

ankylosing spondylitis

A form of arthritis of the spine that occurs most commonly in men between the ages of 20 to 40. It is a chronic, progressive process that causes inflammation of the joints and ligaments in the spine. Over time, these normally flexible ligaments become bone-like in consistency, causing stiffness and loss of mobility. Occasionally, the hips and ribs may become involved, causing further loss of mobility and impairment in the ability to expand the chest. The cause is not known.

The first signs of this disease are lower back pain and stiffness, which are generally worse in the morning. Hip, buttock, and shoulder pain also may be present. In advanced cases there is a characteristic shape to the spine as it becomes fixed in a rigid position, with the neck bent forward.

Treatment in the early stages consists of relieving pain and minimizing the potential of spinal deformities. Non-steroidal anti-inflammatory drugs relieve pain and can assist in allowing a person to maintain an erect posture at all times. Persons are encouraged also to sleep face down, or if this is not possible, to sleep on their backs on a firm mattress. The majority of those with this disease lead relatively normal lives.

anorexia nervosa

A serious eating disorder that mainly affects teenage girls, but may also afflict teenage boys and older women and men. It is manifested by extreme aversion to food, intense fear of gaining weight, and inordinate concern with body image. Often victims lose weight until they are more than 25 percent below ideal weight, yet they continue to maintain they are fat.

Eating may become ritualized, with the anorectic person insisting on the type and amount of food, the manner in which it's prepared and arranged, and the time at which it's eaten. To increase weight loss, victims will claim to have eaten more than they have, hide uneaten food, self-induce vomiting, take laxatives, or exercise excessively. As dietary restriction continues, profound weight loss can lead to emaciation and vitamin and mineral deficiencies.

The nutritional deficiencies, in turn, can have many physical complications, including dry skin, increased body hair, and muscle weakness. Blood pressure may become low normal, and cardiac arrythmias—irregular heartbeats—may develop. The anorectic person may suffer from anemia, an electrolyte imbalance (particularly low potassium levels), impaired kidney function, and hypothyroidism. Left untreated, the condition may prove fatal as the patient literally starves herself to death. Thirty to 35 percent of victims who are more than 20 percent below normal body weight die unless they get treatment. With proper medical therapy, however, the mortality rate is approximately 5 percent.

The exact cause of anorexia is unknown. It appears to be caused by deep psychological problems, including depression, obsessiveness, and unresolved conflicts. The patient may fear sexual development (particularly breast development in females) and feel it can be suppressed or delayed by losing weight. Anorexia may also be a means of rebelling or expressing hostility against parents or other adults. The victims often come from middle- or upper-class families with high expectations and standards; often the parents are overly concerned with weight control and exercise. In some cases, anorectic behavior follows a period of being overly sensitive about adolescent plumpness.

Treatment of anorexia nervosa is in two phases: short term to restore body weight—sometimes to save life—and long term to deal with the personality and family problems. This is a serious disorder, for which hospitalization often is necessary. Management should be carried out by trained professionals. If weight loss is extreme or there are severe electrolyte imbalances, intravenous infusion and tube feeding will be necessary. Psychiatric help often is needed to help the anorectic person overcome underlying psychological problems. Medical self-help groups are sprouting up all over the country that are invaluable in helping victims return to a normal life-style. While prospects for recovery are excellent, relapses are common unless there is some form of supportive therapy.

anthrax

Infectious disease caused by *Bacillus anthracis*, which commonly infects cattle, goats, or sheep. Humans contract the infection from the spores of the anthrax bacillus, which survive for a long time in contaminated wool, hair, or hides. With increasingly hygienic methods of handling these raw materials, the spread of the disease has di-

minished, and it is now rare in the Western world.

The infection can affect the skin, producing a severe localized reaction. The site of infection is marked by an itching "papule" which becomes surrounded by vesicles filled with blood-stained fluid. As the infection spreads, the center of the area dies and becomes black. Symptoms that follow include internal bleeding, muscle pain, headache, fever, nausea, and vomiting.

Infection can also attack the lungs, to produce pneumonia, or it can advance to anthrax bacteremia (blood poisoning), with a high mortality rate if untreated. The old name for anthrax of the lung was "woolsorter's disease." The illness was usually fatal, but now anthrax of both the skin and the lungs responds to treatment with appropriate antibiotics.

antigen/antibody

When certain foreign and therefore potentially harmful substances enter the body, the body reacts to the threat of damage by producing antibodies. An antibody is a chemical compound, a protein, that has the ability to combine with and render harmless a specific foreign substance. The foreign material itself, which initiates the reaction leading to the formation of specific antibodies, is known as an *antigen*.

Most antigenic substances are protein. Proteins have a very complex and almost infinitely variable chemical composition and are constituents of all living matter. For this reason, the antigens that cause the formation of antibodies are mostly substances derived directly or indirectly from living organisms. Common examples of antigens are: the bacteria and viruses that cause human disease; "foreign" blood from an incompatible blood group, inadvertently given during a blood transfusion; and sera from other species injected into humans for the treatment or prevention of infectious diseases. Whatever the situation, the antibody formed in response to a particular antigen is unique to that antigen, reacting with no other (see illustration). The blood of an adult human contains tens of thousands of individual antibodies directed against different antigens, and together they form a distinct group of proteins in the serum, the *immunoglobulins*.

The basic purpose of antibody formation is defensive. One major role of antibodies is to overcome attacks of infectious disease and to prevent future recurrent attacks. Thus, when the person who has never previously had an attack of WHOOPING COUGH comes into contact with the whooping cough bacillus, he will develop symptoms of the disease. The defeat of the invading bacteria depends initially on the action of the *phagocytic blood cells*, which are responsible for the primary defense against bacterial invasion; these cells attack, kill, and engulf the bacteria. As the disease runs its course, however, antibodies against the whooping cough bacilli start to appear in the blood, and the final elimination of the infection is aided by their action. By the time the person is convalescent, a good level of specific antibodies is present in the blood. In many diseases these antibodies persist at such a high level that the person remains immune to a second attack of the disease throughout the rest of his life.

This natural phenomenon forms the basis of *vaccination* and *inoculation* against infectious diseases. Antibodies usually are produced as the result of an infection with bacteria, viruses, or other microorganisms; their production can also be stimulated artificially by introducing a special preparation of these microorganisms or their products into the body. In whooping cough and TYPHOID FEVER, for example, injection of dead bacteria (of the same species that can cause the respective disease) will evoke the identical kind of antibody formation as that seen in the actual disease and will confer lasting immunity. In diphtheria and TETANUS the bacteria produce their effects by means of the toxins (poisons) they produce; injection of the toxin itself, suitably treated to render it no longer toxic though still antigenic, will enable the body to form antibodies against the toxin. Lastly, the inoculation of a specific living virus culture—which has been treated to weaken the virus to such a degree that it no longer can cause symptoms of the disease—will immunize the person against SMALLPOX, YELLOW FEVER, POLIOMYELITIS, and other diseases.

Most antibodies are thus acquired by contact with an antigen, but in a newborn baby some antibodies are already present, passively acquired from the mother; these persist for a few months after birth to provide an early protection against infections.

In rare instances, antibodies may be formed against the body's own cells rather than against invading bacteria, viruses, or other foreign material. In this case, the result is damage to the tissue concerned—a condition known as an AUTOIMMUNE DISEASE.

Transplanted organs or tissues, unless taken

ANTIBODY AND ANTIGEN – how some antibodies work

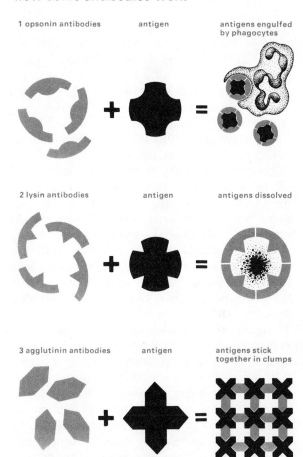

The diagrams show how antibodies produced by the body defend us against foreign substances (antigens). Each antibody can combine only with a specific antigen that has a complementary chemical "shape." Opsonin antibodies cling to antigens such as bacteria and make them more appetizing to certain white blood cells called phagocytes (1). Lysin antibodies kill bacteria directly by dissolving them (2). Agglutinin antibodies cause bacteria or viruses to clump together, rendering them ineffective (3).

from an identical twin, are considered to be foreign invaders by the body and may be rejected unless immunosuppressive drugs are used.

Antibodies also play a major role in allergic diseases. In response to an antigen such as pollen or dog hair, the body can create antibodies. These antibodies are responsible for the symptoms of allergies.

See also IMMUNE SYSTEM.

anxiety

Anxiety is a normal response to a crisis such as an impending examination or a new job; but excessive anxiety can be socially crippling and cause physical illness.

In anxiety disorders a perfectly normal concern about cleanliness, noise, or other everyday circumstance becomes magnified to dominate the thoughts. Typically this leads to obsessional behavior: the sufferer returns repeatedly to his house to check that the door is shut and the gas turned off, or she becomes preoccupied with handwashing or some other ritual. In AGORAPHOBIA, anxiety about leaving the house and meeting strangers may lead to a self-imposed imprisonment in the home. The anxiety may be less specific than this, however. In such cases every minor event is seen as a threat and a cause for apprehension; again, the effect is to restrict behavior to a cautious, predictable routine.

Anxiety is a common component of the *depressive illnesses* that affect a high proportion of all men and women in middle and later life. One third or more of all middle-aged women admit to episodes of depression, often including anxiety about their family relationships and their worth. Anxiety is also frequently provoked in middle age by some episode of illness—such as a heart attack or a head injury—that impairs self-confidence.

The symptoms of recurrent anxiety include loss of appetite and weight, heart palpitations, headache, excessive sweating, and difficulty in sleeping. These symptoms may be suppressed readily following treatment with tranquilizing drugs. Such treatment often is used to control the symptoms associated with isolated life events, such as anxiety about flying or sea voyages.

The symptoms of anxiety might be confused with other illnesses, such as heart or thyroid conditions. The anxious person might undergo many medical tests before being diagnosed as having an anxiety disorder. Many hospitals have specialized anxiety clinics that successfully treat anxiety disorders with medication.

apnea

The absence or cessation of automatic breathing. Apnea sometimes occurs in newborn babies and is usually caused by immaturity of the respiratory control center in the brain. It may also result from a cerebral hemorrhage during delivery, the presence of drugs in the baby's blood, or a congenital malformation.

In later life, cessation of breathing may follow overoxygenation of the blood induced artificially or by overbreathing. Obstructive sleep apnea occurs in obese people with poor lung function. There are repeated episodes of obstructive choking followed by sudden, startled gasping, awakening, and then dropping off to sleep again.

appendicitis/appendectomy

Inflammation of the *vermiform appendix* (commonly called the "appendix"), which is a small structure attached to the blind end of the large intestine (the *cecum*). It is about the size and shape of an earthworm.

Symptoms of acute appendicitis can vary widely and the condition is often difficult to diagnose. In the most typical case, the first symptom is diffuse discomfort felt in the area of the navel (umbilicus) with nausea and perhaps vomiting. There may be constipation or mild diarrhea. The dis-

APPENDICITIS

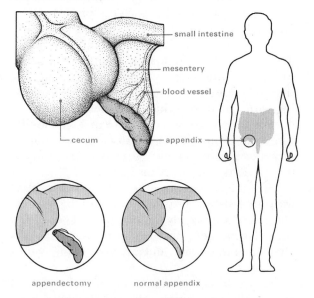

Appendicitis is the most common cause of acute abdominal pain and is a surgical emergency. In some unusual cases, accurate diagnosis may be impossible; a surgeon may then perform an appendectomy unnecessarily rather than risk leaving an inflamed appendix, which could lead to serious complications.

comfort turns into pain, and the pain settles in the lower right-hand part of the abdomen. The wall of the abdomen at first tightens when pressure is applied over the site of the pain ("guarding") and then in time becomes rigid. The temperature is usually only slightly raised.

Treatment is surgical removal of the appendix (*appendectomy*). If this can be carried out within the first twenty-four hours or so, convalescence is usually straightforward; but if the symptoms are not recognized, the appendix may become gangrenous and burst to produce PERITONITIS. Commonly this becomes localized, and an appendix abscess forms, which can be drained after it has been sealed off by natural processes.

The function of the appendix is unknown; it is usually considered a vestigial organ. The operation for its removal is usually relatively easy; surgeons are therefore inclined to perform an appendectomy in most cases where they suspect inflammation of the organ, or to remove it during the course of other scheduled abdominal surgery.

arrhythmias (dysrhythmias)

Abnormalities in the rhythm of the heartbeat, occurring in a healthy person or as a result of cardiac disease.

It can sometimes be felt as an "extra" beat of the heart ("extrasystole"), or it may only be detected by an electrocardiogram (EKG). Arrhythmia may be generated from any location in the heart. The seriousness of the arrhythmia is determined by its location, speed, and the underlying cardiac and medical condition.

In the otherwise healthy person, occasional irregular beats are of no significance; many people experience extra beats, when anxious or after too much coffee or too many cigarettes. However, irregularities of the heartbeat may indicate one of a wide range of heart diseases, including HEART FAILURE, MYOCARDITIS, CORONARY THROMBOSIS, sick sinus syndrome, heart block, and ATRIAL FIBRILLATION. For that reason, persons often are admitted to the hospital for full cardiovascular investigation.

Dysrhythmias may also occur in diseases such as thyroid overactivity (HYPERTHYROIDISM) or as a side effect of drug treatment. Sometimes the rhythm may be restored to normal by drugs or by pacemaker; often, however, the change in rhythm is no cause for concern and no treatment may be needed.

arteriosclerosis

An imprecise term, now falling into disuse, and usually replaced by the term ATHEROSCLEROSIS. It is descriptive of arteries that have become thick, inelastic, and hard. Popular name: *hardening of the arteries.*

It is doubtful that arteriosclerosis ever occurs without some degree of atheroma (fatty patches on the lining of the arteries), so the term ATHEROSCLEROSIS is preferred.

arteritis

Inflammation of an artery.

In *temporal arteritis*, a serious illness that affects elderly persons, the arteries overlying the temples become swollen and painful. If the inflammation extends to the arteries supplying blood to the eyes it may cause sudden and permanent blindness. In most cases, urgent treatment with large doses of corticosteroids suppresses the inflammation and can save the vision.

Other forms of arteritis affect blood vessels in all parts of the body. These include systemic LUPUS ERYTHEMATOSUS, POLYARTERITIS NODOSA, and a number of less well-defined disorders such as POLYMYALGIA RHEUMATICA. The importance of the occurrence of arteritis in these disorders lies in the damage to the organs or muscles supplied by the affected artery or arteries.

arthritis

Joints may be affected by inflammatory or degenerative changes, which cause pain and stiffness described as arthritis. Over one hundred separate conditions can cause arthritis, and these include infection after injury, the onset of age, rheumatic fever, rheumatoid processes which are poorly understood, gout, osteoarthritis, psoriasis, tumors, and diseases of the nervous system.

Injury impairs the efficiency of a joint by damaging the smooth articular surface. *Age* wears out the joint surface, particularly in the joints which have borne the weight of the body for many years—the hips and knees. *Gout* causes the deposition of crystals of uric acid in the joints. *Tumors* derange the anatomy of the joint. *Deficiency in nervous supply* can lead to insensitivity of the joint or abnormality of muscular action; this may

ARTHRITIS

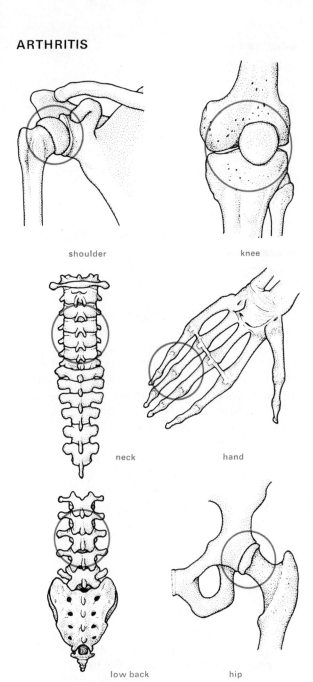

shoulder   knee

neck   hand

low back   hip

The joints most commonly associated with arthritis are painful knee, stiff fingers, and painful hip.

cause bizarre movements or repeated unnoticed injuries which produce mechanical derangement of the joint.

The most common disease affecting joints is OSTEOARTHRITIS, a wearing-out disorder that eventually affects almost all persons. RHEUMATOID ARTHRITIS, the cause of which is unknown, attacks women three times more frequently than men and occurs in at least 3 percent of the population of the United States. The lubricating lining of the joints (*synovial membrane*) suffers chronic inflammatory changes with consequent irreversible damage to the joint capsules and cartilage and formation of scar tissue. Pain, swelling, and deformity of the joints ensue, particularly obvious in the hands, and movement is limited.

Cases of arthritis are differentiated and diagnosed with the help of blood tests and X-ray studies. Treatment depends on the cause; there are specific drugs to treat GOUT, and antibiotics will be used in cases of infection. Anti-inflammatory drugs and aspirin (or similar pain-killers) are of help in cases of rheumatoid arthritis and degenerative arthritis in the elderly, but most of these drugs have the drawback that they tend to irritate the lining of the stomach and must therefore be used with discretion. For many patients with rheumatoid arthritis, the injection of gold salts has been found to be effective in suppressing the disease in its early stages. However, gold has many toxic side effects. The surgical replacement of weight-bearing joints—hips in particular—has proved possible, and such operations relieve pain and restore movement. Steroids (cortisone derivatives) and many other drugs are valuable in arthritis. In nearly all cases physical therapy is invaluable.

Much research is currently in progress on these common and crippling conditions, and the patient suffering from arthritis has a much better prognosis today than in former years.

asbestosis

A life-long lung disease caused by breathing in asbestos fibers over a period of time. Such fibers cause the delicate lung tissue to become scar tissue, and the ease by which oxygen passes through the lungs into the blood is hindered. The person with asbestosis becomes breathless, coughs, loses weight, feels tired, and loses appetite. There is no specific treatment.

A common complication is lung cancer. It is extremely important that persons who work around asbestos not smoke, since smoking increases their risk of lung cancer from sixty- to ninety-fold over that of nonexposed nonsmokers.

Occupations that carry the greatest risk for developing asbestosis are asbestos miners and end-product users such as insulators, textile workers, construction and shipyard workers, and repairers of brake linings and clutches.

It must be stressed that asbestos-containing materials pose no health hazard if they are intact, and they are best left undisturbed.

ascites

The accumulation of fluid, mostly water, in the abdominal cavity. As the fluid collects, the abdomen swells and becomes uncomfortable; to relieve the swelling a needle can be passed through the abdominal wall to draw off the fluid.

Ascites occurs in a number of diseases, including heart failure, abdominal cancer, and some disorders of the liver and kidneys. Treatment is directed toward the underlying condition.

aspergillosis

Disease caused by the fungus *Aspergillus fumigatus*. This microorganism is found almost everywhere and does not normally cause disease in humans; indeed, it often flourishes in the mouths of healthy people. It does, however, sometimes cause disease in birds and occasionally in people who have had intensive antibiotic or antifungal treatment, or who are immuno-suppressed. It can infect the lungs and sometimes the ear or the paranasal sinuses, which drain into the nasal cavities. Infection of the lung produces cough (which may be productive of blood) and fever; parts of the fungus may break off to set up infection in the heart, brain, kidneys, or spleen (carried to these sites in the bloodstream). Sometimes a person with aspergillosis develops ASTHMA.

Treatment involves the administration of intravenous amphotericin B. Except in cases where the infection is widely disseminated, the outlook for improvement is good.

asphyxia

Lack of oxygen in the blood due to the cessation of breathing or to an obstruction preventing entry of air into the lungs. Low oxygen content in the blood leads to loss of consciousness, brain damage, and—if not corrected—death. Common causes of asphyxia are drowning, electric shock, and obstruction of the breathing passages.

asthma

Air drawn into the lungs during breathing is conveyed to the small air sacs (alveoli) in the lungs. It is there that the exchange of oxygen and carbon dioxide (between the inspired air and the blood) takes place. To reach the alveoli, the inspired air must pass through a "tree" of air passages of ever-decreasing diameter (the *bronchi* and the *bronchioles*).

While the larger bronchi are of fixed diameter (their walls contain rigid rings of cartilage which permit no change in their "bore"), the smaller bronchioles have muscular walls and are capable of wide variation in their bore with contraction or relaxation of the muscle coat.

Changes in the bore of the bronchi are usually slight and occur in response to exercise or the secretion into the blood of certain chemically active compounds (hormones). In patients with asthma, however, the bronchioles are sensitive to stimulation by a variety of agents which produce marked contraction of the muscular wall, with narrowing of the bore to a degree that seriously obstructs the entry and exit of air in the lungs.

In an attack of asthma the breathing becomes difficult, expiration often being more affected than inspiration. The patient is short of breath and breathing may become audibly "wheezy," with coughing. The effort to draw breath increases, but despite this the movement of the chest is diminished. The patient may become agitated or confused and his skin color may take on a bluish tinge from insufficient oxygen (CYANOSIS). The attack may be short, lasting only a few minutes, or very long and the patient may become exhausted by his efforts to obtain air.

There are numerous causes of the contraction of the muscular coat of the bronchioles. In some cases a frank allergy exists to a particular material; the patient responds to this by the onset of an attack of asthma, usually within minutes of exposure. Grass and tree pollens, molds and fungi, animal hair and dander, the minute "house-dust mite" (found in all areas of human habitation), and even some types of food may all provoke an asthmatic attack. In other cases a physical or chemical irritant (such as a smoky atmosphere, exhaust fumes, or acid fumes) may bring on an attack. Infections of the lungs, particularly those caused by viruses, may precipitate an attack in susceptible subjects. Prolonged exertion may also provoke an attack, as may a variety of emotional factors (such as stress, tension, or anxiety).

Treatment involves, first, identification and avoidance of the factor that precipitates attacks. Treatment of an acute asthmatic attack involves the administration of drugs such as epinephrine or related compounds that cause relaxation of the contracted bronchioles. In most cases an impending attack can be controlled with the use of one of the new surface-active inhaled steroids. These may be given by a nebulizing inhaler or a pressurized aerosol, both of which produce a fine mist of droplets that are inhaled directly into the affected bronchioles. Dosage must be restricted cautiously or the possibility of a dangerous overdosage may occur. Administration of oxygen may be required in some attacks.

For long-term treatment, drugs may be given by mouth on a regular daily basis. The prognosis is usually good, although very severe untreated cases can be life-threatening. When the condition first occurs in early childhood, there may be a tendency to "grow out of it," but in adults the condition tends to recur.

astigmatism

A common condition of the eye in which the curve of the cornea is increased along one meridian, causing the image seen to be out of focus. To correct this problem eyeglasses or contact lenses are prescribed.

See also VISION.

ASTIGMATISM

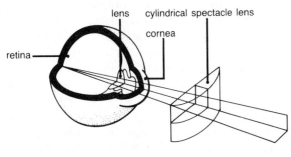

section of eye

An astigmatism is the incorrect curvature of the cornea or lens of the eye, with the result that the image reaching the retina is not correctly focused and appears blurred or distorted. The defect can be corrected by placing a cylindrical lens in front of the eye, thereby focusing the image on the retina.

ataxia

The inability to coordinate movements, especially purposeful movement. Muscular action is impaired, causing unsteady, clumsy movement.

In general, ataxia is caused by lesions within the central nervous system (the brain and spinal cord). Sometimes, the incoordination of voluntary muscular movement results in speech disturbances so that words are slurred and produced slowly.

atelectasis

Incomplete expansion or collapse of a lung or part of a lung. Atelectasis prevents the normal exchange of carbon dioxide and oxygen in the blood. This condition may be congenital or caused by obstruction of the airway by mucus, a tumor, or an inhaled foreign body, such as a tooth. Signs include severe breathlessness, collapse, CYANOSIS, pain, fever, and shock.

atherosclerosis

Atherosclerosis is the number-one killer of the western world. It is the condition underlying myocardial infarction ("heart attack") and STROKE. The smooth internal lining of the arteries develops yellowish fatty patches (atheromas) that narrow the caliber of the vessels. These patches *(plaques)* are often a focus for THROMBOSIS, further narrowing the arterial bore and eventually blocking the vessel completely.

Family history is an important factor in the development of atherosclerosis, but the main established risk factors are excessive consumption of animal fats, high blood pressure (hypertension), cigarette smoking, lack of physical exercise, and psychological stress.

There is no effective treatment for established atherosclerosis, and attention should be directed to limiting its progress by reduction of raised blood pressure and weight loss; a low intake of animal fat is generally advised in an attempt to lower blood levels of fat (lipids, that is, cholesterol and triglycerides). Exercise should be increased and stress reduced. Surgical procedures to overcome failing blood supply in certain specific sites may be helpful (for example, coronary angioplasty and coronary-artery bypass).

ATHEROSCLEROSIS

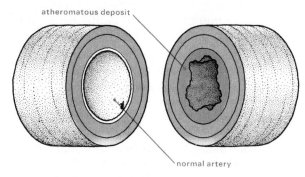

atheromatous deposit

normal artery

Cross sections of a normal artery (left) and one in which atherosclerosis has formed. Atheroma is a fatty deposit of cholesterol and degenerate muscle cells that forms in the inner layer of the wall, narrowing the artery and reducing blood flow.

athetosis

A disorder of the nervous system marked by slow, writhing, continuous, and involuntary movement of the arms, legs, and facial muscles. It is seen in some forms of brain disorders such as *Huntington's chorea* and is caused by dopamine overactivity in the basal ganglia of the brain.

The writhing movements are aggravated by emotion and voluntary action so that they interfere with speech, eating, and other daily activities. Occasionally, athetosis may develop in adult life as a symptom of tumors or infections affecting the basal ganglia.

There is no specific treatment, but drugs such as the diazepams (Valium) may help. Physical training is sometimes of value.

athlete's foot

A fungus infection of the foot, also known as *ringworm of the foot* or *tinea pedis*. See TINEA.

atresia

The abnormal closure or absence of a natural opening in the body due to disease or congenital defect. Among the sites where atresia can occur are the vagina, anus, and internal organs such as the small bowel, heart, and esophagus tube ("gullet"), which leads from the mouth to the stomach. Surgery is the only correction for this condition, and in life-threatening congenital atresia it must be done within the first days of life. For example, in congenital esophageal atresia, where the esophagus does not connect as it should to the stomach, surgery must be done to prevent the newborn from starving.

atrial fibrillation

A consequence of ischemic hypertension (coronary artery disease) and RHEUMATIC HEART DISEASE in which the normally coordinated action of the atria (the upper chambers of the heart) becomes irregular.

The state of atrial fibrillation is quite compatible with life, unlike the state of VENTRICULAR FIBRILLATION; but clots are liable to form in the atria and break off as emboli, hence treatment with anticoagulants ("blood thinners"). The person in atrial fibrillation may become breathless and may develop signs of HEART FAILURE.

Treatment includes the administration of digitalis or other agents (beta-blockers, calcium channel blocking agents) to slow down the ventricular rate of contraction, and possibly the administration of quinidine (or similar agents) to stop the irregular contraction. Defibrillation may be effective in restoring normal heart rhythm in early cases. Anticoagulants may be used for three weeks before restoring normal rhythm.

atrophy

Although literally meaning "lack of nourishment," atrophy has come to mean the wasting away of a body part—most particularly muscles—as a result of disease, inactivity, or interference with blood or nerve supply.

Australia antigen

Hepatitis B surface antigen. It is known to be a "marker" for the presence of the virus causing one type of HEPATITIS (inflammation of the liver). The substance involved probably represents the virus itself and testing for it has become a valuable diagnostic aid; it is also used as one type of screening test before the transfusion of whole blood and other blood products.

autism

A psychosis in children of unknown cause; perhaps related to the adult SCHIZOPHRENIA, from which it differs in a number of respects.

The earliest signs are an indifference to parents and others who try to show affection and care for the child. The baby may not respond to being picked up and nursed and may show ritualistic, repetitive play, even banging his head. He may rock to and fro. Although the child looks healthy and normal, feeding and toilet training become increasingly difficult and ineffective. The child learns to walk, but speaks late or stays mute. If he begins to speak, the words may be inappropriate, repeated, and apparently spoken without meaning. He uses personal pronouns wrongly or not at all, and echoes words or phrases spoken to him.

Autistic children show extreme variability in their intellectual functions. Often they are untestable and if tested their IQ scores usually are well below normal. They are upset by changes in their surroundings—for example, the rearrangement of furniture. They may be particularly fascinated by moving objects and musical sounds. In general, autistic children seem to behave as though they were alone in the world; they cannot perceive others as people, regarding them instead as inanimate objects.

Children may be affected to varying degrees. Some grow up with minimal signs of the illness yet they continue to be socially awkward and inept. Two thirds of autistic children remain severely handicapped as adults.

These children need special training programs to enhance their intact abilities. This disorder is rare and is three times more common in boys than in girls.

autoimmune disease

Many chronic, noninfectious diseases are due to a misdirection of the immune mechanisms, which ordinarily protect the body against infections with bacteria and other microorganisms. Typically, antibodies are formed against vital structures such as the lining of the heart valves or the filtration units (glomeruli) in the kidneys, and the chronic inflammation that results causes fibrosis, scarring, and eventually failure of the organ concerned.

The body deals with microorganisms in two main ways: white blood cells engulf bacteria, destroying and digesting them, and the lymphocytes and other immune cells form antibodies—protein molecules tailored to fit the organism or its toxin and so neutralize it. Both mechanisms come into play in autoimmune diseases, although cellular infiltration is often less prominent than antibody formation. In some cases the misdirection of the immune system operates by the production of severely damaging bodies known as "immune complexes." These are combinations of antigens and antibodies that stick together and circulate in the bloodstream. Substances formed from such combinations attach themselves to various parts of the body causing harm.

However, no such infection seems to be involved in other autoimmune diseases in which antibodies are formed against structures in the liver (causing biliary CIRRHOSIS), the thyroid (causing Hashimoto's disease, or autoimmune THYROIDITIS), the stomach (causing impairment of absorption of vitamin B_{12}, or pernicious ANEMIA), and the joints (causing RHEUMATOID ARTHRITIS). What these diseases have in common is their chronic course, often marked by episodes in which the symptoms improve or become worse for no obvious reason. Treatment with corticosteroid drugs is often effective in damping down symptoms, and immunosuppressive drugs may also be useful, since they slow the formation of antibodies. More specific treatment will have to await a better understanding of the primary disease process in these disorders.

See also ANTIGEN/ANTIBODY.

azoospermia

The lack of living sperm in a given sample of semen.

Azoospermia may be caused by disease, hormonal imbalance, dysfunction of the testicles, or blockage of the tubes in which sperm are stored (epididymis). It may be caused purposely by means of a vasectomy.

backache

Pain in the back may be caused by muscular strain or a "slipped" intervertebral disk, or it may be associated with some disease of the bones and joints of the spinal column.

The twenty-four vertebrae that make up the

spinal column (seven cervical, twelve thoracic, and five lumbar) extend from the base of the skull to the sacrum, the triangular "centerpiece" of the pelvis. The vertebrae are separated by pads of tough, elastic cartilage—the intervertebral disks—which give the spine its flexibility and also act as shock absorbers. The bones are also bound together by strong ligaments and by several groups of powerful muscles that run mainly in two bands on either side of the backbone. The spine acts as the central girder of the skeleton; it also provides a protective tunnel for the spinal cord (which reaches from the brain down to the level of the second lumbar vertebra) and the nerves that branch from it.

Most commonly, backache is caused by strain of the muscles around the lower part of the spine. This may be due to unaccustomed exercise—a weekend spent shoveling snow, for example—or to sitting for prolonged periods in an incorrect posture. Strain on the spine is least when the back is straight; a chair that forces the spine into a curve is likely to provoke chronic back strain.

A separate, acutely painful type of backache also originating in the muscles is LUMBAGO. Here the pain often is localized to one extremely painful spot in the muscles, usually in the lower lumbar region and slightly to one side of the midline. Lumbago is often experienced after a combination of unaccustomed exercise and cold—digging the garden in spring, for example—and may be severe enough for the victim to be unable to move out of bed. The cause is believed to be spasm of a group of muscle fibers. Even with no treatment other than rest and simple pain-relieving drugs, such as aspirin, the condition resolves within a few days; in some cases recovery may be hastened by injection of a mixture of a local anesthetic and a steroid drug into the "trigger spot."

The second common cause of sudden severe backache is damage to one of the intervertebral disks in the lumbar region of the spine. Damage is most likely to occur when the person is lifting a heavy weight while his back is curved. Pressure on the disk, which consists of a tough capsule with a soft, elastic center, may rupture the capsule and allow part of the central nucleus to protrude. If this protrusion extends into the spinal canal it may press on one of the spinal nerves or even on the spinal cord. Typically, this pressure causes pain extending down the main sciatic nerve, which runs from the buttocks to the foot. The pain (SCIATICA) is made worse by coughing, straining, or bending the back. If the symptoms persist there may also be loss of feeling in the foot or lower part of the leg and some muscular weakness.

The basic treatment of prolapsed disk (or "slipped disk") is rest, with the person lying flat on his back in bed. Rest for two weeks, sometimes more, often allows the disk to reabsorb the protrusion and the damaged capsule to heal. If the symptoms from pressure on the spinal nerves are severe, or if they do not resolve with simple rest, TRACTION may be added: Weights are attached to the legs to lengthen the spine, thus pulling the vertebrae apart and promoting return of the disk to its normal condition. The most radical treatment, which may be necessary if the prolapse does not heal or in cases of recurrent prolapse, is surgical excision of the damaged portion of the disk.

Unfortunately, anyone who has suffered a prolapsed disk is at risk of recurrence; once the acute symptoms have settled, some program of preventive treatment is important. This will include exercises to strengthen the muscles that support the spine and instruction on posture and the safe, correct way to lift weights, tie one's shoes, and perform other simple daily activities. Sometimes a physician may advise the wearing of a protective and supporting corset.

The third common cause of sudden backache is a minor displacement of one vertebra relative to its neighbors. Just how frequently this problem occurs is a matter of dispute within the medical profession. Some physicians (and all osteopaths and chiropractors) believe that most episodes of backache can be relieved by manipulation of the spine, thus encouraging the bones to return to their normal alignment. Without a doubt, spinal manipulation often does relieve symptoms, but reliance on this method can be dangerous if the pain is due to one of the rarer causes of backache, such as a tumor or an infection such as tuberculosis.

Chronic backache may be caused also by arthritis of the spinal joints. ANKYLOSING SPONDYLITIS is a severe form of spinal arthritis, especially common in young men and related to RHEUMATOID ARTHRITIS, which may also affect the spine; both diseases cause progressive pain and stiffness of the spine. The common degenerative OSTEOARTHRITIS also affects the spine; most people over the age of 50 have some stiffness of the back from minor arthritic changes. No specific treatment is needed for this form of arthritis unless symptoms develop.

Among the many other causes of backache are infections (TUBERCULOSIS was especially common in the last century and is still a major problem in developing countries), tumors of the bones and of the spinal cord and nerves, and the metastasis (spread) of cancer cells to the spine. For that reason, full investigation—including X-ray studies of the spine and blood tests—is needed before treatment is given in any case in which the cause of the pain is not obvious.

Most episodes of backache are preventable: With correct posture, care in lifting weights, and regular exercise to maintain muscle tone, the joints in the back should remain as trouble-free as those elsewhere in the body.

bacteria

Living one-celled organisms, smaller than yeasts but larger than viruses, found all over the surface of the globe in the air, soil, and water. Many live on or within larger living organisms, including man; some produce disease and are termed *pathogenic*, but not all are harmful. Some are actively useful—for example, the bacteria that produce nitrogen in the soil for plant growth.

Bacteria may be classified by their shape: round (*cocci*), straight rods (*bacilli*), curved (*vibrios*), and wavy (*spirilla*). Most are unable to move, but a few are motile by virtue of their flagellae (tails). The cocci are very often found in typical groups: *staphylococci* in bunches like grapes, *streptococci* in chain formation, and *diplococci* in pairs. Given the right circumstances, all bacteria can multiply very quickly, some doubling their numbers every half hour. In an unfavorable environment most die, but some can form spores—thick-walled cells resistant to heat and drying out (desiccation)—which lie dormant until conditions become favorable again.

Pathogenic bacteria cause disease in two basic ways. They may gain access to the tissues and there multiply to damage their surroundings, or they may release substances called *toxins*, which poison remote parts of the body. *Endotoxins* are contained inside the bacteria to be released when they die, and *exotoxins* are produced by living bacteria. Usually the signs and symptoms of disease are produced by exotoxins—for example, in TETANUS, where the living bacteria multiply in a dirty wound and produce an exotoxin that damages the nervous system.

Dangerous organisms are transmitted from person to person in several ways: by direct contact, by breathing air exhaled from diseased air pas-

BACTERIA

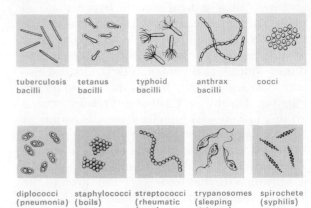

tuberculosis bacilli   tetanus bacilli   typhoid bacilli   anthrax bacilli   cocci

diplococci (pneumonia)   staphylococci (boils)   streptococci (rheumatic fever)   trypanosomes (sleeping sickness)   spirochete (syphilis)

Bacteria are single-cell microorganisms, classified according to their shapes into bacilli, cocci, spirilla, and vibrios. Most are harmless—indeed, many types are beneficial to use—but certain types of bacteria are responsible for infectious diseases that were notorious killers before antibiotics were discovered.

sages, by contact with contaminated excreta, and by insects. In most cases the body is able to deal with harmful bacteria, but if they gain a foothold and produce disease the defensive processes of inflammation and antibody formation can be aided by the use of drugs designed to kill pathogenic organisms or prevent their multiplication. These drugs, antibiotics, are called *bactericidal* if they kill bacteria and *bacteriostatic* if they inhibit their multiplication.

Antibiotics must not be used indiscriminately, since continued exposure of bacteria to a particular antibiotic may result in the development of resistant strains of the bacteria.

Methods of controlling bacteria in the environment include the use of chemical disinfectants, the application of heat (as dry heat or steam), and irradiation.

Baker's cyst

A painless soft cyst at the back of the knee, commonly occurring when the knee joint is damaged by OSTEOARTHRITIS; named after William Morrant Baker (1839–1896), a British surgeon.

In this condition, the synovium (joint lining) produces an excessive amount of joint fluid, which escapes from the joint either by rupturing through the synovium or by pushing the synovium out ahead of it.

The size of the cyst may be reduced by drawing out the fluid with a needle and syringe, and then injecting hydrocortisone (a drug that reduces inflammation) into the affected area. Alternatively, the whole cyst may be removed surgically.

balanitis

Inflammation of the penis.

In infancy the condition is usually of the type called *ammoniacal* balanitis. In such cases the inflammation is due to irritation caused by ammonia produced by the action of bacteria on the urine. Usually it can be prevented by promptly changing wet diapers.

When balanitis occurs in older children and adults, it may be related to sugar in the urine and it may therefore be a warning sign of DIABETES MELLITUS. Other possible causes in adults are an underlying syphilitic sore (chancre) or cancer of the penis.

See also SYPHILIS.

baldness (alopecia)

The loss of hair on the head.

Hair grows from the base (bulb) of hair follicles, tiny tube-like structures in the skin. Although some hair is constantly being shed (as an actively growing hair expels an older one from its follicle), baldness does not usually occur. Hair loss resulting in baldness may occur in disease or as a hereditary phenomenon in healthy individuals.

Skin infections that reach deep enough to affect the base of the hair follicles may cause temporary or permanent bald patches. Other skin diseases, burns, radiation injury, chemical injury, or any injury that causes scarring can lead to permanent bald patches. Some drugs cause an increased rate of shedding of the hair. Chemotherapy (the use of drugs to control cancer) can also cause temporary or permanent hair loss.

Increased shedding may also accompany several illnesses such as prolonged fevers, certain cancers, uncontrolled DIABETES MELLITUS, and diseases of the thyroid, pituitary, and adrenal glands. There is no special treatment for this type of baldness, which is often reversed as the underlying disease is treated.

Some women experience a temporarily increased rate of hair loss after pregnancy.

PATTERNS OF BALDNESS

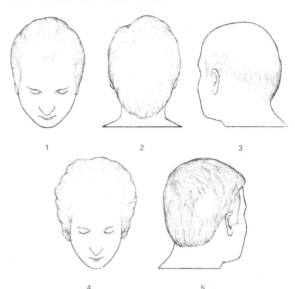

Male-pattern baldness is an inherited condition that usually starts in middle age around the temples (1) and the crown (2). In severe cases only a rim of hair remains around the back of the head (3). Baldness in women is uncommon but sometimes occurs after pregnancy (4). Patchy loss of hair (5) can result either from a skin infection (for example, ringworm of the scalp) or as alopecia areata (see text).

By far the most common type of baldness is *male-pattern baldness*, which starts around the temples and spreads to the crown, leaving behind a rim of hair at the sides and back. As in other types of baldness, the bald areas are seldom completely hairless but are covered with a downy type of hair that is barely perceptible.

The tendency to male-pattern baldness is hereditary and nothing can prevent it. It usually occurs in middle age, although it may start as early as the late teens. It is irreversible and no successful form of treatment exists. In selected cases, however, a course of hair transplantation may improve appearance. Also, the recently available drug minoxidil (for external use) effectively encourages hair growth in previously bald men. However, preliminary reports seem to suggest that it is most effective in men who have been balding for less than a year.

Hair loss of the male-pattern type may also occur in women, but usually results in severe thinning rather than actual baldness.

One type of baldness that can be very upsetting is *alopecia areata*, a patchy baldness that comes on suddenly. The patch may increase in size or new bald areas may form on the scalp, in the eyebrows, or in the beard region. Occasionally there is extensive loss of hair on both scalp and body.

The cause of alopecia areata is not known. Recovery usually occurs without treatment, especially if only a few areas are affected.

Bartholin cyst

The two Bartholin glands, each about the size of a hazelnut, are mucus-secreting glands lying toward the back of the labia majora. They have openings on the inner surfaces of the labia minora, near the vaginal orifice, and become active during sexual excitement, providing a clear, odorless lubricant that facilitates intercourse.

Infection of a Bartholin gland duct is quite common and may lead to blockage. The result is an accumulation of mucus in the gland, which becomes enlarged so that an obvious swelling of the labium occurs. So long as the cyst remains uninfected, the condition remains painless and is no more than a minor inconvenience. Infection, however, leads to abscess formation with pain, redness, great tenderness, and a swelling that may be as large as a hen's egg.

Once an abscess has formed, antibiotics are of little value, and surgical drainage is likely to be necessary. This is a minor operation, usually performed under a brief general anesthetic. In most cases, a drain will be left in place for a few days after the operation.

basal cell carcinoma

One of the most common of all cancers, the basal cell carcinoma, or *rodent ulcer*, mainly occurs on skin that has been exposed to the sun. It is frequently found on the face, often near the angle of the eye or on the nose. It is most common in people who have lived for many years in areas of high sunlight intensity; in some areas, almost half the population has had at least one basal cell carcinoma by the age of 65.

Fortunately, basal cell carcinoma is also the least malignant of all cancers and only very rarely spreads to remote parts of the body. It does, however, gradually spread locally in the skin and, if untreated, tends to penetrate deeply, involving the underlying tissues, such as the bones of the

skull, or even the eye or brain. Only in cases of gross neglect will the condition cause death.

A basal cell carcinoma starts as a small, firm, shiny nodule that slowly enlarges until, after a few months, it develops a circular, raised border bearing small blood vessels. The center of the tumor is dimpled and often crusted. At this stage, cure is easy, and such growing nodules should never be neglected. Examination of a tissue specimen or *biopsy* (see under **Tests**) by a pathologist is mandatory and will positively confirm or exclude the diagnosis.

In many cases the biopsy will consist of the whole tumor, and that will be the end of the matter; but if only a small piece is taken, and the report is positive, further surgical removal will be necessary. The results of treatment are excellent.

battered-child syndrome

A condition in which young children, usually under the age of 3 years, are deliberately injured (often repeatedly) by someone in a position of authority such as a parent or guardian.

The violence occurs on the most trivial provocation and is totally inexcusable. It results in bruising, fractures, injury to internal organs, burns, and even death. Besides being physically injured, the child may be deprived of food, care, and affection, but abuse can occur also in children who are otherwise well cared for.

It has been said that every parent is a potential child abuser; but no matter how exasperating a child's behavior may be, fortunately most parents do not resort to violence.

Child abusers come from all social classes and all levels of intelligence; some may be difficult to detect because they appear concerned over the child's injuries and extremely willing to cooperate with the doctor in every way. There are certain signs that suggest child abuse, however. There may be a few hours' delay before the child is brought to a doctor. The explanation given is that the child had an accident—she fell down the stairs or he bumped into a crib or table—but examination reveals injuries incompatible with the history and may also reveal past injuries. Often there are similar injuries on opposite sides of the body, such as bruises on both legs or on both sides of the neck. The parent may try to explain away bruising by saying that the child bleeds easily.

Many social stressors contribute to the child-abuse syndrome. Social, financial, and emotional problems within the family may contribute to parental stress. Unemployment, multiple pregnancies (the abused child is often an unwanted or unplanned child), and the need to give special care to the child are predisposing factors.

Often, someone was abused as a child will repeat the abuse pattern toward his or her own child. Many abusers are in their 20s. In some cases the father is unemployed or may have a criminal record, and the mother may be in the premenstrual period. Although generally one parent is the abuser, the other usually is aware that the battering is going on. There is no evidence of severe emotional disturbance in all child abusers.

Intervention is aimed at parents of young children, as well as at the child, in order to break the cycle of abuse. Otherwise, in more than half the cases, the child will be injured again.

BCG (bacillus Calmette-Guérin)

A vaccine used in the control of tuberculosis.

The vaccine was developed by two French bacteriologists, Albert Léon Charles Calmette (1863–1933) and Camille Guérin (1872–1961). Their work began in 1906, with a painstaking series of culturing and subculturing of the causative organism of tuberculosis (the tubercle bacillus) until a stable and safe form of vaccine was achieved. The vaccine was first used in the prevention of tuberculosis in 1921 (in a newborn baby whose mother had died of the disease). Culturing the organism in a succession of artificial media removes its virulence, so that while the vaccine can confer immunity or partial immunity against tuberculosis it does not produce the disease in the person vaccinated.

BCG both reduces the incidence of tuberculosis and results in a less progressive form of the disease when it does occur. It is given to persons in high-risk groups and to those in areas of widespread tuberculosis infection.

BCG is now being used experimentally to assist in the treatment of CANCER. The rationale behind this is that the vaccine stimulates the production of antibodies, which are thought to increase the body's general defense system. These antibodies may attack cancer cells and destroy them in the same way they destroy the tubercule bacilli. BCG has proved somewhat effective in the treatment of LEUKEMIA and malignant MELANOMA.

bedsores

Also known as *pressure sores* or *decubiti.* Bedsores are caused by lying or sitting immobile for long periods of time.

The skin and its underlying tissues receive nourishment from very small blood vessels. If these blood vessels are compressed for a long time, as the person lies in bed without moving, the skin is deprived of its nutrition and cells start to die (*necrosis*). Continuing pressure is likely to cause a large area of tissue destruction, and ulcerations in the skin will occur.

Healthy people do not get bedsores because they can move around during sleep and change positions when the pressure area becomes uncomfortable. Pressure sores can develop, however, if a person is unconscious or unable to feel pressure, as sometimes happens in STROKE. Skin can break down after only a few hours of immobility.

The major areas prone to bedsores are the lower spine, the hips, heels, elbows, and shoulders. Very thin persons and obese persons are the most likely candidates for bedsores, but the sores can occur in anyone.

Bedsores begin as a reddening of the skin, which later assumes a bluish tinge. Once an ulcer actually occurs, healing is very difficult. Infection can set in and cause the ulcer to extend into the underlying bone.

Although there are topical medications and therapy for bedsores, the primary treatment is prevention. People who are unable to move themselves need to be repositioned every two to three hours. Regular massages assist the flow of circulation, and a skin-toughening agent, applied to the areas under pressure, will help to prevent tissue breakdown.

bed-wetting (enuresis)

Involuntary urination during sleep. There is no precise age at which bed-wetting becomes abnormal. Most children are dry at night by the age of 2 or 3 years, but others not until age 5 or 7.

Even after good control is achieved, occasional bed-wetting may occur up to the age of 9 or 10, or even older. These lapses of nighttime control usually are associated with fatigue or emotional upset and should not be a cause for concern.

Most cases of bed-wetting persist from infancy, although sometimes regular bed-wetting starts only after a period of good control. There is usually a family pattern for the age at which control is achieved. As a rule, bed-wetting does not require investigation until after the age of 3 or 4.

In rare cases, bed-wetting is associated with some medical condition, such as nocturnal epilepsy, spinal cord disorder, urinary tract disorder, uncontrolled DIABETES MELLITUS, or diabetes insipidus. But in most cases it is considered a temporary emotional or psychological disorder.

The most common cause of persistent bed-wetting extending from infancy is an overvigorous and premature attempt at toilet training. In general, voluntary daytime control does not occur before 15 to 18 months.

Treatment is essentially based on encouragement. Shaming, nagging, scolding, or punishing the child should be avoided, as this may only aggravate the problem. The parents' attitude is extremely important. They should not be overanxious about the bed-wetting and should not make an undue fuss when carrying out measures aimed at preventing it.

These measures include restricting fluids for about two hours before bedtime and waking the child up to urinate. Drugs are of doubtful value, but special devices that ring a bell and awaken the child who starts to urinate in bed may be helpful.

Bell's palsy

A paralysis of the nerve supplying the muscles on one side of the face. This causes a lopsided appearance of the face. Although Bell's palsy refers to cases of unknown cause, inflammation of the nerve is suspected.

Bell's palsy is distinguished from other types of facial paralysis by its sudden onset and usually complete recovery. Characteristics of this condition are onset within two days, slackness of muscles, drooping corner of mouth, and inability to close the eye on one side of the face. Occasionally the faculties of taste, speech, and hearing are affected.

Treatment of this condition is mostly supportive. It includes massaging the affected side, splinting to prevent drooping of low facial muscles, and protecting the eye so that it does not dry out while the eyelid is unable to close.

Recovery usually occurs spontaneously and 80 percent of patients recover completely within a few weeks or months. In some cases, especially when the paralysis persists for a long time, recovery may be partial or absent. In these instances, plastic surgery may be required.

bends

Decompression sickness is a painful, sometimes deadly condition caused by nitrogen bubbles that form in body tissue when a person moves too rapidly from an area of high pressure to an area of low pressure, such as when a scuba diver moves up to the surface too quickly. Permanent neurologic defects, even total paralysis, can result from nitrogen bubbles expanding in the spinal cord. Urgent recompression is needed. If necessary, the subject should be flown by helicopter to a recompression facility.

beriberi

A disease caused by the dietary deficiency of vitamin B_1 (thiamine). This deficiency is usually the result of a diet limited to polished white rice and is common in Eastern and Southeastern Asia. Symptoms include fatigue, constipation, appetite and weight loss, water retention, and disturbed nerve function of the arms and legs, which eventually causes paralysis.

berylliosis

A disease caused by inhalation of the fumes or dust of beryllium, which is a white metallic element. In the past, beryllium was used with other substances to coat the inner lining of fluorescent bulbs. It is still widely used for its hardening properties in ceramics and as an alloy with other metals.

Acute beryllium poisoning causes symptoms resembling bronchitis or pneumonia. The disease can be fatal but most cases are relatively mild and persons recover within one to six months.

Chronic berylliosis adversely affects the lungs and occurs from months to years after exposure. In addition to causing lung damage, the disease can affect the heart and threaten life. The chronic form of the disease is characterized by formation of small masses, or nodules, in the lungs. Medications are used in treatment; supportive measures to aid with decreased lung functioning may also be needed.

The use of beryllium to make fluorescent materials was discontinued in the 1950s. Today, owing to stringent Government controls, beryllium exposure is uncommon, even in the factory environment.

bird breeder's lung

An allergy to substances contained in the droppings of birds. The allergy results in *hypersensitivity pneumonitis*, a lung disease characterized by fever, chills, tightness of the chest, shortness of breath, and cough. It usually occurs a few hours after exposure and needs to be distinguished from asthma by an experienced doctor. Only about 10 percent of persons with this condition will also have asthma.

The disease occurs when inhaled particles reach the alveoli of the lungs, the areas where oxygen exchange occurs. Persons with ongoing exposure develop a chronic form of hypersensitivity pneumonitis that can result in irreversible lung damage.

Primary treatment is avoidance of further exposure. In situations where this is impossible, the person must wear a dust filter over the nose and mouth. Corticosteroid medications are very helpful in relieving symptoms and lung changes if they are started before irreversible lung damage has occurred.

birth injury

Damage to a baby at birth whether avoidable or unavoidable. Birth injuries may be due either to the trauma of delivery (*mechanical* injuries) or to a lack of oxygen at birth (*anoxia*).

Premature babies and those who lie in awkward positions in the uterus are most likely to suffer mechanical injuries, which include bruises, fractures, and nerve injuries.

The most common life-threatening birth injury is hemorrhage into the brain. If the injury is severe, death may occur at birth or within a few days. Those who survive may recover fully, although they sometimes suffer permanent brain damage. It is often difficult to predict the effect the brain damage will have in later years.

The liver is another internal organ occasionally injured during birth. Injury may occur during delivery or as a result of external heart massage during attempts at resuscitation. The prognosis depends on the degree of injury.

Sufficient oxygen is essential because the brain can withstand only a few minutes of oxygen deprivation. Anoxia may result when the placental circulation has been inadequate during pregnancy, as in conditions such as PREECLAMPSIA (toxemia of pregnancy), multiple pregnancy, or hemorrhage before the onset of labor.

Anoxia may occur also when the baby fails to breathe spontaneously at birth. Failure of spontaneous breathing (APNEA) is more likely following some complication of pregnancy such as premature birth, multiple pregnancy, toxemia, or maternal DIABETES MELLITUS. When these complications are present, however, apnea can be anticipated and skilled staff and specialized equipment for resuscitation can be prepared.

Sometimes, however, apnea is totally unexpected. As with brain hemorrhage, it is often difficult to predict how much and what kind of permanent brain damage, if any, will result.

birthmark

A skin blemish present at birth. See NEVUS.

blackheads

Dried plugs of fatty material in the ducts of the sebaceous (oil-secreting) glands. Also known as *comedones*. The black color at the surface of the plugs is not dirt, as often believed; albinos (who lack the pigment melanin) have light-colored "blackheads."

The blackhead is produced by faulty functioning of the sebaceous follicle as it releases *sebum*, the fatty secretion of the sebaceous glands. The consequent obstruction to the gland leads to enlargement of the follicle's opening. Infection by bacteria living on the skin may lead to inflammation and so to the characteristic papules, or "pimples," of ACNE.

Blackheads should never be squeezed; this increases the risk of infection. Gentle bathing with warm water and soap should release most of them.

blackout

A temporary loss of vision or consciousness resulting from a lack of oxygen to the brain. See FAINTING.

bladder problems

Bladder problems can be separated into three types: those arising from infection within the bladder, those due to growths within the bladder, and those associated with loss of bladder control.

Inflammation of the bladder (CYSTITIS) is common and is most often due to bacterial infection. The symptoms of burning pain on urination and increased frequency of urination also may occur without any evidence of infection; this nonbacterial inflammation is especially common in women. Pregnancy and sexual intercourse both increase the likelihood of cystitis in women. Treatment includes the drinking of large quantities of fluids and the administration of appropriate antibacterial drugs. Women who develop symptoms of cystitis in association with sexual intercourse need to pay special attention to regular washing of the genital region.

The bladder is occasionally the site of a growth. The most common is a benign wart-like tumor (papilloma), but only a medical investigation can distinguish these from malignant tumors. In either case the first sign is blood in the urine, occasionally rather than constantly, without associated pain. Later the symptoms may resemble those of cystitis. Small bladder tumors can be removed through a tube passed into the bladder (cystoscope), but regular medical follow-up is needed to watch for any recurrence.

Urinary INCONTINENCE is involuntary urination; it may be caused by a defect in the nervous control of the bladder or by a mechanical problem. Children often have episodes of urinary incontinence, especially during sleep.

Stress incontinence—leakage of a few drops of urine during coughing or straining—is common in women and is most often due to damage in childbirth to the muscles around the neck of the bladder. Surgical repair may be necessary in such cases. (Pregnant women sometimes experience stress incontinence merely as a result of the growing fetus pressing against the bladder.)

Inability to pass urine (*retention*) may be caused by an obstruction, such as a tumor or stone, at the opening of the bladder. In men the most common cause is enlargement of the prostate gland. The early symptoms of prostatic enlargement include increased frequency of urination and slowness and hesitancy of the urinary stream. These symptoms can be relieved by surgical removal of all or part of the prostate gland (*pros-*

tatectomy). Inability to pass urine may be due also to spinal cord injury or disease. In such cases the bladder may need to be emptied by passing a narrow tube (catheter) up through the urethra to the bladder.

blepharitis

An inflammatory and persistent infection of the eyelid margins (lash line) and oil glands of the eyelids.

The symptoms are usually mild, but there may be redness, crusts of dried mucus, swelling, heat, itching, and grittiness, resulting in great discomfort. The eyes may seem tired, unduly sensitive and intolerant to light, dust, and heat. Causes include allergies, bacterial infection, and external irritants (such as foreign particles and wind). The nature of the skin itself (pale-skinned people are generally more susceptible) may also influence the condition. Seborrhea of the scalp is commonly associated with blepharitis.

Squamous blepharitis is a superficial dermatitis in which the area is congested, swollen, inflamed and the skin becomes scaly. The lid looks bleary and swollen as the result of congestion; the scaling skin forms yellow crusts as it adheres to the secretion produced. Later the margins become permanently swollen, thickened, and disturbed in position.

The consequent wetting of the lids, induces rubbing, followed by eczema and eversion of the lid margin. Dirty handkerchiefs and fingers aggravate the infection.

If the condition is chronic the lashes become damaged and may be lost, usually temporarily, but sometimes permanently.

Follicular blepharitis is a less common but more serious form. The inflammation is deeper, pus is produced, and the inflammation may extend outside the hair follicles and form abscesses (resulting in destruction of tissue and ulceration). The lid margins are red and inflamed and the lashes matted. Healing eventually occurs with scarring.

The complications of blepharitis are chronic conjunctivitis, permanently red lids, loss of lashes, and eversion of the lid (exposing its inner surface).

Treatment must include attention to general health and scrupulous cleanliness of the face and scalp. Dandruff must be treated with medicated shampoo. When required, the doctor may prescribe antibiotics (to control any associated bacteria infection) or ophthalmic steroid preparations.

blindness

In the literal sense, blindness is the state or condition of being sightless. But in a legal or practical sense it also includes serious impairment of vision to the extent that certain types of activity or employment may be extremely difficult or impossible. Blindness may be permanent or transient and affect one or both eyes. It may arise suddenly or develop gradually over months or years, and it may affect the entire field of vision or only part of it.

Blindness has many possible causes, but in each case one or more of four basic areas are affected: (1) the optical structures of the eye; (2) the *retina* (the light-sensitive structure at the back of the eye); (3) the *optic nerve* (a bundle of more than one million separate nerve fibers that convey impulses from the retina to the brain); and (4) the *visual cortex* (an area toward the back of the brain that is concerned primarily with interpreting impulses from the retina as visual images).

Sudden loss of vision may affect only part of the visual field of one or both eyes. An unobservant person may at first remain unaware of visual loss in one eye until the other is inadvertently covered up. Total loss of vision that occurs suddenly may be caused by blockage of the artery or vein supplying the retina or by hemorrhage within the eye. Sudden loss of part of the visual field is symptomatic of a DETACHED RETINA or of a blood clot in the blood vessels that supply the nerve tracts from the eye to the brain.

Several conditions may affect the arteries that supply blood to the eyes. These include vessel spasms (which can cause temporary visual impairment), and ATHEROSCLEROSIS, which may seriously impede or block the flow of blood to the eye. Hemorrhage into the eye, sometimes associated with high blood pressure but most commonly as a result of the condition of diabetic RETINOPATHY, is one of the most common causes of sudden blindness.

Blindness can be caused by a congenital defect of the eye, of the optic nerve, or of the visual cortex of the brain. Other causes include injuries or wounds affecting these areas, tumors of the eye or brain, MENINGITIS (inflammation of the membranes that cover the brain), complications that occur as the result of chronic inflammation of the eye, CATARACT, and GLAUCOMA. The three major causes of a gradual loss of vision, mainly affecting the elderly, are cataract, glaucoma, and senile macular degeneration.

Blindness can occur as a complication of certain infectious diseases, including SYPHILIS, TUBERCULOSIS, MEASLES, DIPHTHERIA, SCARLET FEVER, and GERMAN MEASLES.

Some forms of blindness or severely impaired vision (such as cataract) are easily corrected by surgery. Early treatment of other causes of defective eyesight (such as glaucoma and detached retina) can frequently limit or arrest the progress of impaired vision before blindness occurs.

Various institutions and societies exist which offer valuable training and assistance for the blind, including those that provide guide dogs and others that teach the reading and printing of Braille (a system of raised dots, felt with the fingertips, used to represent letters and other characters).

blisters

Fluid collecting under the outer layer of the skin as a result of local damage produces a blister. Blistering may be caused by repeated friction on tender skin (particularly of the hands and feet), by heat (as in the case of burns and scalds), or by irritating chemicals.

Blisters caused by the friction of unaccustomed physical work on the hands or by ill-fitting shoes on the feet will heal easily if the source of friction is removed and the blisters are kept clean so that they cannot become infected. The extensive blistering and broken skin caused by burning or scalding needs careful treatment under medical supervision if infection and subsequent scarring are to be prevented.

blood

There are approximately $10\frac{1}{2}$ pints (5 liters) of blood in the human body. About 40 percent of the blood consists of red blood cells (*erythrocytes*), white blood cells (*leukocytes*), and platelets. The remaining 60 percent consists of plasma, a watery solution of proteins and salts in which the blood cells are suspended.

The functions that make blood so vital to life may be described under three main headings: (1) transport, (2) homeostasis—the maintenance of

BLOOD FILM

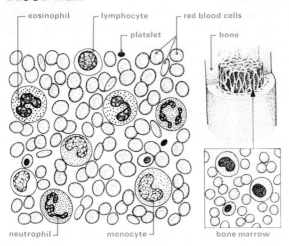

This drawing of a blood film gives an idea of the various cells a hematologist might see when he looks at blood under a microscope. In fact, not all the different types shown here would be present in any one sample. All these blood cells are derived from large primitive cells in the bone marrow.

a stable internal environment and body temperature, and (3) defense against infection and hemorrhaging.

Transport. Its constant movement throughout the body suggests that the principal function of blood is that of a transport medium. All the body's vital processes depend on a supply of oxygen to "burn" sugar and fat and thus produce energy. This oxygen is obtained from the air in the lungs and is carried by the red blood cells to all parts of the body. The principal waste product of energy production, carbon dioxide gas, is also carried in the blood—in both the red cells and the plasma—and is released in the lungs to be expelled in the expired air.

The food we eat, after processing in the digestive tract has reduced it to simpler chemical compounds, is absorbed into the blood mainly through the walls of the small intestine.

All the proteins, fats, sugars, vitamins, and minerals required by the body tissues are carried in the blood—either in simple solution or attached to a transporter protein.

The assimilation of food materials and the replacement and repair of tissues produce waste products, which would be harmful if allowed to accumulate. These are transported in the blood either to the liver for further processing to render them less toxic or directly to the kidneys for excretion from the body.

Homeostasis. Control of the body's functions depends to an important degree on "chemical messengers" (hormones) carried in the blood. These chemicals, produced by the endocrine glands (such as the pituitary and thyroid), are carried by the blood to all parts of the body, giving a rapid and efficient control of its physical and chemical activities; they help maintain the body's systems in a state of balance despite constant physical changes.

Defense. There are at least seven main types of white blood cells that work in combating infection: Of these, the macrophages directly attack bacteria invading the body and remove the debris of dead bacteria and damaged cells that results from infection. The *lymphocytes*, of which there are at least six different types, produce antibodies and other substances that overcome bacteria and viruses and provide a lasting immunity to further attacks. Some lymphocytes provide a cancer surveillance within the body, detecting and destroying cells that have undergone malignant change.

Further, when body tissues are damaged and bleeding occurs, the blood flow through the tissues ensures a continuing supply of platelets and certain protein factors that are responsible for blood clotting and the control of bleeding.

blood clotting

The formation of a blood clot after injury to a blood vessel is the result of a complex series of reactions involving a cellular component of the blood called a PLATELET and a dozen or more (mainly) protein constituents of the blood (*clotting factors*).

Platelets adhering to the damaged wall of the blood vessel release chemical substances that initiate the clotting process. The normal mechanism of blood clotting is disturbed if there is a deficiency in any of the clotting factors or if there is an abnormally low number of platelets (a condition known as THROMBOCYTOPENIA).

See also EMBOLUS, THROMBUS.

Shown right, extremely complex mechanisms interact to maintain and regulate the blood pressure, volume and flow throughout the body's vast network of blood vessels. In addition to the pumping action of the heart, which forces blood through the arterial system, the blood pressure is influenced by nerve impulses to and from the heart and by hormonal control mechanisms.

SOME OF THE FACTORS INVOLVED IN BLOOD PRESSURE CONTROL

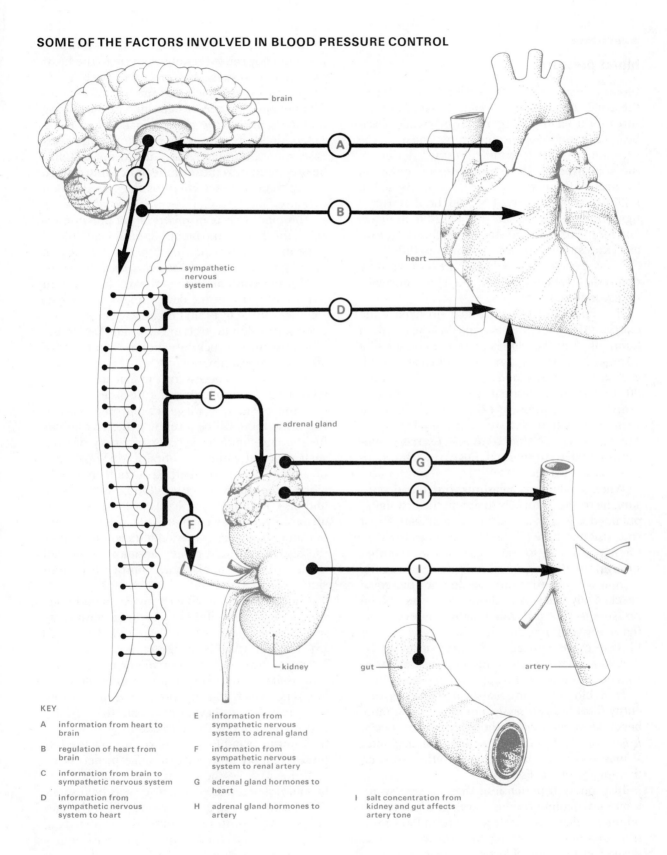

brain

sympathetic
nervous
system

heart

adrenal gland

kidney

gut

artery

KEY

A   information from heart to
    brain

B   regulation of heart from
    brain

C   information from brain to
    sympathetic nervous system

D   information from
    sympathetic nervous
    system to heart

E   information from
    sympathetic nervous
    system to adrenal gland

F   information from
    sympathetic nervous
    system to renal artery

G   adrenal gland hormones to
    heart

H   adrenal gland hormones to
    artery

I   salt concentration from
    kidney and gut affects
    artery tone

blood pressure

Blood pressure normally is defined in terms of the *systolic* pressure, which is the maximum pressure produced in the larger arteries by each heartbeat, and the *diastolic* pressure, which is the constant pressure maintained in the arteries between heartbeats. The blood pressure, measured by means of a SPHYGMOMANOMETER, is expressed in millimeters of mercury. The "textbook normal" figure for the systolic pressure is 120 millimeters and for the diastolic pressure 80 millimeters, usually expressed in abbreviated form as 120/80.

Many people have a blood pressure reading that is slightly below the average. This is normally no cause for concern.

It is important to realize that no fixed value exists for the blood pressure and that the standard figure of "120 over 80" is really the average of a fairly wide range. In a group of normal individuals, few will have a blood pressure of exactly 120/80. In a single individual, considerable fluctuations in blood pressure occur from minute to minute, from hour to hour, and from day to day. The figure may be affected by rest, exercise, emotion, or anxiety; the normal range typically widens with increasing age.

When a physician measures your blood pressure, he or she is unlikely to accept the first figure obtained if it is at all raised, since anxiety about your visit may have affected the reading. The doctor may ask you to wait a few minutes (either sitting down or lying down) before taking it again, or may ask you to return on another day for a check. Only when it is certain that your blood pressure is constantly raised above an acceptable figure for your age, and that this is causing or is likely to cause damage, will the physician decide that you suffer from high blood pressure (*hypertension*) and initiate the appropriate treatment.

High blood pressure may be a primary disease entity (*essential hypertension*) or a result of a number of disorders affecting the kidneys (*renovascular hypertension*), blood vessels, or the adrenal glands. It may also be an unwanted side effect of drug therapy for other diseases.

In primary hypertension, there are no symptoms until complications develop. Contrary to popular belief, uncomplicated high blood pressure does not cause headache, dizziness, fatigue, flushed face, or nosebleeds. Symptoms such as palpitations, shortness of breath on exertion, and changes in eyesight, with blurring of vision in one or both eyes, are caused by hypertension only if it has already caused serious damage to the heart or to blood vessels; they are more likely to be caused by other, much less serious, conditions. The person may need to get up with increasing frequency during the night to pass urine. If the raised blood pressure is the result of another disease, such as kidney failure, the symptoms may be predominantly those of the underlying disease rather than a direct effect of the raised blood pressure.

The main effects of raised blood pressure involve the heart and blood vessels. High blood pressure is one of the major risk factors in the development of *myocardial infarction* ("heart attack") and coronary artery disease. It is also an important factor in the development of a STROKE, whether caused by brain hemorrhage or by blood clots in the blood vessels of the brain. Taking the blood pressure is therefore an important part of any medical examination.

If treatment is necessary, the first step will involve tests to ensure that the disorder is not a symptom of kidney damage or some other disease. Attention then will be given to other risk factors for the development of coronary artery disease, such as cigarette smoking, obesity, or a high intake of animal fat in the diet. Reduction in weight alone often will produce a fall in blood pressure and also a fall in blood levels of fat. If stress or anxiety is present, a change in life-style or the use of tranquilizing drugs may be sufficient to control the disorder in mild cases. Cessation of alcohol or decongestant intake may improve hypertension.

If these measures fail to bring the blood pressure within normal limits for the individual, specific treatment will be required. Untreated hypertension is likely to shorten life.

Specific drugs that lower blood pressure are now available; the most important are the beta-blockers, which act by preventing adrenaline (EPINEPHRINE) from having its usual "fight, fright, and flight" effects. Diuretics alone or in combination with beta-blockers are commonly used. If these fail, more powerful drugs may be necessary.

Unfortunately, these drugs are not always free from unwanted side effects. They may be responsible for producing giddiness on sudden changes of posture (postural hypotension), diarrhea, depression, and (occasionally, in men) impotence. It is important for the doctor to ensure that the drug benefits the person in ways that compensate for any unwanted side effects.

blood types

The surface membranes of human red blood cells contain markers (antigenic determinants) that divide the cells into four classes: A, B, AB, and O. Type A people have antibodies to B antigens in their serum and type B people have antibodies to A. Type AB people have neither A nor B antibodies and type O people have both. So type AB people are "universal recipients" and type O people are "universal donors." All the red blood cells in an individual possess one and only one antigenic determinant. This system for typing blood is called the ABO system.

Other markers on the surface of the red blood cell include (in most people) the Rh antigens, which comprise the Rh blood-typing system. Some individuals—about 15 percent of the population—lack an Rh antigen on their red blood cells. They are classed as "Rh negative."

Although there are other systems for typing blood, the ABO and Rh systems are the most important in determining compatibility for blood transfusions. Blood transfusions can be given only by a donor who has the same blood type as the recipient. For example, a person with A+ blood can get a transfusion only from a donor with A+ blood. Severe reactions can occur if by accident mismatched blood is given to a patient, because the cell antigens react with the serum antibodies.

The blood groups are inherited characteristics passed from parents to their children. A and B are dominant. Blood typing is important in organ-transplant operations as well as in blood transfusion work.

boil

A painful red swelling in the skin (also known as a *furuncle*) caused by bacterial infection of a hair follicle or sweat gland. Usually infection is caused by staphylococci, bacteria normally found on the skin. Boils do not usually occur unless there is some additional factor to provoke infection. This may be an underlying disease (such as diabetes); sometimes the injury from simple friction leads to boils, which is why they appear around the neck, on the forearms, underarms, buttocks, back, and thighs. Boils also can occur as a result of secondary infection during teenage acne.

The first sign of a boil is a red swelling that may be painful and cause itching. In some cases the boil will go no further and will subside after two or three days. But the more usual course is that after six or seven days of enlargement, the swollen boil bursts and releases pus.

It is important to treat boils, because an untreated one can lead to the development of further boils or to generalized SEPTICEMIA (blood poisoning). Treatment consists of antibiotics and, occasionally, incision of the boil to allow drainage.

In diabetics, large boils with multiple discharging openings may develop on the neck and upper back. These are called *carbuncles*.

bone

The substance of which the skeleton is made—a mixture of calcium carbonate, calcium phosphate, and fibrous tissue. There are more than two hundred bones in the human skeleton, all made up of "compact" and "cancellous" bone. Compact bone, found in the shafts of the limb bones, consists of a hard tube surrounded by a membrane (*periosteum*) and enclosing a fatty sub-

BONE

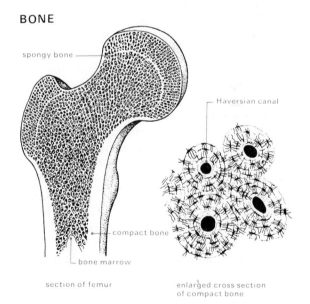

spongy bone

Haversian canal

compact bone

bone marrow

section of femur

enlarged cross section
of compact bone

Bone is a combination of mineral salts and fibrous material that is very resistant to mechanical stresses. The upper end of the femur, or thighbone, has a strongly developed meshwork of "spongy" bone designed to transmit the weight of the body. The shaft of the femur consists of "compact" bone, which is able to resist bending because of its structure—concentric rings of bony tissue.

stance (*bone marrow*). Cancellous bone forms the short bones and the ends of the long bones and has a fine lacework structure (it is also called "spongy" bone).

Bone is a living tissue and even the most dense is tunneled by fine canals in which there are small blood vessels, nerves, and lymphatics by which the bones are maintained and repaired. In children the bones include a plate of cartilage in which growth occurs; in the long bones (such as the femur and humerus) this "growth plate" is at one end only, the "growing end." Following puberty, bone replaces the cartilage, the long bones cease growing, and the skeleton no longer increases in size.

Bone is repaired by cells of microscopic size. One type, the *osteoblast*, lays down strands of fibrous tissue between which calcium salts are deposited from the blood. The other, the *osteoclast*, dissolves and breaks down dead or damaged bone. These processes occur when a bone is broken. The skeletal bones not only determine the body's "architecture," but are also vital because it is in the marrow of cancellous bone that new red blood cells are constantly formed.

botulism

A dramatic, life-threatening form of food poisoning caused by the bacterium *Clostridium botulinum*. This microbe produces seven distinct and powerful toxins that may be absorbed from the intestine or from contaminated wounds.

C. botulinum occurs in soil, in watery environments such as the seabed, in fish, and in many animals. The disease is acquired usually from contaminated food that has not been heated to at least 250°F (121°C), the temperature at which the organism is killed. Thus, smoked or lightly cooked or raw food may be responsible. Home-preserved vegetables are the most frequent cause of botulism in the United States.

Outside the body, the organism exists in spore form, and does not cause disease even when it contaminates fresh food; to do so the spores must germinate and actually produce toxin. Following ingestion of contaminated food, the toxin is quickly absorbed from the intestine. Four hours to a few days later nausea, vomiting, and abdominal pain occur, then weakness and unsteadiness. The nervous system is then attacked by the toxin, resulting in blurred vision, difficulty in swallowing, drooping eyelids, muscular weakness of the

arms and legs, and—potentially much more serious—paralysis of the muscles used in breathing.

Treatment of botulism is directed mainly toward preservation of lung function by use of a respirator, if necessary. Antitoxin is available from the Centers for Disease Control, Atlanta (and other health centers), and a drug called guanidine has proved to be of some value.

bowel and bowel movements

The intestinal tract—the tube that extends from the mouth to the anus—is approximately 26 feet long, although its length will vary, considerably as the muscle fibers in its wall contract and relax. The main sections are the *small intestine*—comprising, from above downward, the *duodenum*, *jejunum*, and *ileum* (together measuring approximately 20 feet in length)—and the *large intestine* or *colon* (about 5 feet in length).

The functions of the intestinal tract are: to digest food particles introduced into it from the stomach; to allow the essential nutrients, which

BOWEL

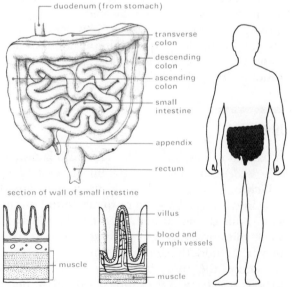

The bowel, or intestine, is a long muscular tube where food is digested and absorbed and waste material is passed to the rectum to be excreted as feces. The magnified sections of small intestine show the villi, *which are important for absorption of nutrients into the blood.*

are broken down into simpler compounds by the act of digestion, to be absorbed into the bloodstream (this occurs mainly in the small intestine); and to excrete the unwanted residue from the body. Bowel contents are moved along by *peristalsis*—waves of constriction passing in the direction of the anus.

The contents of the small intestine are fluid, but after they enter the colon, water is progressively absorbed until, by the time they reach the rectum, they are converted to semisolid (though normally soft) feces (or "stools"). These accumulate in the rectum until increasing distension produces a desire to open the bowels (defecation). The ring of muscle that controls the anus (anal sphincter) relaxes and contraction of the muscular walls of the rectum causes the feces to be passed. In most persons a bowel movement occurs once or sometimes twice daily, but there are wide variations dependent on diet and other factors. There is absolutely nothing abnormal about having a bowel movement only once every two or three days, providing this is regular and achieved without difficulty.

BOWLEG AND KNOCK-KNEE

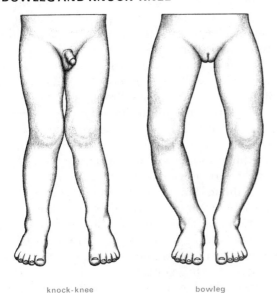

knock-knee   bowleg

Most young babies have bowlegs but the condition corrects itself when they begin to walk. Very rarely, if the deformity persists, it may be necessary for the child to wear corrective splints at night. A mild degree of knock-knee is also very common in children under 6 years of age and only needs active treatment if it is severe. In adults either of these deformities can result from trauma, rickets, or Paget's disease.

bowleg

An outward bending of the legs. It is common during infancy and requires no treatment or undue concern unless the condition persists. A normal posture occurs after the child has been walking for about one year. But abnormal bowleg may arise in various conditions where growth is disturbed, such as rickets or tibial osteochondrosis, and it can occur also in adults as a consequence of PAGET'S DISEASE.

If the bowlegged state of infancy does not improve spontaneously or if disease or other abnormality is clearly evident, then further investigation is necessary.

There is a rare condition, the result of deformity in the fetal stage, in which congenital dislocation of the knee is present at birth. The resulting bowleg deformity is avoided by immediate treatment.

Another condition that causes severe bowing of the legs is known as *tibia vara*. It occurs mainly in infants but is seen sometimes in adolescents and most often affects only one leg. This condition will not improve spontaneously and needs surgical intervention.

Bowlegs seen in infancy and in toddlers do not normally require treatment. If the condition persists, however, and if it is not corrected by the use of nighttime splints, surgery may be indicated. If the child is also obese, it is strongly recommended that a weight-loss program be started as well. In adults, the underlying cause must be treated.

bradycardia

A slowing of the heart rate below 60 beats per minute. It can be a normal occurrence in fit people at rest or during sleep (especially among well-trained athletes). In other circumstances bradycardia may be a sign of acute myocardial infarction ("heart attack"), depressant drug action (from the administration of drugs such as digitalis, morphine, reserpine, beta-blockers, or calcium channel blocking agents), or increased "vagal tone" (the influence of the vagus nerve in slowing heart rate).

In most cases bradycardia requires no treatment. However, in persons who have persistent symptoms of lightheadedness, fainting, ANGINA PECTORIS, or congestive HEART FAILURE as the consequence of an abnormally low heart rate or insufficient acceleration of the heart under conditions of stress, an artificial PACEMAKER may be required.

brain

The control center of the central nervous system, enclosed and protected by the skull.

More than 10 billion cells in the brain receive and transmit messages to and from all parts of the body; they filter, store, and form associations between information received through the senses. The brain is often compared with a computer but is thousands of times more complex than any existing electronic circuitry.

During fetal development the top end of the spinal cord thickens and expands to form distinct areas within the brain. Broadly speaking, the "higher" the center in the brain the more complex its function, culminating in intelligent or "cerebral" behavior.

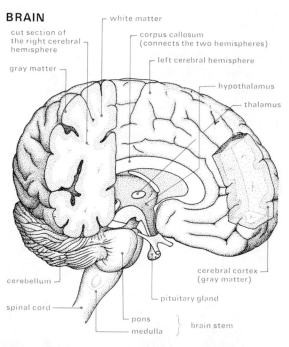

BRAIN

cut section of the right cerebral hemisphere

gray matter

white matter

corpus callosum (connects the two hemispheres)

left cerebral hemisphere

hypothalamus

thalamus

cerebral cortex (gray matter)

pituitary gland

cerebellum

spinal cord

pons

medulla

brain stem

The drawing shows the important structures of the human brain. Centers in the brainstem control the heart and breathing. The cerebellum smooths out our movements. The thalamus relays signals to and from the cerebral cortex, the thin layer of gray matter. The hypothalamus is concerned with "instinctive drives" and with emotions; it has intimate connections with the pituitary gland, controlling the body's hormones.

A diffuse network of cells and fibers called the *reticular activating system* (RAS) extends through the core of the brain stem from the top of the spinal cord up into the HYPOTHALAMUS. The RAS is the seat of consciousness and governs the states of sleep, arousal, and attention. The RAS and the higher centers of the cerebral cortex have extensive two-way connections so that their levels of activity are mutually controlled.

At the back of the skull is the *cerebellum*, which coordinates reflex actions that control posture, balance and muscular activity. Deep within the brain, where the brain mass seems to tip forward, is the center for basic or "uncritical" appreciation of pain, temperature, and crude touch—the *thalamus*. It is the main relay center for incoming sensory impulses (except those of smell), which it transmits to other parts of the brain, including those concerned with consciousness. Vital automatic functions, such as blood pressure, blood circulation, heartbeat, and hormone secretion are in part regulated by the hypothalamus, which is situated just below the thalamus (as its name implies). It also plays an important role in the experiencing of basic drives, such as hunger, thirst, and sex.

Above and billowing out to fill the skull are the convoluted *cerebral hemispheres*, where the nerve centers exist that are responsible for conscious thought and action. In humans, this part of the brain (the cerebrum) is larger in relation to total body weight than in any other animal. A dense layer of nerve cells—the *gray matter* of the cerebal cortex—forms the active "roof" of the brain. Deeper within the cerebrum are insulated nerve fibers of these cells, which intermingle to form the *white matter*. The most important of these nerve fiber tracts pass downward from the surface in two inverted pyramidal bundles—one on each side of the midline—which, after crossing over at a low level in the brain, run down into the spinal cord to supply the voluntary muscles of the body. It is this "decussation" of the pyramidal tracts that explains the common observation that a cerebral hemorrhage or thrombosis (STROKE) affecting the right side of the brain will cause paralysis on the left side of the body, and vice versa.

Distinct areas have been mapped out for many voluntary movements and for sensations from most parts of the body. But the brain's "computer" activity, which is responsible for functions such as reason and memory, is basically a mystery. Indeed, experts still understand little about the phenomenon of consciousness itself.

brain death

An irreversible form of unconsciousness characterized by a complete loss of brain function while the heart continues to beat. Head injury and brain hemorrhage are the most likely causes.

The signs of brain death are: (1) a prolonged failure of the brain to show any evidence of electrical activity (as indicated by electroencephalography); (2) absence of general neurological activity (manifested by fixed, dilated pupils, absence of spontaneous breathing, absence of any response to painful stimuli); (3) a prolonged state of deep unconsciousness.

The legal definition of this condition varies from state to state.

brain tumor

An abnormal growth in any part of the brain.

Brain tumors may be benign or malignant (cancerous). Unfortunately many are malignant, and these may be either primary or secondary—that is, originating in the brain or caused by the spread of cancer cells from another part of the body.

The tumors may appear in persons of any age. As they grow within the enclosed space of the skull they have little room for expansion against the delicate brain cells. Therefore, even quite small tumors in the brain may have serious consequences. They may arise from nerve cells, from the supporting connective tissue, or from the meninges (lining membranes).

The gradually increasing pressure in the brain tissue causes many symptoms. A dull nagging headache and vomiting are common. With some tumors, convulsions sometimes precede other symptoms. Mental changes may occur, such as drowsiness, lethargy, and possibly a change in the personality. Other symptoms—for example, partial paralysis, loss of part of the field of vision, or speech problems—depend on the part of the brain that is affected.

Diagnosis involves specialized X-ray studies, spinal puncture, and EEG tests. In recent years the advent of CAT and MRI (magnetic resonance imaging) scanning of the brain has improved diagnosis. It gives earlier diagnosis and a more accurate picture of the tumor than was possible in the past.

Treatment is mainly surgical; for benign tumors this may be quite successful. In cases of malignant tumors, however, a permanent cure is often difficult to achieve. Surgery radiotherapy, and cancer chemotherapy are all important in treatment.

BRAIN TUMOR

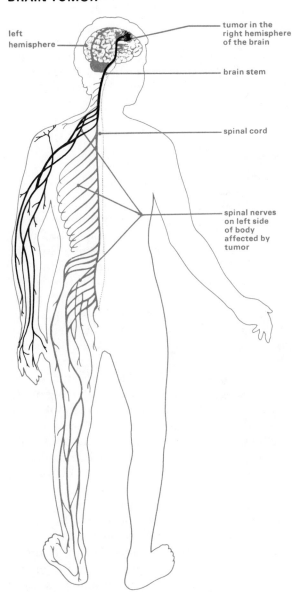

left hemisphere

tumor in the right hemisphere of the brain

brain stem

spinal cord

spinal nerves on left side of body affected by tumor

A tumor or some other disorder such as a stroke affecting the right hemisphere of the brain causes effects on the left side of the body. The reason is that the nerve fibers connecting the limbs and trunk to the brain cross over in the spinal cord or in the brain stem. Depending on the size of the tumor, paralysis or loss of sensation may result in part or all of the opposite side of the body.

BREAST SELF-EXAMINATION

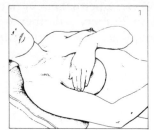 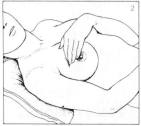 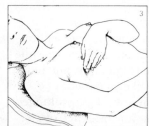 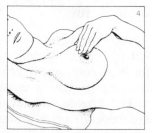

Most breast lumps are not cancerous, but any woman discovering a lump should consult a doctor. The correct method of self-examination is shown above. Feel with the flats of the fingers, not the tips (1). Start with the upper outer quadrant of the breast and remember it extends up into the armpit (2). Then examine the remainder of the outer half and underside of the breast (3). Feel around the nipple and gently roll the inner half of the breast over the ribs (4). Self-examination should be performed monthly. Treatment is more successful in the early stages of breast cancer.

breast

The milk-secreting, or mammary, gland.

Prior to the onset of puberty, there is no difference in the breasts of boys and girls. During puberty in females the breast assumes its adult function in response to hormones produced at this time.

In the adult woman each breast consists chiefly of fibrous tissue radiating from the nipple and dividing the glandular tissue into fifteen to twenty lobes. Under hormonal control, these lobes produce milk following the delivery of a baby. Each lobe has many small ducts draining into a main duct that finally emerges as a tiny opening on the surface of the nipple. Just under the nipple these ducts dilate, forming reservoirs of milk during feeding. Pressure by the infant's mouth on the areola, the distinct circle of dark skin surrounding the nipple, causes milk to be ejected from the fifteen to twenty ducts.

Surrounding the glandular tissue is a large pad of fat cells that gives the breast its shape. The entire breast mass extends over a large area, reaching up into the armpit. (Thus the importance of thoroughness when feeling the breasts during self-examination for early signs of cancer.)

There are no muscles in the breast mass; if the breasts lose their youthful firmness, exercise does not restore it. For this reason, the use of a brassiere is important for both comfort and support. During pregnancy, when the breasts enlarge, support is especially necessary.

Throughout pregnancy the breasts become fuller. This and tingling nipples are, for many women, among the first indications of pregnancy. The areola itself usually darkens in the second month of pregnancy, especially in dark-haired women. The virgin pink color is never restored

Many women worry about the size of their breasts, whether they are too small or too large. Little can be done for either condition, except by plastic surgery. Expensive creams or exercise gadgets are virtually worthless. After the age of 35, fat may be deposited in the breasts, slightly increasing their size.

breast cancer

Most of the lumps that occur in the female breast are not cancerous. Nevertheless, it is essential to seek immediate medical attention at the first sign of any suspicious changes or abnormalities in the breast since early diagnosis and treatment of breast cancer can be lifesaving. Breast cancer continues to be the most common form of cancer in women, especially in those between the ages of about 40 to 45; it claims approximately thirty thousand lives annually in the United States alone.

Warning signs. Among the warning signs of breast cancer are: (1) the appearance of any unusual lump or nodule in either breast (which may or may not be a harmless cyst or other benign growth); (2) changes in the nipple, either by alterations in position or by retraction ("inverted nipple"); (3) puckering of the skin on the breast; (4) bleeding or other discharges from the nipple; (5) an unusual rash on the breast or nipple. Many women may have one or more of these symptoms without having cancer. But because of the rapid growth of many breast cancers, medical attention must be obtained immediately, especially if any unusual lump is evident.

Breast cancer may also be diagnosed at an early stage—before any lump can be detected—by early screening using X-rays (see MAMMOGRAPHY under Tests). At present this form of screening is recommended for women in high-risk groups and for all women aged 50 and over.

Treatment. Treatment of breast cancer may involve a combination of surgery, irradiation, and drug therapy. Controversy still exists within the medical profession regarding the best method of treating various forms of breast cancer. The choice of therapy will depend largely on the extent to which the cancer cells have invaded the breast and surrounding tissues. Most surgeons are now more conservative and avoid radical procedures when possible.

breast-feeding

The natural way of feeding infants, by milk produced in the mother's mammary glands (the breasts). During the first few days, the breasts secrete small amounts of a thick yellow fluid known as *colostrum*—quite adequate for the baby, which has its own initial reserves of food. The milk "comes in" after the colostrum secretion stops. A continued flow of milk depends upon the demands made by the baby. When the baby is weaned, the falloff in the sucking stimulus means that less milk is produced; eventually, the flow ceases. Breast size is unimportant to successful feeding. Even quite flat-chested women may comfortably feed twins.

In this century breast-feeding has largely been abandoned in affluent countries in favor of bottle feeding, while in developing nations the use of a special formula of milk, in bottles, is becoming widespread. Pediatricians are trying to reverse this worrying trend; they are encouraging mothers to give their babies the advantages of breast milk for some time, if only for a few weeks.

A chief advantage is that breast milk protects against infections such as GASTROENTERITIS and PNEUMONIA during the first few months of life when the baby's own immune system is immature. Immunity is passed from mother to baby through the milk. Also, it is believed that breast-fed babies are less likely to become overweight.

Suckling helps to develop close emotional links between mother and baby, demonstrated by the fact that a baby's cry a few rooms away will cause a "let down" of the mother's milk. Nursing also stimulates release of a hormone from the hypothalamus in the brain that promotes the shrinking of the uterus back to normal size following childbirth.

Most women who want to feed successfully can do so. Worry, emotional upset, and illness are major reasons why milk may fail. It is no cause for reproach if a woman is unable to feed her baby, however. Hundreds of thousands of happy adults were bottle fed as infants.

See the extended discussion *Pregnancy and Childbirth* in the section on **Family Medicine and Health.**

Bright's disease

An imprecise term for chronic inflammation of the kidney (NEPHRITIS), accompanied by proteinuria (the abnormal presence of protein in the urine). In modern medical terminology it is basically equivalent to GLOMERULONEPHRITIS.

bronchiectasis

A chronic condition in which one or more of the main airways in the lungs (*bronchi*) lose their elasticity and become permanently widened. Mucus secretions collect in the damaged section of the lung and secondary bacterial infection is a common complication. The disease is characterized by severe bouts of coughing early in the day as the sufferer tries to bring up the infected sputum, which may be blood-stained.

Bronchiectasis may be associated with a congenital defect in the lung. More often it occurs after pneumonia or some other infection, especially WHOOPING COUGH. Bronchiectasis is also common in the genetic disorder CYSTIC FIBROSIS, in which the mucus secreted by the lungs is excessively thick and sticky.

However, with antibiotic treatment readily available for prompt treatment of respiratory conditions, damage is less likely to occur than it once was. In very severe cases, but where damage is confined, an affected lobe of the lung may be removed surgically.

bronchitis

Inflammation of the air passages and mucous membranes of the lung. Bronchitis may be acute or chronic.

Acute bronchitis very often follows a cold or an attack of influenza. First the windpipe (trachea) becomes inflamed; then infection spreads through the bronchial tree to the larger air passages (*bronchi*) and so into the smaller bronchioles. In a severe or untreated case, inflammation may spread into the lung tissue itself to give rise to bronchopneumonia. There is no distinct line between these states.

Initially there is a hard and unproductive cough (no sputum is coughed up), with mild fever, malaise (a general feeling of being unwell), aching muscles, and depression. After a day or two the patient begins to bring up sputum, and the cough is less painful. Treatment includes bed rest, warmth, steam inhalations, and hot drinks; if necessary, antibiotics are given to cut short the duration of the illness and to prevent the development of bronchopneumonia, especially in the aged.

Chronic bronchitis is a different disease, the result of repeated irritation of the lining of the air passages by smoking, dust, fumes, and general atmospheric pollution. It occurs in all industrial communities, and members of the managerial and professional classes are affected less than are unskilled and semiskilled workers. Men are more commonly affected than women.

The patient may be said to have chronic bronchitis when he or she continues to cough up sputum for at least three months in two years. The basic process in chronic bronchitis is excessive secretion of mucus, which interferes with the proper drainage of the respiratory tract and aids the development of recurrent infection. Eventually the lung tissue loses its normal elasticity, the air spaces become disrupted, and there is interference with the blood circulation in the lung, which may lead to increased pressure in the right side of the heart and consequent heart failure.

Symptoms of chronic bronchitis include chronic productive cough, increasing breathlessness, wheezing, and sometimes depression. The patient should stop smoking; usually it is impossible for him to change employment or to move into a more favorable climate free of gross air pollution, but by doing so he may lengthen his life and diminish his discomfort. Acute flare-ups of the disease are treated with antibiotics, since they typically are caused by added bacterial infection. Breathing exercises may help, and in very severe cases the administration of oxygen and the use of bronchodilator drugs under medical supervision may improve the condition.

bronchopneumonia

An inflammation of the lungs and bronchioles characterized by chills, fever, quickened pulse and breathing, cough with bloody sputum, and chest pain. It is usually the result of the spread of bacterial infection from the upper to the lower breathing tract, or it may be due to a viral infection. Treatment includes antibiotics, pain relievers, medications for cough and fever, bed rest, and fluids.

See PNEUMONIA.

brucellosis

A bacterial infection (also known as *undulant fever*) transmitted to man from cattle, hogs, and goats. It is mainly an occupational disease of those in contact with animals or meat, but it can also be contracted from unpasteurized milk.

The bacteria (of the genus *Brucella*) can enter the body through the nose, mouth, or through broken skin. The first symptoms usually appear within two weeks of infection, but the incubation period varies from about five days to several months. Symptoms include fever, headache, chills, fatigue, and depression. Often there are no physical abnormalities except the high temperature, and brucellosis can easily be mistaken for INFLUENZA. The fever sometimes recurs in repeated waves (or undulations) with intervening periods of several days without symptoms.

Even without therapy, the symptoms of acute brucellosis usually disappear within one year. Nonspecific symptoms of chronic brucellosis may persist for many years, however. Treatment of acute brucellosis with antibiotics reduces the chances of a relapse; once established, chronic brucellosis is difficult to cure.

bubonic plague

The most common variety of plague, which killed an estimated twenty-five million people in Europe during the fourteenth century. Today it is more prevalent in unsanitary areas of tropical countries, but limited outbreaks do occur occasionally in the western part of the United States.

The infecting bacteria, *Yersinia pestis*, are transmitted to humans from the bite of infected rat fleas, which abandon rats dying of plague in favor of domestic animals such as cats and dogs.

The characteristic features of the disease are fever and swellings (buboes) of lymph glands in the armpits and groin. Bleeding into the skin results in dark blotches (the source of the historical name, "Black Death"). In addition, the victim suffers high fevers, exhaustion, a high heart rate, low blood pressure, and confusion.

The onset of the disease is very sudden. After a few sporadic cases, the disease may suddenly spread and reach epidemic proportions.

Modern drugs have dramatically changed the outlook for plague victims. Treatment once used to consist of careful nursing and administration of antibubonic serum. Today a combination of sulfonamides and antibiotics is used with great success. Prevention of the disease involves control of the rodent population and the use of insect repellants to ward off the infective fleas.

bulimia

A compulsive eating disorder in which the victim experiences recurrent, uncontrollable urges to eat large quantities of food in a short period of time. Following a binge, many bulimics induce vomiting or purge with laxatives or diuretics to prevent weight gain; others simply go on a strict diet. Some persons may binge and purge or diet about once every few weeks, while others go through the cycle several times a day, with the search for a private place to purge becoming the dominant part of their lives. Bulimics most often are young women from the upper or middle socioeconomic classes, with high school and college students, models, and actresses particularly vulnerable.

It is difficult to recognize the condition because of the secretive nature of binge eating and purging. Bulimia shares many characteristics with AN-OREXIA NERVOSA, and the two disorders may overlap. However, while the anorectic person is obsessed with becoming thin, the bulimic is usually of normal weight and purges or diets for fear of becoming fat. Some victims also claim they induce vomiting or purge to relieve bloating after a binge.

Symptoms are caused by the complications of excessive vomiting or laxative or diuretic abuse. They include chronic sore throat, swelling of the parotid glands or even the whole face, bowel irregularities, dehydration, and electrolyte imbalances. Repeated vomiting can also cause stomach acids to completely erode dental enamel, until the victim is left with small stubs for teeth.

As in the case of anorexia nervosa, patients with severe electrolyte imbalances or dehydration may have to be hospitalized. Physicians may prescribe antidepressant drugs. Individual, family, or group psychotherapy should be sought in order to resolve underlying emotional problems that cause the uncontrollable urges to binge. A national organization called Overeaters Anonymous has helped many bulimics.

bundle-branch block

A defect in the electrical conduction system of the heart. There is a delay or block of the wave of electrical impulses that spreads out from below the region of the heart's atrial chambers.

Normally, the electrical impulses are conducted through a network of fibers known as the *bundle of His*. This bundle forms two branches: A block in the left branch usually means that heart disease is present, whereas a block in the right bundle (although linked with disorders of the heart) may occur in people who have no evidence of abnormality.

Bundle-branch block may occur in people suffering from high BLOOD PRESSURE ATHEROSCLEROSIS, RHEUMATIC HEART DISEASE, cardiomyopathy or congenital heart disease.

Diagnosis usually is made with the help of electrocardiograph (EKG) recordings. The outlook depends on the severity of the underlying disorder.

bunion

Inflammation and swelling of the bursa of the big toe. (Bursas are fluid-containing sacs situated in areas subject to friction; their function is to facilitate movement.) The joint in this case is greatly enlarged and looks dislocated. Bunions are the result of undue pressure on the joint over long periods.

Although injury that has not been treated satisfactorily may cause a bunion, badly fitting shoes are the most common cause. Pointed shoes force

BUNION

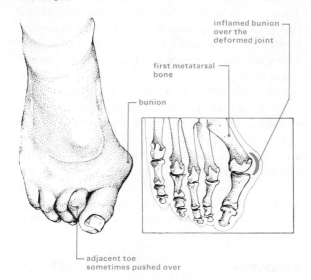

inflamed bunion
over the
deformed joint

first metatarsal
bone

bunion

adjacent toe
sometimes pushed over

A bunion is a painful swelling at the base of the big toe that can result from wearing tight shoes. The primary cause is that the first metatarsal bone deviates from the rest of the foot and the joint becomes prominent. The bursa, a sac of fluid that surrounds the joint, becomes inflamed, tender, or even infected as a result of friction.

the point of the big toe outward, causing a prominence on the inner border. The joint is dislocated, causing the condition of *hallux valgus.* As a result of pressure on the joint, the sac alongside the bones may also become inflamed and tender. Pus may be present.

Strapping splinting, and attention to wearing comfortable shoes may improve matters by reducing pressure. Once the damage is done, the only really effective treatment is surgical removal of the deformity. This operation is usually very successful.

burns

Damage caused to the skin by either dry or wet heat (scalds); the biological properties of the burned skin are destroyed. Anything bringing about this change is said to cause burning—fire, boiling liquid, electricity, acids, alkalis, and other corrosive fluids, extreme friction, or even excessive cold.

The severity of burns is assessed by considering the depth to which the skin is damaged and the surface area affected. A 1 percent burn would cover a surface area equivalent to that of the hand.

Fluid loss is a serious consequence of extensive burns. Plasma leaks out from blood vessels near the burned area. Small burns cause only a little leakage, with local blistering, but very large burns (where skin is severely damaged) may interfere with the circulation to such an extent that large volumes of fluid are lost. There is a danger of a severe drop in blood pressure (shock), and the fluid loss requires prompt replacement through the transfusion of plasma, which may be immediately more important than treatment of the damaged tissue.

A 15 to 20 percent burn may well require transfusions. Burns over 25 percent of the body are virtually certain to require them; burns over 75 percent of the body are nearly always fatal. Children and the elderly are particularly at risk.

Burns are divided into three categories: first-, second-, and third-degree.

First-degree burns involve superficial reddening of the skin with no blistering. This layer of the skin usually is shed and replaced naturally and healing is uncomplicated. Major treatment is unlikely to be necessary, although the victim may suffer some degree of shock.

In *second-degree burns* the outer layer of the skin is actually destroyed and there may be extensive blistering as fluid seeps out of the blood vessels. But enough tissue is left for the surface layer to be fully replaced in time. The chief threat is from infection when the blisters burst.

In *third-degree burns* the entire thickness of the skin is involved and cannot be renewed naturally. New skin will grow at the edges of the wound but destroyed skin must be replaced by skin grafts. These thin layers of skin—taken from other parts of the body—speed up the healing process, help prevent infection, and reduce deformity. Grafts of pigskin sometimes are used as a temporary dressing, but do not "take." Infection is the chief danger and badly burned victims usually are cared for in germ-free isolation units; they may be uncovered in the early stages. Devices such as air beds are used to prevent pressure on the damaged areas.

Although there is still some dispute over the first-aid treatment of burns, most experts advise that burns be cooled immediately. This certainly applies to minor household burns and scalds: The area should be cooled in running cold water for at least ten minutes. Otherwise heat retained in the skin following removal from the source continues to "cook" the tissues. Cooling also helps to relieve and prevent pain. However, concern with this should not prevent rapid transporting of more severely burned victims to the hospital. Smoldering clothing should be peeled off but clothes adhering to damaged skin must be left.

Burns from acid or alkalis or other corrosive liquids should always be flushed with large volumes of water. Acids should not be used to neutralize alkalis, or vice versa. Corrosive liquids in the eye should be flushed with water for some time and the victim encouraged to blink.

Blisters must be left strictly alone. Pricking them gives bacteria entry to a perfect breeding ground. Small trivial wounds may be covered with a sterile dressing, but larger burns should be covered only lightly, if at all. Ointments, creams, or butter should *not* be applied.

Medical attention should be sought where there is any doubt. Burns caused by an electric current may be more serious than they look, as tissue below the surface can be damaged.

bursitis

A painful condition affecting certain joints, caused by inflammation of a bursa.

A bursa is a closed fluid-filled sac that helps muscles and tendons to move smoothly across places where bones are prominent, such as in the knee, shoulder, hip, and elbow. Bursitis can be extremely painful; often the pain starts suddenly, especially in the shoulder—the most common joint to be affected.

The cause of bursitis in most cases is unknown, but it can be caused by injury, inflammatory arthritis, gout, rheumatoid arthritis, inflection, or repeated friction. One popular name for bursitis involving the bursa in the elbow is "tennis elbow."

Acute bursitis often responds to injection of hydrocortisone into the affected bursa. An anti-inflammatory drug, taken by mouth, may also be helpful.

Once the pain has subsided, exercise of the joint will help to restore mobility. This physical therapy, under proper supervision, is important to prevent any permanent loss of joint movement.

byssinosis

A lung disease caused by the inhalation of dust and foreign substances (mold, fungi, bacteria) contained in cotton, flax, and hemp. It primarily

BURSITIS

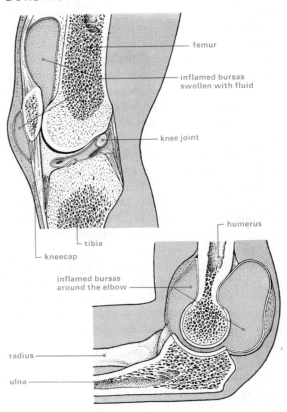

Bursas are small, fluid-filled sacs that allow tendons and skin to move freely over prominent bones. Repeated trauma to these areas leads to bursitis—painful, inflammatory swellings of the bursa. This is particularly likely to occur in bursas around the knee ("housemaid's knee") and at the elbow ("tennis elbow").

affects workers in industries where these materials are processed.

Byssinosis is marked by shortness of breath, cough, and wheezing. It is curable in the early stages, but if left untreated it can lead to EMPHYSEMA, long-term airway blockage, high blood pressure, and lung failure.

cachexia

A severe wasting (atrophy) of the body produced as the consequence of disease. Wasting occurs, of course, in any person who is starved for any reason, but the term *cachexia* usually is reserved for those in whom an underlying illness exists and who usually require treatment in addition to a well-balanced diet in order to regain normal health.

Simple starvation plays some part in many cases of true cachexia. For example, a patient with cancer of the esophagus ("gullet") or stomach may be quite unable, for purely mechanical reasons, to take in enough food to maintain health. In starvation, body fat is lost first; only when this has been consumed for energy production will essential tissue, such as muscles, be broken down. In some debilitating diseases, loss of body fat and muscle wasting often occur simultaneously as a relatively early sign of the disease and cannot always easily be explained by a loss of appetite or diminished food intake. This is particularly true of patients who have cancer (malignant cachexia).

In taking a patient's medical history, a physician often will inquire about any recent loss of weight. If there has been considerable weight loss over the preceding weeks or months, the physician inquires further to find out if the weight loss is associated simply with a reduction in food intake as a result of anxiety or depression, or if there may be some underlying disease. Lastly, certain glandular disorders including overactivity of the thyroid gland (HYPERTHYROIDISM) and a rare disorder of the pituitary gland (known as pituitary cachexia or Simmonds' disease)—may cause severe weight loss and wasting of the tissues, which can usually be corrected by appropriate treatment of the glandular disorder.

calculus

An accumulation of solid material (a "stone") in any of the hollow organs or passages of the body.

Calculi commonly cause symptoms when they occur anywhere in the urinary tract—the kidney, ureter, bladder, prostate gland, or urethra—or the biliary tract (GALLSTONES). The next most common sites for stone formation are the ducts of the salivary glands.

CALCULI

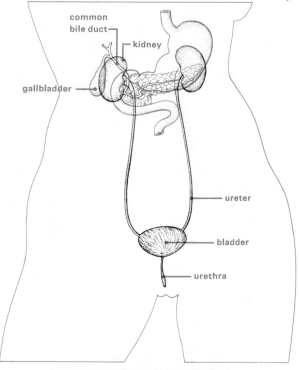

COMMON SITES FOR CALCULI (STONES)

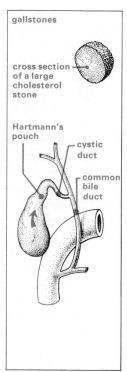

SITES OF IMPACTION
OF A GALLSTONE

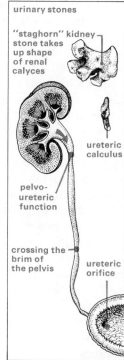

SITES OF IMPACTION
OF A URINARY STONE

Calculi, or stones, form in concentrated bile or urine. Multiple gallstones are often found in the gallbladder. Urinary stones can form anywhere in the urinary system. Large "staghorn" calculi in the kidney may be unnoticed, but tiny stones passing along the ureter cause excruciating pain and blood in the urine.

Urinary calculi usually form as a result of abnormally high blood levels of calcium or other metabolic abnormalities. Stasis of urine, infection, and inadequate fluid intake are sometimes contributing factors.

Most gallstones are caused by an imbalance in the concentrations of cholesterol, phospholipid, and bile salts in the bile; but infection may contribute, and a few cases are due to other diseases, such as hemolytic anemia. For reasons not yet understood, gallstones are becoming more common in Western societies; the most likely explanation is that the modern diet is especially rich in fats and proteins.

Calculi may cause no symptoms, and their presence may first be recognized only on X-ray films taken during a routine health check. However, if symptoms do develop they may be severe. If a stone blocks the bile duct (leading from the liver to the duodenum) or the ureter (leading from the kidney to the bladder) the result is severe abdominal pain. The muscles of the blocked duct go into spasmodic contractions in an attempt to overcome the obstruction, causing repeated bouts of intense pain (COLIC).

Often an attack of colic will be short-lived as the calculus is passed into the bladder or the intestine. Sometimes, however, the obstruction may persist. In the case of a gallstone this will cause JAUNDICE. If the ureter is blocked the kidney cannot function and may be permanently damaged. Even if they do not cause obstruction, the presence of stones in the kidney or the gallbladder encourages inflammation.

When the cause of stone formation is known, as in some types of kidney stone associated with inborn biochemical defects (such as the presence of excessive quantities of uric acid in the circulating blood, which can lead to GOUT), treatment may be given with drugs such as allopurinol (Zyloprim) or with dietary modifications to reduce the chances of further stones being formed. Treatment with the drug *chenodeoxycholic acid* can cause the gradual dissolution of some types of gallstone. However, in most cases in which stones cause repeated symptoms the treatment is primarily surgical. Removal of the gallbladder, called CHOLECYSTECTOMY (see under **Procedures**) can provide a permanent cure of ill health from gallstones in many cases. Removal of kidney stones does not give a guarantee of cure either, but it is usually combined with dietary advice to reduce the risks of recurrence.

A major advance has occurred, in recent years, in the management of stones in the urinary tract. This is known as *extracorporeal shockwave lithotripsy.* Up to 90 percent of stones that, previously, could have been removed only by surgery, can now be dealt with by the new method.

Patients are anesthetized and suspended in a water bath in a controllable cradle. The position of the stone is accurately determined by X-ray image intensifier. Shock waves are then generated in the water by a high voltage spark discharge and focused on the stone by a hemielliptical reflector. Human tissue within water acts as a homogenous medium to the shock waves, which pass through with little obstruction until they reach the stone. When they do, a great deal of energy is liberated and the stone is fragmented. The pieces are then passed normally in the urine.

Lithotripsy has been used also to treat gallstones, but the results are less satisfactory.

callus

1. A local hard growth of the outer layer of the skin. Also known as a *callosity.*

Calluses are a normal reaction of the skin to friction or pressure. For example, many people have a callus on the side of the middle finger of their writing hand, caused by pressure from a pencil or pen.

Calluses usually have a protective function; they prevent damage to the skin and underlying tissues. They must be distinguished from CORNS, which also are pressure-induced but are more localized. (Also, in a corn an apex of the thickened skin points inward and causes pain.)

Calluses rarely require treatment because they are painless and protective. Occasionally they are removed for cosmetic reasons; this is pointless, however, unless the provoking factor also is removed, for they tend to recur. In contrast, corns may need treatment by a podiatrist (foot specialist).

2. The lump of soft, unorganized new bone that forms at the site of a healing fracture and ultimately changes into organized bone that fixes the fractured bone ends firmly together.

cancer

Refers to the uncontrolled growth of cells in any organ of the body.

With the exception of leukemias, certain lymphomas, and multiple myelomas, cancers usually originate in a single isolated growth; at this early stage removal of the solitary tumor will cure the disease. Once the cancer cells spread (metastasize) to the bones, liver, or other major organs, however, the disease is not controllable by surgery alone.

Carried in the bloodstream or in the network of lymphatic channels to distant parts of the body, cells from the primary tumor "seed" themselves and grow, infiltrating and eventually destroying the healthy tissues around them.

Cancers can be divided into four main categories. Tumors that occur in epithelial tissue— such as of the skin, breast, stomach, pancreas, lung, and intestines—are termed *carcinomas.* Tumors of muscle, bone, and other fibrous and supporting tissues of the body are termed *sarcomas;* these are often slower-growing than carcinomas. The *lymphomas* (such as HODGKIN'S DISEASE) are tumors of the lymphatic system, affecting the lymph nodes in the neck, groin, armpits, liver, and spleen; similar in their symptoms and their response to treatment are the *leukemias,* the cancers of the blood-forming bone marrow.

As more of the external causes of cancer are discovered, prevention of the disease becomes possible by protecting people from exposure to these "carcinogens" at work, in food and drink, and by education about the dangers of smoking.

All forms of cancer are better treated in their early stages. Indeed, many of them are curable. Even after a cancer has spread, a combination of drugs, radiotherapy, and surgery may achieve a remission of symptoms for several years.

See the extended discussion, *What Is Cancer?* in the section on **Wellness.**

candidiasis

A genus of yeast-like fungi (*candida,* formerly known as *monilia*) often harmlessly present in the mouths of healthy people. In some circumstances, however, the microorganisms may proliferate to produce a symptomatic infection of the mouth, intestines, vagina, skin, or (rarely) the entire body. The infection is known as candidiasis (or, formerly, *moniliasis*). When the infection involves the mouth, the condition is referred to commonly as "thrush."

Thrush occurs particularly in babies, but it may occur also in debilitated adults or in those who wear dentures. It usually forms a white curd-like

deposit on the tongue, cheeks, and palate which may cause severe discomfort.

Vaginal candidiasis is one of the most common causes of inflammation and itching of the vagina and vulva, typically producing a white, curd-like discharge. Vaginal candidiasis is becoming increasingly common, perhaps partly because of changes in vaginal acidity brought about by use of oral contraceptives, antibiotics, and steroids. It is seen often in pregnant women and diabetics. The condition usually is not acquired during sexual intercourse, but sometimes it may cause a symptomatic infection in the male partner. *Candida albicans* may occasionally infect the entire intestinal tract, causing anal itching and forming a reservoir for repeated accidental infection of the vagina.

The fungus may infect the skin also—particularly in moist areas, such as beneath the breasts of large women and in the finger webs of those who work with water.

Candida infections usually respond to treatment with an antifungal drug such a nystatin— in the form of a mouthwash, lozenge, vaginal suppository, or cream; intestinal infection is treated with oral medication to prevent reinfection elsewhere.

Vaginal candidiasis tends to recur; avoidance of sexual intercourse during treatment reduces the recurrence rate.

Patients with immune deficiency (for example, those with AIDS and those on drugs that suppress immunity) may get a generalized candida infection involving most organs. This is a life-threatening condition that requires the intravenous administration of amphotericin B, a powerful (and quite toxic) antifungal agent used especially in the treatment of persistent, deep-seated infections.

See also VAGINITIS.

cannabis

A drug derived from the flowering tips and shoots of *Cannabis sativa,* a plant that grows wild or under cultivation all over the world. The active substances in the drug are chemicals called tetrahydrocannabinols. Cannabis is known under many names, including hashish, Indian hemp, marijuana, grass, pot, tea, weed, and ganja.

It is one of the oldest known drugs and was used in early surgery to produce drowsiness and euphoria. It has few legitimate medical uses today

INDIAN HEMP (Cannabis Sativa)

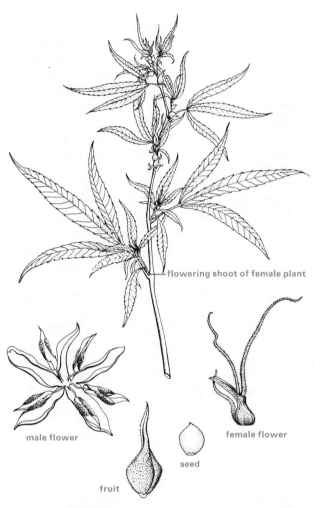

flowering shoot of female plant

male flower

seed

female flower

fruit

Cannabis (marijuana) is obtained from the Indian hemp plant pictured above; it can be taken either by mouth (mixed with food or drink), or smoked in a pipe or cigarette. It is not considered to be an addictive drug, although heavy users may become psychologically dependent.

but is widely consumed throughout the world—illegally, in most Western countries. The plant and its flowers are dried, ground up, and smoked in a cigarette (a "joint"). (It has been used experimentally in the treatment of glaucoma and in the relief of symptoms in patients with terminal cancer.)

In the West, cannabis resin is smoked in a small pipe ("hash pipe"); in some parts of the world (the United Kingdom, for example) it is mixed with tobacco and the smoke inhaled from a cigarette. It can also be drunk as an infusion (bhang), as in India, or eaten in food.

The effects of cannabis vary with the individual. Mild intoxication is characterized by cheerfulness, giggling, and easygoing extrovert behavior. With more severe intoxication there may be irritable outbursts, feelings of unreality, auditory and visual hallucinations, and even frank psychosis. The effect usually wears off within twelve hours or less.

Long-term use of cannabis has not been shown to have major dangers—but neither has it been shown to be safe. Chronic users often appear to be generally apathetic ("amotivational syndrome"), but this could be a reason for the long-term use rather than the result of it. Suggestions of brain damage due to prolonged use have not been confirmed, but decreased sexual function and potency seem to be a real, if slight, hazard.

Physical dependence on cannabis does not occur but psychological dependence may be severe. While cannabis does not directly lead the user toward "hard" drugs or crime, the drug subculture in which it is often used may expose users to greater dangers, and its hallucinogenic activity may tempt them to seek the stronger effects of LSD or other drugs.

Canabis may be no more harmful than alcohol (many experts believe that it is much less so), but it is debatable whether this is a sufficient argument for its legalization.

carbohydrates

A large group of sugars, starches, celluloses, and gums that are the main source of energy for all body functions. Carbohydrates range from simple sugars such as glucose and fructose, known as monosaccharides, to more complex carbohydrates such as starch and dextran, known as polysaccharides.

Each carbohydrate yields 4 calories per gram. Excessive carbohydrate intake is one cause of obesity and dental caries. Diabetics must regulate their intake carefully.

carbuncle

A large boil with multiple openings.

Carbuncles may reach the size of an apple. They cause severe throbbing pain associated with fever and a general feeling of being unwell (malaise).

Carbuncles usually occur where the skin is thick, especially on the back of the neck. Extension beneath the skin is probably favored by the thickness of the skin here, whereas elsewhere the infection would "come to a head." Carbuncles are particularly common in persons whose defense against infection is reduced due to other debilitating illness, such as DIABETES MELLITUS.

Treatment of carbuncles involves the administration of appropriate antibiotics. The application of local heat may relieve pain. Surgical drainage is sometimes performed, but it is often ineffective since there is no single collection of pus.

Before antibiotic therapy was available carbuncles were potentially dangerous, often leading to blood poisoning and even death. Now, with appropriate antibiotic therapy, they usually are cured, although in some cases the infecting microorganisms become resistant to one or more of the antibiotics, making successful treatment more difficult.

carcinoma

Any of various types of cancerous growths composed of epithelial cells—the cells that line the body's organs and ducts.

carpal-tunnel syndrome

A condition that occurs due to the compression of a large nerve, the median nerve, as it passes through a tunnel composed of bone and ligaments in the wrist. The compression can be caused by several things, such as injury or arthritis, but the most frequent cause is an inflammation of unknown origin.

Carpal-tunnel syndrome is fairly common, most often occurring in women over the age of 40. Symptoms include a gradual onset of numbness, a tingling or burning sensation in the part of the hand affected by the median nerve—the thumb, index, and middle fingers, and part of the ring finger. Pain may occur also in the wrist and forearm. Usually, the pain first occurs at night, but it then may progress to the daytime and worsen as a result of the person's normal activities.

Mild cases of carpal-tunnel syndrome usually can be relieved by rest, use of a wrist splint, and pain-control medications. In more serious cases, however, there may be severe pain or loss of sensation in the affected fingers. In these cases, a minor surgical operation can be done to relieve the pressure on the nerve.

CARPAL TUNNEL SYNDROME

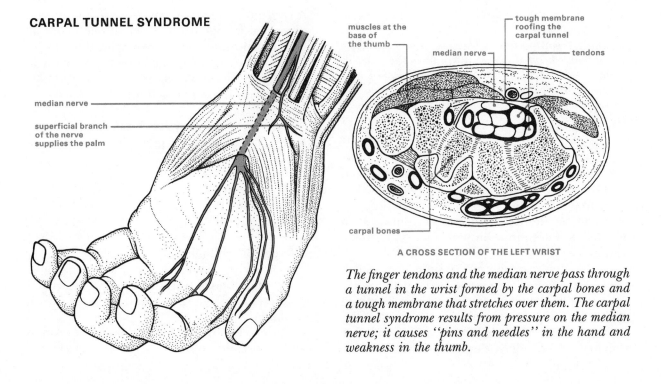

median nerve

superficial branch of the nerve supplies the palm

muscles at the base of the thumb

tough membrane roofing the carpal tunnel

median nerve

tendons

carpal bones

A CROSS SECTION OF THE LEFT WRIST

The finger tendons and the median nerve pass through a tunnel in the wrist formed by the carpal bones and a tough membrane that stretches over them. The carpal tunnel syndrome results from pressure on the median nerve; it causes "pins and needles" in the hand and weakness in the thumb.

CARTILAGE OF THE KNEE

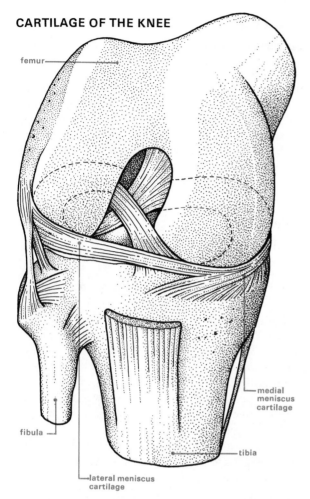

femur

medial
meniscus
cartilage

fibula

tibia

lateral meniscus
cartilage

Cartilage is a tough, bluish-white, translucent material. Its perfect smoothness facilitates movement at the joints. At the knee, for example, the contacting ends of the femur and tibia are covered with a thin layer of cartilage. In addition, two crescent-shaped plates of cartilage, the menisci, help the bones to fit together snugly.

cartilage

A tough, dense, elastic tissue that—together with bone—constitutes one of the two main skeletal tissues of the body. Mature cartilage contains no blood supply of its own, but obtains nutrients for its living cells from the surrounding tissue fluids. (In meat, it is called "gristle.")

In the developing human embryo, the skeleton is formed of cartilage that eventually is transformed into bone by the process of *ossification* (the deposition of calcium within the cartilage). At this stage the cartilage is penetrated by small branching canals containing blood vessels. Cartilage persists until adolescence in the rapidly growing

regions of the skeleton and in particular at the ends of long bones (as *epiphyseal plates*). In adults, cartilage is restricted mainly to the frontal ends of the ribs (*costal cartilage*), the surfaces of joints, and certain areas outside the skeletal system—such as the rim of the ear, the nose, and parts of the respiratory passages (especially the trachea and larynx).

The cartilage on the surfaces of most joints (articular cartilage) acts to reduce friction. The low "friction coefficient" of cartilage (three times more slippery than one ice cube moving across another) aids joint movement; it also has a cushioning effect.

Pads of cartilage mixed with tough fibrous tissue (*fibrocartilage*) are found as intervertebral disks between the bones of the spine. Fibrocartilage pads are found also in the knee; these are called "semilunar cartilages" because of their half-moon shape. These are sometimes injured in contact sports and have to be surgically removed.

Cartilage is occasionally the site of a benign tumor (CHONDROMA) or a malignant tumor (chondrosarcoma).

catabolism

The process whereby cells in the body break down complex chemical substances into simpler ones, providing energy for use by the body (for example, energy from glucose).

In all living cells catabolism occurs side by side with *anabolism* (building-up processes). These two processes in combination are known as *metabolism*.

The energy released in catabolism is used to maintain body temperature, movement, and other functions. This energy is used also in the anabolic process for energy storage, growth, and repair. The normal, healthy adult has a net equilibrium of catabolism and anabolism and is said to be in "metabolic balance."

In severe illness, the patient may enter a hypercatabolic state in which catabolism predominates and body tissues are broken down, resulting in rapid weight loss. Unless this process is stopped with appropriate medical treatment, it leads to severe body wasting and eventually death.

cataract

An opacity in the internal lens of the eye causing defective vision.

CATARACT

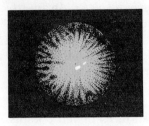 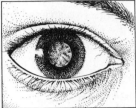

early cataract seen with an
ophthalmoscope

mature senile cataract

A cataract is any opacity in the lens of the eye. Most cataracts are associated with aging ("senile cataract") and are present in both eyes, leading to progressively blurred vision. However, surgical removal of the lens restores vision in more than 90 percent of cases.

Cataracts may be present in one or both eyes and may develop at any age. Fully developed cataracts cause severe impairment of vision. Initially the symptoms include shortsightedness (helped at first by glasses), a change in the perception of colors, and gradually diminishing vision. Cataracts do not cause pain or discomfort. Fully developed cataracts at birth may prevent the normal development of visual ability unless they are treated within a few months.

Cataracts may result also from injury to the lens of the eye, including injury by heat or ionizing radiation. The great majority of cataracts occur in elderly persons (senile cataracts)—where they are considered to be an extreme case of the inevitable hardening of the lens that occurs with age. Some degree of opacity occurs in almost all elderly people. Diabetics often develop cataracts about a decade earlier than others.

The only treatment for cataracts is surgical. The opaque lens is removed through the front of the eye under local or general anesthesia. Complications are uncommon, and it is no longer necessary to wait until the vision is severely defective before operating. Modern anesthesia has made the operation safe in many elderly persons who previously would have been considered unsuitable.

There is no possibility of recurrence in the same eye after the operation. In nearly all cases removal of the cataractous lens is followed by the implantation of a tiny, plastic artificial lens. This gives excellent results and glasses often are needed only for reading. Heavy, strongly-magnifying "pebble" glasses are largely a thing of the past.

catarrh

A term, not strictly medical, for inflammation of the air passages of the nose and throat.

The symptoms under the general heading "catarrh" vary according to what the patient means by the word, but they usually include one or more of the following: blocked nose, runny nose, facial discomfort due to sinusitis, hearing difficulty due to obstruction, sore throat, and cough.

catatonia

A combination of mute withdrawal and abnormalities of movement and posture found in some forms of schizophrenia.

The person may be completely immobile and remain in any position in which his body is placed (a state known as *waxy flexibility*). For example, if his arm is lifted above his head he may leave it there until it is again moved for him. He may also obey verbal orders to move his body to an uncomfortable posture or he may precisely imitate the movements of another person.

Long-continued repetition of a meaningless word or phrase or the same movement (*perseveration*) is also common—for example, repeated eating motions with a knife and fork long after the food is finished. In extreme forms of catatonia the stupor may progress to complete unresponsiveness, with failure to eat and drink (often necessitating tube feeding) and incontinence or retention of urine and feces. Such a phase may last for a few hours to several days.

The cause of catatonia—like that of schizophrenia—is unknown. Treatment is directed at the underlying schizophrenia and may include drugs, electroconvulsive therapy (ECT), or psychotherapy.

catheter

A tube used to introduce fluids into or withdraw them from any of the body cavities or passages.

Early catheters were rigid and usually made of metal. The development of rubber and plastic catheters over the past few decades has greatly extended their uses.

Many catheters with special uses are now available—there is at least one specially made catheter for every space in the body. The following are some of the more common types:

Urethral catheters are inserted through the urethra into the bladder to drain urine in cases of urethral obstruction (for example, when caused by an enlarged prostate gland). They are needed also in certain other medical and surgical situations, such as kidney failure or after gynecological surgery. Most patients require urethral catheters for only a short period, but patients with a paralyzed bladder may need permanent catheterization.

Intravenous catheters, or cannulas, are inserted into a vein to take blood or administer fluids and drugs.

Cardiac catheters are passed via arteries and veins to the heart to measure cardiac function. Cardiac catheterization is often a routine preliminary to HEART SURGERY.

A *peritoneal dialysis* catheter is inserted through the abdominal wall into the peritoneal cavity to allow the exchange of fluid that takes place in this procedure.

A *nasogastric* tube is a catheter passed via the nose to the stomach for the administration or removal of fluid.

An *epidural* catheter is used for the administration of anesthesia into the subarachnoid space surrounding the spinal cord during childbirth.

causalgia

A chronic, severe, burning pain of the skin that can occur after injury to a nerve. It can occur anywhere in the body; the pain is experienced in the area from which the nerve carries impulses.

The condition is common after bones are broken, or in accidents where there are deep wounds. It can occur also in persons with peripheral neuropathy (disease of the outlying nerves). Unfortunately, pain relief may be difficult to achieve since not all cases respond to analgesics (painkillers). Sympathetic nerve block is the most valuable measure. Sedatives may prove beneficial to some persons. Brisk rubbing of the affected part may help, as may *transcutaneous electrical nerve stimulation (TENS)*.

celiac disease

A condition in which the small intestine fails to absorb fats, vitamins, and other nutrients. A prominent symptom is pale, foul-smelling stool that is difficult to flush away because it is frothy, light, and fat-laden. Signs and symptoms include weight loss, a swollen, protruding stomach, vomiting, diarrhea, extreme fatigue, and muscle-wasting.

Celiac disease is caused by a sensitivity to gluten, a protein found in wheat, rye, and other grains. Most patients do well with a high-protein, high-calorie, gluten-free diet. Vitamin supplements may be required.

Although originally described in children, there is an adult counterpart, which can develop at any age, known as "nontropical sprue."

cell

The functional unit of which all animals and plants are composed.

The human body contains an astronomical number of cells. The brain alone has billions of cells, and the total number of red blood cells is around 30 trillion (an average of 5 million in every cubic millimeter). Cells are quite variable in their size and shape. The average cell is around 7 microns (millionths of a meter) in diameter, but some are much smaller. Nerve cells are characteristically long and thin; in fact, some single nerve fibers stretch from the spinal cord to the tips of the toes.

A typical cell is composed of a *nucleus* (containing the genetic material DNA) and *cytoplasm* (which contains the enzymes necessary to translate the genetic information stored in the DNA into chemical action).

The cytoplasm contains a number of "organelles" in which the various metabolic processes are organized. These can be identified clearly with the electron microscope and include the ribosomes, endoplasmic reticulum, mitochondria, and lysosomes. The cytoplasm is surrounded by the cell membrane.

The internal environment of the cell is remarkably constant and differs greatly from the surrounding tissue fluid. This difference is maintained by active processes in the cell membrane. These processes, together with the other metabolic activities necessary for life, require a continuing supply of energy. This is released during the breakdown of sugars, fats, and proteins, and this requires a constant supply of oxygen.

All the cells in the body are derived by division from the original fertilized ovum. As the embryo

CELL

A GENERALIZED CELL

mitochondrion

endoplasmic reticulum

cell wall

vacuole

ribosome

nucleus

lysosome

nucleolus

Golgi body

centrosome

SOME SPECIALIZED CELLS

squamous tissue

ciliated columnar cells

striped muscle cells

bone cells

red (left) and white blood cells

nerve cell

ovum and sperm

Cells form the building blocks of all living tissue. Essentially, they consist of a sac of fluid enclosed by a membrane. Floating in the cell are smaller membranous sacs, or organelles, such as mitochondria and ribosomes, which are the sites of specialized activity. The varied shapes of the cells in the lower part of the drawing show how they adapt to perform many different jobs.

develops, cells take on specialized functions; most remain capable of division in the event of injury. Nerve cells have no such potential, and mature red blood cells have lost their nuclei and are simply envelopes of cytoplasm. Most cells are capable of regeneration if they are partially injured.

The study of individual types of cells has contributed to medical understanding of abnormalities in many diseases, including cancer and metabolic disorders.

cellulitis

A diffuse, spreading inflammation of tissues most commonly of the skin and underlying areas. It is usually caused by bacterial infection that easily

spreads through the tissues causing a feeling of heat in the affected area, together with redness, local pain, swelling, sometimes fever, chills, and a general unwell feeling (malaise). Abscesses and tissue destruction can follow if antibiotics are not taken.

cerebral embolism

Any abnormal matter, such as a blood clot, fatty tissue, air, or cholesterol, which is carried in the bloodstream to a brain artery where it affects and obstructs the blood flow. This results in a lack of oxygen and nutrients in the brain cells beyond the clot.

The onset of illness in cerebral embolism is sudden. There is often a headache for a few hours before the signs of neurologic damage arise, such as paralysis or loss of feeling. Sometimes the illness starts with convulsions. Cerebral emboli usually derive from atheroma (see ATHEROSCLEROSIS) in the arteries of the neck or from clots forming in the heart. Small emboli cause "transient ischemic attack"; larger emboli cause STROKE. About one quarter of persons become unconscious for some minutes, then return to consciousness in a confused state.

cerebral hemorrhage

STROKE caused by bleeding from an artery in or near the brain.

Cerebral hemorrhage starts with a sudden, very severe headache—much more intense than other headaches—which often extends to the neck and back. For a short initial period the person may be able to feel the pain in one particular place, such as the front, back, or one side of the head. This localization can be helpful in detecting the site of the lesion, as the pain quickly spreads throughout the head. Following the headache come dizziness, vomiting, sweating, and shivering, then progression from drowsiness to stupor and unconsciousness. In mild cases the person recovers consciousness, but for many days or even weeks afterward there is lethargy, clouding of intellect, confusion, or delirium. In the first seventy-two hours after the cerebral hemorrhage, the accumulation of blood around the surfaces of the brain and spinal cord leads to irritation of nerves and stiffness of the neck muscles.

Cerebral hemorrhages arise from a ruptured

artery. In the young, the most common cause is "berry" aneurysms—small balloonings of thinned arterial walls—usually in the system of arteries lying at the base of the brain. The aneurysms appear to form at points of weakness that develop in the arterial walls after infancy. Other causes of arterial rupture include high blood pressure, congenital abnormalities of the arteries, and tumors involving the blood vessels.

Cerebral hemorrhage carries a high death rate.

cerebral palsy

An imprecise term applied to various non-progressive motor disorders caused by brain damage occurring during pregnancy or birth. The term covers a wide range of disabilities, including paralysis of the muscles, inability to coordinate their movements, and the occurrence of involuntary movements in an otherwise normal person.

Most cases are the consequence of injury at birth, caused either by surgical instruments or an obstructed delivery, or from lack of oxygen during labor or birth. Other causes include developmental defects of the brain, maternal infection during pregnancy, and RHEUMATIC HEART DISEASE or JAUNDICE in the first few days of life. A quarter of all cases start in infancy after a brain infection, thrombosis, embolism, or injury. The condition is more common in first babies, particularly boys.

Milder cases have spastic paralysis of the legs or of both limbs on one side and normal intelligence. "Scissors gait" and toe-walking are common. More severe cases exhibit widespread loss of muscle control, seizures, mental retardation, and deficiencies in speech, vision, and hearing. Treatment includes the wearing of braces, surgical correction of some deformities, physical and speech therapy, and medication to relax the muscles and prevent convulsions.

cerebrospinal fluid (CSF)

The clear, colorless fluid surrounding the brain and spinal cord and filling the spaces and channels (ventricles and aqueducts) within them. Examination of cerebrospinal fluid is important in diagnosing diseases of the central nervous system (CNS).

Most of the CSF is formed in the ventricles of the brain from tufts of tiny blood vessels in their walls, called *choroid plexuses*. The CSF flows out

CEREBROSPINAL FLUID (CSF)

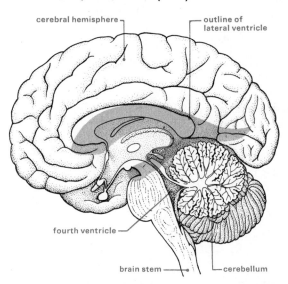

Cerebrospinal fluid (CSF) is produced in the ventricles of the brain. It escapes through openings in the roof of the fourth ventricle to bathe the surface of the brain and spinal cord. If the flow of CSF through the ventricles is blocked, pressure builds up leading to the condition of hydrocephalus. The composition of CSF changes in meningitis and certain other diseases.

over the surface of the brain through openings just above the base of the skull and is later reabsorbed into the venous system. The CSF acts as a "water cushion" between the brain and skull and between the spinal cord and vertebrae.

CSF has a density similar to water's. In a healthy person it is alkaline, almost protein-free, totally free of red blood cells, and with very few white blood cells. Its content of salts (such as sodium, chloride, bicarbonate, and potassium) is similar to that of the blood.

Examination of CSF taken by needle from the lower back (*lumbar puncture*) or from the neck (*cisternal puncture*) helps in the diagnosis of neurological disease. CSF pressure and protein levels may be raised in CANCER; in cerebrovascular disorders blood may be present in the CSF; in MENINGITIS white cells and bacteria are found in the CSF.

cerebrovascular disease

Any disorder of blood circulation in the brain. The most common is ATHEROSCLEROSIS of the blood vessel wall leading to clotting of the blood within the vessels (STROKE). Attacks often recur, and often those who survive are disabled.

The symptoms of paralysis, numbness, apathy, and loss of intellect or memory arise from a reduction of oxygen supply to the brain cells.

See also CEREBRAL EMBOLISM, CEREBRAL HEMORRHAGE.

Chagas' disease

An infectious disease caused by a species of parasitic protozoan (*Trypanosoma cruzi*). The disease (also known as *South American trypanosomiasis*) affects more than seven million people in Central and South America.

The infecting protozoa are transmitted to man by the bite of certain species of bloodsucking insects known as *reduviids* ("assassin bugs"), which often are found in the cracked walls of mud houses or in the roof thatch. They deposit their contaminated feces on the skin of their victims, who then scratch the area and permit the protozoa to gain entrance to the body through the resulting abrasion.

The parasites eventually enter the bloodstream. Many of them reach the heart, where they invade the heart muscle (myocardium). As they undergo developmental changes they can cause inflammation of the heart muscle (MYOCARDITIS). In this stage of the disease there may be enlargement of the heart and eventual HEART FAILURE. Severe damage can also be caused if the parasites migrate to the digestive system, with consequent dilation of the esophagus, stomach, and small and large intestines.

There is no specific treatment as yet for Chagas' disease, although research is being conducted into the development of an effective vaccine. There are no drugs available that can remove the parasites from the heart muscle and other tissues, but some drugs are effective in eliminating them from the blood circulation. Preventive measures involve control of the insects that spread the disease (by means of insecticides) and improved domestic hygiene.

chalazion (meibomian cyst)

A cyst of the eyelid.

Chalazion is caused by blockage of an oil-secreting (*sebaceous*) gland in the eyelid (also known as a *meibomian gland*). The gland slowly enlarges, producing a lump in the eyelid which is more of a nuisance and a disfigurement than a source of pain or discomfort. Small chalazia often are not noticed until the finger is run over the eyelid. Everting the eyelid to show the inner surface reveals a purple or red discoloration over the chalazion in the early stages, which later turns gray.

Pressure building up within the cyst may force the seepage of the contents of the cyst through the inner surface of the eyelid, giving rise to a chronic irritating discharge from the eye. If the gland becomes infected the swelling may be red and painful with a yellowish discharge.

Treatment is surgical removal of the cyst, a minor operation performed painlessly under local anesthesia.

chancroid

A highly contagious, sexually transmitted disease caused by infection with the *Hemophilus ducreyi* bacterium.

The first sign of chancroid is a small pimple that appears on the skin of the external genital organs. The pimple grows and finally bursts, leaving behind a painful pus-filled ulcer.

A skin test is used to diagnose this condition. A ten- to twenty-day course of antibiotics is used to treat chancroid.

cheilitis

A swelling and cracking of the lips due to inflammation.

In *acute* cheilitis the lips become swollen, tender, and painful. In *chronic* cheilitis they are dry and cracked and peel easily. Persons with chronic cheilitis often pull or bite pieces of inflamed skin, thereby increasing the irritation and inflammation. Or they may habitually lick their lips in an attempt to ease the discomfort. Some cases of cheilitis are of nervous origin.

Cheilitis can be caused by allergy to chemicals in lipsticks, dentifrices, perfumes, and—particularly in young children—foods. Deep fissures from chronic cheilitis may be persistent and annoying.

Persons with a protruding lower lip which they constantly expose to sunlight sometimes develop *actinic* cheilitis, a condition that may develop into cancer.

"Cold sore," or herpes simplex infection of the lip, is a common form of cheilitis. Repeated herpes attacks occur in the same places on the lip, suggesting that there may be a dormant virus that is reactivated at intervals, leaving minimal scarring. Such attacks often are precipitated by sunburn or fever.

Nibbling at warts on the fingers may transfer the virus to the lips in *warty cheilitis.*

Chronic cheilitis often responds to corticosteroid ointments, and herpes simplex cold sores can be treated with Acyclovir.

chest pain

Pain in the chest is a common complaint. The pain may be a symptom of a potentially serious heart disease, or it may represent a relatively minor condition such as reflux acidity ("heartburn") brought on by overindulgence in food or alcohol.

Chest pain may arise from the muscles, bones, or joints of the chest wall, or from any of the organs in the chest or the upper part of the abdomen, or it may be "referred" from disease of the spine. Most chest pain comes from the esophagus, trachea, and chest wall, rather than from the heart.

When they suffer severe pain in the chest, most people fear heart disease, and most physicians will first try to exclude the possibility of heart disease before they consider an alternative diagnosis. Pain that actually arises from the heart is produced by *ischemia* of the heart muscle—that is, a deficiency of the heart's blood supply brought about by disease of the coronary arteries, or by inequality of demand versus supply of blood to the heart muscle. It is usually related to effort, coming on, for instance, after walking a fixed distance.

Peptic ulcers and gallbladder disease may both produce pain that is referred to the lower part of the chest, often felt at mealtimes. Hiatus HERNIA (a defect in the diaphragm) can cause pain or discomfort behind the sternum (breastbone).

Pain from the respiratory apparatus may be central, arising from the trachea ("windpipe") as a result of infection by viruses or bacteria, or it may be on the side—arising, for example, from inflammation of the membranes that cover the lungs (PLEURISY). Chest pain may be a consequence of lung inflammation secondary to pneumonia, or it may be associated with a tumor of the lung; in such cases the pain is made worse during intake of breath.

Occasionally, pain in the chest is caused by PNEUMOTHORAX or PULMONARY EMBOLISM, both conditions being accompanied by breathlessness. The skin of the chest may be affected by HERPES ZOSTER (shingles), a painful inflammation of the sensory nerves, characterized by blistering of the skin along the line of the nerve. *Mitral valve prolapse,* which in the majority of patients is a benign anomaly, may be associated with chest pain. In a number of cases no cause for chest pain can be found. A person may be unduly concerned about his or her heart and develop an anxiety state in which the chest pains are experienced, or said to be experienced, without any physical cause (a condition known as *cardiac neurosis*). A thorough physical examination and certain tests (which may include an electrocardiogram, stress test, or angiogram) will help in the diagnosis.

In all cases, treatment of chest pain is directed at the underlying condition. Symptomatic relief can be given with analgesics such as aspirin or other drugs.

chicken pox

A disease most commonly affecting children between the ages of 5 and 10 and usually occurring in limited outbreaks in the winter and spring. It rarely attacks adults or infants in the first six months of life. One attack virtually ensures permanent protection against future infections.

Chicken pox is passed on by inhalation of virus-laden droplets—coughed or sneezed. The incubation period of fourteen to twenty-one days is followed by a short period when the child feels generally unwell, perhaps with a mild fever and headache. Crops of spots appear during the next five days. They are thickest on the trunk and face and relatively sparse on the limbs. Some may appear inside the mouth and throat.

The rash develops from pink, flat spots into tiny single blisters that become dry and encrusted within two to four days. During this stage the patient is highly infectious, although he or she may not appear to be particularly unwell.

The rash often itches severely and younger children are strongly tempted to scratch. Scratching should always be discouraged because it can lead to bacterial infection of the skin and the subsequent formation of scars (pockmarks). Hygienic measures—such as daily baths and close cutting and frequent cleaning of the fingernails—are also useful in preventing such complications.

Crusts may be removed from the skin by compresses or applications of carbolized oil. Once the last crop of blisters has become dry and encrusted, the person is no longer a source of infection. There is no specific treatment for the disease. Chicken pox victims are put on bed rest, fluids, and medications to reduce fever; wet compresses or calamine lotion swabs help to reduce itching. As a rule chicken pox is self-limiting and resolves completely with no adverse effects. Exceptions to that rule are children with LEUKEMIA or those who are immuno-compromised. These children may develop pneumonia or liver problems. Chicken pox pneumonia may occur in adults, leaving many small lung scars, which are seen on chest X-ray pictures after the illness has cleared up.

The virus that causes chicken pox is the same one that causes HERPES ZOSTER (shingles). In fact, shingles—a disease mainly of adults— arises from reactivation of the virus which has remained dormant in the body since an attack of chicken pox during childhood.

chilblain

Hot, red, swollen patches of intensely itchy skin on the toes, feet, fingers, and hands caused by the effect of exposure to cold on small skin blood-vessels. Also known as *pernio*.

Chilblain affects women and children more than men, especially those who are not well protected from exposure to the cold.

Acute chilblain usually disappears after a few days, but it can become *chronic*, with dull violet discoloration of the skin and the appearance of painful blisters containing blood-stained fluid. Ulceration may follow. Repeated exposure to cold may produce several areas of chronic chilblain that leave scars on healing.

Prevention of chilblain is easier than cure; the condition hardly ever occurs in people who wear enough warm, dry clothes (including gloves and footwear) in the colder seasons.

childbirth

The birth of a child either by way of the vagina (vaginal delivery) or by surgical means (see CE-SAREAN SECTION under **Procedures**).

By teaching the expectant mothers the physiology and anatomy of childbirth and how to achieve good muscular relaxation through con-trolled breathing, it is possible to shorten labor, control pain, and reduce muscular tension during labor to such an extent that a minimum of medication is needed—or in some cases no medication at all.

In normal labor there are three stages. The first stage consists of a series of contractions of the muscles of the uterus to allow the cervix (neck of the uterus) to open. The baby starts to descend through the pelvis during the second stage when its presenting part, usually the back of the head, has passed through the fully opened cervix. At some time during this process the "bag of waters" that has enclosed the baby bursts and the fluid escapes.

After the beginning of the second stage of labor the mother is able to aid the delivery by pushing with her abdominal muscles in time with the frequent pains or contractions of the muscles of the uterus. As the baby's head descends through the pelvis it may press upon nerves, causing pain in the back and legs. Pressure of the head on the vaginal outlet gives a sensation of fullness in the anus and a flattening of the outlet. The appearance of the baby's head at the outlet is called "crowning."

In normal childbirth the nape of the baby's neck rests behind the mother's pubis. With the final push the head is expelled, the neck extending as it does so that the narrowest dimension of the skull is presented for passage through the narrow pelvic outlet. The back of the skull is delivered first, then the forehead, face, and chin.

During a brief period of rest, the baby's head slowly rotates, to face one of the mother's thighs. This allows easy delivery of the shoulders with the next contraction, and the rest of the baby quickly follows. With the baby comes the remainder of the amniotic fluid and a little blood. The womb is now contracted and can be felt through the stomach wall as a firm, ball-shaped mass.

The umbilical cord is tied, clamped, and cut. The baby should have gasped and cried on being born. It will be checked briefly by the obstetrician, nurse, or pediatrician, then passed to the cradling arms of the mother (if she is conscious).

Childbirth is not complete until the PLACENTA, or "afterbirth," is delivered, usually ten to fifteen minutes after the baby.

In a number of cases the obstetrician will consider that it is dangerous for the baby to be born through the natural birth passages and will advise delivery by cesarean section. In such cases an incision is made through the lower part of the ab-

CHILDBIRTH

THE THREE STAGES OF LABOR

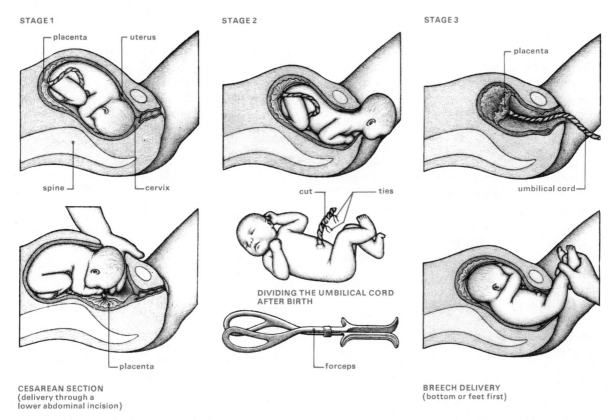

STAGE 1 — placenta, uterus, spine, cervix

STAGE 2 — cut, ties

DIVIDING THE UMBILICAL CORD AFTER BIRTH — forceps

STAGE 3 — placenta, umbilical cord

CESAREAN SECTION (delivery through a lower abdominal incision) — placenta

BREECH DELIVERY (bottom or feet first)

During Stage 1 of labor, which often lasts as long as twelve to sixteen hours, the cervix or exit from the uterus widens so that the baby can pass through. Stage 2, begins when the cervix is fully open and ends, in under an hour, with the delivery of the baby. Stage 3, expulsion of the placenta and umbilical cord, takes only five minutes. The use of forceps or delivery by cesarean section is sometimes necessary to assist childbirth.

domen and the lower part of the uterus, through which the child is delivered.

See the extended discussion under *Pregnancy and Childbirth* in the section on **Family Medicine and Health**.

chill

The popular name for an attack of shivering accompanied by the sensation of being cold, resulting from a disturbance of the nerve centers in the brain that regulate body temperature. Despite the feeling of being cold, the person may have a fever. Typically the chill occurs as the fever rises; when the fever breaks, the chill stops abruptly and the person perspires profusely.

Most "chills" are due to minor viral infections of the nose, throat, or chest; but an unexplained fever may be due, for example, to bacterial blood poisoning (septicemia), to infection of the kidneys or bladder, or to a protozoal infection such as MALARIA.

Whatever the cause of a fever, treatment should include plenty of fluids to replace those lost in sweat. If the temperature rises above 104°F (40°C) the person may be cooled by sponging the chest and forehead with cool but not ice-cold water. Persistence of a fever for more than forty-eight hours or the development of further symptoms provides grounds for seeking medical advice.

chiropractic

A method of treatment that assumes that anatomical faults cause functional disturbances in the body and that, therefore, illnesses can be treated by "manipulation"—particularly of the spine. The specialty of chiropractic began with the ancient techniques of "bonesetting." Eventually, chiropractors began to treat all types of strains, sprains, and dislocations. Well before the end of World War II, the practitioners of spinal or skeletal manipulation considered themselves far more than mere bonesetters; they firmly believed that they had helped to develop a new system of medicine.

As probably the most successful form of nonmainstream medicine (with about 40,000 practitioners in the United States alone), chiropractic has in the past been fiercely opposed by the American Medical Association (AMA). Nevertheless, it has prospered since it was founded a century ago by Daniel David Palmer, and an estimated forty million Americans are receiving or have received treatment from a chiropractor, the great majority for back complaints.

Palmer believed that minor displacements of bones in the spine lead to nerve irritation and that this, in turn, leads to illness. The theory holds that if the chiropractor manipulates the spine to correct the anatomical faults, the pressure on the involved nerves will be relieved. This is maintained to be beneficial for the course of the illness.

Some practitioners make wide and medically unjustified claims for chiropractic (including the ability to treat organic diseases such as cancer); this is one of the main reasons for the AMA's opposition. In virtually every state, however, chiropractic is recognized by insurance companies as a legitimate form of medical treatment.

In addition to straightforward manipulation, chiropractors use such orthopedic techniques as immobilization and traction. They also use a wide range of special electrical or mechanical devices in therapy, including those that employ ultrasonics, vibrotherapy, and electric currents.

chloasma

A localized brown coloration in the skin associated with PREGNANCY or the MENOPAUSE.

Chloasma is most obvious on the face, but it also occurs on the nipples and around the genitals. The cause is thought to be a disturbance in hormone production that leads to a rise in the amount of melanin (brown pigment) formed in the deeper layers of the skin. It may occur in women using oral contraceptives. Although chloasma is sometimes disfiguring, it usually disappears at the end of pregnancy or after the menopause.

In severe or persistent cases, some success in reducing the pigment has been achieved with drugs. Surgical "planing" of the affected area sometimes is performed to remove the discoloration.

Very rarely, chloasma is a sign of an ovarian tumor.

cholecystitis

Inflammation of the gallbladder, usually associated with the presence of gallstones.

Acute cholecystitis is the most common form of the disease and may appear merely as "indigestion" along with tenderness and pain on the upper right side of the abdomen. More severe cases include spasm of the abdominal muscles. When gentle pressure on the spot is released, a flash of pain is experienced—a phenomenon called "rebound tenderness."

The body temperature usually is raised to more than 102°F (38.9°C), and nausea and vomiting are very common. Jaundice occurs in about 25 percent of patients.

The diagnosis can be confused initially with peptic ulcer or acute appendicitis, but it is confirmed by the estimation of several enzymes in the blood and by EKG and X-ray investigations.

Treatment of acute cases is surgical removal of the gallbladder. Most surgeons prefer early excision; others like to wait a few days, during which time they administer intravenous fluids and antibiotics. Tube feeding may be given to rest the intestines.

Chronic cholecystitis is much less common. It is characterized by some tenderness and upper abdominal pain, often felt at night or after eating a fatty meal, but the symptoms are so general as to make the disease hard to diagnose. X-ray studies are essential for accurate diagnosis. Treatment commonly requires surgical removal of the gallbladder.

cholera

A serious bacterial infection of the small intestine.

Cholera is caused by infection with comma-shaped bacteria known as *Vibrio cholerae* (or *Vibrio comma*). It occurs most often in India and other parts of Southeast Asia. Epidemics of cholera arise when people come into contact with water or food contaminated by the feces of infected persons. Outbreaks thus reflect unsanitary living conditions. The severity of the disease can vary widely. On occasion it is fairly mild, but in some outbreaks up to 50 percent or more of those infected have died.

The symptomless incubation period may be as long as six days, but once the illness starts, it is dramatic. The most prominent symptom is watery diarrhea, in which gray "rice water" stools are passed almost nonstop. Fluid loss may be as much as 20 quarts (19 liters) in a day. The liquid stools are flecked with mucus and there is little or no sign of fecal matter. There may also be vomiting, and the catastrophic loss of body fluid causes cramps and collapse. There is little or no output of urine, and without prompt medical treatment, death can occur within forty-eight hours. In the mild case, however, complete recovery typically occurs within one to three weeks.

The key to the treatment of cholera is replacement of water and salts lost in the diarrhea. If treatment is given early the fluid may be taken by mouth, but in severe cases the fluid has to be given by direct infusion into a vein. Once this has been accomplished, an antibiotic is given to overcome the bacteria. Vaccination every six months offers some protection for those who must remain in affected regions.

Control or prevention of cholera involves measures to purify public water supplies and the establishment of modern methods of sewage disposal. Also important is abandonment of the practice of fertilizing crops with human waste.

cholesterol

A substance, technically known as a *sterol*, that is found in animal oils and fats, nervous tissue, bile, blood, and egg yolk. Cholesterol is essential in limited amounts for the production of steroids, which include the sex hormones and the hormones of the adrenal glands.

An increased level of cholesterol in the blood has been shown to increase the risk of ATHEROSCLEROSIS, which is the deposit of fatty plaques on the inside of the blood vessels. These plaques lead to a narrowing of the diameter of the blood vessels and to heart disease. It has been found that if animal fat in the diet is replaced with vegetable oil containing polyunsaturated fats, the blood

cholesterol level will fall and remain low as long as animal fats are omitted from the diet.

Atherosclerosis affects a great many people in the United States. Although diet modification, exercise, and abstinence from smoking can help in limiting the effects of this disease, the best way of controlling it is through prevention. A restricted intake of butter, cream, fatty meat, and eggs, as well as salt and sugar, will assist in preventing the development of atherosclerosis.

Cholesterol is also responsible for the development of gallstones in the majority of cases. Again, diet modification is important.

See extended discussion under *The Healthy Heart* in the section on **Wellness**.

chondrocalcinosis

Also known as *pseudogout*, this disease is an acute or chronic inflammation of a body joint. It is seen in both men and women over 50 years of age. It affects as much as 5 percent of this older population and is caused by the formation of calcium crystals in the joint.

This condition has a rapid onset: In twelve to thirty-six hours the joint becomes swollen, red, warm, and painful. Although it usually occurs in only one joint at a time, most often the knee, it can progress to other joints such as the shoulder, wrist, elbow, or ankle. Fifty percent of these persons, mostly women, will develop a chronic condition that results in degenerative changes in multiple joints.

Although this condition may mimic arthritis and gout, an accurate diagnosis of chondrocalcinosis is made by examining the joint fluid for the presence of calcium crystals. Treatment is based on the severity of the disease, but usually consists of medications to control pain and swelling.

chondroma

A benign tumor composed of cartilage.

chondromalacia

A rare disease of connective tissue especially involving cartilage, the white gristle-like substance that cushions the joints and plays a structural role (for example, in the nose and ear). Inflammation causes the cartilage to soften and produces deformities such as saddle nose and floppy ears. The windpipe, lungs, and joint cartilages (such as in the knees) can all be affected. Chondromalacia of the patella (kneecap) is most often seen in teenagers and is apparently the result of repeated trauma to that area.

Generalized chondromalacia can occur in men and women of all ages. It is a chronic disease which from time to time flares up to produce pain, reddening of the overlying skin, and swelling of the affected cartilage. Fever and a raised white blood cell count are usually present. The softening effect mentioned above is the aftermath of acute attacks of this kind.

Regular administration of corticosteroid drugs may keep inflammatory episodes to a minimum.

chorditis

Inflammation of the vocal cords. Small inflamed fibrous nodules are found on the surface of one or both cords. These are called "singer's nodes."

Chorditis is especially common in people who repeatedly subject their voices to considerable strain. Heavy smokers and drinkers also are at special risk.

Symptoms vary from slight huskiness or hoarseness of the voice to complete loss, together with pain on swallowing and difficulty in breathing. Diagnosis is made by means of the laryngoscope, which enables the doctor to obtain a direct view of the inflamed parts.

The essential treatment is total rest of the voice; any attempt at its continued use makes things worse. If necessary, thickened sections of the cords can be removed by a minor but delicate operation.

In singers and public speakers there may be the underlying problems of incorrect voice production, in which case speech therapy may be required.

chorea

Disordered movements of the body owing to the lack of muscular control. Normal body movements are unpredictably interrupted by rapid, jerky movements: Walking may suddenly be replaced by disorganized lurching, while the face may grimace and the eyes screw closed. Interference with other muscles may affect breathing and

speaking, and the person is often unable to sit still.

Huntington's chorea was first described in 1872 by a physician, George Huntington, who saw several cases in a family in Long Island, New York. It is a chronic, progressive hereditary disease that affects 5 out of 100,000 people. The symptoms are those of chorea, with progressive mental deterioration. The disease usually does not begin until a person is in his 30s or 40s and results in death five to twenty years after onset.

There are some variations in symptoms. If the disease does not begin until old age, there is usually no mental impairment. Also, in about 6 percent of the cases, muscular rigidity is present rather than the typical uncontrolled body movements. In rare cases where onset begins while the person is still a child, as many as half will have muscular rigidity.

Genetic counseling is of vital importance. The child of a parent with Huntington's chorea has a 50 percent chance of developing the disease. Unfortunately, in cases of obscure family history, a married couple may have a child without knowing that he or she is at risk for the disease. Research is currently under way for diagnosing the disease before symptoms occur.

There is no cure for Huntington's chorea, and medications are used only to reduce the severity of the uncontrolled muscular movements.

Sydenham's chorea, also known as St. Vitus' dance, bears no relation to Huntington's chorea. It is not hereditary and does not involve mental deterioration. This is a childhood disease that has become very rare since the decline in incidence of rheumatic fever, with which it usually is associated. Sydenham's chorea is one of the complications that can occur after infection with a type of bacteria known as *hemolytic streptococci*.

The onset of the disease is usually slow and progressive over a period of months, although about 20 percent of cases show acute dramatic symptoms. In half of the cases abnormal movements are restricted to one half of the body only. The age group most commonly affected is between 5 and 20 years. Psychological changes are common, and the child typically becomes emotionally volatile, irritable, and disobedient.

About a third of patients also show evidence of heart involvement at the same time, although this usually subsides within six months.

Treatment consists of rest and sedation. The chorea resolves within about six months; recurrences occur in about a third of cases but eventually the disease is self-limiting. Sufferers should be reassured.

It is worth noting that women who have had *Sydenham's chorea* in childhood have been known to have a recurrence if they take the contraceptive pill.

choriocarcinoma

A malignant tumor arising in the tissues of the placenta. Most choriocarcinomas follow the evacuation of a hydatidiform mole (an abnormality of the placenta that occurs in one out of every 2,000 births), but 25 percent accompany spontaneous miscarriages or ectopic pregnancies. The remainder occur following a normal pregnancy and delivery. About one third of these tumors occur in women after the age of 40. The tumor appears a few months after pregnancy and induces vaginal bleeding. There may be abdominal pain and discomfort; the tumor may spread to produce secondary growths in the lungs or brain.

Choriocarcinomas secrete a hormone called human chorionic gonadotropin (HCG). The diagnosis of this rare tumor can be made by analyzing the blood for HCG.

Choriocarcinomas are extremely sensitive to chemotherapy. Even those that have spread widely can be cured with multiple drug therapy in a high percentage of persons.

chromosomes

The block of genetic material in the nuclei of all cells in the body. Chromosomes carry the genes—the units responsible for the transmission of parental characteristics to the offspring and also for passing on essential information with each cell division during the development of the embryo, during the growth of a baby into an adult, and throughout life. The material that makes up the chromosomes is deoxyribonucleic acid (DNA); this long-chain molecule provides the "templates" for the formation of the protein-building blocks of the cells of every tissue and organ in the body.

Human cells contain twenty-three pairs of chromosomes: twenty-two are identical pairs, but the twenty-third pair, the sex chromosomes, are identical only in females, who have two X chromosomes. In males the twenty-third pair contains only one X chromosome and a smaller Y chro-

CHROMOSOMES

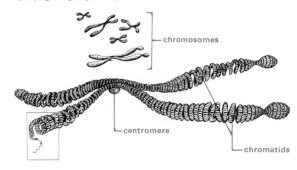

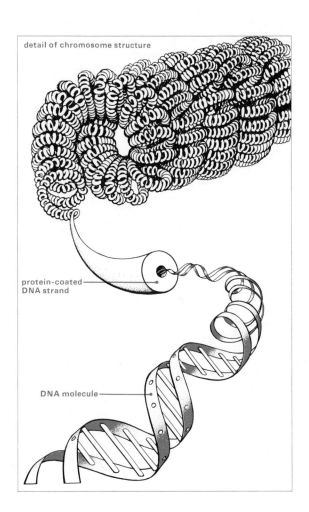

detail of chromosome structure

protein-coated DNA strand

DNA molecule

The chromosomes present in every cell nucleus in the body contain DNA and protein. Each DNA molecule consists of two long chains wound in a double helix. Genes, the units of inheritance derived from both parents, consist of long lengths of DNA chains. By controlling manufacture of the body's proteins, genes are ultimately responsible for each person's characteristics. Except for sex cells (spermatozoa and ova), all human cells contain 46 chromosomes (23 pairs).

mosome. The sex cells themselves (the spermatozoa and ova) contain only half the normal number of chromosomes—one of each of the twenty-three pairs—so that when fertilization takes place, the full complement of forty-six is restored. All ova contain an X chromosome, but sperm may contain either an X or a Y; the sex of a child is thus determined by whether or not the sperm cell that fertilized the ovum carried an X chromosome (giving a girl) or a Y chromosome (giving a boy).

In the process of cell division in the sex organs, which leads to a reduction of the forty-six chromosomes to twenty-three, the chromosomes split and reform so that each sperm or ovum contains a slightly different selection of the genetic characteristics of the parent. This "shuffling of the DNA pack" ensures that children are not carbon copies of each other or of their parents. However, the process is also susceptible to error, and the resulting change or mutation may be either beneficial or harmful. Many congenital defects, such as DOWN'S SYNDROME (mongolism), are due to chromosomal abnormalities. Less obvious mutations are also responsible for disorders such as HEMOPHILIA and MUSCULAR DYSTROPHY, which may then be passed on from one generation to the next.

To determine an individual's chromosome pattern, doctors take a cell sample from anywhere in the body—usually from inside the mouth—and treat it so that the cells divide. On division the chromosomes become visible under the microscope. They are then photographed to be counted carefully later. The technique can be used for prenatal diagnosis of chromosomal abnormality by the examination of fetal cells taken from the womb by AMNIOCENTESIS. (see under **Tests**).

circadian rhythm

Circadian (Latin: *circa*—about, approximate; *dian*—day) rhythm describes an observable daily pattern in the behavior of body processes. For example, temperature, blood pressure, pulse, blood sugar levels, etc., vary slightly within a twenty-four-hour period. Normal body temperature drops at night by a degree or two and climbs steadily during the day to reach a maximum between 6:00 P.M. and 10:00 P.M.

This "internal clock" usually continues to operate even when persons are isolated from time measurements such as clocks and natural sunlight.

The disabling effects of JET LAG have been blamed on the interruption of a person's circadian rhythms, including the important sleep-wake cycle.

cirrhosis

A condition induced in the liver by scarring secondary to the destruction of liver cells by infection, poisoning, or any other cause. The term was coined originally to describe the tawny color of the cirrhotic liver as seen after death. The essential feature of cirrhosis, however, is that much of the liver is replaced with a thick fibrous tissue; the relatively few remaining normal liver cells are left to cope with the vast functions of the organ.

Cirrhosis may follow virus HEPATITIS (infectious jaundice), and it is also commonly seen in association with ALCOHOLISM (*alcoholic cirrhosis*). Cirrhosis may also develop as a complication of HEART FAILURE (*cardiac cirrhosis*). Whatever the cause, the features of the disorder are due partly to the failure of the liver cells to carry out their normal functions and partly to *portal hypertension*—a raised pressure in the veins draining into the scarred liver from the intestinal tract.

In an attempt to compensate for the deficiency of normal liver cells, the organ often initially increases in size; enlargement of the liver (hepatomegaly) is one of the early signs of the disease.

Liver cell failure leads to a whole range of biochemical defects. Accumulation of breakdown products causes the yellow discoloration of the skin (JAUNDICE). The amount of protein in the blood is reduced, leading to retention of fluid and swelling of the abdomen (ASCITES). Blood clotting may be slower than normal. In the later stages of the disorder the breath may have a characteristic sweet smell and an increase in the ammonia content of the blood may cause mental disturbances and eventually coma.

The portal hypertension causes the spleen to enlarge (SPLENOMEGALY), and the raised pressure may lead to bleeding into the stomach from engorged varicose veins at the lower end of the esophagus.

When cirrhosis is due to alcoholic poisoning, the condition may be halted if drinking is stopped. In some other forms of cirrhosis the progress of the disease may be slowed by treatment with drugs. The symptoms may be relieved by a diet containing little protein, and fluid retention may be reduced by diuretic drugs. The complication of portal hypertension may require surgical treatment. In some cases the pressure in the portal vein may be lowered by diverting the blood flow into an alternative pathway, a surgical procedure known as a *portocaval shunt.*

claustrophobia

Fear of closed spaces or of being shut in (see PHOBIA). It is natural for everyone to feel some fear of confined spaces, since there are circumstances in which one might be trapped in a narrow cave passage, a wrecked automobile, or a closet or small room where the door has swung shut and can be opened only from the outside. The claustrophobic person, however, finds it unbearable merely to be in a closed room or the inside of a building, even though he is free to open the door and walk out.

Such a phobic condition may prove severely disabling, preventing the person from entering a vehicle to travel to work or from entering the building in which he works. In such circumstances he may develop over-breathing, rapid heartbeat with palpitations, sweating, and other symptoms of panic.

Treatment of all phobias is difficult. Psychotherapy may be useful if it can uncover the original reason for the development of the phobia.

Another useful form of therapy is *desensitization,* in which the person is either exposed to the feared situation or is instructed to imagine himself in it while being continually reassured and encouraged by the therapist. This process may be assisted by the use of tranquilizing drugs.

There are also anxiety clinics where a combination of medication and supportive counseling has shown promising results. A cooperative and sympathetic relative may also be of great help.

The prognosis remains uncertain, however; many persons subsequently relapse despite initially successful therapy.

cleft lip/cleft palate

Cleft lip and cleft palate are developmental deformities present at birth. Besides the obvious and

CLEFT LIP/CLEFT PALATE

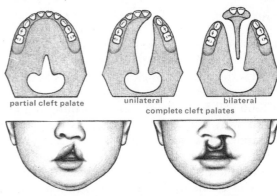

partial cleft palate   unilateral   bilateral
complete cleft palates

unilateral cleft lip   bilateral cleft lip

The face, lips, and palate normally form in the embryo by the fusion of several different components. About one baby in every 500 is born with a cleft deformity caused by failure of this fusion process. There is a wide spectrum of cleft defects ranging from minor lip notching to bilateral complete clefts of the lip and palate.

distressing physical disfigurement, the condition often presents feeding problems as well as difficulties with speech and hearing. However, modern plastic surgery usually can provide remarkable repair of even the most severe deformities.

Clefts of the lip and palate arise because of a flaw in the processes of tissue fusion that normally take place early in the development of the fetus. Defects may vary from minor nasal and lip notching to deep splits running the full length of the roof of the mouth and dividing the upper lip at either side.

Cleft lip and palate occur in two to three liveborn babies in every thousand, with males affected more than females. There may be a family history of deformity.

The treatment of a child with cleft palate involves a team of surgical and other specialists who follow the child's progress into adult life. Normally the lip is repaired at the age of 3 months and the palate at 12 to 15 months; major surgery involving the hard palate usually is postponed until late adolescence. In addition to correcting the deformity of the hard palate (which forms the roof of the mouth), the surgeon also examines the soft palate at the back for less obvious defects.

The child should return to the clinic for regular checkups and correction of any minor defects that may arise with growth. Speech, hearing, and dental problems require special attention and help.

clonus

A rhythmic muscular spasm characterized by alternate contraction and relaxation. It is to be contrasted with *tonus*, in which the muscle is held in a partial but steady contraction.

Clonus of the ankle or foot is encountered in persons with spastic diseases such as PARAPLEGIA and paralytic HEMIPLEGIA. When the foot is forcibly flexed (tipped up) with the knee extended, rhythmic clonic movements occur at the ankle joint. This is one of the tests used in the examination of such persons.

Clonic facial spasm is nearly always confined to elderly people, usually women. Almost without exception it is restricted to one side of the face, and the person suffers from the embarrassing problem of involuntary winking. Botulinum toxin is now being used to treat this condition.

Clonus is one of the possible signs of cramp, experienced as jerky, painful muscle contractions. Cramp is brought on usually by poor blood circulation, as in cases of varicose veins, but it may arise in healthy people engaged in strenuous activity. Treatment of the condition involves stretching the contracted muscles.

Clonus sometimes is found in people who are anxious, and it often affects healthy people who are under stress; they may notice rhythmic contractions of the calf muscles when the foot is pressed on the ground so as to stretch the Achilles tendon. In those cases clonus is of no significance.

clubbing

Clubbing of the fingers and sometimes the toes refers to an overgrowth of hard tissue in the region of the nailbed. It was first described by Hippocrates in the fifth century B.C. in persons suffering from tuberculosis of the lung. Finger clubbing is present in approximately one third of persons with lung cancer, but it is seen also in a great variety of respiratory and other diseases.

The first stage in clubbing involves a filling-in of the angle between the nail and the surrounding skin. The nailbed thickens and the top joints of the finger expand so that the finger resembles a drumstick.

Besides the link with lung cancer, finger clubbing may be a sign of fungal infection of the nailbed or diseases of the heart, liver, and thyroid gland; *in some cases it may be an inherited trait and represent no cause for concern*. Clubbing can arise in *hypertrophic osteoarthropathy,* a condition that produces severe joint pain and in about 80 percent of cases is associated with lung cancer.

The treatment of clubbing necessarily involves treatment of the underlying disorder.

clubfoot

A deformity, present at birth, that prevents the foot from being placed flat on the ground. Boys are affected twice as often as girls. Clubfoot may also be acquired as a result of paralytic disease such as POLIOMYELITIS, or it may be associated with a spinal abnormality.

The main defect is usually in the heel, which is pulled inward and upward so that the afflicted person walks on his toes. In another form, the toes are pulled back and the person walks on his heel. The foot itself may be twisted so that only either the outer or inner edge of the sole touches the ground. The foot arch is often abnormally high. Usually both feet are affected.

The structural faults in uncorrected clubfoot are due to defects in the shape and alignment of the bones of the foot. However, there may be secondary contractures in the soft tissues and shortening and tightening of the Achilles tendon and ligaments. Children with clubfoot can be divided into two main groups: (1) those with flexible clubfoot and less severe deformity and contracture, and (2) those with rigid clubfoot and poorly developed muscles, a small heel, and a deformed forefoot.

The key to successful reversion of clubfoot is early treatment, particularly in cases of flexible clubfoot, where the outlook is good. Manual manipulation of the deformed soft tissue should begin immediately after birth so that the various parts of the foot can be coaxed into proper alignment. If this is not done the rapidly developing bones of the foot may be irreversibly distorted. It is common for the surgeon to teach the various manipulative techniques to the parents so that therapy can continue at home. Correction is maintained by strapping and splinting the foot.

If manipulation is not completely successful, surgical correction of clubfoot is performed usually when the child is 3 months old. The foot is then kept in a plaster cast for about six weeks. Special boots are worn for at least two years thereafter.

Surgery in adolescence usually is reserved for

VARIETIES OF CLUBFOOT

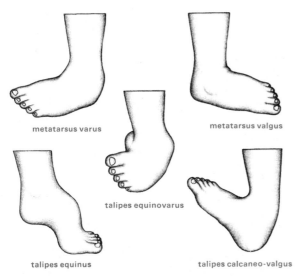

metatarsus varus

metatarsus valgus

talipes equinovarus

talipes equinus

talipes calcaneo-valgus

"Clubfoot" usually refers to talipes equinovarus (center, above), a relatively common congenital deformity of unknown cause. The other varieties are much less common. The deformity can be corrected if treated immediately after birth.

the person with crippling painful deformity. Today the frequency of such interventions is decreasing—evidence of the value of early manipulative treatment.

coccidioidomycosis

A fungal infection that first attacks the lungs and can spread to the skin, bones, and brain. It consistently arises in people living in desert areas of the United States and Central America. The disease is picked up by breathing in dust from soil contaminated with microscopic spores of the fungus *Coccidioides immitis*. For this reason farm laborers often are affected.

Coccidioidomycosis usually produces a mild influenza-like illness; these symptoms disappear for a period of time. Later, new problems develop, which last for weeks to years. These include low fever, appetite and weight loss, bluish skin, and breathing difficulty. In addition, sputum is tinged with blood, skin sores develop, and painful bones and joints are noted.

Dissemination occurs rarely and may result in meningitis or lesions in the organs. These consist of patches of dead tissue surrounded by inflam-

mation. They may involve the lungs, bones, bowels, or brain.

colic

Any severe abdominal pain of a spasmodic nature resulting from muscle spasm in the wall of a hollow organ. Types of colic include biliary, renal, and intestinal colic. It is experienced also in certain types of poisoning and in appendicitis. Treatment involves rest, pain-killing medications, and correction of the cause occasionally by surgery.

colitis

Inflammation of the lining of the large intestine (colon). It begins most often in people in their 30s and is a chronic condition characterized by sudden repeated attacks separated by periods of remission. Colitis should not be confused with the far less serious complaint of *spastic colon*, which is caused by emotional factors.

Among the possible causes of colitis are bacterial infection of the intestine, food allergies (especially milk), and genetic factors. In most cases, however, the cause is unknown or at least not documented.

Colitis may begin insidiously or suddenly. In about half of its victims the first indications are malaise (a general feeling of being unwell), vague abdominal discomfort, and mild diarrhea or constipation. As more severe signs and symptoms appear, such as lower abdominal pain or bleeding from the rectum (indicative of a condition known as ULCERATIVE COLITIS), the person usually seeks medical advice. If the disease strikes abruptly there is worsening fever, bloody diarrhea, loss of appetite, and weight loss. This happens in about a third of cases.

The first step in the diagnosis of colitis is direct visual inspection of the walls of the intestine with an endoscope (sigmoidoscope). A small sample of the diseased tissue is removed for further examination and to test for the presence of infection. X-ray studies of the intestine are done also. Further tests may be needed to rule out diseases such as colonic cancer, diverticulitis, and infectious enteritis, which can coexist with colitis or produce similar symptoms.

Persons with colitis are classified on the basis of the severity of their symptoms. Those with mild disease can be treated at home and allowed a normal diet. A second "moderate" group usually is cared for in the hospital; in addition to the appropriate drug therapy, these patients receive a high-protein diet with replacement of salts and fluids lost during bouts of diarrhea and bleeding. Seriously ill persons may require blood transfusions and surgical removal of all or part of the intestine and a COLOSTOMY (see **Procedures**).

collagen diseases

A group of disorders affecting connective tissue, which is largely made up of collagen, a protein of exceptional strength. These diseases are all associated with inflammation of small blood vessels (vasculitis) and some of them are due to the production of antibodies to cell nuclei, including anti-DNA antibodies. They include systemic LUPUS ERYTHEMATOSUS, POLYARTERITIS NODOSA, RHEUMATOID ARTHRITIS, progessive systemic sclerosis, POLYMYALGIA RHEUMATICA, Wegner's granulomatosis and DERMATOMYOSITIS.

Systemic lupus erythematosus occurs mainly in women between the ages of 20 and 50. It may start with symptoms of arthritis and pain in the muscles, pleurisy and pneumonia, the passage of protein in the urine, myocarditis (inflammation of the heart muscle), anemia, enlargement of the spleen, skin rashes, hepatitis, or a combination of these. The diagnosis is made by specific blood tests. Treatment includes rest, analgesics, and the administration of corticosteroids.

In polyarteritis nodosa the signs and symptoms are varied; they include weight loss, fever, high pulse rate, chronic bronchitis, recurrent pneumonia, abdominal pain, acute diarrhea, passage of protein in the urine, arthritis, and pain in the muscles. The treatment resembles that used for systemic lupus erythematosus.

Women are affected more frequently than men by rheumatoid arthritis; the usual age at onset is between 20 and 50. It is fairly common, but the incidence is lower in the tropics than in temperate climates. Some studies put the incidence as high as 3 percent of the adult population. There is usually a preliminary illness lasting a number of weeks with raised pulse rate, fatigue, loss of weight, sweating, and discomfort in the limbs. This is followed by the development of arthritis in the hands, which spreads to affect the wrists and elbows; the feet, ankles, and knees may also be affected. These joints become hot, swollen, and painful, and there is wasting of the muscles that

act on the joints. There may be anemia, and nodules may be found in the skin.

Treatment includes rest, with physical therapy directed at joints and muscles. Salicylates and other anti-inflammatory drugs usually are prescribed. Gold salts by injection may be used under strict medical supervision, and the drug penicillamine is also useful. In chronic disease, orthopedic surgery may have much to offer; for example, hip joints crippled by chronic rheumatoid arthritis may be restored by hip replacement.

Colles' fracture

This fracture of the wrist is quite common at all ages, but especially in women over 40. Colles' fracture usually is caused by a heavy fall on the outstretched hand.

The fractured bone is the *radius*, which runs from elbow to wrist on the thumb side. Usually

COLLES' FRACTURE

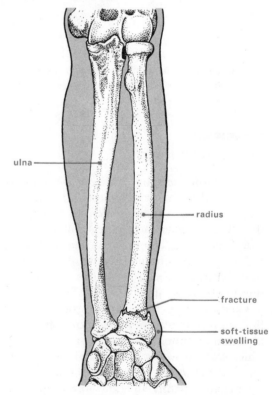

ulna

radius

fracture

soft-tissue swelling

Colles' fracture of the lower end of the radius results from falling onto the outstretched hand and is very common in elderly persons. This is partly because the elderly tend to fall heavily, and also because their bones are brittle.

it is broken across, within 1 inch of the wrist. The force of the blow displaces the separated end a little sideways, toward the thumb side and backward, moving the hand with it. This gives the characteristic "dinner fork deformity"—the forearm being the "handle" of the fork with a depression just before the wrist, and the hand forming the curved "prongs" of the fork. Very often the other bone of the forearm (the *ulna*) is also involved, its lower and outer tip (the *styloid process*) being detached; the cartilage of the wrist joint also may be damaged.

Treatment generally requires an anesthetic, under which the bones are manipulated back to their correct positions. The wrist and the forearm to above the elbow are then immediately immobilized in a plaster cast. The fingers and the further end of the palm are left free so that the fingers can move fully. It is often necessary to take another X ray soon after immobilization to make sure that correction has been maintained.

The cast has to be worn for up to six weeks, after which light work can be undertaken; heavy work should not be resumed for about another six weeks. While the wrist is in a cast, it is imperative that the fingers and shoulders be exercised several times a day to prevent them from stiffening and thereby causing limited use of the entire hand even after the fracture has healed. After the cast is off, the person will need physical therapy for the wrist, to increase both flexibility and strength.

colon cancer

Cancer of the large intestine (colon) is the third most frequent cancer in men, after lung and prostate cancer. In women it is the second most frequent, after breast cancer.

Predisposing factors include ulcerative colitis and papillomatous conditions of the intestine. There may be a hereditary factor, and diet is thought to play a part in the development of colonic tumors.

The most common warning symptom is an alteration in bowel habits. Some colon cancers cause intestinal obstruction whereas others cause discomfort, weight loss, and anemia.

The main drawback to successful treatment is that most lesions do not produce symptoms until late in their course and are usually advanced on initial diagnosis. Earlier diagnosis can be achieved through regular proctosigmoidoscopy and stool tests for occult blood.

Surgery is the primary method of treatment, with the aim of removing the tumor completely and restoring the continuity of the bowel. It may be necessary during surgery to use a temporary colostomy (formation of an artificial anal opening), but the end result is designed to avoid the necessity of permanent colostomy. Overall results are much better than those of surgery for cancer of the lung or stomach.

color blindness

An abnormality of the eye in which a person cannot accurately distinguish colors. The most common forms involve a relative insensitivity to red and green. This form of color blindness affects about 10 percent of men. It is very rare in women. Total color blindness (also called *monochromatism* or *achromatic vision*) is the inability to perceive any color at all. This is extremely rare.

Color blindness is present from birth and persists throughout life. It is a sex-linked condition inherited from the mother, who nearly always has normal color vision but carries a defective "color gene," on one x-chromosome. Congenital color blindness cannot be corrected.

coma

A state of deep unconsciousness marked by the absence of eye movements and of response to pain and sound. The person cannot be awakened. Coma may result from brain damage due to head injury, intracranial bleeding, tumor, infection with brain inflammation, or massive blood loss. Other causes include electric shock, diabetes, poisoning, liver failure, and the ingestion of too much alcohol.

Treatment of coma is directed toward the underlying cause; but in all cases it is imperative that the airway be kept clear.

A patient who is comatose will require artificial feeding by an intravenous infusion of nutrients.

common cold

A viral infection of the upper respiratory passages. If differs from other respiratory infections in that fever is most often absent and the symptoms are generally milder. Modern research has revealed that any one (or a combination) of more than a hundred different viruses can cause a cold. Colds are spread by direct person-to-person contact, although some people can become infected and spread the cold viruses without having any symptoms.

Colds are more widespread in winter: About half the American population picks up a cold during the winter. This figure drops in the summer.

The precise symptoms of the common cold vary from one individual to the next. Some people always seem to get "head" colds whereas others suffer from pharyngitis or cough. The first signs of a cold usually are sneezing, headache, and a general feeling of ill health (malaise). Then come chilly sensations, a sore throat, and heavy nasal discharge. Often, after a brief respite, the person progresses to the classic symptoms of the common cold, chief of which is nasal congestion as the mucus changes from being clear and thin to being thick, tenacious, and yellow-green in color. By this stage the sore throat normally has disappeared, but cough may become an increasing problem and last until the cold has completely resolved (generally in one to two weeks).

Because so many viruses can cause a cold, and because the illness is short and readily dealt with by the body's natural defenses against infection, doctors usually recommend only supportive treatment. This means bed rest and warm clothing to make the person feel more comfortable. If breathing difficulties occur, drugs such as expectorants and nasal decongestants may be used. Aspirin is effective in relieving headache and malaise. Physicians tend to frown on the exotic "cocktails" of vitamins, multiple pain-killers, antihistamines, tranquilizers, and so on, that are widely advertised as the remedy for colds. Antibiotic drugs are helpful only when a secondary bacterial infection closely follows a cold, a relatively common event.

complex

An organized collection of emotions and ideas of which the individual may not be fully aware but which strongly influence his attitudes and behavior.

The *Oedipus complex* is one of the main planks of PSYCHOANALYSIS, Freud's method of psychiatric treatment. It refers to a distinct group of linked ideas, instincts, and fears that are observed most commonly in male children between 3 to 6 years and form a normal part of development. During this period a boy's sexuality is at a peak and is directed primarily toward his mother, accompanied by feelings of hostility toward his father. Baby girls go through a similar phase, but this time sexual interest is centered on the father and aggression on the mother (the *Electra complex*). At the age of 5 or 6, this peak of sexual development subsides and the Oedipus complex normally passes.

In our society it is typical for parents to discourage overly intense expression of infant sexuality. This in itself is not wrong provided that it does not become an excuse for rigorous repression. With firm but loving direction, sexual and aggressive impulses can be channeled into constructive activities such as learning and play. Parents must certainly guard against viewing infant sexuality as abnormal or wicked.

A number of complexes relate to adolescent or adult life. One of the most widely known is the *inferiority complex*, in which the individual experiences an acute sense of inadequacy; this manifests as extreme shyness or compensatory aggressiveness. The *Cain complex* refers to excessive jealousy of a brother, and the *Diana complex* to ideas leading to the adoption of masculine behavior by a female. These terms are essentially descriptive and should not be understood as implying mental disorder.

"Complex" is often used to describe feelings of apprehension or fear directed toward some particular object, person, or social situation. To some extent such tensions are normal, but if they become severe they can cripple an individual's behavior. They are then more properly described as *anxiety states*, *phobias*, or *obsessions*, depending on their exact nature. Persons with these disorders usually need psychiatric help.

concussion

An injury resulting from impact with an object, a common result of a blow to the head. This usually causes temporary or prolonged unconsciousness.

If uncomplicated, the person regains consciousness in a short time; there may be vomiting, rapid pulse, flushed face, restlessness, and headache for twelve to twenty-four hours. In severe cases a loss of memory may follow.

The mechanism of concussion is not fully understood, but it is thought that at the time of injury there is a wave of very high pressure inside the skull that is transmitted to the brain. This may produce many small pinpoint hemorrhages; the concussion is assumed to stop the higher centers of the brain from working for a time, although the lower centers continue to function. It is probable that the injury suffered by the brain in concussion differs in degree rather than in kind from the more severe injuries that result in coma.

condyloma

A flat, moist skin lesion raised from the surface like a wart. They usually affect the genital area of the body and can occur in both sexes at any time.

Condylomas are of two main types: those caused by the common wart virus but spread as venereal warts (*condylomata acuminata*), and those that appear during the secondary stage of syphilis (*condylomata lata*). The latter are not related to common skin warts.

In recent years viral condylomas have become increasingly common. They are infectious and transmitted by direct sexual contact. Beginning as small pinpoint spots, they rapidly enlarge to form soft clusters of red or yellow warts. Condylomas thrive in moist regions of the body, which accounts for their tendency to infect the penis, anus, and vulva. Small condylomas can be treated with applications of a drug called podophyllin, which erodes and destroys the warts over a short period of time. Larger lesions may be removed with cryosurgery, a freezing technique, or with laser surgery. Because of their tendency to recur, treatment may have to be done several times.

Recent research has shown that some forms of condylomata acuminata can lead to cancer. This is especially true for warts that appear on the cervix and underlines the need for prompt treatment and regular medical follow-up. Sexual partners of those with venereal warts also require treatment. Because of the slow growth and appearance of the warts (up to six months after exposure), reinfection with the virus can occur.

The condylomas of secondary syphilis are usually about half an inch or less in diameter and often appear in large numbers grouped closely together on the vulva and around the anus. They have a pink or violet color and may cause the skin surface to break down to form a shallow gray-pink ulcer that exudes a sticky pus-like fluid. Examination of a sample of this fluid under a microscope reveals the presence of the highly mobile *Treponema* spirochete and enables the doctor to distinguish between these and viral condylomas. These lesions are highly infectious.

congenital dislocation of the hip

The hip is a ball-and-socket joint, where the ball (the head of the femur) fits into the socket (acetabulum). Some children are born with hips in which the tough fibrous tissue that surrounds this joint is unnaturally lax, causing the joint to be unstable and easily dislocated. The deformity tends to run in families.

All newborns are given a complete physical examination which includes checking for dislocation of one or both hips. When it is found early in life, relatively simple measures can be taken to correct the deformity. The child is fitted with flexible splints that hold the legs apart so that the femur head rests properly in the socket. This treatment usually cures the condition.

Occasionally, however, the deformity is not noticed until the child begins to walk and develops a characteristic limp and shortened leg. In these cases, a cast may have to be used for months at a time. Older children and adults with this untreated condition may need surgical treatment to repair the dislocation. The older a person is, however, the higher the risk of complications. If left untreated, there is great strain and much wear and tear on the joint, and a complete hip replacement may be needed in later years.

conjunctivitis

Inflammation and swelling of the *conjunctiva*, the membrane that lines the eyelid and covers the front surface of the eyeball. Conjunctivitis is caused by infection, allergy, or an irritant in the eye.

The affected eye feels gritty and burning, the discomfort increasing on movement and blinking. Both eyes soon become inflamed and in most cases there is a yellow, sticky discharge. Antibiotic eyedrops usually are prescribed when bacterial infection is thought to be the cause of the inflammation. The person is warned that the infection can be spread easily through contaminated towels and washcloths, thus he or she must be very careful not to share toilet articles.

In some cases treatment is not immediately successful and the condition becomes chronic. This is sometimes the case in viral infections. Or it may be due to an allergy, since the conjunctiva can become sensitive to a number of cosmetics and drugs.

constipation

A problem in passing stool.

The frequency with which bowel movements occur varies greatly from person to person. It is not necessary to have a bowel movement every day; some quite healthy people have bowel movements every two or three days, others twice or more during the same day. However, when emptying of the rectum is delayed there is increasing reabsorption of water from its contents so that the stools become excessively hard and dry. This in turn may lead to difficulty in passing them at all. The person who has a bowel movement without difficulty every third day has no problem, but if difficulty results, he or she suffers from constipation. In severe cases, the hard feces cannot be passed, but "paradoxical diarrhea" may occur, with fluid feces from the large bowel being passed around the hardened mass of stool.

The causes of constipation include diseases of the bowel itself, an unsuitable diet containing too little roughage or dietary fiber (low-residue diet), and certain neurological disorders resulting in paralysis of the muscular walls of the bowel. Of much greater importance, however, is a failure by the individual to adhere to a regular bowel-opening habit. This may be due to inadequate toilet training as a child, to an unwillingness to open the bowels because of pain from piles or other anal conditions, or, most important, to a willful neglect of the urge to open the bowels because of lack of time, laziness, or other factors.

Treatment of constipation depends on its cause. Any painful condition such as piles must be relieved. A diet containing plenty of dietary fiber should be taken and breakfast should be a meal of adequate bulk. If laxatives have been taken previously, they should be replaced by one of the bulk-producing preparations. In severe cases the bowel may have to be emptied initially by means of enemas or even by manual removal of the dry feces by a doctor or nurse.

contact lens

A small, curved, plastic lens shaped to fit snugly over the cornea. Most contact lenses are used to

CONTACT LENS

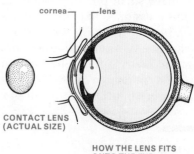

cornea   lens

CONTACT LENS
(ACTUAL SIZE)

HOW THE LENS FITS
ONTO THE EYE

Most of the focusing of light rays takes place at the cornea in the front of the eye, with the lens making further adjustments. Contact lenses, which are placed directly on the cornea, perform exactly the same function as glasses but do so more efficiently.

correct vision problems—which they do more efficiently than glasses. Many are made of polymethylmethacrylate (PMMA), which is a hard, non-permeable plastic, but co-polymers of PMMA and silicon or cellulose acetate butyrate (CAB) are now widely used. Most soft lenses are made of hydroxyethylmethacrylate (HEMA), which is a "hydrogel."

The period for which contact lenses can be worn without interruption depends on the individual and the type of lens; but if the lenses are fitted correctly most people can wear them all day, removing them only at night. Soft lenses can sometimes be left in place longer.

Contact lenses are especially valuable to those with severe refractive errors such as high myopia (nearsightedness) or aphakia (absence of internal lens) following cataract surgery without lens implant. Certain medical conditions are greatly helped by contact lenses. One of these is keratoconus, an abnormality of the cornea.

Most people can wear contact lenses if properly fitted and advised, and if motivation is good.

convulsion

A sudden violent uncontrolled twitching or contraction of a group of muscles in the body caused by an abnormal discharge of electrical activity in the brain. Convulsions are commonly associated with EPILEPSY, being the most disturbing feature of the major epileptic seizure. But they can be brought on by many other disorders, such as

STROKE, MENINGITIS, KIDNEY DISEASE, and HEAT STROKE. In young children convulsions may be caused by high fever.

In the typical convulsive attack, as in the major form of epilepsy, the patient first loses consciousness and falls heavily to the ground, his muscles locked. For a brief period breathing may be impaired, which accounts for a temporary bluish discoloration of the skin. Next comes a series of rapid, jerky, and uncontrolled movements in the trunk and limbs. The jaw and tongue may also be affected, so that sometimes the patient lathers his saliva into a foam and appears to froth at the mouth. The tongue may be badly bitten. This period of frenzied activity usually lasts between two and three minutes. After a few more minutes of unconsciousness the patient generally regains consciousness, often to complain of a severe headache. He may remain in a state of confusion for several hours after an attack.

corns

A painful, localized thickening and hardening of the skin of the foot occurring as a reaction to local pressure, which then forces the hard patch

CORN

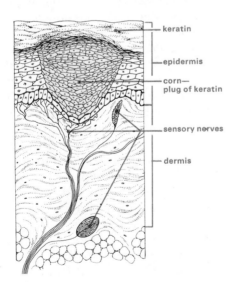

- keratin
- epidermis
- corn— plug of keratin
- sensory nerves
- dermis

A corn is a horny thickening in the skin and may occur at any point of continued pressure. It consists of a compressed mass of keratin (dead skin cells), and usually has a conical shape with a broad base on the skin surface and a point extending down into the dermis. Pain is caused by pressure of the horny plug on nerve endings.

into the skin. (A CALLUS is a thickening over a wider area.)

Corns on the upper part of the toes are caused by wearing tight or badly fitting shoes. Those on the underside of the foot are due to unevenness in the sole of the shoe. Where the skin is pinched or continually rubbed it grows more rapidly and, under the effect of pressure, gradually hardens. Corns between the toes are moist and are referred to as *soft corns.*

The first essential of treatment is to wear sufficiently large and properly shaped shoes (despite the demands of fashion). Shoes should not be pointed; the width of the sole at the level of the little toe should equal that of the bare foot when supporting the full weight of the body.

Corn pads are circular pieces of felt, which, when applied over a corn, give relief by spreading the unwelcome pressure of the shoe over a larger area.

Corns can be removed by soaking the foot in hot soapy water and then carefully cutting away the upper part of the softened corn. The affected area is dried and painted with a salicylic acid solution (included in many corn-removing lotions) to soften the corn even more and break it down. These lotions can damage healthy tissue surrounding the corn and should be used with great care. Corns will inevitably recur unless the causal factors are removed.

If foot problems continue, your physician may be able to recommend a foot specialist.

coronary thrombosis

Blockage by a blood clot forming on a patch of *atheroma* in a branch of one of the arteries that supplies the heart muscle (coronary artery). The obstruction causes myocardial infarction (heart attack). See HEART DISEASE and extended discussion under *The Healthy Heart* in the section on **Wellness.**

cor pulmonale

A condition that can afflict people suffering from lung diseases, such as chronic BRONCHITIS, EMPHYSEMA, and chronic ASTHMA, in which the right side of the heart (leading to the lungs) is overextended.

Acute cor pulmonale often is precipitated by

a lung infection. This worsens an already poor respiratory performance and leads to an oxygen deficiency in the capillary vessels of the lung. These constrict, requiring the right chamber of the heart to pump harder to keep the blood moving. The overall result is a heart working under considerable strain.

The typical signs of cor pulmonale include a bluish discoloration of the skin, especially in the hands and feet (which are often warm to the touch), and there may be swelling of the limbs and ankles.

Stethoscopic examination of the chest may reveal abnormal heart sounds. The electrocardiogram (EKG), which provides a graphic record of the heart rhythm, typically contains various abnormalities.

The main danger in cor pulmonale is failure of the overworked heart, specifically the right side. Treatment is aimed at improving lung performance, and antibiotics such as tetracycline and ampicillin may be administered to overcome the pulmonary infection. Persons suffering from severe breathing difficulties frequently receive oxygen therapy.

cosmetic surgery

Cosmetic surgery has become increasingly popular during the last twenty years; about a million Americans a year now have "image-enhancing" operations.

Disfiguring facial deformities sustained by servicemen during World War I provided a great impetus to the development of *plastic surgery,* from which cosmetic surgery evolved. The public still tends to identify "plastic surgery" only with elective cosmetic surgery, but the subspecialty also deals with cosmetic repair following injuries like burns and removal of tumors. Here, however, we will discuss only those operations designed to improve outward appearance and sought by the patient.

The work falls into three broad categories: (1) removal of blemishes and scars, (2) repair of congenital defects, and (3) improvements in contour. Most cosmetic operations are designed to eliminate wrinkles and pouches of baggy tissue in order to provide a firmer skin and a more youthful appearance, although one procedure—breast enlargement through silicone implantation—adds rather than removes for its enhancing effect.

Theoretically there is no limit to the amount of cosmetic surgery any one person can have. The effects of a procedure like a face-lift usually last about seven years.

Many persons are afraid that cosmetic surgery will scar them. Scars are inevitable, but they can be hidden beyond the scrutiny of the eye. Any reputable surgeon will advise about treatment and the likelihood of noticeable postoperative scars.

The following are some of the more commonly performed cosmetic operations:

Rhytidectomy (standard face-lift). The surgeon separates the facial skin and part of the skin of the neck through an incision just beyond the hairline. He then pulls the skin up to the temples and back toward the ear, cuts away all the excess, and closes the incision. Persons such as film stars, to whom a youthful appearance is often particularly important, may have several operations over the years.

Rhinoplasty (alteration of the nose). One of the most common surgical procedures. A large nose can be reshaped with the removal of cartilage or bone. Conversely, a sunken or flat nose can be remodeled by implantation of a carved piece of bone or cartilage. No scars are visible, since incisions are made from within the nasal cavity.

Blepharoplasty (eyelid correction). A basically simple technique to improve a tired-looking pair of eyes by removing excess skin from the upper and lower creases of the eyelids. Scars can be concealed in the remaining skin folds.

Supraorbital rhytidoplasty (eyebrow correction). Drooping eyebrows can give a tired look to the eyes. The incision is made above the brow, which is raised with the removal of an ellipse of skin. The suture line can be hidden within the upper hairline of the brow.

Mammoplasty (cosmetic breast surgery). Silicone implants can be used to restore the shape of the breasts after mastectomy; this is an extremely valuable procedure in making necessary mastectomy operations a more tolerable prospect to many women. Other operations can be performed to enhance or reduce the size of the breasts.

Many people have unrealistic expectations about what a change of looks will do for them; thus, any responsible surgeon will subject a potential patient to searching questions about motives. It must be fully understood that cosmetic surgery cannot perform miracles and cannot be used as a means of solving some deep-seated emotional problems, wrongly blamed on external appearance.

cough

A sudden, noisy, forceful release of air from the lungs and air passages in an effort to clear them of excessive mucus or irritating foreign matter.

Any condition that increases the secretion of mucus in the lungs will produce a cough. Coughing can be suppressed by drugs acting on the cough reflex, by drinking soothing liquids, or by adding moisture to the air with a humidifier. Coughs that produce blood require immediate medical attention.

Coxsackie virus

A group of common infecting agents (first isolated in Coxsackie, New York) that produce a wide variety of diseases. Thus, they may produce a condition resembling either the common cold or influenza, with a sore throat and painful neck glands. The sore throat may be accompanied by small blister-like lesions in the back of the throat (a condition known as *herpangina*); similar lesions may appear on the feet and hands as well (*hand, foot, and mouth disease*). The pleura (membrane lining the chest cavity and covering the outer surface of the lungs) may be affected, giving a painful chest condition known as EPIDEMIC PLEURODYNIA, or Bornholm disease. In both children and adults, the heart muscle may be affected (MYOCARDITIS) as well as the membranes surrounding the brain and spinal cord (MENINGITIS).

Infections produced by this group of viruses usually are not serious, though they may be painful and distressing to the persons involved. They are rarely fatal, though some deaths occur among young children.

cramp

A sudden, involuntary, and prolonged spasm of the muscles causing severe pain.

It can occur in the abdominal muscles owing to immersion in cold water (*swimmer's cramp*) or in groups of muscles used continually (for example, *writer's cramp*). Hard physical labor in the heat leads to excessive salt losses by sweating and causes *heat cramp*.

Cramps occur in all age groups, but they tend to be more common in the elderly, especially leg cramps. The cause of leg cramps is unknown, although pregnancy, dehydration, diabetes, gout, alcohol abuse, and certain medications are associated with this painful condition.

The treatment of muscle cramp is to relax the spasm and improve the local circulation. Keep the limb warm, rub and massage it, and avoid excessive fatigue. Heat cramps should be treated by drinking plenty of water to which a little salt has been added.

Night leg cramps are quickly and effectively relieved by quinine taken before retiring. Calcium supplements appear to be effective for leg cramps associated with pregnancy.

cretinism

A congenital condition characterized by retarded physical and mental development caused by a deficiency of thyroid hormone.

Inadequate or absent secretion of hormones by the THYROID GLAND in fetal or early neonatal life retards growth of the skeleton and the brain. This underactivity of the thyroid gland can be the result of a lack of iodine in the diet; it may occur when the mother has been taking thyroid-regulating drugs before or during pregnancy; or it may be due to a biochemical abnormality in the thyroid (sporadic cretinism).

In the first months of life an infant with this condition fails to feed properly and has a protruding tongue, thick dry skin, slow reflexes, and poor muscle tone. These signs in a baby may lead to an early diagnosis. If not, then later, delayed dentition (development of the teeth), constipation, yellow scaling skin, and retarded growth indicate the need for biochemical investigations. The tests will show depressed thyroid function and establish the diagnosis.

It is important to diagnose cretinism early before permanent brain damage occurs. Treatment with thyroid hormone has to be continued, with increasing dosage as the child grows. Early treatment and good control can produce normal development and a complete cure.

crib death (sudden infant death syndrome)

This is the most common mode of death for infants between one month and one year of age and accounts for 30 percent of all deaths in this age group. In spite of agonized public concern and intensive study, the causes remain unknown, and the incidence of this tragic event has not declined. In the US, 3 babies in every 2,000 die in this way.

Sudden infant death syndrome (SIDS) is defined as an unexpected death in which a thorough autopsy fails to reveal a cause. Until recent times, all such deaths were attributed to "overlying" by the mother, and it is clear that, throughout the ages, countless women have been unjustly accused of bringing about, either accidentally or intentionally, the deaths of their infants. But in the past 20 years this attitude has changed, for it has been conclusively proved that sudden death commonly occurs in a baby sleeping alone. Overlying is now rarely proposed as a cause of the SIDS.

The tragedy is more likely to affect a boy baby than a girl and is more likely to occur in winter than in summer. Prematurely born babies are at greater risk than the full term. Black babies are more likely to be affected than white, and SIDS affects poorer families more often than the better off. Those whose mothers smoke during pregnancy and those with narcotic-addicted or alcoholic parents are at greater risk of SIDS. Breast-fed babies are less at risk than bottle-fed babies.

Many studies of cases have been published and many hypotheses proposed. Because of the absence of autopsy findings, the diagnosis of SIDS has to be made by excluding all possible causes, and there are suggestions that if the investigation is thorough enough, a cause can sometimes be found. Some of these deaths have been attributed to oversoft bedding, in which the baby's face becomes buried; some to hypersensitivity to cow's milk; some to unnoticed chest or gastrointestinal infection; and some to biotin deficiency. But, by definition, these cases are not SIDS. The current view of some authorities is that SIDS results from a transient disorder of the neurological control of the breathing and the heart beat.

In most cases death occurs during sleep without any suffering on the part of the child, but the effect on the family is devastating and close support is needed.

Crohn's disease

A long-term inflammatory bowel disease of unknown cause that most often affects the lower small intestine, the main part of the large intestine, or both, causing ulceration and thickening of the intestinal wall.

It is characterized by recurrent episodes of abdominal pain (usually on the lower right side), diarrhea, fever, weight loss, and appetite depression.

Crohn's disease mainly affects young adults, and in the early acute attacks it is often misdiagnosed as appendicitis. There is persistent diarrhea. If the disease is not treated, serious complications such as peritonitis and abscesses may occur. It attacks both men and women and most ethnic groups, although it is unusually common among Jewish people.

Initial symptoms include a low-grade fever, recurrent bouts of diarrhea, weakness, and weight loss. As the attacks get worse and more frequent, diagnosis requires investigation by X rays (a barium enema) and biochemical analysis. The typical X-ray picture confirms the diagnosis.

In approximately a third of the cases the disease eventually resolves by itself and subsides. In the remainder it has to be treated by a high-calorie, high-protein diet and special drugs to relieve the stress and diarrhea. Corticosteroid drugs help in overcoming the acute phase and in bringing about a remission; long-term steroids in low dosage will control symptoms in some people.

Surgery is usually necessary for severe cases and for persons over the age of about 50. Excision of the affected area of the intestine can bring short-term relief in all cases and long-term cure for some. The disease can recur after surgery; such persons are treated with a combination of dietary care, medication, and support.

croup

An inflammation of the larynx ("voice box") leading to difficulty in breathing accompanied by a harsh croaking noise. The medical name is *acute laryngotracheo-bronchitis*. The condition is virtually confined to small children.

Croup is usually a complication of a viral or bacterial infection of the upper respiratory tract. Inflammation in the larynx leads to a narrowing of the gap between the vocal cords which obstructs breathing. The attack usually occurs at night when the child is lying down; breathing becomes strident and difficult, and the child will usually be frightened. Croup can be dangerous if the gap between the vocal cords is completely closed, and urgent treatment in the hospital may be needed to overcome the obstruction either by passing a tube down the windpipe (*intubation*) or by making an opening through the neck into the windpipe (TRACHEOSTOMY; see under *Procedures*).

Once a child has had an attack of croup the inflammation is liable to recur, so he should be guarded against cold, damp conditions, which tend to encourage respiratory disorders. If a child suffers from an attack of croup and is having difficulty breathing, a doctor should always be called. In the meantime, opening the window (in a centrally heated house) may bring relief since an excessively hot, dry atmosphere seems to encourage croup. For the same reason, a vaporizer should be placed in the bedroom. (It is potentially dangerous to increase the humidity of the child's bedroom by means of a boiling kettle or pan, as scalding accidents are not uncommon.) The parent should not panic, but instead show a reassuring and relaxed attitude.

Cushing's syndrome

A disease caused by excessive secretion of the hormone cortisol by the adrenal glands.

Among the signs and symptoms of Cushing's syndrome are: protein depletion, causing muscle wasting and weakness; fragility of the blood vessels, causing increased susceptibility to bruising; decalcification of the bones, causing spinal curvature; occasional biochemical disorders such as diabetes; and—most obvious of all—the "moon face" and "buffalo hump" caused by facial obesity and redistribution of body fat. Women also suffer masculinization: Excessive hair grows on the body, the voice deepens, and menstruation ceases.

Cushing's syndrome is relatively rare, is more common in women than in men, and develops most frequently in women over 30, particularly after a pregnancy.

The complicated disorders of the body seen in Cushing's syndrome—all due to an excess of cortisol hormones—are nowadays more commonly seen as a result of long-term treatment with large doses of cortisone or similar steroid drugs. People who depend on steroids to control such conditions as ASTHMA, RHEUMATOID ARTHRITIS, or COLITIS can develop the characteristic "moon face" of Cushing's syndrome as an early sign of chronic overdosage.

Apart from excessive steroid treatment, the cause of Cushing's syndrome is either a small tumor of one of the adrenal glands (which lie just above the kidneys) or a tumor of the PITUITARY GLAND leading to excessive production of the adrenal-stimulating hormone ACTH. In either case, the tumor must be treated. Pituitary tumors must be surgically removed or, if this proves impossible, treated with supervoltage irradiation. Adrenal tumors can usually be treated by surgery.

The diagnosis is made by careful biochemical assessment of hormone output and, in particular, by measurement of the urinary excretion of cortisone breakdown products over a given period. Skull X-ray studies (to reveal a possible tumor of the pituitary gland) and complicated blood tests also are necessary. Once the diagnosis is made, drugs are necessary to compensate for the chemical, mineral, and other hormonal deficiencies.

When the diseased adrenal gland is removed surgically along with the tumor, the remaining gland is often found to be shrunken. Thus, supplements of the correct amount of cortisone-like hormone are necessary until the other gland recovers function; they may be necessary throughout life.

cyanosis

Blue coloration of the skin due to the presence of HEMOGLOBIN without sufficient oxygen in the blood. Normally most of the pigment (hemoglobin) in the blood is combined with oxygen, giving it a bright red color. If for any reason the blood lacks oxygen a substantial proportion of the pigment is in its "reduced" form, giving the blood a dusky blue color. This is most noticeable in the person's lips, face, fingernails, hands, and feet.

Babies with congenital heart defects, children and adults with diseases causing respiratory or cardiac failure, and the elderly with circulatory or cardiac inefficiency may show signs of cyanosis owing to inadequate oxygenation of the blood. Poor circulation in the limbs may also cause cyanosis—for example, in RAYNAUD'S PHENOMENON, VARICOSE VEINS, or exposure to cold.

The condition is a *sign*—not a disease in itself— and may appear whenever an extra demand is made on a circulatory or respiratory system that cannot cope with more than its normal work. A "blue baby" is cyanosed because some of its blood bypasses the lungs and is therefore not oxygenated. A cardiac invalid may become cyanosed when he sustains a respiratory infection.

Treatment depends on the underlying cause, but if cyanosis appears during an illness, hospitalization and the provision of oxygen are usually necessary. Cardiac surgery may be required for the baby with congenital heart disease.

cyst

An abnormal sac or pouch within the body, usually filled with fluid, semifluid, or solid material (gas-filled cysts occasionally occur).

A common example is a SEBACEOUS CYST. Sebaceous glands in the skin secrete an oily material (sebum) essential to the maintenance of normal skin texture. Blockage of the opening of the gland leads to an accumulation of sebum in the duct of the gland. As the duct becomes greatly dilated, a rounded mass develops immediately beneath the skin, with its walls formed by the original lining of the duct. Such cysts are commonly half an inch in diameter but may occasionally be much larger.

Cysts may occur in any organ that produces a secretion if the duct becomes blocked while secretion continues. Cysts of this type may occur in the breast, mouth, genital tract, in the specialized sebaceous glands in the eyelid (CHALAZION), and in many of the internal organs, such as the ovaries, pancreas, and kidneys. Other types of cysts may occur as the result of imperfect gland development before birth, with the gland forming but its duct being absent. A dermoid cyst occurs when a portion of skin becomes buried in the tissues, either as a result of a penetrating injury or before birth with the joining of two developing skin folds. Occasionally, a tumor may develop a cystic area within itself and eventually come to resemble a cyst.

Cysts may develop also as a result of infection with parasitic worms, which form cystic structures in the tissues at certain stages of their life cycles (*hydatid cyst*).

Treatment of cysts may be unnecessary if they cause no symptoms. If they are unsightly, cause pressure on surrounding structures, or are suspected of originating in a tumor, surgical removal usually is required. In some cases, simple aspiration of the cyst contents is performed to establish its nature.

cystadenoma

An ADENOMA containing cysts.

cystic fibrosis

A hereditary disease that affects the mucus-producing glands in the pancreas, lungs, and intestines, causing thick, sticky mucus to be formed. It is one of the most common life-threatening genetic diseases in white people, affecting one in 1,500 to 2,500 births. It is very rare in black people and Orientals.

The pancreas is an abdominal organ responsible for producing insulin and substances necessary for proper digestion. In cystic fibrosis there is obstruction of the pancreatic ducts and therefore a deficiency or total absence of its secretions. This leads to an inability to digest fats and can lead to malnourishment and malnutrition. In most cases insulin is still produced so diabetes is not a common side effect of this disease.

The thick mucus in the lungs can lead to obstruction of airways and frequent infections. A severe hacking cough, with thick mucus production, is characteristic. Overwhelming lung infection leading to respiratory arrest is one of the primary causes of death in persons with cystic fibrosis.

Diagnosis of cystic fibrosis is made, in part, by evidence of the above symptoms, as well as by a "sweat test." This test measures the amount of salt, especially chloride, present in the sweat. In cases of cystic fibrosis, the levels found will be above normal.

In the past, persons with cystic fibrosis died while in childhood. Now, however, with early recognition and aggressive medical treatment, more and more live into their 20s. There is no cure for cystic fibrosis, only treatment of symptoms: antibiotics for infections; medications to thin mucus in the lungs; high-calorie, low-fat diet to help with digestion; and vitamin supplements.

A diagnosis of cystic fibrosis can place a heavy financial and emotional burden on a family. There are support groups and foundations that can be of help to patients and families. Genetic counseling may also be helpful for parents who are considering further family planning.

cystinuria

An inherited defect of the kidneys that causes the urine to contain excessive amounts of an amino acid called cystine and other related substances. This occurs because of the failure of the kidneys to reabsorb these substances in the normal way.

Cystine excretion poses no threat to life. The excess in the urine, however, may lead to stone formation in the kidneys or bladder and surgical treatment may then be necessary. Prevention of stones depends on the regular and frequent drinking of water as a lifetime habit.

cystitis

Inflammation of the urinary bladder. Cystitis is ten times as common in women as in men. It may be caused by a bacterial infection, a stone, or a tumor. Symptoms include pain in the lower part of the abdomen, a desire to pass urine frequently, painful urination, and the passing of urine that may be cloudy, blood-tinged, or foul-smelling. Treatment includes drinking a large amount of fluids to increase urine flow, antibiotic medication, bed rest, and in some cases surgery.

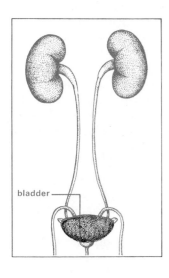

In females, cystitis mainly results from bacteria that have climbed up the urethra; in males, it is often associated with obstruction due to large prostate.

cystocele

A bulging of the urinary bladder backward into the vagina, sometimes occurring as a complication of injury during childbirth or general muscle weakness after multiple childbirth. It may also be a complication of prolapse of the uterus. The bladder forms a pouch bulging down into the front wall of the vagina. A similar situation may occur if the rectum herniates into the vagina (RECTOCELE).

Symptoms of cystocele include difficulty in emptying the bladder completely, with a resulting increase in the frequency of passing urine, a tendency to recurrent bladder infections, and (most commonly) difficulty in preventing escape of urine when the bladder is full, especially on coughing or straining ("stress incontinence").

Treatment usually involves a surgical procedure known as *colporrhaphy*. The ligaments supporting the pelvic floor are tightened, the muscle layers repaired, and the normal anatomic relationships of the bladder, uterus, vagina, and rectum restored. In older women the procedure may be combined with surgical removal of the uterus. See HYSTERECTOMY under **Procedures**.

cytomegalovirus disease

A disease caused by infection with the cytomegalovirus that attacks the salivary glands, liver, spleen, and lungs. The virus is a member of the herpes virus family.

In babies the virus causes pneumonia and a severe blood disorder that leads to hemorrhage in the tissues and death. Newborn babies, who are thought to be infected before birth via the placenta, have insufficient immunity to fight the disease. Most adults have antibodies against the virus, suggesting that infection in a minor form has been encountered and overcome—perhaps as a misdiagnosed attack of a "mumps-like" disease. It is the occasional nonimmune mother, infected by the virus in late pregnancy, who will pass it to the fetus.

In nonimmune adults some cases of virus pneumonia are due to infection with the cytomegalovirus, but they usually recover unless leukemic-type complications occur as a result of damage to the tissues that produce blood cells. Severe and fatal cytomegalovirus infection is common in the terminal stages of AIDS.

No treatment for the disease is known (immunity cannot yet be produced by vaccination), but the presence of antibodies in most of the adult population suggests that many attacks are relatively harmless. The virus is resistant to Acyclovir.

dandruff

A dry, scaly, itchy eruption of the scalp; it may also occur, less commonly, as thick, greasy scales. Dandruff is also known as *seborrheic dermatitis*. It is thought to affect about 60 percent of people to some degree; the condition, although unsightly, is of little consequence. It is sometimes associated with BLEPHARITIS.

There are many shampoos on the market that are designed to relieve this common condition. If the dandruff is not responsive to the medicated shampoos and the condition is a troubling one, the person should seek advice from a physician. There are prescription medications available, including a selenium shampoo, that may be of help.

deafness

Loss or impairment of hearing. From about the age of 10 to 15 years every person begins to lose the hearing acuity of childhood; thus every adult hears slightly less well than children do, particularly in the higher frequencies.

Specialists generally recognize four types of deafness:

1. *Conductive deafness* is caused by disease or injury affecting some part of the hearing apparatus (the eardrum or the tiny auditory bones) that conducts sound waves from the atmosphere to the fluid of the internal ear.

2. *Sensorineural deafness* (also known as *perceptive* or *nerve deafness*) is caused by damage to the part of the hearing apparatus that perceives the sound (from the inner ear to the brain).

3. *Mixed deafness* is a combination of the two above types.

4. *Functional*, or *psychogenic*, *deafness* is caused by psychological upset or shock in the absence of any organic disease.

Conductive deafness may be caused by a plug of wax in the outer ear or by a direct blow to the ear that injures the eardrum. A common cause in wartime is explosions that rupture the eardrum, but traffic accidents are now responsible for many cases. *Otic barotrauma*, damage caused by repeated changes in atmospheric pressure during air travel, can produce a special type of conductive deafness.

Sensorineural deafness can result from injury and also from constant subjection to loud noises, such as those made by machinery or loud rock music groups. Certain classes of drugs, especially the aminoglycoside antibiotics—such as Neomycin, Streptomycin, Gentamycin, and Kanamycin—and some of the diuretics, are known to be ototoxic and cause deafness.

About one in 1,000 of all children are born deaf, due to either heredity, maternal rubella (German measles), or drugs taken during pregnancy. Nearly all cases of congenital deafness are sensorineural.

A large proportion of people over the age of 65 complain of some degree of deafness, owing to degenerative changes in the hair cells of the organs of hearing. This is usually permanent but it can be helped by appropriate hearing aids.

Some of the "miracle cures" of deafness arise from the fourth category.

See also OTOSCLEROSIS, and STAPEDECTOMY under Procedures.

degenerative diseases

A group of disorders caused by aging of the structures of the body, with loss of elasticity, a reduction in the number of active cells, and an increase in the proportion of fibrous connective tissue.

A major difficulty in the consideration of degenerative diseases lies in making the distinction between symptoms (which are indications of disease) and the universal effects of aging. If the rate of decline is faster in one organ than in the rest of the body, the diagnosis is likely to be a degenerative disease. Doctors regard OSTEOARTHRITIS and ATHEROSCLEROSIS as diseases, whereas wrinkling of the skin and changes in the sex organs are accepted as normal processes of aging. In part, this is a difference of degree: While a family is likely to accept some forgetfulness, irritability, and quirky behavior in an elderly parent, they will probably seek medical advice if his mental functioning falls below a certain level (and he may well be diagnosed as having senile DEMENTIA).

In many degenerative diseases there is a hereditary tendency. This factor is difficult to assess in common conditions such as osteoarthritis and atherosclerosis, but it is striking in disorders such as RETINITIS PIGMENTOSA (which often seems to run in families).

Research into degenerative diseases is aimed at alleviating existing symptoms and possibly arresting the progress of degenerative diseases. This would improve the quality of life—although it would probably not significantly increase the human life span.

dehydration

The state produced by abnormal loss of body water; the deprivation or loss of water from the tissues.

Water is an important constituent of the body; in fact, it forms approximately 65 percent of a person's body weight. Most of this fluid (about 41 percent of the body weight) is contained within the cells (intracellular fluid), from which it cannot be removed in any quantity without severe disturbance of cells' metabolic processes. The remaining fluid includes that which lies between the body cells (intercellular fluid), the liquid portion of the blood (blood plasma), the lymph, and the fluid in certain cavities of the body (serous cavities). This extracellular fluid can be subject to greater variation than the intracellular fluid. The plasma component can to some extent use the intercellular water as a reservoir, but to maintain the circulation and other body functions, the total amount of extracellular fluid cannot be greatly reduced.

Dehydration may arise from deprivation of water or from an inability to drink either because of difficulty in swallowing (as, for example, in cancer of the esophagus), or because the person is weak, drowsy, or comatose from any cause.

Vomiting may both prevent fluid intake and increase fluid loss from the body as the secretions of the stomach and intestine are expelled. Diarrhea may act in the same way to increase water loss, and a combination of vomiting and diarrhea will lead to rapid dehydration, especially in infants and children.

Dehydration may also be due to excessive secretion of urine despite falling body reserves of water; this occurs in untreated DIABETES MELLITUS and in certain kidney disorders. Finally, excessive sweating in a hot climate will cause rapid dehydration if water is not freely available.

It is unusual for dehydration to occur as an isolated problem. Vomiting, diarrhea, sweating, and kidney disease frequently cause simultaneous excessive loss of salt from the body, and the gross deficiency of salt may be more serious than that of the water itself.

Symptoms of uncontrolled dehydration are thirst, followed by weakness, exhaustion, and finally delirium and death.

Whereas a healthy adult may survive weeks without food, complete deprivation of water and food may prove fatal within about three days. If food but not water is available, survival time will be longer, since most foods contain some water and additional water is produced during their metabolism in the body. Dehydration in small infants is more serious still, and death may occur very quickly.

Treatment—if dehydration is the result of water deprivation alone—is by the cautious administration of fluids. If complicated by vomiting, diarrhea, or sweating, laboratory tests to determine the extent of any salt deficiency and the administration of intravenous salt solutions may be required.

déjà vu

A feeling that some event or experience has happened before; an apparent familiarity with what are in reality new events or strange surroundings or people.

Déjà vu (French for "already seen") is experienced by normal individuals from time to time, especially when fatigued. However, it can be a prominent feature in the phobic anxiety type of neurosis, or it may precede an attack of psychomotor EPILEPSY.

Déjà vu usually occurs at a time of decreased consciousness and is often described as a dream-like experience. It may be accompanied by other distorted perceptions, such as a feeling of depersonalization. It is probably due to a neurologic "short circuit" to the memory store before the data are registered consciously. It is common in some forms of brain damage.

An analogous phenomenon of "jamais vu" (never seen), where objects appear unreal or very distant, can also be a symptom of temporal-lobe epilepsy.

delirium

A clouding of consciousness in which perception is disordered. The person is often restless, anxious, and inattentive. Hallucinations, both auditory and visual, occur and add to the person's distress.

Delirium can occur as a result of head trauma, infections, acute alcohol withdrawal, drugs, brain lesions, or brain hemorrhages. Onset may be sudden or gradual. Symptoms range from mild, such as occasional wandering of the mind, to the severe, where confusion is so great that the patient is unable to recognize family, respond appropriately, or sleep and is prone to self-injury. There is remarkable variability in the person's mental status from hour to hour.

In some bacterial infections, the accompanying delirium is thought to result from the action of toxins on certain parts of the brain. A similar effect can occur from overdoses of certain drugs such as amphetamines or antidepressants. By contrast, abrupt withdrawal of alcohol or barbiturates—drugs that have a strong depressant effect on the brain—can lead to delirium. Brain lesions or hemorrhages can cause delirium by interfering with the function of certain areas of the brain.

Treatment of delirium involves control of the underlying cause. Removal of the person from noisy, potentially overstimulating areas often is recommended. Depending on the cause of the delirium, sedatives may be ordered to prevent the person from becoming exhausted or hurting himself.

delirium tremens (DTs)

A form of DELIRIUM due to sudden withdrawal of alcohol following a long period of intoxication. It is the most dramatic complication of ALCOHOLISM.

Delirium tremens usually appears one to three days after alcohol intake is stopped, but it may appear as late as seven to ten days after cessation of drinking. The onset of the condition may be preceded by a generalized epileptic seizure, wakefulness, tremulousness, and hallucinations.

In a full-blown attack the person has many symptoms common to other types of delirium, but the special features of delirium tremens are: (1) a fine tremor of the tongue, lips, and hands; (2) an increased pulse rate and profuse sweating; and (3) terrifying auditory and visual hallucinations (often of small animals). The episode usually ends abruptly after one to six days and the person usually sleeps deeply afterward, normally waking up hungry, exhausted, and clear-minded—but with very little memory of the delirium.

Sedatives and anticonvulsants may be given during an attack, but they are only a prelude to the long-term treatment of chronic alcoholism. About 10 percent of cases of delirium tremens end fatally.

delusion

A belief firmly held despite evidence to the contrary. A delusion occurs when a normal perception is abnormally interpreted so that it takes on an inexplicable personal meaning or significance.

For example, a man sitting next to you on a train lights a cigarette and this immediately conveys to you that he is having an affair with your wife. Such delusions appear suddenly and cannot be refuted by rational argument. They are one form of thought disorder typically encountered in schizophrenic persons.

The false belief may also be based on an abnormal initial perception (hallucination), or it might form part of an elaborate delusional system, the origin of which is not clear even to the person himself. Delusions are not specific to the diagnosis of schizophrenia because they are found in most other psychotic diseases, notably manic-depressive psychosis.

A *schizophrenic* person might construct a tortuous system of delusions on the basis of what voices in his head have told him. Often these delusions persecute the person; they may have a political, erotic, or religious theme. Delusions of grandeur also occur in schizophrenia.

In *depressive illness*, delusions are commonly hypochondriacal: The person is convinced that his body is decomposing or that he has cancer. Alternatively, delusions of guilt, unworthiness, or poverty can haunt him. By contrast, in the *manic* phase of depression the delusions are of grandeur and omnipotence.

dementia

Literally, "loss of mind." Dementia can have many possible causes and mechanisms, but the constant feature is loss of memory, particularly for recent events.

The earliest signs of dementia are often very subtle and can be detected only by an observant relative or employer. There may be a mood change or a minor shortcoming at work, often attributed to depression by the doctor. However, as the underlying brain disease of dementia progresses over months or years, the person loses all intellectual powers and emotional control, with the result that his personality is completely degraded. This total deterioration can be prevented in a few cases, so that it is important to try to establish the cause of every dementia.

Senile dementia is a degenerative condition of the nerve cells of the brain, particularly those of the cerebral cortex. The brain shrinks, the natural cavities (ventricles) within it enlarge, and the surface convolutions begin to waste away (atrophy). Senile dementia is not just an exaggeration of the normal aging processes; its effects are more pronounced than the ordinary blunting of intellectual faculties.

ALZHEIMER'S DISEASE is an identical progressive dementia but it begins long before old age and results in early death.

In old people, disease of the brain's blood vessels causes *atherosclerotic dementia*, which can be impossible to differentiate from senile dementia; indeed, the two conditions can coexist.

No specific therapy is available for the above dementias. Conditions such as subdural hematoma (a blood clot beneath the outer covering membrane of the brain), tumors of the frontal lobe of the brain, hypothyroidism, and neurosyphilis can all give rise to a similar progressive intellectual deterioration. In these cases the underlying disease is treated.

demyelination

The destruction and loss of the protective coating (*myelin sheath*) of a nerve fiber.

For the nervous system to function swiftly and efficiently, the nerves have to be insulated from each other. In many nerves this is achieved by a sheath of fatty material, called myelin, around each nerve fiber. Loss of myelin is the common feature in "demyelinating diseases" of the central nervous system.

Such diseases may be acute (where the demyelination can occur within a few days) or chronic (where the condition progresses over several years, as in MULTIPLE SCLEROSIS).

dengue fever

An acute and often epidemic disease caused by infection with the group B arboviruses. (The disease is known also as "breakbone fever.") It is transmitted to man by the Aëdes mosquito and is found throughout the tropics, particularly in the mosquitoes' active season. When the symptoms develop, three to fifteen days after the bite, the broad clinical pattern is one of fever, rash, and headache.

In the *classical* form, a runny nose or conjunctivitis is followed within hours by a severe headache ("breakbone"), pain behind the eyes, backache, leg and joint pains, and depression. The fever may be of a characteristic "saddleback"

DEMYELINATION

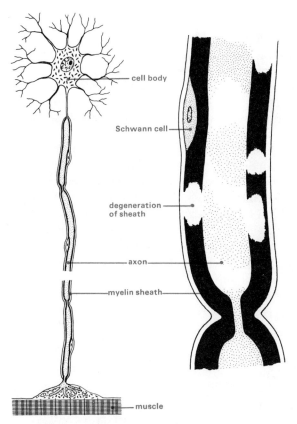

Nerve fibers are wrapped in a fatty myelin sheath that acts as an insulator and allows nerve impulses to travel at high speeds. In certain chronic demyelinating diseases—for example, multiple sclerosis—the loss of insulation causes neurological disorders such as paralysis and numbness.

type: a raised temperature for about three days followed by several hours when the symptoms and fever disappear before returning for another day. During the second phase of fever, swollen glands and a characteristic berry-like rash are frequently present. Classical dengue fever usually lasts only five to six days and is never fatal. Treatment involves only the relief of symptoms (strong analgesics may be required). The person involved commonly feels depressed and tired for several weeks. The *atypical* mild form of dengue fever usually lasts less than seventy-two hours.

Dengue hemorrhagic fever is a severe form affecting mainly children. There is bleeding into the skin and internal organs, and a mortality rate that may be as high as 30 percent.

dental decay

Dental decay is the decalcification of a portion of a tooth, accompanied or followed by the disintegration of the living part of the tooth—resulting in the formation of "cavities" (caries).

Dental decay causes no symptoms during its early stages, but when the living zones of the tooth are affected, toothache results.

Dental decay is a disease of the modern Western world; the major cause is dietary. Unlike primitive societies, the people of modern cultures consume large amounts of refined sugar (sucrose). Sucrose adheres to the surface of teeth and is quickly converted to acid by bacteria. The combination of sucrose, food debris, and bacteria, known as *dental plaque*, covers the area where decay develops.

Sticky sweet foods are more likely to adhere to the teeth than are granular ones; the more frequently the food is eaten, the worse the effects.

Almost all Americans have some caries, but their frequency and severity can be reduced by avoiding sweet foods, by regular use of a toothbrush and dental floss to remove plaque, by fluoridation of the water supply or fluoride supplements given to children, by the direct application of fluoride to the teeth as paints or in toothpaste, and by more modern techniques such as *fissure sealing*. Regular inspection by a dentist and the use of *disclosing tablets* help to reveal areas of plaque.

The development of dental decay can be arrested but not reversed, thus, the proper treatment of the resulting cavities is essential. If left untreated, dental caries destroys teeth completely and poses the added risk of serious infection (OSTEOMYELITIS) of the jawbones.

CARIES

STRUCTURE OF TEETH

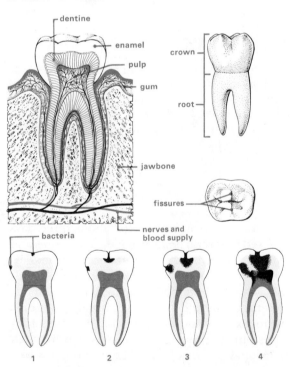

Dental decay is the most common disease in the Western world. Bacteria collect in the pits and fissures of the teeth and produce acid from refined sugar (1). The acid eats into the enamel (2). Decay then spreads more rapidly through the softer dentine (3). When the pulp becomes infected, irritation of the nerve leads to toothache (4).

depilation

The removal of unwanted body hair.

Unwanted hair is a common cosmetic problem, especially affecting women. If hair growth is excessive, a physician should examine the individual

DENTAL HYGIENE

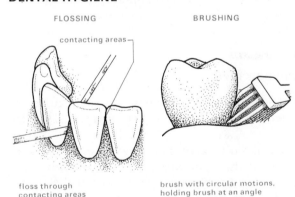

Without adequate dental hygiene, bacteria collect in the crevices and fissures of teeth, setting up caries, or tooth decay. Regular brushing helps prevent tooth and gum disease, while twice weekly use of dental floss helps clear bacteria and debris from between the teeth, particularly the "contacting areas." Your dentist will offer special advice.

before any treatment is undertaken, because occasionally the cause is an underlying disorder of the ovaries, pituitary gland, or adrenal glands. In most cases, however, no such problem exists and hormonal treatment is both ineffective and potentially dangerous.

A variety of local treatments is available to remove hair without unnecessary damage to the skin. Shaving is one method. Depilatory creams can be applied to the area but must be used in the correct concentration and not left on too long. Alternatively, the skin can be dusted with powder and hot wax applied. When the wax has hardened it is pulled off, bringing the hairs with it. Both depilatory creams and wax treatment are only temporary solutions; the hairs reappear within a month or so.

Permanent removal of superfluous hair may be achieved by electrolysis. This technique destroys the papilla that carries nutrients to the hair follicle in the skin. In the hands of a skilled operator, electrolysis should be relatively painless and not leave visible scars.

depression

A mental state characterized by loss of interest in all things normally pleasurable such as food, friends, work, and sex. Depression may be a normal reaction (probably experienced by everyone at some stage in life) or it may be a pathological state. There is no clear-cut boundary between the two; a diagnosis of depressive illness usually is made when the degree or duration of symptoms is out of proportion to the apparent cause.

Psychiatrists traditionally have divided depression into two types. The first type, *reactive depression*, is precipitated by physical or emotional factors such as chronic illness or bereavement. These events would sadden anyone, but some people become overwhelmed by them or even by an apparently trivial event.

In the second type, *endogenous depression*, there is no obvious precipitating cause but a family history of depression may exist. There may be pure depression or mood swings between despair and elation—the condition known as *manic-depressive illness.*

The main symptom of all depression is a persistent unhappy mood. According to a set of criteria established by psychiatrists in 1972, the person should have, in addition, at least five of the following eight symptoms: poor appetite, sleep difficulty, loss of energy, slowness of thought, poor concentration, feelings of guilt, loss of interest in usual activities (particularly sex), and recurrent thoughts of death or suicide.

Treatment depends on an exact psychiatric classification of the depression; both psychological support and drugs are important. There is some evidence that endogenous depression results from a depletion of substances called biogenic amines (particularly norepinephrine) in the nerve cells of the brain.

Two of the most widely used groups of antidepressant drugs—the tricyclics and the monoamine oxidase inhibitors—both conserve norepinephrine, and this is thought to be the basis of their efficacy.

Lithium carbonate, a simple salt, has proved extremely useful in the treatment of manic-depressive illness. Electroconvulsive therapy is used by some psychiatrists in the treatment of depression that is refractory (unresponsive to any other treatment) and severe, but its use is controversial.

dermatitis

An inflammation of the skin. It may be the result of an infection, exposure to an allergen, contact with a strong chemical, or contact with the leaves of certain plants (such as poison ivy, poison oak, or poison sumac). Although the term "dermatitis" covers a larger number of conditions—which in themselves may arise from a bewildering number of causes—the pathological changes are remarkably constant.

Like any other inflammation, dermatitis can be classified as *acute, subacute,* or *chronic.* The initial or acute stage is characterized by redness and swelling of the skin with the formation of vesicles (tiny blisters) in the outer layer. As the acute stage subsides, there are fewer vesicles and the skin becomes thickened and scaly. In chronic dermatitis, where the process has persisted for many weeks or months, there are usually no vesicles but the epidermis often becomes much thicker and leathery in appearance.

Although the classification of many apparently different skin conditions under the heading of dermatitis is an oversimplification, it does avoid a multiplicity of terms that would otherwise be needed to denote minor variations.

Much confusion exists in the usage of the terms "dermatitis" and "eczema." In the United States, chronic recurrent skin inflammations are called "eczema" and more acute self-limited ones "dermatitis." The trend now is to regard the two terms as synonymous.

All of the individual types of dermatitis described below can be aggravated by the following factors: scratching; application of irritating medications, which might have no effect on normal skin; infection due to a change in the bacterial population of an area of inflamed skin; and blockage of the sweat ducts, which can cause a secondary heat rash.

Acute contact dermatitis—probably the single most common type of dermatitis—is a reaction to external agents. The causative agent is often an irritant such as a strong acid or alkali; the skin reaction appears within twenty-four hours of contact. Alternatively, sensitizing agents such as nickel or rubber penetrate the epidermis and link with a tissue protein to form an antigen. The sensitized individual then experiences a delayed allergic response to this skin antigen over a period of days or years, leading eventually to dermatitis.

Primary irritants in sufficient concentrations will cause dermatitis in everyone, but sensitizing agents present in low concentrations over prolonged periods will cause a reaction only in susceptible individuals.

The sensitizing agent can be very difficult to identify, but the site of the dermatitis often gives a clue. For example, hair dyes and shampoo affect the scalp; airborne sprays or dusts, volatile chemicals, and cosmetics involve the face; clothing and deodorants affect the armpits; and glue, industrial chemicals, plants, and rubber produce a reaction on the hands. Many ointments, especially antibiotics, can cause contact dermatitis.

If dermatitis is recurrent and has no known cause, *patch testing* of the person's skin with potential sensitizers can be carried out.

The first step in treatment is the removal of the offending agent. In severe cases a cortisone-like steroid drug, such as hydrocortisone, may be applied to the skin.

Atopic dermatitis runs in families and is closely associated with hay fever and asthma. About 10 percent of the population are *atopic* (that is, allergic) because they are predisposed to form high concentrations of IgE-type antibodies in their serum, although there is little evidence that these are directly responsible for the dermatitis.

Eczema usually starts in infancy and often disappears before adolescence; no cure is available but the intense itching can be relieved with creams. *Nummular* (coin-shaped) *eczema* is a subacute dermatitis that begins in middle age.

Seborrheic dermatitis, often an inherited condition, is characterized by greasy scaling of the skin—not only of the scalp but around the eyebrows, behind the ears, between the shoulders, and in skin folds generally. In mild cases the dandruff can be controlled by more frequent shampooing, but more extensive involvement may require steroid ointment. Since secondary bacterial infection may occur, an antibiotic is sometimes combined with the steroid.

dermatofibroma

A fibroma affecting the skin, most common in middle-aged women. These small hard, slightly elevated lesions are not usually the natural color of the person's skin but are pinkish, brownish, or grayish. Although sometimes confused with more serious skin lesions, they can be diagnosed by experienced physicians.

dermatomyositis

Inflammatory disease of the muscles accompanied by rash over the eyelids, cheeks, chest, and knuckles.

It affects women more commonly than men and may occur at any age, although two thirds of the affected people are over 30 years old.

A slowly progressive weakness develops, particularly affecting muscles around the shoulders and hips, during a three- to twelve-month period. The person may notice difficulty in climbing stairs or in raising his arms above his head. The skin rash may appear before, during, or after the onset of weakness.

Up to 50 percent of persons with dermatomyositis also show signs of a COLLAGEN DISEASE (rheumatoid arthritis, systemic lupus erythematosus, or scleroderma). There is also some association with CANCER, especially among older people.

The exact cause of dermatomyositis is unknown but it is thought to be an autoimmune disorder (see AUTOIMMUNE DISEASE); antibodies against their own muscle have been found in the blood of many affected persons. Most improve on high doses of corticosteroids, and the chances of a cure are good in young persons.

dermatosis

A nonspecific name for any skin disorder.

Skin diseases usually are diagnosed by their visual appearance and the following terms are common:

A *macule* is a flat area of altered color, common to many rashes.

A round solid elevation of the skin is called a *papule* when it is less than $\frac{2}{5}$ inch (1 cm.) in diameter, and a *nodule* when larger than that.

A *plaque* is a raised flat patch of skin of any color; typical plaques occur in PSORIASIS.

A *vesicle* is a small fluid-containing blister; vesicles appear in numbers in the acute forms of DERMATITIS.

Bullae are larger fluid-filled spaces found in conditions such as PEMPHIGUS.

desensitization

1. A treatment used to suppress some forms of allergy such as hay fever or asthma. For uncontrollable hay fever, for example, after determining which variety of pollen is responsible, repeated injections of minute doses of the offending pollen are given for perhaps three to six months before the pollen season. Densensitization works by inducing "blocking antibodies," which in effect neutralize pollen antigens before they reach the cells that produce the reaction. Desensitization is highly effective in some cases but it needs to be repeated each year, and the same result may not be obtained on later occasions. Some individuals find, however, that after several years of treatment their symptoms disappear completely.

2. Desensitization is also the name of a method used by psychiatrists to reduce phobic anxiety by slowly accustoming the person to the source of his fears while he is relaxed—often with the help of an intravenous injection of a tranquilizer. *Deconditioning* is another name for this treatment.

In the first stage the person is asked to think of a small aspect of his phobia until it no longer provokes fear. For instance, if the phobia concerns air travel he might be asked to imagine himself taking a taxi to the airport. Then he has to imagine progressively more frightening situations until he can tolerate the whole idea of air travel. The next stage is to go through the same steps in real life. Desensitization is a painstaking and lengthy technique, but it can be effective in selected cases.

desquamation

Normal loss of scales from the very outer layer of the skin (*epidermis*).

The epidermis consists of several layers of squamous (scale-like) cells covered by a layer of keratin. Squamous cells are thin flat cells that fit together to form a continuous membrane.

The cells in the deepest layer of the epidermis divide and move toward the surface. As they approach the surface, these cells are transformed into *keratin*—a tough, waterproof protein that forms a protective covering for the skin. Keratin is continuously being replaced from below as the superficial layer sloughs off. This sloughing of keratin is desquamation.

detached retina

In this condition there is not an actual detachment of the retina (the light-sensitive "screen" at the back of the eye) from the underlying tissues, but a collection of fluid between two layers of the retina. This fluid can come either from blood vessels or, more commonly, from the *vitreous humor* (fluid within the eye) through a hole in the retina.

When the "detachment" begins, the person

DETACHED RETINA

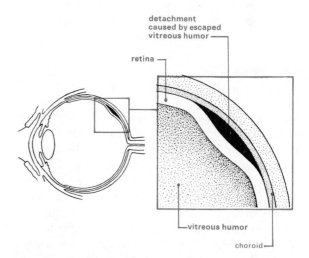

The retina is the film at the back of the eye that contains the light-sensitive receptors of the optic nerve. Detached retina results from a tear in this delicate film; the jelly-like vitreous humor squeezes through the hole and separates the retina from the underlying choroid. Prompt treatment is vital.

may notice flashes or streaks of light, clouding of vision, and large floating spots. The visual loss is characteristic and is as if a black drape were descending, or rising, to obscure the field of vision. Most detachments occur in people with high degrees of myopia or who have had a cataract operation. Injury is not a common cause.

Detachment is treated by indenting the white of the eye with a piece of silicon rubber sponge sewn in place over the detached area. This causes the subretinal fluid to absorb. Inflammation, caused by application of a freezing probe, then causes the retina to adhere. In skilled hands the results are excellent.

Unless surgery is undertaken quickly, the detachment extends progressively and sight in the affected eye may be forever lost. Prophylactic surgery can be carried out in the unaffected eye if it is thought to be at risk for future detachment. The argon laser is useful for this purpose but has no place in the treatment of established detachment.

deviated septum

A displacement of the partition of bone and cartilage that divides the nose so that one part of the nasal cavity is smaller than the other. Occasionally the deviation, which is most often caused by injury, may handicap breathing, block the normal flow of mucus from the sinuses during a cold, and prevent proper drainage of infected sinuses. It is rarely considered serious but can be corrected by surgery if necessary.

diabetes mellitus

A syndrome in which the basic defect is absence or shortage of the pancreatic hormone *insulin*. There are two major types of diabetes, which differ in their cause, onset, and response to treatment.

Juvenile-onset diabetes usually comes on very suddenly with excessive thirst and appetite and an unusually high daily output of urine. In addition to raised blood sugar levels, weight loss is often apparent. These children or young adults are totally dependent on regular insulin injections and a strict diet for control of their blood sugar levels. However, unlike the grim and inevitable fate before insulin therapy became available in the 1920s, their life expectancy is not drastically shortened.

Maturity-onset diabetes has a slower onset, in middle age or later years, and usually can be controlled by diet alone or with oral medication. In fact, the mild symptoms of maturity-onset diabetes mean that it often goes unrecognized.

Diabetes runs in families, although there is no simple pattern of inheritance. Close relatives of diabetics stand a two-and-a-half-times increased chance of developing diabetes. Juvenile-onset diabetes has some genetic basis but this is probably no more than a predisposition to an autoimmune reaction to a virus infection. Early cases recently have been cured by immunosuppressive treatment. Maturity-onset diabetes is the result of obesity and thus has a strong genetic basis.

In a small number of patients diabetes mellitus is associated with some other predisposing disease—such as ACROMEGALY, CUSHING'S SYNDROME, or HEMOCHROMATOSIS—or with the effects of drugs.

Although insulin primarily controls the metabolism of carbohydrates, fat metabolism is also disordered in diabetes. The latter defect leads to the appearance of ATHEROSCLEROSIS at an unusually early age in diabetics and may account for many of the complications (such as diseases of the kidneys and retina, gangrene of the feet, and nerve disorders).

A severely diabetic person will lose consciousness if the diabetes is uncontrolled. HYPERGLYCEMIA (too much glucose) can occur in an undiagnosed diabetic or in one who has neglected to take his insulin; this can lead to a very dangerous condition marked by COMA. HYPOGLYCEMIA (too little glucose) is very common and usually results from undereating or insulin overdose. It produces sweating, nervousness, weakness, irrational behavior, and then rapid loss of consciousness. Sugar given by mouth during the brief period of warning symptoms will prevent the unconsciousness.

Diabetes mellitus is a disease that needs careful monitoring by physicians. Weight loss, diet, and exercise are all important components in controlling the disease.

diarrhea

The frequent passage of loose, watery stools.

A sudden change in bowel habit to voluminous, watery stools, as in acute diarrhea, is an unmistakable symptom. Intermittent bouts of loose stools extending over a period of months (chronic diarrhea) usually present a more difficult diagnostic problem.

Acute diarrhea in a previously healthy person is nearly always due to infection; it is occasionally possible to identify a particular meal as the source of infection, especially when other people contract the same illness. If diarrhea occurs within twenty-four hours of eating the meal, it is probably due to ingestion of a bacterial toxin. "Traveler's diarrhea," the scourge of tourists everywhere, is a self-limiting condition that lasts up to three days. It can be due to a pathogenic strain of the bacterium *Escherichia coli* or might result from the normal bacteria in the bowel being changed to unaccustomed strains.

If the diarrhea is blood-stained, DYSENTERY due to *Shigella* bacteria or the protozoan *Entamoeba histolytica* may be responsible. The *Salmonella* group of bacteria produces either typical food poisoning with diarrhea about seventy-two hours after ingestion or the much more serious TYPHOID FEVER or PARATYPHOID FEVER, in which diarrhea is a late symptom.

The prevention of acute diarrhea by strict hygiene is more effective than its treatment, which in the self-limiting disease consists of salt and water replacement, and medications to add bulk to the feces. Antibiotics are of value only in prolonged illnesses such as typhoid.

In *chronic diarrhea* it is the change in bowel habit that is important, rather than the number of daily visits to the bathroom or the consistency of the stools. Associated signs or symptoms might reveal that the diarrhea is one feature of a generalized disease. In the majority of patients, however, chronic diarrhea results from inflammation or irritation of the bowel. Such irritation occurs in ULCERATIVE COLITIS, CROHN'S DISEASE, diverticular disease, and tumors of the large bowel. In the absence of any positive physical findings, the diagnosis of IRRITABLE BOWEL SYNDROME often is made. Some drugs can cause diarrhea as a side effect.

diastole

Each of the four chambers of the heart acts as a pump, contracting (*systole*) and filling (*diastole*) alternately. Diastole is the period when a chamber passively fills with blood.

The period of ventricular diastole corresponds to the period when the atria are contracting and discharging blood into the ventricles.

When the term *diastolic blood pressure* is used, it refers to the pressure in large arteries during the period between the pulse beats, when the ventricles are not contracting.

diathermy

The generation of heat in body tissues by means of an electric current. Diathermy is one form of *cautery* (the use of an agent to burn or destroy tissue).

The heat produced in tissues by the passage of the current may be sufficient to destroy them. This technique is used in surgery to seal blood vessels as they are cut and in the destruction of certain tumors.

Short-wave diathermy uses current of a much higher frequency than that used in cauterization. It produces insufficient heat to destroy tissue but enough to dilate blood vessels and relax muscles. It is used frequently to relieve the pain and stiffness of rheumatic conditions of joints or muscles. Commonly the heat treatment is applied for about thirty minutes, several times a week.

digestion

The process whereby food is broken down into its constituent nutrients ready for absorption into the bloodstream.

Digestion of complex food molecules into smaller, absorbable molecules begins in the mouth and is completed by the time the food reaches the end of the small intestine. Apart from the mechanical processes of chewing and swallowing, the journey of food through the digestive canal and its digestion take place without any voluntary control, but the activity of the digestive organs is very susceptible to emotions such as excitement, fear, and anger.

Digestive juices are produced in the mouth, stomach, intestine, and pancreas under the control of nerves and hormones, and fat-emulsifying bile is secreted by the liver and stored in the gallbladder. Enzymes in these juices encourage the breakdown of large molecules into smaller ones. Each digestive enzyme is responsible for the chemical splitting of a particular type of nutrient.

Digestion of carbohydrates (starches and sugars) begins in the mouth under the influence of saliva and continues in the stomach and small intestine. The large molecules are split into smaller fragments, eventually yielding simple sug-

DIGESTIVE TRACT

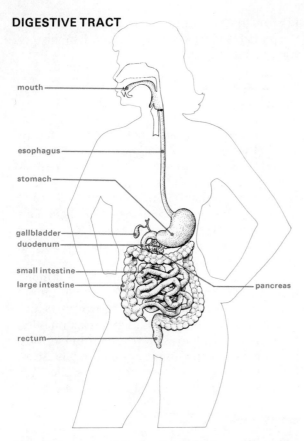

mouth

esophagus

stomach

gallbladder
duodenum

small intestine
large intestine

pancreas

rectum

Digestion starts with chewing in the mouth; in the stomach the food is churned for several hours and mixed with acid and pepsin (a protein-breaking enzyme) so that it becomes liquid. Small amounts of this liquid are released into the duodenum where enzymes from the pancreas complete the digestive process.

ars such as glucose. In the same way, proteins are digested into their constituent amino acids by a series of enzymes secreted by the stomach, small intestine, and pancreas.

Dietary fat is digested into smaller units in the small intestine, where these are mixed with bile salts which enable them to be absorbed as an emulsion.

Almost all the nutrients in the food—including minerals and vitamins as well as the end products of enzymatic digestion—are absorbed in the small intestine. The liquid waste then is passed into the large intestine (colon) where most of the water is absorbed and the solid feces are stored in the lower part of the bowel (rectum) until it is convenient to discharge them.

Apart from the rare cases of absence of one or more of the digestive enzymes, most of the dis-

eases of the gastrointestinal tract are due to physical damage to the organs concerned. The most common cause of indigestion is unwise eating or drinking—especially the excessive consumption of alcohol. The modern American diet is made up largely of highly refined foods—white flour and white sugar—and contains few unrefined cereals or raw vegetables. The lack of vegetable fiber ("roughage") in such a diet is known to slow the movement of food through the intestines and is now thought to be largely responsible for disorders such as CONSTIPATION and diverticular disease. The lining of the stomach and intestine may also be irritated and inflamed by viral and bacterial infections and by toxins (as in some forms of food poisoning). More serious digestive disorders may be due to ulceration of the stomach, the duodenum, or the colon, to chronic inflammation of the intestine (as in CROHN'S DISEASE), and to tumors.

dilatation

The expansion of a cavity or the widening of an opening, tube, or passageway.

Dilatation (or "dilation") may occur naturally under hormonal or nervous control. For example, blood vessels dilate in order to supply tissues with more blood when necessary; and the pupil of the eye dilates when it needs to admit more light in dim conditions.

Dilatation may also be part of a disease process or an adaptation to a disease. In HEART FAILURE the ventricles dilate as the heart is unable to pump blood out of them. When a tube such as the ureter is obstructed, the part of the urinary tube before the obstruction is forced to dilate.

In some circumstances dilatation is used as a therapeutic procedure. A narrowed urethra, which makes passage of urine difficult, may be mechanically dilated; or the cervix may be dilated to provide access for a curette in the procedure of DILATATION AND CURETTAGE (see under **Tests**).

The opposite of dilatation is *constriction*.

diphtheria

An infectious disease, mainly of children, that was once common, highly dangerous, and a terror to parents, but that now, as a result of immunization, has almost been eradicated in developed countries. Indeed, diphtheria is so little known to modern mothers that there is a danger that immunization may be neglected and the condition return, in epidemic form. Present legislation makes this improbable in the U.S.

Diphtheria is an acute contagious disease caused by the *Corynebacterium diphtheriae*. About three days after contact the child develops a low rise of temperature and a slight sore throat, and examination shows a gray membrane spreading over the tonsils, the palate, and the back of the mouth. This is the dreaded diphtheritic membrane, resulting from tissue damage by the Corynebacteria, and the organisms within it send virulent toxins into the bloodstream to attack the heart, the muscles, and the nerves.

Diphtheria toxin is a powerful poison that can damage muscle and nerve tissue to cause heart failure, permanent weakness in the limbs, paralysis of the breathing muscles, or general loss of muscle power. Sudden death from its effects on the heart can occur, but a more common cause of death used to be the blockage of the air passages by membrane and the associated swelling. Many lives were saved by tracheostomy (making an artificial opening into the windpipe), but many victims were left with permanently damaged hearts.

Diphtheria was controlled in the western world, and millions of children's lives saved, solely by immunization. But it should never be forgotten that the causal bacteria are still about, ready to attack the unprotected.

dislocation

The displacement of a part of the body—most commonly a joint—from its normal position.

Injury is the usual cause of dislocation of a joint. The severity of the condition depends on whether the displaced joint presses on a neighboring artery or nerve.

The dislocated joint can be put back in position by skilled mechanical handling, a maneuver that is quick and safe in experienced hands but capable of causing great pain if attempted by the unskilled. The joint may afterward be splinted to help it stabilize in the correct position. Joint dislocation sometimes tends to recur; in such cases an operation may be necessary to tighten the ligaments and thus help hold the joint in place.

CONGENITAL DISLOCATION OF THE HIP, as the name implies, is present from birth. It is due to a genetic or acquired structural deformity or to lax ligaments. All babies today are examined for CDH

DISLOCATION

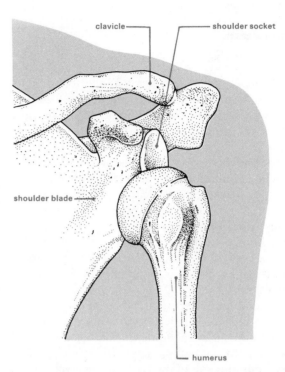

Dislocation is the complete separation of the two bones that make up a joint; it usually results from trauma. The shoulder joint becomes dislocated relatively frequently because the socket into which the humerus fits is shallow. Because of the pull of the muscles, the humerus usually dislocates forward and inward as shown.

so that cases can be corrected immediately. Otherwise they might not be detected until the child attempts to walk, by which time irreversible damage may have occurred. Uncorrected CDH also carries an increased risk of OSTEOARTHRITIS in later life.

Chronic inflammation also can cause joint dislocation, though this is rare.

diuresis

The passing of unusually large amounts of urine. It may be a symptom of disease, or it may be caused deliberately to relieve certain medical conditions in which the body contains too much fluid. Several effective diuretic drugs are commonly used to treat EDEMA from a variety of causes. Certain foods (such as fresh asparagus, pineapple, and citrus fruits), coffee, and tea have a mild diuretic effect.

diverticulitis

Diverticula (small pouches that can form in the walls of a hollow organ) commonly are found in the large intestine of people after middle age. (This condition is known as DIVERTICULOSIS.) *Diverticulitis* is the term for the inflammation of these pouches.

The inflammation may affect one diverticulum or many diverticula along a considerable length of the colon. Attacks tend to be recurrent. Symptoms usually are mild and consist of recurrent attacks of pain in the left side of the lower part of the abdomen, associated with constipation or bouts of diarrhea. This may continue for months or years.

Sometimes an acute attack occurs, characterized by pain and tenderness in the left side of the lower part of the abdomen, often accompanied by fever. In an acute attack a diverticulum may perforate the wall of the colon to produce a generalized PERITONITIS. One complication of recurrent attacks of inflammation is the growth of fibrous tissue and the consequent narrowing of the inside of the colon, which can result in complete obstruction of the colon.

Another complication is that the inflammation may extend to adjacent structures—most commonly the bladder, sometimes other parts of the small bowel, and—rarely—the uterus and vagina. The inflamed areas between these structures may break down, resulting in abnormal passageways (fistulas) between the colon and the organs affected. Hemorrhage is another complication of diverticulitis and can sometimes be massive.

The diagnosis of diverticulitis is confirmed by a barium enema. Treatment consists of giving a bulk laxative to produce bulky and soft stools; pain produced by spasm of the colon may be relieved by the administration of an antispasmodic drug. Acute attacks may require bed rest and antibiotics. Surgery is urgently indicated when signs of PERITONITIS are progressive, when hemorrhage is severe, or when other complications occur.

diverticulosis

The presence of small sacs (diverticula) lined with mucous membrane that pouch outward from the walls of the large intestine. In industrialized countries the condition is found in about a third of the population middle-aged and older. It is thought that the normal contractions of the large bowel exert pressure to such a degree that the mucous membrane is forced through the muscular walls of the intestine at points of weakness where blood vessels run.

The condition is rare in countries where the normal diet contains much roughage (dietary fiber). The part of the large intestine most commonly affected is the sigmoid flexure of the colon, which lies in the lower left-hand side of the abdominal cavity. Normally these pouches do not give rise to complications, but in a minority of cases they become inflamed and give rise to the disease known as DIVERTICULITIS.

dizziness

This is a term loosely used for a variety of sensations, including lightheadedness, faintness, and feelings of falling or of things "spinning." The more precise medical terms, however, are VERTIGO and *pseudovertigo.*

True vertigo is a condition in which the person feels that he, or his environment, is rotating in space. This may be accompanied by headache, nausea, or vomiting and can indicate that there is a disorder in the parts of the nervous system that are involved with maintaining balance. These equilibrium-maintaining structures involve the brain, eyes, and inner ears.

Pseudovertigo is applied to the other sensations listed above. Although unpleasant, this type of dizziness rarely has an underlying physical cause. It may be an indication of a temporary lack of blood supply to the brain. Its occurrence is therefore common when a person suddenly gets up from a reclining to a standing position, when hungry, or when affected by anemia or heart or lung disease. If the pseudovertigo is not associated with an obvious cause, or is unrelieved by rest, medical advice should be sought.

double vision

Seeing two of every image. Also known as *diplopia.* It may be caused by defective eye muscles or by a disorder of the nerve that signals the eye muscles. Temporary double vision is common after a mild concussion. Double vision may be caused by diabetic nerve damage, partial or full STROKE, MYASTHENIA GRAVIS, MULTIPLE SCLEROSIS, and other conditions. It should never be ignored. Pending investigation, it may be relieved by covering one eye with a patch.

Down's syndrome

A congenital disorder that causes mental retardation and a variety of physical abnormalities. Previously known as "mongolism," the scientific name is *trisomy 21*, because of the chromosomal abnormality that is responsible. The normal number of human chromosomes is 23 pairs. In Down's syndrome, however, there is an extra chromosome of the type known as #21, leading to a total of 47, rather than 46, chromosomes.

In most cases this chromosomal abnormality occurs unpredictably rather than by inheritance, although there may be a familial tendency. The overall incidence of the syndrome is one in 600 births, rising to one in 400 in mothers over 40 years old, and one in 40 for mothers over 45 years old.

The mental deficiency in Down's syndrome ranges from mild to severe, but it does not cause aggressive or antisocial behavior. Depending on the degree of retardation, individuals can be taught simple tasks and socially acceptable behavior. The average mental age attained is about 8 years.

There are particular physical characteristics in Down's syndrome: enlarged, protruding tongue; upward-slanting eyes; small, poorly aligned teeth; small, incompletely formed ears; short stature; and broad spade-like hands and feet. Adults rarely exceed the height of a 10-year-old child.

The internal abnormalities in this disease lead to a high death rate in infancy. Cardiac malformation alone accounts for the deaths of one third of all infants born with Down's syndrome. LEUKEMIA and respiratory tract infections are also common causes of death. Many of those who do survive to puberty go on to live until middle age, but these surviving adults have a high incidence of ALZHEIMER'S DISEASE.

There is no cure for Down's syndrome. For those couples with a family history of the disease, or when the mother is of older childbearing years, genetic counseling is important before planning pregnancy.

Aminocentesis is also available for diagnosing whether a fetus is affected: If this is the case, a clinical abortion may be chosen. There are often great physical, psychological, and financial burdens in caring for a Down's syndrome child. There are organizations that provide information on the care of those affected by Down's syndrome.

dreaming

Ideas, thoughts, emotions, or images that pass through the mind during the rapid-eye-movement (REM) stages of SLEEP. If an individual is awakened during REM sleep he usually can remember his dream in vivid detail; if he is awakened some time after a period of REM sleep, he will remember less of it.

drug abuse

In the early years of this century, addiction to opium and hashish was prevalent in the Far East but rare in the United States and Europe. Sniffing cocaine was briefly fashionable in the 1920s, but drug abuse became a major social problem with the growth of heroin addiction. Heroin—an extract of opium that is usually taken by intravenous injection—is the most powerful and destructive of the drugs in addiction, and its use spread very rapidly in economically deprived areas of inner cities after World War II.

The 1950s also saw an explosive growth in the prescription of sedatives and stimulants by doctors. As amphetamines, barbiturates, and tranquilizers came into ever wider legitimate use, their abuse also became common. At much the same time, people began to write of the mind-enhancing potential of drugs such as LSD and mescaline (peyote), derived from the mescal cactus, and the use of mind-altering drugs became more widespread in the United States population.

Experimentation with drugs is now commonplace, especially among high school and college students. Many try CANNABIS (marijuana or "pot") or tranquilizers, especially when these are handed around at a weekend party; experimentation with injected barbiturates or opiates such as heroin or morphine is less common. Increasingly common is the use of cocaine, derived from the coca plant, which is a stimulant and mood enhancer. Its popular use can, in part, be attributed to its rank as a "status drug," owing to its high cost in comparison to other recreational-use drugs. Whether or not experimentation leads to addiction depends on many variables, including the addictive potential of the drug (high for heroin, amphetamine, and tobacco; low or nonexistent for cannabis) and the personality and social environment of the individual.

Psychological dependence on drugs is common. Most people are mildly dependent on coffee or tea; a similar but stronger dependence on sleeping pills or tranquilizers may develop. Dependence on cannabis and cocaine is also psychological, rather than physical. But serious addiction is much more likely when the drug concerned causes physical dependence, when deprivation of the drug causes physical symptoms (see ADDICTION). In the case of heroin, for example, an addict who is deprived of the drug will within a few hours develop severe abdominal pains, sweating, and tremors. Alcoholics have a similar strong physical dependence on their "drug."

Drug addiction causes problems partly from its socially disruptive effects, and in particular from the effects of chronic addiction on an individual's ability to live and work normally. Many addicts turn to crime to find money to pay for their supplies. Addiction to intravenous injectable drugs such as heroin also carries a substantial hazard to health, particularly from injections given without sterile precautions. These addicts have a high mortality rate from HEPATITIS (inflammation of the liver) and blood poisoning, as well as from drug overdosage. Needles shared by intravenous drug abusers commonly transmit AIDS.

Treatment of persons with an established addiction is unrewarding. When heavy physical dependence exists, the risk of relapse is very high. The complex interactions of psychological and social factors that promote drug abuse are still little understood.

See also *Drug Abuse* in the section on **Wellness**.

duodenal ulcer

An ulcer in the first part of the small intestine (*duodenum*), the most common type of peptic ulcer. Peptic ulcers include those that affect the lower part of the esophagus, the stomach, and the first part of the duodenum. They are patches of tissue loss in the lining of these structures produced by the action of digestive juices (acid and pepsin) secreted by the stomach. Normally the lining is able to withstand the action of these digestive secretions.

Symptoms may start at any age but usually begin in young adulthood. Men are affected four times as frequently as women. Symptoms may be vague, absent, or atypical, but usually the patient complains of upper abdominal pain—which has variously been described as gnawing, burning, cramp-like, or boring. Typically the pain starts an hour or two after a meal and is relieved in about half an hour by taking food or milk. Diagnosis is confirmed by a barium meal or by gastroscopy. The aim of drug treatment is to reduce the secretion of the digestive juices, to neutralize the acid after it has been secreted, or to increase the resistance of the gastrointestinal lining to the action of acid and pepsin. Stress and anxiety are thought to play a part in producing ulcers in some patients; thus, a sedative also may be prescribed.

It is no longer considered necessary to adhere strictly to a bland diet. Most persons would know what foods aggravate symptoms in their own cases, and these foods should be avoided. Smoking encourages ulceration and delays healing and should be avoided, as should alcohol. Meals should be regular and frequent to neutralize the acid that is produced.

Treatment with histamine H_2 receptor blocking agents, such as cimetidine and ranitidine, is safe and effective. Symptoms tend to be recurrent despite treatment. In some cases symptoms persist despite drug treatment, and surgery may prove necessary. When complications such as hemorrhage, perforation of the duodenum, or STENOSIS (narrowing or obstruction due to fibrosis) occur, the need for surgical treatment becomes urgent.

Dupuytren's contracture

A relatively common deformity of the fingers in the hand, most often affecting middle-aged men. The cause is not known.

The tendons that flex the fingers lie within the palm side of the hand. In Dupuytren's contracture, the covering of such a tendon contracts and shortens into a fibrous nodule. In so doing, it causes the relevant finger to bend toward the palm. The fingers that are affected are the ring finger, the little finger, or both, and often both hands. The only other changes that occur are thickening and dimpling of the skin on the palm. This is not usually a painful condition.

In early cases, splinting, which forces the finger to remain straight, is used. For all other cases, however, surgical intervention is the only treatment. After surgery, a splint is worn for a short time. It is imperative that physical therapy begin after the splint is off to prevent recurrence of the original condition.

dysentery

An infection of the colon characterized by painful diarrhea with mucus and blood in the stools. Dysentery may be due to bacterial or amoebic infection.

Bacillary dysentery is the result of infection of the large intestine by bacteria of the genus *Shigella*—*S. sonnei, S. flexneri, S. dysenteriae,* and *S. boydii,* the last three flourishing in tropical and subtropical countries. Infection with *S. sonnei* is usually relatively mild, while the other infections tend to produce severe loss of fluids and prostration. The incubation period of all is usually two or three days. Infection is spread by food contaminated by feces, being the result of poor standards of personal hygiene and sanitation. Flies may spread the infection. Diagnosis is made by isolation of the infecting organisms from the stools; treatment depends on the severity of the condition, ranging from simple medications in mild cases to suitable antibiotics and intravenous fluid therapy in those suffering from serious fluid loss.

Amoebic dysentery, also spread by faulty hygiene, results from infection with protozoa of the species *Entamoeba histolytica.* The disease is found all over the world, particularly in poor communities, and produces symptoms of varying severity ranging from mild abdominal discomfort with loose stools to severe and acute bloody diarrhea with frequent abdominal pain. The condition may become chronic and may be mistaken for other gastric and intestinal disorders. But in time large numbers of amoebas spread to and multiply in the liver and may cause an abscess, which may burst into the abdominal cavity, the chest, or through the wall of the abdomen or chest. Diagnosis is made by microscopic examination of the feces for *E. histolytica,* by endoscopy of the large bowel (which, when infected, shows typical ulceration), or by serological techniques. Effective drugs exist. Abscess formation in the liver may require surgical treatment.

It is important to note that both bacillary and amoebic infections can be spread by "carriers," infected persons who show no signs of having the disease but who carry live organisms in their intestines. Unexplained outbreaks of dysentery in institutions sometimes are traced to such a carrier by examination of the stools of apparently healthy kitchen workers.

dyslexia

Word blindness; extreme difficulty in understanding the written word.

Dyslexia covers a wide range of language difficulties; in general, sufferers cannot grasp the meaning of sequences of letters, words, or symbols or the concept of direction.

The condition can affect people of otherwise normal intelligence and of every socioeconomic group. Sometimes there is a family history; sometimes the condition arises from brain damage. Often the cause is obscure.

In severe cases the dyslexic individual is unable to read, makes bizarre errors in spelling, cannot name colors or "left" and "right," and has difficulty putting a name to a picture. Milder cases show less extreme forms of the same difficulties and may go unrecognized.

Indeed, even severe dyslexia is often not diagnosed as the root of a person's problem; the sufferer may therefore be considered lazy, stupid, mentally handicapped, inattentive, or obstinate. In fact, he may be of normal intelligence but frustrated with his inability to comprehend words.

Signs that a child may be dyslexic include late language development, clumsiness, no preference for one hand over the other, a tendency to alter the sequence of syllables in words (like "efelant" for elephant) or of words in a sentence. Any of these signs in an otherwise bright child may raise the suspicion of dyslexia.

Treatment—which is most successful when the condition is diagnosed early—requires painstaking special teaching techniques.

dysmenorrhea

Pain associated with MENSTRUATION.

The most common type is *primary dysmenorrhea,* which is an extreme form of the discomfort most women feel in the first few hours or days of a menstrual period. The lower abdominal pain may be continuous or spasmodic and is accompanied sometimes by pain in the lower back or down the legs. In severe cases the woman may vomit or faint.

Dysmenorrhea is common in women who have not had a pregnancy. The pain is thought to be due to a reduction in blood supply to the uterus when its powerful contractions at the start of a period constrict the blood vessels. Childbirth usually cures the condition because extra blood vessels develop during pregnancy. Even in women who remain childless, dysmenorrhea tends to ease after the age of about 25 and to disappear by 30.

A healthy, active life prevents primary dysmenorrhea. Simple analgesics such as aspirin, acetaminophen, or ibuprofen usually can relieve the pain. Rest in bed with a hot-water bottle is a traditional and often successful treatment.

If such measures are ineffective, a doctor may prescribe the oral contraceptive pill for chronic sufferers, since it prevents ovulation (only periods following normal ovulation are painful).

Secondary dysmenorrhea is a symptom of disease rather than a problem of its own. Diseases causing painful menstruation include chronic PELVIC INFLAMMATORY DISEASE, ENDOMETRIOSIS, and FIBROIDS.

The pain usually starts about a week before menstruation and increases in intensity until the start of the period. It may then be relieved once bleeding starts or may worsen in some cases. Treatment is directed at the underlying disease.

Although many gynecological disorders produce dysmenorrhea, it should be stressed that dysmenorrhea does not necessarily indicate the presence of a disorder; very commonly it can be primary. Therefore it is not a symptom that should cause undue anxiety.

On the other hand, in persistent cases medical advice should be sought; the doctor may be able to relieve the pain and exclude the possibility of any underlying disorder.

dyspareunia

Difficult and painful sexual intercourse experienced by a woman. There is often incomplete vaginal penetration by the penis because of the pain or discomfort felt by the woman.

In most cases, the embarrassment and sensitivity felt by the woman leads to frigidity. There are many causes of this condition, both physical and psychological.

Physical causes include extreme obesity of either partner, injuries of the hip joint leading to difficulty in separating the legs widely, a thick hymen ("maidenhead"), a scarred vagina (as a result of episiotomies or gynecological surgery), and inelastic vaginal walls in postmenopausal women.

Infection or inflammation of the pelvic organs (ovary, uterus, or Fallopian tubes), PROLAPSE of the uterus, and ovarian cysts make intercourse painful. The complaint of dyspareunia may lead to the diagnosis of such conditions when they were previously asymptomatic.

Among psychological causes are clumsiness in the man, previous experience of pain, and fear of pregnancy. In these circumstances the vaginal muscles can go into spasm (VAGINISMUS) and prevent entry of the penis.

Approximately 22 percent of women experience dyspareunia at some time in their lives. The treatment of physical causes is fairly simple: for example, eradicating the infection, correcting the prolapse, or removing a cyst.

Psychologically, confidence may be less easily restored. Education of both partners in sex techniques (including the use of lubricants and vaginal dilators) is necessary and usually successful.

dyspepsia

Literally, "difficulty in digesting," or indigestion.

Dyspepsia is experienced by most people at some time in their lives, since INDIGESTION is extremely common. It is ordinarily not a serious problem unless it is either constant or prolonged for many weeks. It can be associated with irregular meals, alcoholic excess, or eating foods to which one is unaccustomed.

The symptoms include belching, a feeling of distension in the upper part of the abdomen, an acidic taste in the mouth, stomach pains, and sometimes nausea. Common causes include eating fatty foods (especially when fried), foods that contain sulfur (such as eggs, cucumbers, onions, and salads) or strongly acid foods (fruit and wines). Dyspepsia is sometimes associated with smoking on an empty stomach, skipping meals, and chronic anxiety—with consequent excess secretions of gastric acid.

If dyspepsia is continual, regularly causes disruption of sleep, or occurs after every meal, it may be a symptom of a developing ulcer. Prompt medical attention should be sought to confirm the diagnosis and permit early treatment.

In mild cases the most effective treatment is the use of oral antacids—particularly the effervescent types—which usually will relieve the discomfort.

dyspnea

Shortness of breath or difficulty in breathing, sometimes after slight physical activity.

Dyspnea can occur in people who are otherwise healthy, often as a result of obesity, lack of physical fitness, excessive smoking, or high altitude. It is also associated with cardiac and respiratory problems. Sufferers show a varying tolerance that depends on the anxiety level produced by the experience of breathlessness.

Rest, appropriate treatment of any underlying disease, dietary control, and carefully graded physical training may improve the condition.

dysuria

Painful or difficult urination. Dysuria can be a symptom of such conditions as inflammation of the urinary bladder, swelling of the prostate, and urinary tract infections or tumors.

earache

A pain in the ear that may be sharp, dull, burning, intermittent, or continuous. It may come from the hearing mechanisms themselves—the eardrum, inner ear, outer canal, or the deeper bone structure—whenever they are subject to trauma or inflammation; or it may arise from the joint of the *mandible* (jawbone) or elsewhere. The most common causes are OTITIS MEDIA and OTITIS EXTERNA.

Acute earache sometimes is felt during plane trips because of unequal air pressures on the two sides of the eardrum. Blockage of the eustachian tube, which normally equalizes pressure by allowing air to pass into or out of the middle ear, is a common cause of earache. This occurs in upper-respiratory-tract infections.

Because the cranial nerves of the neck, face, jaw, and scalp all collect sensory branches from the ear, earache can be caused by disorders such as dental disease, tonsillitis, nasal congestion, jaw inflammation, and cervical spine (neck) injury. Eruption of the wisdom teeth often is marked by coincident earache in adolescents, and the growth

of teeth in infants frequently is accompanied by earache.

Diagnosis of the cause is important to ensure there is no serious ear disease. Treatment, apart from relief of pain, may include the administration of antibiotic drops for the ear, removal of excess earwax, and dental assessment. In young children with OTITIS MEDIA, appropriate treatment is necessary to prevent the complications of chronic infection that may damage hearing.

earwax

Accumulated secretions of the tiny glands in the skin that line the outer canal of the ear. These secretions protect the eardrum and maintain elasticity. Excessive secretions, however, may form a brownish-yellow mass that can block the canal and cause sudden or progressive impairment of hearing or even deafness. The wax then requires removal.

Usually it is softened first with drops that dissolve fat (or with warm olive oil); later it can be gently and painlessly removed by a nurse or physician.

People who work in a dusty, humid atmosphere or who frequently wear earphones tend to secrete more earwax. Some may require attention regularly.

No object should be put into the ear to remove wax unless this is done by a doctor or nurse.

ecchymosis

A purplish patch of flat bruising caused by bleeding under the skin.

It may occur as a result of minor trauma, blood-clotting defects, or fragility in blood vessels. Ecchymoses are common in the elderly and are a normal part of aging—even when there is no evidence of other circulatory disorders, nutritional deficiency, or blood disease.

In young people ecchymoses are rare unless they are associated with HEMOPHILIA, SCURVY, PURPURA, or the effects of various drugs or chemicals.

Ecchymoses usually resolve themselves without treatment by reabsorption of the "leaked" blood. This gradual reabsorption process usually takes a week and accounts for the color changes of the bruises as they age. Frequent recurrence or the presence of many small ecchymoses (*petechiae*) indicates the need for special blood tests.

ECHO virus

A group of viruses responsible for several mild diseases such as summer flu, diarrhea of the newborn, and certain skin rashes. (The name is derived from viruses belonging to the so-called Enteric Cytopathogenic Human Orphan group.) They attack young children mainly, although not exclusively, and are more active during the warm months of the year. Often they cause minor epidemics in which several children in a neighborhood become infected with the virus. The symptoms include a high fever, headache, pains in the limbs, and a sore throat.

One group of the ECHO viruses can produce blisters of the mouth or soft palate, while another causes PERICARDITIS (inflammation of the outer lining of the heart). Some other ECHO viruses produce ORCHITIS (inflammation of the testicles); a further group is responsible for a serious form of MENINGITIS (inflammation of the membranes that surround the brain). This last type of ECHO virus infection requires hospitalization, as does the highly infectious diarrhea sometimes seen in newborn babies.

Many cases of ECHO virus infection go unrecognized. The person tends to assume that it is a cold, chill, or sore throat. As a result of these mild infections, most people develop immunity to the ECHO viruses by the time they reach adulthood.

The treatment of mild infection is simple home nursing care. The illness seldom lasts more than a few days.

ectopic pregnancy

Pregnancy in which the fertilized egg begins to grow somewhere other than the womb.

Normally the fertilized egg passes down the Fallopian tube and becomes implanted on the inner wall of the uterine cavity. An ectopic pregnancy occurs when the egg starts to develop in another area, such as the abdominal cavity, a Fallopian tube, an ovary, or the ligaments of the uterus. By far the most common site for an ectopic pregnancy is the Fallopian tube; this is called a "tubal" pregnancy.

The space for the embryo to grow is limited

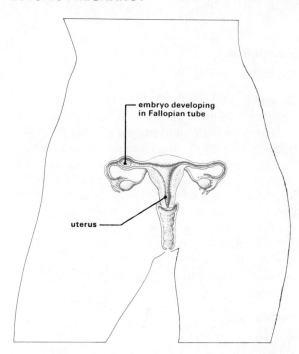

An ectopic pregnancy occurs when a fertilized egg becomes implanted and continues to develop somewhere outside the uterus. A Fallopian-tube pregnancy is the most common variety, and usually occurs following narrowing of the tube by infection.

in ectopic pregnancies, and the result is an acute surgical emergency, with risk of serious hemorrhage, at any time from the sixth week onward. Such pregnancies rarely last beyond the sixteenth week without provoking a crisis.

eczema

A noninfectious inflammatory disease of the skin that takes the form of redness, blistering, crusting, and scaling.

The well-known type of eczema seen in infancy and childhood, medically called *atopic eczema*, tends to run in families where there is asthma or hay fever. The skin typically breaks out in eczematous patches—particularly on the forearms, the backs of the knees, and the face.

There are other types of eczema. *Allergic eczema* usually is due to food allergies. Identification and avoidance of the cause, which may be anything from cow's milk to seafood, cures the problem. *Occupational eczema* may be caused by skin irritants

ECZEMA

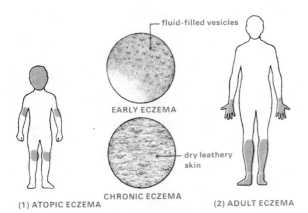

fluid-filled vesicles

EARLY ECZEMA

dry leathery skin

CHRONIC ECZEMA

(1) ATOPIC ECZEMA   (2) ADULT ECZEMA

Eczema can run in families ("atopic eczema") or result from an external irritant. Atopic eczema may start in infancy, when the face is particularly affected, and later tends to be confined to the hollows of the elbows and behind the knees (1). In adults, hands often are affected in certain occupations, and eczema over the legs develops with bad varicose veins (2).

EDEMA

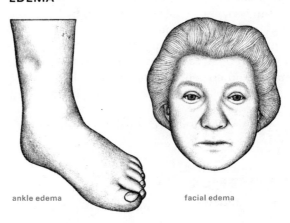

ankle edema   facial edema

Edema is the distension of the soft tissues by excess fluid which has seeped out of the circulation. Ankle edema usually results from poor drainage by the veins and is seen in congestive heart failure and pregnancy. Facial edema is a characteristic of kidney disease and is especially noticeable after a night's sleep.

such as mineral oils, detergents, and degreasing agents. Liquid detergents and soap powders are a common cause of this type of eczema. In other cases the eczema may be caused by the application of ointments that produce a sensitivity reaction.

"Eczema" and "dermatitis" are often interchangeable words, especially in the sensitivity type of inflammation.

Eczema is fundamentally a reaction to irritants. It is common, affecting 20 percent of the population at some time in their lives, and is more frequent in whites than in blacks.

See also DERMATITIS.

edema

A generalized or local swelling of body tissues due to the retention of tissue fluid.

Excess body water normally is removed by the circulation and excreted via the kidneys. Many disorders of the heart or kidneys will result in edema, as the body is unable to rid itself of fluid. A patient may retain 10 to 20 pounds (9 kilograms) of excess water before edema becomes apparent. Swelling in the ankles is often the first sign, although in bed-bound patients the first swelling may appear in the lower back.

If you press a finger into tissues that are edem-

atous, a "pit" mark remains afterward, and this is used to assess the severity of the edema. Edema is a sign of a disorder or disease rather than a disease itself.

Edema often occurs in people with severely incompetent varicose veins, and in hot weather it is seen even in healthy people. In pregnancy, however, edema is often an early sign of toxemia and requires a medical evaluation.

Pulmonary edema is the collection of fluid in the lungs, a potentially life-threatening condition.

Cases of edema need to be evaluated to find their underlying cause. A variety of medications can be used to lessen edema by increasing cardiac output and/or kidney excretion (diuretics). Fluid restriction and low-sodium diets may be used in severe or chronic cases. In using diuretics, potassium often is excreted along with the excess fluid, so potassium-supplement medications or foods rich in potassium (leafy green vegetables, bananas, fresh orange juice) should be given.

electric shock

The effect of the passage of an electric current through the body.

An electric shock sometimes is used to treat mental patients suffering from depression and other disorders. But, in general, electric shocks to the body, especially those caused by high voltage, can be dangerous and even fatal (electrocution). Every effort should be made at all times to avoid contact with live electrical wires, for even household current can give a fatal shock. Much can be done by way of first aid, however, to help victims.

See also *Electric Shock* in the section on **First Aid.**

elephantiasis

Dramatic swelling of the tissues caused by severe blockage of the lymphatic vessels by tiny thread-like worms (*filariae*).

These microscopic worms are transmitted to humans in tropical and subtropical zones of the world largely by a particular species of mosquito (*Culex fatigans*). *Obstructive filariasis*, to use its proper name, is known commonly as elephantiasis because it causes such marked and chronic swelling of the legs, scrotum, arms, breasts, and vulva that the huge deformities look elephantine in their disproportion.

This severe form of filariasis develops slowly only after years of chronic reinfection and is seen in fewer than 0.2 percent of those infected with the worms. Treatment of the early infection is successful with drugs; once chronic obstruction has developed, however surgical removal of the elephantoid scrotum, vulva, or breast may be necessary. Surgery for limb elephantiasis is difficult.

embolus/embolism

Blockage of a blood vessel by material transported in the blood circulation. The condition is called embolism; the blocking material is an embolus.

An embolus is often a piece of solid matter that forces its way through the circulatory system until it becomes wedged in and blocks a small blood vessel. It may be a clot of blood, a globule of fat, or a piece of tumor tissue that has eroded a blood vessel. Or it may be a bubble of air admitted during an intravenous injection.

The most common cause of embolism is the breaking away of a piece of a thrombus, a blood clot that has formed in an artery, a vein, or the chambers of the heart. When a fragment of the thrombus breaks off it becomes the embolus,

which eventually may lodge in a smaller blood vessel.

The effect of an embolism is to deprive the involved tissues of their blood supply (ISCHEMIA), which can cause irreparable damage to or even the death of those tissues.

Pulmonary (lung) *embolism*—obstruction of the pulmonary artery or one of its branches—is so serious as to cause death in approximately 5 percent of cases. Most emboli arise from the veins of the legs and pelvis and are a well-recognized complication of pregnancy, postoperative recovery, or extended bed rest.

Fat embolisms may occur after injury to the long bones and the consequent release of bone-marrow fat into the bloodstream.

Air embolism, as a consequence of unskilled intravenous injection, commonly is seen in drug addicts. It can occur in a serious form in scuba divers who surface too quickly.

Cerebral embolism—where an embolus has lodged in an artery of the brain may produce signs of a STROKE (cerebrovascular accident). In an *arterial embolism* (most often seen in the legs), the area beyond the blockage becomes white, cold, and painful.

Vascular surgeons can often successfully remove an arterial thrombus, especially if they operate soon after the diagnosis. In time small venous embolisms may be bypassed naturally with the development of new channels for the flow of

EMBOLUS

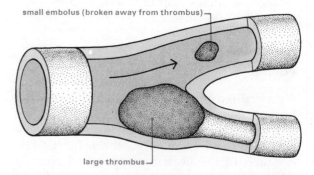

small embolus (broken away from thrombus)

large thrombus

An embolus is any abnormal particle circulating in the blood. The most common type is a fragment of blood clot that has broken off from a larger thrombus, as pictured here. The embolus travels until it blocks a small blood vessel, thus cutting off the supply to an area of tissue. Embolisms can be fatal, especially when they block circulation in the lung or brain.

EMPHYSEMA

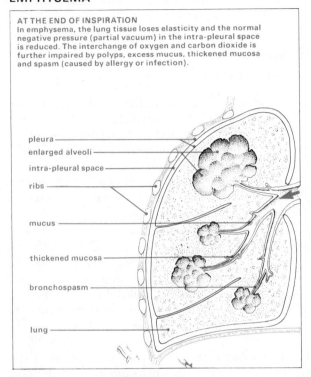

AT THE END OF INSPIRATION
In emphysema, the lung tissue loses elasticity and the normal negative pressure (partial vacuum) in the intra-pleural space is reduced. The interchange of oxygen and carbon dioxide is further impaired by polyps, excess mucus, thickened mucosa and spasm (caused by allergy or infection).

pleura
enlarged alveoli
intra-pleural space
ribs

mucus

thickened mucosa

bronchospasm

lung

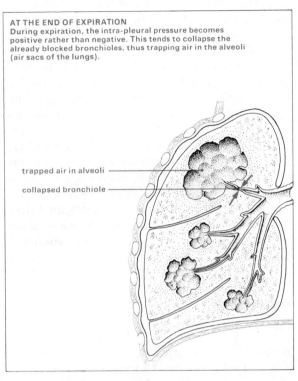

AT THE END OF EXPIRATION
During expiration, the intra-pleural pressure becomes positive rather than negative. This tends to collapse the already blocked bronchioles, thus trapping air in the alveoli (air sacs of the lungs).

trapped air in alveoli
collapsed bronchiole

Emphysema is a progressive disease in which the air sacs (alveoli) of the lungs become overdistended or inflated with trapped air. The condition may be associated with an inherited weakness of the lungs, an infection of the lung tissue, or the prolonged inhalation of polluted air (including smoking).

blood. Their recurrence can be prevented by the use of anticoagulant drugs.

emphysema

A defect of the lung causing overinflation and changes of the air sacs where oxygen–carbon dioxide exchange takes place.

Emphysema is one of the leading causes of death from respiratory illness in the United States. It may occur as a consequence of other diseases such as BRONCHITIS or WHOOPING COUGH, in which the damaged air sacs merge into larger spaces. This results in a decrease in the surface area available for oxygen entry, with a resulting strain on the heart, breathlessness, and EDEMA. The chest may become barrel-shaped, and wheezy breathing is particularly common. Treatment of this basically irreversible condition is to protect the person from infection and to preserve general health as long as possible. For people with emphysema, cigarette smoking is disastrous.

empyema

A collection of pus in a body cavity—most often the chest. It is a fairly rare complication of a primary infection of the lungs (such as PLEURISY, PNEUMONIA, or TUBERCULOSIS).

The natural course of empyema is for the contained pus and fluid to burst and discharge itself outward through the chest wall or inward into the bronchus. Before this happens, however, the condition may be manifested by fever, sweating, and either lung collapse or visible fluid levels in the chest X-ray study.

Empyema has virtually been wiped out by antibiotic therapy.

encephalitis

An inflammation of the brain, usually viral but sometimes bacterial in origin.

Certain viruses that attack human beings—a few of them transmitted by insects—show a tendency to localize their effects in the brain and the membranes (meninges) surrounding the brain. These tissues may become inflammed, swollen, and waterlogged; the resulting vascular congestion sometimes leads to small hemorrhages. The patient is then suffering from encephalitis (sometimes called "brain fever").

Symptoms include headache, neck pain, fever, nausea, and vomiting. Nervous system problems may occur such as seizure, personality changes, short temper, laziness, paralysis, weakness, and coma. Treatment includes antibiotics for infection, steroids to reduce brain swelling, medication to control fever and headache, and prolonged bed rest.

encephalitis lethargica

A disease that occurred in the wake of the pandemic of influenza during and for about ten years after World War I. Also known as *von Economo's disease*. Nothing like this disease is recorded from before 1914 and few if any cases have been recorded in America and Western Europe since 1930.

Although the organism was never identified, the disease was typical of a viral infection. Persons usually suffered from pronounced somnolence together with ophthalmoplegia (paralysis of the eye muscles), although a minority were hyperactive. Headache, insomnia, dizziness, tiredness, confusion, and disorders of movement were common. More than 29 percent of the victims died within a few weeks and a high proportion of the survivors developed PARKINSON'S DISEASE. Some children developed psychopathic personality with compulsive behavior.

encephalomyelitis

Diffuse inflammation of both the brain (ENCEPH-ALITIS) and spinal cord (MYELITIS). It can be caused by a number of agents, including viral infections and syphilis; bacterial encephalomyelitis rarely occurs.

It is characterized by fever, headache, stiff neck, back pain, and vomiting. Problems of the nervous system such as seizures, paralysis, personality changes, a lowered level of awareness, coma, or death may occur.

endocarditis

Inflammation of the surface of the heart valves or of the lining of the heart chambers. Most often endocarditis is caused by bacterial infection; it may also be a complication of a COLLAGEN DISEASE such as systemic LUPUS ERYTHEMATOSUS or RHEUMATOID ARTHRITIS. Endocarditis occurs not infrequently in intravenous drug users and may be caused by unusual organisms like fungi.

Infective endocarditis may be an illness of slow onset, and weeks of unexplained ill health may pass before an accurate diagnosis is made. The initial symptoms include fever, sweating, and weight loss; later, small painful nodules may develop in the hands and feet and there may be bleeding beneath the fingernails. If untreated, the multiplication of bacteria on the surface of the heart valves causes distortion of the valves' shape. Treatment depends on recognition of the condition and laboratory culture of the microorganisms in the bloodstream that are responsible. Prolonged therapy with an appropriate antibiotic should eradicate the infection, especially if begun at a relatively early stage in the disease.

Bacterial endocarditis is unusual in persons who have no heart trouble. The infection starts most often in persons with a heart defect associated with a congenital heart disease or in those with a heart valve that has been scarred by RHEU-MATIC HEART DISEASE (a common complication of RHEUMATIC FEVER during childhood).

Persons known to have valvular heart disease usually are given antibiotics to protect them from bacterial endocarditis on occasions (such as before tooth cleaning or other forms of dental surgery) when bacteria may be released into the bloodstream.

endocrine glands

The ductless glands of the body that secrete hormones directly into the bloodstream. Examples of these glands are the thyroid gland in the neck, the adrenal glands in the abdomen, and the pituitary gland in the brain.

See also ENDOCRINOLOGIST in the section on **Providers**.

endometriosis

The internal lining of the uterus, the *endometrium*, normally is confined to the cavity of the organ, but in some women "islands," or fragments, of endometrial tissue are to be found on the ovary or in various places within the abdominal cavity. These patches of endometrium respond to the hormonal changes of each menstrual cycle in the same way as the lining of the normal uterus. Internal bleeding occurs with each cycle and leads to the formation of blood-filled cysts in the affected organs.

Endometriosis may be silent or it may produce symptoms, usually in women between the ages of 30 and 40. Lower abdominal discomfort or pain (worse at the time of the menstrual period), pain during sexual intercourse (DYSPAREUNIA), and disordered menstruation all suggest the possibility of endometriosis.

The condition is one cause of infertility; but as it is often found in women who marry and conceive later in life and less often in those who have early pregnancies (so that pregnancy may be said to protect against endometriosis), the relationship is obscure. Symptoms certainly improve during pregnancy and almost always disappear at menopause.

Treatment depends on the severity of the disease. In mild cases nothing may need to be done. In more serious cases minor surgery may be needed or medications given to suppress hormone production. In the most severe cases it may be necessary to remove the uterus, ovaries, and Fallopian tubes (complete hysterectomy).

endometritis

Inflammation of the *endometrium* (the lining of the uterus), usually caused by a bacterial infection such as gonorrhea or by the chlamydia trachomatis. Also known as PELVIC INFLAMMATORY DISEASE.

The disease may occur spontaneously or may follow childbirth, septic abortion, or injury involving the pelvic organs. It is especially common in women fitted with the intrauterine contraceptive device (IUD). It may be acute or chronic; the chronic form of the disease is usually the result of repeated acute attacks.

Acute endometritis is characterized by pain in the lower part of the back, low abdominal pain,

ENDOMETRITIS

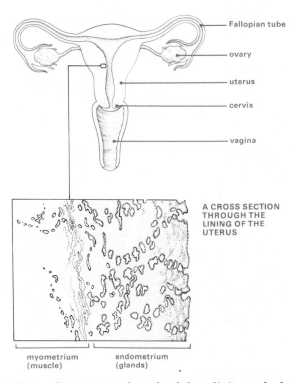

Fallopian tube

ovary

uterus

cervix

vagina

A CROSS SECTION THROUGH THE LINING OF THE UTERUS

myometrium (muscle)   endometrium (glands)

The endometrium—the glandular lining of the uterus—thickens during every menstrual cycle in preparation for a possible pregnancy. Endometritis, inflammation of the endometrium, occurs as a result of bacterial infection.

and disorders of menstruation (such as DYSMENORRHEA or MENORRHAGIA). The fallopian tubes are involved often, and infertility may result.

Diagnosis may require dilatation and curettage (D & C), followed by microscopic examination of a sample of the affected tissues and culture and identification of the causative microorganisms. Once the cause of the inflammation of the endometrium is established, the appropriate antibiotic therapy can be initiated.

enema

A procedure in which fluid (usually water, soapy water, or oil) is introduced into the rectum through the anus for cleansing or treatment. The enema is given through a thin tube lubricated at the tip or from a special container. It is given slowly and the person receiving the enema is asked to retain the fluid for as long as possible before expelling it.

An enema may be necessary to: (1) clear the bowels of feces in severe constipation, or where the feces have become impacted, or before labor; (2) clean out the bowels before an operation on that part of the body; (3) replace body fluid in mild dehydration; and (4) administer drugs, as in the treatment of ULCERATIVE COLITIS.

enlarged prostate

Some degree of prostatic enlargement is extremely common in men over age 45 and is a natural result of aging. However, in some men the enlarged prostate gland becomes rigid and obstructs the passage of urine through the urethra. For an extended discussion, see "prostate problems" in *Common Diseases and Disorders of Aging* under **Senior Living**.

PROSTATE GLAND

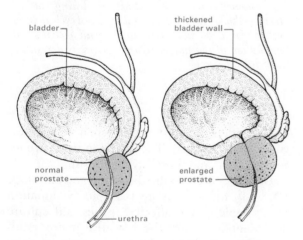

Left, normal prostate; right, enlarged prostate.

enteritis

Inflammation of the intestines, particularly the small intestine.

There are several possible causes. The most usual one is bacterial or viral infection after consuming contaminated food or water.

Outbreaks of food poisoning occasionally pro-

duce serious attacks of GASTROENTERITIS lasting a few days, with headaches, fever, and severe diarrhea. Public health measures may be required to track down the offending organism, which often originates in a specific restaurant or institution. Gastroenteritis in babies is serious since it can cause rapid dehydration.

Acute gastroenteritis may also result from food allergies and immune deficiency.

epidemic pleurodynia

An infectious disease characterized by the sudden onset of severe abdominal pain or chest pain (or both), fever, and headache. Also known as *epidemic myalgia, devil's grip,* and *Bornholm disease.*

Epidemic pleurodynia usually occurs in outbreaks in the summer and fall, but it may also occur in single cases. It is most common in children and young adults and is caused by a virus of the Coxsackie B group. The first symptom is usually chest pain or severe abdominal pain that is made worse by movement. Some persons have a preceding illness—a "head cold," with headaches and muscle pains—for a few days; all eventually have headaches and a fever. The pattern of symptoms varies from one outbreak to another.

In an outbreak the diagnosis is made easily, but single cases are more difficult to diagnose and the condition may be confused initially with serious illnesses such as acute APPENDICITIS or MYOCARDIAL INFARCTION ("heart attack").

There is no specific treatment. Bed rest and the relief of pain and fever by drugs such as aspirin are all that can be offered. Death has never been reported and serious complications are very rare. The disease usually lasts for only a few days, but some people may have lingering after effects of tiredness and weakness, with only a gradual return to full health.

epilepsy

Disorganized electrical activity in the brain leading to transient attacks of disturbed sensory or motor function. Some forms of epilepsy are characterized by convulsions (epileptic seizures).

In what is known as *symptomatic* epilepsy, the convulsions may be traced to one of several definite causes. These include: a structural disorder of the brain—such as a tumor or abscess—that causes pressure on sensitive brain tissue; disease of the blood vessels of the brain; poisoning by drugs; and injury to the brain. Children very often experience seizures during infections that are accompanied by high fever, but these are not epileptic.

More common, however, is *idiopathic* epilepsy, where abnormal brain-cell activity arises for no apparent reason. This is the condition that most people think of as epilepsy.

Warning symptoms may be noticed: headaches, drowsiness, giddiness, yawning. These are followed by the "aura," the actual beginning of the seizure, in which there may be tingling sensations in the limbs and disturbances of taste and smell.

The attack itself falls into one of three main types:

Petit mal, or "absence," attacks are quite difficult to recognize clinically, particularly in children, in whom they mainly occur. The child may appear to be vacantly daydreaming for a few seconds. If he is standing, he may sway slightly and fall to the ground. Observers often are unaware that an attack has occurred.

Grand mal attacks are preceded more often by warning symptoms and the aura. As consciousness is lost, the patient may fall, sometimes emitting a characteristic "epileptic cry" as the larynx goes into spasm. The muscles contract rigidly and the jaws clamp shut with tremendous pressure. Sometimes the person bites his tongue. Then the muscles start to jerk violently, and the person may look blue until the convulsion passes and normal breathing is resumed.

As the fit passes off, the person may fall into a deep sleep (from which he should not be disturbed) or may go into a trance-like state. It is important that an epileptic not be left to lie face upward or in a position where he could inhale his own vomit.

Focal seizures (or "Jacksonian seizures") usually result from organic disease or brain injury. The attack starts in a localized group of muscles and usually does not lead to loss of consciousness.

Many adults, especially those with a mild form of epilepsy, keep the seizures totally under control with drugs. The most effective are phenytoin and carbamazepine. Other useful drugs are ethosuximide, primidone, clonazepam, and diazepam; after a period of trial and error the correct dose is worked out for each individual. If the person has not had a seizure after two years or so, the dose is slowly reduced. Some persons appear to be completely cured, but this is rare.

epinephrine

A hormone secreted by the ADRENAL GLANDS. Also called adrenaline.

epistaxis

Bleeding from the nose. See NOSEBLEED.

epithelioma

A type of tumor of the skin. There are various types with different degrees of severity.

Malignant tumors of the skin may be caused by overexposure to sunlight; their incidence in such people as farmers, sportsmen, and sun worshipers is linked directly to exposure to the sun. Fair-skinned people are more susceptible. See BASAL CELL CARCINOMA.

Tumors known as *squamous cell epitheliomas* may start to grow suddenly after a long latent period. Shaped like papules or plaques, they develop into crusted ulcers or fungal growths. The mucous membranes of the mouth, nose, and vulva may be affected as well as the exposed skin.

Unusual nodules, bumps, and ulcers on the skin should always be reported to the doctor. After early diagnosis, treatment by surgery or irradiation is very successful.

Epstein-Barr virus

A virus, named after its discoverers, that is responsible for causing INFECTIOUS MONONUCLEOSIS. It is strongly implicated also as a cause of Burkitt's LYMPHOMA.

ergotism

A serious but fortunately rare disease caused by eating bread made from rye that is contaminated with the parasitic fungus *Claviceps purpurea.*

The symptoms are severe muscle pains, cold skin, vomiting, diarrhea, weakness, and severe mental confusion.

erysipelas

A dangerous skin disease, caused by infection with the bacterium *Streptococcus pyogenes*. Erysipelas (also known as "St. Anthony's fire") produces a bright red inflammation and swelling of the skin, together with fever, chills, and sometimes nausea and vomiting.

The condition may originate from infection following a minor scratch or from contamination of a surgical wound. Infection with the streptococci causes a red, glistening swelling of the skin with a clearly demarcated edge. The inflammation may spread rapidly and in untreated cases may progress to collapse and death. Antibiotics are highly effective, however, and the disease is now rarely seen in its florid form.

erythema

Redness of the skin caused by congestion of the tiny blood vessels (capillaries) near the surface. The capillaries may become dilated and congested with blood due to any of several possible factors: some emotional mechanism; exposure to an external stimulus such as heat, cold, or ultraviolet rays (as in SUNBURN); exposure to ionizing (high-energy) radiation such as X rays or gamma rays. Among other causes of erythema are reactions to certain drugs, insect bites, or stings; certain viral infections (such as MEASLES) can produce an erythematous rash. Patchy erythema may also occur in chronic diseases such as systemic LUPUS ERYTHEMATOSUS.

Specific types of erythema are indicated in medical practice by a modifying term: for example, *erythema nodosum*, characterized by the formation of red nodules, is an acute inflammatory skin disease, thought to be caused by various types of allergic reactions.

eschar

An area of dead tissue produced by the action of corrosive substances or by burning.

Escharotics are substances employed to treat warts, other skin diseases, and some infected tissues. Their action is unpredictable and the area burned may exceed that desired.

esophageal varices

Enlarged and tortuous veins in the lower part of the esophagus ("gullet") found in association with raised blood pressure in the abdominal veins (*portal hypertension*), a complication of CIRRHOSIS of the liver.

In the United States portal hypertension is caused most commonly by alcoholic cirrhosis, but it may occur in cirrhosis secondary to HEPATITIS or to other causes. The branches of the veins in the esophagus near the stomach form links with the portal vein—which drains blood from the intestines into the liver. Raised back pressure occurs because of the cirrhosis. The varices often bleed. This may be massive and sudden or there may be minor bleeding for days before the condition is discovered.

It is often difficult to diagnose the source of this hemorrhage, since bleeding in the stomach may be due to an acute or chronic peptic ulcer. Treatment also is difficult. Injection of a medication that causes the blood vessels to contract is sometimes effective. If this fails it may be necessary to use "balloon tamponade," a procedure in which an inflatable device is inserted into the esophagus and pressed against the site of the bleeding. Finally, a surgical operation may be needed to seal the veins and thus stop the bleeding directly. In cases of recurrent bleeding, the portal hypertension may be treated by diverting the blood from the portal vein into the vena cava, the vein that brings blood into the right-atrium of the heart.

esophagitis

Inflammation of the lining of the esophagus ("gullet"), often caused by the flow of small amounts of gastric juice up the esophagus from the stomach (see HEARTBURN). Other causes include infection and caustic injury from corrosive liquids taken accidentally or in suicide attempts.

estrogens

One of the two types of female sex hormones secreted by the ovaries. There have been more than twenty different estrogens identified biochemically, but estrone, estradiol, and estriol are the three of greatest clinical interest.

Estrogens are responsible for the regeneration of the uterine lining immediately after menstruation; their withdrawal (as the ovarian follicle degenerates) is what provokes menstrual bleeding and the onset of a period. Estrogen production is considerably diminished after menopause, and many of the unwanted symptoms at this time in a woman's life are related to the reduced amounts of estrogens circulating in the blood.

In pregnancy, estrogens are secreted by the placenta to stimulate breast growth in the mother and to maintain uterine growth and receptivity to the fetal demands. Measurements of estrogen levels in the plasma and urine offer a useful assessment of placental efficiency where the baby is smaller than the norm for its stage of development, or where there is doubt about the prognosis for the pregnancy (for example, after threatened labor or hemorrhage).

Estrogens, synthetically produced, are a constituent of the combination-type of oral contraceptive used to suppress ovulation. They are used therapeutically in hormonal creams or suppositories for the treatment of postmenopausal VAGINITIS, or as tablets in hormone-replacement therapy for the menopausal woman. Used cosmetically to rejuvenate aging skin, they have no value. Excessive doses are associated with an increase in blood clotting, and in recent years the dosage used in oral contraception has been reduced.

Replacement therapy with estrogens is generally recommended in cases where menopause is accompanied by troublesome symptoms, but there is a slightly increased tendency for women who have taken estrogens for a long time to develop cancer of the endometrium (lining of the womb). Most evidence suggests that the incidence of breast cancer is not increased; but mammography (breast X ray) should be done at regular intervals, especially for those taking estrogens.

Menopausal estrogen deficiency often leads to OSTEOPOROSIS, sometimes with serious consequences, such as spine or hip fractures. Estrogens are a valuable part of the management. A history of vein thrombosis or of severe liver disease contraindicates estrogen replacement.

euthanasia

Also called *mercy killing*. The deliberate ending of the life of a person who is suffering from an incurable disease. In recent years, the term has come to include the withholding of procedures and treatments that would prolong the life of an incurably ill patient who could not survive without them, but this is quite a different matter.

exophthalmic goiter

Exophthalmos is an unusual bulging of the eyeballs. This condition develops in HYPERTHYROIDISM and often is accompanied by a GOITER, a swelling in the neck at the site of the thyroid gland. Hyperthyroidism can be caused by several things and needs to be evaluated by a physician. With proper treatment and medication, the bulging of the eyes often can be reduced to normal.

extrasystole

The heart normally beats in a regular rhythm that is controlled by specialized tissue in the heart known as the *conducting system*. The beat is generated by a small mass of tissue belonging to this system and known as the *sinoatrial* (or *sinus*) *node*. From this point, the impulse travels along the rest of the conducting system and through heart muscle to cause other parts of the heart muscle to contract in a well-ordered sequence.

Sometimes, however, impulses are generated outside the sinoatrial node so that extra beats (or extrasystoles) occur. This may happen in normal health, as a result of stress or excitement, or as a side effect of drugs; otherwise the cause may be heart disease.

The extra beat is followed by a longer than usual pause before normal rhythm is resumed. The person may notice a "skipped beat," or a flutter, or extra beats. The significance of extrasystoles depends on their location, underlying cause, and frequency. Too many extra beats prevent the heart from pumping blood around the body efficiently and cause the heart to be overworked. Treatment depends on the cause and on the type (site of origin) of the extrasystole.

fainting

Complete or partial loss of consciousness due to a temporary lack of blood supply to the brain.

Fainting is usually part of a physiological reaction to overwhelming pain, emotional shock, or extreme fear. These cause stimulation and overactivity of the *vagus nerve;* consequently the pulse rate slows, the heart reduces its output, and the blood vessels in the muscles widen. The result is a drop in the pressure of the blood in the circulation to the brain and a temporary reduction in oxygen and glucose supply. Normal brain function is critically dependent on a sustained supply of both.

Fainting can also be induced by a close, hot atmosphere, prolonged lack of food, or by standing still in one position too long so that the blood pools in the vessels of the legs.

The person who is about to faint feels weak and nauseated; the skin breaks out in a sweat and feels cold, and there is yawning or deep sighing. In a little while the complexion becomes pale and consciousness slips away.

Recovery quickly ensues once the person's head is lowered in relation to the rest of the body, permitting a prompt increase in the supply of blood to the brain.

Fallopian tube

The tube through which the female egg cell (*ovum*) travels from the ovary to the uterus; there is one tube on each side of the uterus.

In each menstrual cycle a *Graafian follicle* forms in an ovary and eventually ruptures, releasing an ovum into one of the Fallopian tubes. It is during the passage of the ovum through the tube (which takes several days) that fertilization by a sperm cell occurs. After fertilization the egg continues its journey through the tube and enters the uterus where it becomes implanted in the wall of the womb.

Sometimes, however, the embryo remains in the tube and begins to develop there—a condition known as ECTOPIC PREGNANCY.

Sterilization in women is performed usually by ligation ("tying") of the tubes, which prevents ova from descending from the ovaries. The Fallopian tubes may be blocked by disease with the same effect, making the woman infertile. Surgery to reopen blocked tubes is only occasionally successful.

farmer's lung

A disease associated with prolonged exposure to organic dusts, particularly those given off by moldy hay, grain, and other vegetable matter. It is known also as *acute interstitial pneumonitis,* or "thresher's lung."

Characteristically it begins suddenly with night sweats, cough, fever, difficulty in breathing, headache, and chest pains. Most sufferers recover soon after being removed from the environment in which they are exposed to hay and grain. With repeated attacks, however, more serious lung conditions such as EMPHYSEMA may develop with potentially fatal consequences.

Farmer's lung is thought to be due to sensitivity to antigens in the molds.

fecalith

A hard mass in the large intestine formed from hardened dried feces and calcium salts. This condition is rare but is a potentially serious complication of chronic constipation. If the fecalith blocks the intestine, surgical removal may be necessary.

feces

The solid waste matter eliminated from the body after the digestion of food. Feces, like urine, are often a useful aid in the diagnosis of various diseases.

The process of digestion takes place in the stomach and small intestine. After passing through the large intestine, where its water content is largely reabsorbed, the indigestible residue of this process collects in the rectum—together with large quantities of bacteria that have assisted in the process of digestion and coloring agents such as bile. The normal dark brown color of the feces is derived from a bile pigment known as stercobilin.

For most people, one daily bowel movement is normal; but for other individuals "normal" can range from several times a day to once every several days. A sudden change in bowel habits may be a warning sign of disease.

The shape of feces ("stools") should be cylindrical and the consistency should be firm but not hard. Many physicians believe that modern Western diets lack essential fiber ("roughage") and that added fiber is needed to ensure a healthy digestive system.

The two most common departures from the

norm are DIARRHEA and CONSTIPATION. Each can be a sign of a number of different diseases; if either is prolonged, medical attention should be sought. Blood in the feces can be a sign of conditions as diverse as hemorrhoids and tumors and is an even more urgent reason to seek medical attention.

Fecal fat often is measured during hospital laboratory investigation since it provides an indication of the efficiency of digestion and absorption.

felon

Any acute inflammation of the deep-seated tissues of the fingers, usually one that exudes pus. The term may be applied also to an inflammation of the toes. Also called *whitlow.*

The structure that is affected may be the root of the nail, the pulp of the fingertip or toe tip, the bone, or the sheaths of the tendons that run along the back and front of the fingers or toes. Usually the felon begins either as a small abscess at the root of the nail or as an abscess in the tissues (both fatty and fibrous) that make up the pulp of the digit.

Inflammation of bones in the fingers or toes is rare, but a felon may originate in the sheath of a tendon and, if untreated, it may lead to severe stiffness and disability.

Treatment involves incision and drainage of the lesion (usually by a surgeon who specializes in treating disorders of the hand) and the administration of antibiotics or other appropriate drugs.

fertility

The ability to produce young. Male and female fertility—as measured by the number of children a couple have during the woman's reproductive lifetime—depends on a combination of biological and social factors.

A woman's potential for childbearing is determined by her age at the MENARCHE (the onset of menstruation) and at the MENOPAUSE, on the time spent recovering between pregnancies, and on the frequency of sexual intercourse. A woman in good health in her 20s is estimated to have a 25 percent chance of conceiving from intercourse at the fertile midpoint of a single menstrual cycle.

Male fertility is measured less easily, but most men retain their fertility as long as they remain sexually potent, often well into their 70s or later.

See the extended discussion under *Pregnancy and Childbirth* in the section on **Family Medicine and Health.**

fertilization

The union of an egg cell (ovum) with a sperm cell. The process normally takes place in a FALLOPIAN TUBE, along which the egg cell descends after ovulation. Sperm cells swim up through the uterus into the Fallopian tube to meet the egg. When they meet it they release an enzyme that softens the outer layer of the ovum, thus making it possible for one sperm to penetrate it.

Of the millions of sperm produced during intercourse, only one is required to fertilize the ovum. The entry of the sperm is immediately followed by the formation of a barrier around the ovum to prevent further penetrations. At this point, in a small minority of cases, the fertilized ovum may split in two and so bring about the conception of identical (*homozygous*) twins. Non-

FERTILIZATION

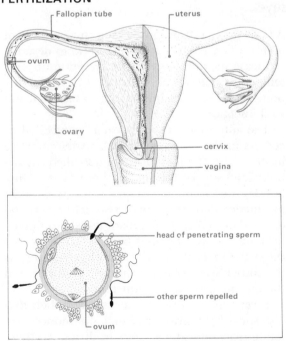

When a sperm meets the ovum, it releases enzymes that digest the membranes surrounding the egg, allowing the head of the sperm to penetrate it. After successful union, no other sperm can penetrate this barrier. The fertilized egg implants itself in the uterine lining about one week after ovulation.

identical (*heterozygous*) twins are conceived as a result of a simultaneous fertilization of two separate ova. (The release of more than one ovum is exceptional, however.)

Upon fertilization, the center of the sperm fuses with the center of the ovum, forming a single cell that contains the 46 chromosomes necessary for human development (see GENES, CHROMOSOMES). Division of the cell proceeds while the ovum is passing along the tube into the uterus, where it arrives as a *blastocyst* containing many new cells. The process of fertilization is complete when the blastocyst implants itself onto the lining of the uterus, where it will develop for the rest of the pregnancy.

fetal distress

The state of a fetus with an abnormal heart rate or rhythm. If possible, the cause is found and corrected. Cesarean section or use of forceps may be necessary to ensure the safety of the fetus.

fever

A body temperature above the normal average of 98.6°F (37°C). The term is used also to describe a disease in which there is an elevation of body temperature above normal. Fever is one of the body's defense mechanisms against bacterial and viral infection.

The autonomic nervous system, controlled by centers in the brainstem, regulates temperature in the body: The part of the brain called the hypothalamus is the biological "thermostat." On a hot day the hypothalamus senses the greater heat production and directs an increased flow of blood to the skin so that the capillaries dilate to radiate heat and the sweat glands become active to cool the skin. On a cold day the hypothalamus directs the muscles to contract rapidly, or shiver, and thereby increase heat production.

Fever can be caused by bacteria and their toxins, spirochetes, viruses, fungi, hormones, immune reactions, and a range of drugs. All these promote the release from macrophages of a substance called interleukin-I. This substance resets the thermostat in the hypothalamus to a higher level than normal, and this may be enough to eliminate the microorganisms responsible for the illness.

The early symptoms of a fever may include a feeling of cold and discomfort, flushed skin or rash, increased pulse and respiration rates, nervous restlessness, and insomnia. The simplest and most effective drug to control fever is aspirin or acetaminophen, but if the fever rises above 104°F (40°C) additional cooling may be provided by ice packs, fans, and sponging with tepid water. Prolonged fevers should be evaluated by a doctor.

fibrillation

The action of the heart muscle is normally coordinated so that the heart can pump blood efficiently. When the muscle relaxes, the chambers of the heart fill with blood flowing into them— on the right side, from the great veins, and on the left from the lungs.

Contraction normally occurs in an ordered sequence: The atria contract just before the ventricles to complete ventricular filling just before the ventricles themselves contract to expel the blood under pressure. Backward flow of blood is prevented by the heart valves.

There is a natural pacemaker in the wall of the right atrium, the *sinoatrial node,* from which a wave of excitation spreads through the muscle of the heart. If contraction becomes disorganized, the muscle contracts and relaxes irregularly (fibrillates) throughout its mass and is effectively paralyzed. Circulation ceases in the part of the heart affected.

Fibrillation may affect the atria or the ventricles. ATRIAL FIBRILLATION is not fatal. VENTRICULAR FIBRILLATION (cardiac arrest) will cause death within minutes unless treatment is immediate.

fibroadenoma

A benign tumor containing a mixture of fibrous and glandular tissue. Fibroadenomas are found in many organs, but they are especially common in the breast.

These tumors occur in the breasts of 10 to 15 percent of women, and the condition is probably much more common than is revealed by cases coming to the attention of surgeons.

Fibroadenomas are usually round, firm, movable, nontender masses. Treatment is by removal under local anesthesia on an outpatient basis. The tumors are sometimes recurrent, and some women will have several removed over a period of years. Even so, any swelling or lump detected in the breast should be examined medically to exclude the possibility of cancer.

fibroids

Tumors of the womb consisting of muscle and some fibrous tissue.

Fibroids are benign and are the most common of all uterine tumors. Their cause is unknown.

They are more correctly known as *myomas*, since they rarely contain much fibrous material and consist almost entirely of smooth muscle. Fibroids are three times more common among black American women than among whites and are also more common in childless women. About one woman in five over the age of 35 has them, but the vast majority of the tumors are benign and cause no symptoms. The fibroids range in size from microscopic lesions to multiple tumors weighing several pounds. Abnormal bleeding is the most common symptom.

In most cases the tumors require no treatment—particularly when there are no symptoms and when the woman is past menopause. Once fibroids have been diagnosed the doctor normally will perform an examination every six to twelve months to check for any increase in size. Some gynecologists have a rule that fibroids should be removed only when they are bigger than a uterus in the twelfth to fourteenth week of pregnancy. However, cervical myomas larger than 1.5 inches (3–4 centimeters) in diameter usually should be removed surgically.

Total hysterectomy (removal of the uterus and ovaries) is rarely necessary; it is performed only when the fibroids are large and multiple. Smaller fibroids often can be removed by "shelling" them out (*myomectomy*).

Surgical removal normally is not attempted when a woman with fibroids is pregnant, unless there is a definite risk that the size of the fibroids may cause spontaneous abortion.

fibrosarcoma

A malignant tumor of the fibrous tissue found in any of the different organs. These malignant tumors are uncommon.

Localized sarcomas generally are treated by surgery.

fibrosis

The formation of scar tissue.

Fibrous repair of damaged tissue restores the continuity of the damaged part, but fibrous tissue cannot function as part of the repaired organ; moreover, it contracts as the scar forms and can interfere with normal function.

Continued irritation of tissue may promote fibrosis. Examples include the fibrosis of lung substance produced by the inhalation of particles of silica in PNEUMOCONIOSIS, and the extensive fibrosis found in cases of ASBESTOSIS, when respiratory function is grossly impaired.

fibrositis

A general term for an aching condition of the muscles. Also called *muscular rheumatism* or *fibromyalgia*.

The condition was given the name because it was wrongly believed to result from inflammation ("-itis") of the fibrous tissue that binds the muscles together.

The pain described as fibrositis is sharp—particularly in the muscles of the back, shoulders, and neck.

The connection between tension or stress and fibrositis is well known. This may be explained by the fact that nervous tension causes muscle tension. Cold is mentioned sometimes as a cause of fibrositis: Tensing of muscles is a natural reflex to cold conditions.

Treatment consists of rest (with occasional moderate exercise if the pain is not too severe) and some form of heat treatment, which may be as simple as warming the affected area with hot towels.

fistula

An abnormal opening or passage between two hollow organs or structures, or between an organ or structure and the exterior. The condition may be present from birth (congenital fistula) or may be a complication of an acquired disorder or disease process.

F!STULA

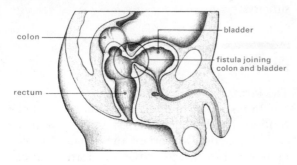

colon

bladder

fistula joining
colon and bladder

rectum

A fistula is an abnormal connection between any two hollow organs or between a hollow organ and the skin. Fistulas occur in Crohn's disease, in cancers, as a result of inflammation (for example, a rectal abscess), and as postoperative complications. A fistula between the colon and bladder, as pictured above, would let air and infecting bacteria into the bladder.

flatulence

The presence of an excess amount of gas in the stomach or intestines.

Excessive swallowing of air (*aerophagia*) is a common cause. This can occur when the person gulps down food, or it can be associated with emotional stress. Flatulence may also be caused by bacterial fermentation of food.

Gas in the stomach may be belched out through the mouth; gas in the bowels causes rumbling, discomfort, and "breaking wind."

Close control of the diet and attention to any air-swallowing habit are essential for the successful control of flatulence.

fleas

Wingless blood-sucking insects of the order Siphonaptera.

Several flea species are of medical importance because they can act as both host and transmitter of disease organisms.

The human flea, *Pulex irritans*, is parasitic on the skin of people. It is a host of the larval stage of *Dipylidium caninum*, the common tapeworm of dogs which can be passed on to humans. It also transmits *Hymenolepsis diminuta*, the dwarf tapeworm. The bites of *Pulex* can cause dermatitis and it may on occasions pass plague from one victim to another. Like all fleas, it is susceptible to DDT and to more recent insecticides.

More important as a disease vector is the rat flea, *Xenopsylla cheopsis*. In addition to the dwarf tapeworm, it passes from infected rats to humans the microorganism that causes bubonic plague, *Yersinia pestis*, as well as *Rickettsia mooseri*, the cause of murine typhus.

Two species of flea commonly infest pet animals: *Ctenocephalides canis* in dogs and *C. felis* in cats. Many pet owners find that these fleas, while normally confined to the coats of animals, make the transition to human hosts quite freely. Frequent use of flea-killing preparations on pets may be necessary to avoid the irritation and threat to health that infestation can bring.

Apart from the general undesirability of harboring a parasite that feeds on human blood, fleas should be eradicated because they are a common cause of papular URTICARIA in children. This condition—a rash of red blotches and white weals—is caused by animal fleas and is an allergic reaction to the protein of the fleas' bodies, whether dead or alive.

Any unduly sensitive child should not be allowed close contact with pets that may be infested. Several proprietary preparations containing the latest effective pesticides against fleas are on sale at any drugstore. Read the directions carefully before using.

Cat or dog fleas are rarely bothersome to hu-

FLEA

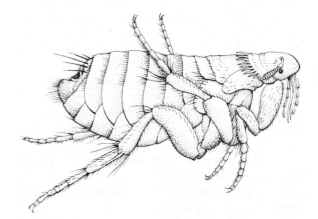

The flea is a wingless parasite that feeds solely on the blood of mammals and birds. More than two hundred different species of fleas are found in the United States, including the common rat flea (illustrated above). During the Middle Ages this little insect (length 0.1 inch) brought about millions of deaths by transmitting from rats to humans the bacteria that caused the Great Plague.

mans where cats or dogs are around (since they really *prefer* cats and dogs); but when a cat or dog dies or is suddenly removed from the house, the house may suddenly appear massively infested and even become uninhabitable without the aid of professional pest control measures on two or three successive weeks. Also, fleas can stay active in an empty house for months without any host being present.

flukes

Minute flatworms of the Trematoda family which may infest humans and other animals as parasites.

Flukes can invade many organs of the body and cause a number of diseases, the most important of which is SCHISTOSOMIASIS (or bilharziasis), which affects about two hundred million of the world's population, most of them in Africa and the Far and Middle East.

Flukes have at least two hosts in their life cycle: Although they develop in invertebrates, usually snails, they live in vertebrates, usually humans. They often leave the snail as free-swimming cercariae, which lie in wait in the water until they are attracted to their next host by the agitation he produces while swimming or walking nearby. They penetrate his skin, leaving an irritating sore ("swimmer's itch") that blisters and then dries up in about two days. Fortunately, flukes do not multiply in the vertebrate host, and the severity of the disease depends on the number of cercariae that are able to gain entry.

Schistosomes become mature and mate in the veins of the host's liver; the eggs, which carry spines, are laid in the veins of the intestines or bladder where, by ulceration, they make their way into the cavity of the organ and pass to the exterior via the excreta. In water the eggs hatch into miracidia (a larval stage), which must gain entry into a suitable snail within thirty hours or die.

Flukes other than *Schistosoma* can cause human disease. Infection may follow after one has eaten raw or pickled freshwater fish in the Far East or Southeastern Europe and parts of Asia. The lung fluke develops in crabs and crayfish. A liver fluke commonly found in cattle and sheep may affect humans, and a similar organism is found in the Far East, usually in pigs.

There are medications to treat the various types of fluke infestations. A common problem, however, is that persons will be reinfected if changes in living or eating habits are not made. This disease is very common in underdeveloped countries.

fluoridation

Addition of fluoride (a compound of the chemical element fluorine) to the public water supply in order to prevent dental decay, especially in children. It is one of the simplest and most effective health measures available today and costs only a few cents per person per year. Yet it has been strongly resisted by some critics who maintain that it represents compulsory medical treatment and that fluoride is poisonous.

The incidence of dental caries is lower in districts where fluoride is a natural component of the water supply than in areas where it is not. Reputable scientific studies have established that adjustment of the fluoride level in water to one part per million can reduce caries by half: The reason is that the fluoride becomes incorporated in the mineral structure of the teeth and strengthens their resistance to caries.

An alternative way to obtain fluoride is in the form of toothpastes, mouthwashes, or tablets. For the maximum protection, fluoride should be ingested with drinking water throughout tooth development.

folliculitis

Inflammation of the hair follicles of the skin or the scalp. It is caused usually by bacterial infection, the commonest organism being *Staphylococcus.*

Folliculitis may take any of a variety of forms. Acute infection originating in a hair follicle may develop into a boil or carbuncle. When the infection affects the hair follicles in the beard area, the person has *sycosis barbae,* or "barber's rash." This condition is now rare.

Pseudofolliculitis gives a similar appearance but is not directly due to infection. It is caused by damage to the surrounding tissues by the sharp tips of shaved hairs reentering the skin around the follicle. Milder cases of folliculitis may occur on the legs or arms as a reddish rash corresponding to the distribution of hair follicles. This condition may be caused by infection, but irritants such as oils or chemicals coming into contact with the skin may also produce it.

Treatment is by attention to skin hygiene and, if severe, by the administration of antibiotics.

food poisoning

Food contaminated by bacteria or bacterial toxins can produce dramatic and swift intestinal disorders characterized by vomiting and diarrhea.

Staphylococci bacteria growing on food—commonly dairy products or cooked meat and fish—release a toxin that reduces the victim to a state of shock in a few hours, but the attack passes off relatively quickly. Bacteria of the genus *Salmonella* can contaminate various sorts of food; the symptoms they produce take longer to appear but last longer than the symptoms of staph poisoning. The person may suffer from headache, shivering, as well as diarrhea and vomiting. The illness may be extremely severe.

A rare but very dangerous disease—BOTULISM— is produced by the organism *Clostridium botulinum*, which grows without oxygen at low temperatures and can survive as spores resistant to boiling. The processes of home canning often are insufficiently stringent to kill this organism, which multiplies in preserved food and releases a toxin that can be absorbed by the intestine and taken up by the central nervous system. Botulism is characterized by double vision, dilated pupils, paralysis of the face, difficulty in swallowing, and eventually paralysis of the respiratory muscles and cardiac arrest. Hospital treatment is essential, but even when this is provided the disease may prove fatal. A small but continuing number of cases have been recorded in recent years in the United States.

Treatment of staphylococcal food poisoning is directed toward relieving the symptoms, for the disease is not caused by the living organism itself. Salmonella food poisoning is a true infection, and severe cases may require the use of antibiotics.

Prevention is more important than cure. In tropical and subtropical climates it is important to remember that all foods, particularly vegetables, may be contaminated and should only be eaten fresh after washing. Food must be stored in cool, well-ventilated places free from flies and dirt. All persons who handle food must be very careful in their personal hygiene. Those with septic skin infection should be kept off work. Home canned and preserved food must not be eaten if there is any suspicion that it has deteriorated, and processed food must not be kept too long.

FOUR TYPES OF FRACTURE

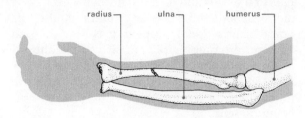

radius   ulna   humerus

1 simple—skin intact over fracture

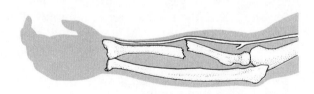

2 open—bone exposed to infection

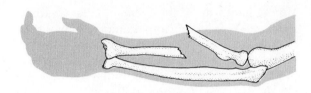

3 complicated—artery torn causing hemorrhage

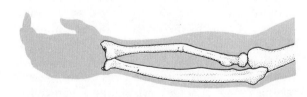

4 greenstick—incomplete break common in children

Bones may break in many different ways, depending on the type of injury and on the age and general health of the person. Children have relatively soft, elastic bones, which often break on one side only—a greenstick fracture (4). Elderly people have brittle bones, which tend to be fractured by relatively slight forces. The most important complications of fractures are infection due to protrusion of bone through the skin (2) and damage to structures adjacent to the fractured bone such as nerves, blood vessels (3), and internal organs.

fracture

A break in a bone.

The signs and symptoms may include pain, swelling, deformity, shortening of the limb, loss of strength, abnormal movement, and a grating noise between the fractured ends. In severe cases there may be shock caused by loss of blood.

The obvious cause is direct violence, such as a blow from a heavy object. But there are indirect causes also. For example, falling on the hand may cause a fracture of the collarbone or wrist as well as of the hand; or a sudden violent contraction of muscles may fracture the kneecap. X-ray examinations are used to confirm the diagnosis.

In young children the break may be incomplete; this is referred to as a *greenstick* fracture.

A *closed* fracture is one in which the skin is not broken, whereas an *open,* or *compound,* fracture is one in which the broken bones pierce the skin. If the fractured end protrudes through the skin, bacteria gain access and may cause severe infection.

The fracture is said to be *complicated* when it is associated with injury to an important structure, such as the brain, major blood vessels, nerves, lungs, or liver, or when the fracture is associated with dislocation of a joint.

Pathological fractures may be the result of bone disease; for example, a cyst or tumor may cause preliminary softening which leads to a break. Postmenopausal OSTEOPOROSIS is an important cause of pathological fracture.

An *impacted* fracture occurs when one fragment is driven into the other and locked into position.

In administering first aid, do not move the person unless he or she is in immediate danger. If there is suspicion of spinal injury or a disabling leg fracture, medical attention should be brought *to* the victim.

frigidity

Lack of sexual response or failure to achieve orgasm; usually refers to women. This inability to experience sexual satisfaction may be a permanent feature, or it may persist for a time and then under favorable conditions be replaced by a more normal sexual response.

The cause is often psychological. Poor general health also may diminish sexual interest.

Ignorance of the basic techniques of sexual intercourse—especially lack of knowledge, in one or both partners, of the essential role of the clitoris in governing the female sexual response—or poor communication about sexual needs may contribute to frigidity. Many women are aroused sexually more slowly than men and may be left unsatisfied and disappointed.

Concepts of femininity and masculinity, attitudes toward marriage, and fear of pregnancy or genital injury can all affect sexual fulfillment.

If a teenage girl receives faulty sexual instruction she can come to believe that sexual matters are shameful or distasteful, and this attitude of mind may be difficult to change.

The amount of time and energy the partners are able to devote to the sexual side of their relationship also may be significant. The pressures of life can seriously dampen a woman's response to intercourse.

Reassurance and education are essential in the treatment of frigidity. A sympathetic interview by a physician may bring to light problems and mistaken attitudes.

In particularly severe cases of frigidity some form of psychiatric counseling or psychotherapy may be useful. In addition, many excellent books exist (which the family physician can recommend) that can help dispel ignorance concerning sexual techniques. One of the best treatment modes, however, is patience, understanding, and tenderness on the part of the partner.

gallstones

Stones in the gallbladder or the bile ducts. They are far more common in women than in men up till the age of 50. Women who have had children are more commonly affected than those who have not. The incidence increases with age; gallstones are very rare in infancy and childhood.

The mechanisms underlying the formation of gallstones are poorly understood, but the stones often are associated with infection of the gallbladder. There are three main types of stones: mixed stones, made of bile pigments, calcium, and cholesterol; pure cholesterol stones; and those made up of bile pigments alone, which are rare. Cholesterol stones usually are solitary and large—up to 1.5 inches (4 centimeters) or more in diameter—whereas mixed stones and those composed of bile pigments alone are small and multiple.

The stones may be silent, producing no symp-

GALLSTONES

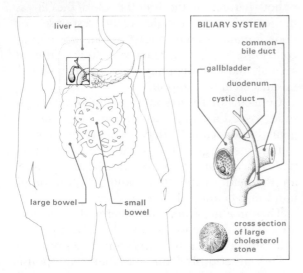

The gallbladder stores and concentrates bile, which is a mixture of substances manufactured in the liver. Most gallstones form because the concentration of cholesterol in the bile is too high, although the pure "cholesterol solitaire" shown above is unusual. If gallstones produce symptoms of jaundice, pain, or fever, the gallbladder should be removed.

toms, or they may be associated with recurrent infection of the gallbladder following obstruction of the cystic duct. Obstruction of the common bile duct by a stone may lead to obstructive JAUNDICE. In obstruction of either duct, the gallbladder first shows a noninfective inflammation of its wall, secondary to the retention of bile under pressure, and then secondary infection by organisms from the intestines. The person develops an acute pain in the upper part of the abdomen, usually traveling from the midline to become concentrated under the right ribs. Pain may be felt in the back and in the right shoulder, and may be accompanied by fever, nausea, and vomiting.

Most cases settle with bed rest, a light fat-free diet, and antibiotics. Subsequent plain X-ray examination may demonstrate radiopaque stones; but only about 10 percent of stones contain enough calcium to produce a strong shadow on the X-ray film, and in most cases it is necessary to carry out "contrast radiography." If the gallbladder is shown to contain stones, and especially if its function is deficient, it may be necessary to remove the gallbladder and the stones by surgical operation. Some acute cases require urgent operation, but often surgery is best left until the

acute attack has subsided and the inflammation has died down.

ganglion

A cyst on the sheath covering a tendon. These soft painless swellings occur most frequently on the hand or foot. Ganglions are completely harmless, but many people have them removed surgically because of their appearance.

gangrene

Refers to an area of dead tissue. Tissue death occurs when the blood supply to the area is compromised by injury or obstruction of the arteries that carry blood to the area. Such arterial disease is seen frequently in the legs of the elderly and of diabetics.

Dead or devitalized tissue easily becomes infected with a number of different types of bacteria. *Moist* or *wet gangrene* refers to dead tissue that is infected. *Dry gangrene* is dead tissue that is not infected.

Gas gangrene occurs in tissue infected by the *Clostridium* bacterium, which actually produces gas in an infected wound. In addition to local symptoms, clostridial infection can cause a severe, generalized blood infection.

Treatment of gangrene depends on the area involved and on whether infection has occurred. Systemic antibiotics and/or surgical removal of the gangrenous part may be necessary as a life-saving measure.

gastric ulcer

An open sore on the lining of the stomach. Gastric ulcer most commonly occurs in the 60 to 70 age group, slightly more often in men than in women.

Indigestion occurs episodically, with acute attacks lasting from two weeks to two months and with free intervals lasting from two to twelve months. Pain usually occurs within two hours of eating. Weight loss is not uncommon and vomiting is a frequent feature.

X-ray examination following a barium meal may assist the diagnosis. The ulcer may actually be seen directly on the stomach lining, however, through a *fiberoptic endoscope* (a special illuminated instrument passed into the stomach through the mouth and esophagus).

Bed rest in the hospital and abstinence from smoking promote the healing of gastric ulcers. Milky diets and antacids do not speed healing but they may help to relieve the symptoms. There has been considerable controversy over the use of special diets. Many clinicians now feel that the person himself is the best judge of what he should eat. It may help to eat regular, frequent meals, avoiding highly seasoned and greasy foods. H_2 receptor blocking agents such as cimetidine are generally considered the treatment of choice. Aspirin should be avoided. Surgery (for example, gastrectomy) may have to be considered in cases that do not respond to medical treatment.

Possible complications of gastric ulceration are hemorrhage, anemia, obstruction, and perforation of the stomach wall.

gastroenteritis

Inflammation of the lining of the stomach and intestine.

It is usually due to infection and begins suddenly with a feeling of general discomfort, loss of appetite, vomiting, abdominal cramps, and diarrhea. Persistent vomiting and diarrhea may result in severe dehydration and shock, requiring immediate medical attention. Other causes include FOOD POISONING, arsenic or mercury poisoning, and the excessive use of harsh laxatives or other drugs such as aspirin or broad-spectrum antibiotics.

In adults the symptoms usually subside. All that may be necessary is bed rest with plenty of fluids to drink until diarrhea and vomiting have stopped; thereafter, a bland diet can be given. If symptoms do not disappear within forty-eight hours, stool examination and culture are needed to discover a possible causative organism.

Organisms called *rotaviruses* have recently been shown to account for about half the cases of gastroenteritis in children. Gastroenteritis often damages the villi (the absorptive cells of the intestine), preventing the absorption of milk sugar which then attracts water into the intestines with consequent frequent and fluid stools.

The most serious danger in infants is that DEHYDRATION may lead to death, which can occur rapidly in a small baby. Signs of dehydration are failure to pass urine, sunken eyes, inelastic skin, and a dry tongue. Prompt admission to the hospital usually is essential. Milk and solids are withheld from the diet initially; instead, clear fluids (such as 5 percent glucose solution) are given.

Gaucher's disease

An inherited disease seen most commonly in Jews of Eastern European origin. The absence of a certain enzyme results in the accumulation of a fatty compound in body organs, including the liver, spleen, and bone marrow.

The progression of the disease is variable. It can cause death in infancy, or the onset of symptoms may be delayed until adulthood.

There is no specific treatment.

genes

That part of the living cell that controls the inheritance of a specific physical characteristic of the organism. Genes are located on structures in the cell called *chromosomes*.

The genes are molecules of deoxyribonucleic acid, and many thousands of them are carried by the chromosomes. All the genes are present in every living cell of the body. Each gene has its specific location on its chromosome and, with the exception of the pair of sex chromosomes, each chromosome has a partner with a corresponding gene at the same corresponding locus. Pairs of genes occupying loci are called *alleles*. These pairs may be identical (*homozygous*) or dissimilar (*heterozygous*). A gene that exerts its effect when present on only one chromosome of the pair is known as *dominant*. When both alleles must be present to cause the effect, the gene is *recessive*.

genetic disorder

Any disease or malformation caused by an abnormality in the composition of the genes (*genome*). Some are due to changes in the genes (*mutation*), some may be passed on from parent to child by genetic inheritance. Examples of genetic disorders include DOWN'S SYNDROME, *Turner's syndrome*, *Triple X syndrome*, and KLINEFELTER'S SYNDROME.

Not all genetic orders take the form of physical malformation. Some involve the absence of a substance the body needs for proper functioning. HEMOPHILIA, a bleeding disorder, is an example of a genetic disorder in which the body fails to produce a factor necessary for normal blood clotting.

A genetic disorder is not necessarily the same as a *congenital disorder*, which means any abnormality present from birth, whether inherited or not.

German measles

An acute viral disease, common in childhood, but in most cases fairly mild. Also known as *rubella*. It is caused by an RNA virus spread mainly by aerosol droplet infection. The importance of rubella as a public health problem is not in its effects on the sufferers but in the fact that if it is contracted by a woman during the early months of pregnancy, there may be congenital defects in the baby.

Defects can be multiple and include congenital CATARACT in both eyes, HEART DISEASE, deaf mutism, MENTAL RETARDATION, and microcephaly (an abnormally small head).

No woman should embark on a pregnancy without having immunity to the disease as a result of a previous infection or of vaccination. However, if infection occurs in pregnancy, an intramuscular injection of *gamma globulin* (a special protein formed in the blood, also available for therapeutic use, which contains specific antibodies to the virus) may be effective in diminishing the risk of abnormalities. The rubella virus appears to cause a major epidemic of the disease every seven years or so; formerly, in epidemic years before strong preventive measures were taken, there may have been as many as 20,000 abnormalities and fetal deaths in the United States.

In children, rubella is a mild disease with an incubation period of fourteen to twenty-one days. Symptoms include slight fever, a moderate rash (which first appears on the face and neck and then spreads to the body and limbs), and some enlargement of the glands behind the ears. Until the fever and rash have subsided, the child can infect others who have not had rubella. The child should get plenty of rest and be given fluids and light meals. One attack of rubella usually provides immunity for life.

Giardia

A genus of common intestinal parasites, found especially in warm climates, which can cause acute attacks of diarrhea and abdominal pain.

The particular microorganism responsible,

Giardia lamblia, is a pear-shaped protozoan parasite. The disease (known as *giardiasis*) is most prevalent in areas of poor sanitation and in institutions, but outbreaks have been reported due to contamination of water supplies.

Infection leads to multiplication of the protozoa within the bowel. There may be no symptoms, but heavy infections produce diarrhea, abdominal cramps, bloating, anemia, fatigue, and weight loss. Undigested fat may be present in the stools. Drugs are highly effective in clearing up the condition.

gingivitis

Inflammation of the gums, causing pain and often minor bleeding when cleaning the teeth or eating hard food such as apples.

Gingivitis is the most common oral disease in adult life (children are more likely to have symptoms from caries, or "cavities"). It is most often due to a combination of a soft, sugary diet and poor dental hygiene, but it may occur also as a

GINGIVITIS

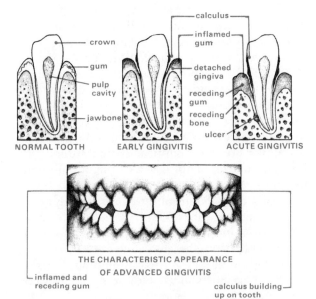

Gingivitis usually results from the buildup of calculus (tartar) near the junction of teeth and gums. It causes varying degrees of redness, swelling, and bleeding of the gums, and contributes to halitosis (bad breath). If left untreated, teeth may eventually become loose and fall out.

complication of debilitating diseases and of vitamin deficiencies.

Gingivitis is best treated by a dental surgeon, who may cut away damaged, overgrown portions of the gum (*gingivectomy*) in addition to giving advice on better dental hygiene and the use of a mouthwash.

glaucoma

Impairment of vision due to a rise in the fluid pressure within the eye. One of the most important causes of blindness in the elderly.

There are several distinct types of glaucoma. The most common is *chronic simple glaucoma*, in which the rise in pressure within the eye occurs over a period of months or years without causing any symptoms. The gradual narrowing of the field of vision (so that only objects directly in front of the eyes are visualized) may pass unnoticed unless the eyes are examined by an ophthalmologist. Without treatment chronic glaucoma eventually causes total blindness.

Acute glaucoma, in contrast, usually develops very suddenly, with severe pain in the eye, which becomes extremely hard, red, and tender. The person may see halos around lights. *Urgent treatment* is needed to lower the pressure within the eye if vision is to be saved.

Glaucoma may also be secondary to some other disease of the eye, such as *iridocyclitis* or *retinal vein thrombosis*.

Whatever the type of glaucoma, the underlying cause is a defect in the mechanism that removes fluid continuously formed in the front chamber of the eyeball. In acute glaucoma there is a physical block due to narrowing of the angle at the root of the iris; in chronic glaucoma the blockage is thought to be in the meshwork of vessels that normally would absorb the fluid.

Treatment depends on the cause: narrow-angle glaucoma usually is relieved by a minor surgical operation, whereas chronic glaucoma is treated with drugs in eye-drop form that reduce the rate of formation of fluid. Anyone with a family background of glaucoma should have regular eye examinations.

glioma

A type of BRAIN TUMOR made up of glial cells.

Most gliomas are malignant (cancerous), but they seldom spread to other parts of the body. As with other brain tumors, the symptoms include headache, vomiting, and pressure on nerve tracts. There may be progressive mental or physical deterioration, such as deafness, partial blindness, or personality change. Other symptoms suggestive of tumor are giddiness and convulsions.

The diagnosis can be confirmed by skull X-ray studies, electroencephalography (EEG), or brain scanning. A glioma cannot usually be removed completely; the usual treatment is partial removal followed by radiotherapy.

globulin

Refers to a kind of protein that is carried in the liquid part of the blood (plasma).

There are three classes of globulin: alpha, beta, and gamma. Each can be subdivided further; for example, there is an alpha I and an alpha II globulin.

Each of the globulin proteins has an important function in the body.

Alpha and *beta globulins* combine loosely with other important body chemicals to carry them around in the blood. Alpha I globulin contains a fraction that binds bilirubin and another one that carries steroids and lipids. Alpha II globulin combines with free hemoglobin in the plasma.

Beta globulins include some that are responsible for transporting lipids and others that bind copper and iron for transport. Prothrombin, one of the blood-clotting factors, is a beta globulin.

The *gamma globulins* are extremely important in the body's IMMUNE SYSTEM: They are known alternatively as immunoglobulins and are subdivided into classes (IgA, IgE, IgM, etc.) according to their function.

The overall pattern of alpha, beta, and gamma globulins may be measured to assess the progress of many different types of disease and treatment, since they quite commonly are affected. The specific immunoglobulins are also useful diagnostic indicators.

glomerulonephritis

Inflammation of the *glomeruli*, the tiny clumps of blood vessels that act as filters to form the urine within the kidney. The condition may be acute or chronic and is an important cause of kidney failure: Glomerular disease accounts for approxi-

GLOMERULONEPHRITIS

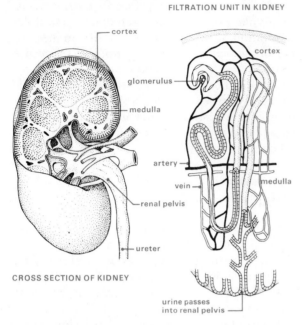

FILTRATION UNIT IN KIDNEY

cortex

cortex

glomerulus

medulla

artery

vein

medulla

renal pelvis

ureter

CROSS SECTION OF KIDNEY

urine passes
into renal pelvis

Glomerulonephritis is a complex disease resulting from the production of immune complexes which damage the glomeruli in the kidney. Blood plasma passes through the glomeruli in the first stage of urine formation. In glomerulonephritis, proteins and red blood cells leak through as well so that the urine is said to resemble cola.

mately two thirds of all deaths from KIDNEY DISEASE.

Acute glomerulonephritis is most often a complication of infection—in the throat or elsewhere in the body—with a *Streptococcus* bacterium. The immune defenses against the infection produce complexes that also damage the glomeruli. This reaction usually occurs two to three weeks after the bacterial infection. The damage to the kidneys reduces the output of urine, which may become dark from the presence of blood. Typically, the ankles swell and the face becomes pale and puffy. Most often the symptoms of acute glomerulonephritis resolve within a few weeks. But in a minority of persons, the kidney failure may become total; without specific treatment by dialysis or a kidney transplant, the outcome is fatal. In another small proportion of cases, although the recovery appears complete, the inflammation within the kidneys persists and the condition then becomes chronic. Over a period of years the kidneys become scarred and contracted, and again there is danger of kidney failure.

The glomeruli may also be damaged by chronic diseases such as DIABETES MELLITUS, by high blood pressure, and by connective-tissue disorders such as systemic LUPUS ERYTHEMATOSUS. Whatever the underlying cause, loss of a substantial proportion of the two million glomeruli (one million in each kidney) leads to kidney failure.

glossitis

Inflammation of the tongue. Glossitis may be caused by an infection as SCARLET FEVER, in which the red taste buds (*papillae*) protrude through a white coating, or "fur." Later the coating disappears, leaving the swollen papillae projecting from a bright red "strawberry tongue."

A type of glossitis marked by a smooth, bald tongue occurs when there is a deficiency of some vitamins—for example, in PELLAGRA (niacin deficiency) and pernicious ANEMIA (vitamin B_{12} deficiency). A similar appearance is seen in CELIAC DISEASE and in the severe anemia of STARVATION.

SYPHILIS causes a chronic superficial glossitis. There are areas of opaque, white, thickened skin; between these areas the surface is scarred and lacking papillae.

In general, glossitis is marked by pain, swelling, and burning of the tongue, especially when eating or drinking.

glycogen storage diseases

The body stores glucose, or sugar, in the form of a substance called glycogen. Normally, glycogen is stored in the liver and muscles. In a rare group of inherited diseases, collectively known as glycogen storage disease (GSD), the body lacks certain enzymes necessary to process glycogen. Twelve separate entities currently comprise GSD; symptoms vary widely and may begin shortly after birth or be delayed until the teens. No treatment is available for GSD; some forms of the disease can be managed through dietary measures, however.

glycosuria

The presence of sugar (glucose) in the urine.

Glycosuria is the major sign of DIABETES MELLITUS, although not everyone with glycosuria necessarily has diabetes.

Doctors can detect glucose in a urine specimen by means of a simple test. Similar tests are used by diabetics to detect and measure glucose in their own urine, thus permitting them to determine if their disease is under control.

Normal urine contains no glucose. It appears when the amount of glucose in the blood exceeds the "renal threshold"—that is, the point at which the kidneys experience an overload of glucose in the blood and cannot prevent it from escaping into the urine. In diabetes the threshold is exceeded because of the high level of glucose in the blood. Glycosuria can occur in a nondiabetic if the person has a low renal threshold.

Once glycosuria is detected, a test called a *glucose tolerance test* is used to determine whether a patient has diabetes or merely a low renal threshold requiring no treatment. In a glucose tolerance test the patient drinks a standard amount of sugar and the quantity remaining in the blood is measured hourly over several hours.

goiter

A swelling of the thyroid gland in the neck. It may be caused by a lack of iodine in the diet, by various drugs, or by an excess of certain foods, such as turnips, that prevent the gland from making the thyroid hormone. It can arise also from unknown causes.

Iodine deficiency occurs in areas of the world where soil and water are virtually free of iodine. It is then called *endemic goiter*. The introduction of iodized salt for table use has caused this disease to become much less common. It is still seen, however, in some parts of the world, especially in mountainous regions.

The early sign of endemic goiter is a gradual enlargement of the neck. When iodine deficiency is slight, the disease usually is confined to young women. Men and preadolescent children are only affected where the deficiency is severe; in these areas, CRETINISM is common.

Simple nonendemic goiter usually occurs as a smooth swelling in the neck. This may disappear in a few years, or it may proceed slowly to become "nodular" (with small lumps) in middle age and "toxic" in old age, when signs of increased thyroid activity arise. In less than 2 percent of patients, simple nonendemic goiter may become cancerous.

The treatment of goiter depends on its cause. In cases of endemic goiter due to the lack of

GOITER

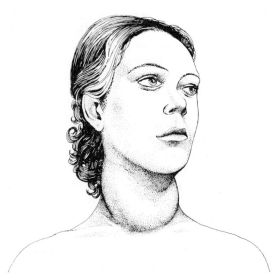

large goiter in a girl aged 20 years

A goiter is a swelling in the neck caused by an enlarged thyroid gland. Surgical removal of goiters is performed only when drug treatment has failed, unless there is an acute emergency such as a respiratory obstruction due to a large goiter (above) or if it seems that a cancer might develop.

iodine, replacement therapy with iodine medication does not have good results, and even may cause thyroid overactivity. Hormone treatment is needed.

In nonendemic goiter, early cases may be treated with thyroid hormone preparations and this is often very successful. In long-standing cases, a hormone replacement medication may actually make the condition worse and needs to be carefully monitored.

Surgical removal of the enlarged gland usually is not done because of the severe effects it can have. In cases in which the goiter has grown large enough to obstruct the airway, modified surgery may be done. In cases in which nodules develop, which may suggest cancerous changes, exploratory surgery may be done.

gonadotropins

Any hormone capable of stimulating the gonads (sex glands); the term refers especially to certain female sex hormones.

The female reproductive system depends on these hormones, which are secreted either by the pituitary gland at the base of the brain or by the placenta. Immediately after menstruation the first of the pituitary gonadotropins—*follicle-stimulating hormone* (FSH)—passes into the bloodstream. The ovary responds by ripening a small area on its surface, called a Graafian follicle, which contains an ovum.

The second pituitary gonadotropin—*luteinizing hormone* (LH)—starts flowing some days after FSH and stimulates the follicle to produce the hormone *estrogen.*

After two weeks a sudden surge of LH induces the Graafian follicle to rupture, expelling the ovum from the ovary into the Fallopian tube. The follicle, now termed the "corpus luteum," produces the hormone *progesterone,* which encourages correct implantation of the ovum into the lining of the womb after fertilization.

The production of progesterone from the corpus luteum depends on continuous pituitary secretion of LH. If conception does not occur, the pituitary secretion of gonadotropins falls, and the ovarian production of both estrogen and progesterone drops correspondingly. This results in the menstrual shedding of the uterine lining, which has thickened in response to stimulation by the hormones.

If the ovum is fertilized, the placenta produces a third gonadotropin—called *chorionic gonadotropin*—which maintains the corpus luteum for the first three months of pregnancy and ensures the safe continuance of the pregnancy. This is the hormone whose presence in the urine confirms pregnancy.

In men, FSH promotes the growth of the sperm-forming tubes within the testicles and of the sperm themselves; LH ensures that the testicles produce androgens, the male sex hormones.

gonorrhea

A common sexually transmitted disease.

Gonorrhea is an infection of the genital organs and urinary outlet by the bacterium *Neisseria gonorrhoeae.* If the infection is left untreated it can spread to other organs—for example, the joints, tendons, muscles, heart, and brain—but this occurrence is relatively rare since the advent of antibiotics.

The true incidence of gonorrhea is unknown, since the disease tends to be under-reported. Many persons treat themselves, and many infected women have no symptoms.

Who gets the disease? Among men, gonorrhea tends to be seen in the armed forces, in men whose occupation requires a great deal of travel (such as migrant workers and seamen), and in homosexuals. In women, similar life-styles may predispose to the disease; prostitutes also are commonly infected.

Although sexual intercourse is by far the most common means of transmission, gonorrhea does spread in other ways. A baby can be infected at birth if the mother is infected. In such cases the disease causes a severe conjunctivitis, which can lead to blindness. Until recently this was a principal cause of blindness, but it was largely eradicated when doctors began the routine procedure of instilling protective ointments into the eyes of the newborn. In very rare cases infants and young children may contract the disease from their parents by close contact.

The incubation period of gonorrhea is between two and ten days. The illness starts suddenly in men, with a repeated, urgent desire to pass urine and severe pain during urination. Considerable quantities of pus are discharged from the penis. At this stage infection is so obvious that the man cannot fail to recognize the need for treatment. If the disease is not treated it can spread to the prostate gland and testicles, giving rise to fever and perhaps involuntary retention of urine. Eventually it will subside, even without treatment, but it may leave strictures (narrowing) of the urinary outlet and cause sterility.

In women the disease may produce no symptoms at all—which is a danger, since the woman may not realize she is infected. In other cases there may be urgency and pain on urination, discharge of pus, and the formation of abscesses. Even when these resolve, the infecting bacteria remain to infect the woman's sexual partners unless she is properly treated with antibiotics.

Penicillin is the mainstay of treatment for persons with gonorrhea, although higher doses and longer courses have become necessary over the years as the gonococcus has developed resistance. Some strains now fail to respond to penicillin at all, in any dosage, and must be treated by other antibiotics. In every case, all sexual partners should be informed and treated.

A condom provides some barrier to the spread of gonococcal infection but is not completely protective.

GOUT

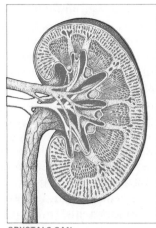 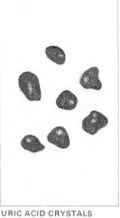 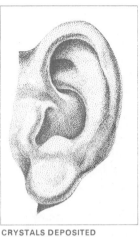 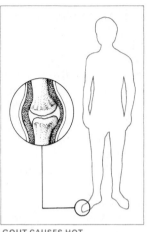

CRYSTALS CAN
DAMAGE KIDNEYS

URIC ACID CRYSTALS

CRYSTALS DEPOSITED
IN EARS AS "TOPHI"

GOUT CAUSES HOT,
SWOLLEN, PAINFUL JOINTS

Gout is an extremely painful condition that predominantly affects men. It is caused by an excess of uric acid, which forms needle-sharp crystals in the joints, ears, and kidneys. Gout is in part a hereditary disease but is also exacerbated by foods with high purine content such as liver, sardines, kidney, and sweetbreads.

gout

A disease that causes painful swelling of the joints. It results from the accumulation in the bloodstream of a body waste product, uric acid. Deposition of the uric acid in the joints is responsible for the symptoms. The uric acid may also be deposited in the skin and kidneys, causing symptoms in these organs.

The first attack of gout usually occurs with the sudden and extremely painful swelling of a single joint—most often the first joint of the big toe. After the first attack, more flare-ups can be expected in the absence of treatment. Acute attacks of gout can be managed with anti-inflammatory drugs such as colchicine or indomethacin. The prevention of future attacks is achieved by the continuous use of another drug, allopurinol.

granuloma inguinale

A chronic bacterial disease, widespread in tropical and subtropical areas, in which an ulcerating infection spreads slowly over the skin of the genital organs and groin.

It is thought to be transmitted during sexual intercourse or other close contact and is caused by microorganisms known as *Calymmatobacterium granulomatis*. In rare cases the disease has been known to spread from the genitals to joints or bones in other parts of the body, owing to invasion of the lymphatics and blood circulation.

Granuloma inguinale usually is not painful, but it is very destructive of tissue as it spreads over the genitals and the surrounding skin. Secondary infection with other bacteria is inevitable. Doctors can distinguish the disease from syphilis by microscopic identification of the Donovan bodies (bacteria).

A two-week course of antibiotic treatment usually cures granuloma inguinale, although severe cases may take longer to heal. The best preventive for this disease is to wash the genital organs thoroughly after sexual intercourse.

growth hormone

Also known as *somatotropin*. This hormone is released from the pituitary gland, in the brain, which regulates growth.

A deficiency of growth hormone in a child will result in an adult of short stature. If there is an overproduction of this hormone in a child who has not yet reached puberty, it will result in abnormal overgrowth (*gigantism*). If adolescence has ended and the person's bones can no longer grow, a production of growth hormone at this stage will cause ACROMEGALY, enlargement of the head, hands, and feet. Synthetic growth hormone is now available; it is used for prepuberty children who are not producing the hormone naturally.

Guillain-Barré syndrome

A patchy loss of the myelin sheath of nerves and (less commonly) the spinal cord, of unknown cause. It usually follows seven to twenty-one days after an infection of the upper respiratory tract (such as the common cold) or after a gastrointestinal infection.

Guillain-Barré syndrome starts slowly, with weakness and abnormal sensation in both legs. Later the weakness becomes a paralysis affecting muscles of the trunk, arms, and occasionally the face.

Eventually the paralysis, and accompanying loss of sensation, reaches a plateau that may last for several weeks. Then a gradual return to normal health occurs, though this also may take weeks or even months.

Intensive care is given in the early stages of the condition because there is a risk of paralysis of the muscles that control breathing.

gynecomastia

Excessive enlargement of the breasts in a boy or man.

Some enlargement of the breasts is a normal,

GYNECOMASTIA

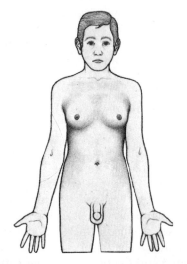

Gynecomastia results from an excess of the hormone estrogen. It is common in newborn boys, and the high estrogen levels in breast milk can prolong it for months. Gynecomastia is also normal around puberty, but at other ages it can be due to one of a number of diseases or drugs.

transient occurrence in a newborn boy whose breasts are engorged and swollen in response to his mother's hormone levels. It may also be seen temporarily during adolescence, when it is of no significance except as a minor embarrassment. Fat boys may appear to have enlarged breasts— but this is not *true* gynecomastia, which is related to hormonal imbalance.

Boys with persisting gynecomastia may have the rare chromosomal abnormality known as KLINEFELTER'S SYNDROME characterized by small testicles, disproportionately long limbs, and a feminine body shape. Similar enlargement of the male breast occurs in hormonal disorders, overactivity of the pituitary or thyroid gland, lung and testicular tumors, and cirrhosis of the liver.

Gynecomastia also occurs occasionally as a side effect of certain drugs.

halitosis

Bad-smelling breath arising from the mouth or from the lungs.

Many people have a faint sweetish halitosis in the morning, accompanied by a bad taste in the mouth; both can be relieved by proper cleansing of the teeth and tongue.

Halitosis can arise from poor oral hygiene (failure to brush away particles of food lodged between the teeth), decayed teeth, or pockets of infection in diseased and overgrown gums. The breath is often foul after dental surgery, particularly when there is bleeding. Less often halitosis can be associated with an oral infection such as trench mouth.

Causes of halitosis outside the mouth include chronic infections of the sinuses or lungs and lung abscesses. More commonly halitosis results from foods such as garlic, whose chemical odors are excreted in the breath.

A fishy odor of the breath is found in people with hepatic failure; a urinary odor is found in kidney failure; and a sweet, fruity odor is typical of severe, uncontrolled diabetes.

hallucination

An experience of sensory perception in the absence of any physical cause.

Hallucinations may be visual, auditory, gustatory (of taste), olfactory (of smell), or tactile. They vary greatly from simple flashes of light to sensations of highly specific and identifiable objects or sounds. Normal people under severe stress may share a hallucination, as when survivors of a sinking ship believe they see a nonexistent shore.

Hallucinations may be a sign of a mental disorder, such as SCHIZOPHRENIA or severe DEPRESSION, or they may occur as a result of physical illness. Epileptics often experience hallucinations just before a seizure. In states of altered brain function—caused, for example, by high fever, alcohol withdrawal, head injury, liver failure, or senile brain degeneration—repeated and often terrifying hallucinations are common. Tumors of the brain can cause hallucinations of taste, vision, or hearing, depending on the site of the brain tumor.

Some drugs, especially narcotics, can be powerful hallucinogens. Mescaline and LSD are classed as hallucinogenic drugs because of the vivid and unpredictable nature of the visual sensations they induce. Stimulants such as amphetamines can cause hallucinations in high doses or with abuse.

To suppress hallucinations the first approach is to treat the underlying disease. The hallucinations seen in delirium associated with TYPHOID FEVER, for example, disappear as the body temperature returns to normal; the alcoholic with delirium tremens stops seeing terrifying images after undergoing sedative treatment.

Hashimoto's disease

An inflammatory chronic disease that causes swelling (goiter) of the thyroid gland in the neck.

It occurs most often in middle-aged women and is thought to be caused by an autoimmune process, in which, for reasons that are not understood, the body begins to attack itself. The disease is known to run in families.

Diagnosis usually is made on the basis of laboratory tests, but occasionally a biopsy of the goiter is done. Replacement thyroid hormone can be given to make up for the low level of hormone produced by the affected gland.

hay fever

Also known as *allergic* or *seasonal rhinitis*. This is an allergy-related disorder that affects the respiratory tract (primarily the nose and the lungs) and the eyes. It is caused by an increased sensitivity to airborne pollens and is often seasonal in na-

ture—occurring when the air contains pollens of a specific type. There are many different pollens and substances that cause reaction in the susceptible persons; hay pollen is only one of them. These substances are called *allergens*.

The term "hay fever" is used primarily for the condition that affects the eyes and nose. Persons who have allergic changes in the lungs have ASTHMA. Hay fever is characterized by reddened, tearing eyes and runny nose, often with nasal sinus congestion. This condition can affect males and females of any age. There is often a family tendency.

Grass and tree pollens are present at different times throughout the spring and summer months. Persons with allergic rhinitis who are sensitive to one or two pollens will have symptoms only for the time these pollens are present in the air. Persons with multiple allergies will have a longer period of affliction. Ragweed pollen causes allergic responses in many; it is present in Eastern and Midwestern areas and occurs in late summer and early fall. Fungus spores are sometimes responsible.

The symptoms come about because of the reaction the allergen sets up in the mucous membrane linings of the mouth, nose, lungs, and eyes. These allergens trigger the release of *histamine*, a chemical substance normally found in the body, which when in excess leads to allergic reactions such as runny nose, tearing, and itching. Symptomatic relief usually can be obtained with the use of antihistamines, which block the release of the chemical. For those with severe allergies or poor response to medications, DESENSITIZATION therapy may help.

Hay fever is generally a lifelong condition but not a life-threatening one. Asthma, however, which can be life-threatening, occurs in approximately a third of these persons.

headache

Encompasses all aches and pains in the head. Headaches represent one of the most frequent human discomforts. The most common type of headache is the *tension* or *nervous headache* caused by contractions of the muscles of the scalp and back of the neck.

MIGRAINE arises from the constriction and dilation of blood vessels in the scalp, temple, and face. Migrainous headaches usually are one-sided, sudden, very intense, and associated with visual disturbances. Mild migraine headaches may require no treatment, but the more severe ones may respond to one of several drugs.

Cluster headache, a migraine variant, combines one-sided headache with sweating, flushing, watering of the eyes, and a runny nose. Usually it occurs two to three hours after the person has fallen asleep. It tends to recur nightly for several weeks or for a few months (hence the term *cluster*), after which there is complete freedom for months or years.

Congestion and inflammation of the nasal sinuses may give rise to pain in the forehead and face. Headaches also can result from disease of the teeth, ears, and nerves, and from disorders of the bones, muscles, and joints of the neck and jaw.

An exhaustive list of the causes of headaches is extensive and complex. Fortunately, the dangerous causes of headaches are rare. Nevertheless, unremitting headaches that are not relieved by simple measures may be a warning of a serious underlying illness.

hearing

The sense that allows sound to be perceived. It is the major function of the ear. Loss of hearing is called DEAFNESS.

Sound waves in the air are converted by the ear into impulses that travel via the auditory nerve to the brain, where they are perceived as sound. The outer ear canal (*external auditory meatus*) conducts the sound waves to the eardrum. On the inner surface of the eardrum (which begins the middle ear) three small bones (*ossicles*) amplify the vibrations and conduct them to the *cochlea* in the inner ear. Nerve endings in the cochlea transmit the vibrations as impulses through the auditory nerve to the brain.

Hearing may be impaired by obstructions (such as wax) in the external ear canal, by disturbances in the middle ear (*conductive deafness*), or by disease of the inner ear (*perceptive* or *sensorineural deafness*).

Hearing is examined by a number of tests that

HEARING

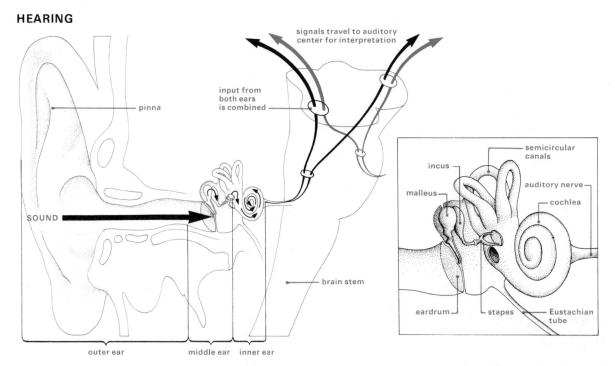

Hearing, the perception of sounds, involves mechanical and nervous mechanisms. Sound waves cause vibrations in the eardrum, which are transmitted and intensified by three small bones in the middle ear called the malleus, the incus, and the stapes (sometimes referred to as the hammer, anvil, and stirrup). The spiral cochlea contains delicate hair cells arranged along a membrane, and they are stimulated by movements of the stapes to send signals up the auditory nerve to the brain.

vary from the simple one of whispering in the patient's ear while the other ear is covered up, through the use of the tuning fork, to the use of the audiometer (an instrument that produces sounds of selected pitch and volume).

Conduction through the air and through the bones of the skull can be measured. For both these means of conduction the degree of deafness is measured in decibels; the measurement represents the increased intensity of sound required for hearing in the deaf ear compared with that required in a normal ear. Speech audiometry is very useful, since it measures the intensity of sound necessary for the understanding of recorded speech. Audiometry can help in the diagnosis between conductive and perceptive deafness.

heart attack

See CORONARY THROMBOSIS and HEART DISEASE.

heartburn

A burning sensation felt behind the breastbone, sometimes radiating into the neck or the back. Technical name: *pyrosis.*

It is a common complaint, produced by the reflux of gastric secretions into the lower part of the esophagus ("gullet"). Usually it is made worse by bending over or lying down. Normally, the contents of the stomach do not back up into the esophagus. Regurgitation is prevented by the shape of the upper part of the stomach and by the muscles of the diaphragm, which act as a sphincter. In some cases, particularly when the person is obese or pregnant, the upper part of the stomach may herniate upward through the opening of the diaphragm and form a hiatus HERNIA. In such cases heartburn is liable to follow a heavy meal, especially if the person goes to bed after eating; it may be relieved by sitting up.

Acid reflux, though, more commonly ocurs without hiatus hernia. Effective measures to relieve the symptoms are the use of antacids and the avoidance of heavy meals. In hiatus hernia surgical treatment may prove necessary.

heart disease

Heart disease affects persons of all ages: the baby born with congenital structural abnormalities of the heart, the teenager and the young adult with rheumatic heart disease, and the older person with ischemic heart disease due to coronary artery blockage or high blood pressure. Coronary artery disease is now the most common cause of death in adult Americans.

Disorders of the heart affect its ability to pump blood around the body. Infants with mild *congenital* heart disease may show this by failing to grow as quickly as other children, or by becoming easily breathless or tired on exertion.

Congenital heart disease is not necessarily inherited. Maternal German measles infection during pregnancy may cause multiple heart abnormalities, but most children born with abnormal hearts have a normal genetic makeup. Their mothers can be reassured that future babies will be healthy.

Rheumatic heart disease in the older teenager and adult stems from throat infections with the bacterium *Group A hemolytic Streptococcus*; the body's reaction to this leads to RHEUMATIC FEVER. Half the persons with rheumatic fever develop an acute heart illness that, on subsiding, leaves a slowly progressing disorder of the heart valves and the muscular walls of the heart. Penicillin by mouth destroys the streptococci; therefore, early and effective treatment of streptococcal sore throats prevents both the rheumatic fever and the subsequent heart disease. Antibiotics have no effect on rheumatic fever itself. Its incidence has fallen steeply since the 1940s, however, so that rheumatic heart disease is becoming rare.

Even those with established rheumatic heart disease can take comfort from the great strides in heart surgery since the 1950s. Narrowed valves often can be reopened or replaced with artificial valves at minimal risk to the individual, and sophisticated drug therapy helps control possible complications.

The symptoms of *ischemic heart disease* arise from failure of the coronary arteries (which supply blood to the heart muscle itself) to deliver sufficient oxygen to the muscle. (See ISCHEMIA.) The result is ANGINA PECTORIS—a deep, aching, crushing, or vice-like pain in the chest, radiating perhaps to the arm or to the neck and jaw. It is fairly common in men in their 40s and older whose arteries have been seriously narrowed by ATHEROSCLEROSIS. The condition may progress to complete blockage of the arteries, with a resultant MYOCARDIAL INFARCTION ("heart attack").

Factors leading to the current high death rate from ischemic heart disease have been investigated all over the world. Smoking, stress, lack of exercise, and obesity are all considered to predispose to heart disease. Widespread recognition that heart disease is largely the result of overindulgence, at least in the Western world, and can only be prevented by people themselves, has led already to fewer "heart" deaths. Americans are exercising more and smoking less, are aware of

A CROSS SECTION OF THE HEART

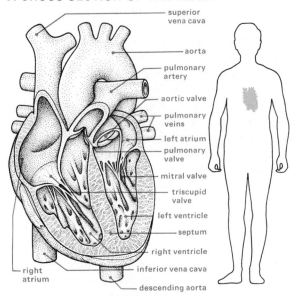

BLOOD FLOW THROUGH THE HEART

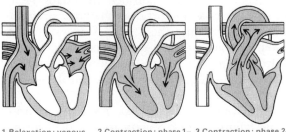

1 Relaxation: venous blood fills atria.

2 Contraction: phase 1— atria contract forcing blood into ventricles, which are still relaxed.

3 Contraction: phase 2— ventricles contract forcing blood into arteries.

The heart pumps out approximately 1.3 gallons (5 liters) of blood every minute, and it can double this amount when necessary during exercise. As the ventricles relax, the valves open (1), allowing blood to flow down from the atria (2). When the ventricles contract (3), the valves are slammed shut, and blood from the right ventricle enters the pulmonary artery to go to the lungs, while the left ventricle pumps blood into the aorta; from there it is transported around the body in the arterial system.

their blood pressure, and are seeking treatment sooner. Once severe ischemic heart disease is present, drugs or surgery can help, but prevention is far more effective than cure.

heart failure

A clinical condition in which the heart fails to maintain adequate circulation of blood. It may result from failure of the right or left ventricle due to congenital or acquired disease.

The most common kind of heart failure is left-ventricle failure following coronary artery disease, high blood pressure, or disease and incompetency of the mitral or aortic valves of the heart. Chronic disease of the lungs and congenital heart disease lead more often to right-ventricle failure.

The first symptom of left-ventricle failure is usually shortness of breath on exertion, which may progress so that the person finds it difficult to make any exertion. He may find it easier to breathe sitting up rather than lying down. He feels tired and may complain of a feeling of tightness in the chest. There may be attacks of severe breathlessness at night.

Right-ventricle failure is characterized by swelling (edema), the site of which is determined by gravity: If the person is up, the ankles swell; if he is in bed, the swelling is most obvious over the base of the spine. The liver may be swollen and the stomach and intestines congested creating discomfort in the abdomen and a feeling of nausea.

The most important single factor in the treatment of heart failure is rest, which must be absolute in very severe cases but in milder cases proportionate to the degree of failure. It is dangerous to let elderly people become completely bedridden, as they may develop bedsores or infection of the lungs. The administration of digitalis is a major component of therapy in treating persons with chronic heart failure. Its primary effect is to increase the force of contraction of the heart muscle and to slow the pulse rate. Excessive use of salt in the diet must be avoided, and in most cases the use of a diuretic helps in the excretion of excess water from the body tissues.

heart murmur

Extra sounds between, or even replacing, the usual sounds from the heart. They do not necessarily denote heart disease. *Functional murmurs*, arising from the flow of the blood through the heart, are not related to structural defects. *Organic murmurs* arise from obstruction to the flow of blood through a narrowed valve, or from regurgitation through an incompletely closed valve. Murmurs in childhood may arise from defects in the walls between the chambers of the heart.

heart rhythms

See ARRHYTHMIA, ATRIAL FIBRILLATION, EXTRASYSTOLE, VENTRICULAR FIBRILLATION.

heart surgery

The first operation on the heart to relieve symptoms caused by a diseased heart valve was attempted on an aortic valve in 1894. An attempt was made to correct the action of a diseased mitral valve in 1924, but it was not until the 1950s that surgeons began to operate successfully for stenosis (abnormal constriction or narrowing) of the mitral valve.

At first, operations were carried out on the beating heart. But the development and use of heart-lung machines, which keep the blood cir-

THE HEART-LUNG MACHINE

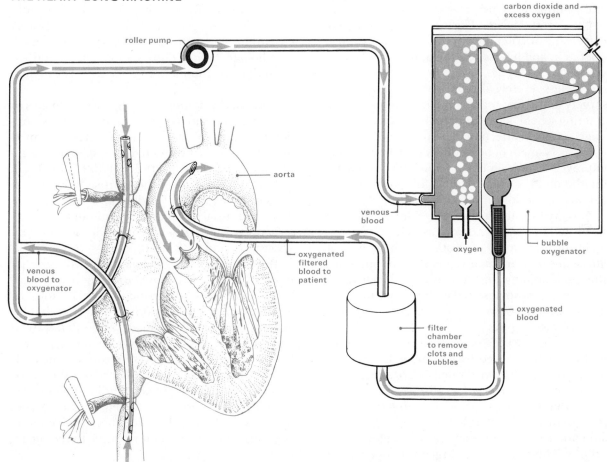

Open-heart surgery was impossible before the development of a safe means of temporarily stopping the heart, so that delicate internal repairs could be made. This is now possible with the use of the heart-lung machine, a device that permits the surgeon to bypass the heart entirely and maintain the blood circulation to the organs and tissues of the body.

culating while bypassing the heart completely, made it possible to operate on a resting heart. Techniques of "open-heart" surgery then advanced rapidly.

It is now possible to replace heart valves with artificial valves, to bypass or widen impaired coronary arteries(*angioplasty*), and to transplant complete hearts—although the problems associated with rejection of grafted heart muscle are far from solved. The correction of congenital heart malformations is possible in many cases, and there has been a remarkable improvement in mortality and morbidity figures.

Surgery involving opening the heart or the grafting of new vessels to its arterial tree requires use of heart-lung bypass technology. In babies with congenital heart malformations who would not survive their first year without surgery, techniques of surface cooling and total circulatory arrest (introduced in 1967 but not adopted generally until the 1970s) have enabled surgeons to operate on still hearts. This has allowed complete correction of complex abnormalities in a single operation and has led to dramatic improvements in results.

The less severely affected child, not requiring surgery in the first year, can wait until just before entering school before undergoing his or her one-stage surgical correction. The diagnosis and ongoing assessment of heart disorders have not only improved technically but are much more humane for the child, so that regular follow-up investigations are no longer a source of fear.

Surgery for valvular heart disease has shown a steady fall in operative deaths as well as improvement in the number of deaths and incidence of illness due to heart disease after surgery. Surgeons still are searching for the perfect artificial valve, but even the valves inserted in the early 1960s and now considered obsolete are associated with very good survival figures.

In the first decade of surgical replacement of mitral valves damaged by rheumatic fever, some deaths occurred from sudden heart attacks due to ischemic coronary artery disease. The recognition that both ischemic and rheumatic disease may occur together has led to routine X-ray examination of the coronary arteries before valve surgery. This has enabled surgeons to operate on both valve and artery and has considerably reduced the risk.

Replacement of diseased coronary arteries by vein grafts has become a frequent heart operation in the United States. Coronary bypass surgery involves replacing a blocked artery with a length of vein taken from another part of the body. Even in the most severe cases, success (particularly in relieving pain) can be startling, and the opportunity it gives to repair ANEURYSMS may prolong life by years.

heat stroke

A medical emergency that usually occurs in very hot, humid, windless weather. It is caused by a breakdown of the body's heat loss mechanisms and is divided into two types, classic heat stroke and exertional heat stroke.

In *classic heat stroke*, of which the cause is unknown, the victim loses the ability to get rid of internally generated heat and his temperature may rise to 105°F (40.5°C) or more. The skin is often hot, dry, and red, but sweating may occur. The victims are frequently elderly, infirm, or otherwise debilitated persons. Those with a history of cardiovascular disease, alcoholism, or obesity, or who are taking diuretics, sedatives, antipsychotic or anticholinergic drugs are also susceptible.

Exertional heat stroke typically strikes athletes or other persons who have exercised strenuously under hot atmospheric conditions. The victim is likely to be sweating and have wet skin; body temperature hovers at 103° to 104°F (39.5° to 40°C).

Regardless of type of heat stroke, other symptoms include rapid pulse, dizziness, nausea, headache, and visual disturbances. Without treatment, lethargy will progress to confusion, loss of consciousness, and even death.

If you suspect someone has heat stroke (either type), medical help should be summoned at once. While waiting for help to arrive, quickly move the victim into the coolest possible place, preferably an air-conditioned or shady area. Remove his clothing, and cool him down by sponging the body with cold water or even by rubbing the body with ice if it's available. Temperature should be lowered as rapidly as possible until it reaches 101° to 102°F (38.5° to 39°C). Keep the victim cool by covering him with a wet sheet and fanning vigorously. If his temperature starts to rise again, resume cooling measures.

In hot, humid weather, one should take certain precautions to prevent heat stroke. Avoid staying in the sun for long periods of time, drink plenty of water, avoid alcohol (which dehydrates the body), and wear light clothing and a broad-brimmed hat. If you feel you are getting excessively hot, rest in a shady or air-conditioned area, or take a cool bath or shower. Avoid strenuous activity, particularly during the hottest part of the day. And, be aware that heat stroke is most likely to strike during the first few days of a heat wave; after that, the body acclimates to some degree.

hematemesis

The vomiting of blood. Hematemesis may be caused simply by irritation of the stomach (for example, by aspirin or alcohol), or it may be a sign of more serious illness, such as ulcers, cancer, or varicose veins at the lower end of the esophagus ("gullet"), often associated with liver disease.

About one third of hmatemeses originate from chronic duodenal ulcers; another quarter are from acute ulcers of the stomach or duodenum. Bleeding from the junction of the stomach and esophagus, or from the esophagus itself, is usually bright red; bleeding from the stomach or duodenum is similar to coffee grounds in appearance. Endoscopy and X-ray studies are used to determine the site of bleeding.

Treatment depends on the diagnosis and may include blood transfusion, medical treatment, or surgery.

hematoma

A swelling composed of blood that has escaped from an injured, diseased, or abnormally fragile blood vessel into the tissues—in other words, a bruise. The vast majority of hematomas subside in their own time, usually about a week, without need for treatment, changing color from purple to brown to green-yellow.

Internal hematomas may follow severe injury; the effects depend on the site of the hematoma. After head injuries hematomas may occur over the surface of the brain or within its substance. Injury-induced hematoma of the lung or kidney can occur also.

hematuria

The abnormal presence of blood in the urine. Hematuria can be caused by kidney disease; by infection of the urethra, bladder, prostate gland or kidney; by a bleeding disorder; or by the pres-

HEMATOMA

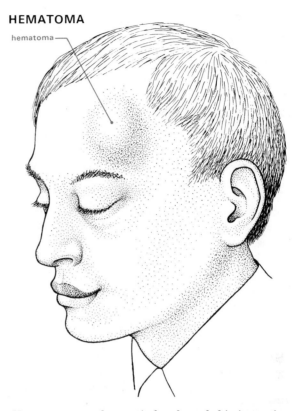

hematoma

Hematomas can become infected, and this is particularly dangerous around the nose and eyes, because it can spread through the skull to cause meningitis. If somebody starts to behave strangely or complain of severe headaches some days after an injury, he or she should be taken to the hospital for immediate medical evaluation.

ence of stones (calculi) in any part of the urinary tract. The most important cause is tumor of the kidney or bladder. Hematuria must *always* be investigated.

hemianopia

Blindness in half the visual field. It may be *bitemporal*, in which both eyes are blind for the outer half of their field of vision; *nasal*, in which the eye cannot see the inner half of the visual field; or *homonymous*, in which each eye is blind for the same half visual field. The type of hemianopia depends on the site of interruption of the optic nerve pathway from the eye to the brain.

Hemianopias may arise from STROKE, injury, congenital abnormality, or tumor, and all require neurological investigation. Recovery of sight is rare.

hemiparesis

Weakness of the muscles on one side of the body, usually the sign of damage or disease affecting the part of the brain that controls the nerves that direct movement (motor nerves).

hemiplegia

Paralysis of one side of the body, the result of damage to or disease of the part of the brain that controls the motor nervous system (the left side of the brain controls the right side of the body, and the right side of the brain, the left).

Damage can arise from injury, either at birth or as the consequence of accidents or wounds, and in such cases recovery is at best partial. The most common cause of hemiplegia is CEREBROVASCULAR DISEASE leading to clotting in the cerebral arteries or bleeding from the diseased arterial wall (STROKE).

hemochromatosis

A chronic illness in which iron is deposited in certain body organs causing them to malfunction. The liver and pancreas are mainly involved, but the heart and skin may also be involved.

Hemochromatosis is caused by the body's inability to prevent the absorption of large amounts of iron in the diet. Treatment usually involves giving a chelating agent that binds the iron; both drug and iron are then excreted by the kidneys. Phlebotomy (bloodletting) may also be used to remove excess iron.

hemoglobin

A complex protein containing iron, present within the red blood cells. Its function is to carry oxygen from the lungs to tissues all over the body. Normal blood contains about 14 to 15 grams (0.5 ounce) of hemoglobin in each 100 milliliters (3.3 fluid ounces), although slightly lower levels are normal in women and children. A fall in hemoglobin below the normal lower limit for the individual constitutes ANEMIA.

In the normal adult, the hemoglobin is of a fixed and unvarying chemical composition almost entirely of one type known as hemoglobin A.

There are very small amounts of two other types—hemoglobin F and hemoglobin A_2.

In certain persons, however, a small chemical and structural abnormality is present in their hemoglobin molecule. Genetic abnormalities can result in the presence of other types of hemoglobins. The diseases that result from these abnormal types of hemoglobin are called *hemoglobinopathies*.

In sickle-cell disease, for example, most of the hemoglobin is in the form of hemoglobin S. This causes the red cells to become distorted (sickle-shaped when seen under the microscope) when they give up their oxygen, and they are easily destroyed. The symptoms of sickle-cell disease include anemia and episodes of severe pain and fever due to the sickled cells blocking the small blood vessels in the bones and other organs.

Other hemoglobinopathies include THALASSEMIA (affecting mainly people of Greek, Italian, or North African origin) and diseases associated with rarer abnormal hemoglobins such as hemoglobins C, D, and E.

hemophilia

Perhaps the best known of the inherited bleeding disorders. Although comparatively rare, it is still much more common than other similar disorders. In addition, its historical association with the royal families of Europe in the nineteenth and twentieth centuries has made it familiar to many.

Hemophilia affects 2 to 3 people per 100,000 of the population. It is caused by an inherited deficiency of a specific clotting factor in the blood (*antihemophilic globulin*, also referred to as *Factor VIII*). The mode of inheritance of this clotting-factor deficiency is unusual: It is "sex-linked recessive," meaning that males are affected; while females are carriers but are not affected.

Clinically, the disorder may occur in either a mild or a severe form; there may also be some variation within a family or a single generation.

Persons with hemophilia bruise easily. Hemorrhage into joints may occur. Small injuries may result in excessive bleeding for long periods. Hemophilia may be revealed first during surgery or after the extraction of a tooth, although in many cases the abnormality will be discovered by means of preoperative tests to determine clotting time. Severe cases may be identified for the first time in infancy when the baby starts to crawl and is more prone to injuries. Diagnosis is based on the person's medical history and on the results of specific blood tests that reveal the absence of the clotting factor.

Treatment is now greatly improved but remains a complex problem that requires the supervision of a unit specializing in the management of bleeding disorders. Replacement of the missing factor with concentrated Factor VIII (obtained from human donor blood) is the mainstay of therapy. An effort is made to arrange home treatment so that the person may lead a more normal life, especially with regard to educational and job opportunities.

hemoptysis

The coughing or spitting up of blood. Hemoptysis can be a sign of certain serious diseases such as TUBERCULOSIS or lung CANCER. In some cases, blood from the nose may trickle down the back of the throat and then appear to have been coughed up from the lung; this is not hemoptysis.

hemorrhoids

A condition (also known as "piles") in which the veins around the anus or in the anal canal are abnormally dilated. In certain cases, as in pregnancy, obstruction to the flow of blood in the veins of the rectum is the cause. In others, factors such as CONSTIPATION, straining at stool, lack of dietary fiber, obesity, heavy lifting, athletic exertions, and a hereditary predisposition have all been implicated.

Whatever the cause, the first symptom of hemorrhoids is usually bleeding from the anus, particularly during a bowel movement. Bleeding may be severe, or only a slight trace of blood may be seen on the toilet paper. Irritation and itching commonly occur. Internal hemorrhoids, if large, may come to project through the anus (*prolapsed piles*), where they are painfully constricted by its contraction.

Although hemorrhoids are a very common condition, the treatment remains as controversial as the cause. In severe cases the dilated veins may be removed surgically and the remaining parts of the veins tied off (*hemorrhoidectomy*); or, in less severe cases, the dilated veins may be injected with chemical solutions that will cause obliteration of the affected vessels by clot formation. The condition may also be treated by local freezing (*cryosurgery*), or the anus may be dilated and stretched

HEMORRHOIDS

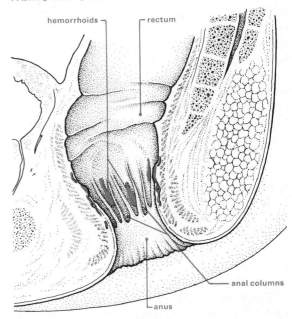

Hemorrhoids are abnormally swollen veins in the lining of the anal canal. They are extremely common in American adults but opinions vary as to their cause. Small hemorrhoids may go unnoticed, whereas large ones protrude through the anus and may require surgical removal.

under an anesthetic to relieve the pressure on the veins and allow them to return to normal.

All these methods of treatment are moderately successful, even though they are often uncomfortable for the patient. Surgical removal of the veins and cryosurgery usually require admission to the hospital, but injection and dilatation may be performed on an outpatient basis. Various suppositories and creams may provide temporary local relief but will not cure the condition, which may, however, regress by itself. Constipation and diarrhea both aggravate hemorrhoids.

hepatitis

Inflammation of the liver; unless further qualified, the term usually is taken to refer to the virus infection of the liver known as "infectious hepatitis."

Viral hepatitis occurs in two basic forms, one of which is called *hepatitis A* and the other *hepatitis B* (or *serum hepatitis*). These two conditions, although clinically similar, are caused by different viruses. There are other differences as well, including the length of the incubation period and the means by which the virus is spread. Hepatitis B appears to be transmitted mainly by the injection or transfusion of contaminated blood or blood products, or by accidental skin pricks or other injuries caused by contaminated needles or other sharp objects. Transmission also occurs from inadequately sterilized hypodermic needles, syringes, surgical and dental instruments, tattooing instruments, and razors. Hepatitis B is common among narcotics addicts and others who use unsterile syringes for drug injections.

The virus that causes hepatitis A, by contrast, is present in the feces; although it can be spread by blood transfusion, the main route is from infective feces to the mouth via the hands or objects contaminated with feces.

There is also a less common form of hepatitis called *non-A non-B hepatitis*, caused by an unknown virus.

The person with hepatitis may notice little or nothing wrong, since many cases are very mild and occur without JAUNDICE (a yellowing of the skin). In more severe cases the person will have fever, headache, nausea, and vomiting, a severe loss of appetite, and aching in the muscles. The jaundice appears after a few days or, in some cases, a week or two from the onset of the symptoms. The liver may become enlarged and tender. With the appearance of jaundice, the symptoms may be increased temporarily but soon diminish. Convalescence may be prolonged and complicated by mental depression.

More acute cases occasionally occur and may eventually lead to death from liver failure. A few persons will remain jaundiced, with an enlarged liver, for some months but in most cases they recover. Some persons may recover but ultimately develop CIRRHOSIS of the liver. This appears to be more common with hepatitis B, as is the condition of *chronic active hepatitis*, in which liver damage continues over a long period and requires special treatment.

An uncomplicated case requires only bed rest at home and care in the handling of infected excreta. Alcoholic beverages should be rigorously avoided. Immunization may temporarily protect against hepatitis A infections in those contemplating travel to high-risk areas.

Toxic hepatitis is caused by poisoning of the liver with various chemicals (such as industrial solvents), drugs, or (rarely) general anesthetics. Bacterial, protozoal, or other microbial infection can also lead to hepatitis. In such cases the treatment is directed toward the underlying cause.

hepatoma

A malignant primary tumor of the liver. It must be distinguished from the much more common secondary tumors of the liver that arise from the spread (metastasis) of cancer cells from other parts of the body, especially from organs within the abdominal cavity.

Cancer of the liver is relatively rare in the United States. It makes up 2 percent of all cancers.

There is a high association between CIRRHOSIS and hepatoma. A similar relationship exists between hepatitis B virus and hepatoma.

hernia

The protusion of any organ or tissue through a covering. Most hernias involve the abdominal cavity. A weakness or defect in the wall allows a knuckle or loop of bowel to pass through.

The most common site for a hernia is the groin, in a man at the point where the spermatic cord passes out of the abdomen to enter the scrotum, and in a woman at the point where the round ligament of the uterus leaves the abdomen to connect with the labium majus. Thus hernia is more common in men than in women, and it may pass down into the scrotum itself to form a considerable swelling.

The hernias that follow the path of the spermatic cord are called *indirect inguinal hernias;* those that make their way through a weakened abdominal wall behind the cord to form a bulge are called *direct inguinal hernias.*

A type of hernia more common in women than in men appears in the upper part of the thigh just below the groin; it makes its way out of the abdomen on the inner side of the canal through which the major blood vessels pass into the leg. This is called a *femoral hernia.*

Less common than both inguinal and femoral hernias is a third type that emerges at the navel—the *umbilical hernia.* It may be found at birth, caused by part of the bowel failing to return to the abdominal cavity from its developmental position within the umbilical cord; or, more rarely, it may be the result of infection of the umbilicus soon after birth. Hernias are found in adults near the umbilicus; they pass through a weak area of the abdominal wall just above or below the umbilicus itself and are called *para-umbilical* hernias.

Incisional hernias are the result of weakening

HERNIA

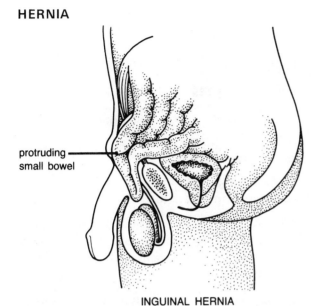

protruding
small bowel

INGUINAL HERNIA

A hernia is any protrusion of an internal organ through the wall of the cavity that normally contains it. Most hernias involve the gut, the most common form being the inguinal hernia, which causes a lump in the groin. Inguinal hernias should always be repaired by surgery.

or incomplete healing of a surgical wound in the abdominal wall, usually in the midline below the umbilicus. It may follow sepsis of the wound and is more likely to develop in obese persons who have weakened abdominal muscles.

The only common hernia in which the abdominal organs escape into another body cavity is the *diaphragmatic*, or *hiatus, hernia*. Occasionally such a hernia forms in the newborn as a result of a developmental defect in the diaphragm, but in adults the protrusion of a part of the stomach through the esophageal opening of the diaphragm is not uncommon, especially in those who are overweight. Usually, this hiatus hernia produces no symptoms, but it may mimic peptic ulcer and result in pain in the upper part of the abdomen or behind the lower part of the sternum (breastbone). It may also lead to uncomfortable HEARTBURN, caused by the reflux of food or gastric juices into the esophagus ("gullet"), especially when the patient is lying down after a heavy meal.

Signs and symptoms of hernias in the abdominal wall include uncomfortable swelling and often pain on straining. Using steady pressure, it is often possible to return a hernia into the abdominal cavity; if this cannot be achieved, it may mean that the hernia has become "trapped." This is potentially dangerous, for the contents of the

protruding hernia tend to swell and if left unreduced they may become gangrenous.

It follows that the best treatment for a hernia is a surgical operation designed to replace the herniated contents into the abdominal cavity and repair the defect in the abdominal wall. The attempt to hold a hernia in place with truss is both insufficient and potentially dangerous.

Management of a hiatus hernia is much the same as that for peptic ulcer, with the added measure of sleeping with the head of the bed raised; it is often possible to gain relief by sitting up when troubled at night. Only in severe cases is an operation justified.

herpes simplex

A virus that causes crusted sores, commonly around the lips and mouth ("cold sores") and the genitalia. "Herpes simplex" also refers to the infectious condition itself.

Many people suffer repeated attacks of cold sores whenever they have a fever or a rise in skin temperature, or are exposed to sunlight. Herpes simplex is intermittently present in the mouths of healthy carriers and is spread by personal contact. Genital herpes is spread by sexual contact with an infected person and is a venereal disease.

An attack begins with itching of the skin in the affected area, quickly followed by redness and swelling. Within a few hours fragile blisters appear and rupture to exude a sticky serum-like fluid that rapidly crusts. Unless secondary infection with bacteria occurs, the lesions heal without scarring within about a week.

The appearance of the rash is so characteristic as to make the diagnosis obvious in most cases of herpes affecting the face. There are no serious complications of oral herpes simplex except for the unsightly appearance. When the conjunctiva is involved, however, there is a danger of corneal ulceration.

Antibiotics may be administered to prevent bacterial infection. The drug Acyclovir is effective in controlling recurrences, but it is unlikely to effect a cure.

Genital herpes infections may cause painful inflammation of the cervix in women, with ulceration and a vaginal discharge. In men the genital infection is usually less severe.

Herpes simplex is very contagious and can be passed when an open sore is on the lip or genitalia and kissing or intercourse takes place.

herpes zoster (shingles)

A disease of sensory nerves caused by the same virus (varicella-zoster virus) that causes chicken pox. It is characterized by a rash preceded by pain and skin irritation, and it affects mainly adults.

Beginning as reddened raised areas, "zoster" develops into blisters that join together and rapidly rupture and crust. The affected areas are always along the course of one or more of the spinal nerves beneath the skin. The rash typically progresses in a band around one side of the chest, trunk, or abdomen. The virus also may attack the ophthalmic cranial nerve, causing a rash that stretches from the eyelid up to the hairline on one side.

Once the rash appears, the diagnosis is obvious and needs no laboratory investigations. It can arise in times of stress, which is believed to reactivate the viruses lying dormant in the nerve ganglia since the attack of chicken pox years before.

The main complaint from people following an attack of herpes zoster is pain (due to irritation of the affected nerve below the skin), which can be severe and particularly distressing in the elderly. The rash usually disappears within two weeks or so, although the pain can persist for many weeks thereafter. The person may require frequent doses of analgesics (pain-killing drugs). As with most viral infections, there is no specific treatment for herpes zoster. Dressings of calamine lotion can help dry up the crusts and antihistamines can help relieve the itching. Recurrent attacks of shingles are uncommon.

hiccup

A sound produced by the involuntary, unintentional squeezing or spasm of the diaphragm followed by a rapid closing of the vocal cords. Causes include eating or drinking too much, indigestion, some types of surgery, and brain inflammation. Hiccup is of no medical significance unless it persists, in which case some disorder of the stomach, diaphragm, or chest may be responsible.

In a normal attack of hiccups the most effective cure is to hold the breath for as long as possible in order to suppress the response of the diaphragm. A number of treatments have been attempted for rare cases of very persistent hiccups, from dry sugar to numerous powerful drugs. A guaranteed treatment, if the hiccup is severe and persistent enough to merit it, is crushing of the phrenic nerve in a surgical operation.

high blood pressure

See BLOOD PRESSURE. Also called *hypertension*.

Hirschprung's disease (congenital megacolon)

A rare congenital disorder involving the absence of nerves in the smooth-muscle wall of the colon, resulting in poor or absent squeezing ability in the affected part of the colon, building-up of feces, and widening of the bowel (megacolon). Hirschprung's disease affects more men than women.

The infant may vomit and appear to have difficulty in passing feces soon after birth. Further trouble may be avoided while the baby is on a liquid diet. But as soon as he starts to eat solid food, the bulkiness of the stools leads to more and more obstruction of the intestine; weeks may elapse without a bowel movement.

The disorder can be distinguished from a normal bout of persistent constipation because the latter responds to alterations in diet or to laxatives. Also, the abdomen of the baby with Hirschprung's disease becomes extremely distended and growth is retarded. Once the diagnosis is confirmed by X-ray examination and biopsy, the affected area of the colon is removed surgically and the remaining ends rejoined. The outcome of the operation is usually excellent.

hirsutism

The growth of unwanted hair on the body. The term is used nearly always to describe excessive hair growth in women, which creates upsetting cosmetic problems.

Typical of hirsutism are growth of the pubic hair up toward the navel, excessive growth of hair around the nipples, and hair in the "shaving" areas of the face. There may be some demonstrable hormone change that can be related to the woman's change of life (menopause), but such hormone problems are found in only about one case in a hundred.

Some rare genetic, hormonal, and metabolic diseases cause hirsutism. In the majority of cases, however, there is no explanation and little point in making detailed hormonal investigations. What is required is skilled treatment for the cosmetic problem of the unwanted hair.

Hormone therapy cannot be used, as a rule, because it would cause too many other undesirable effects. The basis of treatment, therefore, is disguise or removal of the excessive growth of hair.

Unwanted hair can be disguised by bleaching or dying it a light color; shaving the hair is often the most effective method and does not cause stronger growth. Temporary removal can be effected by depilatory creams, abrasives, or shaving waxes; a course of electrolysis is necessary for permanent removal. The advice of a skilled cosmetologist is recommended.

Electrolysis—removal of the individual hairs by cautery of their roots—is expensive and in some cases can leave scars, but for small patches of strong growth it is effective.

histocompatibility antigens

The antigens responsible for an individual's "tissue type," which is an important factor in the success of organ transplantation.

An antigen is a protein substance that provokes an antibody response from the host through the mechanisms of the IMMUNE SYSTEM. All human cells have antigens on their surface, which can be recognized by the body as "self" but which, if transferred to another individual, would be recognized as "nonself." If too many of the antigens (termed "HL-A antigens" or "transplantation antigens") are dissimilar in the recipient of a donated organ, his body is likely to reject it.

Unlike blood group matching—where A, B, AB, and O blood groups can be matched accurately—histocompatibility antigens are far more complex.

When testing the suitability of a donor organ for transplantation, an attempt usually is made to match at least two of the HL-A antigens. The chances of success are known to correspond to the closeness of the match. A minor degree of mismatching is not of crucial importance, however, since treatment with immunosuppressive drugs can dampen the rejection mechanisms.

Several diseases, including PSORIASIS, ANKYLOSING SPONDYLITIS, REITER'S SYNDROME, and DIABETES MELLITUS, are known to be more common in people with particular HL-A patterns.

histoplasmosis

A fungal disease of the lungs caused by the inhalation of contaminated dust.

The parasitic fungus responsible (*Histoplasma capsulatum*) is found particularly in the dust from chicken houses and other areas contaminated by bird feces. Once inhaled it spreads through the lungs to cause a severe and persistent cough, shortness of breath, chest pain, fever, and a general feeling of being unwell (malaise).

Histoplasmosis is usually a mild and self-limiting disease. Some severe and untreated cases can be extremely serious, however. Treatment is by administration of an antifungal agent, usually given intravenously.

Hodgkin's disease

A malignant disease of the LYMPHATIC SYSTEM.

When affected by this cancer, the lymph nodes—which are present in many parts of the body and play an important role in immunity—enlarge, sometimes to the point where they cause pressure on adjacent structures. The cancer cells also may invade the spleen and liver and cause them to enlarge. The disease is not painful in the early stages, although there is fever, weight loss, malaise (a general feeling of being unwell), anemia, and sometimes itching of the skin.

Hodgkin's disease affects two men for every woman and is seen most often between the ages of 15 and 35 and after the age of 50. Why the whole lymphatic system is affected by malignant growth is unknown. A viral cause for Hodgkin's disease has been suspected but not proved.

The nodes in the neck, groin, and armpit first draw attention to the condition, usually because they do not settle after an infection in the normal way. Chest X-ray studies show lymph node enlargement in the chest; superficial lymph nodes feel tense and rubbery as they grow over a period of weeks and become matted together.

The disease is treated with radiation and chemotherapy; newer combinations of anticancer drugs are being tried constantly with increasing success. Most patients can now be cured.

For localized Hodgkin's disease, radiation is

the treatment of choice. Combination chemotherapy is used for more advanced disease.

The prognosis is good, even for persons with advanced Hodgkin's disease.

hole in the heart

A common name for a congenital heart defect in which the two sides of the heart are not properly separated.

The term "hole in the heart" is an accurate description of the condition, which may occur on its own or with other congenital deformities in

HOLE IN THE HEART

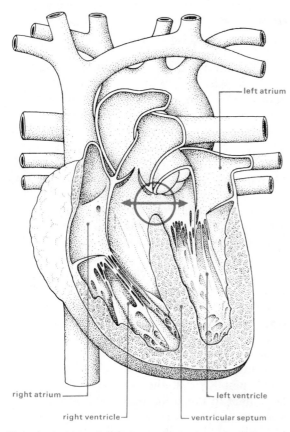

Ventricular septal defect—a hole in the septum between the two ventricles of the heart—is the most common type of congenital heart disease. Fortunately, most of these holes are small and close of their own accord, but larger defects and holes associated with other heart malformations require cardiac surgery to correct them.

the cardiovascular system. The hole may be between the two upper chambers (an *atrial septal defect*) or between the two lower chambers (*ventricular septal defect*). In either case, the hole allows blood to pass directly from one side of the heart to the other without going to the lungs, so that unoxygenated blood circulates. Consequently the person may have a blue appearance due to the high proportion of unoxygenated blood in the circulation.

Congenital heart defects of this kind affect about one child in every thousand in America. The diagnosis usually is made when the pediatrician detects a heart murmur. It must be stressed, however, that there are many different types of heart murmurs and that many of them are not dangerous.

If surgical treatment is planned, the diagnosis will be confirmed and the severity of the defect measured by cardiac catheterization—the passing of a thin, flexible tube through a large vein into the chambers of the heart. The movement of blood within the heart is charted by the pressure in the chambers and by X-ray examination. Many septal defects are isolated defects, but in a minority of cases there are other problems in the heart, making surgical repair more difficult.

With advances in heart surgery, such as the use of the heart-lung bypass that allows the surgeon to work on a resting heart, most cases of septal defect can now be corrected. If the hole is large it is covered either by tissue taken from elsewhere in the person's body or by an artificial knitted Dacron patch. Usually correction of the defect allows the child to return to a normal or near normal life.

homosexual

Homosexuality includes sexual thoughts, feelings, fantasies, and overt sexual acts involving a member of one's own sex. The term *homosexual* is often applied to a person who regularly practices overt sexual acts with members of the same sex past adolescence into adulthood. It has been suggested that there may be hormonal differences between homosexuals and heterosexuals, but this has yet to be validated. The consensus is that all forms of homosexuality are learned and are determined by multiple factors in each society in which they occur.

In some societies, homosexual practices exist

as social ritual; they may be institutionalized by custom, religious practice, or tradition, or used as a means of dealing with isolated maladapted members. In those societies organized around the exclusively heterosexual family, however, all forms of adult homosexuality, derived from whatever cause, generally are considered deviant.

Some researchers believe a predisposition to homosexuality may develop if there is a delayed adolescent period in which the young are kept emotionally or economically dependent. They also say the same may be true if the young are presented with confused or contradictory criteria as to what constitutes an adequate "male" or "female" role.

hookworm

A human parasite common in certain parts of the United States.

The adult hookworm lives attached to the inside of the human intestine, from where it releases as many as 10,000 eggs daily which pass out with the feces. Eggs deposited on warm, moist soil develop into larvae. Many weeks later the larvae may penetrate the skin of another person, enter a blood vessel, and be carried to the lungs.

The larvae break out of the lung tissue and migrate up the bronchi to the throat, where they are swallowed. Eventually they reach the intestine to develop into adults. About six weeks elapse between skin penetration and the first appearance of eggs in the feces, but the adult can remain in the intestine for many years once it is established there.

Hookworm infection is common in many parts of the world where the climate is suitable; usually it is confined to rural areas where sanitation is poor and many people go barefoot. The "hookworm belt" in the United States is along the Atlantic and Gulf coasts from the Carolinas to Texas; the disease is also endemic in parts of Virginia, Kentucky, and Tennessee.

Since the hookworm feeds on blood, it causes a severe ANEMIA. At the site of entry there is severe itching, with local redness and swelling. A heavy larval infestation frequently will cause symptoms of bronchitis.

Any inexplicable case of anemia should be investigated for hookworms. The diagnosis is made by examination of the stools for egg cells.

A single dose of specific antihookworm drugs will kill all the adults in the intestine; it is usual to check the feces two weeks later to be sure. Thereafter, iron therapy progressively corrects anemia.

Prevention of hookworm infestation requires the proper disposal of human excreta, at least by deep burial, and the avoidance of any possibility of skin penetration by the wearing of shoes in all contaminated areas.

hormones

Hormones are protein or steriod substances secreted by the ductless (endocrine) glands to serve as blood-borne "messengers" that regulate cell function elsewhere in the body. They form a communications system in the body and can bring about extraordinary changes in cell activity.

Hormones exert their effects by altering the rates at which specific cellular processes proceed. For example, insulin promotes glucose (sugar) uptake by cells that require energy; follicle-stimulating hormone provokes the ovary into producing an ovum; testosterone enhances the production of spermatozoa in the testes. The hormones do this by combining with enzymes, or by enhancing enzyme production in a cell through a chemical effect on the RNA (ribonucleic acid) of the cell. The result in the body depends on the target organ cell of the hormone and its function. The table below illustrates some of the major hormones and their effects.

The nervous and endocrine systems of the body actually function as a single interrelated system. The central nervous system, particularly the hypothalamus, plays a crucial role in controlling hormone secretion; conversely, hormones greatly alter neural function. No hormone is secreted at a constant rate, and most hormones are either broken down by the liver or excreted by the kidneys. The investigation of endocrine disease therefore depends on measurements of excretion rates and circulating blood levels; but since many of these chemical messengers are bound to protein in the blood, the diagnostic tests are particularly complicated and expensive.

Disease in the endocrine system is revealed by an alteration in the expected effects of the target organ cells. For example, growth fails to occur, ovulation is inadequate, or myxedema occurs because of inadequate function of the thyroid gland. Less frequently the disorder may be that of ex-

Gland	Hormone	Effect
Anterior pituitary	Growth hormone Thyroid-stimulating hormone Adrenocorticotropic hormone (ACTH) Gonadotropic hormones Prolactin	Increase in body size Enhanced metabolism Response to physical stress Growth of gonads (sex glands) Milk production control
Posterior pituitary	Oxytocin Antidiuretic hormone	Uterine contraction Urine excretion control
Thyroid	Thyroxine	Metabolic rate increase
Adrenal cortex	Cortisone Aldosterone	Defense against stress Excretion rate control
Ovaries	Estrogen Progesterone	Maintenance of sexual and reproductive function
Testes	Testosterone	Development of male sexual characteristics
Parathyroids	Parathormone	Calcium uptake by bone
Pancreas	Insulin	Glucose uptake by cells

cessive hormonal secretion, for example, virilization in a woman from a pituitary tumor, or thyrotoxicosis from a thyroid tumor. The treatment of hormonal disorder is undertaken by an endocrinologist and involves the achievement of balance in the supplements administered; diabetic control by the appropriate daily dosage of insulin is the clearest example of this.

In therapy, hormones are used as replacement where the patient is deficient (as with insulin for the diabetic), as treatment to overcome disease (for example, cortisone for arthritis or asthma), and as controlling agents to divert natural functions (for example, sex hormones as contraceptives). Synthetic compounds, designed to resemble the natural products but to achieve enhanced or differing effects, have gradually become available since the 1930s, and in recent years an explosive increase in the knowledge of their benefits—and their disadvantages—has been achieved.

Considerable improvements in the effectiveness of hormone treatment and replacement therapy have been made, but the accurate elucidation of each hormone's multiple influences on human physiology is a continuing challenge.

Hormones are chemical messenger substances secreted directly into the bloodstream by the endocrine glands shown here. They travel in the blood to different "target organs" where they control the rate of cell activity.

HORMONES

ENDOCRINE GLANDS WHICH PRODUCE THE BODY'S HORMONES

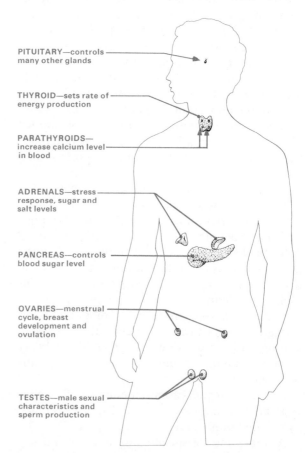

PITUITARY—controls many other glands

THYROID—sets rate of energy production

PARATHYROIDS— increase calcium level in blood

ADRENALS—stress response, sugar and salt levels

PANCREAS—controls blood sugar level

OVARIES—menstrual cycle, breast development and ovulation

TESTES—male sexual characteristics and sperm production

housemaid's knee

Inflammation and swelling of the bursa in front of the kneecap (a form of BURSITIS), caused by prolonged kneeling on a hard surface.

hydatidiform mole

A tumor-like mass in the uterus that originates in and mimics a normal pregnancy. It is most common in Asian women. Typical signs of the condition are extreme nausea, uterine bleeding, the passage of grape-like masses of tissue, an unusually large womb for the expected length of pregnancy, absence of fetal heart sounds, and high blood pressure. Ultrasound scanning will confirm the diagnosis.

The mole will then be removed and the gynecologist will conduct further examinations at regular intervals to make sure that all fragments have been removed. A check of gonadotropin hormone is important. The serious risk with a "molar pregnancy" is that the growth may be malignant, or become so.

It is recommended that a one-year waiting period be observed before trying to conceive again.

hydatidosis

Formation of cysts (*hydatids*) in the internal organs due to infestation with the larval stages of the dog tapeworm (*Echinococcus granulosus*). The condition occurs most often in agricultural communities where dogs mix closely with human families.

The parasite is transmitted to humans by the ingestion of food and water contaminated with the feces of infected animals, by hand-to-mouth transfer of dog feces, and through objects soiled with feces. Eggs may survive for several years in farmland, gardens, and households.

Ingested eggs hatch in the intestine and the larvae migrate to various organs to produce cysts, most often in the liver and lungs. Less commonly they occur in the kidney, heart, bone, central nervous system, and thyroid gland. Humans do not harbor the adult tapeworm, which lives in the intestines of infected dogs.

The symptoms of hydatidosis are variable and depend on the location of the slowly growing cysts. Cysts in the liver may reach a considerable size without causing symptoms. Sometimes there is a "dragging pain" in the abdomen, and pressure on the bile duct may cause jaundice.

When the cyst is in the lungs there may again be no evidence of the disease, except perhaps for a cough and sometimes bloodstained sputum. Long-standing cysts may become calcified. In vital organs the cysts can cause severe symptoms, and may need to be removed surgically.

The most effective preventive measure is education of schoolchildren and the public about the hazard.

hydrocele

An accumulation of fluid in any sac-like cavity or duct, specifically in the bag surrounding the testicles (scrotum) or along the spermatic cord. In some newborn infants the problem may correct itself. Treatment for lasting hydrocele is surgery. Removal of the fluid is only a temporary measure and may cause secondary infection.

hydrocephalus

An abnormal collection of cerebrospinal fluid around the brain or in the brain cavities. The condition is known colloquially as "water on the brain."

Hydrocephalus is caused by obstruction to the circulation of cerebrospinal fluid in the brain or from interference with normal absorption. The condition may be congenital (a defect that prevents the fluid from circulating normally), or it may be acquired due to inflammation of the membranes covering the brain. It is often associated with SPINA BIFIDA.

When hydrocephalus afflicts an infant, the skull is still capable of distension, and rapid enlargement of the head will take place in the first few weeks of life. The forehead bulges outward and the eyes turn down. When the condition occurs in an adult, the fluid pressure rises, causing damage to the brain and especially the visual nerve pathways.

Through surgery it is possible to drain the extra fluid or shunt it to the heart or peritoneal cavity.

Without surgery, hydrocephalus causes brain damage and can be fatal.

hyperemesis gravidarum

A potentially serious, abnormal form of morning sickness in which excessive vomiting during pregnancy may lead to fluid and electrolyte imbalances and weight loss. Treatment involves the administration of replacement fluids and of antiemetic drugs (safe for use in pregnancy) to stop the vomiting. The mother-to-be is placed on bed rest.

hyperglycemia

Abnormally high level of sugar—mainly glucose in the blood.

The level of sugar in the blood is carefully controlled by the action of insulin and other hormones. In DIABETES MELLITUS this control is defective and the blood sugar level rises beyond normal limits, a condition known as *hyperglycemia*.

Above a certain level of blood sugar, the sugar overflows into the urine, producing the condition called GLYCOSURIA.

hyperparathyroidism

Overactivity of the parathyroid glands, causing parathyroid hormone to be produced in amounts greater than normal.

Parathyroid hormone controls the level of calcium in the blood, and overproduction of the hormone leads to a rise in blood calcium. If this is great, the person complains of exhaustion, depression, loss of appetite, weakness, nausea, vomiting, constipation, and occasionally excessive thirst. Calcium is removed from the bones; pain and tenderness may follow, and the bones (being fragile) are more prone to fracture. This may lead to a diagnosis of the condition, since the X-ray appearances of the bones alter.

Increased excretion of calcium in the urine often leads to the formation of kidney stones; about 5 percent of persons with kidney stones are likely to show features of hyperparathyroidism.

There are four parathyroid glands, one pair situated on each side of the thyroid gland, and they are normally about the size of a pea. Overactivity may be due to the development of a tumor of one of the glands (*primary hyperparathyroidism*) or may be the result of a chronically low level of calcium in the blood—such as occurs in kidney disease or deficient absorption of calcium from the intestine. Treatment of primary hyperparathyroidism is surgical removal of the tumor; treatment of *secondary hyperparathyroidism* requires correction of the underlying condition. It is possible to raise the blood calcium level by reducing the phosphate level, so that in chronic kidney failure a diet low in protein and phosphorus, with added aluminum hydroxide and vitamin D, may be recommended.

hyperthyroidism

Excessive activity of the thyroid gland leading to an oversecretion of the thyroid hormone. Also known as *toxic goiter* or *thyrotoxicosis*.

About five times as many women as men are affected; it can occur at any age, with the marked peak between the ages of 20 and 40. The onset of the disease is slow. It may be recognized first when the condition is made worse by emotional stress, hot weather, or an infection. The person feels hot, sweats excessively, and dislikes hot weather and heavy clothes. Sometimes he or she becomes very thirsty, loses weight, suffers from palpitations and breathlessness, becomes anxious and shows a fine tremor of the hands. Emotional instability is common, as is muscular weakness, and the person may be subject to diarrhea or vomiting. The menstrual periods in women may be scanty or absent, and in many cases there is an obvious GOITER. The upper eyelids become drawn up to reveal more of the eye than normal, often being so far retracted that the white of the eye is seen above the cornea. The eyeball itself may be pushed forward in the orbit (its bony casing) and become unduly protuberant; this condition is called *exophthalmos*. Infiltration of the tissues behind the eyeball by white blood cells, as well as edema of the connective tissue, may produce partial paralysis of the muscles that move the eye. It may prove necessary to relieve the condition by a surgical operation to decompress the orbit.

Hyperthyroidism may be treated in three basic ways, all of which are designed to reduce the amount of thyroid hormone circulating in the bloodstream. Part of the thyroid gland may be removed surgically (*partial thyroidectomy*); a proportion of the cells making up the thyroid gland may be destroyed by radioactive iodine introduced into the body; or specific drugs that interfere with the formation of thyroid hormone can be administered. Antithyroid drugs commonly are tried first; but if they fail and the person's condition relapses (as it does in about 50 percent of cases), it may be necessary to remove part of the thyroid surgically, particularly in people under the age of 40. In older persons, the physician may administer carefully calculated doses of radioactive iodine, which enters the thyroid cells to produce partial destruction of the gland over a period of approximately one to three months.

hypnosis

A technique by which a passive state of mind is induced artificially without the use of drugs. The hypnotized subject shows increased obedience to suggestions or even commands.

The hypnotic state is brought about in susceptible subjects by placing them in a quiet environment at rest; they are asked to concentrate on a monotonous stimulus while listening to the voice of the hypnotist, who speaks quietly and insistently. It is possible to hypnotize a subject by making him stare at a pin stuck into the wall while he listens to a recording of the hypnotist's voice.

About 15 percent of people cannot be hypnotized; about one in 20 is exceptionally prone to hypnotic suggestion. It is not possible to make a person under hypnosis carry out any order or suggestion that conflicts with his or her conscious or unconscious wishes (although it may be possible to trick the subject into thinking that some harmful act is harmless).

While many conventional health professionals reject hypnosis, some persons find that it helps them overcome harmful habits of overeating, smoking, or drinking.

hypocalcemia

An abnormal decrease in the concentration of free calcium ions in the blood circulation.

Although 98 percent of the calcium in the body is in the skeleton, the small proportion in the blood is essential to health. Results of hypocalcemia include increased neuromuscular irritability, which may lead to TETANY—cramp-like involuntary muscle spasms, which affect especially the hands and feet. Hypocalcemia may be a sign of HYPOPARATHYROIDISM (a deficiency of the parathyroid hormone), or may arise from kidney failure, acute nutritional deficiency, MALABSORPTION, and PANCREATITIS—although tetany does not appear in all these diseases. The aim of treatment is, first, to restore calcium to normal levels by supplementary dietary calcium and vitamin D, which relieves symptoms of the neuromuscular irritability, and, second, to correct the underlying cause of the hypocalcemia whenever possible.

hypochondria

Preoccupation by a person with his or her general state of health or the condition and function of a particular organ.

Hypochondria often is linked with obsession and depression and may be a symptom of a specific mental illness. Complaints usually involve the abdominal organs; the person insists that there is a malady, against all reassurance by the physician. Often he exaggerates the intensity of normal physical sensations, or describes bizarre discomforts. He cannot admit that his troubles are not due to physical illness and rarely agrees to seek psychiatric help. He is liable to damage himself by taking excessive medication, and in some severe cases there is a risk of suicide.

Hypochondria is a personality disorder that may become manifest from adolescence onward. The origins of the disorder may lie in childhood experiences, however, particularly where illness may have been used successfully as "emotional blackmail" or as a device to secure attention.

hypoglycemia

A condition in which the level of sugar (mainly glucose) in the blood is abnormally low.

The level of sugar in the blood is carefully controlled by a number of mechanisms, including the action of insulin. In DIABETES MELLITUS lack of insulin causes a rise in the blood sugar level, among other metabolic disturbances; treatment by the injection of daily doses of insulin is necessary in many cases.

A potential danger of this treatment, however, is that too large a dose of insulin will produce an excessive fall in the blood sugar level, giving rise to hypoglycemia. The person becomes weak, shaky, and confused, and may, without further warning, lapse into coma.

Reversal of these symptoms can be obtained by giving sugar by mouth in the early stages, but hypoglycemic coma constitutes a serious emergency that requires immediate admission to the hospital or expert medical management.

hypospadias

A congenital defect in which the urinary opening is on the underside of the penis. The farther back the opening, the more serious the condition.

In mild cases the urethral opening is just under the tip of the penis. No surgical treatment is necessary unless the presence of a fibrous band causes a severe downward curvature of the penis.

Other reasons for surgery are cosmetic, urologic, and reproductive.

hypothalamus

An important part of the brain that lies just above the pituitary gland. It is essential in the maintenance of human life, for it is involved with temperature regulation, sexual maturity and function, growth, appetite, fluid balance, blood pressure, and the sleep-wake cycle. Through its action on the pituitary gland, which produces a wide range of hormones, it influences the activity of the thyroid gland, pancreas, parathyroids, adrenal glands, and sex glands. The pituitary gland also produces the hormone by which growth in childhood and adolescence is regulated.

Although the complete functioning of the hypothalamus is not yet completely understood, it is thought that the levels of hormones circulating in the blood are "sensed" by the hypothalamus, which keeps the balance as required through its controlling action on the pituitary gland.

Disease rarely affects the hypothalamus, but it can be affected by injury (trauma to the head or surgical injury) or by tumors growing nearby. The symptoms of disturbed function include excessive urination and extreme thirst, overeating, growth disorders, loss of temperature control, and drowsiness.

HYPOSPADIAS

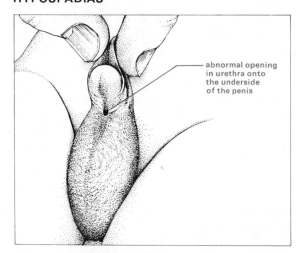

During embryonic life the underside of the penis normally closes up like a zipper; hypospadias occurs where this closure is incomplete. Minor degrees of hypospadias do not require treatment, but an opening well down the shaft of the penis interferes with urinary and sexual functions and needs surgical correction.

HYPOTHALAMUS

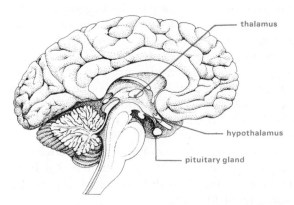

MIDLINE SECTION THROUGH THE BRAIN

The hypothalamus is a structure on the underside of the brain which regulates many bodily functions. It is linked to the higher centers via the thalamus and exerts its influence mainly by controlling the output of hormones from the pituitary gland. Tumors in the hypothalamus can disturb appetite, emotion, sexual behavior, blood pressure, and sleep.

hypothermia

Refers to abnormally low body temperature. The normal body temperature is maintained at 98.6°F (37°C), and fluctuations around this figure usually are small.

Hypothermia often occurs because of immersion in cold water after a boating mishap. It is also a threat to hikers, climbers, and others who spend long periods outdoors during cold, damp weather. Hypothermia can occur at temperatures well above freezing; however, when temperatures fall below 65°F (18.3°C) the risk greatly increases.

Symptoms begin when body temperature falls to 95°F (35°C). The person is listless and confused and makes little or no effort to keep warm. At 86°F (30°C) serious problems appear, with lowered respirations, pulse, and blood pressure.

Many victims of hypothermia are elderly persons living alone in underheated rooms. Such persons should wear several layers of clothing—both in their nighttime and daytime garb—in order to avoid becoming cold.

A person who is suffering from hypothermia should be removed to a warmer environment and wrapped in insulating material until the ambulance arrives. Sudden reheating, as in a hot bath, should be avoided since it could be fatal.

hypothyroidism

Underactivity of the thyroid gland leading to partial or complete deficiency of thyroid hormone in the circulating blood.

The condition may be the result of some congenital defect of the thyroid gland or may be associated with a metabolic disorder. It may be divided into *adult* and *juvenile* types. Adult cases commonly occur in people between the ages of 40 and 60, and in the approximate proportion of six women to one man. Hypothyroidism may be accompanied by a GOITER, and it is common in those parts of the world where simple goiter is endemic because of lack of iodine in the diet. If the condition is not accompanied by a goiter, it is thought to be due to an AUTOIMMUNE DISEASE. Hypothyroidism may occur also as a result of radioactive iodine therapy or surgical removal of part of the thyroid gland in cases of overactivity of the gland (HYPERTHYROIDISM).

Symptoms of hypothyroidism, which are most likely to be felt when the weather is cold, consist of undue tiredness, a feeling of weakness, and a general slowing down of activity. The patient may experience an unusual weight gain, constipation, impaired memory, and shortness of breath. Signs include a gradual change in appearance. The skin becomes thickened, particularly in the hands, feet, and face (which typically becomes swollen and pale), and there is very little perspiration. The hair becomes dry and coarse and tends to fall out. Occasionally, mental processes are affected. The condition, when fully developed, is called MYX-EDEMA; if medical treatment is not provided, the patient becomes cold and eventually may even fall into a coma. Fortunately, if the condition is not too far advanced, myxedema responds to adequate doses of thyroid hormone.

Hypothyroidism in children is more difficult to recognize. Growth is retarded; appearance of the teeth is delayed; and at first the child may be thought lazy and careless. Mental deficiency may occur.

Hypothyroid babies, if untreated, become *cretins*. The face is puffy, the nose snub and obstructed, the tongue too large for the mouth, and the skin yellowish, cold, and thick; intelligence is diminished. The sooner treatment is begun with thyroid hormone, the more likely the infant is to recover; but in many cases lack of thyroid secretion in early development leads to permanent intellectual deficiency.

hypoxia

A deficiency of oxygen in the tissues. Even if oxygen is present in normal amounts in the air, hypoxia may still occur if lung disease is preventing the oxygen from reaching the blood or if the circulation to the lungs is reduced by heart failure.

Treatment involves the administration of oxygen and correction of the underlying condition.

hysteria

In its popular sense, hysteria means any excessive emotional response. But psychiatrists define it as a disorder in which the person develops symptoms of illness (mental, physical, or both) for subconscious reasons. Typically, the development of hysteria allows the person to escape from an anxiety-producing or life-threatening situation.

Dissociative hysteria may take the form of loss

of memory, overreactivity, or sleepwalking. *Conversion hysteria* takes the form of loss of function of some part of the body. There may be sudden and complete paralysis or loss of sensation in the legs or other parts of the body, blindness, deafness, or vomiting. Such effects are dramatic, but they are totally reversible—recovery is just as sudden as the onset of the disability.

The treatment of hysterical symptoms often is delayed while X-rays studies and laboratory investigations are performed to exclude the possibility that there is an underlying physical disease. Once the psychological basis is clear, treatment may be given with psychotherapy, tranquilizers, and more specific measures to remove the emotional stresses that precipitated the illness.

iatrogenic disorder

A problem or disease that develops as a consequence of treatment or oversight by a medical practitioner.

ichthyosis

A hereditary condition characterized by thick, scaly, and very dry skin.

Keratin, the protective substance on the surface of the skin, normally is shed and replaced continuously throughout life. In ichthyosis there seems to be an imbalance in the rates of replacement and shedding: There is either an overproduction of keratin or it sheds relatively slowly.

The condition usually becomes apparent in the first few weeks or months of life. Mild cases may pass off as merely dry skin, but in severe cases the skin looks like fish skin or alligator hide. The scalp may also be affected, but usually not the palms and soles. Warm weather seems to have a beneficial effect.

Treatment consists of measures such as protecting the skin against the cold, avoiding the handling of detergents, and lubricating the skin daily with lanolin or ointments based on petroleum jelly.

In winter it is advisable to have daily or twice daily baths in weak salt water to hydrate the skin, followed immediately by the application of ointments that impede the evaporation of water. Some people claim that vitamin A taken in winter months is helpful.

All these measures may improve the condition of the skin, but a permanent cure is unlikely.

idiopathic disease

Any disease in which the cause is unknown or not clearly understood.

ileitis

Inflammation of the ileum, the third and last part of the small intestine.

By far the most common form of ileitis is a condition variously called *regional enteritis, regional ileitis,* or CROHN'S DISEASE. Although the ileum is the site most frequently affected by Crohn's disease, any other part of the intestine may be affected, especially the colon.

ileus

Paralysis of the intestine. Peristalsis, the wave-like rhythmic movement that propels food along the gastrointestinal tract, ceases and the effect is a nonmechanical obstruction of the intestine.

The most common cause of ileus is PERITONITIS. Cessation of peristalsis in such a situation helps to localize infection, which could spread very rapidly if peristalsis continued. It is not unusual for a temporary ileus, lasting about forty-eight hours, to occur following an abdominal operation.

Ileus may occur also when the blood supply to the intestine is cut off, or following severe injuries to the abdomen or spine. Generally, when there is a mechanical obstruction, that part of the intestine above the site of obstruction contracts vigorously in an attempt to overcome the obstruction; but if this persists an ileus may result.

The symptoms of ileus are abdominal distention and vomiting. Pain is not a prominent feature.

No food should be taken by mouth when there is an ileus. During this time, the person is fed intravenously and a tube is passed into the stomach to remove the digestive juices, which continue to be secreted. Salts lost in this way have to be replaced in the intravenous feeds. If there is peritonitis, antibiotics are essential. Otherwise, treatment is directed toward the underlying cause of the ileus.

immune system

The body surface provides a remarkable degree of innate protection against invasion by infective organisms. The intact skin is a barrier to most infectious agents, but some can gain entry via cuts, scratches, or pricks, and some are able to penetrate the lining membranes of the mouth, throat, lungs, intestines, rectum, genital system, or other structures.

In the absence of immune defensive mechanisms, the interior of the human body—by offering warmth, moiture, nutrients, and darkness—would be an ideal site for the propagation of these organisms. This is strikingly demonstrated in the condition of AIDS, in which much of the normal defense against infection is absent.

Many of these invaders—viruses, bacteria, fungi, and protozoa (single-celled parasites)—damage local tissue, producing a reaction known as *inflammation*. One feature of this is an increase in local blood supply so that large numbers of *white blood cells*—elements of the immune system—can be brought to the area to combat the invasion. Some of these white cells are called *phagocytes* (literally "eating" cells), and many of the invaders which have succeeded in entering the body are destroyed by them. In most cases of minor infection this is sufficient; in others a more complex defense process, involving other cells of the immune system, is necessary.

To perform its functions, the immune system must be able to distinguish between those substances which should be allowed to remain safely within the body (self), and those which must be regarded as dangerous or foreign to the body (non-self). Any such foreign materials entering the body are known as ANTIGENS. One of the main functions of the immune system is to produce appropriate antibodies to neutralize the antigens.

All normal body cells have surface markers—specific chemical molecules that the immune systems can recognize as self and ignore. Foreign organisms or cells have different surface markings, and the highly specialized cells of the immune system are capable of reading these surface markings and acting appropriately if non-self markers are encountered.

In addition to dealing with foreign invaders, the immune system also exerts a constant surveillance over the body's own cells, checking them for viral or other infections and for cancerous changes. Any cells found to show surface evidence of culturing viruses or other pathogens and any with the features of cancerous change, which might develop into tumors, are immediately destroyed. It is probable that without this cancer surveillance, humankind would have perished long ago.

Certain phagocytes, known as *macrophages*, act as identifiers of the foreign material, engulfing them and then expressing, on their own surfaces, the specific chemical markers that can be recognized by other cells of the immune system. These are called *lymphocytes*, and there are two main classes, the T cells responsible for dealing with most viruses, some bacteria and fungi, and for cancer surveillance, and the B cells, which, acting in conjunction with T cells, produce protein substances known as immunoglobulins (antibodies).

After the macrophages and their attendant T cells have completed the recognition process, the existing repertoire of B lymphocytes is scanned to find one capable of producing the most appropriate kind of antibody. This cell is then stimulated to multiply and the resulting "clone" of identical cells starts synthesizing very large numbers of antibodies able to bind to, and neutralize, the antigens. Once this has occurred, the organisms bearing the antigens fall easy prey to other phagocytes. Binding of antibody and antigens may also activate the complement system, which increases the efficiency with which phagocytes engulf the invading organisms.

The T cells are of several types, and these include *helper cells, suppressor cells*, and *cytotoxic killer cells*. The helper cells assist the macrophages to recognize antigens and, among various other functions, activate the killer cells that destroy cells that have been invaded by viruses or other parasites, or are undergoing cancerous change, and which now have the tell-tale markers on their surfaces. They act in a similar way against cells in transplanted tissue.

Lymphocytes that have been activated in this way can survive for many years, providing "immune memory" and preventing us from suffering a second attack of many infectious diseases.

Sometimes the operation of the immune system works to our disadvantage, as in ALLERGY, and in the rejection problems that may arise after organ TRANSPLANTION. In allergy, the immune system mounts an inappropriate response to what are usually innocuous antigens, such as pollen, causing the release of highly irritating substances like histamine.

The rejection of grafted tissue is a normal response of the immune system that would, in other circumstances, be beneficial. If the graft is to take and remain healthy, the immune system must be deliberatedly switched off by drugs. People in this situation are, of course, susceptible to infection, but new drugs are being developed that can prevent rejection while having a less severe effect on the other functions.

In certain circumstances the immune system may itself be a cause of disease. Sometimes certain of the body's own tissues acquire new surface markings so that they are mistaken for antigens and an immunological attack is mounted against them. The resulting diseases are called *autoimmune* disorders. It is now known, also, that many serious conditions are caused by another unfortunate consequence of the immune response. Sometimes, antigens combine with antibodies to form agents known as *circulating immune complexes*. These attach themselves to various sites in the body and cause severe local inflammation. This process is involved in rheumatoid arthritis, systemic lupus erythematosus, some forms of serious kidney disease, drug reactions, aspergillosis, and other diseases.

It is of interest to note that the AIDS virus, HIV, has a specific affinity for the helper T cells, and by infecting and destroying them, gravely interferes with the normal functioning of the immune system.

impetigo

A highly contagious bacterial infection of the superficial layers of the skin. The organism most commonly responsible for the infection is *Staphylococcus aureus*; less frequently, the infection is caused by streptococcus. Impetigo may occur at any age, but it is most common in the newborn and in children.

The lesions start as a reddening of the skin that develops into clusters of blisters and pustules. These break, leaving sores with straw-colored or honey-colored crusts. The only symptom is itching. The lesions may occur anywhere on the body but are most common over the face and limbs.

Treatment should begin promptly or the infection may spread rapidly to other areas of the skin. In babies, especially those who are ill or are premature, the infection may spread to other structures such as the bones or lungs. Occasionally, NEPHRITIS (inflammation of the kidneys) occurs a few weeks after the skin infection has settled.

Treatment consists of rupturing the blisters and pustules and of removing the crusts by washing gently with water and an antiseptic agent. It may be necessary to soak the crusts with wet dressings to make them easier to remove. Antibiotic ointment is applied locally to the lesions, but if there is no improvement in three or four days, or if the infection is severe, antibiotics may have to be given by mouth or by injection.

To prevent the spread of infection to other areas of the skin or to other people, the person should wash his hands frequently and take care not to touch or scratch the lesions.

impotence

The inability to attain or sustain erection of the penis in the presence of sexual desire.

Transient impotence is fairly common and does not imply a physical or psychological disorder. It is often related to mild degrees of anxiety, depression, preoccupation, or fatigue associated with ordinary problems of daily living.

Chronic impotence, on the other hand, is due to either physical or psychological reasons; emotional problems account for a large proportion of cases.

Physical factors should be ruled out first. These include aging (it is not uncommon for men over 65 to be impotent), chronic debilitating disease, alcoholism, drug addiction, diabetic neuropathy, diseases of the nervous system (such as spinal cord damage and multiple sclerosis), endocrine disorders (such as those of the pituitary gland, the thyroid, or the gonads), damage to the urethra, and large hydroceles or hernias. Various drugs, including certain antihypertensive drugs, antidepressants, and tranquilizers, may produce impotence in some men; the problem is solved when the drug is discontinued.

Whether or not impotence due to physical factors can be treated depends on the underlying cause. If it is due to hormonal imbalance, improvement is usually possible; but if nerve damage is present, little can be done.

Psychological reasons for chronic impotence often include guilt and anxiety about the sexual act itself, hostility toward the partner, unwillingness to assume responsibility for all that goes with marriage and children, or various neurotic tendencies. Psychosexual counseling may help.

incontinence

The inability to retain urine in the bladder.

Stress incontinence usually denotes loss of bladder control at times of increased intra-abdominal pressure, as when the person is coughing, sneezing, or climbing stairs. Many elderly women have this problem. In some women, childbirth can weaken the muscles of the pelvic floor, leading to involuntary loss of urine. In men, stress incontinence may be a complication of prostate surgery.

Neurologic conditions and trauma to the spinal cord may lead to loss of bladder control due to interruption of the nerve pathways to the bladder.

Treatment depends on the cause and may involve surgery. In many cases, cure is not possible.

indigestion

A nonspecific term used to describe a number of vague symptoms thought to be associated with food intake or otherwise arising in the digestive system. Also called *dyspepsia.*

"Indigestion" has different meanings for different people: abdominal discomfort, fullness, pressure, pain, heartburn, belching, distension, flatulence, or nausea. Some people even use it to mean constipation or diarrhea.

All of these symptoms may arise from disease in the gastrointestinal tract, and if symptoms are severe or persist, the person should see a doctor. Often, however, the symptoms are the consequence of consistently poor eating habits. Sometimes they are psychogenic in origin, especially in those who complain of "nervousness" or bowel problems. Eating habits that cause indigestion include overeating, gulping down food, or eating when the appetite is depressed by anger or worry.

A person may notice that certain foods bring on symptoms. It could be that the person lacks the enzyme needed for the digestion of that particular food; for example, people who lack lactase may get "indigestion" after drinking milk, which contains lactose. In such cases, which can be confirmed by special tests, the offending food should be avoided. Usually, however, one can avoid indigestion simply by eating regular, unhurried meals.

Often indigestion is due to increased quantities of gas in the gastrointestinal tract. Most of this gas is swallowed, the rest being produced by bacterial fermentation of carbohydrates and proteins—often from raw fruit and vegetables. Swallowing air (*aerophagia*) is normal, but someone who has chronic anxiety or poor eating habits tends to swallow more air than is normal. Fatty meals may aggravate the symptoms of gas because these foods stay longer in the stomach, thereby delaying the passage of gas down the gastrointestinal tract.

If there is no recognized disease causing the symptoms, and if better eating habits do not help, it may be possible to relieve the symptoms with drugs that neutralize gastric acid (antacids) or calm the gut. In rare cases psychotherapy helps.

infarct/infarction

An *infarct* is an area of dead tissue surrounded by healthy tissue and results from a blockage of blood flow to the affected area. "Infarction" has the same meaning but refers also to the formation of an infarct or the process that leads to it.

When the heart muscle is the site of the infarct, the condition is known as a *myocardial infarction* ("heart attack"). Heart infarcts occur when a thrombus or embolus blocks the flow of blood through one of the coronary arteries.

infectious mononucleosis

An acute viral infection, also known as *glandular fever.* It is caused by the EPSTEIN-BARR VIRUS, a member of the herpes group, which is present worldwide. Most infections with the Epstein-Barr virus occur in childhood and usually go unrecognized; the virus may be found in the throats of healthy people.

Infectious mononucleosis can affect persons of any age, but most are between 10 and 35. The incubation period is uncertain. The mode of spread is uncertain also, but there is evidence that it is transmitted in the saliva either by kissing or by sharing drinking vessels. The virus remains in the person's throat for several months after recovery.

The disease affects many parts of the body and manifests itself in a number of ways. Typically the person has a fever, a general feeling of being unwell (malaise), loss of appetite, aches and pains all over the body, enlarged lymph nodes felt as slightly painful lumps (particularly around the neck), and a sore throat. Approximately half the persons have a rash; equally common is an enlarged spleen, which does not produce symptoms although it is big enough to be felt (palpated) by the doctor. Some affected persons have jaundice, and in a smaller proportion the heart, kidney, or lungs may be affected without producing symptoms, although the involvement shows up in laboratory tests. In a smaller proportion still, meningitis, encephalitis, or neuritis may develop.

Because the disease resembles other conditions, blood tests may be required to confirm the diagnosis. As the name suggests, the blood contains atypical *mononuclear cells.* These are B lymphocytes that have been rendered abnormal by the virus.

There is no specific treatment for the disease. Bed rest is advisable until the fever disappears, and aspirin may be given to bring down the fever and relieve aches and pains. Gargle may relieve the sore throat. Ampicillin causes a rash.

In uncomplicated cases, the fever settles in about ten days and the enlarged lymph nodes and enlarged spleen return to normal in about four weeks. In some cases the disease may linger on for months. Those who have had jaundice should avoid alcohol for about six months. Recovery is usually complete.

infertility

Diminished or absent ability to produce offspring. The cause of infertility may lie in the man or the woman. Infertility may be temporary and reversible or permanent and irreversible.

Among the physical causes are immature sex organs, problems in the reproductive system such as low production of sperm or ova, and hormonal imbalance. Infertility may result also from psychological or emotional problems.

Investigations for causes in men are safer and simpler, and normally they are performed first.

Some causes of infertility are treatable with either surgery or medication.

See extended discussion under *Family Planning* in the section on **Family Medicine and Health.**

inflammation

This is the very complex way in which living tissue responds to injury from germs, chemicals, burns, or trauma. It is essentially a protective mechanism by which the body attempts to localize the injury.

The blood vessels around the site of injury dilate and become permeable, so that white blood cells can leave the vessel and migrate to the site of injury, where they either ingest the infecting organism or release chemical substances to digest damaged tissue.

Inflammation produces swelling, heat, redness, pain, and loss of function of the affected part. Sometimes the effects of inflammation are seen beyond the site of the injury, as when there is fever or a change in the number and types of white blood cells.

influenza

An acute viral infection of the respiratory tract, with symptoms present elsewhere in the body. It can affect people at any age. The consequences in the very young, the elderly, the debilitated, and those with heart or lung disease are particularly dangerous. The infection is spread when infected droplets discharged by an infected person during speaking, coughing, or sneezing are inhaled by an uninfected person. There is an incubation period of one to four days before symptoms appear.

Symptoms appear abruptly and include fever, chills, a dry cough, nasal stuffiness and runny nose, aches and pains all over the body, a sore throat, headache, loss of appetite, nausea, weakness, and depression. Mild cases may resemble a common cold, although the weakness and depression usually are greater.

As with viral infection in general, there is no specific drug treatment for influenza. General measures include bed rest during the acute phase, followed by a gradual resumption of normal activity. If required, aspirin or other mild antipyretic/analgesic medication may be taken to relieve symptoms. In uncomplicated cases, symptoms usually subside within a week.

Influenza reduces the person's resistance to bacterial infection; superimposed bacterial bronchitis is a common complication, which if untreated may lead to pneumonia. Other bacterial complications include sinusitis and infections of the middle ear (OTITIS MEDIA).

If the fever persists more than four days and purulent (pus-containing) sputum is brought up on coughing, it is advisable to see a doctor—who may prescribe antibiotics if it appears that secondary bacterial infection has occurred.

The simplest way of minimizing the possibility of an attack is to avoid crowds during an epidemic.

An attack of influenza confers immunity to the particular strain to which the infecting virus belongs. A temporary immunity to one or more strains can be acquired by injection of a vaccine prepared against those strains. Such vaccines take about two weeks after the injection to become effective; it is useless to have the injection once symptoms have appeared. Thus, immunization against influenza usually is given in the autumn to protect against attacks during the winter when influenza is most common.

Routine immunization generally is not advised for everyone. Most doctors advise immunization only for those who are particularly susceptible. Unfortunately, immunization against known strains of influenza virus does not protect against new strains, which crop up periodically and are responsible for the epidemics that appear every few years.

insulin

A hormone produced in the pancreas and responsible for the control of carbohydrate metabolism. The breakdown of carbohydrates produces glucose (sugar). Insulin helps the muscles and other tissues to obtain the sugar needed for their activity. When not enough insulin is produced,

INSULIN

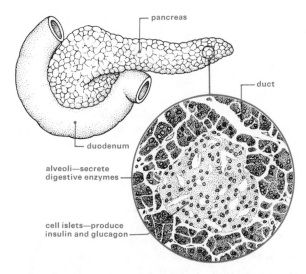

The pancreas is a mixed-function gland. It secretes digestive enzymes through ducts into the intestine where they break down fats and proteins. It also secretes hormones, including insulin, directly into the bloodstream.

the glucose in the blood cannot enter the tissues of the body and builds up to dangerously high levels in the blood. This occurs in the condition known as DIABETES MELLITUS.

Medical insulin, a pancreatic extract, can be administered by injections to keep the blood glucose level under control and to allow the body to utilize the needed sugar. (The reason that insulin is not taken by mouth is that digestive enzymes in the bowel destroy it before it can work.) Many types of insulin are available; they differ in the duration of their action and in their source, which can be beef, sheep, or pig pancreas. Such insulin can be modified so as to be closer in chemical composition to human insulin. Human insulin is now being produced by genetic engineering. Before the introduction of insulin, most cases of severe diabetes mellitus led to death.

For mild diabetes that does not need insulin therapy, oral medications can be used to combat the mild glucose elevations. Called *hypoglycemics*, these medications are not related to insulin.

intermittent claudication

A cramping pain, usually affecting the calf muscles, that comes and goes during walking. It is caused by an insufficient supply of blood to the muscles owing to narrowing or obstruction of the arteries that supply the leg, usually by ATHEROSCLEROSIS.

The compromised blood supply to the leg can produce damage to the tissues of the limb in addition to causing pain. If the pain worsens or if the condition of the leg deteriorates, the narrowed or obstructed artery may have to be replaced with a synthetic graft.

This condition affects more men than women and is most common after the age of 50. Diabetics are particularly at risk as well as persons with high blood levels of cholesterol.

intertrigo

Chafing of the skin where two surfaces, usually moist, rub together.

As a result of the chafing, erythema (redness) or dermatitis (skin inflammation) may occur. Intertrigo may be a particular problem in young infants, since the child does not detect the chafing. The most common sites are the natural folds of skin in the groin, armpits, and elbows. Elderly obese people with a greater than normal overlap of tissues are also especially susceptible. Diabetics are also at increased risk.

In general, the condition may be encountered whenever obese individuals sweat profusely, especially in extremely hot weather.

Retroauricular intertrigo is an inflammatory condition of the skin that develops in the fold where the ear joins the scalp. A painful crack may appear and is sometimes extremely persistent.

Seborrheic intertrigo, a condition similar to retroauricular intertrigo, arises from chafing under heavy breasts or in the folds of the buttocks. The skin between the scrotum and the thigh is another common site where intertrigo may appear.

Monilial intertrigo is a yeast infection that develops in skin folds. It is characterized by bright red areas of raised skin and commonly occurs under the arms, breasts, and in the groin area of obese adults, particularly diabetics.

Prevention of intertrigo is best accomplished by keeping the skin clean and dry. Mild soaps should be used and after drying the skin, medicated powder can be applied. Obese persons should be encouraged to lose weight. Clean, comfortable, loose-fitting clothes and underclothes should be worn.

intrinsic factor

A substance, produced by the lining of the stomach, that is essential for the transport of vitamin B_{12} through the lining of the intestine.

Because the daily requirement of vitamin B_{12} is very small, symptoms of B_{12} deficiency are almost invariably due to a breakdown of the absorption mechanism. The cause may be a failure of the stomach to secrete intrinsic factor or loss of the secreting cells due to tumorous growth or surgical removal.

Lack of intrinsic factor for any of these reasons, by preventing B_{12} absorption leads to the type of anemia known as *pernicious anemia*—which can be fatal if the person is not treated with vitamin B_{12}, iron, and a balanced diet.

intussusception

A condition in which one part of the intestine becomes pushed or telescoped into the adjoining portion.

It occurs mainly in infants under one year and usually starts at the lower end of the ileum. It may result when overactive wave contractions (peristalsis) of the intestine drive a segment of the bowel inside the adjacent segment. Further peristaltic movements may aggravate the condition so that more of the intestine becomes involved. The sudden intestinal obstruction causes severe abdominal pain. The infant has attacks of screaming and draws up its legs. The face becomes very pale when the pain is most intense and brightens in the intervals between spasms. Vomiting starts early and is severe and repeated. After the first bowel movement, the infant passes only red jelly-like clots of pure blood and mucus from the bowel.

Examination of the abdomen by the doctor usually reveals a sausage-like mass.

Prompt surgical treatment is necessary to pull the telescoped portion of the intestine back to its normal position. If the intestine is gangrenous, as happens in some cases, surgical removal of the affected part is necessary.

iritis

Inflammation of the iris, the colored part of the eye; characterized by pain, contraction of the pupil, and discoloration of the iris itself. Some temporary or permanent decrease in vision may also be involved.

The causes are often not found. Iritis can be associated with injury to the eye, TUBERCULOSIS, SYPHILIS, COLLAGEN DISEASE, REITER'S SYNDROME, ANKYLOSING SPONDYLITIS, and juvenile RHEUMATOID ARTHRITIS.

Swelling of the upper eyelid and pain radiating to the temple are common symptoms. There may also be excessive secretion of tears, intolerance of bright light, blurring of vision, and transient nearsightedness.

The eye becomes bloodshot and pus may appear in the front chamber of the eye or cover the surface of the lens. Adhesion may form between the iris and the lens, and may be permanent.

The *acute* form of the condition usually lasts several weeks and tends to recur. *Chronic* iritis may last considerably longer, with the outcome depending on the severity of the complications.

Early treatment is important. A drug is used to dilate the pupil so that adhesions are less likely to form between the iris and the lens. Steroid

A CROSS SECTION OF THE EYE

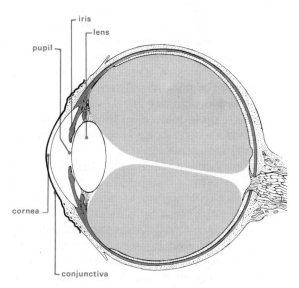

The iris is the colored part of the eye that surrounds the pupil. Iritis, inflammation of the iris, causes a painful red eye with a constricted pupil and blurred vision. Although iritis can occur in isolation, it can be a feature of many systemic dieases, for example rheumatoid arthritis, sarcoidosis, and syphilis.

drugs frequently help to suppress the formation of exudates. The underlying causes of the inflammation should be investigated and eliminated if possible.

iron

A common metallic element necessary for blood formation.

Approximately two thirds of the body's iron is found in HEMOGLOBIN, the oxygen-carrying component of red blood cells. The body of an adult contains 3 to 4 grams (0.10 to 0.14 ounce) of iron. Iron is lost in small quantities in the urine, feces, and sweat, and in larger quantities during menstruation. Hemorrhage results in a more serious loss.

Children and pregnant women require a higher intake of iron than does the average adult. Foods rich in iron include liver, lean meats, and green leafy vegetables. Supplementary iron is commonly prescribed.

irritable bowel syndrome (IBS)

The name given to a common group of disorders of the digestive tract. The most widely accepted definition is based on the presence of two symptoms: abdominal pain and alternating bouts of constipation and diarrhea without detectable organic disease. Other symptoms include abdominal cramping and bloating. The symptoms are usually made worse by tension, anxiety, or emotional disturbance.

This group of disorders has many names, including irritable colon, spastic colitis, mucous colitis, intestinal neurosis, and spastic colon.

Irritable bowel syndrome is the most common disorder of the digestive tract in the United States. Its onset is usually gradual; more than 50 percent of victims experience their first symptoms before reaching 35. Women are more likely to have the syndrome than men.

While the cause of IBS is still unclear, a number of factors—including emotional stress, allergic response to certain foods, and lactose intolerance—have been implicated. Some medical professionals believe that the lack of fiber in the American diet predisposes us to the disease.

Diagnosis of IBS is not simple, since many of its symptoms are characteristic of other disorders. The physician will perform numerous medical tests, including a barium enema and a sigmoidoscopic examination, to preclude the possibility of organic disease. Medical history is of paramount importance in diagnosis, so patients should tell their doctors everything they can about their eating and bowel habits, use of laxatives, and the type and frequency of abdominal pain.

Treatment often centers on increasing one's intake of dietary fiber ("roughage"). Fiber retains water and makes intestinal contents soft, aiding in motility. Good sources of fiber are raw fruits and vegetables and whole-grain breads, flour, and rice.

If lactose intolerance is a factor, milk and milk products must be restricted. In other cases, regular hours and meals, adequate sleep, exercise, and restriction of alcohol may help. Sometimes, the doctor may prescribe sedatives or antispasmodic drugs.

Since emotional factors exacerbate symptoms, it helps to avoid situations that produce anxiety or stress. Just assuring oneself that there is no organic disease (though uncomfortable, IBS is not medically serious) can be of great benefit in relieving symptoms. If depression or anxiety are severe, the physician may recommend psychological counseling.

ischemia

A reduction in the supply of blood to a part of the body due to a narrowing or complete obstruction in the artery that normally carries blood to that part of the body.

Ischemia may cause pain and in severe cases even the death of the affected tissue. For example, narrowing of the arteries supplying the heart can cause heart pain called ANGINA PECTORIS. Complete obstruction causes death of heart muscle, a condition known technically as MYOCARDIAL INFARCTION but more commonly as "heart attack." Ischemia of the arteries of the brain can lead to a STROKE.

islet cell tumor

A tumor of the insulin-secreting cells in the "islets of Langerhans" of the PANCREAS. These tumors rarely are malignant. They may produce excess insulin for the body to cope with, causing HYPOGLYCEMIA, or they may be nonfunctioning.

Islet cell tumors are very rare. The vast majority of pancreatic tumors are malignant ADENOCARCINOMAS, which are not associated with the production of insulin.

itching

A sensation of tickling and irritation in the skin, producing a desire to scratch. Itching is known medically as *pruritus.*

The degree of itching can vary widely and may be experienced in one place only or body-wide. A mild itch may almost go unnoticed; at the opposite extreme, severe and unrelenting pruritus may cause the person lasting torment. The sensation arises in nerve endings in the skin, which are stimulated by released enzymes; substances such as histamine and prostaglandins are thought to be involved in the reaction. Itching can be caused by chemical, mechanical, thermal, or electrical stimuli. For example, by rubbing an insect bite you may prolong the itching for a considerable time after the original stimulus has been removed, because the skin is in a state of increased excitability.

Vigorous scratching of an itch leads to an enlargement of the area involved, and thus the threshold is lowered further. The damage to the skin may lead to a secondary infection and the formation of fissures or crusts.

Apart from outside stimuli, the root of the problem may be parasites such as scabies or lice, or skin diseases such as ECZEMA, LICHEN PLANUS, and PSORIASIS. Or there may be an underlying disease such as MYXEDEMA, JAUNDICE, KIDNEY DISEASE, LYMPHOMA, or internal malignancy.

Pregnancy, menopause, and drug and food allergies are other possible causes. Psychological elements are commonly associated with itching.

Treatment can be very difficult, especially in cases caused by internal disease; often the itching can only be relieved through treatment of the disease. When the itching obviously is due to a particular stimulant, it can be controlled by removing that cause. In other cases, more general measures may have to be used, such as the avoidance of very hot baths or a change in the brand of soap or cosmetics. Noninfected areas of skin can be treated with external steroid preparations. Drugs such as aspirin, antihistamines, tranquilizers, or sedatives also may be valuable.

jaundice

A yellow discoloration of the skin and whites of the eyes caused by deposits, in these tissues, of a substance called *bilirubin.* Normally, bilirubin is excreted into the bowel by the liver and never builds up in excess amounts to cause jaundice. In several disease states, however, jaundice may be seen.

When a great many liver cells are damaged, as in HEPATITIS, the bilirubin level rises, causing jaundice. In the absence of liver cell damage, obstruction of ducts in the liver prevents the normal excretion of bilirubin into the bowel and thus leads to elevated blood levels and jaundice.

There are other causes of jaundice but they are rare. Frequently, the yellow skin discoloration is accompanied by very dark urine and chalk-colored stools.

jet lag

The symptoms that many people experience when they cross several time zones during air travel.

During a long flight—such as one across the

Atlantic Ocean—the physiological functions of the body become "desynchronized" from man's artificial time system.

When traveling from east to west, for instance, an airplane may leave one time zone at noon, fly for seven hours, and land in another time zone at 2 P.M. The passenger then usually resumes his activities as if only two hours, rather than seven, have passed. He may carry out normal activities for the remainder of the day until he goes to bed; but his CIRCADIAN RHYTHMS are those that would have been appropriate for the period between 7 P.M. and 3 A.M, rather than the 2-to-10-P.M. period of his new time zone. Symptoms include a dry mouth, racing pulse, disorientation, insomnia, and often a loss of appetite.

"Circadian rhythms" are fluctuations in the body's biological system that operate on a period of approximately twenty-four hours. They include slight changes in body temperature, minor changes in blood levels of salts such as potassium and sodium, and changes in hormone secretion. The question of how long it takes to return to normal circadian rhythms is one that is still being debated by scientists; it is certainly true that some people are more adaptable than others. However, there is a rough rule of thumb that a passenger should rest for one day after a flight lasting seven hours. West-to-east flights are more taxing than east-to-west flights because they result in a longer day; passengers therefore often lose sleep in addition to disturbing their circadian rhythms.

There is some evidence that jet lag affects performance. Some companies insist that executives not make important decisions until a few days have passed after a long flight.

Passengers in pressurized airplanes tend to become dehydrated. This is associated with both the extremely dry atmosphere of the cabin and (often) the consumption of alcoholic drinks. The dehydration aggravates the symptoms of jet lag. To minimize problems a passenger should drink plenty of fluids (without alcohol), sleep as much as possible (preferably without sedatives or sleeping pills), and retire to bed at the end of any long journey rather than undertake strenuous activity immediately.

keloid

A large, pinkish scar elevated above the surface of the skin. It results from an excessive growth of the cells known as *fibroblasts* in a wound, and it may invade the subcutaneous tissue as well as the skin. "Keloid"—from the Greek for crab claw—refers to the scar's characteristic claw-like projections.

Persons with burns often become victims of keloid when raw granulating surfaces in deep burns are not resurfaced with a skin graft. Keloid also may appear in accidental or surgical wounds, or even in such slight traumas as the scar of a boil or abscess, a smallpox vaccination, or an ear prick. It is more common in people with dark complexions, in tubercular patients, and in pregnant women.

Keloid tissue frequently itches and may ulcerate in places. Unlike more common forms of hypertrophied scars, it may grow for months or even years and it is notorious for recurring after surgical removal, but it rarely develops into a malignancy. In its early stages it may be relieved by the application of hydrocortisone medication. The conventional treatment is to subject the scar to deep X rays in order to diminish the blood vessels and to stop the proliferation of the fibroblasts. If surgical removal is undertaken, it is usual to cover the area with skin grafts, but there is no guarantee that the keloid will not grow back.

keratitis

Inflammation of the cornea, the transparent front lens of the eye. Worldwide, the most common cause is deficiency of vitamin A, but keratitis may also be due to chemical injury or to infection with viruses or bacteria. Exposure to sunlight or ultraviolet light may cause a transient keratitis.

Treatment clearly depends on the cause. Correction of the vitamin deficiency will produce a dramatic cure if the condition is not too far advanced. Bacterial infections usually respond to the appropriate antibiotic, and viral infections to an appropriate antiviral drug, used under the close supervision of a specialist. If the condition is allowed to progress untreated, however, it may eventually lead to severe corneal scarring and loss of vision.

keratosis

Thickening of the outer horny layer of the skin. This layer, called *keratin*, acts as a protective layer for the skin.

In *senile keratosis*, multiple warty lesions covered by a hard scale form on the forehead, cheeks, lips, and on the backs of the hands and forearms as a consequence of repeated and prolonged exposure to sunlight. The condition also is called *actinic* or *solar keratosis*, and those who spend their lives working outdoors may develop the lesions relatively early in life. These lesions may be precancerous and therefore usually should be removed. Persons with this disease should guard against further sun exposure.

Keratosis follicularis is a rare hereditary disease marked by multiple growths that form large patches on the head, neck, armpits, and trunk.

kernicterus

A condition in which the brain of infants suffering from severe jaundice becomes yellow, the nerve centers at the base of the brain (basal ganglia) in particular being susceptible.

If areas in the medulla oblongata are affected the baby may have difficulty in breathing and show twitching of the face and limbs; damage to the basal ganglia is manifest as abnormal writhing movement of the limbs and retarded psychomotor development. Mental defects may become apparent in consequence of damage to the higher cortical centers. The infant may be floppy, feed poorly, and may suffer seizures.

As there is no known treatment for the condition once it has occurred, excess of bile in the blood of an infant must be dealt with by exchange transfusion in the period immediately following birth. About 75 percent of cases are due to hemolytic disease (see RH FACTOR), the others often being associated with birth before full term. Preventive treatment requires the early diagnosis and treatment of conditions in the newborn that can cause hemolysis. Amniocentesis can give early warning.

Before the introduction of exchange transfusion, about one in 1,000 babies born alive was liable to develop kernicterus.

kidney disease

Persons with kidney disease may either develop problems related to urine formation or present a more confusing picture in which the symptoms at first do not seem to involve the kidneys.

The main signs and symptoms of disease of the urinary tract are the presence of abnormal constituents in the urine (such as blood and protein), a large increase or decrease in the volume of urine, frequency of urination, and pain. The pain may either be a burning sensation on passing urine or low back pain (which has many causes other than kidney disease). Manifestations of kidney disease unrelated to the urinary system include anemia, hypertension, edema, loss of appetite, nausea, weakness, stunted growth in childhood, itching, convulsions, coma, and bone disorders.

Apart from URINARY TRACT INFECTION (UTI), most of the kidney diseases discussed here are uncommon. UTI is predominantly a disease of women and is caused by bacteria from the anus spreading up the urinary passages. If the infection is not effectively treated with antibiotics, the kidney eventually is involved in PYELONEPHRITIS, marked by fever and lumbar pain. In low-grade pyelonephritis there may be no symptoms, yet the disease can progress insidiously to produce small scarred kidneys and chronic renal (kidney) failure.

Chronic renal failure has many possible causes, pyelonephritis being the second most common. The chief cause in children and adults is GLOMERULONEPHRITIS—an inflammatory disease of the kidney that results from disorders in the body's defense mechanisms. Damage to the blood vessels of the kidneys, whether from ATHEROSCLEROSIS, hypertension (see BLOOD PRESSURE), or DIABETES MELLITUS, also can result in chronic renal failure. Various congenital abnormalities such as POLYCYSTIC KIDNEY can produce chronic renal failure in adult life. Among the other causes is the ingestion over many years of large doses of analgesics such as aspirin.

Most persons who are developing chronic renal failure, from whatever cause, do not notice any symptoms until they have the equivalent of half a single kidney left functioning. The complications that then follow depend on a number of pathological mechanisms: (1) the failing kidney can no longer concentrate urine, leading to frequent voiding and imbalance in the blood levels of sodium, potassium, and hydrogen; (2) at a later stage, urine formation falls dramatically so that toxins normally cleared from the blood by the kidney are retained; this state is called UREMIA and is marked by cardiac and neurological disorders; (3) the kidney normally activates vitamin D, which is important for calcium absorption, and when this process fails, bone disorders can occur; (4) hypertension is a common feature of chronic

THE KIDNEYS

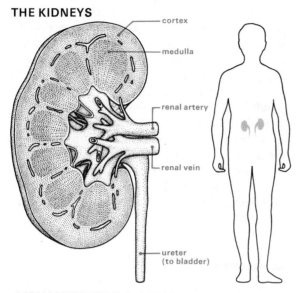

A CROSS SECTION THROUGH A KIDNEY

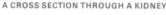

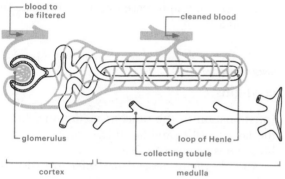

MAGNIFIED DIAGRAM OF A NEPHRON

The kidneys are paired organs, each about four inches long, lying alongside the backbone. Each kidney contains about one million functional units or nephrons. Blood is filtered through glomeruli in the cortex to produce urine, which then flows through the rest of the nephron to the collecting tubules, with great changes in its concentration and chemical composition being made on the way.

renal failure and the blood pressure may increase rapidly to cause fatal cerebral hemorrhage; (5) the healthy kidney secretes erythropoietin, a hormone that stimulates the bone marrow to produce red blood cells, this mechanism is depressed in chronic renal failure, causing anemia, which is further exacerbated by the state of uremia.

Until recent years the above complications of chronic renal failure were invariably fatal within a short time. Now with techniques of dialysis and surgical TRANSPLANTATION it is possible to prolong life, often for many years, although the problems are formidable.

Acute renal failure—in contrast to the long, insidious buildup in chronic renal failure—is a state where the production of urine falls suddenly to less than a pint every twenty-four hours. An abrupt reduction in renal blood flow following hemorrhage, crushing muscle injuries, burns, or overwhelming infection can cause such a drop in urine output. If prompt action is taken to restore the blood pressure, the volume of urine produced soon returns to normal. Otherwise, prolonged lack of oxygen kills cells in the kidney tubules and acute renal failure is established. The same picture can result from a variety of drugs and toxins and from the transfusion of incompatible blood. A person who suddenly stops producing urine completely probably has an obstruction in the urinary tract due to a CALCULUS (stone), blood clot, or tumor.

If a person with acute renal failure survives, he passes little urine for the first few weeks and then has a "diuretic phase" when the urine output increases to 6 to 8 pints (2.8 to 3.7 liters) per day. With good medical care, renal function usually returns to normal.

There are two main types of *cancer of the kidneys.* *Wilms's tumor* affects young children and is thought to originate in the fetus in many cases. Combination treatment with surgery, irradiation, and drugs has recently improved the prognosis for these children. *Nephroma* accounts for less than 2 percent of all adult cancers and usually affects people over 45 years of age.

NEPHROTIC SYNDROME is mainly a disease of children and is caused by heavy loss of protein in the urine.

Klinefelter's syndrome

A chromosome disorder in men which in its classic form is marked by small testes, infertility, enlargement of the breasts, and sometimes mild retardation and antisocial behavior.

kraurosis vulvae

A condition in which the vulva becomes dry, shriveled, red, sore, and itchy. The fatty tissue on the mons (the pubic bone) and the labia withers and atrophy of the clitoris occurs.

Some atrophy of the vulva is normal after the menopause, and kraurosis vulvae probably represents an extreme degree of these normal changes. It is caused by a decrease in the level of circulating estrogens following the menopause; younger women rarely are affected.

Kraurosis vulvae needs treatment for two reasons: It may cause discomfort, and it increases the risk of both vulval infections (with CANDIDA or bacteria) and vulval cancer. Treatment is with estrogen, best given in the form of a cream to reduce the risk of side effects.

kyphosis

An abnormal curvature of the spine in which its normal curves are exaggerated. It results in the condition commonly referred to as *hunchback* or *humpback*. The condition may be worsened by OSTEOPOROSIS.

labor

The processes that occur during CHILDBIRTH, from the beginning of cervical dilation to delivery of the baby and the placenta.

lacrimation

The normal production and discharge of tears. The term also is used sometimes to imply excessive tear production.

Tears wash the eyeball constantly, removing dust and foreign particles. They contain an enzyme capable of killing many types of bacteria.

Tears are produced by the lacrimal glands, situated behind the outer part of each upper eyelid. They flow over the eyeball to the inner part of each lower eyelid. From here they drain through tiny ducts (the lacrimal canaliculi) into the lacrimal sac, which in turn drains through the nasolacrimal duct to the nose.

Excessive production of tears may be caused by emotional factors as well as by any condition that irritates the surface of the eyeball—such as conjunctivitis, foreign bodies, or chemical irritants.

Tear production may appear to be excessive when the drainage apparatus is blocked: The tears spill over to run down the cheeks (a condition known as *epiphora*). Blockage is due commonly to infection, but it may also be due to a congenital defect, for example, the failure of the drainage apparatus to develop properly. Epiphora may also be caused by a fungus in the lacrimal sac, or by paralysis or eversion (outward turning) of the lower lid, which prevents normal drainage.

Blocked ducts may be treated by antibiotic eyedrops. Surgery sometimes is required.

Lacrimation is decreased in certain rare conditions. Damage to the surface of the eye may be avoided in such cases by the use of "artificial tear" eyedrops.

lactation

The production and secretion of milk by the female breasts.

laryngitis

Inflammation of the mucous membranes lining the larynx, with swelling of the vocal cords and hoarseness or loss of voice.

Acute laryngitis arises from infection (usually influenza or another virus) and often occurs in association with inflammation of the throat (PHARYNGITIS) or TONSILLITIS. It usually causes a harsh dry cough; in young children it may cause obstructed noisy breathing and CROUP. As in most infections, the person has a fever and feels ill.

Humidified oxygen treatment may be necessary in very young children; steam inhalation may also help to relieve symptoms. A cough suppressant may control the dry cough. Antibiotics are often prescribed, but are indicated only in the minority of cases where the infection is bacterial. Acute laryngitis commonly resolves spontaneously within a few days.

Chronic laryngitis most often results from overuse or abuse of the voice and is common in preachers, actors, politicians, and singers; it is aggravated by smoking. Treatment is absolute rest of the voice for a few days. Rarely, chronic laryngitis may be due to infection with tuberculosis, and the symptoms may also be due to a tumor on the vocal cords. Anyone with persistent change or weakness of the voice should be seen by a doctor.

LARYNX

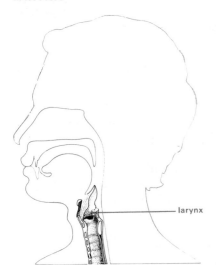

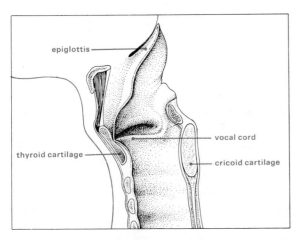

The larynx is the "voice box" in the throat. It is an arrangement of cartilages connected by ligaments and muscles. Movements of the cartilages set the tension in the vocal cords, and this determines the pitch of the voice.

lead poisoning

Usually symptoms are due to chronic poisoning, since lead acts as a cumulative poison. Because lead is not readily excreted in the urine or feces, anyone who regularly absorbs even traces of the metal slowly builds up the lead content of the body. Water running through lead pipes can absorb enough of the metal over time to cause problems. In areas of antiquated housing, where lead-containing paints may still cover walls, children sometimes swallow flaking paint. Poisoning has resulted from the use of lead-glazed pottery to store wine or cider. Pollution from industrial plants such as smelters may cause lead poisoning in the surrounding communities.

In adults, lead poisoning may cause crampy abdominal pains, discoloration of the gums, and damage to the nerves leading to muscle weakness.

In children, lead poisoning may cause mental irritability and mental retardation.

Once suspected, lead poisoning is diagnosed by laboratory tests of the blood. Treatment, apart from prevention of further exposure, consists of removing the lead from the body by chelating agents—drugs that become chemically bound to the lead to form compounds that are readily excreted in the urine.

left ventricular failure (LVF)

Failure of the left ventricle (left lower chamber) of the heart to pump blood adequately for the needs of the body.

Left ventricular failure is caused most commonly by coronary artery disease, hypertension (high blood pressure), or disease of the heart valves.

The major symptom is breathlessness due to the pooling of blood and fluid in the lungs. At first the person is short of breath only on exertion, but the condition gradually worsens. Shortness of breath is often most acute when the person is lying down; sudden and terrifying episodes of breathlessness may occur during sleep. The victim may feel the need to sit or stand to catch his breath.

Acute or *severe LVF* requires urgent treatment with drugs that make the heart beat slower and more effectively and with diuretics to get rid of excess body fluid. The individual should sit up and receive oxygen. Other drugs are sometimes needed.

Chronic LVF requires treatment with the same drugs and an adjustment of the person's life-style to suit his condition; control of hypertension is particularly important. Diseased heart valves and blocked coronary arteries may require surgical treatment.

If left untreated, both acute and chronic LVF may lead to the point when a person's lungs become so full of fluid that he no longer can breathe adequately and may lapse into a coma from lack of oxygen.

Effective treatment of hypertension has reduced the frequency of LVF, and heart-valve disease associated with previous rheumatic fever is becoming far less common. Coronary artery disease, however, is all too common and is now the major cause of LVF in the Western world.

legionnaire's disease

An acute bacterial infectious disease usually producing a form of PNEUMONIA. Legionnaire's disease is characterized by an influenza-like illness followed by high fever, chills, muscle aches, headaches, and diarrhea approximately one week later. The illness is usually self-limiting but deaths do occur.

The diagnosis is made by finding the organism in specimens of sputum, lung biopsy, or from the pleural fluid or by detecting antibodies to legionnaire's agent in the blood.

Contaminated air-conditioning cooling towers and moist soil may be a source of organisms. Treatment includes supportive care such as bed rest, fluids, antibiotics, and medication to lower fever.

lens

Any device that causes a beam of light to converge or diverge as it passes through.

The lens of the eye (*crystalline lens*) consists of elongated fibers enclosed in a transparent elastic capsule, suspended by a ligament behind the iris. The ligament is attached to the circular ciliary muscle. Contraction and relaxation of the muscles change the shape of the lens, altering its focusing power; this is the mechanism that allows us to make a sharp image of objects at variable distances from the eye.

The lens becomes stiffer with age and the range of focusing decreases. Most people over the age of 45 need glasses for reading to compensate for this. The lens normally becomes slightly opaque from the age of 60 onward, but impaired vision due to opacity of the lens (CATARACT) may occur at any age.

A penetrating injury of the lens can cause opacity. The lens also may be dislocated from its ligament by external injury to the eye.

Artificial lenses made of glass or plastic are the chief component in glasses and contact lenses. They compensate for the inadequacies in the focusing ability of the lens of the eye (*presbyopia*),

for an uneven curvature of the cornea or lens (*astigmatism*), or for long or short sight caused by abnormalities in the shape of the eyeball.

leprosy

A chronic but only mildly contagious disease caused by infection with bacteria of the species *Mycobacterium leprae*. Also known as Hansen's disease.

Leprosy occurs mainly in countries between the 30th parallels of latitude, but also in Japan, Korea, South China, and South Africa. In the United States the disease occurs mainly in those states bordering the Gulf of Mexico and Hawaii.

Leprosy damages the cooler tissues of the body: skin, superficial nerves, nose, pharynx, larynx, and occasionally the eyes and testicles.

There are two main types of leprosy: lepromatous and tuberculoid.

In *lepromatous leprosy* the victim's resistance to infection is low. Many red painful swellings appear on the skin of the face and elsewhere. These swellings harden and coalesce, causing the great disfigurement that has been feared and loathed since Biblical times. The victim has chronic ill health; he rarely dies from leprosy itself, but death from a secondary infection is common.

In *tuberculoid leprosy* the victim's resistance to infection remains high; his main reaction to the disease occurs in nerves, marked by numbness, tingling, and loss of sensation in the areas these nerves supply. Deformities such as wrist-drop, foot-drop, or claw-toes may result; these areas may be painlessly damaged, with ulceration and even the gradual disappearance of the ends of fingers and toes.

Tuberculoid leprosy is not contagious; even lepromatous sufferers are infectious only to those with whom they are in prolonged intimate contact. Contrary to popular belief, isolation of the diseased is unnecessary. The medical emphasis now is on early detection and treatment.

Leprosy usually is treated with medication. Tuberculoid leprosy responds well, but lepromatous leprosy is not so predictable. Surgery sometimes is needed to correct deformities.

leukemia

A progressive malignant disease (or cancer) of the white cells in the circulating blood and in the bone marrow. Proliferation of the cancerous cells crowds out the normal healthy white and red blood cells and blood platelets, causing ANEMIA and bleeding disorders and lowering the natural defenses against infection.

Leukemia is still relatively rare, but it has become somewhat less so over the past fifty years. Its causes are poorly understood. Exposure to ionizing radiation increases its incidence, but this cannot account for all cases. Viruses can cause leukemia in some animals, and a virus has been linked to some T cell leukemias in humans.

Leukemia is classified as *acute* (short course) or *chronic* (long course), as well as by the type of cells involved: *myeloid, lymphoid* (or *lymphatic*), and *monocytic.*

Acute leukemia occurs most commonly in children and, at any age, is commoner in males than females. Usually the onset of the disease is sudden, with fever, sore throat, and often bleeding from the nose or mouth; it quickly becomes apparent that the person is very ill. Examination of the blood and a bone marrow biopsy confirm the diagnosis.

Without treatment death usually occurs within a few days or weeks in all types of acute leukemia. Steady progress in treatment has occurred over the past twenty years, however; a remission of the disease can now be induced in most persons, especially in children, by a combination of anticancer drugs and radiation therapy.

Many persons relapse after a period of remission, but further treatment may then be effective. Some persons may be permanently cured by modern treatment, and in the most common leukemia of childhood, *acute lymphoblastic leukemia,* the cure rate is now approaching 50 percent of all cases.

Chronic myeloid leukemia (*CML*) comes on much more gradually than acute leukemia. Symptoms include tiredness caused by anemia and abdominal discomfort associated with massive enlargement of the spleen. Diagnosis again is confirmed from the results of blood tests and a biopsy of the bone marrow. Treatment is with drugs. Persons with CML may survive for several years, but despite treatment the disease often leads to fatal acute leukemia. Bone marrow transplantation, during the early stages, can probably be curative.

Chronic lymphatic leukemia (*CLL*) occurs particularly in men of late middle age. Symptoms are similar to those of CML, but the spleen is not as large and there is a general enlargement of the lymph nodes. Treatment is with drugs, and persons often survive in reasonable health for several years; a few persons have lived for twenty years or more from the time the disease was first diagnosed and treatment begun.

leukoderma

A patchy deficiency of pigmentation of the skin, the patches often being milk-white. Leukoderma is another name for VITILIGO.

leukodystrophy

A group of disorders characterized by progressive degeneration of the white matter of the brain. These disorders are due to an inborn metabolic error, with a breakdown in the enzyme systems concerned with the metabolism of lipids (fats or fat-like substances) in the nerve cells.

There is progressive destruction of the protective and insulating myelin sheaths of the nerve fibers, which usually begins in the back part of the brain and spreads throughout the white matter of the cerebral hemispheres.

Some forms of leukodystrophy begin in early childhood; there are also late childhood forms, which usually confine the child to a wheelchair in adolescence.

The symptoms include paralysis, generalized fits, speech difficulties, disorganization of movement, and mental deterioration. There is no known treatment.

leukoplakia

A localized patch of abnormal thickening and whitening on the tongue, the lining of the mouth, the lips, or the genital area. Affected areas may be yellowish white and leathery. The lesions may be precancerous. By the time pain is present, there is usually an advanced lesion.

Leukoplakia may result from chronic irritation in the mouth caused by tobacco, highly seasoned food, alcoholic drinks, excessive heat, trauma, jagged teeth, or dentures.

The first step in treatment is to remove the cause of the irritation. Good oral hygiene must be established.

Early, thin leukoplakia that fails to respond to conservative measures should be removed completely after a biopsy has been performed. Larger lesions may require more than one operation for surgical removal. Regular reexamination of treated areas is advisable in case there is a serious recurrence.

Leukoplakia can also occur in the vulvar or vaginal area in women or on the penis in men.

leukorrhea

An abnormal whitish discharge from the vagina, which may occur at any age. It affects most women at some time in their lives.

The amount of normal vaginal secretion varies among women and in the same woman during the menstrual cycle. Excess mucus production may occur normally as a result of sexual and emotional stimulation, at the time of ovulation, and during pregnancy. Secretions are greater just before and after menstruation.

In leukorrhea, the abnormal vaginal discharge may just be excessive or it may be purulent (pus-filled) as the result of an infection by *Trichomonas vaginalis* (a protozoan), *Candida albicans* (see THRUSH), or *Gardnerella vaginalis*, which causes a "fishy" odor, worse after washing with soap. A purulent discharge may be due also to disease of the cervix or uterus, to senile VAGINITIS, or to the presence of foreign objects.

Any prolonged or foul-smelling discharge needs to be attended to by a physician. Treatment depends on the cause; many medications, in cream and suppository form, are available by prescription. Genital hygiene is important, but douching is more likely to treat the symptoms rather than the cause and is therefore of limited value.

libido

A drive usually associated with the sexual instinct—that is, for pleasure, and the seeking out of a love object. In Jung's original sense of the term, the energy designated "libido" was of a general kind and applied to any instinctive force.

Freud maintained that in early life the individual obtains instinctive satisfaction largely from his or her own body. As development proceeds, the person obtains instinctive satisfaction increasingly from without, and the libido becomes directed toward external objects.

According to Freudian theory, the infant's oral and anal cravings give rise to guilt feelings. In the ensuing so-called phallic stage, satisfaction is concerned with the genital zone. In the final stage, the person may attain complete "object-love."

lice

Three kinds of lice affect humans; infestation with lice is known as *pediculosis*. The louse itself is a small wingless flattened insect.

Pediculosis capitis, head louse infestation, affects the scalp, although sometimes it involves the eyebrows, eyelashes, and beard; it is particularly common in children. The lice feed on blood from the scalp, having infested it by direct contact with hair and with items such as combs, towels, and headgear. The bites cause severe persistent itching and the lesions may become infected. The glands of the neck may sometimes enlarge.

Adult lice may be noticed around the back of the head and behind the ears. The small ovoid eggs, or nits, are easier to detect, being firmly attached to hair shafts. These hatch in three to fourteen days unless removed with a nit comb. In addition to combing, the scalp should be treated with benzyl benzoate or gamma benzene hexachloride (GBH). Members of the same household also should be examined for infestation.

Pediculosis corporis, body louse infestation, occurs when lice inhabit the seams of clothing worn next to the skin and feed on the skin. Under good hygienic conditions it is uncommon. The bites of the lice appear as small red marks, and itching may lead to severe scratch marks with secondary bacterial infection. Lesions are especially common on the shoulders, buttocks, and abdomen. Both the parasites and nits show up readily in clothing.

Laundering and hot ironing of seams will kill the lice. The skin should be rubbed with GBH. Lotions may soothe inflammation.

Nits remain viable in clothing for as long as one month, hatching when they are reexposed to body heat. Dissemination of lice occurs through contact with infected persons, clothing, or bedding.

Pediculosis pubis is crab louse infestation of the area of the genitals and anus and sometimes other hair regions. Infestation may be venereal or acquired from clothing, bedclothes, or toilet seats. Severe irritation, with scratch marks, occurs. Application of benzyl benzoate or GBH is an effective treatment. Prolonged use of such chemicals should be avoided, however.

Lice are known to transmit typhus fever, re-

HUMAN LOUSE

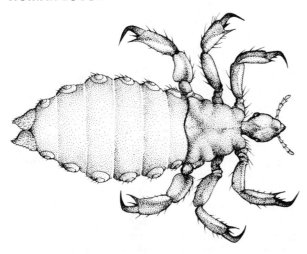

Human lice are small, wingless insects that spend their whole existence on man. They lay their eggs on hair and spread from person to person by direct contact. The species of louse pictured above lives in hair and underwear and causes itching. More important, it transmits the microorganism that causes typhus.

lapsing fever, and trench fever, but these infections are rare.

lichen planus

A fairly common benign inflammatory disease of the skin and the lining of the mouth, which often gives rise to itching. There are small discrete raised areas of skin which at times coalesce into rough scaly patches. The raised areas are angular and have a flat shiny surface of pink or violet hue.

Certain drugs may produce an identical eruption. The initial attack persists for weeks or months and may recur intermittently. Children rarely are affected.

The condition typically affects the wrists, arms, legs, and trunk, but is rarely seen on the face. Occasionally the lesions are widespread.

The cause of the disease is unknown. Sedation may be necessary in severe cases, but usually all that is required is the application of a soothing lotion or hydrocortisone ointment.

lipoma

A soft, round swelling or tumor composed of fat cells, occurring in the skin. The fat tissue is en-

closed in a fibrous capsule. Usually solitary, but sometimes multiple, lipomas vary in size from minute growths to huge masses weighing several pounds.

They may occur from early age to advanced age, but from 40 to 50 percent appear between the ages of 30 and 40, when the body begins to accumulate excess fat, at which time the incidence of these benign tumors is about twice as high in women as in men. In some cases they are associated with endocrine and neurological disturbances.

Lipomas occur typically on the neck, back, shoulders, and abdominal wall; they occur only rarely on the face, scalp, hands, and feet. As a rule such lumps cause few symptoms, but in areas such as the inner surface of the thighs they may form pendulous masses.

Lipomas may be associated also with muscles or with the larger joints. Internal lipomas—on the intestine, for instance—are relatively uncommon. Malignant change is rare.

Since lipomas do not infiltrate adjacent areas, surgical removal is usually a simple procedure.

liposarcoma

An extremely uncommon malignant tumor composed of fat cells. They arise primarily in deeper structures, especially in the thigh, leg, and buttock. Liposarcomas rarely arise from lipomas.

Beginning as inconspicuous swellings, they usually attain an appreciable size before they are diagnosed and treated. Treatment involves surgery.

liver disease

To understand the consequences of liver disease, it is first necessary to appreciate some of the normal functions of the organ. They may be considered under three main headings: blood, metabolism, and detoxification—the removal of drugs and toxic substances.

Blood. Red blood cells stay in circulation for 120 days on average and are then removed by the spleen and other tissues. Most of the HEMOGLOBIN from these cells is converted into bilirubin, which is then transported to the liver. Enzymes in the liver cells modify the chemical structure of bilirubin to make it soluble in water—a process called "conjugation." The conjugated bilirubin is se-

THE LIVER

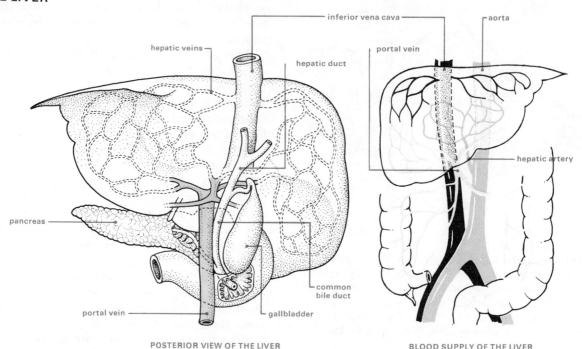

POSTERIOR VIEW OF THE LIVER   BLOOD SUPPLY OF THE LIVER

The liver develops in the embryo as an outgrowth of the intestine and always retains a close link with the digestive system. The portal vein drains blood from the intestine into the liver, where nutrients are utilized and toxic products removed. The liver also secretes bile which is then stored in the gallbladder; after a meal, the gallbladder contracts, squeezing bile into the duodenum where it helps in the digestion of fats.

creted into the bile ducts and eventually passes to the intestines. Here bacteria convert the bilirubin into a number of pigments that form the coloring matter of feces.

The total level of bilirubin in the blood does not normally exceed 10 milligrams per liter; if this concentration doubles for any reason, bilirubin is deposited in the skin and whites of the eyes to produce the characteristic yellow appearance of JAUNDICE. There are numerous causes of jaundice and they do not all originate in the liver itself. *Gilbert's disease* is a common harmless condition that runs in families and is marked by a mild, fluctuating jaundice due to inefficient transportation of bilirubin into the liver cells. Jaundice is found almost universally in newborn babies because their conjugating enzymes are limited in capacity.

HEPATITIS, inflammation of the liver due to viruses, alcohol, or drugs, reduces the number of functioning liver cells and blocks the bile ducts as a consequence of tissue swelling.

The other functions of the liver concerned with blood are the manufacture of plasma proteins

(particularly albumin) and factors necessary for blood clotting. Both these processes fail in chronic liver diseases such as CIRRHOSIS, when large numbers of cells have been destroyed. The major consequences of these failures are easy bruising and ASCITES (collection of free fluid in the abdominal cavity).

Metabolism. The portal vein carries nutrients from their sites of absorption in the small intestine to the liver, where they are extensively processed according to the body's needs. Carbohydrates and other foods are converted into glycogen by the liver. Glycogen is stored in many body cells and can be broken down into glucose (sugar) when energy is needed. Blood glucose levels can be significantly altered in the presence of severe liver disease. If the liver fails to process and eliminate the by-products of protein breakdown, the buildup of ammonia and amino acids can damage the brain and is an important cause of COMA.

Cirrhosis not only leads to the death of many liver cells but also distorts the "architecture" of the organ, blocking the blood flow through it. This leads to back-pressure down the portal vein—*portal hypertension*—and the blood is forced to take alternative routes. The easiest but potentially most dangerous alternative route is through the veins around the esophagus ("gullet"). These become dilated and eventually may burst, leading to massive vomiting of blood (HEMATEMESIS). Drastic measures then have to be taken, and if the victim survives there is a great risk of brain damage.

Detoxification. The final major role of the liver is the removal of drugs and toxic substances from the blood. As mentioned above, some toxins (for example, ammonia) are derived from proteins in the diet. The liver deals with many drugs in the way it does with bilirubin: It conjugates them into water-soluble substances that can be excreted in the urine or feces. In persons with liver disease, drug therapy presents major problems, and common drugs like diuretics (given to reduce fluid load in ascites) can precipitate coma. Diets must be strictly controlled, with protein and fluid restrictions and limited amounts of salty foods.

Primary cancer of the liver, HEPATOMA, is the most common cancer in Africa and the Orient, but accounts for only about 2 percent of all cancers in the United States. On the other hand, secondary cancer, which has spread from elsewhere in the body, is very common.

lumbago

The popular name for a condition marked by acute and severe pain in the lower part of the back for which no definite cause can be found. Treatment includes bed rest (on a hard mattress), analgesics (pain-killers, such as aspirin), and the local application of heat.

lupus erythematosus

A chronic skin disease, thought to be associated with an immunological disturbance, that manifests itself in two ways: One is confined to the mucous membranes and the skin, the other is a systemic disorder that may affect the skin. Many medical experts believe that lupus occurs in persons with a genetic predisposition to the disease after they have contracted a viral infection. Many more women than men develop this disease.

There are two types of lupus. *Discoid lupus erythematosus* is a relatively mild condition, characterized by a red patch on the face—or on other areas exposed to the sun—which slowly spreads to become a well-defined disk covered by gray scales. As the lesion spreads, the center atrophies and, as it scars, small vessels become prominent (TELANGIECTASIS). Individuals need to be cautious of sun exposure and use sunscreens. Some of these individuals will go on to develop the second type of lupus—*systemic lupus erythematosus (SLE)*.

SLE is a progressive and potentially serious disease, classed among the COLLAGEN DISEASES. It can affect nearly every organ in the body. Among the possible complications are pleurisy, kidney lesions, disorders of the central nervous system, and inflammation of the membrane lining the heart and of the smooth membranous sac enveloping the heart.

There is no cure for SLE but there are drugs available to control it. Among these are antimalarial medications and steroids. These drugs do have some major side effects, however, and all persons need to be under close medical supervision.

lupus vulgaris

Tuberculosis of the skin. It is a slowly developing disease, fortunately now rare. When it does occur it often affects the face or neck. The tubercle bacillus—the responsible bacterium—may invade the skin directly or spread to it from underlying infected glands or joints or (via the lymphatic system) from a respiratory tract infection. It is more common in women than in men.

The shape of the lesion is always irregular and the surface may be covered with a crust. Eventually the lesion may ulcerate. The mucous membranes of the nose and mouth frequently are affected, and in these cases the ultimate effect (if the condition is left untreated) is serious deformity with tissue loss and scarring. The tongue when attacked has large painful fissures.

Antituberculosis drugs may have to be continued for many months.

Lyme disease

A disorder new to the textbooks and named for Lyme, Connecticut, where a group of cases occurred in the small community in 1975. It is caused by a previously unknown *spirochete* (spiral-shaped organism) transmitted by ticks. The disease now has been reported in half the states in the U.S. Most patients are children and young adults living in wooded areas.

The disease begins as a small, slightly raised, red spot at the site of the bite, which enlarges, as the spirochetes move outward, to form a circle well over a foot in diameter, often with a clear center. This persists for several weeks, and the affected person feels feverish and experiences tiredness, headache, stiff neck, and aches in the joints and muscles.

Some weeks to months later, in about 50 percent of cases, the disease begins to affect some of the large joints, usually the knees, causing pain, redness, severe swelling, and stiffness. These episodes of joint swelling tend to recur, and in some cases the arthritis lasts for up to six months at a time. The spirochetes, which have, by now, spread throughout the body, produce these effects by exciting a strong immunologic reaction with high levels of *antibodies* and circulating immune complexes.

Fortunately, the spirochetes are sensitive to antibiotics, such as tetracycline, penicillin and erythromycin, and the results of treatment are good, especially if given early. Antibiotics are effective in about half the cases with established joint involvement.

lymphadenitis

See ADENITIS.

lymphangitis

Inflammation of a vessel in the LYMPHATIC SYSTEM.

It is caused by the spread of infection to the lymphatic vessels, causing prominent red streaks under the skin. Inflamed vessels may throb painfully; in many cases the person also has a fever and chills. The infection can spread rapidly. Antibiotics are given to avoid the possibility of SEPTICEMIA.

lymphatic system

The vast network of vessels throughout the body (similar to the blood vessels) that transports a watery fluid known as *lymph.*

Lymph is formed from the clear fluid that bathes all tissues of the body, largely by filtration from the blood capillaries. It also carries cells— LYMPHOCYTES—and other substances concerned with the IMMUNE SYSTEM.

Tiny lymphatic vessels are found in all organs except the heart and brain. Protein, bacteria, and other foreign particles enter the lymphatics, which unite to form larger vessels. Like veins, lymphatic vessels have valves to prevent a backflow of fluid. If for any reason a lymphatic vessel becomes obstructed, the buildup of lymph is called LYMPHEDEMA.

Eventually all the lymphatics drain their contents into two large ducts; from there the lymph reenters the blood circulation through veins at the base of the neck.

Lymphatics draining the small intestine (known as *lacteals*) have a function apart from clearing debris and defending the body: Fat is absorbed from the small intestine into the lacteals and so eventually into the bloodstream.

The lymphatic system is interrupted at intervals by groups of *lymph nodes*—often incorrectly called lymph *glands*—which have two main functions: (1) They have a role in immunity, producing both lymphocytes (defensive white blood cells) and antibodies; and (2) they also act as a second line of defense against infection by bacteria, filtering off and destroying any that bypass the inflammatory response at the site of infection. In the case of cancer cells, the lymph nodes act as a temporary but only partially effective barrier to metastasis (spread of cancer cells from one site to another).

When a lymph node is stimulated into activity—for example, by infection—it swells and becomes painful. This swelling may be noticeable even before the infection itself is apparent (swelling of the "glands" in the neck during a throat infection is a common experience).

Apart from those in the back and sides of the neck, the main groups of lymph nodes are in the armpits and groin; either of these groups may be felt as swollen and painful during a limb infection. Other lymph nodes lie at the base of the lungs and around large veins in the abdomen and pelvis.

The tonsils and spleen are composed of lymphatic tissue and usually are regarded as part of the lymphatic system.

The lymphatic system (shown right) is a network of vessels that drain most of the body's tissues and return excess fluid from between the cells back to the bloodstream. During this journey the lymph fluid filters through lymph nodes, where any foreign particles such as bacteria will be trapped.

THE LYMPHATIC SYSTEM

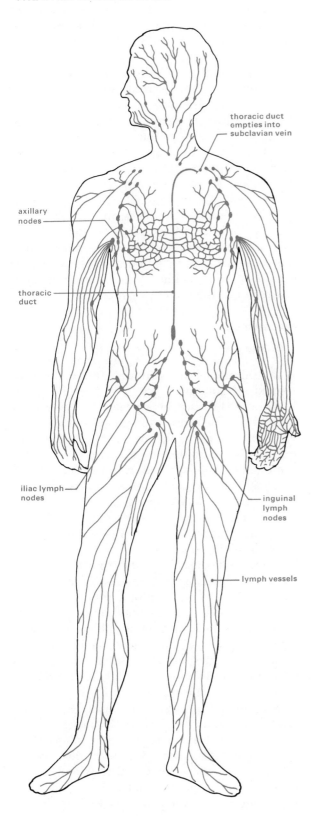

thoracic duct
empties into
subclavian vein

axillary
nodes

thoracic
duct

iliac lymph
nodes

inguinal
lymph
nodes

lymph vessels

lymphedema

Throughout the body there is a vast network of tiny vessels (the LYMPHATIC SYSTEM) that transport a watery fluid known as *lymph*. These vessels can become blocked in certain areas of the body. When this occurs in a limb, the entire extremity can swell.

Although there are a number of possible causes of lymphedema, in the United States population it occurs most often as a consequence of surgery and radiation therapy involving the armpits and groin.

See also ELEPHANTIASIS.

lymphocyte

A type of white blood cell, comprising between 20 and 50 percent of white blood cells in an adult. Lymphocytes are produced in the lymphoid tissues of the body (see LYMPHATIC SYSTEM). They play an important role in immunity by recognizing and producing antibodies against "foreign" substances. The so-called B lymphocytes produce antibodies that are released into the bloodstream. The T lymphocytes, on the other hand, carry antibodies on their own surface and produce cellular immunity—for example, in the rejection of organ transplants. The AIDS virus (HIV) attacks certain kinds of T lymphocytes—the helper T cells—and this leads to severe immune deficiency.

In persons with chronic infections, large numbers of lymphocytes are present both in the blood and at the site of the infection. There may also be excessive numbers of these white cells in LEUKEMIA, but in such cases immunity is depressed because the lymphocytes are abnormal.

lymphogranuloma venereum

A sexually transmitted disease caused by virus-like organisms of the genus *Chlamydia*. It is uncommon in North America.

After infection, through sexual contact, there is an incubation period of five to twenty-eight days. A blister then forms on the genital area, often unnoticed. It disappears and the infection spreads to the lymph nodes, which enlarge, soften, and eventually break down. In women and in homosexual men the rectum may become inflamed. Fistulas (abnormal openings) may form and the rectum and the anus may be permanently narrowed.

Elsewhere in the body the infection leads to fever, joint pains, skin eruptions, and conjunctivitis.

Early treatment with an appropriate antibiotic (usually tetracycline) cures the condition and prevents the later complications. Pain over the enlarged lymph nodes can be relieved by hot compresses and analgesics.

lymphoma

A group of malignant diseases of the lymphoid tissue of the body. These include HODGKIN'S DISEASE and non-Hodgkin's lymphoma. There are several types, of varying degrees of malignancy, which can be distinguished by microscopic examination of a sample of tissue.

There are about 8,000 new cases of non-Hodgkin's lymphomas each year in the United States, and about the same number of new cases of Hodgkin's disease.

The usual symptoms include persistent lymph-node swelling, weight loss, and sometimes fever.

The type of treatment depends on the appearance of the lymphoma under the microscope as well as the extent of the spread of the lymphoma.

Treatment can involve either radiotherapy or chemotherapy, or a combination of both. In most cases of Hodgkin's disease and about 50 percent of non-Hodgkin's lymphoma, treatment can result in a cure.

malabsorption

A term applied to a number of conditions in which normal absorption of nutrients is impaired. Malabsorption causes disturbed intestinal function and disorders of the body due to deficiencies of substances necessary for health.

The body's failure to absorb fat from the intestine produces offensive pale stools that are larger than normal and tend to float in water; sometimes there is diarrhea with colic, sometimes constipation. If the malady involves failure to absorb carbohydrates, the abdomen becomes enlarged and uncomfortable and there is a frothy diarrhea. Various deficiencies may show themselves. In children and infants there is failure to thrive and perhaps loss of weight.

Persons suffering from malabsorption are weak and may be anemic. Vitamin deficiencies may lead to RICKETS, TETANY, a low level of calcium in the blood, dry skin and sparse hair, sore mouth and tongue, and various neurological signs. If there is a loss of water and salts, there may be a low blood pressure, cramps, thirst, weakness, and abnormalities of sensation.

Malabsorption occurs in many conditions, ranging from diseases that block the lymphatic vessels draining the intestine to the operative removal of parts of the intestine or stomach. The best-known causes, however, are CELIAC DISEASE, TROPICAL SPRUE, CROHN'S DISEASE, LIVER DISEASE, chronic ENTERITIS, infestation by worms, and atrophy (wasting away) of the stomach that leads to pernicious ANEMIA. Diseases of the gallbladder and pancreas may produce malabsorption syndromes, as may the effects of radiation. In each case, treatment is directed at the underlying disease.

malaria

A parasitic infection occurring mainly in the tropics and subtropics.

Malaria is caused by a protozoan parasite of the genus *Plasmodium*, which requires two different hosts during its life cycle: human and mosquito. It is transmitted from person to person by the bite of an infected *Anopheles* mosquito. The mosquito sucks blood from an infected person, taking in the parasite which can then continue its life cycle within the mosquito. Later, when the mosquito bites another human, the parasites enter with the insect's saliva.

Once inside the human, the parasites continue to develop in the liver. From there they reenter the bloodstream and multiply inside red blood cells, causing them to rupture within two or three days. This rupture of the red cells is responsible for the characteristic chills, fever, and sweating of malaria. Parasites released into the bloodstream when the cells rupture can enter other red cells, and the life cycle is repeated.

Four species of *Plasmodium* cause human malaria. Three of them (*P. vivax*, *P. falciparum*, and *P. ovale*) repeat the cycle every forty-eight hours and produce symptoms every third day (tertian malaria); *P. malariae* repeats the cycle every seventy-two hours (quartan malaria).

Among other consequences of the parasitic infestation and rupture of blood cells are ANEMIA, JAUNDICE, enlarged spleen, obstruction of small

MALARIA

LIFE HISTORY OF *Plasmodium* PARASITE

A female Anopheles *mosquito (1) injects* Plasmodium *parasites into a human (2); they develop in the liver (3) before reproducing asexually inside red blood cells (4). These cells periodically burst, releasing parasites that attack more red cells, causing fever (5). Some red cells become filled with sexual forms of* Plasmodium *(6), which reproduce in the stomach of a mosquito (7) after it has sucked blood from the man. Infective forms then migrate to the mosquito's salivary glands (8), ready to enter the next victim when the mosquito bites.*

blood vessels in the brain, and kidney failure.

Quinine was the classic antimalarial drug, but it has been largely superseded by less toxic drugs such as chloroquine and primaquine. Other drugs can protect against malaria if taken for two weeks before the person enters a malarious area and for a month after he leaves it. The inhabitants of malarious regions have to take regular doses of drugs to protect themselves against infection.

At a public health level, eradication of malaria is best attempted by attacking the mosquito in order to break the life cycle of the parasites. Partial success has been achieved by draining swamps and other breeding places and by the use of special insecticides (unfortunately, mosquitoes tend to develop resistance to these chemical agents). Despite prolonged efforts by the World Health Organization, malaria is still a major public health problem in Africa and Asia.

Malaria may be seen in temperate areas, since it can develop in travelers after their return from the tropics. Symptoms may be delayed for weeks or even months. The parasite can also be transmitted directly from human to human by the transfusion of contaminated blood. A history of malaria may disqualify a person as a blood donor.

malnutrition

Any nutritional disorder resulting from an unbalanced diet, too much or too little food, or improper use of food by the body.

Causes of malnutrition include poverty, fam-

ine, natural disasters, diseases such as malabsorption syndrome, neurological deficits affecting the ability to swallow or feed oneself, and psychological disorders such as ANOREXIA NERVOSA.

Provided there is an adequate supply of drinking water, a healthy adult can go without food for approximately two weeks with little effect other than weight loss. The effects of prolonged undernutrition include swelling of tissues (most obvious in the legs and abdomen); weight loss; lowering of blood pressure, pulse, and temperature; diarrhea; anemia; apathy; and emotional instability.

mania

A disordered mental state characterized by a mood change to excitement and elation. Often the mood swings between mania and depression—the *manic-depressive psychosis*.

The sufferer becomes optimistic and overconfident and has a general feeling of euphoria. He becomes talkative yet changes subjects frequently and is easily distracted. He has little insight into his condition and rarely will admit that he is unwell.

The manic person often gets into difficulties—by overspending, for example, or making rash promises or unwise business deals, or becoming violent when thwarted.

The severity of the mania varies widely; in mild cases it is necessary to have an idea of the person's previous personality to be sure of the diagnosis.

Mild mania is known as *hypomania* and severe mania as *acute mania.* In acute mania mental activity may be so "high" that the person's speech is incoherent and his constant restlessness and failure to sleep can lead to total exhaustion. Acute mania is a medical emergency.

The outlook for persons with recurrent attacks of mania (with or without depression) has been transformed by the discovery that regular treatment with *lithium salts* can prevent or reduce the severity of the episodes. The dose has to be carefully adjusted to avoid toxic side effects (tremor, mental confusion, and eventually coma); regular measurement of the blood content of lithium is an essential part of treatment. Major tranquilizers may also be indicated for treatment.

mastitis

Inflammation of the breast.

Its most important manifestations occur in lactating (milk-producing) women. In one type, the woman may have a raised temperature and congested, painful breasts; there is no pus present and the inflammation is hormonal rather than infective in origin.

By contrast, in *acute suppurative mastitis* the breast becomes infected with *Staphylococcus aureus* or (less frequently) *Streptococcus pyogenes.* The bacteria gain access to the breast either via the ducts or through a crack in the nipple. If appropriate antibiotic treatment is not begun, an abscess may form, resulting in considerable pain and possibly scarring of the breast.

Chronic mastitis describes certain hyperplastic and cystic conditions of the breast. The condition is extremely common and is caused by an imbalance in the hormonal cycle associated with menstruation. As a result the breast tissue feels more nodular than usual and may be tender. Inflammation plays no part in the cause and the major pathological changes are of fibrosis, cystic change, and an increase in the number and size of fatty lobules in the breast. It usually occurs in older women still in their child-bearing years.

mastoiditis

Infection of one of the mastoid bones, usually a complication of a middle-ear infection. It is marked by earache, fever, headache, and pain.

Prompt treatment of middle-ear infections with antibiotics usually is effective in preventing this once common complication, but surgery (*mastoidectomy*) may be required if infection becomes established in the bone itself.

masturbation

The practice of sexual self-stimulation, masturbation is a normal and natural activity. Contrary to old wives' tales, it will not cause madness, blindness, pimples, warts, or any other physical problems.

Many studies have shown that most Americans—regardless of age, sex, or marital status—masturbate. It is a means of giving oneself pleasure and releasing sexual tension.

If a child tends to fondle his or her genitals in public, you should explain to him or her that masturbation, although normal, is a private activity that should be restricted to an appropriate time or place. Scolding or punishment will result in unnecessary guilt that can lead to emotional problems.

While it will not cause physical disorders, excessive masturbation may be a symptom of emotional stress or feelings of inadequacy. In such cases, professional counseling may be needed for the underlying psychological problem.

measles

A highly contagious viral disease (also known as *morbilli* and *rubeola*), common in childhood.

Before the introduction of active immunization, measles epidemics used to occur every two or three years. In affluent countries the illness mainly involves children aged 3 to 5 years and is usually mild; in underdeveloped countries, where nutrition is poor, children under 2 years predominantly are affected and there is a high mortality rate.

The measles virus is extremely small. Infected individuals shed the measles virus in droplet secretions from the nose, mouth, or throat for four to five days before their skin rash appears and for three to five days after the rash disappears; throughout this time they can pass the infection to susceptible people.

The incubation period from exposure to the onset of symptoms is usually ten to fourteen days. The first symptoms are a fever, cough, runny nose, red and watery eyes, and general irritability. During the period just before the rash appears it may be possible to notice what are known as *Koplik's spots*, which resemble coarse grains of salt on a red background; these often appear on the mucous membranes of the mouth opposite the molars.

The rash first emerges behind the ears and along the hairline and quickly involves the whole face. It then travels downward to reach the feet on about the third day. Initially the rash consists of dusky red spots, but these coalesce to form irregular blotches. After three days the rash begins to fade, the fever subsides, and the individual's condition rapidly improves.

Complications do occur and mainly involve the respiratory and central nervous systems. Secondary infection with bacteria leading to bronchitis or ear infection is relatively common, and should be suspected if fever persists; it is treated with antibiotics. More seriously, one in 1,000 cases develops a postinfectious encephalitis (inflammation of the brain) three to four days after the onset of the rash. Its symptoms can vary from transient drowsiness to coma and death.

Immunity against measles can be induced by giving a live attenuated virus vaccine by injection. This vaccine is effective about 95 percent of the time, unless the patient already is infected with the virus. Immunity to the disease, both from an attack and from vaccine, is lifelong.

melanoma

Malignant tumors of pigment cells (*melanocytes*). These cells are most plentiful in the skin, but they do exist in other tissues as well, and malignant melanomas occasionally arise in these sites.

Pigment cells in the skin can form *nevi* (moles), but melanocytes are distributed throughout the skin even where no moles or freckles exist.

Melanomas can arise either at the site of preexisting moles (pigmented nevi) or at apparently unblemished sites in the skin. Although malignant transformation in a mole is very rare (one in 1 million), any changes in shape, size, or pigmentation, or the appearance of itching, ulceration, or bleeding in a dark spot should arouse strong suspicion.

Early diagnosis and treatment of a malignant melanoma is vital because it spreads cancer cells to other sites and can be fatal. Malignant melanoma is responsible for about 2 percent of all cancer deaths in the United States, and nearly all affected persons are over 30 years old. Factors thought to predispose to malignant melanoma are excess exposure to sunlight in fair-skinned persons, X-ray exposure, and contact with tar.

A definite diagnosis can be made only after examining a specimen of tissue microscopically. Surgery remains the most effective treatment for the early localized lesion.

For an extended discussion see "Sun, Skin and Cancer" in Chapter 18 in the section on **Wellness**.

melena

The passage of black, tarry stools, indicative of bleeding from the upper gastrointestinal tract. It may occur independently of or in conjunction with HEMATEMESIS (vomiting of blood). The altered color of the blood in melena is due to the action of gastric juice; if the hemorrhage originates below the small intestine, red blood may be passed with the stools.

Melena can be due to swallowed blood from nose bleeds or dental extractions; however, the three most common sources of blood are PEPTIC ULCER, gastritis (inflammation of the stomach lining), and varicose veins in the lower esophagus.

Other sources of upper gastrointestinal hemorrhage are esophagitis (inflammation of the esophagus) and cancer of the esophagus or stomach. To distinguish between these causes, it is usually essential to pass a fiberoptic endoscope through the mouth and into the stomach to observe any lesions. Once the site of bleeding has been identified, it is possible to initiate the appropriate treatment.

Finally, it should be remembered that black stools can be caused by ingestion of iron, charcoal, or bismuth.

memory

The ability to recall past experiences, ideas, and sensations.

In human beings, memory is an integral part of the mental processes of learning and thinking and depends on perception, language, attention, and motivation. Thus, memory is not only a complex process in itself, but it is extremely difficult to study in isolation. Nevertheless, the problems of memory have been addressed at various levels by philosophers, psychologists, neurologists, and biochemists. In recent years the advent of computer science has led to the analysis of memory in terms of information storage.

The key steps that need to be explained by any theory of memory are: (1) how the information to be remembered is encoded by the brain; (2) how and where this coded information is stored; (3) how the information is retrieved from storage when required. Despite intensive research for many years, any ideas we have about these stages remain largely speculative.

Human memory has two phases, usually referred to as *short-term memory* and *long-term memory*. Short-term memory is operative for a few minutes after new information has been received and is of limited capacity.

Unless the information transiently held in short-term memory is consolidated and transferred to long-term memory, it is totally lost. Memory not regularly rehearsed tends to fade. That is why students who "cram" for exams may have little knowledge of the subject matter days later. Information that has been learned properly tends to be forgotten, but can be refreshed with less effort than new learning. To explain such storage over many years, stable complex molecules such as nucleic acids and proteins have been suggested as the repositories for information in long-term memory, but this has not been proved. The exact sites of memory storage also are unknown, but lesions in the front part of the temporal lobes of the cerebrum frequently are found to impair memory.

menarche

The time of the first menstrual period, at puberty. In the United States the average age of a girl at the menarche is about 13 years; it has fallen steadily during the twentieth century, most likely because of the general improvement in nutrition.

The timing of the menarche is much influenced by genetic factors, but body weight is also important. The natural variation in the age of onset is so wide that menarche is not considered to be abnormally delayed until it has failed to appear by the age of 17.

Normally, in girls 8 to 11 years old estrogen production by the ovaries gradually increases and becomes cyclical in nature about one year before menarche. Secondary sexual characteristics, such as breast development and pubic hair growth, also usually precede the menarche. The initial menstrual periods tend to be irregular and painless.

Nevertheless, their occurrence can be a frightening experience for the girl if she has not been psychologically prepared for her menarche.

In rare cases a girl experiences the symptoms of menstruation, but no menstrual blood is passed. This may indicate a vaginal obstruction due to an imperforate hymen ("maidenhead") and should be corrected surgically.

True primary *amenorrhea*, a delay in the menarche beyond the age of 17, may be due to a malfunction or disease of the ovaries, the pituitary gland, or the hypothalamus. It may also occur in malnutrition anemia or in generalized debilitating disease. Precocious menarche may result from a hypothalamic disorder, and the child should be evaluated by a physician.

Ménière's disease

A disease of the inner ear characterized by dizziness (VERTIGO), deafness, and buzzing or ringing in the ears (TINNITUS).

The first attack of vertigo is profoundly disturbing to the victim, who feels that either he or his surroundings are spinning. Such an attack may last up to two hours and often is accompanied by vomiting.

The attacks of vertigo recur irregularly, but often every few weeks. During a period of remission the hearing and tinnitus may improve, but they become progressively worse with each attack. Ménière's disease tends to run its course over several years; the attacks tend to decline in severity and finally cease, but the victim is left with severe deafness.

The cause of Ménière's disease is unknown, but the major pathological change is an accumulation of excess fluid in the inner ear (*endolymphatic hydrops*) that damages the delicate nerve endings. Treatment for Ménière's disease may be medical or surgical, but there is no definitive cure. Drug treatment largely comprises sedatives and antiemetics (to prevent vomiting). Surgery is rare, however, as many patients have only mild and occasional attacks and require relatively little treatment.

meningioma

A tumor of the meninges, the membranes that cover the brain and spinal cord.

Characteristically, a meningioma is a single,

large tumor that is clearly separate from underlying brain or spinal cord. These tumors are classified pathologically as benign because they do not invade the adjacent brain or spread to other parts of the body. Meningiomas usually occur in persons middle-aged and older and are slightly more common in women than in men.

Although meningiomas are classed as benign, their presence within the skull or spinal canal displaces the normal tissue and can have serious consequences. *Spinal meningiomas* initially cause sensory symptoms such as pain and can progress to complete paraplegia. Because meningiomas grow slowly, the brain can often adjust and accommodate large tumors with little or no evidence of symptoms (*intracranial meningioma*). When symptoms do occur they may include paralysis or weakness of limbs, convulsions, headache, impairment of speech, interference with vision, and subtle mental changes.

Unless an intracranial meningioma can be removed surgically it may eventually be fatal. The techniques of COMPUTERIZED AXIAL TOMOGRAPHY (CAT scan) and MAGNETIC RESONANCE IMAGING (MRI) (see both under **Tests**) are very effective in displaying small meningiomas, and early diagnosis should improve the chances of successful surgery.

meningitis

Any infection or swelling of the membranes covering the brain and spinal cord.

The brain and spinal cord are covered by three

MENINGITIS

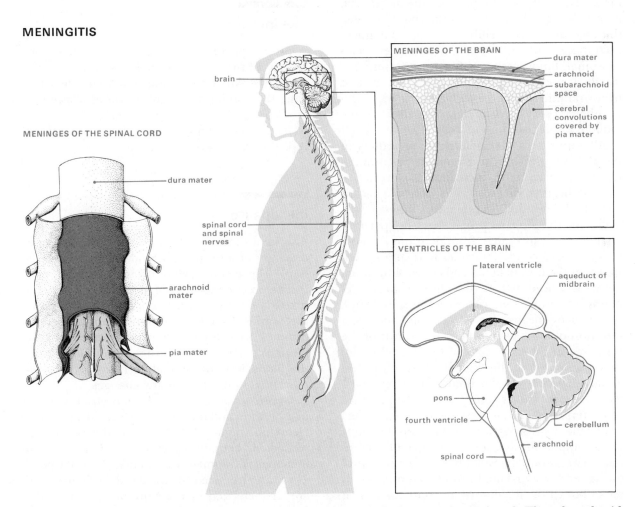

The meninges are three layers of protective membranes that cover the brain and spinal cord. The subarachnoid space between the two inner layers contains cerebrospinal fluid (CSF), which is produced in the ventricles of the brain. Meningitis, inflammation of the meninges, results from bacteria or viruses multiplying in the CSF.

membranes called the *meninges*: the *dura mater* (the outermost and toughest, in contact with the inner surface of the skull), the *arachnoid* (the middle membrane), and the *pia mater* (the innermost membrane, directly in contact with the surface of the brain).

Meningitis is caused most commonly by a bacterial or viral infection. The microorganisms can reach the meninges from the exterior (for example, by means of a severe head wound), from the bloodstream, from the nose and sinuses, or (rarely) directly from the brain itself.

In the United States cases of acute pyogenic ("pus-forming") meningitis are caused by infection with any one of three species of bacteria: *Neisseria* (or *Meningococcus*) *meningitidis*, *Diplococcus* (or *Pneumococcus*) *pneumoniae*, or *Hemophilus influenzae.*

When any of these bacteria infect the lining membranes of the brain, the meninges can quickly become inflamed and the space between the two innermost membranes (the "subarachnoid space"), which normally contains clear cerebrospinal fluid, becomes filled with pus. Pus usually is not formed in acute meningitis caused by a viral infection or by the causative organism of tuberculosis (*Mycobacterium tuberculosis*, or the "tubercle bacillus").

All forms of acute meningitis, regardless of their cause, give rise to a number of common symptoms. Headache, increasing in severity, is usually the first symptom. The person typically has a high fever and pronounced stiffness of the neck. As the disease progresses, the person's mental state can change from delirium through drowsiness to coma. PHOTOPHOBIA (extreme sensitivity of the eyes to light) and convulsions often are experienced also. A definitive diagnosis depends largely on a study of the cerebrospinal fluid, obtained by means of a lumbar puncture (the insertion of a hollow needle between two of the vertebrae in the lower part of the back through which a sample of the fluid is drawn off). The visual appearance of this fluid (cloudy or clear), its protein and sugar contents, and the presence of bacteria (which can be stained and examined under the microscope for specific identification) are all important diagnostic evidence of meningitis. Diagnostic confirmation by bacterial culture of the cerebrospinal fluid takes about one or two days, but it is imperative to start treatment immediately.

Both *Meningococcus* and *Pneumococcus* usually are sensitive to penicillin. Typical initial treatment involves the intravenous injection of benzyl penicillin (penicillin G) every four hours. Meningococcal meningitis normally responds particularly well to penicillin, but, increasingly, penicillin-resistant strains are arising. Pneumococcal meningitis is typically slower to improve and occasionally is associated with permanent neurological complications (such as impairment of hearing).

Meningitis caused by infection with *Hemophilus influenzae* usually can be cured in the majority of children by prompt treatment with ampicillin or chloramphenicol.

With the exception of HERPES SIMPLEX infections, there is no specific treatment available for viral meningitis, which comprises the majority of the remaining cases, but most individuals make a full spontaneous recovery.

meningocele

A protrusion of the covering membranes (meninges) of the brain or spinal cord through a defect in the skull or vertebral column. In the latter case, the condition is known also as a *meningomyelocele.*

It does not contain nerve tissue and can be repaired by surgery.

menopause

Also known as *climacteric.* Menopause marks the cessation of a woman's sexual cycles (menstruation). The average age of occurrence is 50.

The precise mechanism underlying the menopause is not fully understood, but it seems that the ovaries become unresponsive to the gonadotropic hormones (GONADOTROPINS) secreted by the pituitary gland at the base of the brain. Therefore, the blood level of circulating ESTROGEN falls significantly, resulting in many changes.

In normal menopause the menstrual periods may be scant and infrequent before the cessation. Heavy or irregular bleeding should always be investigated. Perhaps as many as 70 percent of menopausal women experience "hot flashes." These are produced by vascular disturbances and are characterized by a feeling of warmth in the face, neck, and the chest; they may be accompanied by blushing or sweating. It is not known exactly what causes this flashing, but it is thought to be related to fluctuating hormone levels. Flashes usually last for only a few minutes at a time but may occur several times a day. Other symptoms that may occur, such as nervous tension and irritability, may be psychological in nature or may be due to the lack of estrogen.

Other characteristics of menopause include a thinning and drying of the skin of the genital area and a decrease in breast size. The main health hazard is OSTEOPOROSIS. The decreased amount of estrogen is responsible.

Estrogen replacement is the only effective treatment for OSTEOPOROSIS, hot flashes, vaginal atrophy, and urinary tract atrophic changes. Estrogen administration should be cyclic. Estrogen vaginal cream can be used for KRAUROSIS VULVAE. There is no conclusive evidence that estrogen therapy increases the risk of coronary thrombosis or cancer, but it should not be taken if there is a history of estrogen-dependent cancer, vein thrombosis, or severe liver disease. All women on long-term therapy should be closely supervised. It is unlikely that short-term therapy is dangerous.

Postmenopausal bleeding (vaginal bleeding that occurs a year or more following the onset of the menopause) must always be investigated.

menorrhagia

Excessive or prolonged menstrual bleeding. In menorrhagia, up to 6.5 ounces (195 milliliters) of blood can be lost during each menstrual cycle, and as a result the woman can easily become anemic. In a normal period only about 2 ounces (60 ml.) of blood would be lost.

Menorrhagia has many possible causes and should always be investigated fully by a gynecologist. Pelvic lesions that can give rise to this condition include FIBROIDS, POLYPS, and ENDOMETRIOSIS. In many cases, however, no specific cause can be found; "dysfunctional bleeding," as it is called, is possibly related to a disorder of the production and release of the hormones that control menstruation.

Dilatation and curettage (D & C) is often the only way to establish the cause of menorrhagia. In addition to providing diagnostic information, D & C is frequently a curative procedure. Hormonal therapy with PROGESTINS (or, more commonly these days, with the oral contraceptive pill itself) is sometimes successful in controlling dysfunctional bleeding. In severe cases, HYSTERECTOMY

or surgical removal of the uterus (see under Procedures) may be required.

menstruation

The normal monthly discharge of blood and cellular debris from the vagina which accompanies the periodic shedding of the lining of the uterus (womb) in nonpregnant women.

By convention, the first day of menstruation is taken as "day 1" of the menstrual cycle (which is an average of twenty-eight days long). Only human females and other female primates menstruate; other mammals have an "estrous cycle" characterized by a period of "heat" when the sexual interest of the mature female is aroused.

In women the time of the first menstrual period (MENARCHE) is generally about the age of 13; the menstrual cycle continues (in the absence of pregnancy or of certain other influences) until the MENOPAUSE.

Normally menstruation lasts for about four days, but it can vary from two to seven days. On average, about 2 ounces (60 milliliters) of blood is lost, and at the end of the menstrual cycle all but the deepest layers of the uterine lining have been shed. The lining of the uterus is restored during the latter part of the first, or "follicular," phase of the menstrual cycle (days 1–14). During this phase the ovarian follicle is ripening and secreting estrogen. One ovarian follicle develops during each cycle, and at about fourteen days before the next menstrual period begins, the follicle ruptures and releases an ovum (egg) which makes its way down the FALLOPIAN TUBE where it is ready to meet the male's sperm cell. This is OVULATION, the second phase of the monthly cycle. (A simple, although rather unreliable, indicator of its occurrence is a temporary rise in the woman's body temperature.)

Shortly after ovulation the empty ovarian follicle is transformed into the *corpus luteum*, which secretes ESTROGEN and PROGESTERONE for the remainder of the menstrual cycle. This period is the third, or "luteal," phase in which the corpus luteum prepares the lining of the uterus to hold the fertilized egg. If fertilization of the ovum does *not* take place, the corpus luteum begins to decay on about the twenty-fourth day, and the lining of the uterus prepares to be shed. Menstruation then occurs. (If fertilization *does* take place, the corpus luteum enlarges and maintains the uterine lining

THE MENSTRUAL CYCLE

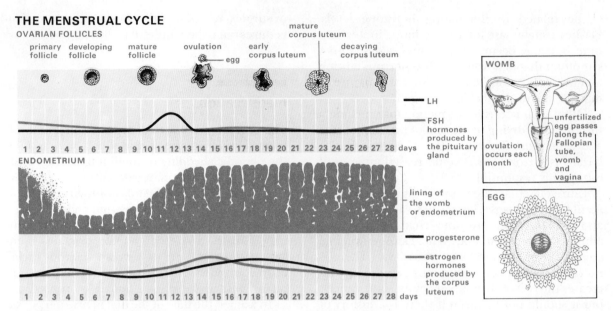

The human menstrual cycle is a monthly fluctuation in the state of the endometrium (lining of the uterus), and depends on hormonal changes governed by the pituitary gland in the brain. Day 1 is the first day of menstruation, when the old endometrium starts to slough off. Although the length of the cycle can vary from 23 days to 35 days in normal women, ovulation nearly always occurs 14 days before the end of the cycle.

in a suitable condition for the nourishment of the fertilized egg, and, thus, menstruation does not occur.)

mental illness

The term "mental illness" covers personality disorders, drug dependence, psycho-sexual disorders, NEUROSIS, and the psychotic states of SCHIZOPHRENIA and DEPRESSION.

The nature, cause, diagnosis, and treatment of mental illnesses are more controversial than is the case with diseases caused by microorganisms or those related to an obvious physical abnormality such as a tumor. That so many different views of mental illness are defended reflects our basic collective ignorance about many facets of the subject.

Psychiatrists are divided in their opinions as to the origins of mental illness. Some believe that it originates primarily as a result of a structural or biochemical disorder in the brain. Others attach primary importance to the influences in infancy and childhood and to psychological reactions to conscious and unconscious stresses. These two basic approaches are not mutually exclusive, however: Neurological and psychogenic influences may *both* be involved in most mental problems.

When it comes to treatment, psychiatrists also fall into one "camp" or the other. Those who believe in an organic cause of mental illness will treat the afflicted ones with the use of appropriate physical techniques, including drugs, surgical procedures, and electroconvulsive therapy (ECT). Those who favor a "psychogenic" cause will lean toward various psychotherapeutic techniques—which are often expensive and time-consuming. However, when specific, effective drug treatments are available (such as the use of lithium in manic-depressive psychosis), there is usually a consensus of opinion.

See also MANIA.

mental retardation

An inclusive term used to describe retarded intellectual development resulting in low intelligence. The cause may be present at birth as a constitutional trait or childhood environmental insult, such as trauma or infection, may lead to it.

Although there may be a clear-cut genetic cause for retardation, it is always important to provide the retarded person with an environment that allows fullest expression of potential, however limited it may be. The deterioration of mental powers later in adult life is classified as *dementia* rather than as mental retardation, because a normal level of intelligence has been attained at some stage.

To understand the concept of mental retardation, it is first necessary to form a working definition of intelligence and to understand how it can be measured. Psychologists have defined intelligence in many different ways, but most would agree that it involves the individual's ability to adapt successfully to his environment and his capacity to learn and manipulate abstract ideas.

There is much controversy about the worth of intelligence tests, but they do provide a standardized means of comparing one person's mental capacity with that of the general population. Many tests are designed so that if the average *intelligence quotient* (IQ) is 100, then approximately 68 percent of the population will have an IQ between 85 and 115, and about 95 percent will have one between 70 and 130. In fact the distribution of intelligence among the population is not quite symmetrical: there are more people with IQs of less than 70 than there are gifted people with IQs above 130.

As a crude measure, an IQ of less than 70 often is taken as the criterion for mental retardation, although this varies with the type of IQ test used. Obviously there is no clear-cut boundary between high-grade mental handicap and the lower levels of "normal" intelligence. Moreover, while subnormal intelligence is the essential factor in mental handicap, it is often the social incompetence and emotional inadequacy of the individual that present the greatest problems.

In the majority of cases, intellectual deficit is not associated with any known organic disease. However, many mentally retarded people show physical signs of a brain defect and this is nearly always the case in the most severely retarded. For practical purposes it is useful to grade mental retardation into four groups: the mildly, moderately, severely, and profoundly retarded.

The *mildly retarded* have IQs of approximately 50 to 70 and constitute the largest group with mental retardation. They are often the children of parents who themselves are intellectually dull. Their constitutional disadvantage is often compounded by poor living conditions and inadequate parents. As infants they tend to lack curiosity and are quiet and well behaved. For this reason they are often undetected until they go to school, where their performance falls progressively further behind that of their peers. It is especially important to identify these children, because with special training they can be helped to lead independent lives. Unfortunately, many do not receive appropriate education.

By contrast, the *severely* and *moderately retarded* (with an IQ of approximately 20 to 50) are incapable of independence and are more likely to be diagnosed earlier because of an associated physical abnormality. Their developmental milestones are delayed and typically they show impulsive, infantile behavior throughout their lives. Parents of these children usually have normal intelligence and accept that their child will benefit from special education. DOWN'S SYNDROME is by far the most common syndrome associated with this degree of mental subnormality.

The *profoundly retarded* are estimated to have an IQ below 20. They are differentiated from the other groups by their need to be protected constantly against common physical dangers. The majority are stunted in growth, have severe brain damage, and may suffer from epileptic seizures. Many are bedridden and do not survive childhood.

See also INTELLIGENCE TESTING under **Tests**.

mercury poisoning

Mercury can cause acute or chronic poisoning. Metallic mercury is not dangerously poisonous in very small doses: The child who bites through a clinical thermometer and swallows a few drops of the metal will probably come to no harm. However, *mercuric chloride ingestion*, either intentional or accidental, results in acute poisoning. The initial symptoms are nausea, vomiting, diarrhea, and abdominal pain. Cardiovascular collapse may occur after several hours.

Chronic mercury poisoning is most often due to occupational exposure or to industrial pollution of the environment. Depending on the amount and length of exposure and the age of the victim, symptoms include weakness, tremors, progressive incoordination, and paralysis. Numbness in the fingers and toes is an early sign of poisoning. Mental changes include lethargy and intellectual dullness.

Mass outbreaks of chronic mercury poisoning have occurred in the past few decades: Minamata disease in Japan was due to contamination of fish by industrial effluent. More recently, industrial contamination of fishing lakes in northern Quebec caused an epidemic of mercury poisoning, and in several countries there have been epidemics of mercury poisoning resulting from the human consumption of chemically treated wheat seed.

mesothelioma

A rare malignant tumor of the pleura and peritoneum, the membranous sacs lining the chest and abdominal cavities, respectively.

In 1960 a relation was established between mesothelioma and exposure to asbestos. It was found that exposure to asbestos need only have been for one to two months to account for the development of a mesothelioma twenty to fifty years later. Thus, although protective measures are now taken against environmental pollution with asbestos, new cases of mesothelioma will still be presenting themselves at the end of the twentieth century.

While radiation therapy occasionally prolongs survival in cases of *pleural mesothelioma,* most persons die within a year of diagnosis.

metabolism

This term, literally meaning "change," refers to all the chemical and energy transformations that are carried out in an organism or in a single cell.

The first specific function of metabolism is to extract chemical energy from the environment. The cells of all higher animals derive energy by the chemical breakdown of complex nutrients, principally into carbon dioxide and water. This chemical degradation is called *catabolism.*

Besides, the complete catabolism of ingested nutrients to yield energy, the body's metabolic processes have to convert foodstuffs into molecular building blocks and assemble them into the components of cells, such as proteins, nucleic acids, and lipids (fats or fat-like substances). This synthesis of cellular macromolecules is called *anabolism.* Finally, some of these macromolecules have to be broken down for use or for excretion, as do drugs administered to the body.

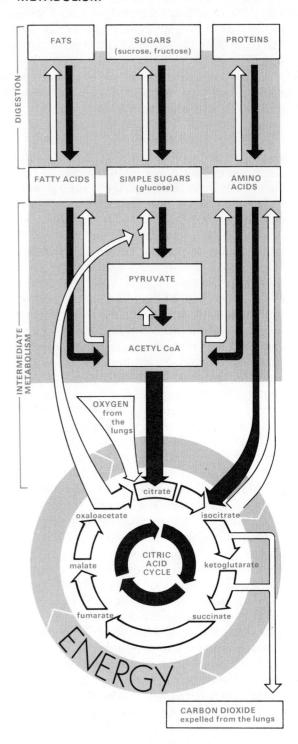

METABOLISM

The diagram shows the pathways of metabolism. Sugars, fats, and proteins are broken down into simple chemicals in the stomach and small intestine; the chemicals are absorbed into the blood and transported to the tissues. Within each cell they are transformed into a key substance: "acetyl CoA." Then follows the "citric acid cycle," where controlled combustion with oxygen leads to the production of energy; carbon dioxide is released during this process.

The *basal metabolic rate* (*BMR*) is the amount of energy consumed by a person in a day to maintain essential bodily functions. In an average adult under conditions of mental and physical rest, the BMR is about 2,000 kilocalories/day; someone in a sedentary job consumes about 2,500 kilocalories per day. The BMR is raised by anxiety but decreased in depression. Metabolic processes are sensitively regulated by hormones, and increased levels of epinephrine, norepinephrine, and thyroid hormone raise the BMR.

The end products of digestion in humans are mainly amino acids, fat derivatives, and sugars such as glucose. These digestive products are catabolized to simpler, intermediate molecules, which constitute the common "metabolic pool." The intermediate molecules then either undergo anabolism into proteins, fats, or carbohydrates, or they may be catabolized further into hydrogen atoms and carbon dioxide. This final catabolism, the consequence of a biochemical process known as the *citric acid cycle*, occurs in the specialized mitochondria of cells. The energy thus liberated is not used directly by the cell but is stored in high-energy phosphate compounds, the most important being adenosine triphosphate (ATP).

metastasis

The spread of cancer cells from one site in the body to other parts of the body.

See CANCER.

migraine

A throbbing headache, usually occurring on only one side of the head.

Classically, a migraine starts with visual disturbances. Jagged brilliant streaks of light may be seen on one side; an expanding blank area may obscure the vision in one half of the field. This may be followed by numbness or "pins and needles" in the hands or face, and sometimes weakness of a limb or of half the body. After fifteen to thirty minutes these symptoms give way to a boring pain on one side of the head, which typically reaches a peak of intensity after an hour or so. The headache becomes throbbing in character and is often accompanied by nausea and vomiting.

Migraine usually appears first around the age of puberty and recurs with gradually diminishing frequency through adult life. It may begin during early childhood or in middle age, however. Women are more susceptible than men and it often runs in families.

Sufferers from migraine are more prone to allergies, and it is not uncommon for attacks to be linked to certain dietary factors, such as red wine, oranges, cheese, or chocolate. Migraine sufferers are treated with several types of medications, ranging from aspirin to mild tranquilizers.

miliaria

Miliaria ("heat rash" or "prickly heat") is an acute itching eruption of the skin that commonly occurs in hot summer weather and in tropical and subtropical areas.

The condition results from excessive sweating and blocked sweat glands. Prolonged exposure to heat and moisture causes the skin to swell enough to block the openings of the sweat glands. Newly produced sweat is then deposited in the skin and not on it; this results in local irritation and in the formation of minute blisters. Pimples may develop as well as itch due to inflammation, and the involved area may become infected. Sites that tend to be involved are the chest, back, waistline, groin, and armpits. The best treatment involves moving the person to a cooler, less humid atmosphere. Lotions, cold compresses, and cool showers or tub soaks also may help. Anything that causes irritation—such as unsuitable clothing, medications, or harsh soaps—should be avoided.

If fungal infections develop in the affected areas, they require separate treatment with antifungal ointments or other preparations.

In cases of severe itching, antihistamines may be given.

miosis

Contraction of the circular muscle of the iris, causing the pupil of the eye to become smaller. Constriction of the pupil cuts down the amount of light reaching the retina but improves the depth of focus, so reading may be easier in bright light.

Drugs that constrict the pupil are used in the treatment of some eye diseases such as GLAUCOMA.

miscarriage

The spontaneous expulsion of the embryo or fetus (technically known as a *spontaneous abortion*) before the twentieth week of pregnancy. The woman undergoes a miniature labor with dilation of the cervix and experiences some pain. The most common time for a miscarriage to occur is about the twelfth week.

The cause of spontaneous abortion often cannot be determined, but the following factors can play a part:

Many early aborted fetuses have abnormalities. Maternal disease may be a cause, such as hypertension, kidney or heart disease, diabetes, or thyroid abnormalities. Uterine and placental abnormalities, a "lax" cervix, severe vitamin deficiencies, or possibly violent exercise also tend to interrupt pregnancy.

A threatened miscarriage is indicated by bleeding and pain. If it progresses and the cervix becomes dilated, loss of the fetus becomes inevitable. If placental tissue is retained in an incomplete miscarriage there is a danger of hemorrhage and sepsis. Thus, prompt medical attention—usually including a dilatation and curettage (D & C)—following a miscarriage is essential.

mites

Small organisms (technically known as *arachnids*, the group to which spiders belong), some species of which burrow into the skin and cause irritation. They may transmit serious disease, and some varieties may cause allergic reactions such as asthma.

The human parasite *Sarcoptes scabiei* is the cause of SCABIES, an irritative skin disease. Scabies itching is intense, especially at night. The penetration of the mite (smaller than a pinhead) causes scratches, small blisters, or pimples. Scabies parasites are transmitted by direct contact, especially sexual contact, and from shared towels and bed linen. Bathing and applications of gamma benzene hexachloride or benzyl benzoate are effective treatments.

House mites are responsible for passing on *rickettsialpox* in North America and Europe. Mice infected with RICKETTSIAE (microorganisms intermediate in size between bacteria and viruses)

maintain the infection. Treatment is with tetracyclines.

Mites living in house dust do not infect humans directly, but their presence in the dust is an important cause of hypersensitivity and asthmatic reactions, especially in children. Removal of dust-laden mattresses may bring dramatic relief of symptoms.

mole

A blemish on the skin that may be present at birth or may develop subsequently. Moles are composed of clusters of *nevus* cells, which are specialized epithelial cells containing the pigment melanin.

Moles may be small or large, flat or raised, smooth, hairy, or warty. They vary in color from yellow-brown to black. A mole also is classified as a type of pigmented NEVUS (birthmark).

In rare cases a mole undergoes cancerous change to become a malignant MELANOMA. These can be classified according to where they arise, which gives some indication of the likelihood of malignant change occurring in a mole. About a quarter of malignant melanomas do not develop from a preceding mole.

Intradermal, or "common," moles—in which the melanin-forming cells are in the lower layer of the skin or dermis—are benign. They are elevated and often have a hair in them. These intradermal nevi need not be removed except for cosmetic purposes since they are not precursors of melanomas.

Another type known as *junctional nevi* arises from nevus cells at the junction between the outer layer of the skin (epidermis) and the dermis underlying it. They may be flat and are deep brown or black in color. Though more susceptible to activation, only a small percentage become malignant. They do not require removal unless they show a recent change, are situated in the nail matrix, are the site of frequent trauma, or are on surfaces such as the lips, anus, penis, or vulva. Bleeding, ulceration, or a sudden increase in size or color is an indication for surgical removal of junctional nevi.

In general, malignant melanomas develop more readily from moles on the lower legs and on mucous membranes than from those elsewhere. Pigmented moles subjected to constant irritation or trauma show a relatively high incidence of malignant changes.

During pregnancy a benign increase in mole size and color is common. Children tend to develop more junctional nevi than intradermal nevi, yet they rarely acquire malignant melanoma. Large, speckled, flat, rough lesions resembling junctional nevi are common on exposed parts in the elderly; they are best removed surgically because of their potential for malignant transformation.

molluscum contagiosum

A viral disease of the skin, characterized by one or more firm, dome-shaped nodules with a central dimple and containing a cheese-like substance.

The virus is transmitted by sexual contact as well as by shared use of clothing, linen, and towels or other items that have been contaminated with the virus; outbreaks in schools are not uncommon.

For cosmetic purposes, the nodules may be unsightly, but they are not dangerous. Once diagnosed, they can be removed by a dermatologist with a curette or by electrodesiccation. The nodules can recur if the infected items are not sanitized or if a sexual contact is not treated.

morning sickness

Nausea and vomiting of varying severity that occur in pregnancy, usually in the early months.

Morning sickness occurs in about half of pregnancies from about the end of the first month, usually ceasing by the end of the third month. As the name implies, it tends to occur in the early part of the day but can develop at other times.

The symptoms begin with a feeling of nausea on arising. Often the expectant mother is unable to retain her breakfast, but by midday the symptoms decrease. In some cases the condition evolves into prolonged bouts of vomiting with a resultant weight loss (HYPEREMISIS GRAVIDARUM).

Most women with morning sickness can keep it under control by taking only small meals with generous amounts of fluid between meals. Nausea can sometimes be averted or minimized by getting out of bed slowly. Drugs not prescribed by the doctor should be avoided if possible, but antinauseants and sedatives may be necessary in the more severe cases.

mosquitoes

Approximately 2,500 different species of mosquitoes have been identified. The bloodsucking habits of the females of a few of these species are responsible for transmitting various diseases to humans and other mammals. In obtaining their "blood meal," the females use their specially modified mouth parts to pierce the skin of their victims and suck their blood.

The female mosquito first injects saliva containing an anticoagulant into the skin of its victim to prevent the blood from clotting. It also injects a "sensitizing" agent, which may cause severe irritation in some people. Soothing lotions and creams may be applied to alleviate the itching.

As a mosquito feeds it may transmit various disease-causing microorganisms from one person to another. Several diseases are spread in this way, including MALARIA, YELLOW FEVER, and DENGUE FEVER.

Many "arboviruses" are known to cause diseases in humans. Most of these diseases are acquired accidentally through the bite of an insect such as the mosquito. The diseases can be divided into three basic categories: (1) acute central nervous system diseases, usually with ENCEPHALITIS; (2) acute benign fevers; and (3) hemorrhagic fevers.

Of the mosquito-borne infections in the first category, *eastern equine encephalitis* carries one of the highest mortality rates. Cases are recognized in the eastern and north central United States and Canada. Mosquitoes usually acquire the infection from wild birds or rodents.

Dengue fever comes within the second category. During the twentieth century, epidemics of dengue fever have occurred in the southeastern and Gulf sections of the United States and elsewhere. The fatality rate is low. Mosquitoes can pick up the pathogenic viruses from an infected person from the day before the onset of the person's fever to the fifth day of the disease; eleven days after the mosquito takes its blood meal it becomes capable of infecting another person.

Yellow fever belongs to the third category—hemorrhagic fevers. Except for a few cases in Trinidad, West Indies, in 1954, no urban outbreak has been transmitted by mosquitoes since the 1940s. Jungle yellow fever is present from time to time in mainland countries of the Americas from Mexico to South America.

The bite of a mosquito harboring infective larvae of a worm parasite transmits the tropical condition known as *filariasis*.

Preventive measures against all these conditions involve keeping the mosquito under control. Besides the drainage of mosquito breeding grounds, these measures include the use of insecticide sprays in homes and outbuildings, mosquito repellants for personal use, screens on doors and windows in homes or mosquito netting where screens are not practical, and sufficient clothing, particularly after sundown, to protect as much of the skin surface as possible against bites.

multiple myeloma

A malignant growth of certain cells in the bone marrow (plasma cells). It occurs most commonly in people over 40 and affects men twice as often as women. The condition may be accompanied by anemia and kidney damage.

The most common initial symptom is bone pain, often in a rib or vertebra. (The bones most frequently affected are the ribs, spine, and pelvis.) There are multiple well-defined areas where bone is destroyed.

Fractures in the ribs and long bones and collapse of the vertebrae may occur. X-ray studies may show general demineralization of the bones or characteristic punched-out lesions.

Anemia, from impaired production of red blood cells, is usual. The disease gradually disseminates through the body, although a single lesion may be involved initially. The excess plasma cells produce an abnormal protein. The tubules in the kidneys may become blocked by coagulated protein.

The drug melphalan may be used in treatment alone or combined with steroids. The pain from local involvement of bone can be relieved by radiotherapy. Transfusion may be required to correct anemia.

multiple sclerosis (MS)

A disease marked by patchy loss or destruction of the protective myelin covering of the nerve fibers of the brain and spinal cord.

Symptoms of multiple sclerosis usually appear first in young adulthood and continue throughout life. Early signs are numbness or tingling in the arms and legs or the face. Other signs are muscle weakness, loss of vision in one eye, dizziness, and slowed speech. As it progresses there may be loss of bowel and bladder control, extremes in emotion, and increasing disability. The severity of the symptoms is likely to change over time, with periods of remission and exacerbation.

There is currently no specific cure, but wide claims have been made for a number of treatments. Spontaneous remissions make any treatment difficult to evaluate. Massage of weakened limbs and muscle training are of some benefit.

Prompt treatment of infections and an adequate diet with vitamin supplements, where necessary, are sensible measures. In the later stages of multiple sclerosis, good nursing will help in the prevention of bedsores. Medications are used to alleviate symptoms.

mumps

A contagious viral disease common among children which usually causes painful inflammation and enlargement of the salivary glands, particularly the parotid glands. There is fever, and swelling develops in front of the ears, making the chewing of food difficult. Also called *epidemic parotitis.*

In young children mumps is a relatively trivial illness, but if contracted after puberty it may affect the testicles and ovaries.

The disease is spread by droplet infection through the respiratory tract. The incubation period is twelve to twenty-eight days, but the great majority of children develop it about eighteen days after exposure.

The initial symptoms may be a high temperature, headache, and sore throat; these may arise a few days before the characteristic swelling of the parotid glands, but often the swelling is the first symptom. It usually subsides within seven to ten days.

A child with mumps can usually be cared for at home. He is infectious until the swelling subsides. A child who has once had the infection is unlikely to contract it again because of the long-term immunity that develops.

Occasionally the virus invades tissues other than the salivary glands, notably the testicles, ovaries, pancreas, and the meninges (membranes covering the brain and spinal cord). About a quarter of boys over 14 years of age having mumps develop inflammation of the testicles (orchitis) as a complication; this may sometimes cause permanent sterility. Sterility rarely occurs in girls.

Live mumps vaccine was introduced in the late 1960s and it may be useful in those who have

MUMPS

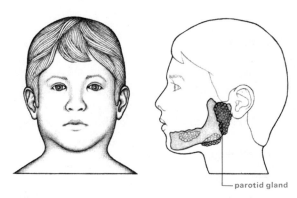

parotid gland

Mumps is one of the common viral diseases of childhood. The virus attacks the parotid gland in front of the ear, producing a painful, swollen face.

reached puberty without contracting the illness, or for administration to younger children. The vaccine must not be given to pregnant women.

Munchausen's syndrome

A strange type of complaint named after the eighteenth-century Baron von Munchausen, who was a traveler and the reputed teller of a collection of preposterous, fanciful stories.

Persons with this syndrome travel from one hospital or doctor to another telling untruthful stories about their medical condition, describing dramatic but false symptoms, or simulating acute illness. They may eagerly submit themselves for countless operations (having scars that bear testimony) or undergo what they know to be unnecessary medical investigations.

They often leave a hospital without notice (or payment) and resume their travels.

muscle

Tissue composed of fibers that have the ability to contract.

There are two types of muscle: *Voluntary*, or striated, muscle is under the direct control of the will; *involuntary*, or smooth, muscle cannot be controlled consciously. Leg and arm muscles are examples of voluntary muscles, while involuntary muscles are those found in the heart, blood vessels, the walls of the stomach and intestines, and most internal organs.

Since voluntary muscles are activated and controlled by the brain through nerves that pass down and out of the spinal cord, an injury to the brain, spinal cord, or nerves can result in the paralysis of certain muscles.

When muscles are exercised vigorously, their oxygen supply is consumed. When muscle oxygen is completely depleted, the muscle derives energy by a process called *anaerobic metabolism*. This process results in the production of a substance called lactic acid. Pain in the muscles after sustained vigorous exercise is due to the buildup of lactic acid.

muscular dystrophy

A group of hereditary diseases that result in progressive weakness due to degeneration of muscles. Muscle fibers are replaced by fat cells and connective tissue. Onset is usually in childhood or adolescence, with loss of muscle power that is symmetrical and slowly progressive.

Several types of muscular dystrophy are seen only in infancy or childhood. Of these, the most frequent is the *pseudohypertropic*, or Duchenne, form that affects only boys. The disease becomes evident between the ages of 2 and 6. The pelvic and hip muscles are affected first, resulting in frequent falls, difficulty in climbing stairs, an awkward gait, and an inability to run properly. Paradoxically, the muscles appear unusually large and firm, in contrast to their weakness (pseudohypertrophy).

The other childhood muscular dystrophy is the *facioscapulohumeral*, or Landouzy-Déjerine, type, which starts later in adolescence. Both sexes are equally affected. Muscle weakness and degeneration begin in the facial muscles. Weakness of the shoulder girdle is more prominent than leg weakness. Some persons with the condition are scarcely aware of the symptoms throughout a normal life span; in others, disabilities gradually increase. An affected child may lack normal facial expressions and be unable to raise his arms above his head.

Other forms and intermediate conditions exist. For instance, there is an arm-and-shoulder variety and a rarer form known as *distal myopathy*. In the latter condition weakness starts in the hands and spreads inward.

There is no specific drug treatment for these diseases. Muscle-strengthening exercises, corrective surgery, and the use of braces may be helpful in some cases.

myasthenia gravis

A form of muscle weakness characterized by abnormal fatigue of muscles after exercise and rapid recovery of strength after a period of rest. It is a slowly progressive disease that affects approximately 6 in 100,000 persons. Although it can occur in both men and women at any age, twice as many women are affected as men—women usually in their 30s, men usually after age 60.

In this condition there is a disorder of conduction at the point where the nerves meet, and normally activate, the muscle cells; the muscles thus fail to respond to the signal from the nerve endings. Myasthenia gravis is thought to be caused by a lack of formation of the "neuromuscular transmitter" chemical *acetylcholine.*

Typically the paralysis produced is minimal in the morning and worse at night. The disease most often affects the eyes, face, shoulder girdle, and (less often) the legs.

Onset of the disease is gradual, with drooping of the eyelids often being the first indication. As the disease progresses, double vision and eventually paralysis of the eye muscles can occur. Weakness of facial, chewing, and swallowing muscles causes difficulty in eating. In severe cases, respiratory paralysis also may occur.

Not all cases progress to become life-threatening. There is spontaneous remission in some persons, and others manage on medications that improve neuromuscular transmission. In severe cases the removal of the thymus gland, located in the chest, has been found to bring improvement in a majority of patients. An excessive formation of tissue in the thymus gland has been associated with many cases of the disease.

mydriasis

The widening or dilation of the pupil of the eye. Mydriasis occurs when the light falling on the eye decreases in intensity or when the lens focuses from a near object to a distant one. The widening pupil permits more light to fall on the retina, thus improving vision in poor light.

Stimulation of sensory nerves may cause a dilation of the pupil. In conditions such as excitement, fear, pain, or asphyxia (which lead to the release of epinephrine from the adrenal glands), the pupils dilate, as they do when the sympathetic nerves to the eyes are stimulated. Certain drugs can produce mydriasis. Alcohol intoxication has the same effect.

myelitis

A swelling or inflammation of the spinal cord, sometimes linked with motor-nerve or sensory-nerve dysfunction.

myiasis

Invasion or infection of a body area or cavity by the larvae (maggots) of flies. Many fly species have been implicated. Some are termed *obligate parasites*—that is, they cannot survive without involving humans in their life cycles. Others, known as *facultative parasites,* are capable of being free-living as well as acting as parasites. A third category of parasites infests humans only by chance.

Myiasis usually involves the skin or mucous membranes, especially the nasal passages and the throat. Lesions in the skin may be shallow or deep, leading to "boils" containing the larvae.

In some infestations the larvae burrow deep and reach the membranes or cavities of the nose, throat, ear, eye, and vagina, where they can cause extensive damage.

Gastrointestinal myiasis arises from the accidental swallowing of larvae in contaminated food, which may occasionally lead to invasion of the intestinal wall.

Surgical removal of deep-burrowing skin larvae may be necessary, but a more superficial type can be treated with an ethyl chloride spray or the application of ice (which kills the larvae before they are removed).

Larvae in a deep boil are best extracted surgically. Eggs of the screwworm fly, which is found in the southern United States, are laid in an open wound from which they may invade tissue extensively.

myocarditis

Inflammation of the muscle tissue of the heart. This sometimes serious condition may arise owing to an unknown cause, or it may be a complication of a number of illnesses such as RHEUMATIC FEVER, SCARLET FEVER, diphtheria, and TYPHOID FEVER. Apart from being associated with bacterial, fungal, or viral diseases (especially COXSACKIE VIRUS B), myocarditis may be due to toxic chemicals, alcohol, or drugs, to electric shock, or to excessive X-ray treatment.

The most common symptoms of acute myocarditis are pain in the area of the heart and stomach and shortness of breath. Examination by a physician may reveal a cardiac arrhythmia and a rapid, soft, and irregular pulse. Once the condition is suspected, complete bed rest, sedation, and continuation of therapy for any underlying illness may help to prevent a sudden increase in the severity of the disease. Anti-inflammatory drugs also may be used.

Myocarditis may leave a residual effect on the efficiency of the heart after recovery.

myopia

A condition of nearsightedness: Close objects are seen clearly, distant objects appear blurry.

The normal eye is shaped so that rays of light from distant objects are brought to an exact focus on the retina. Nearer objects are brought into focus by a contraction of the ciliary muscle of the eye, allowing the lens to become more spherical.

In the large majority of cases, myopia is simply a variation in the shape of the eyeball. It usually progresses while body growth is continuing, and then stabilizes. In some cases the eyeball may continue to enlarge throughout life (*progressive myopia*), leading to a retinal degeneration or even to DETACHED RETINA.

Myopia is corrected with eyeglasses fitted with concave lenses. Contact lenses also may be used to correct myopia.

myxedema

A condition caused by malfunction or surgical removal of the thyroid gland. Subsequent lack of circulating thyroid hormone in the body gives rise to a series of signs and symptoms, which represent a severe form of HYPOTHYROIDISM.

There is swelling of the face and limbs because of fluid being deposited under the skin. This may particularly affect the area around the eyes, hands, and feet. The skin becomes dry and rough and there may be some hair loss. The person exhibits slowness of action and thought, and this mental dullness is accompanied by slow speech, with a voice that may become hoarse. Lethargy and

MYOPIA

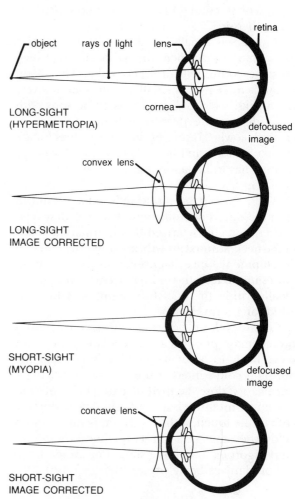

LONG-SIGHT (HYPERMETROPIA)

LONG-SIGHT IMAGE CORRECTED

SHORT-SIGHT (MYOPIA)

SHORT-SIGHT IMAGE CORRECTED

Myopia, or short sight, can result from either an elongated eyeball or from a lens that is too powerful. The outcome, as shown above, is that rays of light are focused in front of the retina so that the image is blurred. Long sight is the reverse optical error and usually results from the lens weakening with age. Both conditions can be corrected by wearing eyeglasses with lenses of the correct prescription.

weakness may be associated with slowed reflexes, a slow pulse, lowered metabolism, and subnormal body temperature. The person sometimes experiences poor tolerance to cold and (especially in the elderly) HYPOTHERMIA. The appetite may be poor, yet there is often a mild weight gain. Shortness of breath and constipation are not uncommon. Personality change, amounting to frank psychosis ("myxedema madness"), may occur.

The condition may arise through primary disease of the thyroid or as a consequence of the removal of the gland for treatment of life-threatening GOITER conditions such as cancer or overactive thyroid.

Recovery is usually excellent with the administration of replacement thyroid hormone, which must be continued throughout life. The medication is increased by small amounts about every two weeks, as necessary. In older persons with heart disease the thyroid hormone level is increased slowly, since a rapid rise can precipitate angina pectoris and heart failure. Each person's therapy has to be tailored to his or her own particular needs.

When thyroid hormone deficiency occurs in infancy (different from myxedema) it may lead to CRETINISM, characterized by abnormal thickness of the neck, stunted growth, and imperfect mental development. Once diagnosed, this condition requires immediate thyroid replacement therapy—ideally within the first three months of life—to avoid long-term damage.

COMA developing in a person suffering from myxedema represents a medical emergency. It is more likely to occur in the elderly (particularly during a cold winter) if they are not receiving a satisfactory dose of thyroid extract. Treatment should be intensive but not hasty. The sufferer is cold to the touch, with a body temperature often below the range of a standard clinical thermometer. Vigorous rewarming should be avoided, the use of blankets being preferable.

nausea

A feeling of wanting to vomit, with a characteristic sensation that passes through the upper part of the abdomen.

Normally the stomach contracts regularly to empty its contents into the duodenum. If this reflex action temporarily ceases and the abdominal muscles contract in such a way as to threaten to compress and empty the stomach upward, the individual experiences nausea.

Nausea can be brought on by virtually anything that affects gastrointestinal function directly or indirectly.

necrosis

The death of areas of tissue surrounded by healthy parts. It can occur in any part of the body.

Necrotic tissue is seen, at the simplest level, in the pustular content of even the smallest infection, where the yellow fluid discharged is composed of dead bacteria, the body's dead white blood cells, and skin cells that have failed to survive the ravages of an infective agent. Necrosis takes place even where infective agents are not present when any tissue is deprived of its blood supply: for example, in small areas of the heart muscle after MYOCARDIAL INFARCTION a ("heart attack"), in the center of tumors that have outgrown their blood supply, and in areas of the body where GANGRENE (another name for a wide area of tissue necrosis) has occurred.

When OSTEOMYELITIS occurs in bone there is necrosis of the bone cells (*sequestrum*) because the inflammation has caused the blockage or thrombosis of the minute arteries supplying these bone cells. In ATHEROSCLEROSIS the blood vessels may be partially blocked by fatty deposits (atheromas), and the blood supply to the peripheral parts of the lower limbs may be insufficient to maintain nutrition of the tissues, so that necrosis—or gangrene—may occur in the toes. In frostbite, necrosis of the tissues may occur because the peripheral blood vessels have frozen.

Treatment depends on cause. Most often, however, the necrotic area must be removed so that tissue regeneration can occur, if possible. This can result in amputation of limbs in severe cases if deep-tissue death has occurred. Necrosis, when occurring internally or over large areas of the skin, can be life-threatening and requires prompt medical treatment.

neoplasm

An abnormal new growth of cells or tissues; tumor.

nephritis

Inflammation of the kidney. Nephritis falls into two principal groups: (1) PYELONEPHRITIS, a bacterial infection that spreads from the bladder and ureters, and (2) GLOMERULONEPHRITIS, a noninfective disease usually affecting both kidneys.

nephrotic syndrome

A kidney disease resulting from excessive loss of protein (albumin) in the urine. There are low levels of albumin in the blood, increased blood cholesterol, and collection of fluid in body tissues (EDEMA). Many conditions can result in the leakage of protein from the blood through the kidney into the urine.

Nephrotic syndrome can be due to diseases confined to the kidney itself, including various forms of GLOMERULONEPHRITIS. It may also be a secondary manifestation of generalized systemic diseases such as HEPATITIS, MONONUCLEOSIS, and DIABETES MELLITUS. Certain drugs can cause nephrotic syndrome (for example, gold, penicillamine, and X-ray contrast medium).

neuralgia

A condition, caused by a variety of disorders, leading to pain experienced along the course of a nerve. The pain may be severe, dull, or stabbing. Usually nothing can be seen, but sometimes there is evidence of inflammation or damage to the affected nerve.

neurasthenia

A term previously used to describe a vague condition of nervous exhaustion and physical fatigue. An inability to concentrate, impairment of memory, and complaints such as "pressure in the head," "eyes ache when reading," palpitations, constipation, and impotence would lead to a diagnostic label of neurasthenia.

The condition was commonly diagnosed after a debilitating illness, particularly in the era before antibiotics, and was especially applied to professional or curious patients who required an "explanation" for their symptoms of fatigue. Nowadays it would be considered a normal convalescent stage in which the patient recovers spontaneously and progressively with rest.

neuritis

The inflammation or swelling of a nerve or nerves, usually associated with a degenerative process.

Degeneration of the nerve tissue occurs with consequent loss of sensation, impairment of muscular control, and symptoms that vary from severe pain to tingling and "pins and needles" brought about by movement of the involved part of the body—particularly if the nerve is stretched. A single nerve or multiple nerves may be involved and the causes may be *infective* (as in TUBERCULOSIS or LEPROSY), *mechanical* (as in compression, ARTHRITIS, or obstetric injury), *chemical* (as in arsenic poisoning or antibiotic sensitivity), *vascular* (as in ARTERIOSCLEROSIS or DIABETES MELLITUS), or *nutritional* (as in BERIBERI or ALCOHOLISM).

Treatment is aimed at relief of the cause, if it is specific, combined with rest, physical therapy, and analgesics (pain-killers). Correction of dietary inadequacy achieves a cure of the neuritis where malnutrition is the cause.

neurofibroma

A tumor of the connective tissue that forms the covering sheath of nerves. It may occur as a single swelling and reach a considerable size. Normally benign, the tumor may become malignant, but it usually gives rise to symptoms because it exerts pressure on neighboring structures, for example, the spinal cord or the nerve upon which the tumor lies. A neurofibroma may be evident as a swelling in the skin; treatment of the solitary tumor is surgical removal.

Neurofibromas may occur in considerable numbers as part of VON RECKLINGHAUSEN'S DISEASE (*multiple neurofibromatosis*). The tumors are associated with irregular brown-pigmented patches on the skin (*café au lait spots*), and they represent a defect in the development of the supporting tissue of the nervous system. When they give rise to symptoms they may require surgical treatment.

neuropathy

Any abnormal condition marked by swelling and wasting of nerves. Fragmentation of the nerve fibers can be seen on microscopic examination. The effects are variable but include loss of sensation of touch, pain, or temperature, muscle weakness and atrophy, and loss of tendon reflexes.

Management of neuropathy is mainly control of pain and protection of the weakened muscles from stretching and from excessive wasting (ATROPHY). Bed rest is recommended, and aspirin or a stronger analgesic is used to control the pain. Heat from lamps or warm baths is helpful. Splints and limb supports may be necessary to prevent deformity; when local muscle tenderness subsides, passive action, massage, and other forms of physical therapy are advisable. A well-balanced diet should be maintained and, where malnutrition was responsible for the neuropathy, vitamin supplements may be prescribed. Recovery depends on the extent of the original damage.

neurosis

A personality disorder in which a person has difficulty adapting to anxiety and internal conflict. The neurotic person maintains contact with reality, and his or her behavior does not violate social norms. However, behavior traits, thought processes, emotional responses, and some body functions may all be influenced by the neurosis.

A neurosis may be traced to the early learning experiences of life and to childhood in particular. The individual may suffer great conflict and discomfort in not being able to recognize his own failure to adapt to the anxiety that is the cause of his neurosis. Neuroses develop in the predisposed individual from childhood onward, and appear at the particular times of life when society and community living demand adaptation of the personality. For example, in adolescence when a sexual identity is being sought, in adult life when vocational demands or choices provoke stress, and in parenthood when responsibility for the dependence of others is felt as a challenge—in all these common circumstances of life, neurosis is prone to occur in the insecure individual.

Neurosis may appear as a response to the stress of a career and the responsibilities of marriage; it may occur in women at the menopause, when adjustment to a new life is required. In elderly couples the approach of retirement can sometimes provoke neurosis. It may appear anew in a middle-aged individual who has shown no previous neurotic tendencies.

Neurosis commonly takes the form of an exaggerated response to physical illness, which is a threat to security. In answer to fear, and as a consequence of exposure to anxiety-arousing situations, neurosis can become phobic, obsessive, compulsive, hysteric, or psychosomatic in its character. Recent thinking emphasizes the importance of an individual's feelings of loneliness and the shallowness of his interpersonal relations with other individuals. The neurotic person's expectations of helpers and physicians are often immature and demanding of immediate relief; thus these persons face a lifetime of disappointments and frustrations that further entrench the neurotic personality.

Acute and severe attacks may provoke psychosomatic symptoms that cause severe distress; *hyperventilation* (overbreathing) is one example another is the *panic attack* marked by an overwhelming sense of impending death. PHOBIAS with regard to crowds, open spaces, heights, dirt, or insects can be occupationally disabling, as can *compulsive neuroses* that involve ritual handwashing. *Genitourinary neurosis* can produce DYSPAREUNIA (pain experienced by a woman during sexual intercourse) or FRIGIDITY; a dermatological expression of neurosis may be a chronic skin RASH; gastrointestinal manifestations may include PEPTIC ULCERS or COLITIS; and, in particular, coronary ISCHEMIA (reduced blood supply to the heart muscle) is complicated by anxiety.

Diagnosis involves psychological testing and a careful medical history to ensure that physical illness is not causing the problem.

Treatment has to be skilled, prolonged, and supportive. Psychotherapy and behavioral techniques can assist in adjustment; medication may be prescribed, depending on the specific symptoms. Professional supportive therapy may help the individual to adjust to life's demands and largely overcome psychological discomfort.

neurotransmitters

Chemical substances that transmit nerve impulses between nerve cells.

The basic unit of the human nervous system is the nerve cell (*neuron*), which has a long extension called an *axon* that comes almost in physical contact with muscle fibers, glands, or other nerve cells. Across this microscopic gap (the *synapse*) an electrochemical impulse is transmitted from the axon of one neuron to the dendrites of an adjacent neuron, or to a gland cell to cause secretion, or to a muscle to cause contraction. The transmission of the impulse is achieved by the release of neurotransmitters from special parts of the nerve cell membrane.

Neurotransmitters are not all identified chemically, but they include such substances as acetylcholine, dopamine, norepinephrine, serotonin, beta-endorphin, gamma-aminobutyric acid (GABA), and glutamate. The neurotransmitter is stored on one side of the synapse with the reactive site on the other side. The signal ceases when the neurotransmitter is chemically changed, diffuses away from the synapse, or is reabsorbed.

The neurotransmitter is vulnerable to drugs or

THE PERIPHERAL NERVOUS SYSTEM

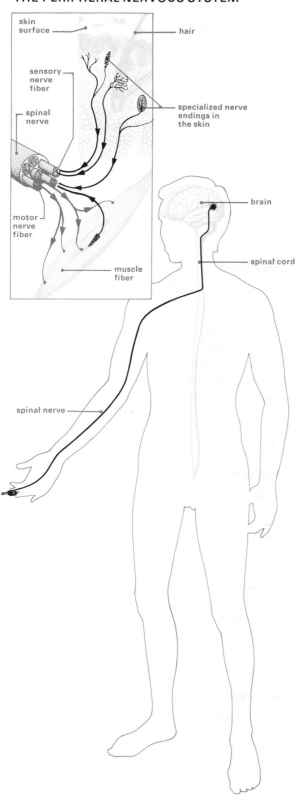

skin surface

hair

sensory nerve fiber

spinal nerve

specialized nerve endings in the skin

motor nerve fiber

muscle fiber

brain

spinal cord

spinal nerve

toxins that modify its synthesis or action. Anything that interferes with its breakdown will cause prolonged action (as in TETANUS), while substances that delay its release have equally dramatic effects (as in paralysis due to curare poisoning). Many drugs act by their effect on neurotransmitters, for example, certain drugs used to control blood pressure.

nevus (birthmark)

A type of skin discoloration. It is due to an anomaly in the embryonic development of the skin, particularly affecting the blood vessels of the subcutaneous layer in small or wide areas.

Nevi vary considerably in size and appearance. The most commonly recognized type is the "strawberry" birthmark. Others are the "spider" nevus, a tiny star-shaped discoloration commonly seen in adults, and the quite disfiguring "port wine stain" (*nevus flammeus*) that can occupy half the face of the newborn.

Nevi affect the sexes equally. They may appear at birth or soon after; occasionally they develop within the first two years of life. They affect all ethnic groups, from the "blue" nevus seen in Mongolians to the "pale" nevus seen in blacks. There is no known cause and the suggestion that nevi are intrauterine "pressure" marks is untrue.

Nevi may be single or multiple, faint in discoloration or very obvious. *Pigmented nevi*, containing an excess of melanin that makes them much darker than normal skin, may grow hairs that are thick, black, and profuse. *Vascular nevi*—those containing blood vessels—deepen in color when a child cries or exercises, as the incomplete blood pathways become engorged with blood. Nevi usually have demarcated borders and rarely increase in size.

The "strawberry" birthmark usually disappears as the child grows, since deposits of subcutaneous fat tend to hide it; such a nevus therefore requires no treatment. Pigmented nevi with hairs also may

The illustration (left) shows how the central nervous system (brain and spinal cord) connects with the peripheral nervous system—in this case a spinal nerve supplying the fingers. When receptors in the skin are stimulated, signals travel up the sensory nerve fibers to the spinal cord and brain. The brain processes this incoming information and then sends a return message down a parallel motor pathway to the muscles of the fingers so that an appropriate movement is made.

NEVUS

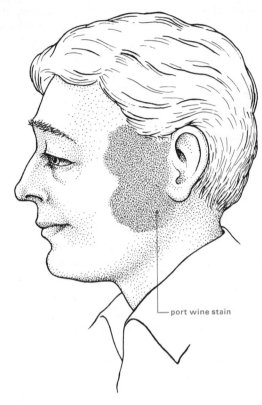

port wine stain

A nevus, or birthmark, is an area of discolored skin that results from a congenital malformation of surface blood vessels. Certain types of nevi have descriptive names, such as "strawberry nevus" and the "port wine stain" (illustrated here).

be left; in time they may fade or disappear, but occasionally they require surgical excision or other treatment such as electrolysis, diathermy cauterization, or "freezing." Spider nevi respond to electrolysis. There is no truly effective treatment for a port wine stain, but a cosmetician can prepare a special cream that matches the person's skin to provide a means of concealing the flaw.

Any nevus that begins to bleed or undergoes a sudden change—such as a darkening in color or a change in shape—must be seen by a dermatologist. These changes may indicate a cancerous process.

night blindness

A condition in which vision is fairly normal in good light but defective in dim light. The technical term is *nyctalopia*. It is primarily a symptom of severe vitamin-A deficiency, but it occurs also in RETINITIS PIGMENTOSA, an inherited degenerative disorder of the retina.

The ability of the eye to adapt to varying degrees of light and dark depends on photoreceptors in the retina. One type of photoreceptor, the rods, mediates vision in dim light. The rods contain pigment known as rhodopsin, or "visual purple," which is temporarily bleached by light. The speed of the eye's adaptability to dark depends on the speed with which rhodopsin is reformed in darkness, which in turn depends on vitamin A.

If night blindness is due to vitamin-A deficiency, treatment is by vitamin-A replacement; if it is due to retinitis pigmentosa, there is no effective treatment.

nonspecific urethritis

A sexually transmitted inflammation of the urethra that cannot be attributed to GONORRHEA. The symptoms include pain and burning on urination and urinary frequency. There is a urethral discharge. The start of symptoms is linked to sexual intercourse and is confined to the sexually active. Nonspecific urethritis, which is more conspicuous in men, is caused by *Chlamydia trachomatis* and *Ureaplasma urealyticum.* Tetracycline is effective.

nosebleed

Known medically as *epistaxis*, nosebleed is a fairly common occurrence and usually results from simple trauma to the nose, including picking. Other much less common causes include high blood pressure, abnormalities in the blood-clotting system, and tumors of the nose and sinuses.

Frequent and recurrent attacks may require cauterization of the affected blood vessel by a specialist.

See also *Bleeding* in the section on **First Aid.**

nystagmus

Involuntary, rapid, rhythmic flickering movements of the eyeball—back and forth, up and down, around, or mixed.

Normal nystagmus occurs when a person is looking at scenery from a moving vehicle. Otherwise, the causes of abnormal nystagmus fall into four main groups: (1) defects in vision in which the eye does not receive sufficient visual stimuli for it to fix its gaze; (2) disturbances of the elaborate balance-maintaining mechanisms in the ear which have nervous connections to the eye; (3) diseases of the nervous system; and (4) the common congenital nystagmus, usually of no medical importance.

Nystagmus usually does not produce symptoms, but it may sometimes produce vertigo or double vision. Treatment depends on the cause.

obesity

The excessive accumulation of body fat, mainly under the skin and in the abdomen. Generally a person is considered obese when his weight is more than 20 percent above the ideal weight for persons of his build and height. Another commonly used method for assessing obesity is the measurement of skinfold thickness, because a large proportion of the fat in storage is found just beneath the skin.

Obesity predisposes humans to conditions such as DIABETES MELLITUS, ATHEROSCLEROSIS, BACKACHE, and OSTEOARTHRITIS.

Most cases of obesity are due to an energy input (in the form of the caloric value of food eaten) that is greater than the energy expenditure. Obesity runs in families, and juvenile-onset obesity is associated with an increase in the actual number of fat cells, possibly as a result of injudicious overfeeding. Such people have life-long problems. Maturity-onset obesity is not associated with an increased number of fat cells and is easily controlled by forming healty eating habits.

Often there is an emotional component to obesity, comfort being found in eating; PSYCHOTHERAPY may then be required to help achieve weight loss.

For an extended discussion, see *The Wellness Diet* in the section on **Wellness**.

obsession

A repetition of irrational thoughts, doubts, actions, or fears of which the person is aware but which he cannot conquer, however hard he tries. One obsession may lead to another. For example, an obsession with contamination may result in repeated handwashing; the obsession drives the person to wash his hands repeatedly even though he knows they are already clean.

Obsession may be a symptom of several psychiatric disorders or of organic brain disease. It may also exist alone—in which case it is referred to as an *obsessional trait.*

Treatment is essentially by PSYCHOTHERAPY, but if the symptom has led to anxiety, tension, or depression, appropriate drug therapy may be required.

occult blood

Small quantities of blood in the feces that are not apparent to the eye and are detectable only by special laboratory tests.

If occult blood is detected it suggests that there is bleeding somewhere in the gastrointestinal tract, and further tests will be necessary.

Since the bleeding may be intermittent, the laboratory tests have to show no occult blood in the stool on several occasions before the physician can be fairly certain that there is no bleeding in the gastrointestinal tract. Blood from ingested meat (even if cooked) can give a positive result to the test; thus, the patient should go on a meat-free diet for about three days before the test.

occupational diseases and disorders

Refers to a group of disorders related to repeated exposure to one or more factors in the working environment.

Almost any organ system in the body can be adversely affected by conditions at work. Hearing can be impaired by continued contact with very noisy machines such as jackhammers, jet engines, or heavy construction equipment.

The eyes need protection wherever grinding is being done or caustic chemicals are in use. Skin rashes can be caused by contact with irritants or with substances that cause allergic reactions.

The most common types of occupational diseases involve the lungs. Lung disorders such as PNEUMOCONIOSIS, SILICOSIS, and ASBESTOSIS occur when very fine dust particles in the environment pass through the body's physical defenses (for example, the hairs in the nostrils or the cilia in the bronchi) to reach the air sacs of the lungs. There, over a number of years, they may induce fibrous reaction that in some cases impairs breathing and produces chronic disability. In other cases they may produce no symptoms and be detected only by X-ray studies.

Industrial poisoning was once a fairly common occupational disorder. It may be acute, as with a leak of noxious fumes (for example, ammonia) into the environment; or it may occur insidiously, such as occurs in lead poisoning—although this is less common now since many high-risk industries have begun testing their workers at regular intervals for the presence of lead.

Some cancers may result from occupational hazards. For example, cancer of the scrotum was recognized more than two hundred years ago to be an occupational disease of chimney sweeps. Scrotal cancer is still seen, mainly in those who work with cooling oils in the engineering industry. Cancer of the bladder was at one time quite common in those working with aniline dyes; some of these dyes are no longer produced, but cases have been reported in persons working with other amines. Recently there has been medical interest in investigating the incidence of liver tumors occurring in those who work with vinyl chloride and of MESOTHELIOMA in those exposed to asbestos.

The most important aspect of occupational disease is prevention. Workers should take care to minimize exposure to any factor likely to cause an occupational disease.

Newer and safer equipment is constantly being designed, and safer substitutes for materials such as asbestos are being developed. Unfortunately, new developments often bring new and unforeseen hazards. More and more occupational diseases are being recognized, although many conditions may not easily be recognized as occupational diseases because of the long time they take to develop. A disease may sometimes appear several years after a person has ceased contact with the alleged causal agent.

Oedipus complex

Excessive love of a boy for his mother, persisting into adolescence and beyond. It is named after the mythical Greek king who killed his father and married his mother.

Freud suggested that between the third and sixth years, an Oedipal situation may arise in a boy, who experiences sexual desire for his mother but hostile and aggressive feelings toward his father. These feelings must be repressed, and may cause conflict and symptoms later in life. The corresponding situation for girls, who are said to be sexually attracted to the father, is the *Electra complex.*

oliguria

A reduced ability to make or excrete urine. It may be caused by KIDNEY DISEASE or a urinary tract blockage.

onychia

Inflammation of the nailbed. The most common cause of the inflammation is infection of the root. The nail often is lost but it will regrow if the matrix is not permanently injured. If the matrix is chronically inflamed, the nail that forms is discolored and cracked.

Onychia is common among persons whose hands have to be immersed in water for long periods. The skin around the nails becomes red, swollen, and painful, while the nails themselves lose their natural gloss, become opaque, and—in severe cases—may become loose and drop off.

onychomycosis

Fungal infection of the nail. It is the most common inflammatory nail disorder and may be caused by a number of fungal species, which are identified by examining nail scrapings in the laboratory.

Fungal infection is common in people whose resistance to infection is low, such as diabetics or anyone taking corticosteroid drugs. It is also common in sufferers of PARONYCHIA (inflammation of skin around the nail), usually people whose work involves immersing the hands in water for long periods, or people with ingrowing toenails.

Onychomycosis is chronic but painless. The nail lacks luster and is opaque and brittle. It may show striations, have a "worm-eaten" appearance, or have a surface of heaped-up flakes. Paronychia of the surrounding soft tissues may cause pain and tenderness, with the oozing of blood serum or pus—especially if there is a superimposed bacterial infection.

Onychomycosis is treated with grisofulvin (an antifungal drug) applied to the nail or taken orally—the more effective method. Treatment usually has to be continued for months or years and even then may not achieve a permanent cure. Filing the affected nails may shorten the course of the disease by removing infected nail. Sometimes the entire nail has to be removed. Any underlying condition should also be treated, as should any superimposed bacterial infection. Persons should keep the nails clean and dry and footwear should never be shared.

ophthalmoplegia

Paralysis or weakness of the muscles that control eye movements, and dilate and contract the pupil. If there is only mild weakness, the earliest symptom is double vision. If the muscles are actually paralyzed, it may be obvious to an observer that the eye does not move in certain directions.

Ophthalmoplegia can be produced by any condition affecting the muscles themselves or the nerves that supply them. Head injuries, STROKE, MENINGITIS, ENCEPHALITIS, brain tumors, and DIABETES MELLITUS are the usual causes. The condition also occurs in HYPERTHYROIDISM and MYASTHENIA GRAVIS. The treatment depends on the cause.

orchitis

Inflammation of one or both testicles.

Acute orchitis usually is the result of a generalized infection such as MUMPS, SCARLET FEVER, or TYPHOID FEVER. In other cases it may result from the spread of infection from neighboring structures such as the epididymis, the seminal vesicles, or the prostate, or from other distant structures via the bloodstream.

Chronic orchitis may be caused by SYPHILIS; it is often unnoticed since it is painless. TUBERCULOSIS is another cause of chronic orchitis; here the testis is hard and nodular and may be mistaken for a tumor.

In orchitis the testis enlarges and there is severe pain in the scrotum, which is tender, red, and swollen. The person usually has a fever and a general feeling of being unwell (malaise). Severe acute orchitis may result in some wasting away of the testis (occasionally enough to cause sterility).

In treatment the scrotum is supported and raised and ice packs are applied during the acute phase. Analgesics such as aspirin and codeine will relieve pain. There is no specific treatment for mumps orchitis, but other infections may be treated with appropriate antibiotics.

orgasm

The climax of sexual activity.

The normal response to sexual stimulation can be divided into four phases: excitement, plateau, orgasm, and resolution. In the first two phases a number of physiological changes occur; these include not only changes in the breasts and genitals of both sexes but also flushing of the skin and a rising pulse rate and blood pressure.

During the *orgasmic phase*, which is the shortest of the four phases, there is intense physical activity: involuntary contractions of various muscles, thrusting movements of the pelvis, a further quickening of the pulse and breathing rate, and a further rise in blood pressure. In the male orgasm, there is contraction of the prostate, seminal vesicles, and urethra. In the female, the vaginal muscles contract, but this may be inapparent. The female cervix dilates and the male ejaculates semen.

Orgasm is followed by the phase of resolution during which there is a relaxation of sexual tension and a reversal of the physiological processes of sexual excitement. Restimulation of the woman during this phase may induce another orgasm, but in the man there is a variable period during which restimulation does not produce another orgasm.

orthodontics

The branch of dentistry concerned with the study of the growth and development of the jaws and teeth and with the correction of irregularities of the teeth (such as abnormal alignment).

Orthodontic treatment may be required for several reasons—in addition to the obvious aesthetic and psychological value of having regular, symmetrical teeth. Some positions of teeth may result in poor coordination of the chewing muscles, giving rise to symptoms in the joint between the jaw and the rest of the skull. If teeth are overcrowded, the teeth and gums cannot be cleaned effectively (naturally or artificially), and the person may become prone to gum trouble and cavities. Finally, orthodontics may be required to facilitate other forms of dental treatment—such as certain types of oral or dental surgery, and the fitting of dentures, bridges, or crowns.

The basic principle of orthodontic treatment is to apply pressure to the teeth to direct their growth into the position required. Teeth may be tipped, rotated, or repositioned entirely. Some dentists use devices that exert a small pressure continuously, while others prefer to exert stronger pressure with intermittent periods of rest.

Pressure is applied by a variety of devices, such as wires, braces, screws, wedges, and rubber bands. Some can be attached entirely within the mouth, whereas others need "extra-oral" attachments by bands around the head or neck. Some are fixed, whereas others have to be removed and replaced by the person for cleaning. Treatment usually has to be continued for months or even years, and several courses of treatment may be needed as a child grows.

There are limits to what orthodontics can achieve: It is not the solution to every speech defect or to all types of malalignment of the upper and lower jaws. Even so, children should be encouraged to cooperate with orthodontic treatment since good results are more likely while the jaws and teeth are still growing.

orthoptics

For the development of normal vision it is essential that during infancy and childhood clear visual images be focused on the retinas of both eyes. The *retina* is the sensitive membrane inside the back of the eye, corresponding to the film of a camera. Retinal images cause complex messages to be passed back along the optic nerves to the brain. Later in life, these nerve impulses merely carry visual information to the brain, but in the early years of life they have an additional function. It is this function with which orthoptics is primarily concerned.

Although the nerve connections with the brain are present at birth, they are not functionally fully active. Correct nerve impulses "switch on" these connections. If this is prevented—by barriers to proper visual input—normal vision will not develop. These links can be made only during the period of neurological "plasticity" that lasts from birth until the age of seven or eight years. Thereafter, no further development is possible.

In general, it may be said that the maximum level of visual acuity achievable cannot exceed the level experienced during this "plastic" developmental period. Plasticity is not, of course, lost suddenly at the age of eight. It is maximal soon after birth and then declines progressively. So the longer the barrier to clear vision exists, the poorer

will be the ultimate result. Visual defect caused in this way is called AMBLYOPIA (Greek: *ambly*, "dull," + *ops*, "eye").

Failure to form normal retinal images may result from several causes, with all of which the orthoptist is concerned: congenital CATARACT, uncorrected severe eyelid droop with coverage of the pupil (*blepharoptosis*), severe focusing errors, especially ASTIGMATISM, or a large inequality in the focus of the two eyes so that the better eye is used preferentially. The most common cause of amblyopia is squint (STRABISMUS) and much of the time of the orthoptist is taken up with the management of children suffering from strabismus.

In medical usage, the term *squint* does not mean "screwing up" or narrowing the eyelids. Nor does it mean that both eyes consistently turn inward or outward. Squint is the condition in which the neuromuscular control of the eyes is so out of balance that only one eye can be directed at the object of interest. The other eye may point inward (*convergent squint*) or outward (*divergent squint*) or even upward or downward (*vertical squint*).

If both eyes are perceiving while looking at different objects, the result will be double vision. When squint begins in adult life—usually as a result of disease or injury—there is almost always severe and distressing DOUBLE VISION (*diplopia*), which unless treated by surgery or other means is permanent.

But when an otherwise normal young child develops a squint (and this occurs in about 4 percent of children) another factor operates. Double vision certainly occurs, and one can often, for the first few days after onset, observe the child deliberately shutting or covering one eye. But because of the plasticity of the nervous system, the brain makes a rapid adaptation to relieve the doubling. Within a very short time the child ceases to show any signs of discomfort and carries on happily, apparently quite unconcerned by the squint. The child is now using one eye only, and the brain has ceased to accept impulses from the squinting eye.

This adaptation is called *suppression*, and from the moment it starts, the visual development in the squinting eye stops. If untreated, the result is permanent amblyopia. Ironically, and unfortunately, the greatest input disturbance is caused by very small-angle squints and it is in these that the suppression, and the resulting amblyopia, is worst. This is not really surprising. If one eye is just looking at the side of the nose, the brain has little to ignore, compared with an overlapping doubling of two images.

In general, the earlier the onset of squint, the more serious is the failure to provide treatment. There is, however, one exception to this rule. Double vision is possible only if the power of simultaneous perception with the two eyes (*binocular vision*) has developed, and this does not occur until some time after birth. Babies *born* with squints are unable to develop binocular vision, so they never have double vision and the squint does not cause amblyopia. Instead, these babies learn the trick of using whichever eye happens to be pointing in the required direction and transiently suppressing the vision in the other eye. They are never, at any time, capable of simultaneous perception.

Squint should *never* be ignored and treatment should always be sought at the earliest possible stage. Early treatment is usually successful. It consists of a full history taking and a careful examination of the eyes, including a refraction after atropine drops have been instilled. Glasses are often necessary. The most important part of the treatment is the judicious and well-timed use of patching (firm covering) of the straight eye so as to force the child to use the amblyopic eye. This is often difficult as the child naturally resents being forced to see badly for a time. Failure to achieve effective occlusion is almost always due to parents being inadequtely informed of the full implications.

Patching, if done early enough, will almost always restore vision, and the aim is to achieve balanced vision and an "alternating" squint. Double vision commonly recurs, and this is a good sign. Surgical correction is often needed at this stage to complete the treatment.

osteitis

Literally, inflammation of bone.

Inflammatory disease of bone commonly is due to infection and often affects the marrow as well, in which case it is known as OSTEOMYELITIS. The term *osteitis* tends to be used for a number of other bone disorders, not necessarily inflammatory in nature. Some are the result of biochemical disorders, while others are inherited or of unknown cause.

Osteitis deformans, also known as PAGET'S DISEASE, is of unknown cause. There is excessive bone destruction and subsequent spontaneous repair; the

repair takes place in a disorganized fashion leading to deformities. Often there are no symptoms at first, but some individuals suffer pain. Later the back may become hunched, the legs bowed, and the skull enlarged; often a waddling gait develops and bones fracture easily.

Complications include kidney stones (the calcium coming from the destruction of bone) and bone deformities that may press on nerves and cause blindness or deafness. In a few cases, cancer of the bone may develop. Several drugs are now available to suppress the excessive activity of bone.

Osteitis fibrosa cystica is a bone disease caused by the overactivity of the parathyroid glands (HYPERPARATHYROIDISM). The excessive amounts of parathyroid hormone remove calcium from the bone so that cystic demineralized areas develop throughout the skeleton. Symptoms range from back pain, joint pain, and other bone pains to fractures, loss of height, and a hunched back. Treatment involves correction of the parathyroid disorder, which often is due to benign tumors in the gland. They can be removed surgically.

SYPHILIS, whether congenital or acquired later in life, can cause a type of osteitis. In children, inflammation of the bone, cartilage, and periosteum (outer lining of the bone) may pass unnoticed because it produces no symptoms. In some cases, however, fractures may occur and pain may prevent the child from moving the limbs. In adults the bone involvement usually takes the form of localized areas of destruction by "gummata" (the characteristic syphilitic lesions).

Osteitis fibrosa disseminata and *osteitis condensans generalisata* are two rare bone disorders. The former is of unknown cause and is characterized by fibrous overgrowths in bone. The latter is an inherited condition in which the bone becomes very dense.

osteoarthritis

A degenerative, "wear and tear" disease of the joints, usually accompanied by pain and stiffness.

X-ray studies show that more than 80 percent of people between the ages of 55 and 64 show changes characteristic of the disease; of these, about 20 percent complain of symptoms. Osteoarthritis causes a great deal of pain and discomfort to a large number of people of both sexes, although women tend to suffer more severely than men. The cause of the disease is not fully understood, but it may be described as a degenerative disorder developing with age.

Many sufferers give a history of prior injury, sometimes many years before; any fracture or joint disease that results in injury to the joint cartilage or misalignment of the joint predisposes a person to the development of the disease. The large weight-bearing joints of the lower limbs are particularly affected, but osteoarthritis also can affect the fingers, elbows, shoulders, and the vertebrae. Occupations involving the use of other joints may, in time, produce signs of the disease in unexpected places.

The basic change in the affected joints is loss of the *articular cartilage*, which normally protects the ends of the bones and provides a smooth working surface for movement. The exposed ends of the bones become hard and shiny, and at their margins small spurs of bone develop that are known as *osteophytes*. The changes are evident in X-ray examinations which show the osteophytes and the narrowing of the joint space where the cartilage has been lost. The membranes lining the joint (*synovial membranes*) become thickened, and there may be an effusion of fluid into the joint, which causes it to swell.

The person suffers increasing pain on movement of the joint, and the joint becomes stiff. Usually the pain becomes worse as the day progresses, and the affected limb is difficult to use. In advanced cases of the disease, joint function may be lost and the muscle acting on the joint may waste (atrophy). Grating (*crepitus*) may be felt in the joint on movement. Where the fingers are affected, small swellings may develop beside the finger joints. As the disease progresses, the hands may become deformed. In the back and neck, degeneration of the intervertebral joints with osteophyte formation may involve the spinal nerves as they leave the spinal cord and produce neurologic symptoms.

The treatment of milder cases includes reduction of body weight in those who are obese. As with all common diseases that are difficult to relieve, a great many drugs are offered on the market, but most of them have an irritant action on the stomach, which may provoke the development of a peptic ulcer. They must, therefore, be used with caution. The most useful drug is aspirin, but it too has undesirable side effects and cannot be used in all cases. Orthopedic surgery has improved the treatment of severe cases with the introduction of artificial joints. It is now often possible to replace a painful, diseased hip joint

with success. Also, in many cases the knee can be replaced, although the operation is not yet as uniformly satisfactory as a hip replacement.

osteoma

A benign tumor composed of bone.

Osteomas usually arise from normal bone, but they also may occur in other structures anywhere in the body. They commonly occur in the bones of the skull (including the sinuses) and the lower jaw.

The cause of osteomas is not known. The common symptom is the presence of a hard, painless lump. Other symptoms may result from pressure of the tumor on nerves or other structures, although these symptoms are quite rare.

Osteomas are not malignant. Treatment is surgical removal, which is indicated only when there are troublesome symptoms, such as pain due to pressure, or for cosmetic reasons.

osteomalacia

Also known as *adult rickets*, this disease primarily affects women and is characterized by a softening of the bones, causing them to be painful and liable to distortion.

Osteomalacia is caused by lack of vitamin D and occurs as a result of inadequate diet, inadequate absorption in the intestine, abnormal metabolism, inadequate sun exposure, increased vitamin requirements during pregnancy, or long-term anticonvulsant drug therapy. The lack of vitamin D leads, in turn, to decreased absorption of calcium from the intestine and to low levels of calcium in the blood. The lack of calcium causes the parathyroid gland in the neck to produce a hormone that stimulates the removal of calcium from the bones. The resulting lack of calcium in the bones is responsible for the softness of the bones seen in osteomalacia.

Osteomalacia causes bowing of the long bones, shortening of the vertebrae, and flattening of the pelvis with narrowing of the outlet. The calcium deficiency also causes muscle weakness and loss of appetite and weight. Blood levels of calcium and other substances may help to confirm the diagnosis.

Treatment of this disease depends on the underlying cause. In cases due to lack of sunlight exposure (ultraviolet light in sunshine synthesizes the production of vitamin D in the skin), anticonvulsant therapy, or lack of vitamin D in the diet, vitamin supplementation can be given. For cases of malabsorption, either much higher doses of medication should be given or ultraviolet light therapy should be used. Persons with other underlying diseases that lead to vitamin-D deficiency need to be evaluated and treated on an individual basis.

Vitamin-D deficiency can be and is prevented in most Americans by adding the vitamin to dairy products; but osteomalacia is still quite common in the elderly and the poor, and in those with disease of the kidneys or small intestine.

osteomyelitis

An infection of the bone and bone marrow.

Acute osteomyelitis can be caused by bacteria from an infection in the body, the bacteria reaching the bone via the bloodstream. It is usually a childhood disease—most often seen in boys—and primarily affects an area in a long bone in the arm or leg. When this disease is seen in adults, it can be the result of surgery, urinary tract infections, or long-term SICKLE-CELL DISEASE. Osteomyelitis often occurs at the site of recent trauma, such as a sharp blow.

The infection takes hold in the bone and leads to extreme pain, tenderness, swelling, and fever. If appropriate antibiotic treatment is not begun, the condition may become life-threatening. In cases of much pus formation, the area may need to be surgically drained.

Chronic osteomyelitis is a condition in which the acute stage is over but the person continues to have a local infection with pain and pus formation and drainage. In long-standing cases, when treatment has not healed the infection, major surgery may be needed. This can involve removal of dead bone tissue or complete scraping of tissue and skin down to the bone. In severe cases, amputation may be necessary. Some persons with acute osteomyelitis appear to recover completely only to develop the chronic form years later.

osteoporosis

A disease in which the bones are generally thinned, owing to a loss of organic matrix with a corresponding decrease in calcified tissue.

After the age of about 20, bones become progressively thinner. When this thinning proceeds faster than normal, it leads to osteoporosis. The disease is common in old age—especially in women, in whom it is due to estrogen deficiency.

Osteoporosis also occurs in a number of other conditions at any age. These include complications following corticosteroid therapy, CUSHING'S SYNDROME, HYPERTHYROIDISM, ACROMEGALY, RHEUMATOID ARTHRITIS, and other diseases that lead to immobilization.

The disease may be symptomless, or it may cause pain—commonly in the back, ribs, or limbs. Vertebrae may collapse suddenly, causing severe back pain; in any case, they contract gradually as the disease progresses, leading to a loss in height and an increased curvature of the spine (KYPHOSIS). Osteoporosis of the femur is the underlying cause of most hip fractures in the elderly.

The main treatment for pain is the administration of analgesic drugs. Support of the affected spine by a corset may also help, and physical therapy and exercises may aid the muscles of the spine in supporting the vertebrae, thus minimizing or preventing pain.

Osteoporosis that occurs as the result of another disease demands treatment of the primary disease. Corticosteroid therapy should be avoided or stopped if possible.

Specific therapies for osteoporosis include the administration of estrogens in women, androgens in men, calcium, fluoride supplements, and a diet high in calcium and protein. (Chicken and fish should be emphasized over red meats.) The range of treatments used shows that none is entirely satisfactory. Prevention is the best treatment.

Osteoporosis itself does not shorten life expectancy; but fractures, especially of the hip, and underlying diseases may lead to premature death.

osteosarcoma

A highly malignant bone tumor.

Osteosarcomas may occur at any age, but are more common in children and young adults. They usually occur in the limbs but may affect any bone.

The usual symptom is pain. Sometimes there is swelling and tenderness; occasionally the diagnosis is made only when the affected bone fractures.

Osteosarcomas are malignant, and the major spread of the cancer cells (METASTASIS) occurs to the lungs. X-ray examinations are helpful in making the diagnosis and in determining whether metastasis has occurred.

Diagnosis is made by biopsy of the tumor. Osteosarcomas are managed best by a combination of surgery, radiotherapy, and chemotherapy.

The prognosis for persons with malignant bone tumors is not hopeless. In many cases these lesions respond well to aggressive treatment.

ostomy

Literally, an artificial stoma (pore) or opening in an organ. In practice, the term is used to refer to a surgical procedure in which an artificial opening is made between two hollow organs or between an organ and the skin. Examples of the latter are the common COLOSTOMY and ILEOSTOMY (see under **Procedures**). Other types include *cecostomy* (a type of temporary colostomy) and *cystostomy* (opening into the urinary or gall bladders).

In a colostomy, the artificial opening is made in the large intestine. Colostomies can be temporary or permanent.

A *temporary* colostomy usually is performed when only the lower part of the colon (large intestine) is affected by cancer or another disease and the surgeon wishes to divert the bowel contents to facilitate treatment. The temporary procedure is indicated also if severe inflammation of the intestinal wall is present. In the operation, the surgeon creates an opening in the abdomen and connects it to the tip of the loop of the transverse colon (the middle portion of the large bowel). About three months after the disease responsible for the temporary colostomy has been successfully treated, the continuity of the bowel is restored and the opening is closed.

If cancer affects the upper or entire large intestine, or if inflammation is so severe that the entire rectum must be removed, a *permanent* colostomy is performed. In this procedure, the lowest section of healthy intestine is fastened to an opening in the abdominal wall. The opening is positioned to one side of the midline so that the collection bag for intestinal contents is in a comfortable site. Recently developed bags need to be changed less often and cause less skin irritation than in the past. Medications are available to improve adhesion and reduce odor. With careful attention to diet to minimize problems with excess gas production or diarrhea, most persons with a permanent colostomy can lead normal lives.

An ileostomy is the surgical formation of an opening through the abdominal wall into the ileum, the lower part of the small intestine. Ileostomies are necessary when the colon or the colon and rectum have to be removed; the opening then acts as an artificial anus through which the contents of the small intestine leave the body instead of passing along the colon to the natural anus. As with a colostomy, an external bag collects excreta. With proper diet, patients can perform normal physical and social activities.

otitis externa

Inflammation of the outer canal of the ear. It is a common and usually trivial condition.

Otitis externa causes pain in the ear that may be severe and a discharge of matter. It may be worsened by movements such as chewing and yawning, but hearing seldom is affected.

Causes include foreign bodies in the ear (and unskilled attempts to remove them), moisture (for instance, if ears are not dried after swimming), cosmetics, hair sprays, and allergy to drugs contained in eardrops. The ear often is infected with bacteria or fungi, but this infection is frequently a *consequence* of otitis externa and not the primary cause; it may lead to a painful boil in the outer ear.

Most cases of otitis externa resolve spontaneously without treatment, but a doctor should be consulted if the condition persists or grows worse for more than a day or two. The ear may be made more comfortable by moistened gauze or bland eardrops. Antibiotics may be required by mouth for an infected otitis externa. Drops containing antibiotics or other drugs are commonly prescribed.

Otitis externa tends to recur, so the person should try to discover the cause and avoid it in the future. Children with otitis externa should not swim until the condition is fully healed, and even then recurrence is common. Otitis externa caused by a fungus infection may take months of treatment to eradicate.

otitis interna

Inflammation of the inner ear. Also called *labyrinthitis.*

The inner ear, or labyrinth, contains the organs of balance and of hearing, both of which may be affected by the spread of infection from the middle ear (see OTITIS MEDIA); the person suffers from VERTIGO. The main danger is spread of infection to the meninges, the membranes covering the brain. Treatment is bed rest with the administration of appropriate antibiotics and perhaps with the addition of medication to relieve the vertigo.

otitis media

Inflammation of the middle ear (the part just behind the eardrum).

Acute otitis media is most common in infants and young children; about 20 percent of children under a year of age have at least one attack.

The middle ear is connected to the back of the nose by the Eustachian tube. In children the tube is short and wide, and the lower end is easily blocked by enlarged ADENOIDS. Infection spreads freely from the nose and throat to the middle ear.

In acute otitis media the eardrum is red, inflamed, and swollen. In severe cases it may burst, or the doctor may incise it to relieve pressure (*myringotomy*). The condition can cause severe illness with fever, vomiting, diarrhea, and failure to feed. In infants there is often no reason for the parents to suspect that the ear is the site of infection; older children usually complain of earache. Deafness may occur during the attacks, but it usually resolves with treatment. The infection may give rise to complications such as MENINGITIS or MASTOIDITIS, although this is rare with current therapy.

Acute otitis media usually responds rapidly to treatment with antibiotics—commonly penicillin—although many cases resolve spontaneously within forty-eight hours or so. Analgesics are needed for the pain; soothing eardrops also may be helpful. In children, ephedrine nose drops help to reestablish drainage of the ear through the Eustachian tube. Successfully treated otitis media has no long-term complications. Attacks may recur, however, and sometimes removal of the adenoids is helpful in preventing them.

Chronic otitis media usually is the result of repeated attacks of acute otitis media. The eardrum is scarred, thickened, and often perforated. The person may be partially deaf in the affected ear, from which there is usually a discharge. The main risk is the development of a *cholesteatoma*, a progressive accumulation of debris that may erode bone and cause further damage to the ear and even to the brain. A cholesteatoma requires skilled surgical treatment.

Secretory otitis media ("glue ear") is a painless condition, most common in children, in which the middle ear fills with viscous fluid. Usually this is the result of recurrent or untreated otitis media, but in a few cases the cause may not be known. The condition leads to deafness and there is a risk of permanent ear damage. Treatment involves long-term drainage of the ear by myringotomy or by the insertion of tubes through the eardrum to drain the fluid.

otosclerosis

A condition that occurs and causes deafness in about 1 percent of the U.S. population. Otosclerosis is the abnormal formation of spongy bone in the inner ear which causes the stapes, one of the tiny sound-conducting bones in the middle ear, to become immobilized. The amplification of sound, normally achieved by these small bones, is thus halted and deafness results.

Otosclerosis often runs in families as part of some rare disease complex. Otherwise its cause is unknown.

Deafness usually starts in the teens or early 20s and progresses slowly. It may remain static for many years or it may progress more rapidly for a

OTOSCOPE

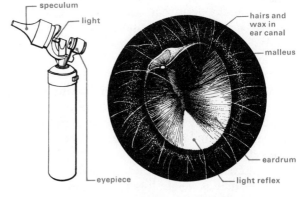

speculum
light
hairs and wax in ear canal
malleus
eardrum
light reflex
eyepiece

VIEW OF LEFT EARDRUM

Otoscopes are instruments for visualizing the eardrums. A healthy eardrum has a pearly appearance and strongly reflects light from the otoscope as a conical "light reflex." In middle ear infections, the eardrum looks red, a fluid level might be seen through it, and the light reflex is absent.

period, especially in pregnant women. Usually it affects one ear before the other and shows itself first by a ringing sensation in the ear (TINNITUS). The diagnosis is suggested by the results of hearing tests.

Otosclerosis cannot be prevented, but usually it can be treated successfully by a surgical procedure called STAPEDECTOMY (see under **Procedures**). The stapes is removed and replaced by a Teflon or wire substitute that restores the vibration characteristics of the chain of tiny bones. The operation is extremely delicate—these tiny ear bones are the smallest bones of the body—and carries a 2 percent risk of causing total deafness in the ear, but thc other 98 percent of persons treated achieve greatly improved hearing within two or three weeks. It is impossible to predict which persons will become deaf, but most sufferers are prepared to accept the risk.

ovarian cyst

A swelling of the ovary, containing fluid.

Ovarian cysts are very common, particularly in women between the ages of 30 and 60. They may be single or multiple and can occur in one or both ovaries. Most are benign, but approximately 15 percent are malignant.

Some ovarian cysts are related to the persistent changes that take place in the ovary during the menstrual cycle. They may result, for example, from retention of a Graafian follicle (developing ovum) or corpus luteum (old ovum)—structures that normally disappear with each cycle. Others, such as *dermoid cysts* or those seen in a "polycystic ovary," are due to developmental abnormalities in the ovary. The cause of most cysts, however, is unknown.

Cysts may grow quietly and go unnoticed until they are found on routine examination. On the other hand, they may become large enough to cause abdominal distension or even obstruct venous drainage, causing swelling of the legs. Malignant cysts may cause the general symptoms of cancer, such as weight loss and wasting.

Bleeding may occur in some cysts and others may rupture. Both these complications are painful, as is twisting of a cyst (torsion), which may occur when the cyst is on a "stalk." These diagnoses may all be confused with acute appendicitis and other abdominal emergencies and may only become apparent on *laparotomy* (examination

through an incision in the abdomen). A further possibility is infection in a cyst, which may cause pain and high fever.

Ovarian cysts usually are removed surgically to prevent further complications. The type of operation depends on the individual case but may include removal of the cyst alone or removal of the entire ovary (*oophorectomy*). Removal of both ovaries results in sterility and artificial MENOPAUSE; it is performed usually only in the treatment of ovarian cancer or in postmenopausal women. Ovarian cancer may require follow-up radiation or drug treatment, but surgery alone is sufficient for most ovarian cysts.

OVULATION

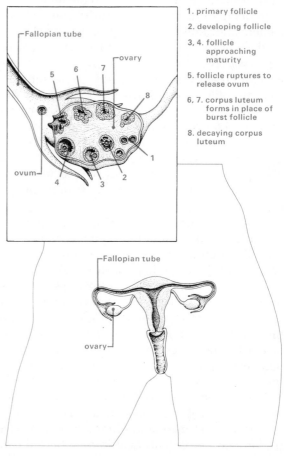

1. primary follicle
2. developing follicle
3, 4. follicle approaching maturity
5. follicle ruptures to release ovum
6, 7. corpus luteum forms in place of burst follicle
8. decaying corpus luteum

At birth the ovaries contain many primary follicles, each containing an immature ovum, or egg. After puberty, one or more of these follicles ripens and releases an ovum (ovulation) at the midpoint of each menstrual cycle. If the ovum is not fertilized, menstrual bleeding ensues.

ovulation

The release of an ovum (egg) from an ovary.

Ovulation occurs around the middle of the menstrual cycle and is followed either by fertilization and pregnancy or, after fourteen days, by MENSTRUATION. The ovum travels down the Fallopian tube to the uterus; if it meets and accepts a sperm cell during its journey down the Fallopian tube, the fertilized ovum becomes implanted in the wall of the uterus. There it grows and develops into a human embryo.

Ovulation depends on the secretion of hormones by the pituitary gland (at the base of the brain), which is itself under the control of the hypothalamus, the region of the brain concerned with basic sex drives, hunger, and sleep. The *hypothalamic releasing factors* stimulate the pituitary to secrete the *follicle-stimulating hormone (FSH)*, which causes a single ovum to ripen and leave the ovary. Fertility depends also on other pituitary hormones—luteinizing hormone and prolactin—which interact with the estrogen and progesterone secreted by the ovaries themselves.

Minor impairment of the hormonal cycle may be enough to suppress ovulation while not interfering with menstruation: A woman may have regular periods but be infertile because she does not ovulate. It is for this reason that the investigation of infertility may require careful measurement of hormone levels in the blood and urine and assessment of the woman's response to hormone treatment. When the cause of infertility is shown to be failure of ovulation, there is a good prospect of successful treatment: Ovulation may be induced either by drugs that alter the hormone balance, or by specific hormone treatment.

pacemaker

An electrical stimulator that sends a specific electrical current to the heart muscle in order to control or maintain heart rate.

In a healthy heart a group of specialized muscle cells, the "sinoatrial node," sends electrical impulses that control the rhythmic beating of the heart. If these cells or their connections do not function properly, the heart may beat too fast, too slow, irregularly, or not at all. In these cases, a temporary or permanent pacemaker may be indicated.

A pacemaker has three major parts: (1) the generator that provides the electrical impulse; (2) the sensing and firing system that determines if and when the pacer should fire; and (3) the electrode that delivers the electrical impulse.

The electrode through which the impulses

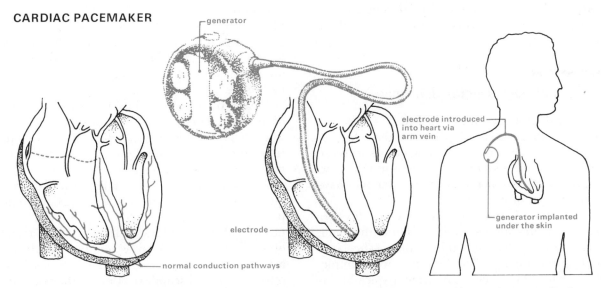

CARDIAC PACEMAKER

generator

electrode introduced into heart via arm vein

generator implanted under the skin

electrode

normal conduction pathways

Heart disease sometimes involves the conduction pathways, causing the pulse to become dangerously slow or irregular. A cardiac pacemaker may then be inserted, temporarily or permanently, to correct the heartbeat.

reach the heart may be on the outside surface of the heart ("external") or on its inside surface ("internal"). External pacemakers require surgical implantation, whereas internal pacemakers can be maneuvered into the right ventricle of the heart via the veins.

Pacemakers may be outside the body if the device is temporary; however, if the device is permanent the generator must be implanted beneath the skin of the chest wall to prevent infection. Most permanent pacemakers use lithium batteries that last for ten to fifteen years. A minor operation is needed to change the battery of a permanent pacemaker.

Most pacemakers in use today will "fire" at a faster rate if the wearer is walking or exercising. These "demand" pacemakers make it possible to live a relatively normal life. Some current pacemakers are also able to correct life-threatening arrhythmias.

The main complication of pacemaker therapy is failure of the device to function—due to battery failure, displacement of the electrode, or fibrosis around the electrode. Other complications include infection in the blood or around the battery box, ulceration of the skin above the box and, rarely, perforation of the heart by the pacemaker. Coming into the vicinity of poorly shielded microwave ovens or other microwave devices can interfere with the pacemaker's function.

Pacemakers are generally safe and effective. Their development during the last twenty-five years has completely changed the previously poor prognosis of many persons with heart block and other cardiac arrhythmias. Many persons in their 80s and 90s are now equipped with pacemakers.

Paget's disease (osteitis deformans)

A bone disease that causes thickened, soft bones. It affects approximately 3 percent of the U.S. population, usually men, and rarely occurs in those under 50. The onset of the disease is usually slow, and some persons may never realize that they have a mild form of it.

The spine is most commonly affected; other common sites for the disease include the skull, breastbone, pelvis, and thigh bones. The bone enlargement may lead to deformity, for example, bowed legs or an enlarged head (typically discovered by the need for a larger hat size).

The softened bones are often painful and prone to fractures. Enlargement of the skull may compress the nerves that pass through it, leading to deafness or other forms of nerve paralysis (occasionally including blindness). Affected bones have an increased blood flow, which may lead ultimately to heart failure. If a person with Paget's disease is immobilized he may develop increased calcium levels in the blood and urine, which may lead to urinary stones. Finally, there exists the risk of developing a type of malignant tumor (OSTEO-SARCOMA) in the affected bones.

The severe bone pain in advanced cases does not always respond to analgesics (pain-killers). Although there is no cure, drugs have been developed that can halt the process and also control the pain.

See also OSTEITIS.

pain

A sensory and emotional experience of severe discomfort occurring anywhere in the body and usually caused by disease or injury.

Pain is difficult to define accurately because it means different things to different people at different times. Since pain cannot be measured objectively, the physician must rely on a combination of the person's medical history and his own experience of pain to assess its nature and the need for treatment.

Pain may be caused by many types of conditions, including trauma, infection, cancer, degenerative changes, and ischemia (inadequate blood supply to an organ or part). In addition, pain commonly is caused or modified by psychological factors. The causes for many types of pain are not diagnosed easily and, in fact, may never be found.

Ideally, pain is treated by removal or treatment of its cause. This is not always possible, and even when it is possible it may take time. It is thus frequently necessary to relieve the pain itself. This may be achieved in several ways:

Analgesic drugs (pain-killers) are the most frequently used treatment for acute and chronic pain. Mild analgesics—including aspirin, propoxyphene hydrochloride (Darvon), and many others—are taken in large numbers for headaches, menstrual pain, flu-like symptoms, and other common discomforts. Despite the potential hazards involved in their long-term use, many people take them as a habit. Narcotic analgesics (such as morphine or codeine) are very effective in the treatment of severe pain, but they are addictive. In the case of terminally ill cancer patients, the addictive potential of narcotic analgesics is not a problem. However, the abuse of this class of pain-killer is a major medical and social issue in the United States today.

Nerve blocks as used by dentists can be an effective short-term and even long-term solution to pain when the affected area can be identified clearly and the relevant nerve blocked with drugs like lidocaine hydrochloride (Xylocaine) or destroyed with alcohol.

TENS—or *transcutaneous electrical nerve stimulation*—sometimes is used in chronic pain situations. It consists of a small battery-operated unit worn on the hip. Electrodes are placed over the spine on the skin. A gentle current of electricity is fed from the battery pack to the electrodes. Theoretically, the electrical impulses from the TENS unit block pain impulses going up the nerves in the spinal cord.

Acupuncture is an ancient Chinese method of pain relief, effective in some circumstances and now fashionable in the West.

Neurosurgery can be employed to cut nerves in the spinal cord or ablate areas of the brain responsible for the perception of pain. Clearly, such invasive techniques are used only after all other methods have been exhausted and only for severe, intractable pain.

Where the cause is not clear or the underlying condition cannot be treated satisfactorily, pain relief is probably best achieved with the help of a physician who specializes in solving the problem of intractable pain—since he is likely to be most familiar with the range of possible techniques.

palsy

Paralysis. A condition involving a loss of motor function. Two examples of different types of palsy are Bell's palsy and cerebral palsy.

BELL'S PALSY is a paralysis of the muscles of one side of the face, caused by damage to the facial nerve. This commonly is caused by a virus, and complete recovery frequently occurs.

CEREBRAL PALSY is a permanent disorder of movement associated with paralysis, caused by a defect or disease of the brain and typically occurring within the first three years of life. Affected individuals are called *spastics* and they may also have

sensory and mental handicaps. Cerebral palsy may be caused by infection or damage during development in the womb, during birth, or in infancy.

pancreas

A large gland situated at the back of the abdominal cavity, behind the stomach and between the duodenum and the spleen.

The pancreas has two main functions. As an *exocrine gland* it produces various enzymes necessary for digestion which flow through the pancreatic duct to the duodenum (the beginning of the small intestine). As an *endocrine gland* it produces hormones that are released into the bloodstream. These include INSULIN and glucagon, which are essential to normal carbohydrate metabolism, and also more recently discovered hormones that are related to digestion.

The pancreas may be damaged by infection (PANCREATITIS) injury, tumor, or alcoholism, and such damage may lead to abnormalities of its endocrine or exocrine functions.

PANCREAS

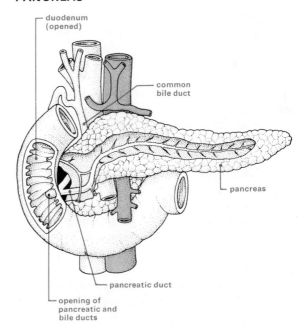

The pancreas is a digestive gland that lies behind the stomach and in front of the major abdominal blood vessels and the left kidney. It secretes digestive enzymes down the pancreatic duct into the duodenum where they break down proteins and fats. The pancreas also produces the hormones insulin and glucagon.

pancreatitis

Inflammation of the pancreas; the condition may be acute or chronic.

Acute pancreatitis is a disease in which the pancreas appears to "digest itself" owing to the liberation of its digestive enzymes into the tissues. It may be provoked by infections (such as mumps), trauma, regurgitation of bile up the pancreatic duct, ALCOHOLISM, and some vascular disease. Affected persons have severe abdominal pain and rapidly become seriously ill. Intensive supportive treatment in the hospital is required, although there is no specific treatment.

Chronic pancreatitis may result from repeated attacks of acute pancreatitis or directly from alcoholism or diseases of the biliary tract. It causes recurrent abdominal pain and MALABSORPTION, with fatty, offensive stools and, less often, DIABETES MELLITUS.

Chronic pancreatitis is common in Western countries, including the United States, where alcoholism is a widespread problem. Treatment involves prohibition of alcohol, a low-fat diet, pancreatic enzymes by mouth, and INSULIN if necessary, but the disease cannot be cured.

papilloma

A benign tumor growing on the outermost layer of cells of the skin or of a mucous membrane, commonly as a mass on a stalk. Papillomas, which include growths such as warts and polyps, are found most often in the mucous membranes that line the intestinal and urinary tracts. Only rarely do they become malignant.

Papillomas may occur on any part of the skin and are especially common in the elderly. Usually they remain small, but occasionally they reach the size of an egg or an orange. Papillomas normally are treated by cautery; the larger ones can be removed surgically by cutting through the supporting stalk.

Intestinal papillomas are most common in the colon and rectum, where they sometimes bleed. They may be single (of unknown cause) or multiple—a condition known as *familial polyposis coli,* which is inherited. The latter form must be regarded as premalignant, since malignant change in this type of papilloma is quite common. Single papillomas can often be removed by using a proctosigmoidoscope a special instrument inserted into the lower part of the large intestine via the rectum; multiple polyps are best treated by surgical removal of the affected portion of the bowel.

In the urinary tract, papillomas are most common in the bladder, though they can occur anywhere from the kidney to the urethra (the passage through which urine is voided). The cause usually is not known, but they are particularly common in persons who have worked in the rubber industry and in persons who smoke. These papillomas are all potentially malignant, and thus should be removed. In the bladder this is usually done through a cystoscope (a special instrument for examining the interior of the urinary bladder). Recurrence is common, and life-long regular cystoscopy usually is necessary once the diagnosis is made.

paralysis

The loss of muscular function in a part of the body, caused by damage to the muscles themselves or to a part of the nervous system. Paralysis may vary in severity from affecting a single small muscle to affecting most of the body.

Disease of the muscles themselves leads more commonly to weakness than to total paralysis. However, some forms of MUSCULAR DYSTROPHY, most of which occur in childhood, can progress to severe and eventually fatal paralysis. There is no effective treatment for these conditions.

Any block in the transmission of impulses from nerves to muscles also may result in paralysis. This occurs in MYASTHENIA GRAVIS, in BOTULISM, and in some other types of poisoning (for example, with "nerve gas").

The peripheral nerves may be injured directly or damaged by disease, including DIABETES MELLITUS, POLYARTERITIS NODOSA, CANCER, ALCOHOLISM, vitamin deficiencies, LEPROSY, PORPHYRIA, and some drug reactions. This damage may lead to weakness or to total paralysis of the muscles supplied by the affected nerves.

The spinal cord may be damaged by a number of conditions, including POLIOMYELITIS, MULTIPLE SCLEROSIS, and trauma. The pattern of the resulting paralysis depends on its cause. Severe damage to the spinal cord results in PARAPLEGIA—complete paralysis of the legs and the lower part of the body, usually including bladder paralysis. If the spinal cord damaged is in the region of the neck, the arms may be paralyzed as well as the legs —*quadriplegia.*

Brain damage also may result in paralysis. The most common cause here is a STROKE, caused by hemorrhage, thrombosis in the brain, or impairment of cerebral blood flow. The extent of the paralysis is variable, but the most common pattern is partial or complete paralysis of the arm and leg on one side—HEMIPLEGIA. Other causes of brain damage include MENINGITIS, ENCEPHALITIS, SYPHILIS, and brain tumors. Transient paralysis (Todd's paralysis) may occur in a part of the body following an epileptic attack.

Paralysis resulting from division of a major nerve tract in the spinal cord or brain is permanent and irreversible, but that resulting from other diseases may have a more variable prognosis. In "acute infective polyneuritis" (the GUILLAIN-BARRÉ SYNDROME), more or less total paralysis may be followed by complete recovery if the patient survives. In some diseases (such as strokes) the extent of recovery is extremely variable, while in others (such as motor neuron disease) recovery is unknown.

Survival in paralysis depends on the underlying disease and whether or not it affects the respiratory tract muscles and heart muscles. Artificial ventilation may keep alive patients with some diseases (for example, poliomyelitis or acute infective polyneuritis) until the paralysis improves or remits. In some cases a person may never recover the ability to breath on his own and will remain dependent on respirators for life.

paranoia

A chronic personality disorder in which the individual develops systematized, sometimes permanent, and mainly persecutory delusions in a setting of otherwise undisturbed thought. Paranoia must be distinguished from *paranoid schizophrenia,* in which the same delusions occur but accompanied by hallucinations and disturbances of thought processes and personality.

Paranoid reactions are displayed by most people at one time or another in response to severe disappointment or humiliation. The reaction is the mistaken belief that the sufferer is the center of attention and that he is being talked about, usually in a critical way that invades his privacy and embarrasses him.

Paranoia is a state in which the person experiences constant "paranoid reactions" and where these reactions cannot be dispelled by others. Suspicion and resentment of others arise, and the

person takes innocent matters to be a direct attack on himself. He usually feels that his true worth is not recognized, and he often has grandiose ideas about what his true worth is.

Temporary paranoid reactions are fairly common and usually harmless—providing they are not associated with other thought disorders or personality changes—although they may be irritating for the family and colleagues of the sufferer. In contrast, true paranoia is relatively rare and can cause considerable annoyance and harm to innocent people outside the sufferer's immediate circle. It is not easy to treat, but is sometimes helped by PSYCHOTHERAPY.

paraplegia

Paralysis of the lower limbs, often accompanied by dysfunction of the rectum and bladder.

Paraplegia usually is caused by trauma to or a lesion of the spinal cord. The extent of the paralysis is dependent on the position and severity of the lesion or trauma. Complete severance of the spinal cord will lead to total paralysis of the legs and fecal and urinary INCONTINENCE. Lesser damage may affect the legs and leave bladder and rectal function unimpaired. Recovery will take place sometimes if the damage to the cord is minimal, but lifelong paralysis is more often the result.

Care of the paraplegic patient should be designed to relieve symptoms often associated with paralysis, such as pressure sores and urinary tract infections. As soon as possible a program of physical therapy and retraining should be started—if necessary, in a special center devoted to the care of paraplegics. The provision of special equipment will greatly ease the problems of incontinence and immobility. Many paraplegics, although confined to wheelchairs, live active and useful lives.

parasite

An animal or plant that lives inside or upon another living animal or plant without extending any benefit to it in return for the advantages gained.

A large number of organisms find humans ideal hosts. Bacteria, viruses, fungi, and protozoa are said to "infect" humans, but worms and insects are said to "infest" people and are what is normally meant by the term *parasites*. They may be quite harmless, or they may produce symptoms of disease.

In general, the hotter the climate and the lower the standard of hygiene, the more parasites flourish. Among the most common in temperate climates are TICKS, LICE, FLEAS, MITES, and bedbugs. They are not usually important carriers of disease, but they are disagreeable. They can be controlled by the use of modern insecticides.

More harmful are worms, which range from the PINWORM, which is more of a nuisance than a threat to life, to the flatworm (trematode) of SCHISTOSOMIASIS, which makes life miserable for more than 200 million people in tropical countries and is responsible for untold morbidity and mortality.

Strict attention to personal hygiene will prevent problems with most parasites, but travelers and others who are not accustomed to the conditions in less developed tropical and subtropical countries may inadvertently lay themselves open to infestation by worms. It is important to avoid uncooked food and to avoid bathing or wading in water that may be the habitat of the freshwater snail that causes schistosomiasis. It is also sensible to wear shoes in the tropics and to avoid drinking from village wells and rivers.

The average traveler is in no great danger of becoming infested with parasites, and those whose lives lead them into the remoter parts of the world usually are well informed about such dangers. Nevertheless, one should keep the possibility in mind.

The control of parasitic diseases is one of the great tasks of the future for developing countries; it depends to a large degree on improving the standards of public and private sanitation.

See also ROUNDWORMS, TAPEWORMS.

paratyphoid fever

An acute generalized feverish disease caused by bacteria of the genus *Salmonella*.

Paratyphoid fever is so called because it resembles TYPHOID FEVER, but in most cases the symptoms are less severe and the course of the disease is less harmful.

The onset of the disease may be more rapid than in typhoid fever, but the symptoms are much the same. The person may complain of discomfort, lassitude, and headache and suffer from insomnia as well as a high temperature. As in the case of typhoid fever, the fever may be greater in the morning but the daily peak gradually rises until about the eighth day, when it levels out. The person feels restless, hot, and uncomfortable; there may be pain in the abdomen, which, however, is not as extreme as in typhoid fever. Rose-colored spots are common in typhoid fever, but less common in paratyphoid fever (although they may occur).

Treatment consists of alleviating the symptoms as far as possible. Drugs such as aspirin to lower the fever may be given under medical supervision, and antibiotics may be useful in shortening the period of illness.

The diet should be bland and nutritious, but little solid food should be given while the gastrointestinal tract is irritated by the bacteria. Convalescence may be prolonged; as in typhoid fever, the attack cannot be regarded as over until six consecutive stool and urine specimens are found to be negative for the presence of the causative bacteria.

Prevention of paratyphoid fever is possible, not only through vaccination but also through the application of measures relating to public hygiene—including a pure water supply—that are common in advanced nations. Travelers to places where paratyphoid fever is still common, such as India, should consult a doctor about vaccination. The TAB vaccine incorporates protection against both typhoid and paratyphoid and commonly is given to children, but the immunity so gained is not permanent. It is prudent to have shots to boost the immunity before going to any country where paratyphoid fever exists.

Parkinson's disease

A disease, especially of the elderly, characterized by tremor (the person's head and limbs shake) and stiffness (muscular rigidity). The person is unable to initiate movements quickly and has a characteristic bowed posture and immobile face.

Parkinson's disease (also known as *Parkinsonism*) is associated with degeneration of nerve centers deep within the brain that are known to be closely linked with the control of posture and movement. The reason for the changes in the brain are not known. Some cases arise from the use of certain drugs, but in these instances the signs and symptoms of the disease are reversible when the drugs are withdrawn.

Research has drawn attention to the importance of *neurotransmitters* in Parkinson's disease.

PARKINSON'S DISEASE

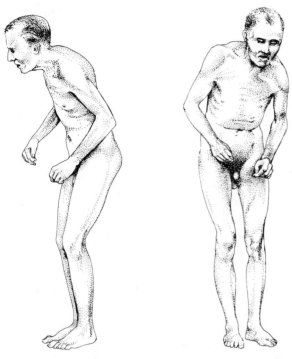

Patients with Parkinson's disease are characterized by muscle tremors affecting the head and extremities, staring eyes, and expressionless face, rigidity of some muscle groups, and a slow gait marked by short shuffles. Often there is also an involuntary "pill-rolling" movement of the thumb against the first two fingers.

These are chemicals that facilitate the transmission of impulses across the junctions between nerves. Sufferers of Parkinson's disease show depleted levels of one of these neurotransmitters, *dopamine.* Since the 1960s, treatment of Parkinson's disease has concentrated on remedying this deficiency. The most important drug now used is *levadopa* (or L-dopa), which is the immediate chemical precursor to dopamine. Levadopa is given to help the body make its own supply of dopamine. About 75 percent of persons with the disease show an improvement of their condition when given levadopa.

Some persons cannot take advantage of levadopa because of severe side effects, which may include nausea and vomiting. More sophisticated preparations, in which the side effects of the levadopa are countered by other drugs, are now being administered. Some persons, particularly those under the age of 50 who are resistant to drugs, can be helped by brain operations. Encouraging results have been claimed for the implantation of fetal tissue into the brain. Another important element in Parkinson's disease is physical therapy,

since any break in physical activity can be disastrous and lead to immobility. Approximately 300,000 people in the United States suffer from Parkinson's disease, and about 40,000 new cases occur each year.

paronychia

A superficial infection of the skin next to a fingernail, usually as a result of tearing a hangnail.

Paronychia is caused most often by infection with the bacteria *Staphylococcus.* The skin becomes red, swollen, and painful, and sometimes the infection burrows under the nail to form an abscess there. These infections have the tendency to recur, especially in nail biters, because of the contamination of an exposed area of the skin with saliva. Paronychia is not a minor condition: If the infection becomes systemic it has the ability to cause severe disability; medical attention should be sought.

Exposure to HERPES SIMPLEX, which infects small cuts or openings on the skin, can lead to herpes *whitlow* of the hand. Whitlow is characterized by the appearance of very painful small lesions that spread along the finger; it is seen most commonly in medical personnel who have not worn gloves when exposed to herpetic infections.

In DIABETES MELLITUS, various fungi can cause chronic paronychial inflammations, and similar lesions are seen sometimes in PSORIASIS and some kinds of PEMPHIGUS.

paroxysm

A sudden increase of symptoms of a disease or an exacerbation of the disease itself; also, a sudden attack, usually of convulsions, spasm, or TACHYCARDIA.

pasteurization

The process of applying heat to milk and other foods to slow or kill the growth of harmful bacteria, without significantly affecting the taste of the food. Pasteurization generally is achieved by heating milk for approximately forty minutes (not less than thirty minutes) at 140°–160°F (60°–70°C). This is followed by a rapid cooling.

patent ductus arteriosus

A congenital heart defect in which the prenatal circulation of the blood persists after birth.

In a fetus, the lungs are immersed in fluid and do not function for breathing. The blood is oxygenated instead through the placenta. To bypass the lungs, the circulation is augmented by the *ductus arteriosus*, which connects the left pulmonary artery with the aorta. Occasionally, the ductus arteriosus fails to close after birth and instead remains *patent* (open).

The result is a mixing of arterial and venous blood, which can lead to respiratory infections and failure to thrive. Once patent ductus is diagnosed, it is possible to treat the condition by use of medications to control symptoms, or by surgery to tie off the open duct.

pediculosis

Infestation with LICE.

pellagra

A deficiency disease caused by a lack of niacin (or nicotinic acid), a B-complex vitamin, in the diet. Symptoms include swelling of the mucous membranes of the mouth, diarrhea, loss of appetite, headache, skin changes causing scaly sores on areas exposed to the sun, and mental problems ranging from depression and confusion to hallucinations.

Treatment includes establishing a balanced diet with niacin supplements if necessary.

pelvic inflammatory disease (PID)

Inflammation of the FALLOPIAN TUBES. Symptoms include fever, chills, foul-smelling vaginal discharge, pain in the lower abdomen, abnormal vaginal bleeding, and painful sexual intercourse.

Some cases have been noted to follow the use of an intrauterine contraceptive device (IUD) but the condition most commonly follows inadequately treated gonorrhea or chlamydia infections or septic abortion.

PID is treated with bed rest and antibiotics.

Failure to take the full course of antibiotics may result in long-term PID, which can yield scars, blocked Fallopian tubes, and sterility.

pemphigus

A group of diseases of the skin and mucous membranes characterized by the formation of blisters. It is thought that they may be autoimmune disorders, since during the active stages of the disease an immunoglobulin may be found in the circulating serum.

Pemphigus vulgaris occurs usually in persons between the ages of 40 and 60. Large blisters suddenly form on the skin, often subsequent to blistering in the mouth or nose. The blisters occur most often on the trunk of the body, in some cases covering very large areas.

In the past, this condition ended in death; now, however, with the use of steroids, this disease usually can be controlled.

Other forms of pemphigus exist but generally they are not as severe as the vulgaris form.

peptic ulcer

An ULCER involving those areas of the digestive tract exposed to pepsin—acid gastric juice. The most common are those involving the stomach (GASTRIC ULCER) and the first portion of the duodenum (see DUODENAL ULCER).

pericarditis

Inflammation of the pericardium, the membrane surrounding the heart. It is usually secondary to inflammation elsewhere. The pericardium may become involved through trauma, cancer, infection (bacterial, viral, or fungal), or from an unknown cause.

The main symptom is pain felt in the center of the chest, which may radiate to the neck, shoulders, and upper arms; the symptoms of the causative disease often predominate, however.

Pericarditis may lead to an accumulation of fluid in the sac surrounding the heart and this may seriously impair the heart's pumping action. The fluid is removed by aspiration through a needle inserted into the fluid-filled sac.

perifolliculitis

Tiny abscesses (*white heads*) involving hair follicles and the surrounding inflammation.

FOLLICULITIS is caused either by staphylococci or streptococci and may be treated with antibiotics.

periodontics

The branch of dentistry dealing with the treatment of gum diseases such as GINGIVITIS.

In adults, disease of the gums is the primary cause of tooth loss. Much of the work of periodontists involves the removal of calcified deposits from around the teeth and their roots. Periodontists also perform operations to remove pockets of pus in the gums and to make other soft-tissue repairs.

PERIODONTITIS

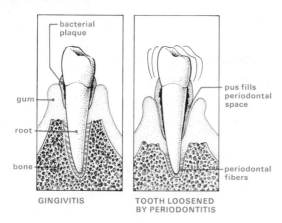

GINGIVITIS   TOOTH LOOSENED
                    BY PERIODONTITIS

If gingivitis (inflammation of the gums) is not treated, bacterial plaque forms between the gums and the roots of teeth. The inflammation progressively destroys the periodontal fibers and bone that hold the teeth in place. Pus forms in the deep periodontal spaces (a condition called pyorrhea), and eventually the teeth fall out.

peritonitis

Inflammation of the peritoneum, the membrane lining the abdominal cavity.

Most acute cases are caused by the perforation of one of the hollow abdominal organs or by infection spreading from an inflamed organ. Occasionally in children no obvious source of infection is found. Peritonitis may remain localized, especially when it arises from inflammation of the gallbladder or the appendix, but in severe perforations—for example, of a peptic ulcer or gangrenous appendix—the whole peritoneal cavity may be involved. Peritonitis resulting from the perforation of a peptic ulcer is at first chemical, but soon bacterial infection spreads and the abdominal cavity becomes filled with pus.

The main symptom of peritonitis is severe pain and tenderness of the abdominal wall, which becomes rigid. The person may experience nausea and vomiting; soon the intestines become paralyzed and the abdomen distends. The pain makes the person lie still with his legs drawn up. The temperature may be raised or may be subnormal, but the blood pressure may fall. The pulse is quickened and may be weak.

In most cases a period of resuscitation with intravenous therapy and the administration of antibiotics precedes the operation necessary to drain the peritoneal cavity and treat the cause of the peritonitis. The postoperative course is likely to be difficult.

personality

The sum total of all the characteristics of a person—including the mental, moral, physical, and social qualities—as they are perceived by other people. The word may be used either in a popular sense, in which the meaning is linked simply to the type of person as seen by others, or in a psychological sense, in which the meaning is more complex and sometimes less obvious.

Psychoanalysts regard personality as the result of the interaction between instinct and the environment. Other schools of psychology and psychiatry have more complicated explanations, combining the effects of heredity, upbringing, experience, and biochemical factors.

One of the most widely followed divisions is Jung's categories of *extroverted* and *introverted* personalities. The distinction in technical terms is that the extrovert directs his LIBIDO and instinctual energy toward the environment, whereas the introvert has weak instinctual energy and directs it inward toward himself. Most persons combine aspects of both personality types, and the extreme examples of either can be recognized by their behavior.

Personality may have no medical connotations at all. To describe a person as having an "unpleasant" personality or a "miserable" personality is not to suggest that he is in any way mentally ill. On the other hand, there are various defects in behavior or life-style that are regarded widely as *personality disorders*. These are characterized by pathological trends in personality structure, with or without anxiety—in most cases manifested by a lifelong pattern of abnormal action or behavior.

Sociopathic personality disturbance, for instance, may be a pathological relationship between the person and the society in which he lives, manifested by irresponsibility, inability to feel guilt, impulsiveness, and poor interpersonal relationships.

Various mental disorders often are expressed in terms of personality. Sufferers will be categorized as *paranoid personalities*, borderline personalities, schizoid personalities, or dependent personalities. There are also authenticated cases of *multiple personality*, which most authorities believe are delusional in character. In all these cases personality is distorted into an abnormal type by the underlying mental or emotional disorder.

pessary

1. Any device placed in the vagina to support the uterus or to provide contraception. 2. Any form of medication (especially a vaginal suppository) placed in the vagina for therapeutic purposes.

petechiae

Minute hemorrhagic spots on the skin, ranging in size from pinhead to pinpoint.

Petechiae are formed by the escape of blood into the skin or mucous membranes. They appear for a variety of reasons when there is a rupture in the junction between the capillary and the artery from which it is fed. There are a large number of conditions and diseases that cause these ruptures.

Petechiae are a sign of many illnesses, ranging from ROCKY MOUNTAIN SPOTTED FEVER to MEASLES, and from SCARLET FEVER to PURPURA. They can also accompany cerebrospinal meningitis, and (especially in older people) they may be an external sign of vitamin-C deficiency. Their appearance after surgery or after the fracture of a long bone can be a sign of a fat embolism.

Peutz-Jeghers syndrome

An inherited disease characterized by gastrointestinal POLYPS and the appearance of small brown lesions on the gums, palate, lips, nose, hands, and feet.

These lesions, which usually appear first when the patient is a child, do not cause physical discomfort. In time, the skin lesions may fade but the mouth lesions remain. Internally, polyps develop in the stomach, small and large intestines, and rectum, with the largest percentage of polyps developing in the small intestine. Polyps in the gastrointestinal tract can cause abdominal pain, vomiting, and bleeding.

This disease is related to the more serious *colonic polyposis*, a hereditary disease affecting mostly the large intestine and in which the polyps have a very high rate of cancerous change. Although Peutz-Jeghers syndrome also is inherited, the percentage of polyps that become cancerous is only 2 to 3 percent. It has also been noted that 5 percent of women with this disease also will develop ovarian cancer.

Peyronie's disease

A disease of the penis in which fibrous tissue grows on the erectile tissue causing bending or angulation of the organ on erection; also known as *corpora cavernosa* or *fibrous cavernitis*. There is no known cause, and treatment is difficult. Surgery or steroid injections may be effective.

phantom limb syndrome

Following amputation of the whole or part of a limb, it is fairly common for the person to feel that the part is still there.

The person may experience feelings of touch, heat, cold, and position in the phantom limb, but often the most serious problem is pain. A person who has lost a hand, for example, may complain of pain in his thumb or at his fingertips.

Most cases of the phantom limb syndrome are mild and disappear within days or weeks of amputation. Severe persistent pain may be relieved by drug treatment. With modern methods of pain relief the phantom limb syndrome can sometimes be treated successfully.

pharmaceutics/pharmacology/pharmacy

Pharmaceutics and *pharmacy* are alternative terms for the art and science of preparing and dispensing medicines. "Pharmacy" also is used to describe the place in which drugs are prepared and dispensed; "pharmaceutic" or "pharmaceutical" also is used as a term for a medicinal preparation or drug.

Pharmacy is concerned principally with the accurate preparation and presentation of drugs. In the past, most medicines were prepared from their basic ingredients by the physician or by the pharmacist in the drugstore. While this is still true of some drugs, most are now formulated and prepared in bulk by the pharmaceutical industry. The pharmacist often simply dispenses already prepared drugs in the dosage and form prescribed by the physician or recommended by the manufacturers. Pharmacists receive a full professional training, however, and are capable of preparing many medicines from their basic ingredients and of aiding patients in choosing appropriate self-medication.

Pharmacology can be divided into two areas: *basic* pharmacology and *clinical* pharmacology. Basic pharmacology is the study of drugs—their sources, chemistry, uses, and actions on living organisms at any level from bacteria to humans, or on isolated biochemical pathways within these organisms. Clinical pharmacology is that branch concerned with the use of therapeutic drugs in the prevention and treatment of disease in humans. Clinical pharmacologists, unlike basic pharmacologists, are physicians who have undergone training in basic pharmacology, clinical pharmacology, and one of several specialties of medical practice.

"Polypharmacy," the prescription of multiple drugs to the individual, although sometimes essential, runs the risk of causing drug interactions that may endanger the person. These risks are a major field of current study for clinical pharmacologists.

See also PHARMACIST under **Providers**.

pharyngitis

Inflammation or infection of the throat (*pharynx*), usually causing symptoms of sore throat.

Pharyngitis is a common component of upper respiratory tract infection, usually caused by viruses (such as those responsible for the common cold) or by bacterial infections.

Chronic pharyngitis may be caused by heavy smoking or by the "postnasal drip" associated with allergic or other diseases of the nose. In immunocompromised, patients, pharyngitis may be caused by THRUSH or by several species of microorganisms that ordinarily cause no problems in those who are otherwise healthy. Some blood diseases (including LEUKEMIA) sometimes cause pharyngitis.

Viral pharyngitis usually resolves spontaneously within a few days. No curative treatment is possible, but the sore throat sometimes may be relieved by gargles containing aspirin or other pain-killing substances. Penicillin and the other antibiotics are of no value in viral infections (but are necessary in streptococcal and other bacterial infections).

Tonsillectomy may be required for severe recurrent pharyngitis involving the tonsils.

Culture of microorganisms obtained by means of a throat swab can identify most of the dangerous causes of pharyngitis, but it is not practicable to perform this test on all patients with sore throats.

phenylketonuria (PKU)

An inherited disease caused by the absence of an enzyme necessary for the breakdown of phenylalanine, which is an amino acid, one of the building blocks of proteins. Phenylalanine accumulates and leads to damage in the brain.

In affected infants, the disease is present from birth, but is not suspected by parents or medical personnel until the early symptoms appear (mental dullness, irritability, vomiting). If phenylketonuria is untreated, it can result in mental retardation. The condition can be diagnosed by a simple urine test applied to the diaper.

When diagnosed, the disease is treated by a special phenylalanine-free diet. Since most foods contain phenylalanine, major modifications must be made in the diet. If diagnosed early and treated properly, the disabling effects of the disease do not occur.

The incidence of this inherited disease in the United States is one per 10,000 live births. Mandatory testing for PKU is practiced in all U.S. hospitals.

PHIMOSIS

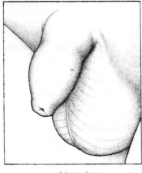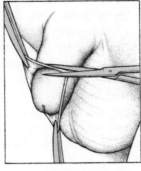

phimosis   circumcision

Phimosis is a tight foreskin which cannot be pulled back over the head of the penis. In boys under the age of 4 years, the foreskin normally adheres to the penis and should not be forced back during washing. Such attempts are likely to cause a true phimosis by scarring the foreskin. Phimosis is relieved by circumcision.

phimosis

Tightness of the foreskin of the penis, which prevents it from being drawn back. Removal of the foreskin is the usual treatment.

See CIRCUMCISION under **Procedures.**

phlebitis

Inflammation of the wall of a vein, commonly associated with THROMBOSIS within the vein.

Phlebitis occurs most frequently in varicose veins in the leg, where it may be spontaneous or may follow trauma or infection. It also may occur elsewhere in the body in abnormal veins (such as hemorrhoids) or in normal veins. It may occur at the site of an intravenous infusion or injection or may be induced deliberately by "sclerosing agents" in order to cure varicose veins or hemorrhoids.

Symptoms vary from mild discomfort over the affected vein to severe pain associated with tenderness and swelling of the surrounding tissue and sometimes a high fever.

Treatment involves supporting and elevating the affected part to prevent painful swelling and movement. Elevation of the leg helps to drain blood efficiently through the deep veins, but a similar effect often can be obtained in the ambulant person by the use of supportive elastic stockings or dressings. Infection may require antibiotic treatment. Drugs containing aspirin may help to suppress both the inflammation and the pain.

Most cases of phlebitis are harmless and resolve spontaneously. Pulmonary EMBOLISM occurs very rarely following *superficial venous phlebitis*, in contrast to the high risk of this complication following *deep-vein thrombosis*. When phlebitis is associated with infection, there is a risk of blood poisoning, but this should be rare with adequate treatment.

phlebothrombosis

The development of a blood clot in a vein without accompanying inflammation.

phobia

A persistent excessive fear of an object or situation that is not of real danger. Examples include CLAUSTROPHOBIA (fear of confined spaces), AGORAPHOBIA (fear of being in the open), specific phobias (as for spiders, mice, thunder, or darkness), and social phobias (such as excessive anxiety in the presence of other people).

Phobias, especially specific phobias, may be isolated abnormalities in an otherwise normal person, or they may sometimes be a manifestation of underlying anxiety or depression of a more general nature. It is theorized that phobias may represent a prolonged response to an unpleasant experience in childhood; the original stimulus usually has been forgotten.

Phobias of all kinds are more common in women than in men, but many individuals have some degree of phobia for some situation.

Phobias produce three main kinds of response: (1) a subjective experience of fear for the object or situation; (2) physiological changes such as palpitations or blushing in response to it; and (3) behavioral tendencies to avoid or escape from it. Some truly phobic persons rarely experience symptoms because they avoid the feared situation, and persons with a severe phobia may have difficulty seeking treatment.

Persons with underlying anxiety or depressive states often benefit from drug therapy or psychotherapy, but most other phobias are resistant to these techniques. Here the most effective therapy is often "desensitization," a form of behavior therapy in which the person is taught gradually to relax while imagining the feared object. An alternative technique is "flooding" or "implosion" therapy, in which the person is confronted by the feared object or situation and encouraged to remain in contact with it until his anxiety disappears.

Therapy for phobias is not always successful, and "cures" are not always permanent, but most sufferers can be helped by current treatments. The understanding and patience of family and friends are essential.

photophobia

1. Abnormal sensitivity of the eyes to light. It is a feature of various conditions, including MIGRAINE, MEASLES, MENINGITIS, CONJUNCTIVITIS, IRITIS, and KERATITIS. Photophobia may be experienced by persons who are taking or are addicted to certain drugs. It occurs also in albinos owing to a lack of eye pigmentation.
2. A morbid or irrational fear of light or of being in well-lighted places. Photophobia is an anxiety disorder more often seen in women than men.

physical therapy

Treatment that assists in the rehabilitation and restoration of normal function and in the prevention of disability following disease, injury, surgical procedure, or loss of a body part.

Physical therapy is practiced to some extent by all who are involved in the care of patients, but those paramedical personnel who are specially trained in the field are known as *physical therapists* (or *physiotherapists*).

Physical therapy usually is prescribed by a doctor and carried out under medical supervision. The methods used include the following:

Therapeutic exercises are of value before and after any significant operation, in prenatal and postnatal care, for any person who has been confined to bed by illness, and (more specifically) for those with disabilities resulting from injury or disease. "Active" exercises are those carried out by the individual; "passive movements"—made on the person's body by the therapist—are of value in unconscious patients and some others, especially to prevent the development of muscle contractures.

Massage and *manipulation*, properly carried out, may be of value in a number of musculoskeletal diseases.

Movement in a pool of water (*hydrotherapy*) is easier than movement in air, for persons with different kinds of arthritis, and this may help to strengthen muscles.

Heat therapy may aid in restoring joint and muscle function. Heat may be applied in a number of ways, including lamps, pads, hot water, and hot wax.

A number of other techniques, including *ultrasound* and *electrotherapy*, have special applications in different areas of medicine and may be administered by physical therapists. Many of these forms of therapy can be carried out anywhere, but some need the facilities of a well-equipped hospital department.

See also PHYSICAL THERAPIST under **Providers**.

pica

The craving for, or habit of, eating substances that are not normally taken as food, such as clay, earth, starch, chalk, or paint chips. It may occur with poor diet, in pregnant women, in mental illness, and—most often—in children.

pinworms

The most common worm PARASITES of humans in the United States, particularly among schoolchildren. The worm is known also as the "threadworm" (scientific name, *Enterobius vermicularis*). The infestation they cause is known as *enterobiasis*.

The adult worms live within the human intestine. Females are about half an inch long; males are much smaller. Mature females crawl out through the anus to the perianal skinfolds where they lay up to 10,000 eggs each, typically at night. This process usually causes intense itching at the anus. Within six hours the eggs turn into infectious larvae. If swallowed by the host the larvae develop into adult worms in the small intestine and the cycle starts again.

The severe itching at the anus causes great discomfort and scratching, and it may lead to irritability and insomnia, but other symptoms are unlikely to be due to pinworms. In particular, it is doubtful if they ever cause the abdominal pain or weight loss so often blamed on them. Female worms may wander into the vagina, uterus, and Fallopian tubes, but serious consequences are very rare.

Transmission of the parasites occurs by self-infection from anus to mouth as a result of

PINWORM(THREADWORM)

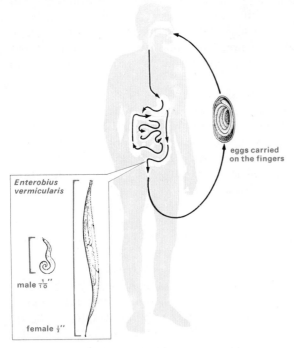

Enterobius vermicularis

male $\frac{1}{10}''$

female $\frac{1}{4}''$

eggs carried on the fingers

Enterobiasis, pinworm infection, is characterized by intense itching around the anus. This is due to the female worm migrating down the intestine at night and laying eggs on the anal skin. Scratching contaminates the fingers with eggs, which are then carried to the mouth and ingested.

scratching in sleep or poor hygiene, by cross-infection from anus to hand to the hand of another individual, or by dust in homes or classrooms.

The worms may be seen in the stools, or the eggs may be taken from around the anus, using transparent cellophane tape which is then examined under the microscope.

Pinworms can be killed by drugs taken by mouth, but reinfection is extremely common and repeated treatment often is necessary. Although irritating, the infection is harmless; complications of infection and treatment are very rare. When one member of a family is infected, all members of the family should be treated at the same time.

pituitary gland

A pea-sized ENDOCRINE GLAND at the base of the brain, which is enclosed within a bony cavity in the skull (the pituitary fossa) situated just above and behind the nasal cavity. The gland is connected to the HYPOTHALAMUS of the brain by a thin stalk and is divided into two parts, the *anterior* and *posterior* lobes.

The pituitary gland produces a number of hormones that influence the function of other endocrine glands and organs throughout the body. But it has become clear in recent years that the anterior pituitary is itself strongly influenced by hormones that issue from the hypothalamus and travel directly to the pituitary through special blood vessels. The hypothalamus in turn is influenced by a complex of factors including the rest of the nervous system and the concentration of various substances in the blood.

The anterior lobe of the pituitary gland releases a number of hormones into the blood:

Growth hormone (SOMATOTROPIN) is necessary for normal growth and has other metabolic actions. Deficiency in childhood leads to dwarfism; an excess, usually caused by a tumor of the pituitary, leads to gigantism in childhood and ACROMEGALY in adult life.

Thyroid-stimulating hormone (TSH) stimulates the thyroid gland to produce thyroxine and triiodothyronine.

Adrenocorticotropic hormone (ACTH) maintains normal activity in the cortex (outer portion) of the adrenal gland, stimulating the normal secretion of corticosteroid hormones.

Luteinizing hormone (LH) and *follicle-stimulating hormone* (FSH) regulate the secretion and activity of the testes and ovaries. Abnormalities of secretion may result in abnormal sexual characteristics and infertility.

Prolactin regulates milk production and breast development in pregnancy. Recently, high levels of secretion have been recognized as a factor in some women with infertility, but the output from the pituitary can be diminished by drugs.

The posterior lobe of the pituitary gland releases two hormones into the blood. Both are produced in the nerve cells in the hypothalamus and pass through the stalk to the far end of the cells in the posterior lobe:

Antidiuretic hormone (or *vasopressin*) acts on the kidneys to prevent excessive water loss in the urine. If the secretion is low because of hypothalamic or pituitary diseases, diabetes insipidus develops, a condition marked by excessive urination and extreme thirst.

Oxytocin makes the uterine muscle contract in labor. Its role in men and at other times in women is less well defined.

The pituitary gland may be damaged by trauma to the head, by infections of various kinds, and

PITUITARY GLAND

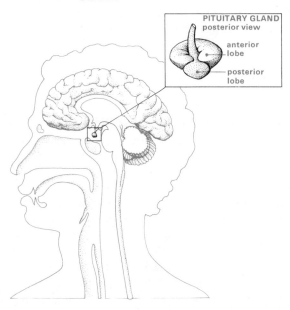

The pituitary, the master gland at the base of the brain, regulates much of the body's hormonal system. Its anterior lobe secretes hormones that stimulate many other glands to produce hormones of their own. Occasionally benign tumors grow in this anterior lobe, causing disturbances in the body's growth, in its response to stress, and in many other functions. The posterior lobe secretes only two hormones known to science; the first acts on the kidneys to retain body water, and the second makes the womb contract in labor.

by tumors. Where deficiencies of hormones occur as a result, those produced by the "target organs" may often be used in treatment, rather than those produced by the pituitary itself, which are difficult to obtain in large amounts.

ACTH is available in large amounts, however, and human growth hormone is used for the treatment of pituitary dwarfism. Oxytocin and antidiuretic hormone are synthesized and generally available.

pityriasis rosea

A mild inflammatory skin disease, probably caused by a virus. It produces a characteristic skin rash and there are rarely any other symptoms. The disease is quite common in the United States, especially in winter.

The rash starts with a single flat red spot, an oval area about 1 inch (2.5 centimeters) across with a ring of tiny scales near its edge, usually on the front of the chest. After a few days smaller but similar oval patches appear, mainly on the chest and abdomen, but also sometimes on the back, upper arms, and thighs. The number of patches ranges from a few to hundreds.

The patches increase in number for two to three weeks and the disease then resolves spontaneously over six to ten weeks. Itching is occasionally troublesome and may require treatment, but there are no other symptoms. Recovery is complete within ten weeks; there are no long-term effects and relapses or second attacks are very rare.

placenta

A blood-rich structure through which the fetus takes in oxygen, food, and other substances and

PLACENTA

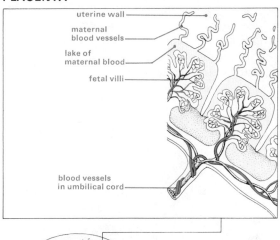

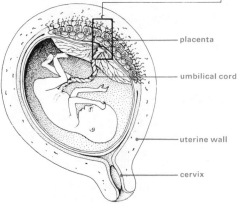

The placenta develops early in pregnancy and normally occupies an area high in the uterus. The maternal and fetal circulations do not mix, but they are able to exchange nutrients and waste products across the placenta. Maternal blood is pumped into "lakes" that surround the villi containing delicate fetal blood vessels. The placenta also secretes hormones.

gets rid of carbon dioxide and other wastes; following delivery it is shed as the "afterbirth."

The placenta begins to form on approximately the eighth day of pregnancy, and at the time of its expulsion weighs about one sixth of the weight of the baby.

placental insufficiency

An abnormal condition of pregnancy in which the fetus fails to grow normally owing to inadequacy of the PLACENTA.

placenta previa

A condition in which the PLACENTA is positioned abnormally in the uterus so that it partly or completely covers the opening of the cervix. The major complication is painless bleeding, usually in the last three months of pregnancy. Diagnosis is made with ultrasound scanning.

PLACENTA PREVIA

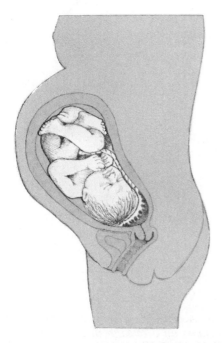

In placenta previa, the placenta (afterbirth) lies over the neck of the womb. This often necessitates cesarean delivery, especially if the placenta lies centrally over the cervix, as otherwise heavy bleeding may occur when labor begins.

Treatment is rest and, if necessary, blood transfusions. If bleeding persists, or if the fetus is in danger, a cesarean section is performed.

plague

An infectious disease caused by the bacterium *Yersinia pestis.* The disease is endemic in the western United States and in South America, China, and parts of Africa.

The causative bacteria normally infect rodents and spread via the rat flea. If a rat is dying from plague, fleas may leave their rodent host and have the opportunity to bite a human.

There are three forms of plague: BUBONIC PLAGUE, marked by general enlargement of lymph nodes and a rash; *pneumonic plague,* a pneumonia of the lungs that can be spread to others by coughing; the *septicemic plague,* where there is rapid spread of the organisms throughout the body in the blood.

The "Black Death" in fourteenth-century Europe was a plague pandemic. Epidemics are now rare, and the precautions can be taken to limit their spread. The disease is still extremely dangerous, however, and antimicrobial treatment usually is effective only if started within a few hours of onset. Treatment involves the administration of sulfonamides, streptomycin, chloramphenicol, or tetracyclines.

plantar wart

A wart occurring on the sole of the foot.

Like other WARTS, plantar warts are caused by a virus. They are common and contagious and are spread particularly by close contact with bare feet—as occurs in swimming pools and locker rooms. Some individuals seem completely immune whereas others may develop large numbers of warts. Plantar warts, unlike most other types, tend to be painful because pressure forces them into the foot.

There is no reliable treatment that will work in all cases. Warts usually can be removed by cautery and curettage or by the application of liquid nitrogen. Special plasters are sometimes effective. Recurrence is common but, equally, the warts may disappear suddenly and permanently for no obvious reason.

platelets

A component of the blood. Platelets (also known as *thrombocytes*) are colorless disks, much smaller than the red and white cells. They are not cells but are cellular fragments produced by large cells (*megakaryocytes*) in the bone marrow. They have a normal life span in the blood of about ten days.

The best-understood function of platelets is their role in the formation of blood clots. The platelets stick to the walls of damaged blood vessels and release substances that initiate the formation of a clot. Although they are not essential for all blood clotting, a deficiency of platelets may lead to abnormal bleeding, especially in the skin (thrombocytopenic PURPURA).

Several diseases lead to a fall in the number of platelets in the blood. Also, some conditions (such as kidney failure) may impair the function of the platelets. Some persons develop a low platelet count for no obvious reason—a condition known as *idiopathic thrombocytopenic purpura*.

Platelets can be separated from blood and transfused into persons who have a deficiency; the effect is temporary but may be of value if such a person is bleeding or requires surgery.

Platelets also are involved in the formation of abnormal and dangerous venous thromboses and are implicated in the formation of the fatty plaques of ATHEROSCLEROSIS. Platelet function can be suppressed by aspirin.

pleural effusion

An abnormal buildup of fluid in the space between the membrane covering the lungs (the *pleura*) and the chest wall. Fluid may accumulate because of cancer of the lung, breast, or ovary, or because of pneumonia, tuberculosis, heart failure, or injury. Symptoms include fever, chest pain, cough, and difficulty in breathing. Fluid may be removed by suctioning, draining through a needle, or via medication.

pleurisy

Inflammation and swelling of the pleurae, the membranes that envelop the lungs and line the chest cavity. A person can have pleurisy with fluid

PLEURISY

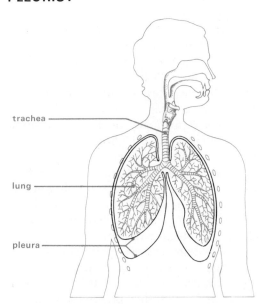

trachea

lung

pleura

The outer surface of the lungs and the inner surface of the chest wall are covered with shiny, lubricated membranes—the pleura. Pleurisy is the condition in which the pleura are inflamed and no longer slide over each other smoothly.

buildup or without. Causes of pleurisy can include tuberculosis, pneumonia, chest injury, viral infection, or lung cancer. Some of the symptoms of pleurisy are breathlessness and stabbing chest pain made worse by coughing or attempts at deep breathing. Treatment of pleurisy involves bed rest, pain-killing medications, and treatment of the underlying cause.

pneumoconiosis

The inhalation of particular forms of dust, over long periods, can lead to changes in the lungs that are nonreversible. This disease is called pneumoconiosis. Mineral dusts, notably silica, asbestos, and coal are the most common causes. Vegetable fiber dusts from sources such as hay and grass can cause what is known as "farmers' lung." Workers exposed during many years in the sugar cane and cotton industries can also contract pneumoconiosis.

There is no treatment for this disease. Prevention requires effective ventilation in the industries of mining, stonecutting, and sandblasting, the wearing of face masks, and the suppression of dust by every means possible.

pneumonia

Inflammation of the lungs from bacterial, fungal, or viral infection or from chemical damage. The outflow of fluid and cells from the inflamed lung tissue fills the airspaces, causing difficulty in breathing; in severe cases the disease can be fatal.

The lungs are unusually open to infection, since the air inhaled with each breath always contains microorganisms. Their defenses include: the filtration of air by the nose; the trapping of dust particles and bacteria by the mucous lining of the air passages; and the operation within the lung tissues of the IMMUNE SYSTEM—the combination of antibodies and protective white blood cells (phagocytes). If these defenses are impaired by old age, by a virus infection such as measles, or by *immunosuppressive* drugs (given to prevent rejection of a transplanted organ) then pneumonia is more likely.

Before the era of antibiotics the most common type of pneumonia was *lobar pneumonia*, due to one species of bacterium, *Pneumococcus*. Pneumococcal pneumonia usually is confined to one lung or one lobe of a lung, which is so heavily inflamed that it changes from a normal spongy, air-filled consistency to a heavy, "consolidated" state. Lobar pneumonia causes a high fever, often with delirium; if it is extensive, the lack of normal lung tissue means that oxygenation is inadequate and the patient becomes very short of breath and cyanosed and may lose consciousness. There may be associated inflammation of the membrane covering the lung chest wall—PLEURISY—causing a sharp pain in the chest with each breath. The sputum coughed up may be bloodstained.

Before antibiotics lobar pneumonia was often fatal, especially when it affected both lungs (*double pneumonia*). Nowadays, however, penicillin typical produces a dramatic cure in up to 95 percent of cases.

In *bronchopneumonia* patches of inflammation and consolidation are scattered through the lungs. The symptoms are usually less dramatic than in lobar pneumonia, but again there will be cough, difficulty in breathing, and fever. Bronchopneumonia may be fatal, especially in the elderly and in anyone weakened by another illness such as advanced cancer, and it is indeed a common cause of death in such diseases.

Bronchopneumonia may be due to a bacterium such as *Hemophilus*, to mycoplasma, and to viruses. It is a common complication of influenza. Treat-

THE LUNGS

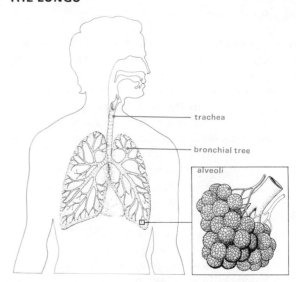

Pneumonia is inflammation of lung tissue usually caused by bacteria or viruses. Fluid and cells pour into the alveoli (air sacs) so that the air is excluded and breathing is impaired. Pneumonia can be life-threatening in the very young and very old.

ment with antibiotics is usually effective in the bacterial pneumonias, but there is still no effective specific treatment for viral pneumonias. However, the symptoms may be relieved by oxygen therapy and drugs to lower the temperature and relieve chest pain.

Pneumonia may also be due to chemical damage to the lungs from inhalation of gases such as sulfur dioxide in industrial accidents, or from inhalation of vomit by an unconscious or semi-conscious person. The treatment of chemical pneumonias depends on the removal of inflammatory fluid from the lungs by suction, anti-inflammatory drugs, and oxygen therapy.

Some forms of pneumonia may be prevented by vaccination against the virus or bacterium responsible. Vaccines against influenza and the pneumococcus are available, and their use may be recommended in the elderly and patients with debilitating illness.

pneumonitis

An inflammation of the lung tissue, pneumonitis occurs in the development of any infection of the lower respiratory tract. In the absence of infection, pneumonitis can occur as a result of inhaling noxious gases or extremely frigid air. The major symptom is a cough that is initially dry and non-productive. Treatment is directed at the underlying cause.

pneumothorax

The presence of free air or gas in the *pleural cavity*. (The pleural cavity is a narrow space between two layers of the *pleura*, the serous membrane that lines the chest cavity—*thorax*—and surrounds each lung.) When this occurs it may cause the lung to retract from the wall of the thorax and even collapse. The condition may be barely detectable or massive and threatening to life.

Spontaneous pneumothorax usually is associated with EMPHYSEMA, ASTHMA, and other chronic lung diseases. *Traumatic pneumothorax* usually results from a penetrating chest wound such as a stabbing.

Pneumothorax may begin with sharp chest pain followed by shortness of breath. Normal chest movements may stop on the affected side. There may be rapid heartbeat, a weak pulse, low

PNEUMOTHORAX

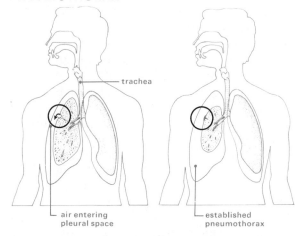

trachea

air entering pleural space

established pneumothorax

The pleural space—between the lung and chest wall—normally is only a potential one. Pneumothorax occurs when air enters this space from the lung or air passages. This may be caused by a penetrating chest wound, a congenital lung weakness, or emphysema. The abnormal pressure of air in the pleural space prevents the lung on that side from expanding effectively and in time may impede the function of the other lung. Pneumothorax may be treated by inserting a drain through the chest wall to release the air.

blood pressure, sweating, fever, dizziness, and pale skin.

The person with pneumothorax should stay in bed in an almost sitting position. In less serious cases no special treatment is necessary. In serious cases a tube may be inserted through the chest wall as part of a draining system and be removed only when air is no longer coming out. Pain-killing medication may be required.

podiatry

A medical specialty concerned with the diagnosis and treatment of diseases, injuries, and defects of the foot; formerly called *chiropody*. A podiatrist is licensed to prescribe drugs, physical therapy, and corrective devices, as well as to perform surgery according to the laws of the state in which he or she is practicing.

There are several conditions for which one might seek the skills of a podiatrist. PLANTAR WARTS on the sole of the foot may be removed by a process of electrocautery and curettage followed by DIATHERMY to the base to discourage regrowth. *Calluses* (areas of hardened skin) will require more gentle treatment. *Ingrowing nails* frequently require prolonged attention to overcome the infection at the side of the nail until the soft tissues are healthy; surgical treatment may be required if other measures fail to overcome the problem.

Flatfoot, or reduction of the longitudinal arch of the foot, commonly calls for podiatric attention. All children for the first two years of walking have "flat" feet, where the middle of the arch almost presses on the ground; but the choice of correct footwear with a heel and arch support in the shoe helps to overcome this. *Foot strain* in middle-aged persons commonly is caused by stress on the longitudinal arch ligaments and sometimes by weakening of the muscles of the foot due to inadequate exercise. Foot-strengthening exercises and electrical stimulation of the affected muscles can overcome this, in addition to the use of appropriate arch supports in the shoe.

For the elderly person deprived (by arthritis, fragility, or dizziness on bending) of the opportunity to maintain normal foot care, podiatric attention can be essential to prevent deformities occurring in uncut nails. Similarly, foot deformities due to OSTEOARTHRITIS, in-turning of the big toe, and BUNIONS are common in the elderly; podiatry then becomes necessary for foot comfort and to permit normal physical activity and mobility. Those who are diabetic require similar attention and care because of the hazard of foot infections, especially in elderly diabetic persons.

poisoning

For emergency measures, turn to *Poisoning* in the section on **First Aid**.

The accidental (or deliberate) ingestion of substances that may be poisonous in small or large doses. Fortunately, because of the increase in sophisticated medical techniques for supporting life's vital functions during hospitalization, death from poisoning is not as common as it once was.

Poisoning can produce abdominal pains, vomiting, delirium, loss of consciousness, suppression of respiration, and death. During this progression a multitude of other symptoms also can occur that are specific to or characteristic of the noxious substance. The effects of some poisons (for example, alcohol) are reversible given time; the human body is capable of excreting them or of changing them biochemically to substances that are less toxic. Other poisons (such as lead) are cumulative in small doses and are stored by the body until they destroy vital functions. Still others (such as the toxic elements of FOOD POISONING) may be evacuated rapidly from the body, although survival and prompt recovery depend on the person's initial state of health.

In all cases, the finding of an unconscious person must initiate certain *first aid procedures*. Because of the danger of choking to death on inhaled vomit, the unconscious person must be turned to the "recovery position"—lying prone, one knee bent, and face pointing sideways and down—while transport to the hospital emergency room is arranged. Should breathing cease, mouth-to-mouth resuscitation should be undertaken. Provided that the physician knows what has recently been ingested, the conscious person may be encouraged to vomit, after which he should be transferred to the hospital, again in the recovery position.

Identification of the poison may depend on finding medicine bottles or other substances near the victim, retaining a specimen of vomit for hospital laboratory analysis, or the questioning of relatives and friends. Such information can greatly aid the physician in the treatment of the poisoned person. Barbiturates (sleeping pills), opiates (morphine, cocaine, heroin), tranquilizers, and antidepressants are the most common pharmaceutical agents used in deliberate overdosage or poisoning. The danger from overdosage with these drugs is respiratory suppression. Thus, delay in hospitalization can prove fatal, for only with the proper facilities can respiration be maintained until full recovery occurs.

Metallic poisons (such as cadmium, lead, mercury, and other substances) are an industrial risk even though their effects may take many months or years to produce symptoms. Herbicides and pesticides can be inhaled accidentally or absorbed through the skin in crop-spraying; the use of respirators and protective clothing prevents poisoning for those handling these substances. Poisoning by gas inhalation (for example, carbon monoxide car exhaust fumes) may be deliberate or accidental; it requires oxygen administration for recovery as well as respiratory support.

Children are particularly prone to accidental poisoning from the ingestion of medicines found in the home, from the eating of poisonous berries, and from contact with household cleaners (especially lye) or other household or agricultural chemicals that are left unguarded or unsafely stored. In all circumstances, if it is suspected that the child has ingested or come into contact with poisonous substances, he must receive immediate hospital care. Small doses of poisonous substances that might not harm an adult may be lethal to a small child.

The prognosis for many cases is good. Some antidotes may be specific (as in barbiturate poisoning), but in general the prevention of death depends on maintaining respiration and sometimes on "washing out" the poison by dialysis—thus ensuring the victim's survival until the poison is excreted. Ingestion of caustic materials by children may require prolonged medical or surgical treatment to repair burned tissue.

Every home, especially where there are children, should have the telephone number of the local poison control center posted by the telephone for quick reference in emergencies.

See also LEAD POISONING, MERCURY POISONING, and Poisons in Chapter 21 in section on **Wellness**.

poliomyelitis

Once called "infantile paralysis," poliomyelitis is an acute viral infection of the gastrointestinal tract that may attack the central nervous system to produce motor nerve paralysis. It is found worldwide and occurs in epidemics during the summer months in temperate zones. It is transmitted by dust and fecal contact, particularly in areas of poor sanitation and hygiene.

Artificial immunity can be acquired by the injection of the "killed virus" developed by Dr. Jonas Salk or by the oral administration of a "live attenuated" (weakened) virus vaccine developed by Dr. Albert Sabin. Poliomyelitis can be acquired by the unvaccinated susceptible person by inhaling or ingesting the virus. The first symptoms may fall into any of three patterns: sore throat and fever; diarrhea; or aching in the limbs and back. These symptoms may resolve within three to five days (*nonparalytic polio*), or the virus may spread through the bloodstream to invade the central nervous system.

Signs of irritation of the covering membranes of the brain develop (stiff neck, PHOTOPHOBIA, HEADACHE) as well as painful muscle cramps and spasms. The virus causes most damage to the nerve cells controlling the muscles (the motor neurons), and within forty-eight hours there is obvious paralysis of the muscles. This may be limited to the muscles of the limbs or it may affect respiration and swallowing (*bulbar polio*). Diagnosis is made clinically and by virus culture or by determination of increases in the specific antibodies. Treatment involves hospitalization and nursing care to rest the affected muscles, and (if necessary) artificial maintenance of respiratory function. No medication is effective against polio virus. The overall mortality rate is about 5 percent. Many persons recover with a return of some degree of muscle function, but a few remain severely or even totally paralyzed.

Prevention depends entirely on immunization. The live oral vaccine confers 100 percent immunity by producing antibodies in the intestine. A policy of infant immunization has virtually eradicated the disease from the United States and other developed countries, but booster doses are recommended every eight years in childhood and before foreign travel for adults, since polio is still a major public health problem in much of Africa, Asia, and southern Europe.

polyarteritis nodosa

This disease is characterized by areas of inflammation that develop in the walls of blood vessels—both arteries and veins. These areas can lead to blockage of the affected vessels with ISCHEMIA and death of the tissues supplied by them. These inflamed areas appear most frequently in the arteries of the heart, kidneys, liver, and muscles. Polyarteritis nodosa occurs primarily in adult men, and the cause is not well understood.

This is an extremely grave disease. Any organ of the body may be affected, with consequent symptoms or function disorders such as high blood pressure, kidney disease, and abdominal complications—that can lead to death. Persons often complain initially of loss of appetite, weight loss, fevers, general weakness, and muscle pains. Diagnosis is made by physical examination; in some instances a biopsy may be necessary. Although steroids are used with good results initially, there is a high recurrence rate.

polycystic kidney

This inherited disease causes dilation of the tubules in the kidney and leads to obstruction, infection, CYSTS, and kidney failure (see KIDNEY DISEASE). It may appear in infancy or be delayed until adult life. The extent of the disease may vary, with the more severely affected cases occurring early in life. Cysts also may occur in the liver, and about 10 percent of patients have ANEURYSMS in the arteries of the brain. Progressive kidney failure occurs but may be delayed by continuous medical care that reduces infection. Death from UREMIA is prevented by an "artificial kidney" machine (see DIALYSIS under **Procedures**) or by a kidney transplant, provided that the disease has not seriously affected other organs.

polycythemia

An increase in the number of circulating red blood cells.

Polycythemia may occur as a result of a decrease in the oxygen available to red blood cells in the lungs. This occurs at high altitudes (*relative polycythemia*) and is normal in healthy people living in the Andes, the Rockies, or in other high mountain areas, and in people with chronic lung diseases such as EMPHYSEMA.

In *polycythemia vera*, the bone marrow, for unexplained reasons, begins overproducing red blood cells irrespective of the amount of oxygen available. Incidence is highest among men in middle and later life—especially males of Jewish ancestry.

A ruddy engorged complexion, abdominal

pain due to spleen and liver enlargement, headaches, and bleeding from mucous membranes may occur. The diagnosis is made by blood tests and a biopsy of the bone marrow. Complications of the disease include THROMBOSIS and hemorrhages in the gastrointestinal tract. Treatment is by blood removal (PHLEBOTOMY; see under *Procedures*) to balance the overproduction and by the administration of radioactive chemicals or cytotoxic drugs to suppress the bone marrow. Prognosis is a chronic recurrence over many years with ultimate anemia and cardiovascular or kidney complications that may lead to death.

polymyalgia rheumatica

Muscle pains throughout the body—appearing abruptly in the neck and shoulder muscles and spreading down the back to the buttocks and thighs—with stiffness, headache, fever, and loss of appetite and weight. Characteristically it attacks middle-aged and elderly persons and is more common in women.

The course is one of remissions and recurrences, but the disease is usually self-limiting, with relief occurring after a few months. Although disability may be severe, bed rest and medication with anti-inflammatory agents or steroids usually produce rapid relief. The symptoms may recur when treatment is stopped, but the prognosis (with treatment) is good. Thirty percent of patients have an associated temporal ARTERITIS, which may cause blindness unless immediately treated.

polyp

A polyp is tissue growth that projects (often from a stalk-like connection) into a body cavity or passage. Multiple polyps occur frequently in the nose, cervix, and uterus; they are rarely malignant in these sites but do cause symptoms owing to obstruction or deformation of the anatomical cavity and to excessive stretching of the mucous membrane. Chronic superficial infections predispose to the development of polyps, which usually are seen only in adults.

Persons with allergies or chronic RHINITIS are more prone to develop nasal polyps. Excess mucus formation, nosebleeds, and loss of the sense of smell may occur, and the polyps are recognized easily on examination as glistening extrusions of

POLYPS

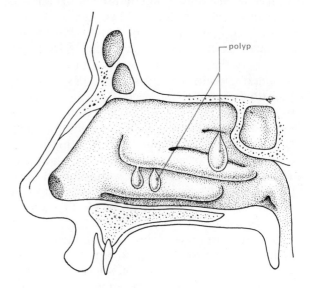

MULTIPLE POLYPS IN THE NASAL CAVITY

Nasal polyps are areas of the membrane lining the nose that become distended with excess tissue fluid and hang down into the nasal cavity. They are usually due to an allergy. Since they can cause nasal obstruction, they may have to be removed.

the nasal lining. In the cervix or uterus, bleeding between menstrual periods is a possible sign of polyp development; some FIBROIDS of the uterus may resemble polyps in shape.

The intestines are another frequent site of polyps, especially in the colon. There are various reasons for their occurrence and they can be benign (noncancerous) or malignant (cancerous). Frequently, the first indication of their presence will be changes in bowel habits (either constipation or diarrhea) and weight loss. These symptoms must be evaluated by a physician who can test the stool for the presence of OCCULT BLOOD and, if necessary, examine the bowel by a variety of tests. If indicated, a biopsy will be done on the polyp or it will be removed surgically so that a diagnosis can be made. Polyps, both benign and malignant, have a tendency to recur, so periodic medical examinations are very important.

porphyrias

A group of rare inherited disorders of porphyrin metabolism caused by gene mutation.

Porphyrins are complex chemical compounds

found in heme, the red pigment that contributes its color to the hemoglobin in red blood cells. In the porphyrias there is an abnormal accumulation in the tissues of various types of porphyrin pigments. There are at least six different porphyrias.

Symptoms of the porphyrias include excessive sensitivity to sunlight, with blistering, pigmentation, and various types of skin eruptions. Discoloration of the teeth and bones is also typical. There may be nerve damage from the toxic effects of the porphyrins on nerve fibers, marked by muscle weakness and paralysis, severe abdominal pain, and other neurological symptoms. Psychological disturbances may occur with MANIA, DELIRIUM, or COMA; in some cases death occurs. Other cases, however, are very mild, with no symptoms except a slight sensitivity to sunlight.

Diagnosis is confirmed by the presence of porphyrins in the urine; it may be reddish ("port wine urine") or may darken on standing in the light. Excessive amounts are also present in the feces, where they can be identified by means of chemical tests.

There is no satisfactory treatment, but persons must be protected from sunlight. Certain drugs may be used to control the psychological manifestations.

Drugs such as barbiturate "sleeping tablets," which can precipitate an attack, must be avoided.

postnasal drip

The trickling of mucus from the back portion of the nasal cavity onto the surface of the throat, usually caused by a common cold or an allergy.

postpartum depression

Some sort of "let-down" feeling is experienced by many mothers in the first week after childbirth. However, true depressive illness—with insomnia, tearfulness, irrational fears, irritability, guilt, and psychic disturbances (which may include rejection of the baby and even infanticide in extremely severe cases) is much more rare. But at least 15 percent of women experience some symptoms of depression within the first six months after birth.

Hormonal origins are suspected and menstrual irregularity is a frequent accomplishment; but environmental, social, and sexual difficulties also predispose the woman to the development of postpartum "blues." In addition, any emotional disorder prior to pregnancy frequently is magnified or exacerbated in the postpartum stage. (Depression following MISCARRIAGE or abortion is similar in its pattern.)

Suicide is extremely rare, but neglect of or physical harm to the baby is a common manifestation. The diagnosis is made by health professionals when family problems emerge that cannot be overcome by support from husbands, relatives, and close friends.

Treatment may include psychotherapy with or without antidepressant medication. Admission to a psychiatric hospital may be necessary in a very few cases. Fortunately, however, most cases of postpartum depression are mild and transient.

posture

Position of the body, usually referring to the upright position of a person when standing. The multiple vertebrae of the spinal column are maintained in position, flexibly, by what are (normally) strong ligaments over which the spinal muscles lie.

Disease of the spinal column, congenital or acquired disorders of the spinal bones, and injury or weakness of the spinal ligaments or muscles can also result in compensatory postures—often leading to curvatures, pains, or lack of flexibility. Normally, with the shoulders held back and the head upright looking forward, there are two natural curves in the spine (the sacrolumbar and the cervicothoracic) which look roughly like an "S" bend when viewed from the side and straight when viewed from the front or rear. If there is hip disease or leg-shortening, then the pelvis tilts and the spinal column curves laterally to compensate—a condition known as *scoliosis.* KYPHOSIS ("humpback" or "hunchback") is an excessive curvature due to disease, abnormal development, or injuries of the upper spine. *Lordosis* is exaggeration of the normal curve in the lower part of the back (the lumbar region) due to obesity, a heavy abdomen, and lax muscles. Minor degrees of spinal deformity and postural abnormality are quite common.

Encouragement of habits of good posture in children is important, not only for a pleasing physical appearance but also to prevent the possible development of permanent deformities. In the adult, *postural backache*—caused by lifting in-

POSTURE

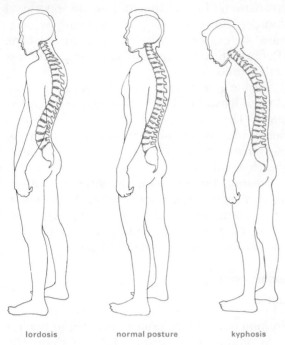

lordosis   normal posture   kyphosis

The illustration shows how the curvature of the spinal column determines posture, whether correct or incorrect. Abnormal postures such as lordosis and kyphosis can result from disease, spinal deformities, and poor posture habits. Poor posture can affect internal organs and lead to such symptoms as low back pain.

juries, strain, and a tendency to slouch when sitting (especially in poorly designed furniture)—is the most common single reason for referral to an orthopedist (specialist in bones and joints). The spinal ligaments loosen with childbirth, debilitating illness, and obesity, and this may lead—in tall persons especially—to pain in lower back. Postural backache, which is worse on stooping, causes great and often recurrent distress. Treatment typically involves physical therapy (heat, massage, and special exercises), manipulation of the lower spine, or the wearing of an external support (corset).

See also SPINAL CURVATURE and SPINE.

post-Vietnam stress syndrome

A disorder observed in veterans of the Vietnam war, attributed to the extreme stresses of their combat experience. An estimated half million Vietnam veterans had problems readjusting to civilian life during the first five postwar years. These problems included vocational and legal difficulties, depression and other emotional upsets, alcoholism, drug abuse, and a high rate of suicide. Many veterans had recurrent, intrusive flashbacks of events that occurred during the war or nightmares about these experiences. In a subconscious effort to avoid such emotional reinvolvement, patients with posttraumatic stress disorder tended to become numbed, isolating themselves from current events or reactions. In many veterans the symptoms persist despite the passage of time.

Pott's fracture

A fracture dislocation of the ankle. This type of fracture usually results from the foot being caught while the body is moving forward (for example, during walking or skiing). As a result, the foot is twisted outward, producing a spiral fracture at the lower end of the fibula (the bony prominence felt on the outer side of the ankle).

This type of fracture is treated by immobili-

POTT'S FRACTURE

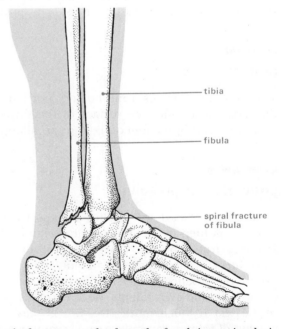

tibia

fibula

spiral fracture
of fibula

Pott's fracture results from the foot being twisted violently outward. The basic injury is a spiral fracture of the fibula, as pictured above, but in addition the inner side of the ankle may be damaged and the bottom of the tibia fractured.

zation in a plaster cast from below the knee to the base of the toes; the cast usually is left in position for about six weeks. However, more severe twisting can pull a flake of bone from the inner side of the ankle and also fracture the bottom of the tibia, or shin bone. In such cases the bones have to be realigned under anesthesia and sometimes held in place with screws; the plaster cast is left in position for up to three months.

preeclampsia

An abnormal condition of pregnancy marked by high BLOOD PRESSURE, abnormal presence of protein in the urine (PROTEINURIA), weight gain, and swelling, especially of the ankles. It occurs most often in young women in their first pregnancies. Early detection is essential. Untreated, the pregnant woman can go into a coma, have seizures, or have problems with premature separation of the placenta. Bed rest, restricted salt intake, sedatives, and medications to control high blood pressure may be required.

See also under *Disorders of Pregnancy* in section on **Family Medicine and Health**.

pregnancy

Conception, the fertilization of an ovum by a sperm, can occur in a woman from the menarche to the menopause and takes place in one of the FALLOPIAN TUBES. Pregnancy occurs when the fertilized ovum moves down into the uterus and implants itself in the wall. Pregnancy normally lasts until labor takes place, on average, forty weeks after fertilization. The initial signs of pregnancy are breast engorgement, blue coloration of the vagina, and absence of the expected menstrual period. The early symptoms are nausea and frequency of urination. To confirm the diagnosis, tests are undertaken on a sample of urine to detect the excess of hormones that are present only from the second week of pregnancy on.

In the first three months the breast signs are the most obvious, with enlargement of the areola (the dark ring of tissue surrounding the nipple) and prominence of the sebaceous glands around it. In the fourth month the uterus enlarges and is able to be felt above the pubis; thereafter the abdominal swelling is plainly visible. Fetal move-

PREGNANCY

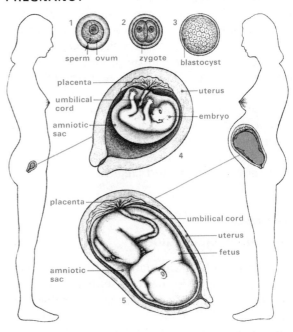

Conception occurs when a sperm fertilizes an ovum (1) and a zygote (2) forms. The zygote divides into many identical cells and becomes a blastocyst (3) which embeds itself in the lining of the uterus. During the first three months the embryo takes shape (4) with the appearance of all its major organs. In the last six months the fetus increases in size dramatically (5).

ments are felt at this time by a woman experiencing her first pregnancy (twenty weeks), a little earlier by those who have previously experienced childbirth. In the eighth month there is a "lightening" as the fetal head descends into the pelvic brim. The onset of labor in the ninth month is announced by a "show" as the mucous plug of the cervix is discharged into the vagina, after contractions of the uterine muscle have been experienced as regular cramp-like pains.

An average weight gain of 30 pounds is associated with minimal complications; most of this is put on after the twentieth week, but many women experience appetite variations in pregnancy—in particular, bizarre or obsessional tastes in the first three months. Constipation is a frequent problem in the later months, and hemorrhoids may be a complication; both need to be dealt with by dietary advice and appropriate medication.

The position of the fetus changes frequently in the last three months of pregnancy, but after the thirty-second week the head should be entering the pelvis. Many women experience backache due to loosening of the ligaments in the last three months. Correct posture, exercise, and antenatal relaxation are helpful in preventing such problems and in preparing the woman for effective labor.

Pregnant women should avoid taking any drugs except under medical supervision, particularly during the first three months.

See also *Pregnancy and Childbirth* in the section on **Family Medicine and Health.**

premature ejaculation

The ejaculation of seminal fluid from the penis at an earlier stage in intercourse than is desired, or even before insertion. This may be a subjective judgment if the achievement of the partner's orgasm is the criterion, and retention and delay of ejaculation will depend on the sexual partner's level of excitation (which is obviously variable). This is a common condition in perfectly normal men who are relatively inexperienced or inactive sexually and who are excessively stimulated by their sexual partner.

Control over ejaculation is acquired with experience. However, infrequency of coitus in middle age may cause the return of premature ejaculation and lead to sexual difficulties. In any age group, the level of control is affected by fatigue, fantasy, and drugs such as alcohol.

Treatment is necessary when premature ejaculation provokes marital problems, especially if it occurs with greater frequency after relative control had been established for some time. An isolated occurrence may be compensated for by resuming intercourse after a period of delay, in order to achieve a second orgasm. Repeated occurrences may lead to psychic IMPOTENCE as a way of avoiding exposure to the risk. In this case, treatment may be beneficial.

Medication has little to offer. Sexual counseling of both partners is recommended—in particular, instruction in the "squeeze" technique. After erection and just prior to the overwhelming desire to ejaculate, the tip of the penis (glans) is firmly compressed—more effectively by the woman—by fingers and thumb placed above and below the coronal ridge. This counteracts the reflex of ejaculation and may be repeated periodically when the desire to achieve orgasm returns.

Effective control is reestablished in a high percentage of cases when this technique is employed mutually.

premenstrual tension

Also known as *premenstrual syndrome.* The condition of mental tension, irritability, headache, depression, and a feeling of "bloatedness," with some evidence of EDEMA, that begins in the week prior to menstruation and resolves completely the day after the period starts.

It is a common condition that causes a good deal of distress to those affected by it—which includes women of all ethnic groups. Hormonal changes are thought to be a cause, with water and salt retention being the consequences of a hormonal imbalance; but psychogenic causes play their part in initiating a behavioral response to physical changes in the body.

Conditions believed to have a *psychosomatic* component—such as eczema, migraine, and allergic responses—may be exacerbated in the premenstrual period. Various events not clearly associated with the menstrual cycle also can occur: Admissions to psychiatric hospitals, suicides, accidents, and misbehavior in schools are all found to occur more frequently during the premenstrual time.

There have been some advances in the treatment of this syndrome but much research continues. It is not known why some women experience premenstrual tension and others do not.

priapism

A painful condition of continuous erection of the penis. It is seldom related to sexual excitement and usually indicates a serious disorder. The cause is often unknown but priapism has been associated with LEUKEMIA and SICKLE-CELL ANEMIA, as well as with neurological damage following spinal cord injury.

Priapism is thought to occur when blood clots in the penile blood vessels, rather than flowing normally. Blood is, therefore, unable to leave the penis and causes continued erection. The condition often is treated by sedation and anticoagulation medications (medicines that prevent clotting).

proctitis

Swelling and inflammation in the area of the rectum and anus caused by infection, injury, drugs, allergy, or radiation. Symptoms include pain, itching, urge to defecate without being able to do so, and pus, blood, or mucus in the stool.

progesterone

One of the two major types of female sex hormones secreted by the ovaries, and the main hormone of the progestogen group.

During the menstrual cycle, progesterone—in combination with estrogens—is secreted by the corpus luteum, which develops in the ovarian follicle after OVULATION. If the ovum (egg) is not fertilized, there is a decline of both hormones; this decline is associated with the onset of menstruation. Progesterone, like estrogen, thus maintains the uterus in a state of receptivity for the implantation of a fertilized ovum.

In early pregnancy the corpus luteum secretes progesterone, as does the developing PLACENTA. Initially the greatest quantity comes from the corpus luteum, but by the tenth week of pregnancy placental secretion is fully established and rises steadily as pregnancy advances.

progestin

The name originally given to the crude hormone of the corpus luteum (which develops in the empty ovarian follicle following OVULATION), now known as *progesterone*. The function of this hormone is to prepare the uterus for the reception and development of the fertilized ovum.

The term "progestin" is now applied generally to *progestational agents*, a group of hormones secreted by the corpus luteum and the PLACENTA. The synthetic analogs of these hormones are the basis of the ovulation-inhibiting effect of oral contraceptives ("the Pill"). In these, progestational agents are combined with estrogens to prevent conception, with a minimum of side effects such as breakthrough bleeding.

prognosis

A prediction regarding the likely course and outcome of a disease or disorder, especially one based on the judgment of the attending physician.

prolapse

The "falling down" of any organ, usually applied to the uterus (womb) and the rectum.

Prolapse of the uterus is relatively common, particularly in elderly women. It is associated with the progressive weakness of muscle and of other supportive structures in the pelvic area in later life. Often this is caused by injury to or overstretching of the pelvic floor in childbirth. Injury to the perineum (the area of tissue between the anus and the vulva) and to the vagina may contribute to the prolapse.

Prolapse of the *first degree* implies the presence of the cervix (neck of the womb) at the vaginal opening. In *second-degree* prolapse the cervix protrudes through the vaginal opening; in *third-degree* prolapse the entire uterus protrudes through the vaginal opening. In some cases there are no symptoms apart from the mechanical discomfort of the movement of the uterus; but there may be some feeling of "bearing down" or heaviness in the lower part of the abdomen and back.

Surgery is the ideal treatment in many cases. The laxness in the ligaments and muscles is taken up and the uterus is returned to its proper position. In women past childbearing age, the more radical operation of removal of the uterus (*hysterectomy*) may be preferred. Another form of treatment in elderly women or in those who are poor operative risks is the insertion of a rubber ring to take up the slack in the vagina and to support the neck of the womb.

In *prolapse of the rectum*, the rectal wall turns inside out and may protrude through the anal opening; this is a *complete* prolapse. In *partial* prolapse, only the mucous membrane protrudes. The latter is much more common, especially in old age, and the protrusion is rarely more than 1 inch long.

Complete rectal prolapse is approximately five times as common in women as in men and is associated with repeated pregnancies and consequent weakening of the pelvic floor. Any condition, such as chronic constipation, that leads to straining at stool may lead to prolapse, but the most common cause is hemorrhoids ("piles"). Again, surgical treatment is necessary if the prolapse is not to recur. Attention must be given also to the predisposing causes.

prophylaxis

Prevention of disease or of an undesired consequence, or various measures that prevent the development and spread of disease.

proptosis

A bulging or outward displacement of a body organ, such as the abnormal protrusion of the eyeball (bilateral or unilateral.)

prostaglandins

Every cell in the body contains enzymes for the synthesis of a range of highly active substances known as prostaglandins. These are formed and released from the cell when it is injured or otherwise stimulated. These substances were first isolated from the prostate gland.

Prostaglandins stimulate smooth muscle, change the heart rate, affect the motility of the intestine, influence blood pressure, and cause the uterus to contract. They also act upon HORMONES, antagonizing the action of epinephrine, glucagon, vasopressin, and ACTH; it seems that they also play a part in metabolic processes. They alter the stickiness of the blood PLATELETS and prevent clotting in arteries.

So far more than twenty different prostaglandins have been isolated, and research in the field is active. Among their possible uses, besides their use to induce abortion or labor at term, may be an application in depressing male fertility, which could make a male contraceptive pill practical.

prostatitis

Inflammation of the prostate gland. The prostate is a gland in men that surrounds the urethra where it exits from the bladder. It produces the fluid that mixes with sperm to produce semen. The prostate is also partly composed of muscle.

The prostate can become inflamed for a number of reasons, and this condition can be chronic or acute. *Acute bacterial prostatitis* is an infection of the gland, often with high fever, urinary frequency and urgency, great difficulty in voiding urine, burning pain, and, sometimes, blood in the urine. Hospitalization and intensive antibiotic treatment, after the identification of the causative organism, are usually required. Treatment is often continued for about a month, so as to avoid *chronic prostatitis*.

Some cases occur as a result of infection with gonorrhea.

prosthesis

Any device used to replace a body part, organ, or limb, usually taking over all or part of its function.

The most common prosthetic device (and the only one that the vast majority of the population are likely to need) is the *artificial denture* ("false teeth" or a "false tooth"). More than 50 percent of the American population over the age of 50 have dentures of some sort, either complete or partial, or have had teeth crowned.

The design of *artificial limbs* has been much improved in recent years. At one time an artificial leg was little better than the old-fashioned wooden leg; but the use of lightweight materials and improvements in joint movement have now made it possible for amputees to pass undetected in company. The most recent advance is the development of artificial limbs that are controlled by nerve impulses fed from the stump of the natural arm. These prostheses look like normal limbs, and their internal power systems enable the user to pick up and manipulate objects.

A third common use of prostheses is in the treatment of ARTHRITIS. Replacement of the hip joint in cases of both rheumatoid arthritis and osteoarthritis is now commonplace, using stainless steel and plastic materials. As a result of the success of this type of operation, surgeons have gone on to design elbow, knee, shoulder, and finger joints that can be implanted to replace joints in persons with severe arthritis.

A prosthesis that has gained much attention in recent years is the artificial heart. It has been used as total heart replacement in a small number of persons with severe, life-threatening, end-stage heart disease who, because of their age and other factors, are not good candidates for heart transplants, and for those in need of a heart transplant but for whom a donor heart is not yet available. So far the results have been so poor that many experts have condemned the procedure. It is still considered experimental.

One of the most common reasons for open-heart surgery is the implantation of artificial heart valves in those whose valves are distorted or damaged from conditions such as RHEUMATIC HEART DISEASE.

Other prostheses in current use include acrylic lenses (to replace those affected by CATARACT) and artificial eyes (whose purpose is entirely cosmetic). An artificial larynx ("voice box") is still under trial, and attempts are being made to miniaturize an artificial pancreas for use by diabetics. In the case of many complex internal organs, however, TRANSPLANTATION has so far proved more practicable than the development of mechanical prostheses.

proteinuria

A condition in which protein is present in the urine; known also as ALBUMINURIA.

Protein in the urine is often a symptom of serious KIDNEY DISEASE or HEART DISEASE. The detection of proteinuria may, in fact, be the earliest and most conclusive evidence of kidney disease. The condition can, however, be without significance.

prurigo

A chronic inflammatory eruption of the skin, usually characterized by the formation of small whitish papules (solid, circumscribed elevations of the skin) accompanied by severe itching. The papules, which are deeply seated, are most prominent on the extensor surfaces of the limbs.

The eruptions characteristically begin early in life. There are two main forms: *prurigo mitis*, which is comparatively mild, and *prurigo agria*, which is severe. The condition may be permanent or it may come and go. In young children the nonpermanent form may be associated with problems of teething or with ECZEMA.

Summer prurigo is another name for *hydroa vacciniforme*, a skin disease usually affecting adolescent boys and young men; it appears in the summer on exposed parts of the body probably as a reaction to insect bites. It is characterized by the formation of ulcers (which may become encrusted) and vesicles. Following the onset of puberty, this disease gradually disappears.

pruritus ani/pruritus vulvae

A continuous itching in the region of the anus (pruritus ani) or the vulva (pruritus vulvae).

Pruritus ani usually is found in men and is quite common. It can be intensely irritating and should be treated if it reaches the point of acute discomfort. The first line of treatment is to find the cause of the pruritus and if possible remove it. One common cause is parasites, particularly PINWORMS, which lay their eggs around the anus and so cause itching. CANDIDA infections also cause itching.

Both lack of cleanliness and excessive sweating can contribute, and the latter may be due to unsuitable underclothes that prevent proper evaporation. In the past, woolen underwear was to blame, but now in many cases it is nylon and other synthetic fibers that are the cause of pruritus. It occurs sometimes in persons who sit for long periods on plastic seats, either at home or at work, since these do not give sufficient ventilation. (A seat pad made of woven material will help air to circulate.) Some pruritus is undoubtedly caused by wearing garments that have been washed in harsh detergents, especially enzyme detergents.

Discharge from the anus or the vagina, as in HEMORRHOIDS ("piles") or VAGINITIS, can be a potent cause of itching.

Pruritus vulvae has similar causes, complicated by the fungus and yeast infections that the vagina is prone to; the modern habit of wearing nylon panty hose has exacerbated the problem.

Persons with pruritus should pay particular attention to personal hygiene. After using the toilet, they should carefully wash and dry the area around the anus. They should avoid the use of harsh detergents in washing their clothes, and wear underclothes made of cotton rather than synthetic materials.

Medication ointments are available—over the counter and by prescription—that will relieve the itching. In instances of prolonged itching and irritation, a physician should be consulted to find if there is a more serious underlying cause.

psittacosis

A disease (also known as *ornithosis* or *parrot fever*) caused by a strain of the microorganism *Chlamydia psittaci*, which is transmitted to humans by a variety of birds. It was first detected in parrots—thus the name, which comes from the Greek word for parrot. But it is now known that several species of birds harbor the microorganisms and can pass them on to humans.

In humans the disease usually takes the form of pneumonia, with fever, dry cough, and perhaps an enlarged spleen. It has been compared with TYPHOID FEVER in its manifestations, and may cause HEPATITIS, MYOCARDITIS, DELIRIUM, and COMA.

Besides parrots, other possible carriers are pigeons, parakeets, budgerigars, ducks, turkeys, pheasants, and chickens.

Treatment with antibiotics is effective.

psoriasis

A skin disease that can affect persons of either sex at any age. Although much research is being done to find the cause of this disfiguring condition, the only treatment at this time is directed toward symptomatic relief.

Psoriasis is not contagious, and the skin lesions take many forms: chronic scaling plaques, ringed lesions, smooth red areas, acute pustules, and drop-like lesions. Most often the condition becomes apparent for the first time in adolescence; sometimes, however, it does not appear until old age. The disease is often complicated by severe ARTHRITIS.

There are many medications, both oral and topical (applied to the skin) for the treatment of psoriasis. Each case may respond differently and

PSORIASIS

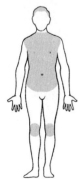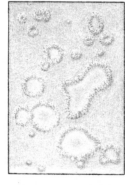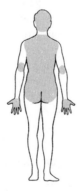

The center figure shows the characteristic skin changes in psoriasis: a clearly defined, red, raised plaque topped by silvery scales. These plaques usually are present over the elbows, knees, and scalp, but may spread more extensively to involve the trunk and hands, as illustrated here.

so treatment is designed for each individual. Drugs, ultraviolet light, and creams made up of a tar mixture or of steroids may all be tried.

Acute, body-wide outbreaks of psoriasis should be treated in a hospital because of the extent of the treatment needed.

Psoriatic persons often need encouragement from their families and physicians, since the chronic nature and unsightly appearance of the lesions can cause depression. Although the cause of psoriasis is still unknown, many of the symptoms can be alleviated by new methods of treatment. This should be emphasized to counteract the stress, anxiety, and emotional extremes that tend to cause a recurrence or worsening of the disease. Persons with psoriasis may need counseling to help them deal with their self-image.

psychiatry

The study and treatment of mental disturbances of all kinds.

Mental illness is present in society in varying degrees. People who suffer from emotional problems may seek the assistance of a *psychiatrist.*

During the twentieth century, classification of mental abnormalities has become more scientific, and psychiatry has developed methods of treating them—methods ranging from chemotherapy to PSYCHOSURGERY and from PSYCHOANALYSIS to ELECTROCONVULSIVE THERAPY (ECT) (see under **Procedures**).

The environmental stresses of life are great enough to cause anxiety, depression, and behavioral disorders in many persons who are not psychotic (that is, who do not suffer from serious mental disturbances). Although psychiatry set out in the modern era to deal with the psychoses (such as SCHIZOPHRENIA and manic-depressive illness), at present psychiatrists spend considerable time treating persons for neurosis and substance abuse.

Psychiatry has evolved into many groups whose rationale and methods are often mutually contradictory. It can be said in general that at one extreme are the psychiatrists who try to treat illness by altering body chemistry, while at the other extreme are those who postulate that psychotherapy without drugs is the most likely course to be successful. In practice, few psychiatrists adopt an extreme position; a psychotherapist, for example, will often prescribe tranquilizers to lower a person's level of anxiety.

Psychiatrists are all medically qualified doctors,

although there is a school of thought that maintains that a full medical training is unnecessary. In the United States there has already been some reduction in the amount of medical training required of a qualified psychiatrist, and the trend may be toward an even greater specialization.

See also PSYCHIATRIST under **Providers**.

psychoanalysis

The system, devised by Sigmund Freud (1856—1939), of analyzing emotional patterns and developments in persons. It is used to bring out valuable information from the unconscious mind and so make it available for manipulation by the conscious mind.

Psychoanalysis is an accepted method of treating emotional disorders such as neuroses. Essentially, it consists of allowing the person, usually lying on a couch, to relax mind and body, to give free expression to his thoughts, ideas, and fantasies. The analyst meanwhile adopts a neutral attitude, withholding judgment on everything that he or she is told, but encouraging the flow of words.

The object is to persuade the person to go further and further back into his childhood and reenact his early emotional attitudes. It is hoped that this will release various infantile emotional tensions, which, according to Freud's theories, can affect the whole of one's emotional development. Theoretically, once enlightenment about the cause of one's mental symptoms has been reached (such as hatred of one's father or guilt about sex), the symptoms should be relieved. Freud's theories were based on the concept that much of our later development is based on the experience of the first five years of life, thus the interest in the earliest memories.

The psychoanalytic theory is based on a three-fold division of the human personality: the *id*, the *ego*, and the *superego*. The id is the "instinctual self" that is concerned with the immediate discharge of energy or tension; the ego regulates the interactions of the person with his environment; and the superego is the "superior being" representing the moral aspects of personality or "conscience."

Freud postulated that there are two great groups of instincts that provide energy for the id. The first, serving the purposes of *life*, provides the energy known as *libido*. According to Freud, all activities of the mind are driven by the need to reduce or eliminate the tension caused by the painful impact of the life instincts. The second group of instincts, such as aggression, sadism, masochism, and the urge to suicide, is in the service of *death*.

To protect itself from anxiety, the ego develops many defense mechanisms, and it is the task of psychoanalysis to break down the barriers that conceal these mechanisms, which often cripple the personality. One should point out, however, that this treatment is lengthy and costly, especially in comparison with the therapeutic usefulness of several new psychoactive drugs and short-term psychotherapy. Freud originated psychoanalytic theory and technique, but his theories have been modified by modern Freudian analysts.

psychoses

Mental disorders of a severe kind in which there is an extensive disorder of thinking, feeling, and behavior. They are usually more severe and more disabling than other psychiatric syndromes and often are accompanied by impaired perceptions of reality.

One of the main psychoses is SCHIZOPHRENIA, a description given to a group of illnesses marked mainly by disordered thought processes, DELUSIONS, and HALLUCINATIONS. The consequences of this disorder include difficulty in communication and in interpersonal relationships. In the United States, the prevalence rate for schizophrenia is estimated to be 1 percent of the population.

Affective disorders may amount to psychosis, although the main symptom is a severe disorder of mood. An example is MANIA, or manic psychosis, characterized by elevated mood, hyperactivity, and disordered thinking. Lithium salts and other medications are used to treat this disturbance.

Paranoid disorders (see PARANOIA) are a group of mental illnesses in which psychosis is manifested in delusions. Typical symptoms are delusions of grandeur and persecution. These disorders may be treated with psychotherapy and medication.

psychosomatic illnesses

Disorders with physical symptoms that are thought to be caused by emotional factors. When modern medicine began to evolve, developments led to an early belief that illness was mainly, if not entirely, physical in origin. With greater understanding of disease processes, it is now realized that the body (or *soma*) and the mind (or *psyche*) are linked intimately in ways that can lead to a wide variety of illnesses.

When a person is put under stress he will react in one of several ways: *normally, neurotically* (when his defense against the stress becomes ineffective), or *psychotically* (when the defense is based on distorted perceptions of the stress). A fourth possibility is that he may react in a "psychophysiologic" way: The alert is translated into an effect on somatic systems, causing changes in body tissues (blushing is a simple example of how the emotions can have a physical manifestation). What is happening is that the physical changes are normal for the emotional states involved, but they are either too sustained or too intense. The individual may not be aware of his emotional state.

An example that is widely known is the PEPTIC ULCER. Tension in one's work or home can produce or exacerbate ulcers, although it is now believed that persons with ulcers may also be predisposed genetically to the complaint by a chromosomal fault that gives them too little of an enzyme necessary for a healthy stomach. Stress can be caused by such factors as success, failure, puberty, aging, parenthood, and conflict. Suppression of anxiety or rage may lead to cardiovascular problems and to "vascular headache."

Irritable colon (IRRITABLE BOWEL SYNDROME) is now regarded as psychosomatic, but in these cases as well there may be a congenitally high sensitivity to nervous system stimulation. ASTHMA is a general description for a group of respiratory disorders, some of which are made worse by psychological stress.

In general, it may be said that some individuals seem to be predisposed by the nature of their personality structure to react to a life situation that threatens their security not by adequate action but by emotional conflict. If the conflict is not discharged by action or speech, it persists and can create a state of acute or chronic emotional tension that seeks another outlet and leads to physical symptoms.

psychosurgery

Surgery that cuts certain nerve pathways in the brain, designed to cure or lessen some symptoms of severe mental illness. Psychosurgery is used only after other methods of treatment have failed to bring about any improvement over a long period of time and only with the informed consent of the patient.

psychotherapy

A method of treating a psychiatric disorder based mainly on verbal communication between the therapist and his patient.

The object is to cure or alleviate the symptoms of the disorder by making the emotionally distressed person feel better and helping him learn how to live more effectively. A feature of many types of psychotherapy is the person's relief at being able to talk to a noncritical listener. Apart from being able to obtain relief through discussing thoughts and feelings, the person may be able to experience the emotional discharge known as *catharsis* by recalling significant incidents and sensations that had been forgotten or repressed. It is also possible through psychotherapy to "desensitize" a person by referring repeatedly to a disturbing topic and to clarify the person's feelings by exploring them.

The role of the therapist is often to interpret the recurring patterns of behavior and enable the person to experience improved relationships with others.

Psychotherapy, which normally is carried out on the basis of weekly interviews, employs PSYCHO-ANALYSIS, HYPNOSIS, conditioning, and aversion therapy. *Group therapy* enables persons to develop skills in interacting with others and to overcome feelings of isolation and alienation. It is a popular and growing form of psychotherapy that is within the financial means of many people.

ptosis

Prolapse or drooping of an organ, often used to describe the drooping of an upper eyelid. In many cases paralysis of the third cranial nerve causes this condition, but it may be congenital.

In young children, *congenital ptosis* is due to malformation of the levator muscle and requires urgent attention if AMBLYOPIA is to be avoided. *Hysterical ptosis* is a drooping of the eyelid caused by a spasm of the orbicularis oculi muscle. *Mechanical ptosis* is due to the thickening and consequent increase in the weight of the upper eyelid that arises in diseases such as TRACHOMA or *blepharo-chalasia.*

Ptosis may be a sign of MYASTHENIA GRAVIS or, more seriously, of an ANEURYSM on a brain artery. In the latter case, eye movements may also be affected. Ptosis can also be caused by DIABETES MELLITUS. It may be caused by skull fracture with involvement of the third nerve, or by severe facial injury in which the levator muscle of the eyelid may be damaged and subsequently be unable to control the eyelid correctly. It is possible to correct the condition surgically to some extent by resecting the levator muscle; but the eye surgeon has to be careful not to raise the eyelid so high that the eye cannot be closed, and also to make it match the other lid as closely as possible.

puerperal fever

Blood poisoning (SEPTICEMIA) caused by bacterial infection of the genital tract shortly after childbirth or abortion. The disease is also known as *puerperal sepsis.*

The raw surface of the womb after separation of the placenta provides ideal circumstances for the growth of bacteria. One of the more common bacteria found to cause this infection is *Streptococcus,* which frequently is found in the nose, throat, rectum, and vagina of healthy adults.

Prior to mid-nineteenth century, death from puerperal fever was very common. The high death rates dropped sharply after the concept of germ transmission was developed. Strict observance of the rules of hygiene and the use of antiseptics greatly improved survival rates, but the development of antibiotics has done even more to control this life-threatening condition. Abortions performed under poor sanitary conditions were also a prime cause of puerperal fever. With the advent of the 1972 ruling that legalized abortion, the infection rate dropped as hospital-style environments could safely be used.

Today any woman found to have an elevated temperature in the fourteen days after delivery or abortion is treated with the appropriate antibiotics. Septicemia following childbirth and abortion has become a rare occurrence.

pulmonary diseases

Any disease affecting the structures necessary for breathing (trachea, bronchi, bronchioles, al-

THE LUNGS

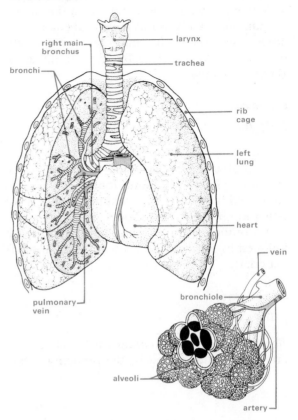

RESPIRATORY UNIT OF LUNG

The lungs are delicate and complex organs. Their function is to allow oxygen to enter the bloodstream and to remove carbon dioxide. Respiration is impaired either when the bronchi are obstructed (for example, by foreign bodies, cancer, or inflammation) or when the alveoli are diseased (emphysema, pneumonia, or fibrosis).

veoli). Pulmonary diseases are either of a blocking (obstructive) nature or a tightening (restrictive) nature. These diseases often involve cough, chest pain, shortness of breath, bloody sputum, abnormal breathing noises, wheezing, fatigue, and loss of appetite. Examples of these diseases are BRONCHITIS, PNEUMONIA, ASTHMA, EMPHYSEMA, and CANCER of the lung.

pulmonary embolism

The blockage of a pulmonary artery (those arteries that take blood from the heart to the lungs) by foreign matter such as fat, a blood clot, a tumor, or any other solid object. Symptoms are similar to those of a heart attack: breathing difficulty, sudden chest pain, shock, and bluish skin tone.

Pulmonary embolism is a medical emergency. Some cases may require immediate surgery; others may be treated with blood-thinning drugs (anticoagulants).

pulpitis

Inflammation of the soft central part of the tooth. Cavities almost always lead to the inflammation. Symptoms include extreme tooth sensitivity to cold liquids and foods. Treatment consists of either tooth extraction or root canal therapy (removal of the contents of the central tooth space followed by sterilization and filling with an inert material).

pulse

The palpable and sometimes visible change in arterial pressure caused by the pumping action of the heart.

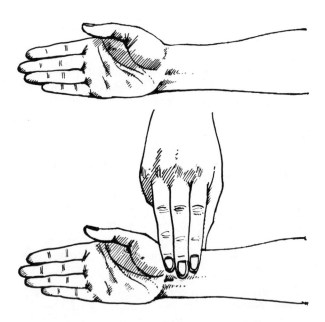

This diagram shows the correct way of feeling a patient's pulse at the wrist. Fingertips, not the thumb, should be used and it is important to count the beats accurately for exactly 30 seconds. Multiply the result by 2 to get the pulse rate.

When the heart contracts, pumping blood through the arterial system, the arteries expand slightly during the increased blood flow. It is this periodic expansion that is felt when a finger is placed on an artery close to the skin surface. Normally, the *radial artery* (in the wrist) is used to take the pulse, but several others in the body and the limbs may also be used.

The pulse is a useful indicator of several aspects of health, disease, and injury. The "normal" pulse rate is said to be about 72 beats per minute, but in healthy individuals at rest it may be anywhere from 50 to 100 beats per minute. While undergoing severe exercise, or while under mental stress, the pulse rate can go far above this range (even above 200) without harm.

The pulse rate is quicker in children than in adults and slows down progressively throughout life. When a person is suffering from a fever the pulse rate usually is elevated. The absence of perceptible pulse is not a definite sign of death; a person suffering from disease or injury may exhibit no pulse, and this startling fact does not always mean that the heart has stopped beating. Persons with heart disease often exhibit irregular pulse rhythms; irregularities and variations are a diagnostic aid in diseases of the heart and arteries.

purpura

A condition in which tiny red or purple spots appear on the surface of the skin, in mucous membranes, and elsewhere owing to the escape of blood from the vessels.

Purpura appears either when the capillaries become more permeable or when there is a shortage of blood PLATELETS which normally seal off damage to the walls of the capillaries.

Several diseases and conditions can cause purpura. It may follow an infection such as SCARLET FEVER; it sometimes appears in wasting diseases; and it can be caused by toxic drugs or malnutrition. In addition, the signs and symptoms occur in what is known as *thrombocytopenic purpura*—when there is a shortage of platelets (THROMBO-CYTOPENIA)—and in *anaphylactoid purpura*, which is thought to be associated with an allergic reaction. *Henoch-Schönlein purpura* is a form of allergic purpura that appears in the walls of the intestine and in the joints. It is seen most commonly in children.

The symptoms of purpura are usually feverishness and exhaustion, followed by characteristic spots on the trunk and limbs. The spots may change color from red to purple until they are nearly black; they finally disappear in much the same way as a bruise. The most serious form is *purpura hemorrhagica*, in which bleeding occurs from mucous surfaces in the nose and also in the mouth, digestive organs, and womb; this form may be fatal.

Thrombocytopenic purpura responds to steroid drugs, but in some cases surgical removal of the SPLEEN (splenectomy) may be necessary. Where purpura follows infection or other disease, treatment is directed at the underlying condition.

pus

A yellowish or creamy white collection of sticky fluid that forms at the site of a wound or infection. It is made up of normal and damaged white blood cells and other cellular debris. White blood cells are used by the body to fight off infections.

pyelitis

Inflammation of the pelvis of a kidney, the funnel-shaped expansion that collects urine and conveys it to the ureter (the passage from each kidney leading to the bladder).

Pyelitis alone is extremely uncommon, since almost invariably the main body (or *parenchyma*) of the kidney also is infected. Inflammation of both the pelvis and the parenchyma of the kidney is known as PYELONEPHRITIS. The term "pyelitis" sometimes is used loosely to mean pyelonephritis.

pyelonephritis

Inflammation of the parenchyma and pelvis of the kidney due to infection. It is a very common condition, women being more often affected than men.

The infecting microorganisms may reach the kidneys by means of the bloodstream or may travel upward from the bladder via the ureters and the lymphatic vessels around the ureters.

Pyelonephritis can be acute or chronic. An attack of pyelonephritis is characterized by fever accompanied by chills, pain in the loin, the need to pass urine very frequently and urgently, and burning pain at the urethra (the urinary outlet from the bladder) on passing urine. The last two

symptoms on their own usually suggest infection of the bladder and infection of the urethra, respectively.

Treatment consists of the administration of antibiotics. The urine will have to be examined in the laboratory to determine which microorganisms are responsible for the infection, so that the appropriate antibiotic can be given. Repeated laboratory examinations of the urine will have to be carried out in the first few months after completion of a full course of antibiotics to ensure that the kidney is completely free of infection. If the infection recurs, or if another infection occurs, a predisposing cause for the condition must be sought.

The steps taken to prevent or delay further damage which could lead to kidney failure include vigorous treatment of any low-grade urinary tract infection (determined by laboratory examination of the urine) and thorough investigation to discover treatable conditions that predispose to pyelonephritis.

pyoderma

Any of the various pus-forming skin infections. The group of conditions known collectively as the pyodermas includes the following: (1) IMPETIGO—a common, contagious, superficial, bacterial infection seen most often in children. The lesions vary from small to large blisters that rupture and release a honey-colored liquid. New lesions can develop very rapidly (within hours). Crusts form from the discharge. (2) *Ecthyma*—similar to impetigo, but affecting slightly deeper layers of the skin. (3) FOLLICULITIS—which affects hair follicles anywhere on the body, including the eyelashes (to form a STY). (4) *Furuncle* (or boil)—a more extensive infection of the hair follicle involving deeper underlying tissues. (5) CARBUNCLE—an extensive infection of several adjoining hair follicles; the carbuncle drains from multiple openings onto the skin surface. (6) *Sweat gland infections*—not a common condition. (7) ERYSIPELAS—an uncommon infection caused by streptococcal bacteria; it results in a characteristic type of CELLULITIS (inflammation of the loose connective tissue under the skin) which appears as a red, warm, raised, well-defined plaque; blisters may form on the skin. (8) PARONYCHIA—painful infection around the nailbed.

The general principles of treatment include: (a) administration of the appropriate antibiotic;

(b) general isolation of the person, with frequent changes of clothing and bedding (towels should not be shared), and strict hygiene; (c) if the furuncle or carbuncle comes to a "head"—that is, when an abscess has formed with a definite point—the pus should be drained by an incision (to be done only by a physician). If pyodermas recur, investigations should be carried out to rule out DIABETES MELLITUS (which makes a person prone to infections).

pyorrhea

An outmoded term meaning the discharge of pus from under the gum margin. Severe gum disease is the cause.

See also GINGIVITIS.

pyrexia

The technical name for FEVER. The condition of an exceptionally high fever is known as *hyperpyrexia.*

Q fever

An infection caused by the microorganism *Coxiella burnetii* (rickettsia), a parasite of cattle.

Cattle excrete the microorganisms in their milk or feces. Humans become infected usually by inhaling dust that is contaminated by infected animal material; sometimes infection comes from drinking infected milk, since the rickettsiae are somewhat resistant to pasteurization.

After an incubation period of two to four weeks, symptoms appear suddenly. These consist of fever, headaches, prostration, cough, and muscle and chest pain. X-ray studies usually show an inflammation of the lung, although the cough may be slight. Occasionally the heart may be affected, sometimes months after the original infection. In severe cases, HEPATITIS is common. The disease may be acute, or chronic and relapsing, but is rarely fatal.

Prevention is by avoiding contact with infected cattle. If the disease develops, symptoms may be suppressed by the administration of antibiotics, although this will not necessarily eradicate the infection.

quarantine

The detention or limitation of freedom of movement of persons (or domestic animals) who are apparently well but who have been in contact with a serious communicable disease (one that can be transmitted directly or indirectly from one individual to another). The reason for quarantine is that such persons or animals may have become infected (although they have not yet shown signs or symptoms of the disease)—that is, they are in the *incubation* stage of the disease, during which time they may be able to pass the disease on to others. To prevent this they are quarantined for the incubation period of the disease in question, at the end of this period it should have become clearer who has been infected and who needs to be isolated or nursed by *isolation* techniques.

Quarantine need not be carried out in the hospital. The person can be quarantined anywhere as long as he does not have unlimited contact with unaffected persons.

There are various degrees of quarantine. *Complete quarantine* means the quarantine of all persons who have been in contact with the communicable disease. With *modified quarantine,* it may be that only those who are likely to pass the disease on to particularly susceptible people are held in quarantine. For example, if children are particularly susceptible to the disease, children who have been exposed to the disease may be asked to stay away from school, since they are the ones most likely to have caught the infection and be "incubating" it.

The least strict form of quarantine is *personal surveillance,* in which the exposed individual's movements are limited only to the extent that health officials should be able to get in touch with him daily or at frequent intervals to ensure that he has not fallen ill.

The type of quarantine applied varies, depending on the seriousness of the disease, the closeness of the contact with the disease, and the state of immunity of the susceptible people within the community.

rabies

A viral disease of animals and humans. It is characterized by irritation of the nervous system followed by paralysis and (in virtually every case) death. The virus is found in the saliva of infected animals, who transmit the disease by their bites. The disease (also called *hydrophobia*) may also be spread if open wounds are contaminated by infected saliva.

Vaccination of dogs in the United States has controlled canine rabies. Most cases that occur are the result of bites from infected wild animals such as skunks, foxes, and bats. Infected animals may have the "furious" form of the disease (in which they become very agitated and aggressive) or the "dumb" form (in which change of habits or paralysis predominates). The diagnosis requires examination of the nervous tissue of the animal obtained at autopsy. If a wild animal bites without provocation, the victim must seek medical attention so that a decision can be made about vaccination.

In humans the incubation period varies from approximately ten days to over a year, but most often it is from thirty to sixty days. The incubation period is shorter if the bite is extensive or nearer to the head. Once the first symptoms appear, the disease is almost inevitably fatal (although at least one documented case of survival exists).

The initial symptom in humans consists of sensitivity of the area around the wound to changes in temperature. This is followed typically by a period of mental depression, restlessness, and fever. The restlessness may increase to states of rage and violent convulsions. Attempts to drink result in an extremely painful spasm of the larynx so that the victim eventually refuses to drink (becomes "hydrophobic") despite great thirst. Spasm of the larynx is also easily precipitated by mild stimuli such as a gentle breeze. The attacks of asphyxia produced by laryngeal spasm can lead to death. Death also may result from exhaustion and paralysis of the muscles that control respiration.

People working with animals should be immunized against rabies. A course of rabies vaccinations should also be started immediately after a person is bitten by an animal suspected of being rabid. If possible, the animal should be confined and observed for symptoms of rabies so that the diagnosis can be confirmed and appropriate treatment begun. The local wound should be washed thoroughly for ten minutes with soft medicinal soap.

No cure currently exists once the first symptoms are experienced. Supportive treatment is the best that can be offered.

radiation therapy

Treatment of disease by radiation; also called *irradiation*. The radiation may be given in the form of a beam, or radioactive material (such as radium) may be contained in various devices that can be inserted directly into the tissues or into a body cavity. The radioactive material may also be given by injection into a vein or as a drink.

The most common condition for which radiation is used is CANCER. Some cancers respond well to radiation therapy alone; others are treated best with radiation therapy in conjunction with surgery or anticancer drugs (or both). When a cancer is too far advanced for surgery, radiation therapy can often help to relieve symptoms.

In addition to killing cancer cells, radiation can also have a harmful effect on normal cells. But cancer cells are more susceptible because radiation acts best on cells that are dividing (multiplying) rapidly. The normal cells most commonly affected are those that divide rapidly—such as those of the skin, the gastrointestinal tract, the reproductive organs, and the bone marrow.

Depending on where the beam of radiation is directed on the body, side effects from radiation can include diarrhea and vomiting, mouth ulcers, hair loss, and suppression of the bone marrow. Most of the side effects quickly disappear if the dose of radiation is reduced or if the treatment is stopped briefly. Modern techniques and equipment have reduced the frequency of side effects.

rash

A skin eruption that typically takes the form of red patches or spots and is often accompanied by itching. The rash may be localized in one part of the body, or it may involve extensive areas. A rash may be the result of a number of conditions, including certain communicable diseases (such as MEASLES and CHICKEN POX).

Diaper rash is the skin inflammation (DERMATITIS) that occurs in infants on the areas covered by diapers and is due to irritation by wet or soiled diapers. A fungal infection (CANDIDIASIS) may be superimposed in diaper rash; if it develops, antifungal treatment is required. In most cases, however, diaper rash can be controlled by keeping the diaper area dry and clean and by prompt changing of wet diapers.

MILIARIA ("heat rash" or "prickly heat") is a form of rash caused by blockage of sweat ducts. The function of the sweat ducts is to moisten the skin surface for cooling; they become very active in hot weather. As a result of the constant irritation of the skin due to the wetness around the sweat pores, the ducts become blocked. The part of the duct behind the blockage swells up.

An *allergic rash* usually appears as wheals, which are well-defined elevated lesions caused by local accumulation of fluid in the tissues. It is the type of rash seen with insect bites or STINGS, allergies to food or drugs, or URTICARIA ("hives"). Drug eruptions, however, may take on a number of other forms ranging from a measles-like rash to sloughing off of the skin. The treatment for allergic rash is to stop contact with the agent causing the rash; if the eruption does not clear up, antiallergic agents such as antihistamines and corticosteroids may be required.

Many *viral infections* produce a rash, which in some infections are fairly characteristic of the particular infection. In measles and GERMAN MEASLES the rash usually starts around the ears or on the face and neck before spreading to the trunk and limbs. In mild cases, the limbs may be unaffected. In chicken pox, the rash usually starts on the trunk and later spreads to the face and extremities; blisters soon form. In ROCKY MOUNTAIN SPOTTED FEVER the rash appears on the wrists, ankles, palms, and soles, and then extends to the neck, face, buttocks, and trunk.

Bacterial infections may also produce rashes; for example, secondary SYPHILIS is characterized by a temporary skin eruption.

A rash may be seen also in the group of conditions known as the AUTOIMMUNE DISEASES. With LUPUS ERYTHEMATOSUS, a "butterfly rash" may form (so named because of the typical pattern it forms across the bridge of the nose and over the adjacent areas of the cheeks).

Raynaud's phenomenon

First described by Maurice Raynaud in 1862, Raynaud's phenomenon is most common in young women: First the fingertips, then the rest of the fingers, go white and cold; the fingers feel numb and may become stiff, and it is evident that their blood supply has temporarily been cut off. On recovery the blood slowly comes back to the fingers, which turn bright red and become painful.

These symptoms result from spasm of small arteries and this is precipitated by cold or emotional upset.

The condition may be slight or severe; in severe cases small ulcers may form on the fingertips and the nails may be affected. If there is no underlying cause, the condition usually improves and eventually subsides. But in some cases the phenomenon is a complication of more widespread disease such as SCLERODERMA or systematic LUPUS ERYTHEMATOSUS.

All sufferers should avoid exposing their hands to the cold. Treatment includes keeping the whole body warm as well as the hands and feet and relieving pain with analgesics. In severe cases it may be useful to block part of the nerve supply to the affected limb or to interrupt it by a surgical operation called SYMPATHECTOMY (see under **Procedures**).

rectocele

A forward protrusion of part of the wall of the rectum into the vagina. It is the result of weakening (during CHILDBIRTH) of the fibrous connective tissue that separates the rectum from the vagina. It may be due to a rapid delivery or to a difficult one. Sometimes the diagnosis is made soon after delivery, but usually symptoms do not appear until a woman is 35 to 40 years old.

Factors affecting the development of a rectocele include the state of the pelvic muscles, the degree of damage, and persistent straining at stool. There is a vicious cycle here, because one of the signs of a rectocele is CONSTIPATION due to collection of feces in the pouch; this leads to straining, which further aggravates the herniation. Persons may complain of a sense of rectal or vaginal fullness and the constant urge for a bowel movement.

Treatment consists of good dietary habits to avoid constipation or straining at stool. Laxatives or suppositories may be necessary. Surgery is required to achieve a cure, the chances for which are good if subsequent vaginal delivery and straining at stool can be avoided.

reflex

An involuntary action or movement that occurs in response to a stimulus. Examples of reflex actions are the quick closure of the eye when an object approaches it or when the eyelash is touched, or the sharp recovery of balance when a person begins to slip. There are also reflexes of which one may not be conscious, for example, the secretion of gastric juices at the sight of food, or the movement of the pupil of the eye in response to a change in the intensity of light.

Some reflexes can be conditioned—that is, learned or modified. The classic example is the experiments with dogs conducted by the Russian physician and physiologist Ivan Pavlov (1849–1936). A bell was rung whenever the dog was given food. The normal response to food is salivation. After a number of times, the dog salivated when the bell was rung without food being given at the same time.

Many reflexes may be tested during a general medical examination. When an appropriate stimulus is provided by the doctor, the reflex response is involuntary; any change in the expected reflex is a sign of disturbed neurologic function. One common test is the "knee jerk" reflex. This is elicited usually by a firm tap with a rubber-headed mallet on the tendon just below the kneecap. The normal response is for the lower leg to jerk outward suddenly and then return to its former position.

Reiter's syndrome

A combination of symptoms occurring after sexual contact or after a bout of bacterial dysentery. An uncommon disease for which the cause is not known, Reiter's syndrome occurs most often in young men, and 90 percent have the HLA-B27 tissue type.

Typically, a young man will develop URETHRITIS that is not caused by GONORRHEA. Urethritis is an inflammation of the urethra (the passageway for urine and semen). It is characterized by painful urination and a pus-like discharge. From a week to a month afterward, ARTHRITIS, CONJUNCTIVITIS, and, sometimes, skin and mouth sores will develop. The arthritis is of abrupt onset and lasts for several weeks, affecting more than one joint (most often the knees, ankles, or toes). Although the initial urethritis can be treated with antibiotics, and the eye inflammation and skin and mouth lesions eventually heal, the arthritis has a tendency to recur periodically. It seldom causes lasting joint damage.

There are exceptions to the general rule in Reiter's syndrome. Not every patient gets all the same symptoms. For example, in cases caused by bacterial dysentery, the only symptom is arthritis. In other cases, some persons may not get the skin or mouth lesions or may not develop the eye inflammation. Women who get the disease after sexual contact will have an inflammation of the cervix rather than of the urethra.

The only therapy for Reiter's syndrome is treatment of the symptoms: antibiotics for urethritis or dysentery, pain-killers and anti-inflammatory drugs for arthritis.

relaxation therapy

A form of behavior modification in which a person is taught to do breathing and relaxing exercises and to think soothing thoughts whenever anxiety, fear, or pain threatens to overcome him.

When a person is able to relax all his muscles voluntarily, certain physiological changes occur (such as a slight reduction in the rate of the heartbeat and a slowed rate of breathing).

The Lamaze method of childbirth uses relaxation therapy to help a woman through the pain of giving birth without drugs.

resection

The surgical procedure of cutting out, especially the surgical removal of a segment or section of an organ.

respiration

The exchange of oxygen and carbon dioxide between the atmosphere and body cells. Oxygen combines with carbon and hydrogen furnished by food. These reactions generate heat and provide the living organism with energy for physical work as well as for the many other processes essential for life, such as digestion, growth, and brain function. The carbon dioxide that is produced during respiration has to be eliminated; accumulation of carbon dioxide in the body disturbs body function by causing the tissue fluids to be too acid.

In an adult at rest frequency of respiration is about 14 to 20 breaths per minute; children tend to breathe at a faster rate. Atmospheric air breathed in contains approximately 21 percent oxygen and 0.03 percent carbon dioxide. Air breathed out of the lungs contains approxi-

RESPIRATION

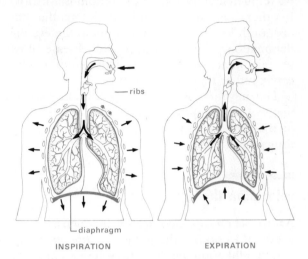

INSPIRATION   EXPIRATION

At rest, a normal adult breathes about 14 to 20 times per minute. Oxygen enters the blood in the capillaries of the lungs, and carbon dioxide is carried away in the expired air. Muscle action lifts the ribs and pulls down the diaphragm, thus increasing the volume of the chest cavity; the lungs expand, drawing in air through the nose or mouth. When these muscles relax, the lungs recoil, and air is expelled.

mately 14 percent oxygen and 5.6 percent carbon dioxide.

All the air in the lungs is not expelled with each breath. The amount of inspired air that actually reaches the lungs with each breath (during normal quiet breathing) is known as the *tidal volume;* it represents only about 1/18 of the total capacity of the lungs. The *vital capacity* is the amount of air the lungs can hold after trying to force out as much air from the lungs as possible and then taking the deepest possible breath. The *residual volume* is the amount of air the lungs hold after trying to breathe out as hard as possible; it is impossible to empty the lungs of all their air in this manner, and approximately 1,200 cubic centimeters (cc) remain—compared with approximately 500 cc of air drawn into the lungs with each breath during normal breathing.

The act of breathing is accomplished by the action of the diaphragm (which moves down) and the muscles between the ribs (which expand the chest upward, outward, and sideways). As air is drawn into the lungs (*inspiration*), the pleural cavity—the airless space between the lungs and the chest wall—becomes larger; this creates a suction effect on the lungs and causes them to expand. As the volume of the lungs increases, it creates a

partial vacuum within the lungs; air rushes in through the nose, mouth (if open), and air passages to fill this space. Breathing out (*expiration*) is a passive action caused by the escape of air temporarily held in the lungs at a slightly higher pressure than the atmospheric air.

There are three components involved in the transport of oxygen and carbon dioxide between the cells and the external environment. Exchange of the two gases between the body cells and the atmosphere takes place in the lungs. Breathing consists of alternate acts of inspiration and expiration; during inspiration, atmospheric air is taken into the lungs, while during expiration the air that is relatively poor in oxygen and rich in carbon dioxide is expelled into the atmosphere.

In the lungs, exchange of gases takes place by diffusion across the walls of the air sacs (*alveoli*); oxygen from inspired air diffuses across the lining of the air sacs and enters the circulation, while carbon dioxide moves in the opposite direction. The gases are transported between cells and the lungs by the blood circulation.

Any disorder that affects transport of the gases can impair respiration, and if the impairment is severe enough, death occurs; death may be of the whole organism or localized, such as occurs in heart attacks (myocardial infarction) or STROKES when the blood supply to specific tissues is cut off. Other disorders that can affect transport of gases include nervous or muscular disorders that impair the movement of chest and abdominal muscles required for breathing, or disorders that affect the lining of the air sacs, such as PNEUMONIA or collapse of the lung (ATELECTASIS).

respiratory tract infection

Any infectious disease of the upper or lower breathing tract.

The respiratory tract extends from the nostrils down to the air sacs in the lungs (pulmonary alveoli). For convenience, the respiratory tract is divided into the *upper respiratory tract* (above the larynx) and the *lower respiratory tract* (below the larynx). Infections (producing inflammation) of specific parts of the respiratory tract are known as RHINITIS (inflammation of the nasal passages); PHARYNGITIS (inflammation of the pharynx, or throat); LARYNGITIS (inflammation of the larynx, or "voice box"); TRACHEITIS (inflammation of the trachea, or "windpipe"); and BRONCHITIS (inflammation of the bronchi or major air passages below

RESPIRATORY TRACT INFECTION

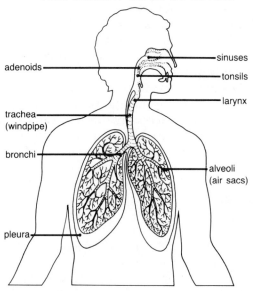

adenoids

sinuses

tonsils

larynx

trachea
(windpipe)

bronchi

alveoli
(air sacs)

pleura

Infections of the respiratory tract cover anything from the common cold to pneumonia. The illustration shows the possible sites of infection; symptoms may include cough, excessive phlegm, chest pain, and breathing difficulties.

the trachea). Inflammation of the lungs is known as PNEUMONITIS. Untreated infection of any part can spread readily to other parts.

The infecting microorganisms—usually bacteria or viruses—most commonly enter the respiratory tract by inhalation of infected droplets exhaled (or coughed or sneezed out) by someone with an existing respiratory tract infection. Sometimes a respiratory tract infection spreads from a previously localized infection in the mouth or is introduced from other parts of the body by means of the bloodstream.

The body has a number of defense mechanisms specifically designed to ward off or attack respiratory tract infections. The nostrils have lining hairs that act as filters for the air breathed in. There are also a number of "turbinates" (intricately shaped bony ridges) in the nasal passages which have mucus-covered surfaces that act very much like "fly-paper" to trap irritants and infective organisms. Furthermore, nasal secretions contain enzymes and antibodies that can kill or interfere with the growth and multiplication of some bacteria and viruses. Irritation of the nose and nasopharynx (the part behind the nose just above the roof of the mouth) also initiates sneezing, which expels irritants; similarly, irritation

of the larynx or upper part of the trachea triggers the cough reflex. Lower down, the volume of the air passages progressively increases so that the velocity of air is gradually reduced as it passes down the respiratory tract, allowing particles to fall out of the airstream and stick to the mucus-covered walls; these walls bear cilia (hair-like structures) on their surface. The cilia move in such a way as to sweep the mucus upward and out of the respiratory tract. Obstruction of the respiratory tract by a foreign body or by a tumor will prevent the mucus from being effectively swept upward. The action of cilia is impaired also by chronic inflammation, such as that associated with chronic bronchitis and the common cold, and by some anesthetics. When the mucus is abnormally thick, and thus unable to flow easily, infection is common.

A number of factors make a person more susceptible to respiratory tract infection; these include the extremes of age, debilitation by chronic illness, immune deficiency, and DIABETES MELLITUS.

Symptoms of an infection of the respiratory tract depend primarily on the severity of the attack and on the site affected.

Treatment is primarily the administration of the appropriate antibiotic.

restless legs syndrome

A relatively common condition characterized by an uncomfortable feeling in the muscles of the lower limbs, accompanied by a desire to move the legs. It is most common in middle-aged women.

The onset of symptoms typically occurs at the end of the day when the person is resting, especially when in bed, and the person may be compelled to get up and walk about to obtain relief. The condition may be familial and in such cases no organic disease is found, but the syndrome often occurs in UREMIA and other conditions causing NEUROPATHY (nerve damage). The treatment is that of the underlying condition. In other cases, there may be benefit from the administration of an appropriate tranquilizer just before bedtime.

resuscitation

Also known as *cardiopulmonary resuscitation* (CPR), the emergency measures performed to restore breathing and the heartbeat in someone who has just stopped breathing. There are three essential measures in resuscitation, most easily remembered by the letters A (keep the *airways* clear), B (restore *breathing*), and C (restore the *circulation*).

To prevent blockage of the airway by the victim's tongue (which may have fallen back and obstructed the upper part of the airway), the head should be tilted back. If the airway is blocked by vomit, mucus, mud, or dentures, this matter should be "hooked out" very rapidly with a finger.

If the patient is not breathing spontaneously, mouth-to-mouth breathing should be initiated at once. This consists of the first-aider taking a deep breath and then immediately blowing air into the patient's mouth, taking care to pinch the patient's nostrils at the same time so that the air blown in does not escape through the nostrils. This should be repeated about 12 times per minute.

If after the first three or four breaths the victim's color has not improved, and there is no detectable pulse or heartbeat, then *cardiac massage*, also known as *external cardiac compression*, is indicated. This procedure should be carried out *only by an experienced person*, otherwise it can fracture ribs and cause damage to internal organs. When cardiac compression is given, it must be accompanied by continued artificial respiration. The precise technique for CPR is taught by many local community hospitals.

See also *Resuscitation* in the **First Aid** section.

retention of urine

Inability to empty the bladder may be caused by obstruction of the urinary passages or by neurological disorders that disturb the neuromuscular mechanisms of urination. Retention of urine may be acute or chronic.

Obstruction to the outlet of the bladder may be caused by enlargement of the prostate gland in men, by benign or malignant tumors, fibrosis of the bladder neck, stones, blood clots, or pressure from outside by fibroids of the uterus or a pregnant uterus. The urethra may be obstructed by strictures (usually the result of previous venereal infection or injury), stones, foreign bodies, or acute inflammation.

One of the most common causes of acute urinary retention is postoperative pain; other conditions disturbing neuromuscular reflexes are diseases of the spinal cord, tumors, injuries, and inflammations. Hysteria may produce acute or chronic urinary retention, and in the elderly the

bladder may not be emptied because of confusion and loss of awareness.

Acute retention is painful except in neurological disorders. The pain is felt above the pubis at the lower part of the abdomen; chronic retention is usually painless.

Treatment includes the use of catheters and surgical relief of obstructions. In chronic conditions it may be necessary to use a catheter permanently; in some cases permanent drainage may be carried out through the lower part of the abdominal wall.

retinitis

Inflammation of the retina, the light-sensitive lining at the back of the eyeball.

The retina forms the innermost of the three coats (tunics) of the eye. True inflammation of the retina does not often occur on its own, but rather together with inflammation of the *choroid* (the middle coat), a condition known as *chorioretinitis*. This may be caused by infections such as TOXOPLASMOSIS, TUBERCULOSIS, or SYPHILIS. The condition is painless and the only symptom is blurring or loss of vision. If the cause is known, specific treatment is administered; if not, corticosteroids may help.

Chorioretinitis can also be caused by the parasitic worm *Toxocara canis*, which may be acquired by children when fondling puppies. The larval worms are carried to the eye in the bloodstream and, in dying, excite an acute inflammatory response. This may produce a tumorlike appearance and the eye may be unnecessarily removed.

Two degenerative (not inflammatory) conditions also are known as retinitis: RETINITIS PIGMENTOSA and *retinitis proliferans*. The latter is a complication of DIABETES MELLITUS and is characterized by the formation of masses of new blood vessels in the vitreous gel in front of the retina.

retinitis pigmentosa

An inherited disorder characterized by a slowly progressive degeneration of the retina of both eyes.

Symptoms may be noticed from early childhood, the earliest signs usually being defective night vision; this is because the degeneration first affects the rods, which are receptors that mediate vision in dim light. Later the central field of vision becomes lost; this gradually progresses until (in some cases) total blindness occurs.

There is no effective treatment for retinitis pigmentosa. Genetic counseling may help to prevent passing on the disease.

retinopathy

Damage to the retina (the light-sensitive layer at the back of the eye) caused by disease of the blood vessels.

In advancing age the blood vessels in general become hardened and narrow (ARTERIOSCLEROSIS). In some people the condition may be severe enough to lead to small hemorrhages into the retina, but usually hemorrhages occur if the blood pressure is above normal and undue strain is put upon the aging blood vessels. These hemorrhages may produce defects in vision.

Retinopathy is one of the most serious complications of advanced DIABETES MELLITUS; it can be treated, however, if caught early.

THE RETINA

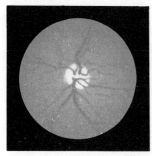 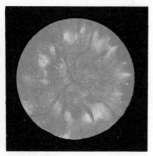

Normal retina as seen through an ophthalmoscope

Hypertensive retinopathy as seen through an ophthalmoscope

Examination of the retina and its blood vessels is a routine feature of most general medical examinations. The ophthalmoscope is a simple optical instrument with a light source, by means of which the general physician—as well as the ophthalmologist—can detect not only primary disorders of the eye but also signs of various bodily disorders, including evidence of high blood pressure and changes associated with diabetes.

Reye's syndrome

This serious but rare condition affects children recovering from various virus infections, such as CHICKEN POX and INFLUENZA. It nearly always occurs in children under the age of 15 and affects about 6 children in 100,000. The condition causes severe brain swelling and HEPATITIS (inflammation of the liver).

Reye's syndrome starts with severe vomiting, lethargy, loss of memory, disorientation, or even DELIRIUM. This is rapidly followed by indications of progressive brain damage with SEIZURES, deepening COMA, and heart and breathing disturbances. Death may occur within a week of onset.

Because the effect on the brain is mainly due to swelling within the unyielding skull, corticosteroids, which reduce inflammation, and the infusion of strong sugar solutions into the blood to draw water from the brain are essential measures in the treatment. The effects of liver malfunction must also be dealt with, often by DIALYSIS (see under **Procedures**) of the blood, or even total replacement. If the breathing is paralyzed, a tube must be passed into the trachea (windpipe) and the respiration maintained by a pump.

With increasing knowledge of the condition and of its management, the death rate in Reye's disease has fallen from 50 percent to about 10 percent. Regrettably, some surviving children are left with permanent brain damage.

Although clearly related to virus infection, there is growing evidence that Reye's syndrome is also connected with taking aspirin. This evidence is now so strong that the Committee on Infectious Diseases of the American Academy of Pediatrics has advised that children suspected of having chicken pox or influenza should not be prescribed aspirin. In Britain, aspirin has been withdrawn as a childhood medication.

Rh (Rhesus) factor

One of the major markers on the surface of human red blood cells. The other major marker system is the ABO classification (see BLOOD TYPES). About 85 percent of people have the Rh factor on their red blood cells (Rh positive); 15 percent lack the Rh marker (Rh negative).

The Rh factor is particularly important during pregnancy. For many years doctors sought to explain why certain women were prone to bear children who were born jaundiced and anemic and who sometimes died soon after birth, or, in severe cases, were stillborn. Eventually such women were found to be invariably Rhesus negative while their husbands were Rhesus positive. Incompatibility between the Rhesus positive baby and the Rhesus negative mother was responsible for these "Rhesus babies" suffering from *erythroblastosis fetalis* (a hemolytic disease of the newborn, characterized by anemia, jaundice, and enlargement of the liver and spleen).

To prevent newborn babies of Rh-incompatible parents from getting this hemolytic disease, the mother is immunized against the Rh marker.

rheumatic fever

A once common disease of childhood and adolescence which is rare today. It occurs as a complication of untreated throat infection caused by *Streptococcus* bacteria ("strep throat"). The exact cause of the damage done by this disease is not known, but evidence indicates that it is an AUTO-IMMUNE DISEASE reaction.

Rheumatic fever occurs in about one in 50,000 children and affects the joints, heart, skin, and (sometimes) the brain. The acute attack produces painful swollen joints, skin rashes, nodules in the tissues just beneath the skin, and fever. The effect on the heart is variable. There may be a persistently raised heart rate, minor irregularities in the heartbeat, or even acute congestive heart failure, but recovery is the rule. Damage to the heart valves may reveal itself many years later in RHEUMATIC HEART DISEASE, with serious disturbance of cardiac function.

Treatment involves the administration of penicillin to clear up the streptococcal infection, and cortisone-like drugs (steroids) and aspirin to relieve symptoms. Better and earlier treatment of streptococcal infections (and of rheumatic fever itself) has reduced the chance of subsequent heart problems.

rheumatic heart disease

A complication or end result of an attack of RHEU-MATIC FEVER.

The interval between the original rheumatic fever (usually occurring in childhood or adolescence), and the appearance of symptoms of rheumatic heart disease may vary from a few years to many decades. Rheumatic fever attacks the heart muscle and the heart valves; while the damage to the heart muscle usually is repairable, changes in the heart valve subsequently may cause the valves to become deformed or to stick together at their edges. The heart valves most affected are the *mitral* and *aortic* valves. Two main types of defect can be produced: (1) narrowing of the valve opening with obstruction to the flow of blood (*stenosis*), and (2) *incompetence* and *regurgitation*, in which the valve fails to close properly and allows a reverse flow of blood.

Symptoms depend largely on the type of defect present and its severity. For many years the heart may continue to compensate for a defectively functioning valve.

Mitral stenosis is characterized by shortness of breath after exertion. It is rarely seen in childhood. It is, however, the most common manifestation of rheumatic heart disease.

Aortic stenosis is typically a complication seen later in life. Eventually incompetence of the valves also will produce symptoms; these may include increasing shortness of breath on exercise, chest pain, palpitations, attacks of shortness of breath on lying down at night, or fainting attacks.

Treatment involves first increasing the strength of the heartbeat with suitable drugs and the avoidance of overexertion. If the problem is severe, surgical repair of the valve or its replacement by a grafted or plastic valve may be required.

rheumatism

A general term that indicates any of the various diseases of the musculoskeletal system characterized by pain and stiffness of the joints.

rheumatoid arthritis

A chronic inflammatory disease affecting the connective tissue of the joints. The incidence is considerably higher in temperate climates, but the symptoms are more pronounced in cold damp places.

Women are affected more often than men, and the usual age of onset is between 25 and 55. The cause of the disease is not known; both immunologic and infectious factors have been implicated. It has been suggested that a "slow virus" infection may be a cause.

The onset of rheumatoid arthritis usually is slow, but in some cases it may be acute and accompanied by fever and weight loss. In others, there may be malaise (a general feeling of being unwell) and fatigue for some weeks, with pains and stiffness in the joints. In time, ARTHRITIS appears, often beginning in the joints of the fingers and spreading to involve the wrists and elbows; less commonly the feet are affected first, with the disease spreading to the ankles and knees. The shoulders and hips may be involved. The joints become swollen, tender, and hot, and movement is painful. The joints are stiff, particularly in the morning and after rest. When the large joints of the shoulder and hip are affected, the resulting disability may be serious. Often, the joints will be affected in a symmetrical pattern. Once a joint is involved, it will stay affected. This is in contrast to other forms of arthritis that may afflict the joint only sporadically, or once and then not ever again.

The joints of the spinal column may be affected, especially in the neck, and the patient may have pain and tenderness in the joint of the lower jaw just in front of the ear; this interferes with eating. Nodules may develop under the skin, and disturbances of the circulation are common in which the hands may sweat to an abnormal extent or may become cold and blue. The lymph nodes draining the affected joints often are enlarged, and in about 5 percent of persons the spleen also is enlarged. ANEMIA is common, its severity being proportional to the severity of the disease; the eye may be inflamed or dry.

Diagnosis of the disease usually is not difficult. In a typical case, X-ray examination will show characteristic changes in the joints; these, together with multiple joint involvement, a positive test for rheumatoid factor, and the ruling out of other forms of arthritis, will lead to a diagnosis of rheumatoid arthritis.

Several drugs are used in the treatment of rheumatoid arthritis. The least expensive and most effective is aspirin. About one third of persons find that aspirin gives them indigestion, in which case it is possible to use special preparations of the drug. Other anti-inflammatory drugs, such as indomethacin and ibuprofen, are used, but they sometimes have adverse effects on the blood and the digestive system. Gold salts have been shown to produce symptomatic relief, but they have a number of serious adverse effects and therefore must be used with caution under close medical supervision. Corticosteroids are not advised for long-term treatment and are not used in short-term treatment except under special circumstances. They may be injected into inflamed joints to relieve pain. Penicillamine is useful in selected cases not responding to anti-inflammatory agents. Immunosuppressive drugs such as azathioprine and cyclophosphamide are being used increasingly in severe cases.

Surgery has a considerable part to play in the treatment both of acute cases and of the deformity

RHEUMATOID ARTHRITIS

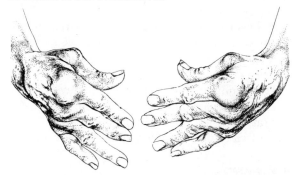

Chronic rheumatoid arthritis is a progressive inflammatory disease which can cause painful swelling and sometimes crippling deformities of the hands. The disease can affect persons of any age, although the most common age at onset is between 30 and 50. No specific treatment exists, but the pain can be relieved by aspirin and other analgesics.

that may result in chronic disease. In the acute stages where there is much pain and thickening of the synovial membranes, excision of the affected membrane may be most beneficial; in chronic disease, arthroplasty and tendon surgery may be employed in selected cases.

Although approximately 10 percent of persons with rheumatoid arthritis will develop a chronic progressively disabling disease, most go on to live relatively normal lives with only some modifications in life-style.

rhinitis

Inflammation of the mucous membrane that lines the nose (nasal mucosa). Rhinitis may be caused by the common cold virus (of which there are more than a hundred species) or by an allergic reaction to substances such as grass pollens, in which case it is a symptom of hay fever. Repeated attacks of acute rhinitis may lead to a chronic form.

rickets

A deficiency disease resulting from a lack of vitamin D, calcium, and phosphorus. It is seen most often in infancy and childhood and is marked by abnormal bone growth.

Signs and symptoms of rickets include soft bones causing defects such as bowlegs or knock-knees, swollen joints, muscle pain, a swollen skull, chest deformities, a curved spine, swollen liver and spleen, sweating, and a generalized tenderness of the body when touched.

Rickets can be prevented by a diet rich in vitamin D or by the routine use of milk fortified with vitamin D. Exposure to sunlight is also preventive.

Treatment of rickets most frequently consists of calcium, phosphorus, and vitamin-D supplementation. Care should be taken to avoid overdose of vitamin D, which can be dangerous.

rickettsiae

A group of microorganisms that are between viruses and bacteria in size; like viruses, they grow within cells, but like bacteria they are sensitive to appropriate antibiotics. Rickettsial disease is transmitted to man by lice, fleas, ticks, and mites. ROCKY MOUNTAIN SPOTTED FEVER is an example of a human rickettsial infection.

rigor mortis

The stiffening of the muscles that occurs after death as a result of molecular changes in the muscle cells. It begins four to ten hours after death in the muscles at the back of the neck, spreads to the rest of the body in a few hours, and lasts approximately two to four days.

Rocky Mountain spotted fever

A tick-borne typhus fever. There are a number of typhus fevers caused by infection from various species of RICKETTSIAE. Rabbits, chipmunks, squirrels, rats, and mice as well as dogs may carry the organisms responsible for Rocky Mountain spotted fever; however, the disease can be spread to humans *only* through the bite of an infected tick.

About twelve days after the tick bite the victim develops fever, with pains in the muscles and joints. The fever may rise high enough to produce delirium; there is a cough, and on the fourth or fifth day a rash appears. Between the twelfth and fourteenth day the condition improves. Treatment consists of appropriate drug administration.

Rocky Mountain spotted fever shows a seasonal incidence, being prevalent from May to September; it occurs throughout the continental United States, being most prevalent in the southern states. Persons in tick-infested areas should use insect repellent on their skin and clothes, and check their body, especially the scalp, every four hours for biting ticks.

See also the instructions for *Tick Bites* in the section on **First Aid**.

rosacea

A chronic disease (formerly known as *acne rosacea*) affecting the skin of the face. The skin has blotchy red areas and the nose is flushed. Often there are raised, reddened areas (papules) and, sometimes, weeping or pus-filled sores (pustules). Dilation of the small blood vessels (capillaries) on the surface of the skin is responsible for the reddened color of the face.

The condition is most common in women in their 30s and 40s but is found in men and women of all ages. Men who neglect the condition may develop the more severe form of the disease, known as *rhinophyma*, in which the nose becomes grossly swollen and deformed.

The cause of rosacea is not yet fully understood, but excessive use of stimulants and vasodilators (substances that cause dilation of blood vessels, such as alcohol, coffee, and tea) appears to play a part. Hormonal imbalances also may play a part.

Antibiotics such as tetracycline can be remarkably effective. Rhinophyma is easily treated by surgery.

roundworms

A human parasite (*Ascaris lumbricoides*) found all over the world, especially in the tropics. Its life cycle is bizarre.

The human host swallows the eggs; larvae hatch in the small intestine, make their way through the intestinal wall into the bloodstream, and become lodged in the lungs. Here they pass through the walls of the capillary blood vessels into the air spaces of the lungs and wriggle up through the air passages into the throat. They then move toward the intestine again through the esophagus ("gullet") and on reaching the small intestine develop into adults. They may live in the intestine for a year.

If their numbers are few they may produce no symptoms. But if they are present as a heavy infestation they produce a cough and spasm of the air passages as they pass through the lungs and interfere with the absorption of food from the

ROUNDWORM

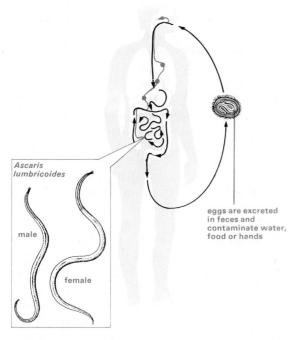

Ascaris
lumbricoides

male

female

eggs are excreted
in feces and
contaminate water,
food or hands

*Ascariasis, infestation with the roundworm pictured
above, is due to poor hygiene and is estimated to affect
one quarter of the world's population.*

intestine. They may wander up the esophagus to
emerge at the mouth or the nose, or may be
vomited up or passed from the rectum. They may
entwine to form a ball of worms that obstructs
the small intestine.

Treatment consists of appropriate drug administration.

salpingitis

Inflammation of a FALLOPIAN TUBE, often accompanying widespread PELVIC INFLAMMATORY DISEASE.
The inflammation sometimes results from GON-
ORRHEA, either immediately or months or years
after the infection. Another kind of salpingitis is
caused by streptococci or staphylococci bacteria,
which may reach the Fallopian tubes following
childbirth or abortion. The infection typically
produces EDEMA in the mucous membrane that
lines the tubes, and a discharge of pus may leave
the tubes and cause PERITONITIS or an abscess.

Among the consequences of salpingitis are sterility, as a result of the tubes becoming blocked
so that ova can no longer reach the womb, and
ECTOPIC PREGNANCY, in which the fertilized ovum
does not reach the uterus but grows in the tube
itself, eventually causing it to rupture and requiring emergency surgery.

Most early cases of salpingitis can be controlled
by administering an appropriate antibiotic. In advanced or long-term cases, surgical incision and
drainage or removal of the Fallopian tube may
be needed.

sarcoidosis

A disease of unknown origin affecting mainly
young adults. It is marked by small round bumps
in the tissue surrounding various organs in the
body, usually the lungs, liver, spleen, skin, and
tear and saliva glands. In many cases there are no
symptoms and the disease is discovered only by
routine X-ray examination. Eye involvement,
sometimes with serious consequences, is fairly
common.

There is often no need for treatment in these
cases and spontaneous remissions are common;
steroid drugs may be effective in relieving any
troublesome symptoms. Sufferers have a normal
expectation of life.

sarcoma

A malignant tumor originating in connective tissue, including bone or muscle.

Sarcoma is distinguished from the other main
type of malignant tumor, *carcinoma*, which is composed mainly of cells similar to skin or mucous
membrane cells. There are about twenty cases of
carcinoma to every one of sarcoma. The most
common sarcomas are the malignant bone tumors, some of which (such as *osteogenic sarcoma*)
are especially common in childhood.

scabies

A skin disease caused by infestation with the parasitic "itch mite" (*Sarcoptes scabiei*). The disease
is spread by close contact with infested persons.

The female of the parasite burrows into the

skin, particularly on the front of the wrist, the sides and webs of the fingers, the buttocks, the genitals, and the feet. Eggs are deposited in the small tunnels she makes, while the male remains on the surface of the skin.

The burrowing activities of the parasites cause intense itching and the original small blister-like lesions may be made much worse by scratching. Treatment will be successful only if all of the person's sexual contacts and household members are treated also. Clothes and towels and linens should be disinfected.

There are many scabies-killing applications available by prescription.

scar

The mark on the skin or an internal organ left by a healed wound, ulcer, or other lesion.

Scar tissue consists essentially of fibers that, in the case of scars on the skin surface, are covered by an imperfect formation of cuticle. The fibrous tissue is produced by cells of connective tissue brought to the lesion by the bloodstream.

At first the scar is soft because the fibrous tissue is supplied with ample blood vessels, so that the scar appears more red than the surrounding skin. As fibers contract and harden, the scar loses its blood vessels and becomes whitish.

There is wide variation in the amount of scar tissue that appears, depending on the extent to which the wound is allowed to gape during the healing process. The smaller the distance between the edges of the wound, the less will be the amount of scar tissue. That is one of the reasons that it is considered essential to close a wound with stitches to make the resulting scar as thin and faint as possible.

In general, scars do not regenerate specialized tissue, such as the hair follicles and sweat glands in the skin, although damaged muscles and nerves do regenerate specialized fibers in scars.

When large areas of skin have been damaged, as in burning, the resulting scars may contract so much that movement becomes restricted. In such cases plastic surgery is indicated, as it is for disfiguring facial scars.

Blacks are very prone to a type of disfiguring scar known as a KELOID. For an unknown reason, the response to a wound is out of proportion to what is needed and results in overformation of scar tissue. These appear as firm, raised scars.

scarlet fever

Some of the streptococci bacteria that cause sore throats produce a poison (*toxin*) that creates a characteristic scarlet rash on the skin.

Scarlet fever is seen most commonly in children of school age, who develop symptoms of fever, rapid pulse, headache, sore throat, and perhaps abdominal pain and vomiting. After one or two days a rash starts on the neck, spreads to the chest, and then covers the abdomen and the limbs. It leaves a pale area around the mouth and lasts for a few days, after which the skin becomes scaly and the scales begin to flake off. While the rash is present the tongue is covered with a white "fur." This peels off to leave the tongue red, with prominent papillae ("strawberry tongue").

In the last century scarlet fever was a serious disease, complicated by infection of the middle ear, rheumatic fever, and inflammation of the kidneys. But with the advent of drugs like penicillin its importance has declined.

schistosomiasis

A chronic illness caused by parasitic worms that live in the blood vessels around the liver and bladder. Schistosomiasis is one of the most important causes of ill health, lethargy, and premature death in tropical countries. Worldwide more than 200 million people are infested.

The complex life cycle of the parasite starts when an infected person excretes eggs in the urine or feces. If the eggs reach fresh water in a lake, canal, or irrigation ditch they hatch into *miracidia*, which may infect a particular form of snail. After multiplication inside the snail the *schistosomes* are released into the water as *cercariae* and this larval form is highly infectious. The cercariae readily penetrate the skin of anyone swimming or wading in contaminated water for even a few minutes.

Once in the bloodstream, the cercariae migrate to the lungs; then, depending on their subtype, they move either to the veins leading to the liver or to the veins around the bladder. Having reached the network of veins, the cercariae mature into adult worms: The male is about 2 centimeters (0.8 inch) long, and the thinner, longer female lives in a cleft in the male's body. Schistosome worms may live for as long as thirty years and some varieties lay up to 3,000 eggs daily. The eggs

SCHISTOSOMIASIS

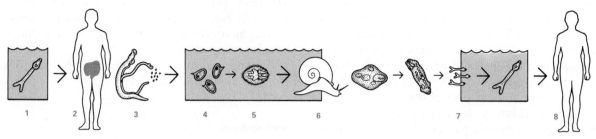

LIFE CYCLE OF *Schistosomatidae* FLUKES

Schistosomiasis affects 200 million people throughout the world. Infective larvae (1) abound in fresh water in many countries and penetrate the skin of bathers (2). They develop into flukes which enter the human bloodstream and damage many organs. Adult flukes lay eggs (3) which are excreted into water (4). The eggs hatch into miracidia (5). These penetrate a snail host (6) and change into thousands of larvae which are released into the water (7), where they can reinfect humans.

penetrate the lining of the bowel and are passed out of the body with the excreta.

Schistosomiasis may cause few or no symptoms, but when the infestation is heavy the victim may pass blood in the urine or have repeated attacks of diarrhea. Weakness, lack of energy, and repeated attacks of abdominal pain cause chronic ill health, eventually leading to failure of either the liver or the kidneys.

Schistosomiasis can be treated by drugs that destroy the worms, but long-term control depends on public health measures. The life cycle of the parasite can be interrupted by providing safe disposal of sewage, together with elimination of the snails from irrigation channels and watercourses.

schizophrenia

A mental illness characterized by false beliefs, irrational thinking, and a retreat from contact with the normal world. Over half the long-term patients in mental institutions have schizophrenia.

The illness typically begins in adolescence; the onset may be abrupt or gradual. Early symptoms include *hallucinations*, especially the hearing of voices critical of current actions, with the patient discussed in the third person; *delusions*, typically of persecution (PARANOIA); and *flight of ideas*, rapid and apparently meaningless changes in the topic of conversation. Often the schizophrenic withdraws from his family and friends to spend hours and days on end in solitary silence. He may become convinced that his thoughts and actions are being controlled by outside influences. Among other common variants of schizophrenia are

CATATONIA, in which the person spends minutes or hours motionless and mute, often in a bizarre posture; and *hebephrenia*, with incoherent speech, outbursts of crying and laughing, and extreme social withdrawal.

The cause of schizophrenia is unknown but there is a genetic factor: The disease is found more frequently among family members; also, individuals with schizophrenia who were raised by adoptive parents were found to have schizophrenia in their biological family. There also seems to be an environmental factor: Schizophrenia may possibly be provoked by excessive emotional conflicts with the family. Theories of biochemical disturbances in the brain are helping to advance the treatment of schizophrenia.

There are many drugs used to treat symptoms of schizophrenia. Drugs of the large group called *neuroleptics* reduce the severity of schizophrenic symptoms and help individuals avoid hospitalization. Many persons with chronic schizophrenia are able to live in the community or with their families with the support of community mental health programs, psychotherapy, and medication.

sciatica

Pain in the area of the body supplied by the sciatic nerve, including the buttocks, hip, back and outer part of the thigh, leg, ankle, and foot.

It is caused by irritation of the spinal nerve roots that go to make up the sciatic nerve. The most common reason for the irritation is disease of the joint between the fourth and fifth lumbar vertebrae. The pulpy inner part of the intervertebral disk—a cushion of cartilage between the vertebrae—may protrude and encroach on the space through which the nerve root passes (the condition inaccurately termed SLIPPED DISK), or the space may become narrowed by arthritic changes in the bones and ligaments of the joint. Sciatica is rarely a symptom of a more serious disease of the lumbar part of the spine.

The pain down the leg is aggravated by straining, coughing, sneezing, or bending, and the part of the leg affected may become numb. The ankle reflex disappears, and the sensation produced by a pinprick is blunted. The muscles may be weakened and, in consequence, the foot may drop in severe cases. The lower part of the back is stiff and loses its normal contour (it becomes flat), while the muscles along each side of the spine go into spasm. Sciatica usually is accompanied by lower back pain, and raising the straight leg makes the pain in the back and leg worse.

The first line of treatment is rest in bed. The bed must be firm (in most cases this is best assured by putting boards under the mattress). Analgesics (pain-killers such as aspirin) are useful, as may be the local application of heat. Resistant cases may need physical therapy followed by special exercises and perhaps manipulation of the back.

Only in severe cases of demonstrable disk protrusion is an operation advisable; but when the protruded disk material is removed in a well-chosen case, the relief is usually immediate and lasting.

scleroderma

Also known as *progressive systemic sclerosis.* A rare disease that produces hardening of the skin, which becomes smooth, shiny, and tight. The skin of the face may shrink so much that it becomes difficult to open the mouth widely; movement of the fingers is hampered and they may develop contractures. The condition is very similar to the toxic oil syndrome, which affected 20,000 people in Madrid in 1981.

The skin manifestations are part of a general systemic disturbance that affects the connective tissue of the joints, intestine, lungs, and kidneys, and may affect the heart. The cause of the disease is not known with certainty, but it is thought to be an immunological disorder.

Scleroderma affects four times as many women as men, and usually occurs in women in their 40s and 50s. Persons with a mild form of the disease have a slow progression of symptoms and a more favorable prognosis. Those with a more severe case will have widespread disease with internal involvement of the heart, lungs, and kidneys, which can cause death.

There is no known cure for this disease, but steroids may bring some relief.

scoliosis

A side-to-side curvature of the spine.
See also POSTURE and SPINE.

scotoma

A blind spot in the visual field, which may be caused by a variety of disorders affecting the retina or the optic nerves. A "blind spot" may be one-sided or bilateral and sometimes not appreciated until a specialist performs full visual-field testing.

Color scotoma may occur when certain areas of the retina are insensitive to color vision. This may be acquired through damage to the nerve fibers brought about by optic neuritis—itself caused by a large number of conditions: diseases such as ANEMIA, MULTIPLE SCLEROSIS, and DIABETES MELLITUS; abuse of tobacco or alcohol; chemical toxicity; and vitamin deficiencies.

Treatment of the neuritis is directed toward the cause, and in some cases recovery is possible if the condition is not progressive.

scurvy

A disease caused by a prolonged dietary deficiency of vitamin C (ascorbic acid). It is characterized by weakness, anemia, bruising of dry scaly skin, and bleeding spongy gums, often with loosening of the teeth.

The average person needs 75 milligrams of ascorbic acid per day, and a normal diet contains an excess. Elderly persons, however, frequently suffer from deficiencies because of inadequate diet. Scurvy can be cured by the administration of ascorbic acid (1,000mg./day) until all signs have disappeared. Treatment is continued for several months. Thereafter a balanced diet must be maintained.

sebaceous cyst (wen)

An accumulation of the fat-like secretion (*sebum*) from sebaceous glands.

The sebaceous glands of the skin secrete sebum, a greasy lubricant that helps maintain the health of the skin. These glands are present throughout the surface of the body except for the palms and soles. They are most common on the face, scalp, shoulders, genitalia, and trunk.

If the outlet on the skin surface becomes blocked, the gland may continue to secrete and thus form a *retention cyst* distended with sebum. Typically, it is a hemispherical swelling, firm, and discrete. The cyst may proceed, if uninfected, to reach a considerable size.

Sebaceous cysts frequently become infected, after which they may discharge and collapse. If a cyst remains or poses a problem it can be removed surgically.

See also CYST.

seizures

A sudden, violent, uncontrollable contraction of a group of muscles. These CONVULSIONS can be caused by EPILEPSY, high fever (especially in children), poisoning, or hysteria. Seizures are controlled with medication after their cause is diagnosed.

senility

Progressive impairment of mental functions. More appropriately known as DEMENTIA.

In the past, mental impairment, characterized by markedly decreased intellectual performance and loss of memory, was thought to be part of the natural aging process. It is now known, however, that such deterioration is abnormal.

Some changes in the brain are to be expected in elderly persons; the weight and size of the brain do decrease (atrophy). However, in some people the brain atrophies to such a degree that intellectual capacity is severely impaired. In these cases, they cannot feed, dress, or care for themselves; they cannot remember what happened from moment to moment, cannot recognize family members, and often lose control over bowel and urinary functions. When this occurs in some-

one who is not considered elderly, it is known as presenile dementia, which is now called ALZHEIMER'S DISEASE. There is also an extremely rare form of rapid-onset senility caused by a slow-growing virus that infects the brain. This is called Creutzfeldt-Jakob disease.

Dementia is considered a degenerative disease, but it is not known why it occurs in some persons and not in others. As modern medical treatment continues to develop, the average age of our population continues to rise. Consequently, more research is being directed toward the problems of aging. As of now, however, there are no treatments or cures for this debilitating condition. Death, when it occurs, is not due to the dementia itself, but to concurrent medical diseases.

septicemia

The presence and persistence in the bloodstream of disease-causing bacteria. If the bacteria are not destroyed with the administration of an appropriate antibiotic, they can multiply and cause a massive infection of the body (systemic infection), possibly leading to death.

The signs and symptoms of septicemia include prostration, high fever, and, sometimes, the formation of pustules and abscesses.

serum sickness

When sera were widely used for the treatment of microbial disease, some persons developed reactions to the injections. Usually these were reactions to foreign proteins of the animals from whom the sera had been prepared—the horse, in particular—and they usually occurred when the serum was given more than once. An example was the use of horse sera to make antitetanus injections.

Serum sickness produces swelling of the face, itching of the skin, and severe joint pains; there may be nausea, vomiting, and fever. It should be noted that very similar allergic reactions may occur in some persons given drugs or receiving blood transfusions.

The condition has become rare since most microbial diseases are now treated with antibiotics; sera prepared from human sources, less likely to cause allergic reactions, are widely available when their use is unavoidable.

The best treatment for serum sickness is the

use of cortisone-like drugs (steroids), though antihistamines may also help. Response usually is rapid.

sex hormones

Chemical substances, secreted by the testes in men and the ovaries in women, which determine sexual characteristics and function.

In men the secretion of *androgens* (the most potent of which is *testosterone*) from the testes aids the development of the male sex organs, stimulates the secretion of semen, and is responsible for the masculine sexual characteristics.

In women the secretion of *estrogen* and *progesterone* from the ovaries stimulates the development of the breasts, the uterus, and the external genitals, and maintains the menstrual cycle and the capacity of women for reproduction. In both sexes the sex organs (gonads) are under the control of the PITUITARY GLAND, which initiates their development at puberty and maintains their function in adult life.

Deficiencies of the sex hormones may occur when the glands themselves are abnormal or when pituitary secretions are insufficient. In contrast, premature sexual development in either sex may be associated with tumors of the gonads, pituitary gland, or ADRENAL GLANDS.

Treatment with sex hormones is effective for identified deficiencies, but the tailoring of the dosage to the individual is essential and requires complicated biochemical analysis. Moderate supplementation is used in either sex for treating some types of infertility and for treating menopause in women. Sex hormones also are used sometimes in the treatment of certain types of cancers.

shock (cardiovascular)

Shock is the medical term for collapse due to inadequate circulation of the blood. Whatever the cause, the symptoms include pallor, sweating, nausea, restlessness, confusion, weakness, and finally loss of consciousness.

Shock may be caused by: (1) failure of the heart to pump sufficient blood through the body because of damage from CORONARY THROMBOSIS; (2) loss of blood as the result of hemorrhage (internal or external); (3) plasma loss associated with severe burns; or (4) loss of body fluids from excessive vomiting or diarrhea (as in CHOLERA). FAINTING may be caused by the blood pooling in some veins and arteries that have suddenly lost their reflex tone; the consequent loss of consciousness is caused by impaired circulation to the brain.

When shock occurs the victim should be placed at rest, kept warm with light coverings, and positioned with the legs raised to encourage the return of blood to the brain. Shock due to diminished circulatory volume—as in hemorrhage, trauma, or dehydration—requires urgent restoration of the volume to normal by the intravenous administration of fluids. Prevention of shock depends on proper evaluation of the factors causing circulatory failure. In cases of trauma, the prompt initiation of therapy by teams of medical or paramedical personnel has done much to save lives that would have been lost otherwise through irreversible damage to the heart, brain, or kidneys brought about through sustained circulatory collapse.

sickle-cell anemia

Within the red blood cell is a substance called HEMOGLOBIN, whose function is to carry oxygen. Hemoglobin has a certain chemical structure known as hemoglobin A.

In about 0.3 percent of U.S. blacks, there is an inherited disease in which an abnormality occurs in the structure of the hemoglobin. This abnormally configured hemoglobin is called hemoglobin S, or sickle hemoglobin.

Two forms of inheritance occur. The abnormal hemoglobin may be present in only one of the parents and the child can only inherit a single gene and its cells will contain only a small proportion of the abnormal pigment. In such cases little harm will result. If both parents carry the gene, however, the child may be homozygous, causing the red blood cells to contain a large amount of the abnormal pigment. Serious illness may then follow.

The presence of large amounts of hemoglobin S in the red blood cells results in a tendency for the red blood cells to become distorted in a crescent shape ("sickle cells") if the level of oxygen in the arterial blood falls. This sickling can be identified by microscopic examination of the blood.

Sickle-cell anemia refers to the inheritance of hemoglobin S from both parents with large amounts of sickle hemoglobin in the cells. Even slight degrees of oxygen lack will result in a marked "sickling" change in the blood and consequent obstruction to the circulation in various parts of the body by masses of sickled cells ("sickle-cell crisis"). During a sickle-cell crisis (and, to a lesser extent, at other times as well), the sickle cells are destroyed and liberate hemoglobin into the blood plasma in great quantity—sometimes enough to produce jaundice and to lower the red cell count seriously. Severe pain, dangerous organ damage, and even death may result.

Inheritance of a single dose of hemoglobin S from just one parent results in a condition called "sickle-cell trait." Although abnormalities can be noted on careful examination of the blood, usually sickle-cell trait rarely results in symptoms.

siderosis

A condition caused by inhalation of iron oxide dust, or by the presence of metallic iron particles in the body. Iron in the lungs causes abnormal-looking X-ray appearances, but is not serious. In the eye, however, a penetrating iron foreign body causes gradual but severe chemical damage, which may lead to blindness.

silicosis

A disease of the lungs caused by the prolonged inhalation of fine particles of silica; the mechanical and chemical irritant effects of silica provoke a response of FIBROSIS (permanent scarring) in the pulmonary tissues.

The most common form of silica is quartz, which is distributed abundantly in the earth's surface. Thus, miners, rock cutters, sandblasters, and those who work in the ceramics and glass industries are especially at risk for silicosis.

In the areas in the lung where the particles accumulate, nodules of fibrosis develop; in advanced cases, both lungs may be heavily scarred. The characteristic feature of silicosis is loss of the normal elasticity of the lungs, so that breathing requires more effort.

The earliest symptom is shortness of breath on exertion (DYSPNEA); this may be followed by coughing, wheezing, and other features similar to BRONCHITIS. There is danger of tuberculosis. Diagnosis is made by chest X ray which reveals the characteristic changes, although exposure to the dust over a period of ten to twenty years may occur

before the symptoms develop. The changes in the lungs are irreversible, and treatment is limited to the relief of symptoms. Prevention of the disease includes the use of efficient ventilation in modern industry, the avoidance of smoking, regular use of respirators, and techniques of dust control.

sinusitis

Inflammation of the lining of one or more of the nasal sinuses.

The sinuses are cavities in the bones of the face and skull. They reduce the weight of the skull and add resonance to the voice. The largest of the sinuses are the *frontal sinuses* in the forehead and the *maxillary sinuses* (antroms) in the cheeks. The sinuses communicate with the nasal cavity; because of the extension of infections from the nose, they are liable to become infected. The symptoms of pain and tenderness over the sinuses (frequently with a thick nasal discharge) are the classical signs of sinusitis.

Sinusitis occurs most frequently as a complication arising from the common cold. Obstruction of normal sinus drainage by thickened mucus produces intense pain in the sinus itself as the fluid level rises. The affected side of the face may

SINUSITIS

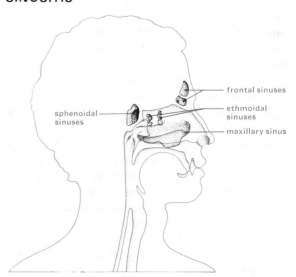

Sinusitis is caused by bacterial infection of the air sinuses which connect with the nose. It usually follows a head cold and causes a heavy feeling in the face and a blocked nose.

swell, as well as the lower eyelid. X-ray studies of the skull may reveal fluid that requires drainage.

Acute sinusitis may resolve rapidly with the administration of antibiotics and steam inhalations. *Chronic sinusitis* may require surgical drainage and "sinus washout" to remove the accumulated pus. To achieve a permanent cure, it may be necessary to perform surgery to remove the lining membrane of the affected sinus.

skin diseases

The skin may be affected by diseases that involve the whole body, but it is also especially vulnerable to external factors such as heat, radiation, and contact with chemicals and other irritants.

Structurally, the skin is divided into two distinct layers: the *dermis* and the *epidermis*. The inner layer (dermis) consists of connective tissue that contributes to the support and elasticity of the skin. The dermis is made up of different types of cells, all of which have their special function—some to produce connective tissue, some to fight infection, and so on. The dermis is also the layer in which the sweat and the sebaceous (oil-secreting) glands and the hair follicles originate. The coils of some sweat glands and the follicles of some of the hairs lie in the fatty layer of tissue just under the skin.

The epidermis is made up of layers of cells that form keratin (a tough protein substance found in hair, nails, and other "horny" tissues) and cells that produce the pigment responsible for skin color (melanin). The epidermis constantly renews itself by shedding old layers as new ones are formed.

Any structure of the skin may be the primary structure affected by a particular disease. A malignant MELANOMA, for example, arises from the melanin-producing cells.

Exposure of the skin to the sun may cause burning, and in pale-skinned persons prolonged exposure to strong sunlight increases the risk of skin cancer. Soap powders, solvents, dyes, and cosmetics all may damage the skin, causing DERMATITIS. Some people develop an allergic sensitivity to metal (especially nickel) or other substances and are affected by a localized inflammation where the skin is in contact with the sensitizing agent (*contact dermatitis*).

Among the more common diseases are ECZEMA, in which the skin is reddened, weeping, and intensely itchy; PSORIASIS, in which patches of silvery

STRUCTURE OF THE SKIN

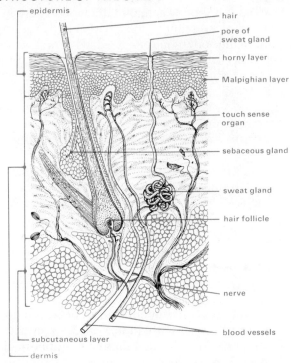

Skin encloses our entire body and provides a barrier against the entry of infection and the loss of tissue fluid. Although we think of skin as being extremely thin, the magnified section shown here reveals that it has many layers.

gray scales appear on the knees and elbows, sometimes affecting the whole body; LICHEN PLANUS, in which there is a thickening and roughening of the skin; infection with bacteria and fungi, such as TINEA ("ringworm"); and a large spectrum of rashes associated with generalized infections, from MEASLES to TYPHOID FEVER.

Identifying the cause of a skin disease often allows the irritant or the cause of an allergy to be removed. But even when the cause remains unknown (as in psoriasis), the symptoms often can be relieved by treatment with a wide variety of medication.

sleep

A recurring state of inactivity accompanied by loss of awareness and a reduction in responsiveness to the environment. Unlike a COMA, or unconsciousness caused by general anesthesia, a sleeping person can easily be aroused. Sleep is not

SLEEP

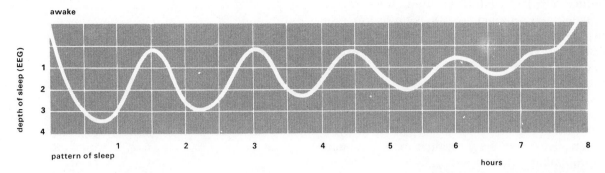

This diagram shows the fluctuations in the depth of sleep during a typical night as reflected by an EEG recording of brain waves. These waves change through stages 1 and 4 as the person becomes more deeply asleep. About every 90 minutes, the sleeper makes rapid eye movements (REMs); it is believed that these coincide with periods of dreaming.

a single state: Electroencephalographic (EEG) studies, which measure the electrical activity in the brain, show that there are two basic alternating states.

The first is known as *nonrapid eye movement (NREM) sleep*, during which the heart and respiratory rates slow down, the muscles are greatly but not completely relaxed, and the eyelids remain quite still. This can be divided into four general states of increasing depth of sleep. If awakened during the NREM sleep, the individual may say that he was "thinking" at the time of waking up.

During *rapid eye movement (REM) sleep*, the eyeballs move jerkily under closed lids, the heart and respiratory rates quicken (but this is variable), and the muscles (especially the neck muscles) are completely relaxed. This is the stage during which dreams occur, and dreams are more likely to be remembered if the individual wakes up or is awakened during REM sleep.

On going to bed, drowsiness is followed by NREM sleep of progressively increasing depth. After about ninety minutes, REM sleep takes over; during this first cycle of sleep, the REM stage may last only about five to ten minutes. There are also fewer eye movements in the first cycle. During a night's sleep there may be four to six cycles of sleep, each lasting eighty to hundred minutes; the duration of REM sleep increases with each successive cycle and may make up about thirty minutes of the later cycles.

The amount of sleep required by an individual and the pattern of cycles vary according to age. The young adult who has about six to eight hours of sleep spends about twenty to twenty-five per-

cent of the night in REM sleep. The baby, whose sleep cycle is short (about forty to forty-five minutes) spends about 50 percent of the sleep in REM sleep. In the elderly—in whom the total sleep time required gradually diminishes—the proportion spent in REM sleep also reduces gradually toward 20 percent.

Despite these general patterns of sleep, the amount required varies greatly from person to person. The function of sleep is not entirely clear, but it is thought to be a time that the body uses to catch up with the processes of growth and repair. Some sleep certainly is required, but how much is difficult to say. Extreme sleep deprivation (used as one method of "brainwashing") can lead to HALLUCINATIONS and PARANOIA. Most people manage to adapt to small amounts of sleep deprivation; they may complain of irritability and loss of efficiency (but again it is difficult to quantify how much of this is caused by the loss of sleep and how much to worry about loss of sleep and lack of efficiency). When they do get a chance to catch up on the lost sleep, they do so not only by longer hours of sleep but also by spending a greater proportion of it in REM sleep.

Sleep disorders may be *primary*—the inability to fall asleep or stay asleep for very long (insomnia), or the abnormal tendency to fall asleep or have uncontrollable attacks of drowsiness in the daytime (narcolepsy)—or they may be *secondary* to various emotional or mental disturbances, chronic alcoholism, disease of the thyroid gland (HYPERTHYROIDISM), or brain disease.

The treatment of primary sleep disorders is the administration of the appropriate drug: stimulants (such as amphetamines) to control narcolepsy, and sedatives or hypnotics (drugs that induce sleep) to control insomnia. It should be remembered, however, that it is unwise to take hypnotics for prolonged periods. Most of these drugs lose their effectiveness when used excessively, and they may make the person psychologically and physically dependent on them. Withdrawal of most of these drugs may cause the individual to react by having more than usual amounts of REM sleep; this leads to vivid dreams, which then make the individual more reluctant to stop taking hypnotics.

sleeping sickness

Another name for ENCEPHALITIS LETHARGICA. The term is applied also to TRYPANOSOMIASIS (African sleeping sickness).

slipped disk

The intervertebral disks act as "shock absorbers" between the vertebral bodies and are responsible for flexibility of the spine. Each consists of a pulpy nucleus contained in an outer fibrocartilaginous ring. The disk cannot "slip" but the soft nucleus may herniate through the outer ring, producing a bulge forward or sideways into the spinal canal. Usually this is due to trauma (80 percent of cases) associated with changes in the fibrous consistency of the disk's outer wall. Typically, the disk "slips" while the person is lifting a heavy weight with the body bent. (The risk of a disk injury can be reduced by keeping the back straight while lifting.) This condition, known technically as *herniated disk, ruptured disk,* or *prolapsed disk,* occurs most often in persons in their 30s and 40s.

Protrusions of the lumbar disks (in the lower part of the back) are approximately fifteen times more common than cervical protrusions (in the neck); thoracic disks (in the chest region) rarely are affected. Protrusion backward may impinge on the spinal cord or the nerves leading from it, causing pain (SCIATICA), weakness, and numbness, especially in a leg.

X-ray examination of the spinal area usually will show loss of disk space between particular vertebral bodies; it will not show the disk itself. Injection of a radiopaque dye (a *myelogram*) is required to define the precise extent of a disk's backward protrusion. Treatment depends largely

SLIPPED DISK

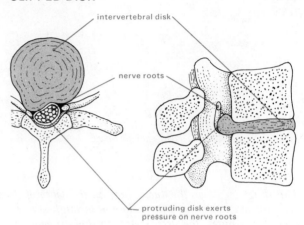

VERTEBRA SEEN FROM ABOVE   VERTEBRAE SEEN FROM SIDE

The picture shows a "slipped disk," where the pulpy center of the disk herniates into the spinal canal. Such herniation results from excessive strain or degeneration of the disk. The rupture presses on nearby nerves, causing backache and pain in the legs.

on the severity of the symptoms and the nature of the injury.

The first treatment for slipped disk is for the person to rest in bed, lying on a firm mattress supported on a wooden base. Complete rest often leads to relief of symptoms within a few days and to healing within a few weeks. If rest alone is ineffective, then the bones of the spine may be stretched apart by TRACTION, under medical supervision.

Persons who have experienced a slipped disk are at higher risk for developing more, either in the same spot or elsewhere. Treatment is aimed at controlling pain and enabling the person to continue to work, but it is not a cure.

If these measures fail, or if the symptoms recur on several occasions, then surgical treatment may be necessary to remove the protruded section of disk.

smallpox

A highly contagious viral disease that at one time was a major cause of death throughout the world.

Smallpox is characterized by a high fever of three or four days' duration followed by a generalized skin eruption. This consists of crops of pink-red spots (1–2 mm. in diameter) that typically appear first on the face and about the mouth. Within a few hours they begin to spread to the neck, arms, and trunk. After a day or so the clear fluid in the center of the spots turns to pus, and this later dries to form scabs. The pustules (pus-filled sores) involve the deeper layers of the skin and after the crusty scabs fall off, they may leave pockmarks on the face or neck.

Because of worldwide vaccination programs, smallpox was eradicated from the world. The last case of naturally acquired smallpox occurred in Somalia in 1977 and the World Health Organization confirmed in May 1980 that the disease no longer exists.

smell

The specialized nerve filaments (olfactory receptors) that give rise to the sense of smell lie in a small patch of the mucosal lining of the upper part of the nasal cavity. This part is above the path of the main air currents, which enter the nose with normal breathing; odorous molecules must either float up to the receptor cells or be moved up by eddy currents caused by sniffing in order to be detected.

To stimulate the sense of smell, an odorous

SMELL

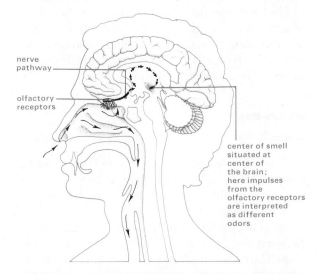

nerve pathway

olfactory receptors

center of smell situated at center of the brain; here impulses from the olfactory receptors are interpreted as different odors

Although our sense of smell is poorly developed compared with that of most animals, we are capable of distinguishing thousands of different aromas. Without it, our appreciation of food, our ability to enjoy numerous pleasant odors, and our capacity to react to important signals from the environment—including dangerous fumes—would be lost.

molecule has to dissolve in the mucus that covers the receptor and set up a particular chemical change; this, in turn, electrically excites the nerve fibers of the two olfactory nerves.

Sensitivity to smell varies with the state of the nasal mucosa. It decreases during the common cold (especially if the nose is stuffy or runny), is impaired by smoking, and is increased in conditions of hunger. In general, females appear to have a slightly more acute sense of smell than males. Damage to nasal bones—in particular, fractures of the frontal base of the skull—may permanently impair the efficiency of the olfactory nerve; in some cases the sense of smell may be totally lost.

smoking

Smoking affects health in three basic ways: (1) Nicotine and other chemical constituents of tobacco smoke have an immediate effect on the body; (2) Repeated exposure to smoke damages the lungs; and (3) Regular smokers have a much greater susceptibility to HEART DISEASE and several common forms of CANCER.

Nicotine is a brain stimulant, although habitual smokers often find it also has a calming effect. It speeds the heart rate, raises the blood pressure, produces a rise in cortisol and adrenaline in the bloodstream, and reduces the appetite.

The irritants in tobacco smoke narrow the air passages in the lungs. Smoke slows the action of the hair-like cilia that line these passages, reducing their efficiency in removing the inhaled dust from the lungs. Smoking also accentuates the normal loss of lung elasticity with age. These two effects account for the frequency of BRONCHITIS in smokers, who often accept a chronic cough as inevitable. EMPHYSEMA, the end result of chronic lung disease, is also directly attributable to smoking in the vast majority of cases. Smokers also have a much higher rate of PNEUMONIA, INFLUENZA, and other lung conditions.

Smoking is a major factor in death from myocardial infarction ("heart attack"). In men aged 40 to 55 who smoke, coronary attacks are three times as common as in male nonsmokers in the same age range—and sudden death from coronary disease is five times as common. As yet the mechanism by which smoking increases the risk of heart disease is unknown—thus claims that some cigarettes are "safer" than others cannot be justified.

Lung cancer is the best-known disease associated with smoking; it is extremely rare in those who have never smoked. Many studies have shown that the risk of the disease is proportional to the amount smoked. Smoking cigarettes carries a higher risk than smoking cigars or a pipe. Smokers also have a higher than average risk of bladder cancer, laryngeal cancer, and stomach ulcers.

Taken together, the association of smoking and disease makes tobacco the single most important cause of death so far identified in Western society. In recognition of this fact, the number of smokers overall has decreased. Social awareness of the ill effects of smoking has in recent years spawned a major campaign to eliminate smoking from public areas. Nonsmokers do not want to breathe air that has been contaminated by smoke. Recent studies have shown possible health hazards for persons who are "passive smokers," who, through proximity to smokers, inhale their smoke.

No other decision will affect a person's life more than to stop smoking. Although it may be difficult because of the addictive nature of nicotine and because of the willpower needed to overcome an often years-long habit, it can be done!

If a person feels he cannot do it by himself, there are numerous organizations that will help. Contact your community American Cancer Society or American Lung Association for information. There is also available a nicotine-based chewing gum that can be prescribed by a doctor. This medication is only prescribed for short periods; it is not meant to be used as a nicotine replacement.

somatotropin

The human growth hormone, released by the anterior lobe of the PITUITARY GLAND.

The physiological effects of this hormone are numerous. They are associated with bone growth and cartilage extension; with the release of stored body fat and its conversion to energy; with increased protein absorption by muscle cells (thus muscle development and growth); and with accelerated use of the body's glucose (sugar). The hormone itself is inextricably linked with the release and the effect of thyroid, adrenal, and sex hormones.

When pituitary disease or damage has occurred and somatotropin is deficient, growth is defective. Children born with a pituitary defect may grow

very slowly (*pituitary dwarfs*), but if the condition is recognized early enough, treatment with the hormone will permit them to reach a normal height. Excess growth hormone production during childhood causes *gigantism*. Excess growth hormone secretion caused by a tumor in later life produces ACROMEGALY; the condition can often be cured by treatment of the pituitary tumor, either surgically or by radiation therapy.

spasticity

Uncontrolled tightening of the skeletal muscles causing a lack of smooth movement. The term "spasticity" is used most often in connection with the birth handicap CEREBRAL PALSY.

In particular, spasticity involves increased resistance to passive movement, exaggerated reflexes, spasms and uncontrolled movements of the limbs (ATHETOSIS). There is considerable variation in severity and in the defects (and, therefore, of muscular control), but it is important to remember that intellectual function and intelligence may not be impaired.

There is no cure for what is essentially an irreversible defect of neurological control; but with physical therapy, bracing of limbs, and the use of other appliances, considerable benefits can be achieved. Surgical intervention can be helpful to minimize deformities, and tendons can be transplanted so that the controllable muscles can achieve voluntary movement and overcome involuntary spasm. Drugs to overcome reflex spasticity are occasionally helpful.

speech

The use of sounds produced by the mouth, tongue, and respiratory system to communicate specific thoughts from one person to another or to many others.

Speech develops slowly in the normal child. Between the ages of 9 months and 5 years the child learns a simple vocabulary and the basic elements of sentence construction, but the acquisition of full language skills takes the whole of childhood. Even in normal children there is great variation in the pace at which speech develops, but a child may be slow to speak because of low intelligence, extraordinary shyness, a physical defect such as deafness, or lack of stimulation in a

SPEECH

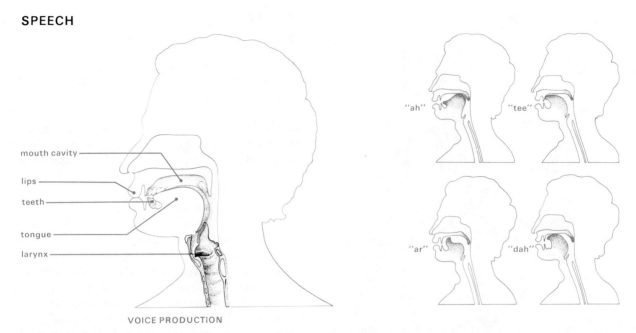

VOICE PRODUCTION

Vibrations of the vocal cords in the larynx produce the basic sound of the voice. The different elements of speech are produced by modifying the shape of the mouth cavity, position of the tongue, and the use of the teeth and lips.

deprived social environment. Speech defects such as lisps and stammering are due more often to psychological than to physical causes.

Once speech has been developed it may be lost again due to physical injury or disease of the larynx or tongue, or more commonly due to damage to the brain from a STROKE (a cerebral thrombosis, embolism, or hemorrhage), a tumor, or any other lesion.

spherocytosis

A condition in which red blood cells have an abnormal shape. It is a rare inherited disorder, found in northern European ethnic groups, with an incidence of 20 to 30 per 100,000 of the population.

The abnormal cells are unusually fragile, so that their life span is reduced, and the spleen enlarges owing to its role in destroying the defective cells. There may be no symptoms, or the high rate of cell destruction may cause a chronic ANEMIA. Diagnosis of the condition, which usually is not obvious until adulthood, is made by a blood test. Treatment is surgical removal of the spleen. This does not prevent spherocytes from still being made, but it reduces the anemia and the incidence

of complications from the increased rate of destruction of red blood cells (*hemolysis*).

sphygmomanometer

A device for measuring BLOOD PRESSURE.

The most common instrument consists of an upright glass column filled with mercury and calibrated in millimeters. To this is attached, by a length of plastic or rubber tubing, an inflatable cuff designed to be wrapped around the patient's upper arm. Inflation of the cuff by compression of a rubber bulb applies pressure to the arm and the pressure in the cuff is recorded by the height to which the mercury rises in the calibrated glass tube (manometer).

The STETHOSCOPE is applied over the main artery of the arm just below the cuff. The cuff then is inflated to about 180 mm., as shown on the manometer. The pressure in the cuff now exceeds the highest pressure generated in the arteries with each heartbeat. No blood will pass through the artery and no sound will be heard. Lowering the pressure slowly, a point is reached at which the blood begins to flow through the vessel with each heartbeat but the vessel collapses between beats. The coming together of the vessel walls

SPHYGMOMANOMETER

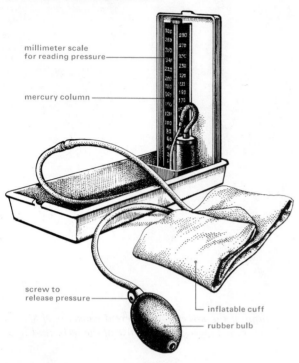

millimeter scale
for reading pressure

mercury column

screw to
release pressure

inflatable cuff

rubber bulb

*The familiar sphygmomanometer is a simple but ac-
curate device for measuring blood pressure. The cuff
is wrapped snuggly and evenly around the person's
arm and inflated to a high pressure by pumping the
rubber bulb; this stops blood flow through the arm.
The examiner then slowly reduces the pressure and
listens with a stethoscope over the artery for the sounds
of the pulse. The levels of the mercury at which these
sounds appear and then disappear are taken as the
person's blood-pressure reading.*

results in a sharp tapping noise, heard by the
examiner. This point is described as the *systolic
pressure*—the highest pressure generated by each
heartbeat.

Lowering the pressure still further, a point is
reached where the blood flow becomes continuous and no sound can be heard. This point is
described as the *diastolic pressure*. It represents the
steady pressure remaining in the arteries between
heartbeats.

The final result of the measurement is recorded
in millimeters of mercury pressure—often expressed, for example, as 120/80 (indicating a systolic pressure of 120 millimeters of mercury and
a diastolic pressure of 80).

Modern variants of the instrument use direct-
reading manometers or the pressure may be electrically recorded, but the underlying principle
remains the same.

spina bifida

During the third and fourth weeks of embryonic
life, the *neural groove*, which runs along the back
of the embryo, fuses to form the *neural tube*. This
tube is the forerunner of the central nervous
system (the brain and spinal cord). Spina bifida
results when closure of the neutral tube is incomplete and is accompanied by a similar defect in
the closure of the bony vertebral canal. The site
most frequently involved is the lumbosacral region (at the bottom of the back), although higher
regions occasionally are affected. Three varieties
of spina bifida are recognized: spina bifida occulta, meningocele, and meningomyelocele.

Spina bifida occulta, the least severe form, results
from incomplete fusion of the bony vertebral arch
and usually is of no medical significance. The site
may be marked externally by a tuft of hair, but
often it is detected only by chance on X-ray examination.

The other two varieties of spina bifida are far
more serious and involve the protrusion of a sac
through the vertebral defect. In *meningocele* the
sac contains meningeal tissue (the *meninges* are
the membranes that cover the spinal cord); in the
more common *meningomyelocele*, the sac contains
spinal cord tissues or nerve roots as well as
meningeal membranes. These forms frequently
coexist with other congenital abnormalities,
especially HYDROCEPHALUS (accumulation of fluid
within the brain).

Severe degrees of spina bifida may be incompatible with life, the baby being stillborn or surviving for only a few hours. Neurologic defects
commonly found in those who survive include
mental handicap, variable motor and sensory loss
in the limbs, and impaired control of the muscular
ring that controls the opening of the anus (anal
sphincter).

The cause of spina bifida is unknown, but a
woman who has had one affected child stands an
increased risk of having another. Recently it has
become possible to diagnose meningocele and
meningomyelocele before birth by detecting increased levels of ALPHAFETOPROTEIN in the amniotic
fluid that surrounds the fetus.

spinal curvature

The SPINE, or spinal column, is shaped somewhat
like an "S." It curves forward in the neck, back-

ABNORMAL SPINAL CURVATURES

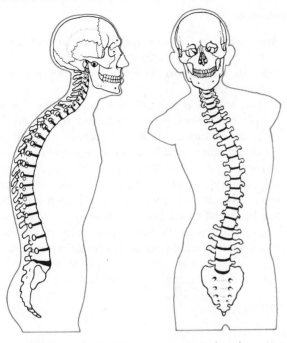

kyphosis—exaggerated convexity
of the spine

scoliosis—lateral curvature
of the spine

Illustrated above are two of the most common spinal deformities. Kyphosis, or "humpback," may result from poor posture (in which case it is often reversible) or from structural abnormalities in the vertebrae. Likewise, scoliosis may be postural, a congenital deformity, or the result of a neurological disease such as poliomyelitis. The two deformities are sometimes combined in a condition called kyphoscoliosis.

ward in the thoracic region, forward in the lumbar region, and like an elongated "S" it curves again in the sacrum to finish pointing downward and forward at the coccyx. Vertically, in correct posture, the uppermost cervical vertebra is in a direct gravitational line above the end of the sacrum. Abnormal curvature may be an exaggeration of the normal curves (KYPHOSIS), or an abnormal lateral curvature on either side of the vertical (SCOLIOSIS), or a combination of both (*kyphoscoliosis*).

Lateral curvature—scoliosis—often is associated with a compensatory twisting of the spine and may be due to congenital abnormalities of the vertebrae, bad posture in a child, paralytic disease affecting the muscles (such as POLIOMYELITIS), or pulmonary disease, particularly where the effects on one lung have caused contraction of the chest wall on that side. Cases that develop in puberty are more common in girls and require constant supervision involving serial X-ray ex-

aminations, physical therapy, exercises, spinal jackets, and (if necessary) spinal fusion to prevent the development of permanent deformities.

Excessive convexity of the spine—kyphosis—may result from trauma (particularly mild compression fracture of a dorsal vertebra), from OSTEOPOROSIS that softens the vertebral bodies, especially in postmenopausal women, and from secondary growths of a tumor.

spine/spinal column

The spinal column consists of twenty-six bones which provide a strong but flexible "backbone" for upright locomotion and which encase the spinal cord and its nerve roots.

There are 7 *cervical vertebrae* (supporting the skull and the neck), 12 *thoracic vertebrae* (providing anchorage for the rib case), 5 *lumbar vertebrae* (the largest), 5 *sacral vertebrae* fused into one bone (the sacrum), and 4 *coccygeal bones* fused into one bone (the coccyx).

The spinal vertebrae are separated from each other by disks of cartilage (*intervertebral disks*). From the second cervical bone to the first sacral bone the vertebrae are held in close proximity by ligaments and muscles that permit a limited range of bending and twisting while also protecting the spinal cord. Although the range of movement between the spinal bones is small, the somewhat elastic nature of the disks also permits them to be compressed. This ability to absorb compression stresses, aided by the natural curves of the spine, means that the effects of the weight of the upright body and the impact of the feet—whether light (as in walking) or more heavy (as in running or jumping)—are smoothed out by this system of "shock absorption."

The anatomy of the spine is complicated in that each vertebral bone is different from the others, but each has a thick and substantial *body* with extensions outward that form protective arches for the nerves. Injury to the spine may be direct, causing fracture of one or more of these vertebral bodies, or excessive bending may cause a *compression fracture* of a vertebral body. In either case, the pressure on the spinal cord can result in paralysis in body parts served by nerves branching from the spinal cord below the site of the injury. Deformities associated with disease, chronic bad posture, or malignancy may occur, and treatment is required at the first sign of abnormality.

See also CHIROPRACTIC, SLIPPED DISK.

SPINAL COLUMN

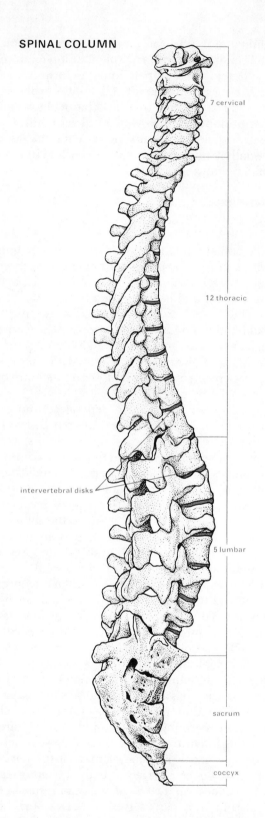

7 cervical

12 thoracic

intervertebral disks

5 lumbar

sacrum

coccyx

The spinal column consists of twenty-four separate vertebrae plus two composite bones—the sacrum and coccyx. Our upright posture has led to the characteristic curvature of the column seen from the side, and means that the skull sits supported on a springlike structure.

spleen

An organ lying within the abdominal cavity, situated under the margin of the ribs on the left side. In shape and size it roughly resembles a cupped hand.

The spleen is similar in structure to a large lymph node such as those found in the neck, armpits, and groin. It is, however, the largest of these structures and has special features not seen in the lymph nodes. It is a vascular organ, having a large arterial blood supply. On entering the spleen, the blood flow slows greatly as it enters a meshwork of dilated blood vessels, or "sinuses." These sinuses lie between large masses of LYM-PHOCYTES, one of the more common types of cir-

SPLEEN

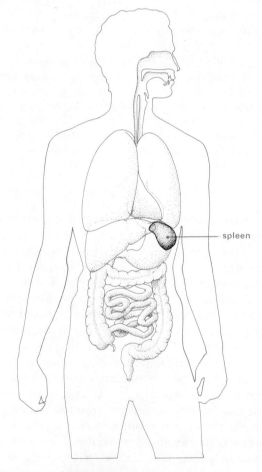

spleen

The spleen is an abdominal organ that lies underneath the lower ribs on the left of the body. It cannot be felt during a physical examination unless it has become enlarged by disease.

culating white blood cells. The walls of the sinuses contain other cells (*phagocytes*) that are capable of engulfing dead cells and foreign particles in the blood and removing them from the circulation. The relatively large volume of arterial blood that enters the spleen leaves it via the *splenic vein* and passes to the liver via the *portal vein.*

Like the lymph nodes, the spleen is an important source of antibodies, which are part of the body's resistance to infection. To a greater extent than the lymph nodes, however, the spleen is concerned with the removal of abnormal or normally worn out ("dying") blood cells from the circulation. Its function in antibody formation can readily be taken over by the lymphocytes in the lymph nodes, and removal of the spleen (following an injury, for example) is without serious effects except in very small children. In certain blood diseases, however, the spleen enlarges and removes blood cells more rapidly than usual from the blood; its removal may then be beneficial (splenectomy).

Enlargement of the spleen (SPLENOMEGALY) also occurs in a number of other conditions, including some infections, parasitic disorders such as malaria, diseases of the liver, and malignant tumors affecting the LYMPHATIC SYSTEM.

splenomegaly

Abnormal enlargement of the spleen, an organ lying in the abdominal cavity under the margin of the left rib and forming part of the LYMPHATIC SYSTEM.

A spleen of normal size cannot be felt by the doctor when examining the abdomen since it lies wholly beneath the rib margin. An enlarged spleen can be felt more easily if the person lies on his right side and takes a deep breath; descent of the diaphragm will then displace the spleen downward so that (if enlarged) it can be felt protruding below the left rib margin.

Many different conditions may cause enlargement of the spleen. Enlargement occurs in some blood disorders (including the chronic leukemias), and a grossly enlarged organ may occupy much of the abdominal cavity. More common causes of enlargement, however, are certain infectious diseases; the detection of an enlarged spleen may be an important diagnostic finding in such conditions as INFECTIOUS MONONUCLEOSIS, TYPHOID FEVER, and MALARIA.

splint

A rigid appliance for the immobilization of a part of the body's musculoskeletal system, or for the correction of a deformity.

A splint may be a simple plaster of Paris cast on the lower forearm and wrist to protect against excessive movements of an injured wrist bone or tendon, or it may be a whole-body plaster jacket, also encasing part of the head, to secure immobility of a fractured spine. Following the correction of some bone injuries or joint disorders, bandages impregnated with quick-setting plaster can be applied after wetting. They can be molded to fit the individual's needs, and they can be left on as long as necessary to secure healing. X-ray pictures can be taken through them and they are easily removed by cutting, using special plaster shears or saws that do not cut the skin.

When a plaster splint has been applied over a fresh fracture, careful observation is necessary in case swelling of the limb in a close-fitting splint impairs the blood circulation. The period of greatest potential danger is from about twelve to thirty-six hours after injury; severe pain or swelling of the exposed limb beyond the splint is a sign for reassessment and perhaps splint removal and replacement, or merely cutting open the splint. In emergencies a splint can be made from any material—a piece of wood or a tree branch—or an injured limb can be splinted to another part of the body by binding (for example, the legs can be bound together or an arm can be bound across the chest). Inflatable splints, which fit like a glove over an injured limb and stiffen when inflated—are a relatively recent invention of great benefit to emergency services. Specialized splints (such as supports for the legs, back braces, or cervical collars) are "tailor-made," frequently from steel or inflexible plastic. Internal splints for fractures and deformities are achieved by the use of metal plates and screws, or rods and nails; this method is used where external splintage would be unsatisfactory.

spondylosis

A degenerative spinal disorder that leads to narrowing of the spinal canal. It can occur in the neck or lower back area and leads to pressure on the spinal nerves or spinal cord.

Initially the cause can be trauma whose effects are felt only in middle life or old age, producing symptoms chiefly in those between the ages of 50 and 60. Degeneration of the nucleus of the intervertebral disk and the surrounding fibrous tissue leads to a reaction of the adjacent areas of vertebrae (see SPINE). Variable calcified outgrowths from a vertebra may then protrude to press on the spinal cord or occlude a spinal nerve's exit from the cord and so cause considerable neurological discomfort. This slow progression of disk degeneration followed by bony overgrowth of the vertebrae may take place over many years and be the result of former sporting injuries, whiplash, or trauma.

Commonly pain is the initial symptom, with some loss of comfortable spinal movement. Muscle weakness may occur in the specific areas supplied by the spinal nerves and, where spinal cord compression occurs, sensory deprivation over wide areas of the body (below the affected level) is experienced.

Diagnosis is by X-ray examination of the spine and by myelography. Treatment consists primarily of rest by immobilization of the affected area of the spine in a plaster or plastic jacket or collar. Surgery to relieve compression may be necessary in cases where pain or paralysis is severe.

CERVICAL SPONDYLOSIS

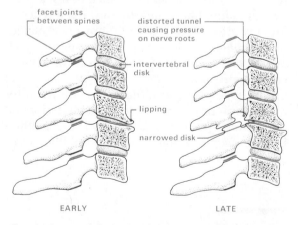

Cervical spondylosis is simply osteoarthrosis of the spine in the neck: As the intevertebral disk deteriorates, the neighboring vertebrae come together. Spurs of bone grow and encroach into the spinal canal and nerve tunnels. The condition results from years of wear and tear on the spine.

sporotrichosis

A fungus infection that may gain entry to the body through inhalation, ingestion, or inoculation from a contaminated environment. The fungus, *Sporothrix schenckii*, exists in soil, peat moss, and decaying vegetation, and the disease is contracted mainly by laborers, farmers, and florists. Outbreaks commonly occur in Mexico and Florida.

Pustules on the exposed skin enlarge and lead to involvement of the lymph nodes, which themselves may ulcerate. Internal absorption of the organism produces the same lymph-node response, and the disease, if untreated, may be fatal.

Diagnosis is made by blood tests and culture of the organism from the gland or pustule. Treatment is usually effective with antifungal medication, which may need to be continued for several weeks.

sprain

The incomplete tear of a ligament. Sprains are not serious injuries, but it is important to distinguish between sprains and complete disruption of a ligament, which may lead to subsequent instability of the affected joint. Complete tears are recognized by abnormal mobility of the joint, and the diagnosis may rest on radiological (X-ray) appearances.

The ligaments of the knee and ankle are most commonly sprained (the ankles more often than the knee), although it is not uncommon for the wrist to be sprained in a fall. The injury is often very painful and is accompanied by considerable swelling and bruising. Movement is painful.

At first the joint will probably be more comfortable if it is bandaged to limit movement and help keep the swelling down, but as soon as possible the joint should be moved and used.

stammering/stuttering

A disturbance in which speech is abruptly interrupted or certain sounds or syllables are rapidly repeated.

It is much more common in men than in women and is said to be more common in left-handed or ambidextrous persons as well as in those who have attempted to become ambidextrous though originally left-handed. It occurs in up to 1 percent of schoolchildren, usually before the age of 10, and tends to run in families.

Whether speech is disturbed by repetition of sounds or syllables, or is interrupted completely because the person "cannot get the word out," a degree of shame or embarrassment is usually present. Persons may thus often appear to have psychological problems or to be shy or withdrawn; but these features may be the *result* of the condition rather than its *cause*. Most persons who stammer or stutter do not have an underlying psychological disturbance.

Treatment involves speech training, the restoration of confidence, and the overcoming of any psychological problems that may have arisen as a result of the disorder. A skilled speech therapist (or speech pathologist) will employ relaxation exercises, breathing exercises, and carefully controlled speech exercises. A slow, syllable-by-syllable type of speech may be cultivated and confidence restored by singing or shouting words that are difficult to speak. Stressful situations are avoided until confidence returns. Tranquilizing or sedative drugs may be helpful. The enthusiastic encouragement of therapist and family plays an essential role.

Prognosis is good with proper treatment. The less the person is disturbed by his speech problem, the better the outcome. Only 1 adult in 300 stammers.

starvation

A condition caused by lack of proper food over a long period of time and marked by numerous disorders of the body and metabolism. In acute starvation the person's intake of calories falls seriously below his normal energy requirements. Loss of body weight occurs first from loss of fat and then muscle protein.

When the last reserves of fat have been mobilized, the patient's condition deteriorates rapidly, since only essential protein-containing tissues can now be drawn on for energy supplies.

There may be swelling of the tissues as the result of an accumulation of fluid, especially in the legs and feet. Lethargy, weakness, lowered blood pressure, and death soon follow.

See also ANOREXIA NERVOSA.

steatorrhea

Greater than normal amounts of fat in the feces, marked by the frothy, foul-smelling fecal matter that floats in water.

stenosis

The abnormal narrowing or constriction of a hollow passage or orifice (the entrance to a cavity or tube). For example, *mitral stenosis* is a narrowing of the mitral valve in the heart.

stethoscope

The common instrument used by medical personnel to listen to the sounds made by a person's heart or lungs (*auscultation*). It can also be used to listen to sounds produced in blood vessels in the neck and limbs and to sounds produced by the movements of the intestines during digestion. Together with a SPHYGMOMANOMETER, it is an essential piece of equipment for taking the blood pressure.

The general shape of the stethoscope will be familiar. The chest piece, which is applied to the patient's chest wall, may be one of two types: either

STETHOSCOPE

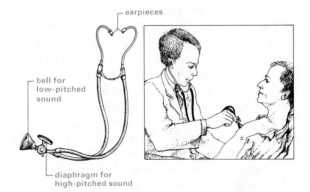

earpieces

bell for low-pitched sound

diaphragm for high-pitched sound

The stethoscope is a very simple instrument that has been in use for many years but still retains an important place as a diagnostic tool in modern medicine. Doctors use it to listen to sounds from the heart, lungs, and elsewhere.

bell-shaped and open, or flat and covered with a plastic or metal diaphragm (Bowles type). The chest piece is attached to a Y-shaped connector that transmits the sounds to the earpieces by means of two lengths of thick-walled rubber tubing.

Modern variants include electronic detection and amplification of the sounds.

stings

Two major groups of stinging creatures exist: (1) fish and other types of marine life, and (2) the venomous or biting arthropods (a group of animals without backbones consisting of more than 700,000 species, including the insects, spiders, and crustaceans).

Among the marine group are the venomous fish that carry poisonous spines. These include the stonefish, scorpion fish, lion fish, and the weever fish. They all inhabit shallow waters and lie concealed in sand or among rocks. Swimmers and skin divers may be stung by them, and fishermen may be injured while removing them from nets and lines. Pain from their stings may be very severe, body-wide symptoms may occur, and death in some cases results. In the case of the stingrays, the fish carries the sting in its tail and drives it into the victim when disturbed.

Jellyfish can cause painful stings and both the Portuguese man-of-war group and the true jellyfish may produce severe pain, extensive rashes, or even death. Contact with them occurs accidentally among swimmers and skin divers.

The stinging insects include the many varieties of wasps and bees. The effect of stings from bees and wasps depends on the person's sensitivity. Lethal reactions are rare but do occur. Often a person who is allergic to the insect's sting will develop difficulty in breathing, hives, and/or facial or body swelling. (See ANAPHYLACTIC SHOCK.) In the case of the potentially dangerous scorpion sting, the mortality rate may be as high as 5 percent.

Two spiders whose bite can produce serious symptoms are the black widow spider and the brown recluse spider. The black widow is identified by a red hourglass marking on its black, shiny abdomen. It is found largely in undisturbed woods and old buildings. Its bite may go unnoticed until the start of symptoms, which occur anywhere from ten to sixty minutes after the bite. Symptoms include severe pain at the site of the bite, headache, nausea, vomiting, and muscle spasms. Anyone bitten by a black widow spider should seek immediate treatment.

The brown recluse spider is found under rocks and woodpiles as well as in clothes piles, closets, and attics. It can be recognized by the dark violin-shaped area on its back. Like that of the black widow, the bite of the brown recluse spider may not be noticed at first. Pain at the site begins one to four hours later, followed by a hemorrhagic blister. A physician should be consulted if bitten.

Bee stings may be treated by removing the venom sac, washing the area, and applying cool compresses. Prompt medical treatment must be sought in serious life-threatening cases. Medications can be given to prevent body-wide systemic collapse. For those who are highly sensitive and who know they will be in a situation that may put them at risk for a sting, there are prescription medications that a person can carry and administer to himself until he can get to a hospital for more complete care.

stoma

A small opening, pore, or mouth; an opening created artificially between two body cavities or passages and the surface of the body (such as the surgical opening created by a COLOSTOMY).

stomach

A digestive organ that lies centrally in the upper part of the abdomen, to which food passes immediately after it has been chewed and swallowed. Food enters the stomach at the *cardiac sphincter*, a valve-like ring of muscle at the lower end of the esophagus ("gullet"), and leaves it by the *pylorus* (a similar structure at the lower end of the stomach) to pass to the duodenum and small intestine.

The stomach has a thick muscular coat and can contract to force food through the pylorus or, in vomiting, up through the esophagus. It is lined by a mucus-secreting membrane (the *gastric mucosa*), which is also responsible for the digestive secretions produced by the organ.

As its contribution to the digestive process, the stomach produces *hydrochloric acid* and an enzyme, *pepsin*, both of which break down protein. The food, already broken up and partially digested by chewing and mixture with saliva, mixes with the acid and pepsin in the stomach and protein digestion begins—although no major ab-

STOMACH

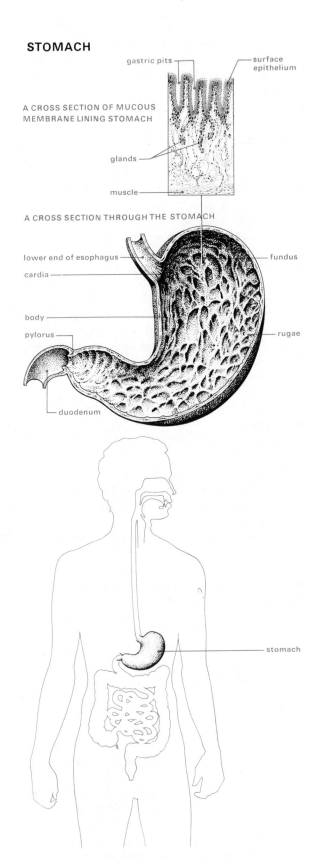

gastric pits — surface epithelium

A CROSS SECTION OF MUCOUS
MEMBRANE LINING STOMACH

glands

muscle

A CROSS SECTION THROUGH THE STOMACH

lower end of esophagus — fundus

cardia

body

pylorus — rugae

duodenum

stomach

The stomach acts as both a reservoir for food and a site for its digestion. The inner surface of an empty stomach is marked by prominent folds (rugae) that flatten as the stomach expands after a meal. When seen under a microscope, the surface is marked by numerous small openings—the gastric pits. Digestive juices well up from these pits when the stomach is stimulated by food.

sorption occurs in the stomach. Contractions of the stomach wall, while the pylorus remains closed, mix the food thoroughly with the digestive juices. When digestion with pepsin is completed, the pylorus opens and allows the food to pass on into the duodenum—where it meets other digestive juices from the liver and pancreas.

Another very important secretion produced by the stomach wall is known as *intrinsic factor.* This substance is required for the normal absorption of vitamin B_{12} from the diet. In "pernicious anemia," thinning and degeneration of the mucosa occur with loss of intrinsic factor secretion, failure of vitamin B_{12} absorption, and the development of a characteristic type of ANEMIA as the result of lack of the vitamin.

stomatitis

Inflammation of the lining membrane of the mouth (*oral mucosa*). It often involves the tongue as well, and the victim complains of a sore mouth.

Many conditions can produce a sore and inflamed mouth. Scalding by hot fluids, smoke from pipes or cigars, irritation from "hot" or spicy foods, and damage from jagged teeth or ill-fitting dentures can all cause stomatitis.

Local infections that produce a sore mouth include CANDIDIASIS ("thrush") and infections with bacteria known as "Vincent's organisms" (see VINCENT'S ANGINA). Some virus infections—including HERPES SIMPLEX ("cold sores"), CHICKEN POX, and MEASLES—may involve the mouth. Prolonged antibiotic therapy, by altering the balance of normal bacteria that inhabit the mouth, also can produce stomatitis.

Certain vitamin deficiencies cause stomatitis. A prolonged lack of riboflavin and niacin (in the vitamin-B group) produces a characteristic clinical picture (a purplish tongue, or a creased and scalloped tongue, respectively); SCURVY, the result of a lack of vitamin C, can produce swelling and hemorrhage in the gums. Vitamin-B_{12} deficiency in "pernicious anemia" is accompanied by a sore mouth and tongue, which is also the case in persons with folic acid deficiency and iron-deficiency anemia.

Other blood disorders—including LEUKEMIA, AGRANULOCYTOSIS (loss of circulating white blood cells, sometimes as a side effect of drug therapy), and "aplastic anemia" (failure of the bone marrow to produce all blood cells)—may be accompanied by severe stomatitis, often with ulceration of the oral mucosa. A condition of unknown cause is *aphthous ulceration* (or *aphthous stomatitis*), in which recurrent crops of small ulcers ("canker sores") appear spontaneously on the oral mucosa.

Treatment of stomatitis is directed toward the underlying cause. Milder cases clear up spontaneously with antiseptic mouth washes or good dental hygiene, and aphthous ulcers usually disappear spontaneously within a few days. Conditions caused by vitamin deficiencies will respond to appropriate supplementation.

strabismus

An abnormal condition in which one or the other eye diverges from the direction in which the gaze is directed; also called "squint."

In strabismus a tendency exists for one eye to become the "master eye," and when the person looks at an object, it is fixed by the master eye while the other is seen to be directed in a slightly different direction. Squints may thus be *divergent* if the squinting eye looks away from the line of the master eye ("walleye"), or *convergent* if it looks toward the line of the master eye ("cross-eye").

Squints may be divided also into the *concomitant* squints (commonly seen in childhood), in which an imbalance exists in the strengths of the paired muscles that move the eyeball, and the rarer *paralytic* squints, in which there is a complete or partial paralysis of one or more muscles in the affected eye.

The appearance of a squint may lead the person to seek medical advice; double vision may occur, especially in paralytic squint. Squint in young children is an important condition, since the brain suppresses the image seen by the squinting eye; if correction of the squint is delayed the eye may become functionally blind (AMBLYOPIA). In such circumstances the child will never develop binocular vision.

Treatment of concomitant squint is by correcting any causal refractive error with glasses, patching the normal eye to force the use of squinting eye and reverse amblyopia, and, if necessary, correcting residual deviation by surgical adjustment of the eye muscle balance. Treatment must be started early and, in such cases, excellent results are usually obtained.

stridor

An abnormal, high-pitched harsh rattling or musical breathing sound made while awake or during sleep. Stridor is caused by partial obstruction and usually occurs when breathing in. It may be due to a swelling in the throat, an inhaled foreign body, or a tumor. In the infant and young child, simple infection can produce the type of stridor commonly known as CROUP.

If the obstruction is severe and cannot otherwise be relieved rapidly, a temporary opening (TRACHEOSTOMY) must be made into the windpipe below the obstruction to provide an artificial airway.

See also *Tracheostomy* under **Procedures**.

stroke

The common name for a sudden paralysis or loss of sensation resulting from a blockage in or bleeding from one of the arteries supplying the brain (CEREBRAL HEMORRHAGE).

Sometimes there is warning of threatened stroke—an episode that lasts only a few minutes, or less than twenty-four hours, with complete recovery (a "transient ischemic attack"). At the other extreme there may be sudden loss of consciousness progressing to death within a few hours. More typically, the onset of symptoms takes a few minutes, with gradual loss of power and feeling in an arm or leg.

The most common form of stroke is caused by a clot (THROMBOSIS) in one of the main blood vessels of the brain (the middle cerebral artery). The resultant partial or total paralysis affects the arm and leg (HEMIPLEGIA) on the opposite side of the body and the facial muscles on the same side. If the right side is affected there may be loss of speech (*aphasia*) as an added disability. Other equally distinctive stroke syndromes, due to thrombosis in different arteries, may affect balance, vision, sensation, memory, or any other brain function. Loss of muscular control may occur without any effect on mental alertness or intelligence, and a stroke patient who has difficulty

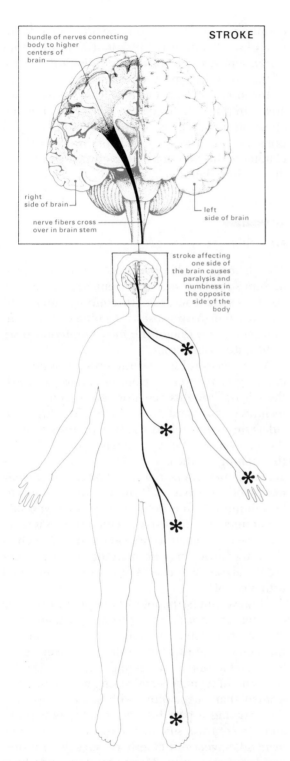

A stroke results from damage to brain cells, following a prolonged interruption to their blood supply. Each artery in the brain is responsible for nourishing a particular territory and the severity of a stroke depends on which vessel is involved. The general arrangement of nerve fibers means that when the right side of the brain is damaged, symptoms of paralysis and numbness affect the left side of the body and vice versa.

in speaking may retain normal understanding.

There is no specific curative treatment for the common forms of stroke, but physical therapy can be very helpful in speeding the recovery of muscle power and control. More specific help may be needed with walking, speech, and the relearning of day-to-day tasks.

Stroke is caused by the arterial disease, ATHEROSCLEROSIS, by the rupture of cerebral ANEURYSMS, and by raised BLOOD PRESSURE (hypertension). Predisposing factors are DIABETES MELLITUS and any condition that makes thrombosis or EMBOLISM more likely (including use of oral contraceptives and POLYCYTHEMIA). The best prospects of reducing the ill-health due to stroke lies in the detection and treatment of the conditions that increase the risk.

sty (hordeolum)

A common type of inflammation of the eyelid, often the upper lid.

Each eyelash follicle is accompanied by a sebaceous gland, which secretes an oily material (*sebum*) that keeps the skin of the lids soft and pliable. Infection (usually with staphylococcal bacteria) starts in a sebaceous gland and spreads to the follicle of the eyelash. Swelling and redness are evident and considerable pain is felt at the margin of the lid. The infection may "come to a head" with a spontaneous discharge of pus.

Special treatment is not often required. If the condition is severe, however, treatment may include removal of the affected eyelash, the local application of medicated ointment, and warm compresses to the eye. Administration of antibiotics rarely is required.

STY

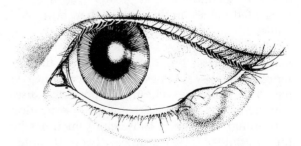

A sty is a bacterial abscess in the follicle of an eyelash. It appears as localized red swelling on the upper or lower lid. The main symptom is pain, which can be helped by warm compresses.

In recurrent cases, a local source of infection (such as boils on the neck or face) should be sought. Inadequate personal hygiene may predispose to infection, and certain diseases such as DIABETES MELLITUS—in which there is a special susceptibility to infection—must be ruled out.

sudden infant death syndrome (SIDS)

This is the most common mode of death for infants between one month and one year of age and accounts for 30 percent of all deaths in this age group. In spite of agonized public concern and intensive study, the causes remain unknown, and the incidence of this tragic event has not declined. In the United States, 3 babies in every 2,000 die in this way.

Sudden infant death syndrome, also known as crib death, is defined as an unexpected death in which a thorough autopsy fails to reveal a cause. Until recent times, all such deaths were attributed to "overlying" by the mother, and it is clear that, throughout the ages, countless women have been unjustly accused of bringing about, either accidentally or intentionally, the deaths of their infants. But in the past 20 years this attitude has changed, for it has been conclusively proved that sudden death commonly occurs in a baby sleeping alone. Overlying is now rarely proposed as a cause of SIDS.

The tragedy is more likely to affect a boy baby than a girl and is more likely to occur in winter than in summer. Prematurely born babies are at greater risk than the full-term. Black babies are more likely to be affected than white and SIDS affects poorer families more often than the better off. Those babies whose mothers smoke during pregnancy and whose parents are narcotic addicted or alcoholic are at greater risk of SIDS. Breast-fed babies are less at risk than bottle-fed babies.

Many studies of cases have been published and many hypotheses proposed. Because of the absence of autopsy findings, the diagnosis of SIDS has to be made by excluding all possible causes and there are suggestions that if the investigation is thorough enough, a cause can sometimes be found. Some of these deaths have been attributed to over-soft bedding, in which the baby's face becomes buried; some to hypersensitivity to cow's milk; some to unnoticed chest or gastrointestinal infections; and some to biotin deficiency. But, by definition, these cases are not SIDS. The current view of some authorities is that SIDS results from a transient disorder of the neurological control of the breathing and the heartbeat.

In most cases death occurs during sleep without any suffering on the part of the child, but the effect on the family is devastating and close support is needed. Help is available from the local chapter of the National Sudden Infant Death Syndrome Foundation.

suicide

The deliberate taking of one's own life, which accounts for less than 1 percent of all deaths in most Western countries. In contrast, attempted suicide from an overdose of sleeping pills or tranquilizers is now one of the most common causes of hospital admission.

Most successful suicide attempts are by persons entering or recovering from DEPRESSION, in which the suicide thoughts were dominated by irrational feelings of guilt and unworthiness. The high suicide rate in severely depressed persons justifies the opinion that the condition is a potentially life-threatening medical emergency warranting urgent treatment. Persons who refuse treatment may need close supervision if the risk of suicide is to be minimized. The belief that people who talk about suicide do not carry out their threats is false. Men are more likely to use violent means such as shooting, drowning, or hanging; women commonly take an overdose of drugs, often combined with alcohol.

However, most people who take an overdose of drugs are not suffering from depression and have no real determination to die. These nonlethal suicidal gestures are a means of seeking attention at a time of emotional conflict. It is most common in teenagers and young adults, more in women than men, often with some personality disorder and a past history of behavioral problems. In contrast, suicide occurs more commonly in middle-aged and elderly persons, with a preponderance of men. Many countries now have organizations that offer a twenty-four-hour telephone counseling service for anyone contemplating suicide; many individual communities have "crisis lines" for the same purpose.

Anyone found having recently taken an overdose of pills should be taken to a hospital emergency room; loss of consciousness may develop quite suddenly in such circumstances, and immediate treatment may be needed.

sunburn

A reaction of susceptible skin to exposure to the ultraviolet rays of the sun. Sunburn can range from slight redness and tenderness to severe blistering. It is common among swimmers, skiers, and outdoor workers (if unprotected).

Blond-haired persons are more susceptible than brunettes. The effect of exposure to sunlight is greatest when the sun is high in the sky (between 10 A.M. and 2 P.M.) and in midsummer. Reflection increases the effect: Snow, water, and sand reflect many of the burning wavelengths of sunlight. Scattered rays also may produce sunburn, even in the presence of haze or thin fog.

The symptoms of simple sunburn need no description; when sunburn is severe, however, there may be a marked constitutional disturbance with nausea, chills, and fever, and the symptoms may be mixed with those of HEAT STROKE and heat exhaustion. Sunburn also may bring on or aggravate other conditions, notably cold sores on the lips and a variety of skin disorders. However, ACNE and some other skin conditions may actually be improved by cautious exposure to the ultraviolet rays of the sun.

Treatment usually is limited to the application of cold compresses to the skin and administration of emollient lotions to counteract dryness and pain-killing drugs to relieve the discomfort. In severe cases medical advice should be sought and admission to the hospital may even be necessary if the person becomes ill.

Prevention is by avoidance of exposure to the sun when it is directly overhead. "Sunscreen" and "sun-blocking" lotions and creams are available which provide varying degrees of protection by interfering with the ultraviolet rays responsible for sunburn.

Certain medications may make persons more sun-sensitive, causing them to become sunburned with relatively little sun exposure. Also, persons with melanin deficiency, the tan-forming pigment of the skin, can be severely sunburned with very little exposure.

Repeated exposure to ultraviolet light increases the risks of BASAL CELL CARCINOMA, malignant MELANOMA, squamous EPITHELIOMA, chronic eye irritation, pterygium, wrinkling of the skin in old age, and other complications.

For an extended discussion see also *What Is Cancer* in the section on **Wellness**.

syncope

FAINTING, a temporary loss of consciousness due to an inadequate flow of blood to the brain.

synovitis

Inflammation of the synovial membrane, a fine membrane that lines the inner surfaces of a joint.

Synovitis may be acute or chronic. Usually it occurs as a result of disease affecting the joint as a whole. Thus, *acute synovitis* occurs in cases of bacterial or viral infection of the joints, after injuries, and in conditions such as HEMOPHILIA in which hemorrhage into joints may occur. *Chronic synovitis* occurs in RHEUMATOID ARTHRITIS and OSTEOARTHRITIS and in infection of the joints by TUBERCULOSIS. The presence of loose fragments of bone or cartilage in a joint may cause acute or chronic synovitis; it occurs in a condition of torn cartilage in the knee.

Treatment depends on the cause. In synovitis associated with rheumatoid arthritis, for example, generalized treatment of the primary disease is required; in osteoarthritis, drugs are administered for the relief of pain. In both these conditions, surgical treatment of the joint (including joint-replacement) may be necessary. Infections are controlled by administering antibiotics. Loose fragments of bone or a torn cartilage in the knee will require surgical exploration of the joint.

syphilis

The most serious of the sexually transmitted (venereal) diseases, which may prove fatal if not treated. It is caused by infection with the spirochete bacterium *Treponema pallidum*; the disease is transmitted only by sexual contact or (very rarely) by the transfusion of contaminated blood.

The first sign of syphilis, which appears after a silent incubation period of two to six weeks, is the *chancre*—a hard, painless ulcer on the penis, the female genitalia, or (less frequently) on the lips, tongue, or finger. There is some swelling of the lymph nodes nearest to the chancre, which subsides slowly in about one month. As the chancre heals, however, syphilis moves into its "secondary stage" with fever, a generalized rash (usually consisting of pale red spots), a sore throat, and swelling of lymph nodes throughout the body. Occasionally the infection may inflame the brain coverings (MENINGITIS), the membranes that surround the bones (*periostitis*), and the iris of the eyes (IRITIS). Even without treatment this stage will resolve after some weeks, leaving the individual apparently cured; but months or years later "tertiary" syphilis lesions will appear. These may damage the heart valves or weaken the main blood vessels, causing stretching, swelling (ANEURYSM), and eventually rupture of an artery. The brain and spinal cord may be affected, marked by mild to severe personality changes, PSYCHOSES, and loss of muscular coordination. Indeed, tertiary syphilis may involve any organ and mimic virtually any other chronic disease.

Syphilis can be cured by a full course of treatment with penicillin. Inadequate treatment may only suppress the symptoms, however, and careful medical follow-up is needed to ensure that the infection has been eliminated. Furthermore, although penicillin treatment will stop syphilis from progressing, it cannot repair the damage to the heart valves, nerves, or other organs caused by chronic infection.

An unnoticed syphilitic infection may be suppressed by a short course of antibiotics given as treatment for gonorrhea or any other venereal disease. However, tests on the blood will establish whether or not an individual has syphilis. Anyone who suspects he may have acquired a venereal disease should be examined and treated by an accredited clinic or specialist.

See also TABES DORSALIS, VENEREAL DISEASE.

systole

The period when a chamber of the heart contracts and ejects blood. (DIASTOLE is the period when the heart muscle is relaxed and a chamber fills with blood.) During *atrial systole*, blood is pumped from the atria into the ventricles; this period corresponds to ventricular diastole. During *ventricular systole* the right ventricle pumps blood to the lungs where the blood becomes oxygenated, while the left ventricle pumps blood to the rest of the body.

The term "systolic blood pressure" refers to the pressure in the large arteries during ventricular systole. *Asystole* means cardiac standstill or absence of a heartbeat. If it lasts more than four minutes, deterioration of brain cells begins.

tabes dorsalis

A form of tertiary SYPHILIS, affecting men more frequently than women, which appears some years (five to thirty) after the primary infection. It is now very rare.

Degeneration occurs in the sensory nerves, which originate in the spinal cord, producing impairment of sensation of temperature and pain and loss of tendon reflexes. Episodes of sudden, severe pain may develop in the arms or legs for no apparent reason. Loss of the ability to feel pain and temperature occurs on the underside of the forearm and arm and spreads over the chest. The abdomen is usually normal, but there is loss of sensation in the legs.

The victim cannot tell where his legs are when his eyes are closed, and he has to keep his eyes open in order to maintain his balance. He develops a characteristic gait with the feet wide apart, and because he has lost sensation in the soles of his feet he picks them up high when he walks and stamps them down. The same loss of sensation leads to damage of the joints and painless ulcers on the soles of the feet. Sensation from the bladder may be lost, so that the person suffers from painless retention of urine, and he may be constipated. In some cases there are attacks of acute abdominal pain, with vomiting, which may mimic an acute abdominal emergency.

The difficulty in walking gives the disease its alternative name, *locomotor ataxia*.

tachycardia

A marked increase in the rate of the heartbeat, which can be either sudden or gradual in onset. It may arise from some malfunction of the heart, from the action of a drug, from exercise, or from excitement or anger.

Tachycardia is considered to be a heart rate of above 100 beats per minute.

taeniasis

Infestation of the body with TAPEWORMS.

tapeworms

Intestinal PARASITES found in virtually every animal

TAPEWORM   *Taenia solium*

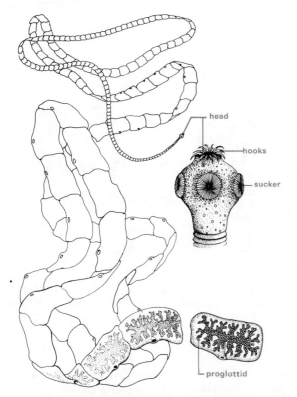

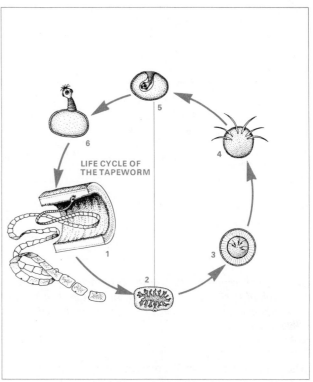

LIFE CYCLE OF THE TAPEWORM

The adult form of Taenia solium, *the pork tapeworm, is found only in the gut of human beings, where it may reach a length of 13 feet (4 meters); it attaches itself by the hooks on its head (1). Segments full of eggs (2) are excreted in the feces, and embryos in the soil (3) are eaten by pigs. Oncospheres with six hooks (4) pass into the pig's bloodstream and become encysted larvae (5), which reproduce in the pig and develop into adult worms (6) after the human host has eaten infected pork that has not been cooked properly.*

species. The two common human tapeworms are acquired from infected pork and beef; a third variety is found in societies that eat infected raw fish. Humans may be parasitized also by the larval forms of tapeworms, including some that affect other animals such as dogs (see FLEAS). Infestation of the body with tapeworms is known as TAENIASIS.

Infection with pork tapeworm *Taenia solium* is acquired by eating undercooked pork, when one or more of the tiny cysticerci (the encysted larval forms of the tapeworm) become attached to the small intestine and develop into adult tapeworms which may attain a length of up to 13 feet (4 meters). A single worm causes few symptoms, but a multiple infestation may cause some loss of weight. For the whole of its thirty-year life span the worm throws off segments packed with eggs that are excreted with the feces. These eggs are infectious for pigs—and for humans. If they are swallowed and partially digested in the stomach, the eggs develop into *oncospheres* (the embryonic

stage in which six hooks exist on the head, or "scolex," of the tapeworm); these penetrate the host's intestinal wall and pass into the bloodstream to form cysts in the muscles, brain, and other organs. This condition (known as *cysticercosis*) is by far the most dangerous aspect of tapeworm disease, for the cysts in the brain frequently cause EPILEPSY.

The beef tapeworm, *Taenia saginata*, is common in countries where beef is eaten raw. Despite its length—16 to 20 feet (5 to 6 meters) or longer—it rarely causes serious symptoms and the eggs are rarely infectious for humans.

Both beef and pork tapeworms shed proglottids, which are white egg–containing segments of the worm's body. They are excreted from the anus and may be found in bedclothes.

The fish tapeworm, *Diphyllobothrium latum*, is the longest human tapeworm, reaching a length of up to 60 feet (18 meters), although the average length is approximately 20 feet (6 meters). Unlike

TASTE

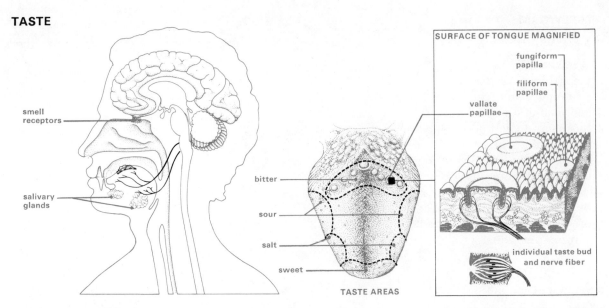

The tongue is covered with thousands of taste buds (tiny onion-shaped receptors containing special nerve endings) that respond to substances dissolved in saliva. The buds are found in the fungiform and vallate papillae. All the subtle flavors we distinguish are different combinations of the four basic tastes—sweet, salt, sour, and bitter—with the sense of smell.

other tapeworms, its presence may lead to serious malnutrition, since the worm competes with its host for vitamin B_{12}; persons infected with the parasites may become profoundly anemic.

Tapeworms may be ejected from the intestines by treatment with special drugs. The only treatment for cysticercosis is the surgical removal of any cysts causing symptoms.

taste

The sense of perceiving different flavors that contact the tongue and send nerve impulses to special taste centers in the brain. Taste sensation is divided into four categories: sweet, sour, salty, and bitter.

The sensation of taste is produced by tiny taste buds on the surface of the tongue and palate in response to the chemical nature of various substances. Each bud is oval or round and consists of a large number of spindle-shaped cells. Although they appear identical, certain buds (distributed on the tongue in groups) are particularly sensitive to specific tastes. The taste buds at the tip are particularly sensitive to sweet substances, those on the edges to sour (acid) and salt, and those on the back of the tongue to bitter substances. At the same time, there is evidence that all taste buds are sensitive in some degree to all

four sensations. Taste sensitivity also has an intimate connection with the sense of smell.

Loss or reduction of the ability to taste may be brought about by smoking or the common cold.

tattooing

A method of obtaining a permanent mark or design on the skin by puncturing and the introduction of color. It is of ancient origin and is found worldwide. Various methods are used to produce tattooing, the most common being with needles and pigment, though special knives also are used.

Tattooing has become increasingly popular in the Western world, despite its permanence. It is not a benign procedure, and when done by unskilled persons it can lead to severe infection. HEPATITIS and AIDS can result from use of unsanitary instruments. Tattoos have been implicated also in some kinds of skin cancer.

It is extremely difficult, and in some cases impossible, to remove a tattoo. Depending on the depth of the pigmentation, dermabrasion may be able to remove some of the coloring. A drastic method would be to remove the entire skin section and graft on new skin, but this is not an ordinary procedure.

Tay-Sachs disease

A rare metabolic disorder, most often found in Ashkenazi Jews, that starts at about the age of 6 months and affects the nervous system. Victims of the disease, which is inherited, show retarded physical and mental development and blindness by the age of about 18 months to 3 years.

About one in 30 Ashkenazi Jews carries the gene that determines the disease, which is a disorder of fat metabolism. Those who feel they may carry the gene should be screened for the trait before starting a family; the gene can be identified by chromosome tests.

telangiectasia

Small vascular malformations consisting of a group of dilated blood vessels (usually capillaries). They are seen in the body as reddish patches of skin and are most common on the thighs and face. The spots sometimes are present as birthmarks or may appear in young children.

There is also a form known as *hereditary hemorrhagic telangiectasia*, where small areas of bleeding occur on the skin, in the mouth and nose, and internally. This bleeding is due to the fragility of the blood vessels. It affects both men and women.

temperature

In humans the temperature of the body remains almost constant despite the temperature of the surrounding environment. Human beings have a normal body temperature of about 98.6°F (37°C).

If the body becomes overheated (for example, by exercise), the blood vessels of the skin dilate and sweat is produced. The sweat evaporates on the skin, producing a cooling effect that results in a lowering of the body temperature back to normal. When the surrounding atmosphere is very cold, the body conserves body heat by contracting the smaller blood vessels, especially those near the body surface. In old people and infants the body is less efficient in maintaining a constant temperature, and both HEAT STROKE and extreme loss of heat (HYPOTHERMIA) are more common in those age groups. Hypothermia is especially dangerous in the elderly since its onset may be slow; an old person living in an unheated house in the

TEMPERATURE

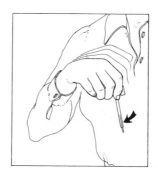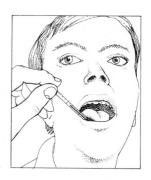

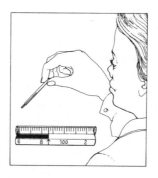

To take a patient's temperature, the mercury must first be shaken down. The thermometer is then placed under the tongue for 3 minutes with the mouth closed. Remember that hot or cold drinks consumed beforehand will cause false readings.

winter may lose heat over several days and eventually pass into a fatal coma.

In disease the temperature of the human body may vary from about 90°F (32.2°C) to 110°F (43.3°C) for a time, but there is danger to life should it drop and remain below 95°F (35°C) or rise and remain at or above 106°F (41°C). Unconsciousness typically occurs when the temperature of the body drops below about 80°F (26.6 °C). Prolonged high fever (*hyperpyrexia*) can cause irreversible damage to the brain.

The Fahrenheit scale normally is used in the United States; in Europe the Centigrade (or Celsius) scale is preferred.

temporomandibular joint syndrome (TM syndrome)

The temporomandibular joint, which lies just in front of the ear, is the hinge joint between the jawbone (*mandible*) and the temporal bone of the skull. The most common disorder of this joint is the TM syndrome in which there is complaint of a dull aching pain on one side, just in front of the ear, spreading to the temple, the angle of the jaw, and even to the back of the head. Sometimes the pain is associated with a clicking or popping noise heard, or felt, in the region of the joint.

In a small proportion of cases, temporomandibular joint syndrome is caused by actual arthritic changes in the joint, but in the great majority it is due to a habit of tooth grinding or clenching of the jaw in response to stress. Occasionally it may due to poorly aligned teeth or badly fitting dentures. The condition is more common in women than in men. When the pain is present on waking in the morning, it results from tooth grinding during sleep (*bruxism*).

The treatment of this condition is directed at the cause. Stress factors must be investigated, understood, and, if possible, eliminated. Psychological help may be needed. It is important that physical responses of this kind be recognized as clear signs of stress, similar to the muscle contraction that causes most headaches. Often the cause of the stress is obvious and sometimes it can be removed. But even if it cannot, a deliberate effort at relaxation and the abandonment of the habit of responding in this way may be helpful in reducing the significance of the stressor.

In some cases muscle relaxants and tranquilizers may be necessary.

tenesmus

Constant ineffectual spasms of the rectum along with the desire to empty it. Usually nothing is passed except mucus (sometimes mixed with blood). The condition is spasmodic and extremely distressing. It is likely to be encountered in such disorders of the large intestine as ULCERATIVE COLITIS, DYSENTERY, HEMORRHOIDS, or tumor. It can occur when the lower bowel is packed with very hard feces or it may be provoked by fissure of the anus or by a growth. In young children tenesmus may be caused by the presence of worms in the bowel. A similar condition can affect the bladder.

Relief of tenesmus depends on treatment of the underlying condition.

tenosynovitis

Inflammation of a tendon sheath—in particular, one of the hand, wrist, or ankle.

Tendons are white, fibrous bands of varying lengths that connect muscle to bone. They are ry strong. Some tendons consists of round bun-

dles of fibers whereas others are flat. Most tendons are encased in a sheath similar to the synovial membrane that lines joint cavities; this ensures that the tendon glides smoothly over the adjoining bone when contracted.

Tenosynovitis may occur as the result of repeated injuries where frequent and rapid movements of the wrist or ankle are involved. Initial treatment consists of rest and the application of heat. Should this fail, local injections of cortisone may be of value. In extreme cases it may be necessary to operate on part of the synovial sheath.

teratogenesis

Giving birth to an abnormal, physically deformed fetus. This may be the result of a maternal infection during pregnancy, most often GERMAN MEASLES (rubella), or it may be caused by the action of certain drugs taken during pregnancy.

The drug thalidomide is the best-known example of a teratogenic drug. Prescribed in the late 1950s as a tranquilizer for pregnant women, it resulted in the birth of many children with serious physical defects.

testosterone

Testosterone is a male sex hormone responsible for the development of the sexual organs and for the growth and maintenance of the sexual characteristics of puberty. These secondary characteristics include the maturation of sex organs, development of body hair, and deepening of the voice.

Testosterone is produced in the testicles under a complicated feedback system involving the PITUITARY GLAND and HYPOTHALAMUS in the brain. Women also are able to produce testosterone, to a far lesser extent. When excess production occurs (for example, as a result of a pituitary tumor), a woman will develop symptoms of masculinization such as excess growth of body hair.

Medications containing testosterone are used for a variety of diseases, such as *hypogonadism*—the failure to develop secondary sexual characteristics. Testosterone is used sometimes also in the treatment of breast cancer that has spread to the bones. Although not a cure, it can limit the spread of cancer in the bone.

tetanus

An acute infectious disease of the nervous system (also known as *lockjaw*) characterized by spasms of the voluntary muscles and painful convulsions. The disease is caused by the bacillus *Clostridium tetani.*

Spores of the bacillus commonly are found in earth, especially when it is contaminated with manure from horses or cattle. These spores may survive in the earth undisturbed for many years and may enter the body when a wound is contaminated with soil. However, the bacteria cannot multiply in the body in the presence of oxygen, so they grow only in dirty wounds or in dead, bloodless tissues around a deep wound. Once multiplication begins, however, the bacilli produce toxins that destroy the tissue around them, providing ideal conditions for further bacterial growth. The toxins also enter the nerves, spreading up the nerve fibers to reach the spinal cord, where they cause generalized muscle spasms.

The first sign of tetanus is stiffness felt around the site of the wound followed by stiffness of the jaw muscles, irrespective of the location of the wound. The spasms gradually extend to the muscles of the neck and eventually affect the muscles of the chest, back, abdomen, and extremities. During such spasms the body may be drawn to the left or right, backward or forward, causing extreme pain and distress to the person, who remains conscious throughout. In the early stages such convulsions are intermittent, but they may be precipitated by any minor disturbance (such as the banging of a door or a sudden exposure to bright light). The person may die eventually from sheer exhaustion due to prolonged spasms.

The treatment of the illness consists of eliminating the infection by cleaning the wound and giving antibiotics, blocking the action of the toxin with specific antitoxins, and reducing the muscle spasms by means of sedatives. In severe cases the spasms may be abolished altogether by the administration of muscle-paralyzing drugs such as curare with artificial maintenance of respiration by a TRACHEOSTOMY (see under **Procedures**) and the use of a respirator. This form of treatment has cut the mortality rate of severe tetanus from about 90 percent to 10 percent.

Tetanus is one of the diseases (including polio and diphtheria) that is entirely preventable by immunization. Children receive lasting immunity against tetanus toxin when they receive the DPT vaccine (the "triple vaccine"), which is effective also against WHOOPING COUGH (pertussis) and DIPHTHERIA. Immunity should be boosted with another shot of tetanus toxoid as part of the treatment of any dirty wound. If these precautions are followed there is no need to fear tetanus.

tetany

A state characterized by spasms and twitching of muscles, particularly of the arms and hands. The elbows are bent and the fingers squeezed together. Sometimes the lower limbs and even the face are affected similarly. (This condition should not be confused with TETANUS.)

Tetany occurs due to a fall in the calcium content of blood and tissue fluids. It is most common in infants, where it may be associated with RICKETS, excessive vomiting, or certain disorders of the kidney. It occurs following accidental removal of the parathyroid glands during thyroid surgery and with vitamin-D deficiency. Tetany can occur also as the result of metabolic disturbances created by hyperventilation (one form of which is hysterical overbreathing).

Treatment involves the intravenous administration of calcium.

tetralogy of Fallot

One of the most common congenital multiple defects of the heart. About a fifth of all cases of *cyanotic congenital heart disease* ("blue babies") are in this category.

The four changes of the tetrology are: (1) transposition (displacement) of the aorta so that both ventricles empty into the aorta; (2) a narrowing of the pulmonary artery (which goes to the lungs); (3) a ventricular septal defect (HOLE IN THE HEART), which allows the blood that cannot get through the narrowed pulmonary artery to pass to the systemic circulation; and (4) enlargement of the right ventricle of the heart caused by the increased force required of the right ventricle.

These infants have a loud heart murmur and are often *cyanotic* (blue) from lack of oxygen in their red blood cells. If untreated, they will grow slowly, will develop swollen (clubbed) fingers, and be susceptible to attacks of bacterial ENDOCARDITIS and heart failure. However, surgery is widely and successfully used to improve the circulation through the pulmonary artery and to repair the heart defects, restoring the child to near-normal health.

thalassemia

A group of inherited disorders affecting the red blood cells and resulting in ANEMIA. The severity of thalassemia varies from mild to life-threatening. The disease is most common in people of Mediterranean origin.

In individuals with the mild form of the disease, diagnosis is generally made as the result of the evaluation of mild anemia.

There is no cure, and in those with the severe form of the disorder, frequent blood transfusions are necessary.

thirst

The instinctive craving for fluid. The sensation of thirst, felt as dryness of the throat and mouth, occurs when there is a deficiency of water in the body.

In the course of twenty-four hours the kidneys excrete about 2.5 pints (1.2 liters) of water, while the lungs and skin also lose considerable quantities through respiration and sweating. To make good this loss, fresh supplies of fluid are required, and thirst is the signal that this has become necessary. In particular, thirst arises from vigorous muscular exercise, owing to the loss of water by the secretion of sweat. Thirst also becomes intense when the body loses a considerable amount of fluid, as in hemorrhage or DIARRHEA.

Thirst is a common symptom in FEVER owing to increased body heat and sweating. The thirst that follows the intake of salt or sugar is an indication of the need to dilute these substances in the digestive tract and bloodstream.

See also DEHYDRATION.

thromboangiitis obliterans

A chronic and recurring vascular disease (also known as *Buerger's disease*) that affects the arteries and, to a lesser extent, the veins. A thickening appears in the inner lining of the affected blood vessel, and this progresses until the diameter of the vessel becomes severely reduced and finally bliterated (*obliterative endarteritis*). The disease v take months or years to reach this stage. The cause is unknown, but the disease definitely is worsened by smoking, is much more common in men than in women, and is seen more often in certain ethnic groups (young Jewish men are particularly susceptible).

A decrease in circulation leads to complaints about the limbs, particularly the legs; this is accompanied sometimes by reddened and painful areas over the veins. This decreased circulation often causes pain when walking. The pain characteristically occurs in the calf of the leg after the person has walked a certain distance, but disappears again rapidly on standing still (a condition known as INTERMITTENT CLAUDICATION). If the blood supply becomes seriously impaired, ulceration of the foot or leg and gangrene of the toes or foot may occur.

Treatment initially is conservative (nonsurgical). Tobacco in any form is forbidden since it aggravates the condition. In severe cases the development of better circulation through unaffected tributaries of the vessels may be encouraged by a sympathectomy, an operation that causes dilation of those vessels that remain unobstructed.

Prognosis for life is good, but amputation of toes, the foot, or even the lower leg is possible if gangrene occurs.

thrombocytopenia

A condition in which there is a deficiency of *thrombocytes* (also known as PLATELETS) in the blood, resulting in the failure of the blood to clot adequately so that hemorrhages occur into the skin and organs. This is one of the forms of PURPURA.

Platelets are minute, colorless particles existing in the blood in great numbers; one cubic millimeter of blood contains about a quarter of a million of them. When a blood vessel is damaged, the platelets fuse together at the site of the injury, effectively plugging the breach. Platelets also release the hormone *serotin*, which causes the blood vessels to contract, thus reducing blood flow.

Insufficiency of platelets can result either from their underproduction in the bone marrow or from the destruction of existing platelets. Certain diseases that inhibit the production of white blood cells also can stop the production of platelets. This can happen through RADIATION, diseases of the bone marrow, or LEUKEMIA. A deficiency may arise also through a massive transfusion of banked blood, since platelets do not remain viable in banked blood.

Underproduction of platelets may occur also on its own and not as the result of another disease. In such cases it is known as *idiopathic thrombocytopenia*. This is rare but is sometimes seen in children and premenopausal women.

Treatment, according to the type of thrombocytopenia involved, is either by drugs (prednisone), removal of the spleen, or by platelet transfusion. The last method is used only in extreme cases because of the danger of developing subsequent resistance to further treatment.

thromboembolism

The blockage of a blood vessel by a THROMBUS (clot) that has become detached from its site of origin so as to become an embolus.

See also EMBOLISM.

thrombophlebitis

Thrombosis (clotting) in veins is divided into two classes, depending on whether or not the wall of the affected vein is inflamed. If it is inflamed the condition is called *thrombophlebitis;* if it is not, the condition is known as *phlebothrombosis.*

In thrombophlebitis, clotting in the vein follows inflammation of the wall of the vein. The affected vessel is red, tender, painful, and hard. The clot sticks to the wall of the vein and there is little danger of it breaking away and producing an embolus. Infection of the vein may be a complication of varicose veins, may be secondary to THROMBOANGIITIS OBLITERANS, or may have no obvious cause. Damage to the walls of varicose veins may be done intentionally by the injection of sclerosing medications in an effort to eliminate the varicose veins.

Treatment of thrombophlebitis is initial rest, analgesics, and support stockings. After the initial resting period, the person should start walking to improve the flow of blood through the veins.

thrombophlebitis migrans

This is a condition in which symptoms of THROMBOPHLEBITIS occur in various parts of the body at different times. They may appear in the neck, abdomen, or pelvis as well as in the legs. Small

THROMBOPHLEBITIS

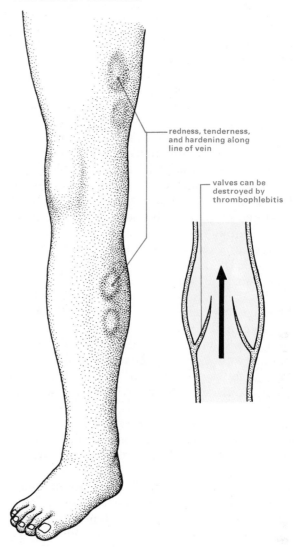

redness, tenderness, and hardening along line of vein

valves can be destroyed by thrombophlebitis

Thrombophlebitis (inflammation of a vein followed by blockage of the vein due to the formation of a blood clot) usually is marked by pain, heat, and redness along the course of the involved vein. The illustration shows this process in the long saphenous vein of the leg. The condition is dangerous only if it extends into the deep leg veins: A piece of blood clot that breaks loose here could travel up to the lungs.

red nodules, which are very tender to the touch, can be seen along the veins immediately under the skin.

This form of thrombophlebitis sometimes arises during the course of an infectious or malignant disease, but can occur also spontaneously for no apparent reason.

thrombus/thrombosis

A *thrombus* is a blood clot; *thrombosis* is the process of formation of a blood clot.

Normally, the inside walls of the blood vessels are smooth; although the blood clots readily when outside the vessels, it remains fluid in normal arteries and veins. If, however, the walls of the vessels are damaged by disease or injury, the blood will clot as it comes into contact with the damaged area. This clotting mechanism prevents blood loss in the case of injury, but in disease it can lead to the formation of blockages inside the vessels.

Moreover, parts of the clot may break off and travel through the circulation until they are trapped in a smaller vessel, blocking the passage of blood. This may occur close to the original clot formation or at a distant site. Pieces of clot that break off in this way are called *emboli*, and the blockage they cause when they become lodged in an artery is an *embolism*.

It is possible for arteries to be completely blocked without causing too much disturbance as long as the part of the body affected has a rich blood supply, since the needed blood can still find its way to the tissues by means of bypasses (collateral circulation). If, however, there is no alternative circulation, the tissues normally supplied by the blocked vessel will die. The area of tissue so affected is called an *infarct*, and the process is known as *infarction*. The effects of thrombosis are therefore more serious in some parts of the body than in others. Examples are: (1) the heart, where thrombosis of a coronary artery (CORONARY THROMBOSIS) may lead to the death of part of the heart muscle (*myocardial infarction*); and (2) the brain, where collateral circulation is poor and a *cerebral thrombosis* leads to loss of function which is manifested by paralysis or weakness of the side of the body opposite to the side of the brain that was damaged by the vascular blockage. Intellectual and sensory loss may also occur. (See STROKE.)

Arterial thrombosis is the end result of atherosclerotic disease of the vessels; but thrombosis of the venous system—commonly seen in the vessels of the lower limbs—may be caused by a number of conditions. Superficial thrombosis of the leg veins is not often of consequence, but thrombosis of the deep veins may be a dangerous condition since emboli may break off and become lodged in other parts of the body, notably the lungs.

Thrombosis of the deep veins occurs principally after childbirth and after surgical operations. It may occur also in women who take oral contraceptive pills and in elderly people who are confined to bed. If the development of deep-vein thrombosis is suspected, anticoagulants are used to minimize the risk of the blood clots breaking off and traveling through the circulatory system.

thrush

A fungal infection of the mouth or throat characterized by the formation of white patches and ulceration of the affected tissues. It is caused by infection with *Candida albicans*, and the condition is known technically as CANDIDIASIS.

thyroid gland

The thyroid is an endocrine, or ductless, gland situated in the neck. It has two lobes, one on each side of the larynx, joined by an isthmus. Two *parathyroid glands* lie in each lobe.

The thyroid gland affects the rate of body metabolism, the process by which energy is made available. This is done by the secretion into the blood of two HORMONES, *thyroxine* and *triiodothyronine*, which are produced from tyrosine and inorganic iodine. These hormones stimulate metabolism and increase the consumption of oxygen. They are also essential for normal development and growth.

Deficiency of thyroid hormone, brought about by failed gland development, disease, or surgical removal, results in HYPOTHYROIDISM. Oversecretion of thyroid hormone results in HYPERTHYROIDISM. The controlling factor in thyroid activity is the *thyroid-stimulating hormone* of the anterior part of the PITUITARY GLAND.

Deficiency in the supply of iodine, normally present in the diet in the small quantities needed, causes the thyroid to enlarge and to form a GOITER.

thyroiditis

Inflammation of the THYROID GLAND. It is a relatively rare condition that can be caused by viral or bacterial infections or by an autoimmune process.

Bacterial infections of the thyroid can cause reddening and swelling and even pus formation. Treatment consists of antibiotic therapy and, if needed, drainage of the infection.

THYROID AND PARATHYROID

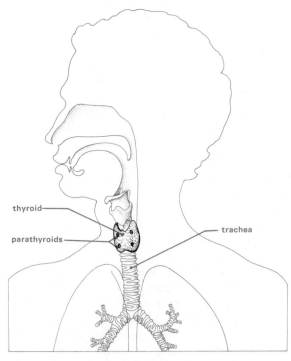

The thyroid gland lies in front of the trachea in the neck and secretes thyroxine, a hormone that controls the rates of many bodily activities. The four pea-sized parathyroid glands embedded within the thyroid secrete another hormone (parathormone), which is essential for maintaining correct levels of calcium and phosphorus in the blood.

Viral thyroiditis usually occurs after an upper respiratory tract infection and causes pain along the jaw and lower ear rather than in the thyroid itself. This disease is often difficult to differentiate from other types of thyroid disorders. Treatment usually consists of aspirin or steroids. Normal thyroid function will return.

HASHIMOTO'S DISEASE is a chronic inflammatory thyroid disease that occurs most often in middle-aged women. It is thought to be caused by an autoimmune disorder, in which—for reasons that are not understood—the body attacks itself. GOITER, swelling of the thyroid, is seen in this disorder.

thyrotoxicosis

A complex variety of body changes that occur in the presence of an excessive supply of thyroid hormone. Also known as HYPERTHYROIDISM. Thyrotoxicosis can result from a variety of diseases that cause the thyroid gland to produce excess hormone. It can result also from inflammation of the thyroid gland, which causes inappropriate leaking of the hormone into the body.

The general symptoms of thyrotoxicosis are inability to sleep, restlessness, tremors, weight loss, heat intolerance, excessive sweating, loss of strength, heart palpitations, eyelid changes, and a staring gaze. Graves' disease is hyperthyroidism with GOITER (increase in size of the gland) and eye and skin changes. This is a common disease, especially among women.

The multiple changes that can occur in so many of the body's functions need to be carefully evaluated by a physician so that the precise underlying cause is found. Proper treatment, whether medication or surgery, is strongly dependent on age, symptoms, severity of disease, and a host of other factors.

tic

An involuntary movement or twitch of part of the body that is repeated time after time for no apparent reason.

A tic usually represents a movement that would be useful in its proper place. For this reason it is sometimes called a *habit spasm*. As an example, a tic of blinking may have come about originally as a result of poor eyesight; even after this has been corrected by glasses, the tic (or habit) of blinking continues, particularly if the person concerned is of a nervous disposition.

A tic may be a sign of overwork or ill health, and is not usually present during sleep. The movement may be mild, such as blinking, coughing, or sniffing, but in some cases whole limbs are affected. The movements are generally sharp and quick, resembling the results of an electric shock. A tic may respond to psychotherapy.

ticks

Small PARASITES belonging to the spider class (arachnids) that depend on an intake of blood for their growth and development.

Ticks, which are found in fields and undergrowth, attach themselves to the skin of their victim, which may be animal or human. They do this by means of sharp and tenacious teeth and with a probe that sucks the host's blood into their body. Both male and female ticks engorge themselves

TICK

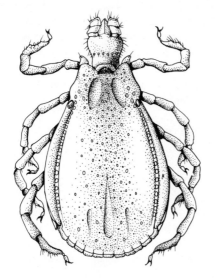

male brown tick *Rhipicephalus appendiculatus*

Ticks are blood-sucking arthropods that transmit harmful microorganisms to humans through their bite. Diseases spread in this manner include tick-borne typhus, relapsing fever, and Rocky Mountain spotted fever.

with blood; the male usually remains unchanged during the process, whereas the female swells up and resembles a red or purple berry on the skin.

A large number of infections are carried by ticks, including ROCKY MOUNTAIN SPOTTED FEVER, LYME DISEASE, tick-borne TYPHUS, and relapsing fever. Ticks can cause Texas fever in cattle.

Ticks usually cannot transmit infection to humans unless they have been on the skin for several hours. In tick-infested areas, therefore, it is a wise precaution to examine the body thoroughly at least twice daily and to remove any ticks found. The tick should *not* be rubbed off or pulled off for fear of further damage to the skin or tissue. It can either be removed by "drowning" with a heavy oil such as salad oil or machine oil, or it can be killed by carefully applying a lighted cigarette to its body. The use of tick-repellent chemicals on skin and clothing reduces the risk of infection in tick-infested areas.

tinea (ringworm)

A group of common fungus infections of the skin, hair, toenails, and fingernails caused by three types of fungus: *Microsporum*, *Trichophyton*, and *Epidermophyton*. The skin lesions tend to spread outward while the central part heals, thus creating the appearance of a ring (the source of the common name of *ringworm*). The infection is also known as *dermatophytosis*.

Tinea capitis is ringworm of the scalp. It is found primarily in children under the age of 10. The scalp develops round scaly patches from which the hair falls out.

Tinea cruris (popularly known as "jock itch") is ringworm of the crotch, seen mainly in young men. A red itchy patch of inflammation extends from the crotch down the inner side of the thighs for about 2 or 3 inches. It is most common in hot weather, and sweating athletes are particularly vulnerable.

Tinea pedis ("athlete's foot") is an extremely common infection, most often occurring in young adults. It is so common that it affects about half the population at one time or another. The skin between the third, fourth, and fifth toes becomes sodden and irritating and peels off. The infection may be found on other parts of the feet and may spread to the hands. In some cases the presence of athlete's foot produces skin changes in the hands, although the fungus cannot be demonstrated there. The fungus may also infect the nails (*tinea unguium*); it is one form of ONYCHOMYCOSIS.

Ringworm is spread by direct contact, and clothes, socks, and towels should not be shared. In tinea capitis the hairs that break off are infectious, so combs should not be shared.

Treatment for ringworm in the past included local applications of fungicidal ointments. However, the development of the drug griseofulvin, which is taken in pill form, has become the usual treatment of choice. The dosage and the length of time one must take it depends on the severity of disease. In cases of deep-seated toenail infections, griseofulvin may have to be taken for a year or more. Fingernails respond more quickly to the medication.

tinnitus

A constant or intermittent hissing, buzzing, or ringing noise in the ear. It most commonly arises from a disorder of the "hair cells" of the cochlea in the inner ear; it may also occur through blockage of the Eustachian tubes or excessive wax in the ears. Damage to the hair cells often results from exposure to loud noise, and it may follow large doses of certain antibiotics, quinine, or other drugs. Tinnitus is a common feature of MÉNIÈRE'S

DISEASE, in which it is accompanied by gradually increasing deafness. Almost all cases of tinnitus are associated with some degree of deafness. In most cases the cause of tinnitus is unknown.

tonsillitis

Inflammation of the tonsils, which are masses of lymphatic tissue lying on each side of the entrance to the throat at the back of the tongue. Almost all cases are caused by infection.

The infection is very common, particularly in children, and usually is caused by a streptococcus. Very often the infection is self-limiting, but in many cases it spreads to involve the lymph nodes that drain the tonsils, and a painful swelling develops behind the angle of the jaw.

Children can become quite ill and run a high temperature during an attack of tonsillitis. In addition to fever, the individual has a very sore throat, headache, difficulty swallowing, earache, and large tender lymph nodes in the neck.

The organisms causing tonsillitis are usually

TONSILLITIS

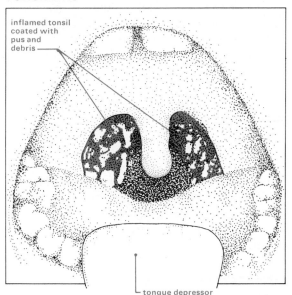

inflamed tonsil coated with pus and debris

tongue depressor

Tonsillitis occurs most often in children and may be caused by bacteria or viruses. The child has a high fever and if old enough will complain of a sore throat and difficulty in swallowing. If the fever does not abate after two days' rest with regular doses of acetaminophen and plenty of fluids, a course of penicillin is necessary. Repeated attacks may require tonsillectomy.

sensitive to antibiotics, and attacks of any severity generally can be controlled with their use. Occasionally, infection goes on to form an abscess, which may need surgical relief (tonsillectomy).

See TONSILLECTOMY under **Procedures.**

torsion of the testis

The twisting of the spermatic cord, resulting in a cut off of the blood supply to the testicle and other structures. Complete cutting off of the blood supply for a prolonged period may result in gangrene of the testis; a partial loss of blood supply may cause wasting away (atrophy). Torsion of the testis can occur during descent into the scrotum in the newborn infant or as a sudden, devastating event in the adult male. There is intense pain and tenderness, often accompanied by nausea and vomiting. Fast medical and/or surgical intervention is needed to save the testis.

torticollis

A condition in which the neck is bent to one side or the other, often accompanied by uncontrollable spasms. There are several causes.

Congenital torticollis usually affects babies who were breech presentations or difficult deliveries, and is usually caused by damage to the sternocleidomastoid muscle on one side of the neck. This is the most prominent muscle of the neck, and scarring prevents growth on one side. Fortunately, it is often possible to correct the condition in young children by repeated stretching of the neck in the opposite direction.

Spasmodic torticollis is a condition of painful spasm of muscles on one side of the neck. The cause is usually inapparent. Average age of onset for this condition is 40 years. It appears about twice as often in women as in men and rarely occurs in adolescents or young adults. It is not believed to be inherited. Some cases are, however, a feature of *torsion dystonia,* a hereditary disease affecting mainly Ashkenazi Jewish families.

Torticollis can also result from imbalance of the eye muscles, so that the head is tilted to correct vertical double vision. Early eye muscle surgery will correct this form.

Treatment of torticollis is directed to the physical cause, if such can be found. In other cases, psychotherapy may be helpful.

tourniquet

A band placed tightly around a limb to control severe arterial bleeding. There are several kinds of tourniquets, but basically they consist of a wide band or pad placed around the limb, with an appliance or lever that tightens it enough to stop the flow of blood through a main artery. (*Tourniquet* is also the term for a short piece of flexible tubing used to constrict the arm to facilitate drawing blood from a vein.)

Modern medical opinion has discouraged the use of tourniquets except in special operative techniques and for the control of severe bleeding at the end of a limb that has been accidentally amputated.

The use of a tourniquet is no longer considered acceptable in first-aid work. Either it is inefficient or it will—in addition to controlling blood loss—do much damage (because of blood deprivation) in the area applied.

toxemia of pregnancy

Another term for PREECLAMPSIA.

toxic shock syndrome (TSS)

A sudden, sometimes fatal infection that was first reported in 1978. Menstruating women are the most frequent victims but TSS can strike any age group of either sex. The use of tampons appears to elevate the risk, but a direct connection between tampon use and TSS has yet to be proved. By 1981, the incidence had dropped sharply after the withdrawal of some tampons from the market.

The major causative factor is a toxin secreted by the *staphylococcus aureus* bacterium, which can invade virtually any part of the body. Symptoms include generalized malaise, muscle pain, severe nausea and vomiting, diarrhea, high fever, a mild cough, and a purulent nasal discharge. Treatment involves the administration of antibiotics as well as the intravenous infusion of nutrients designed to offset the loss of electrolytes and low blood pressure resulting from the disorder.

toxoplasmosis

An infection with a protozoan parasite, *Toxoplasma gondii*, which is common in both animals and humans. Most human infections cause few or no symptoms, but infection during pregnancy may spread to the fetus, causing serious damage to the brain or eyes. This congenital toxoplasmosis occurs in about one in every 2,000 newborn infants.

Adult toxoplasmosis has assumed new importance in recent years since the disease may be a serious threat in persons whose natural immunity has been lowered by the acquired immune deficiency syndrome (AIDS), or by receiving treatment with immunosuppressive drugs after TRANSPLANTATION or anticancer (cytotoxic) drugs.

Toxoplasmosis often reponds to treatment with antimalarial and sulfonamide drugs, but suppression of the disease should be based on public health measures, since the chief sources of human infection are animal excreta (from infected cats) and contaminated meat.

tracheitis

Inflammation of the trachea ("windpipe"), the vertical tube extending down from the larynx to immediately above the heart, where it divides into two main *bronchi*, one extending to each lung.

Tracheitis causes pain in the upper part of the chest, accompanied by a dry painful cough. Often it occurs as a complication of a more general respiratory infection, such as INFLUENZA or BRONCHITIS. The symptoms may be relieved by inhalation of steam, by cough syrups, or by antibiotics.

trachoma

An infectious disease of the eye. Trachoma is contagious and is caused by a microorganism, *Chlamydia trachomatis*. It is marked by swelling, pain, and intolerance to light. Antibiotics are used to treat trachoma; if left untreated, blindness can result.

traction

A technique used in orthopedics for treating FRACTURES and SLIPPED DISKS and for straightening the SPINE.

When a bone has fractured, the resulting inflammation and irritation around the fracture cause the muscles in the area and those attached to the bone to go into spasm. This may result in some overriding of the broken ends of the bone or in their being pulled into an unsatisfactory position. If untreated, the end result would be a shortening of the limb. Traction is applied by fixing weights and pulleys to the broken limb so that the bones are pulled into the correct alignment. Traction, skillfully applied, can overcome the effects of the muscles that have gone into spasm. Overzealous traction, on the other hand, may pull the fractured ends apart and so delay healing.

Persons with SCOLIOSIS, a type of spinal curvature, may also be treated by traction applied to the head and pelvis or to the spine and pelvis; the steady push and pull of the spine in the desired directions slowly results in some straightening.

Traction sometimes is used for treating slipped disks, in which the symptoms are due to pressure of the pulpy center of a ruptured intervertebral disk on the nerves coming off the spinal cord; traction prevents further compression and may allow the pulp to retract. However, some experts believe that traction relieves symptoms by enforcing bed rest.

Traction also may be applied by gravity. This is used, for example, in treating upper arm fractures, or congenital dislocation of the hip in children. With upper arm fractures the wrist is held in a sling so that the weight of the limb pulls on the humerus (the bone in the upper arm).

Skin traction also may be used. With hip and thigh injuries, elastic devices may be applied around the upper thigh and traction exerted on the elastic by connecting it to weights that run over pulleys at the foot of the bed. Similarly, the weights may be connected to pins or wires inserted into the bone to which traction is to be applied.

transplantation

The surgical replacement of a diseased organ or tissue with a healthy one taken from another individual. The donor may be living (usually a close relative) or the part may be removed from a body shortly after death.

The technique of transplantation began with grafting of a small disk of cornea (the transparent layer at the front of the eye) as a treatment for some forms of blindness. When attempts were made to transplant skin, however, it soon became clear that the grafts survived for only a few days:

The body's immune defenses reject grafts from another individual in the same way that they destroy invading bacteria. The bloodless cornea is the exception to this general rule.

Successful transplantation had to wait for the development of immunosuppressive drugs, which temporarily suppress this immune rejection reaction. As these drugs became available, surgeons began the grafting of major organs—including the kidney, liver, heart, and lungs. A major transplant operation usually is considered only in cases of life-threatening illnesses, since the administration of immunosuppressive drugs has potentially dangerous side effects (it lowers the body's defenses against bacteria and viruses, making serious infection a risk during this period in transplant patients).

Experience worldwide with tens of thousands of transplants, mostly of kidneys, has shown that many factors affect the chances of success. The best results have come when the grafted kidney has been taken from a volunteer who is a close relative (ideally, from the patient's own twin brother or sister). Just as successful blood transfusion depends on matching the blood groups of the donor and recipient, so does successful transplantation depend on close matching of the "tissue types," as characterized by their HISTOCOMPATIBILITY ANTIGENS.

There are four sets of transplantation antigens; among the thousands of possible combinations, the best possible match must be found. Good matching is most likely within a family, but many transplant centers now use computers to select the best match among waiting patients when a kidney becomes available from a dying patient. Other factors that affect success of the operation are the age of the recipient, the number of blood transfusions that have been given, and the amount of immunosuppressive medication that is needed. In the early years of transplant surgery another factor was delay between the death of the donor and the removal of the organ. Now, however, with the advent of organ donation control centers and programs that allow people to will their vital organs for transplantation after their death, this is no longer a major problem.

Kidney transplantation is now routine in many specialist centers. The operation is successful in about 70 percent of the cases, and many patients are alive and well more than five years after surgery. If the grafted kidney is rejected or ceases to function it may be removed, and second or third transplants are by no means rare. Even so, the operation carries a substantial mortality rate from complications such as infection in the immediate postoperative period, but this is falling steadily in hospital centers that have extensive experience in kidney transplants.

Today, organ transplantation is commonplace for certain diseases of the heart, kidney, and liver.

The most recent advancements in this area of medicine are the heart-lung transplantation and the pancreas transplantation.

travel sickness

Also known as *motion sickness*. Nausea or vomiting (or both) experienced when moving in a car, ship, aircraft, train, or other vehicle of travel. This is the result of the intermittent and erratic stimulation by the movement of the vehicle on the sensory receptors in the organ of balance in the inner ear.

The organ of balance is made up of a continuous system of passages (the *semicircular canals*) and chambers (the *utricle* and *saccule*) filled with a fluid called *endolymph* and containing sense organs. Movement or a change in position of the head causes movement of the endolymph, which stimulates the receptors. Nerves pass from these receptors to various parts of the nervous system. These connections with the nervous system serve to start off reflex movements that enable the individual to regain equilibrium when for some reason he is thrown off balance. However, some of the nerves also connect with the vomiting center in the brain.

Travel sickness may be to some extent a conditioned reflex, so that a person who expects to be sick is more likely to be sick; it may also be aggravated by psychological or emotional factors. Keeping oneself occupied is one method of attempting to prevent travel sickness. Tranquilizers or drugs that contain scopolamine or antihistamines may help to prevent travel sickness. They are best taken about an hour before the start of a journey. It must be remembered, however, that they can cause drowsiness; a person who has taken them should be careful not to drive while the drug still has its effect.

Other measures that help prevent the severity of an attack include adjusting the ventilation to get some fresh air, sitting with the head tilted back as in a dentist's chair, and having small but frequent meals rather than no meals.

traveler's diarrhea

A brief attack (usually lasting one to three days) of DIARRHEA usually caused by common bowel organisms, such as Escherichia coli, to which local inhabitants are adapted. Viruses may also be responsible. When it affects tourists it often is referred to humorously by such terms as *Montezuma's revenge* and *la turista.*

Besides diarrhea, there may be nausea, vomiting, rumbling noises in the abdomen, and abdominal cramps. The severity varies, but most cases are mild.

Treatment consists of rest and a bland diet. If the diarrhea persists after twelve to twenty-four hours, antidiarrheal agents may help. Antibiotics generally are avoided since they may adversely affect the intestinal flora and even prolong symptoms.

Most important is the prevention of the condition, expecially when traveling to areas where modern standards of hygiene have not been imposed. Drinking water and milk should be boiled, fresh foods should be well cooked, fruit should always be peeled, and shellfish probably should be avoided.

tremor

A series of involuntary rhythmic, quivery movements, with no purpose, caused by the uncontrolled tightening and relaxing of groups of muscles.

Tremor may indicate a disturbance in the *extrapyramidal system*—that is, in those parts of the brain and spinal cord involved in motor activities, especially the control and coordination of postural, static, supporting, and locomotor mechanisms. The disturbance may be due to a variety of causes.

Hunger, cold, physical exertion, fatigue, or excitement may produce a transient tremor that is of no special significance. Tremor may be present also as a benign hereditary condition, which becomes apparent during or after adolescence and is found in several successive generations. Other diseases in which a tremor is quite characteristic are PARKINSON'S DISEASE, HYPERTHYROIDISM, Wilson's disease, diseases of the cerebellum, and MULTIPLE SCLEROSIS. Tremor may be due to the effect of toxins (poisons) on the nervous system, the most common being alcohol; mercury poisoning also produces tremor. It may also accompany emotional disorders such as anxiety states or hysteria.

The cause of the tremor may be identified to some extent by its characteristics and by the accompanying signs of the underlying condition that produces it. Tremors may be rapid and fine (the type usually seen in THYROTOXICOSIS) or coarse and slow (as in Parkinson's disease); they may occur at rest (as in Parkinson's disease) or worsen when an attempt at a voluntary movement is made (as in cerebellar disease), or they may appear when the person is attempting to maintain the position of the affected part without support.

Treatment depends on the cause of the tremor. In toxic states, removal of the toxin is the treatment.

The tremor of Parkinson's disease may respond, in part, to some drugs. Tremor caused by anxiety and emotional disorders usually responds to sedatives, tranquilizers, or antianxiety agents, but that due to multiple sclerosis does not respond to drugs. However, the person can be taught certain postures and maneuvers that may reduce the tremor brought on by a particular movement.

trichomoniasis

Infection with a parasitic protozoon, *Trichomonas vaginalis*, which lives in the vagina and urethra of women and also in the urethra of men (in whom, however, it rarely causes symptoms). Infection is related directly to sexual activity.

Symptoms of an *acute* infection consist of the sudden onset of an intensely irritant discharge, which may be yellowish, greenish, or frothy; the amount of the discharge varies. The vagina feels sore and there is usually pain during sexual intercourse. There may also be a frequent urge to pass urine and painful urination.

In *chronic* trichomoniasis, symptoms come and go, usually appearing around menstruation.

The diagnosis is made by examining the discharge under the microscope for the presence of the parasite. Treatment involves the administration of appropriate drugs such as metronidazole. Both the victim and her sexual partner (even if he is symptomless) should receive the treatment.

trichophyton

A genus of fungi that attacks the hair, skin and nails. The disease that these fungi cause is known as *dermatophytosis*, or ringworm (TINEA).

trismus

A persistent spasm of the muscles of the jaw, sometimes called lockjaw. Trismus can be caused by a mouth infection, abscesses, rabies, and irritation of the trigeminal nerve, which supplies the jaw, face mouth, and nasal cavities.

tropical sprue

A tropical disease of unknown cause, characterized by MALABSORPTION of fats, protein, vitamins, iron, and calcium. Its clinical features include sore tongue, weight loss, fatty stools, and DIARRHEA.

Treatment basically involves the initiation of a balanced diet high in protein (but with only normal amounts of fat) and the administration of folic acid and the antibiotic tetracycline for a period of up to six months.

Nontropical sprue is a term used to describe the adult form of CELIAC DISEASE.

truss

A device for retaining in position a hernia that has been reduced into the abdominal cavity. It is most definitely *not* an adequate substitute for surgical repair. A truss is most commonly used for an inguinal hernia. Essentially, it consists of a pad joined to a belt made of various types of material, such as a leather-covered steel spring. The pad is positioned so as to cover the site of the hernia. In infants it is best to use a washable rubber truss. Correct fit is important, and wearers should be carefully measured for their truss.

A truss is used usually when a person is not fit for surgery or refuses surgery. It is used also for babies with inguinal hernias, who usually are not operated on until they are about 3 months old.

To be effective, the wearing of a truss requires some degree of intelligence and perseverance on the part of the individual. The truss has to be put on while the person is lying down and the hernia is completely within the abdomen; the truss is then applied with some pressure over the hernia site. The skin underlying the truss should be kept clean and powdered to prevent chafing.

trypanosomiasis

Any of the various diseases caused by infection with protozoa of the genus *Trypanosoma*. This organism causes African sleeping sickness, a severe form of ENCEPHALITIS (brain inflammation).

See also CHAGAS' DISEASE.

tube feeding

The feeding of a person through a tube that has been passed into the stomach, either by way of a nostril or through an artificial opening made into the stomach through the abdominal wall. Most of the tubes used now are made of plastic and come presterilized.

Tube feeding is required in unconscious persons; in persons who, because of neurological disease, may be conscious but unable to swallow; and in persons in whom the esophagus is partially obstructed so that solids cannot be swallowed.

In a conscious person the tube usually is introduced while the person is sitting up comfortably in bed with the head supported. The nostrils are cleaned with absorbent cotton plugs soaked in a bland antiseptic. As the tube is passed in through a nostril the person is encouraged to swallow, if necessary by simultaneously sipping water. A conscious person may be very anxious when the tube is being passed and may retch so that it becomes extremely difficult for the tube to reach the stomach. A mild sedative given beforehand, or some local anesthetic sprayed on the throat, may minimize the person's anxiety and discomfort.

Once the tube has reached the stomach, the end protruding out of the nostril is taped to the person's nose or cheek. Liquid food can then be syringed through the tube. The tube has to be checked frequently to see that it is functioning properly, that it is unblocked, and that its tip is still in the stomach. Blockage is checked by injecting air into the tube; the aspiration of gastric juice will confirm that the tip is still in the stomach.

In another method the tube is inserted directly into the stomach by means of a *gastrostomy* (the formation of an artificial opening into the stomach); this is done when a person is unable to swallow the tube, or when the obstruction in the esophagus is complete.

tuberculosis

An infection caused by the bacterium *Mycobacterium tuberculosis* (it may rarely be caused by *Mycobacterium bovis*, which normally infects cows).

In general, human tuberculosis affects the lungs, bovine tuberculosis affects the glands and bones, but practically any organ in the body may be affected by the infection (which may be acute or chronic); however, the most common site is the lung. At one time, tuberculosis was a common cause of death all over the world, but with infection control, antituberculosis immunization, and chemotherapy, mortality due to tuberculosis has decreased dramatically in most developed countries.

Apart from the few cases in which the disease is spread across the placenta from mother to fetus, tuberculosis is acquired mostly by inhalation or ingestion of infected material in the form of droplets, dust, food, and milk. Once the infection has set in, the disease may spread from its primary site directly to adjacent structures, or it may be carried by the lymphatic system or bloodstream to distant sites.

Symptoms of tuberculosis include malaise (a general feeling of being unwell), lassitude, tiredness, loss of appetite, fever, and night sweats. Other symptoms depend on the site affected. For example, with infection of the lungs there may be cough, sometimes with bloodstained sputum. An infection of the intestine (most commonly the small intestine) may produce a malabsorption syndrome or intestinal obstruction. There may be a tuberculous MENINGITIS, PERICARDITIS, ARTHRITIS, and so on. Very often the lymph glands draining an infected area enlarge, and it may be the enlarged lymph nodes that draw attention to the presence of an infection.

The infection may often be present for a long time without producing symptoms. In areas where tuberculosis is prevalent, persons in close contact with tubercular patients sometimes are screened for the disease by a Mantoux test.

Diagnosis is made by X-ray studies and by examining various body tissues and fluids for the causative organisms. Treatment consists of the administration of a combination of bactericidal drugs, usually for at least nine months. Sometimes surgery is necessary. Healing typically results in the formation of a scar at the site of infection. Sometimes organisms in the scar remain viable for a long time and become reactivated at a later date. In most cases the scar itself produces no symptoms; occasionally, however, the scar has some effects. For example, Fallopian tubes that have been infected may become fibrosed and thus induce infertility.

Immunization with BCG gives some protection against tuberculosis in susceptible people. Such an immunization, however, renders the person permanently positive to tuberculin tests in the future, meaning that they cannot be used for diagnostic purposes.

twins

Two offspring produced in a single pregnancy.

There are two ways in which twins can be produced. Normally only one ovum, or egg, is fertilized. If two ova are fertilized at the same time, the result is a pair of *fraternal* (or *nonidentical* or *dizygotic*) twins, who may be as different from each other as any pair of siblings. If only one ovum is fertilized and the resulting embryo divides at a very early stage to produce two embryos, the result is *identical* (or *monozygotic*) twins. Since identical twins form from the same ovum and sperm, they have the same genetic makeup: they will be of the same sex and have the same blood group, same build, same color of eyes, and even the same pattern of hair whorls.

Twins occur in about one in 80 births. The tendency to have nonidentical twins is inherited, especially through the mother's side. Nonidentical twins also appear more frequently after the second pregnancy and with advancing maternal age; mothers who are 35 to 40 years old are three times more likely to have twins than 20-year-old mothers.

Twins have a slightly higher early death rate than single children. For a start, life in the uterus is more difficult, and twin pregnancies bring more obstetrical complications. Twins also are more prone to fetal growth retardation; this may affect one twin more than the other if the distribution of blood supply to the two embryos is uneven. The difference in growth and development may persist after birth.

There is also a higher rate of mental subnormality, CEREBRAL PALSY, and congenital abnormalities in twins. Identical twins may have a higher risk of certain tumors.

Less is known about the psychological development of twins, although they certainly can be different psychologically; even identical twins reared in the same environment may have quite different psychological makeups.

Twins should be treated as individuals, each with his or her unique traits and abilities, and be encouraged to develop apart. Otherwise emo-

TWINS

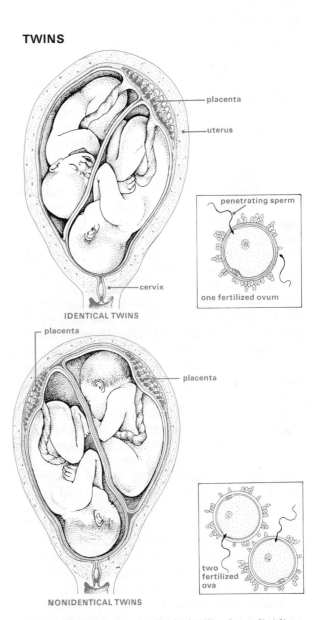

Identical twins are the result of a fertilized egg dividing into two identical cells that then separate and develop independently. Since both twins are derived from one sperm and one egg they are genetically identical. Nonidentical twins are no more genetically similar than ordinary brothers and sisters; they develop from two different eggs (each fertilized by separate sperm) and have separate placentas.

tional disturbances may develop later, especially when the twins begin to lead separate lives.

Siamese twins, or conjoined twins, are twins who at the time of birth are physically joined to each other at some part of the body.

typhoid fever

A bacterial infection acquired from food or water contaminated with particles of human sewage containing the causative microorganisms. The bacteria responsible, *Salmonella typhi,* may be found in dairy produce such as milk and cream as well as in undercooked meats. The disease received its name because of the similarity of its symptoms to TYPHUS.

The incubation period for typhoid fever is from about five days to five weeks (usually eight to fourteen days) between the eating of contaminated food and the onset of illness. Early symptoms include headache, loss of energy, and fever; cough is common and there may be nosebleeds. After seven to ten days the fever becomes steady, the abdomen is swollen, and the person may become profoundly weak, confused, and delirious. In the second or third week a pink "rose-spot" rash appears; at about this time also serious complications may occur, including perforation or hemorrhage in the intestines. In most cases, however, the fever begins to subside at this time and slow recovery follows.

With early diagnosis and antibiotic treatment the course of the illness is cut short. However, a few persons will recover to become symptomless "carriers" who pass typhoid bacteria in their excreta. These persons are the source of further infections, especially if they are employed in the food industry. The inapparent infection is in the gallbladder and CHOLECYSTECTOMY (see under Procedures) will usually correct the situation.

Prevention of typhoid depends on good sanitation, proper hygiene among food handlers, and the tracing and treatment of carriers.

Typhoid fever used to be one of the most dangerous of the "enteric fevers" affecting adults. It remains a threat to health for people who travel to countries with inadequate sanitation, and there are still a few deaths each year among tourists returning to the United States from Europe, Africa, and the Far East. Vaccination gives valuable protection for travelers outside the United States. A course of two or three injections is required,

but the effect lasts for only one to two years, when a further booster dose will be needed.

typhus

Any one of three related infectious diseases caused by a species of *rickettsia* (microorganisms intermediate in size between bacteria and viruses) and transmitted to humans by body lice, rat fleas, or mites. Prior to the era of modern medicine the disease was prevalent wherever people were crowded together in conditions of poor hygiene.

The microorganisms that cause epidemic typhus can multiply in both lice and humans. Lice acquire the infection by biting someone who has typhus; the microorganisms then multiply inside the louse, eventually killing it—but not before it has had a chance to pass the infection on to another human.

The incubation period between infection and the onset of symptoms is about fourteen days. The illness begins abruptly with fever and a severe headache; after three to four days a pinkish rash appears. Typically the high fever is accompanied by confusion and delirium; in untreated cases the mental state may become increasingly stuporous, with eventual coma and death. The mortality rate ranges from 10 to 50 percent, varying with the age of the victim and his previous health.

Early treatment with antibiotics is highly effective. A protective vaccine also exists, but prevention is essentially a matter of personal hygiene. Other forms of typhus are murine typhus (rat-flea typhus), scrub typhus (mite-borne typhus), and ROCKY MOUNTAIN SPOTTED FEVER (tick typhus).

ulcer

An open sore that occurs on the surface of the skin or on a mucous membrane, exposing tissue normally covered by epithelial cells.

Ulcers may develop as the result of several factors, all of which interfere with the proper nourishment of the tissues. These factors include poor blood supply, poor venous drainage leading to waterlogged tissues, infection, damage by physical agents such as heat and cold, continual pressure, malignant growths, and disease of the nervous system leading to loss of sensation and repeated minor trauma. Examples are varicose ulcers,

ULCERS

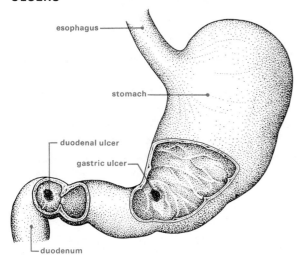

esophagus

stomach

duodenal ulcer

gastric ulcer

duodenum

TWO TYPES OF PEPTIC ULCER

Peptic ulcers are erosions in the lining of the digestive system caused by the action of gastric acid. Many factors—age, sex, occupation, diet, blood group—appear to influence one's likelihood of developing either gastric or duodenal ulcers. Both types of ulcers usually can be managed by drugs and dietary measures.

where the venous drainage is inadequate; syphilitic ulcers from infection; frostbite; and BED-SORES. PEPTIC ULCERS form in the stomach and duodenum when the mucous membranes lose their ability to withstand the action of hydrochloric acid and pepsin. Occasionally peptic ulcers occur as the result of a malignant growth.

Treatment of an ulcer is by removing the cause. Persons with varicose ulcers must elevate the leg as much as possible to promote venous drainage; areas with the potential to develop bedsores must be subjected to as little pressure as possible; malignant growths must be removed. Treatment, however, cannot hope to succeed unless the circumstances that originally led to ulcer formation are rectified. This is particularly true of varicose ulcers and peptic ulcers.

ulcerative colitis

A chronic inflammatory condition of the large bowel (colon) of unknown cause. It is slightly more common in women than men and appears to be more common among Jews. It has been suggested that the disease has an immunological basis and that it is an inherited disorder.

The lining of the large bowel is ulcerated and

has a tendency to bleed, so that the symptoms include incessant bloody diarrhea as well as abdominal discomfort. The loss of protein may be severe enough to produce symptoms of protein malnutrition, and there may be ANEMIA. Complications can occur: The bowel may bleed severely, chronic inflammation may produce a stricture of the intestine, and in some cases the intestine may suddenly distend (toxic dilation)—a condition that requires immediate surgical treatment. The wall of the bowel may perforate, producing PERITONITIS. The risk of developing a malignant growth is significantly greater than it is in the general population.

Diagnosis is based on the person's medical history and is confirmed by endoscopic examination of the large bowel plus a barium enema X-ray study. Treatment is difficult; general measures include rest and the correction of any nutritional deficiencies. In severe cases close collaboration of surgeon and physician is essential, as the need for operative treatment may become urgent.

unconsciousness

A state of unawareness or lack of response to stimuli. Sleep is such a state. Unconsciousness can be caused by breathing difficulty, shock, drugs, poisons, or electrolyte imbalance. It can occur as a result of a lack of oxygen to the brain. Other causes are injury, seizures, stroke, brain tumor, or infection. Unconsciousness can range from simple FAINTING to COMA.

undescended testis

The development of the testis in the male fetus takes place inside the abdomen near the kidney. It descends into the scrotum before birth, but the descent may be imperfect.

There are three varieties of imperfect descent: (1) retractile testis; (2) incompletely descended testis; and (3) ectopic testis. The retractile testis can be manipulated into the scrotum; it descends completely into the scrotum at puberty and requires no treatment, unless a hernia defect remains.

The incompletely descended testis lies somewhere along the normal path of descent: it may be in the abdomen, in the inguinal canal, or at the neck of the scrotum. It cannot be manipulated into the scrotum and it will not descend at pu-

UNDESCENDED TESTIS

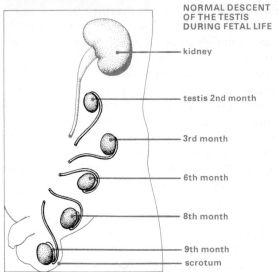

NORMAL DESCENT
OF THE TESTIS
DURING FETAL LIFE

kidney

testis 2nd month

3rd month

6th month

8th month

9th month
scrotum

The downward migration of the testes in the fetus can become arrested at any point, trapping the testis in the abdomen. If it does not descend into the scrotum during early childhood, it should be brought down surgically, preferably before the age of 5.

berty. Such cases usually require operative treatment between the ages of 1 and 3. The affected testis is smaller than usual and there is virtually always an associated inguinal hernia.

The ectopic testis has wandered from the normal line of descent and lies somewhere near the inguinal canal, perhaps in the perineum or near the root of the penis. It is usually of normal size, but because of its abnormal position it is particularly liable to damage. Like the incompletely descended testis, it will not produce spermatozoa unless it is surgically replaced in its normal position in the scrotum by the time of puberty. If it proves impossible to replace the testis in the scrotum it should be removed, for ectopic and undescended testes—if left in their abnormal positions—are liable to develop tumors.

uremia

A general term used to describe a variety of conditions that exist in the body after loss of normal kidney function. The name was given many years ago because an excess of the substance urea was detected in cases of kidney failure. Actually, there are many substances that abnormally accumulate in the body when kidney function deteriorates. Uremia adversely affects virtually every organ sys-

tem in the body and eventually will lead to death if not treated.

The condition is often of gradual onset. The person may be tired and unable to concentrate. As the condition worsens, confusion results. Neurological changes, hypertension, fluid buildup, gastrointestinal disorders, and blood abnormalities all occur in uremia, as do psychological changes. There are many causes of uremia, and when possible the underlying cause should be treated. In severe cases of uremia, the blood must be cleansed of the accumulated waste products by the use of an artificial kidney machine or by a technique called peritoneal dialysis. Kidney transplantation is used when kidney function is irreversibly lost.

urethritis

Inflammation of the urethra (the tube that brings urine from the bladder to the outside of the body). Urethritis is usually a venereal infection, most commonly caused by the gonococcus or the chlamydia trachomatis.

See also CYSTITIS, URINARY TRACT INFECTION.

urethrocele

One form of genital PROLAPSE in women, in which the urethra is displaced downward and backward as a consequence of CYSTOCELE (prolapse of the bladder into the vagina). Often the displaced urethra is also dilated. Like other forms of genital prolapse, it arises from damage to or weakness of the ligaments supporting the uterus—childbirth being the most common cause.

The urethrocele may not form until many years after the initial damage. Usually symptoms do not arise until about the MENOPAUSE, when there is some degeneration of the muscles and connective tissue in the pelvis.

Symptoms include a feeling of discomfort or weakness in the vagina, especially after the woman has been standing all day. There may be urinary symptoms, especially stress INCONTINENCE (involuntary release of urine during such activities as sneezing or laughing), and a tendency to recurrent URINARY TRACT INFECTION.

Treatment involves supporting the prolapse with a pessary, an internal vaginal support, which may relieve symptoms. An operation is required to cure the condition.

urinary frequency

The passage of urine more often than usual without an increase in the total daily volume. Urinary frequency may be a sign of inflammation in the bladder, pregnancy, lowered bladder capacity, structural problems of the urinary tract, or infection. Treatment may include medication or surgery.

urinary tract infection

An infection of the urinary tract, which includes the urethra, bladder, ureters, and kidneys. The condition is more common in women than men and may lack symptoms. Most of these infections are caused by gram-negative bacteria, usually *Escherichia coli.*

Urinary tract infection is marked by urinary frequency, pain on urination, fever, chills, and, if the infection is severe, visible blood and/or pus in the urine. Diagnosis is made by microscopic examination of a urine sample, physical examination of the individual, culturing a urine sample,

URINARY TRACT INFECTION

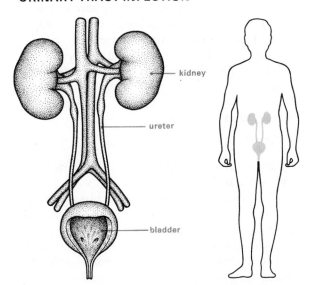

The urinary system is a common site of bacteria infection. Nearly all cases are "ascending" infections caused by bacteria from the anus entering the urethra and then moving up the urinary tract into the bladder. Women have considerably shorter urethras than men, and are therefore much more likely to be affected.

and possibly by more invasive tests such as cystoscopy. Treatments include several different types of medication.

See also CYSTITIS, PYELONEPHRITIS, and URETHRITIS.

urticaria

Also known as *hives.* A skin eruption of raised red and white patches on the skin, which cause irritation and ITCHING. It occurs most commonly on the face and the trunk of the body. If the swelling extends to the throat, there may be difficulty in breathing. The attack may subside within hours or may last several days.

Urticaria is an allergic reaction that can be caused by certain protein foods (especially fish or shellfish); by drugs, especially penicillin; by contact with certain plants; and by insect bites or stings.

As in other allergic disorders, emotional stress and anxiety may be important factors; the condition tends to run in families. In severe cases emergency treatment may be needed; injections of epinephrine or corticosteroids give dramatic relief. Usually, however, itching may be allayed by antihistamines or by any of the many generic "anti-itching" lotions or ointments on the market. The only certain way of eliminating the possibility of future outbreaks is for the factor causing the allergy to be identified and avoided.

See also ALLERGY, IMMUNE SYSTEM.

uterine cancer

Malignant tumors of the UTERUS include CANCER of its body and cancer of the cervix (the neck of the womb). Cancer of the body of the uterus usually originates in the lining. There may be no symptoms or the growth may cause intermittent and irregular blood loss. For that reason, any unusual uterine bleeding should be investigated without delay. When surgical removal of the uterus is performed early in the disease, the outlook is excellent: 75 to 90 percent of early cases of this cancer are cured by surgery.

Cancer of the cervix is the most common form of cancer in women—and the most preventable, since the condition can be detected in its preliminary stage by examining a sample of cells taken from the cervix (cervical smear, or "Pap smear"). Wherever Pap smears have been used by women as a regular screening test, the death rate from the disease has fallen precipitously in the last thirty years.

The cancer starts with a small "ulcer" or bleeding point on the cervix, but spreading to lymph nodes in the pelvis may occur early. Treatment is surgical, sometimes backed up by radiotherapy. Again, the prospects for cure are good in cases treated early in the course of the disease.

uterus (womb)

A pear-shaped hollow organ of the female reproductive system that holds the embryo and fetus from the time of fertilization to birth. It is situated deep within the pelvis between the bladder and the rectum and is about $3\frac{1}{2}$ inches (9 cm.) long, 2 inches (5 cm.) wide, and 1 inch (3 cm.) thick. Its narrow neck (cervix) opens into the vagina. On the upper side of the uterus the Fallopian tubes, one on each side, connect with the ovaries. Underneath, the uterus is supported by ligaments attached to the muscular floor of the pelvis.

In nonpregnant premenopausal women the interior lining of the uterus (endometrium) is shed every month (menstruation) and replaced by a new lining unless fertilization of the ovum occurs, in which case the endometrium is not expelled, there is no menstruation, and the uterus begins to expand in order to accommodate and nourish the developing embryo.

The muscles that form the outside wall of the uterus have remarkable powers of adaptability: During pregnancy they increase from 1 ounce (28 g.) in weight to $2\frac{1}{4}$ pounds (1 kg.). After birth the uterus returns to its normal size within a few weeks, and the process of the monthly shedding of the endometrium (menstruation) begins anew.

Owing to its structure and position, the uterus can suffer from downward displacement, or PRO-LAPSE. Another common condition is the growth of benign tumors (FIBROIDS), but these often can be removed successfully.

uveitis

Inflammation and swelling of the uveal tract (the iris, ciliary body, and choroid—the pigmented, vascular layer of the eye). Signs may include an irregularly shaped pupil, cloudy deposits on the cornea, pain, and tearing. There is pain, redness of the eye, and clouding of vision. Uveitis is usually an autoimmune disorder, but the cause often remains obscure. GLAUCOMA may be a major complication.

vaginal cancer

CARCINOMA of the vagina is a disease of older women, with a peak incidence between the ages of 50 and 70.

There is a recently recognized association of "clear-cell" ADENOCARCINOMA of the vagina in young women whose mothers used the hormone drug diethylstilbestrol (DES) during the first trimester of pregnancy. HERPES virus may also be a causal factor. Treatment is by surgery and radiation therapy.

vaginismus

Uncontrolled, painful spasms of the muscles surrounding the vaginal opening, resulting in painful intercourse (DYSPAREUNIA) or preventing penetration by the penis.

It may be due to anxiety, local tenderness, or an unduly small vaginal opening. The anxiety may arise from previous traumatic sexual experience, ignorance of sexual matters, fear of pregnancy, excessive modesty, dislike or distrust of a sexual partner, or dislike of the act of sexual intercourse itself; it may be allayed by psychiatric treatment. Local conditions producing tenderness can be treated as required. In most cases of vaginismus the cause is fairly clear, and the family physician can be of great help. Graduated dilatation often is successful.

vaginitis

Inflammation of the vagina, usually characterized by a vaginal discharge.

The inflammation may be due to a variety of causes, of which infection is the most common—especially that caused by the fungus *Candida albicans* (which produces CANDIDIASIS) and that by the parasite *Trichomonas vaginalis* (which produces TRICHOMONIASIS). Because the vagina is related anatomically to the cervix, cervical infections (such as that caused by gonorrhea) also may cause vaginitis. In children, vaginitis sometimes is due to a pinworm infestation.

Foreign bodies are another cause of vaginitis in children. In adults, the types of foreign bodies that typically cause vaginitis are devices inserted for the treatment of prolapse of the cervix or tampons still in place after menstruation. Vaginitis due to a foreign body causes an acute, highly offensive discharge which usually responds well to the removal of the foreign body.

Chemical vaginitis usually is caused by the use of an unsuitable chemical for douching or for contraception. Often the chemical solution is too highly concentrated, or the woman is allergic to it. *Senile vaginitis* is seen in postmenopausal women, or premenopausal women in whom the ovaries have been removed or are not functioning. It is due to a deficiency of the ovarian hormone estrogen. The lining of the vagina becomes smooth, thin, shiny, and dry, and small hemorrhages may appear. The vagina normally has a slightly acidic secretion that helps protect it against infection; this protection is lost in senile vaginitis, which is treated by administering therapeutic amounts of the hormone.

Valsalva's maneuver

Named after Antonio Mario Valsalva (1666–1723), an Italian physician and professor of anatomy at the University of Bologna. Valsalva's maneuver is the act of breathing out hard while holding the mouth and nose tightly closed, thus raising the pressure inside the chest. The rise in pressure inside the abdomen may help to empty the bowels or bladder in certain conditions where these functions are impaired.

However, as a result of Valsalva's maneuver, the return of blood to the heart is slowed, the heart itself slows, and the blood pressure rises. Straining to empty the rectum may, therefore, cause a dangerous rise in blood pressure in someone who has vascular disease, with stroke or heart attack ensuing.

varicocele

Enlargement of the veins of the spermatic cord. The condition occurs most often in adolescent boys and affects the left side more often than the right. The affected scrotum feels like a bundle of worms. Varicocele may be accompanied by a dull ache along the cord and a dragging sensation in the groin. The condition usually requires no treatment but may cause infertility, in which case ligation of the internal spermatic vein may be helpful.

varicose veins

Enlarged, knotted superficial veins, which are induced and aggravated by PREGNANCY, OBESITY, and occupations that require prolonged standing. The cause of this condition is poorly operating valves in the veins, which may be acquired or inherited.

The blood supplied to the limbs via the arteries is returned to the heart via the veins. The veins contain one-way valves that allow blood to flow only toward the heart. The blood is forced toward the heart by the contraction of muscles with each movement of the limb. Blood that has passed through a valve cannot return. When this valvular mechanism becomes defective, the veins of the lower part of the leg become swollen by the pressure of the column of blood in the veins higher up the leg. This swelling eventually causes them to become dilated and knotted; they are then described as *varicose*.

In a minority of cases the condition may result from a blockage in the vein. This may occur when a major leg vein undergoes THROMBOSIS, or when the flow of blood from the leg through the lower part of the abdomen is obstructed by pressure on the veins during pregnancy or a tumor in the pelvis. In the majority of cases, however, the cause is incompetence of the valves in the veins.

Varicose veins are a relatively common condition. Many methods of treatment are used, including the use of elastic stockings or bandages to support the veins. The injection of various chemical substances into the veins will cause them to become thrombosed and in due course obliterated by scar tissue. Alternatively they can be removed surgically or tied off at a number of points.

Complications of the condition include the formation of varicose ulcers on the lower leg and a tendency to thrombosis in the dilated vein (superficial THROMBOPHLEBITIS), resulting in a painful, red swelling along the course of the vein.

vasoconstriction

The arteries contain muscle tissue in their walls; contraction of the muscular coat of a blood vessel, reducing its diameter and the amount of blood

VARICOSE VEINS

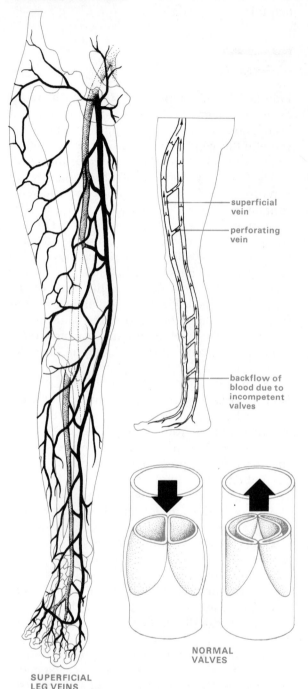

- superficial vein
- perforating vein
- backflow of blood due to incompetent valves

NORMAL VALVES

SUPERFICIAL LEG VEINS

The veins in the legs are arranged into superficial and deep systems, which are connected by perforating veins. If the valves in the perforating or superficial veins leak, blood flows back down the superficial system causing dilated, tortuous vessels. Varicose veins may be symptomless or may cause aching, swelling, eczema, and ulceration as they become distended, enlarged, and twisted. Veins almost anywhere in the body can be involved, although those in the legs are most commonly affected.

that can flow through it, is referred to as *vaso-constriction*. It has a valuable biological function in controlling the flow of blood through tissue. Under certain circumstances, however, an inappropriate constriction of the arterial supply to a tissue can cause serious problems. (See RAYNAUD'S PHENOMENON.)

The degree of contraction present in the muscular wall of an artery is under involuntary nervous control and is also affected by a number of biologically active chemicals (HORMONES) circulating in the blood. It can also be increased or decreased by the action of certain drugs.

A common example of the effect of vasoconstriction is the marked variation in blood supply to the hands in hot and cold weather, causing either extra heat loss (when it is hot) or reduced heat loss (when it is cold).

vasodilatation

Whereas VASOCONSTRICTION refers to the contraction of the muscular wall of an artery, thus reducing the diameter of the vessel and the blood flow through it, *vasodilatation* is the relaxation of the muscular coat. This permits the vessel to increase its diameter, thus also increasing the blood flow within it.

As with vasoconstriction, vasodilatation is under involuntary nervous control and is affected also by circulating drugs and biologically active chemicals (HORMONES) in the blood. Common examples of vasodilatation are seen in the flushing of the skin of the face in response to embarrassment or excitement and the general increase in blood flow to the skin when the body is overheated—allowing more heat to be lost, especially from exposed areas such as the hands.

vegetarianism

The practice of abstaining from all flesh foods of animal origin and eating mostly vegetables. An extreme form of vegetarianism prohibits even the consumption of eggs, milk, and dairy products because they come from animals. Upholders of this extreme practice are known as vegans (especially in Britain) to distinguish them from less radical vegetarians.

Vegetarians who also eat eggs and dairy products have no difficulty in obtaining the required dietary balance, because these foods contain adequate amounts of protein and B vitamins. Vegans, however, find it more difficult to maintain an adequate diet, for the minerals and vitamins present in eggs and dairy products must be replaced from vegetable sources. Their diet must include nuts, whole-grain cereals, and a wide variety of vegetables or there is a risk of mineral-deficiency diseases.

One of the strongest arguments for vegetarianism is that such a diet does not lead to excessive formation of CHOLESTEROL in the blood. Cholesterol has been linked to cardiovascular disease.

venereal disease (VD)

Disease transmitted by sexual intercourse.

The organisms responsible vary a great deal, but most depend on the warmth and moisture of the sexual organs for survival, for organisms die when the temperature drops much below that of body heat. The most serious veneral disease is AIDS. Other common diseases are GONORRHEA, genital HERPES SIMPLEX, and NON-SPECIFIC URETHRITIS; the category also includes CHANCROID, LYMPHOGRANULOMA VENEREUM, GRANULOMA INGUINALE, REITER'S SYNDROME, genital warts, TRICHOMONIASIS, genital CANDIDIASIS, MOLLUSCUM CONTAGIOSUM, and pediculosis pubis (see LICE).

Despite better diagnosis and treatment, the incidence of venereal diseases has continued to increase, mainly because of public ignorance and unconcern. The emergence of resistant strains of organisms has contributed to the increase.

Wider awareness of the altogether more serious risks of HIV infection (AIDS) is, however, having a significant effect on behavior.

ventricular fibrillation

A rapid and uncoordinated contraction of the muscle fibers of the ventricles without a recognizable rhythmic heartbeat. (See ARRHYTHMIA.) Since the effect of this is to prevent the heart from performing its normal pumping action, circulation ceases immediately and—unless immediate measures are taken—sudden death will result.

Ventricular fibrillation can occur as a result of damage to the heart or its valves by drugs, infections, electrical shock, or interference with its blood supply via the coronary arteries (*coronary insufficiency*). Its greatest importance, however, is its occurrence as a complication of a CORONARY THROMBOSIS, where it is often the cause of sudden death.

Treatment is a matter of extreme urgency. If the situation cannot be remedied within two or three minutes, permanent or fatal damage to the brain from lack of oxygen may occur. Drugs are of limited value; the only effective treatment is to apply electrodes to the chest wall and give a short and controlled direct-current shock to the heart from a machine known as a *defibrillator*. This may lead to restoration of a normal heartbeat in a proportion of cases.

While a defibrillator is being set up, maintenance of the blood circulation by means of chest compressions and mouth-to-mouth RESUSCITATION is essential. If efficently performed, it can greatly prolong the normal interval of two to three minutes between cessation of the circulation and BRAIN DEATH and will allow defibrillation to be performed even if the defibrillator is not immediately available.

vertigo

A condition in which the subject feels dizzy, with a definite sensation of movement, and feels that he is or his surroundings are rotating in space. This last factor is an essential ingredient of true vertigo and distinguishes it from simple DIZZINESS. It is often accompanied by nausea, headache, or vomiting.

The loss of balance experienced in vertigo may be caused by motion (as in seasickness), ear disease such as OTITIS INTERNA (labyrinthitis) or MÉNIÈRE'S DISEASE, damage to the acoustic nerve (eighth cranial), cerebellar disease (the *cerebellum*, a major division of the brain beneath the back part of the cerebrum, is concerned with maintaining balance and coordinating muscular movements), or the effects of some drugs (such as streptomycin).

Vertigo also may be a symptom of certain stomach and digestive disorders. In some people it is brought on merely by standing on a height and looking down.

While the attack lasts the person should lie flat on his back with the clothing around his neck loosened. Sedatives may be administered by a physician if the person remains conscious. If attacks occur frequently, the individual should consult his doctor to find the cause and permit the appropriate treatment to be given.

Vincent's angina

A noncontagious infection of the gums and throat caused by either of two types of bacteria or a combination of both: a *fusiform bacillus* and a *spirochete*. Also known by its World War I nickname of *trench mouth*.

Symptoms include painful bleeding gums, excessive production of saliva, and foul-smelling breath. In the untreated disease, ulcers form on the gums and sometimes on the palate and throat, and the affected tissues may be covered with a gray membrane. The irritation or removal of this membrane typically causes bleeding.

Both types of bacteria are found in healthy mouths, but are normally dormant. In cases of poor oral hygiene, poor general health, prolonged exhaustion, or nutritional deficiencies the infection suddenly may establish itself.

Treatment consists of cleansing the mouth and throat with appropriate antiseptic lotions, rest, and attention to the reestablishment of adequate nutrition and good general health. Antibiotics usually are not required.

viruses

The smallest known infectious organisms; with certain exceptions, they are too small to be seen under the ordinary light microscope. The smallest virus is about $\frac{1}{100}$ the size of a bacterium, and about $\frac{1}{750}$ the size of a red blood cell. They are unable to live or multiply outside a host cell since most do not possess the means to synthesize protein.

Structurally, a virus consists of a core of nucleic acid (its genetic material) surrounded by a protein coat. This protein coat is antigenic—that is, it will cause production of antibodies in the blood of the host; each type of virus has an antigenic property specific for its type.

Viruses are classified according to the type of nucleic acid they possess and their appearance. The main groups of medically important viruses are the *pox viruses, adenoviruses, herpes viruses, papovaviruses, myxoviruses, rhabdoviruses, enteroviruses, picornaviruses, reoviruses, arboviruses* (also known as *togaviruses*), and *arenoviruses*.

All forms of life (animals, plants, bacteria) are susceptible to virus infection. Viruses affect the

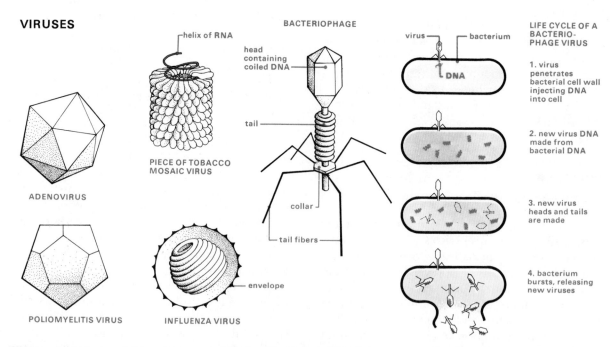

VIRUSES

helix of RNA

PIECE OF TOBACCO MOSAIC VIRUS

ADENOVIRUS

POLIOMYELITIS VIRUS

envelope

INFLUENZA VIRUS

BACTERIOPHAGE

head containing coiled DNA

tail

collar

tail fibers

virus — bacterium

DNA

LIFE CYCLE OF A BACTERIO- PHAGE VIRUS

1. virus penetrates bacterial cell wall injecting DNA into cell

2. new virus DNA made from bacterial DNA

3. new virus heads and tails are made

4. bacterium bursts, releasing new viruses

Viruses, seen here as they appear magnified many thousands of times by an electron microscope, have a wide variety of striking, even beautiful, geometric shapes. They are parasitic microorganisms that can reproduce only by taking over the functions of a host cell (animal, plant, or bacterium).

cells that they inhabit in several ways. They may kill the cell; they may transform the cell from a normal cell to a cancerous cell; or they may produce a latent infection, in which the virus remains in the cell in a potentially active state but produces no obvious effects on the functioning of the cell.

Most viruses are inactivated by heat (100°F/ 37.7°C for thirty minutes, or 212°F/100°C for a few seconds), but most are stable at very low temperatures (for example at −95°F/−70°C). The effect of drying on viruses is variable.

Viruses are important causes of human disease. Most virus infections are mild and may go unnoticed by the person concerned, although the viruses may multiply in the body and be passed on to another susceptible person. In children, the elderly, and those who are debilitated, a viral infection that is normally mild can produce severe effects. Some virus infections (such as smallpox) are severe and have a high mortality rate.

Viruses usually enter the body via the respiratory tract by inhalation, but some enter by ingestion or by inoculation through tears or abrasions in the skin. The disease produced may be systemic—for example, MUMPS, in which the virus travels through the bloodstream and invades many organs and tissues—or it may be localized and invade only tissues near the site of entry, as in respiratory viral infections. The AIDS virus attacks the body's immune system, making the person prey to opportunistic infections that eventually prove fatal.

Unlike some bacteria, viruses do not produce toxins; they produce their effects directly by multiplying in the tissues.

The body attempts to protect itself against viral infections by producing *interferon*, a protein (released from infected cells) that, when taken up by other cells, renders them refractory to viral infection. The body also can produce antibodies to specific viruses; these antibodies may persist for several years.

Although there are a few drugs that exhibit a degree of antiviral activity, they act only against a few types of viruses. Most viruses are resistant to the antibiotics available. Viral diseases are prevented by avoiding contact with infected persons or by vaccination, when the specific vaccines are available.

vision

The ability to see; viewing objects. The structures concerned with vision are the eyes, optic nerves, and the occipital lobes of the brain.

Light enters the eye through the *cornea*, the transparent part of the outer covering of the eyeball that overlies the pupil. The *pupil* is the center of the *iris*, the colored diaphragm that controls the amount of light admitted to the interior of the eye; the radial muscles of the iris contract so that the pupil enlarges when the intensity of the light is low. In conditions of increased light the pupil is small because the circular muscles of the iris contract. The light reflex (or pupillary reflex) is controlled in the brainstem and is sometimes affected by disease.

Behind the iris is the *lens* of the eye (also known as the *crystalline lens*), a transparent biconvex structure with the front curved slightly less than the back. Because it is elastic, its shape can be changed by the action of the *ciliary muscle* on the suspensory ligament that supports the lens; in this way the image of objects near the eye can be brought to a focus at the retina. With age the elasticity of the lens decreases and the ability of the eye to bring near objects into focus fails; glasses for reading then become useful.

EYE

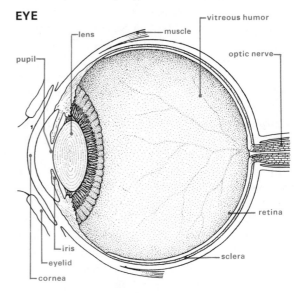

A CROSS SECTION THROUGH THE EYE

The eye is often likened to a camera because it has an adjustable lens and aperture (the pupil) with a light-sensitive film (the retina) behind. The optical images are encoded and transmitted along the optic nerve to the brain, where the simultaneous signals from both eyes are coordinated.

The image of external objects is focused on the *retina*, which consists of receptors sensitive to light. These receptors are of two kinds—*rods* and *cones*. There are about 120 million rods and about 6 million cones. Nerve fibers run from them to gather at the optic disk (the "blind spot") where they form the *optic nerve*, which passes from the eyeball to the brain. Behind the eyes some of the fibers of the optic nerves cross at the optic chiasma so that some of the images entering the eyes from the right are conducted to the left side of the brain (and vice versa).

If the shape of the eyeball is abnormal, objects cannot be brought to a sharp focus on the retina: A long eyeball produces nearsightedness, while a short eyeball cannot produce a sharp image of near objects. Both conditions may be remedied by eyeglasses, as may aberrations of shape of the cornea; if the eyeball is not truly round, parts of an image will not be in sharp focus at the retina, producing a defect in vision known as ASTIGMATISM.

Defects in the cones of the retina produce COLOR BLINDNESS, for the cones are sensitive to three primary colors. Rods contain only one pigment (rhodopsin), whose adsorption is greatest for blue-green light. The retina itself may be affected by diseases resulting in DETACHED RETINA, hemorrhage, or exudation—all of which obscure vision.

Behind the eye, disease may affect the optic nerve or the crossing of the nerves (optic chiasma) causing defects in the field of vision; disease also may interfere with the nerve fibers as they pass through the brain to the occipital cortex at the back of the cerebral hemispheres. Examination of these visual-field defects is of great value to the neurologist, who can often (by considering the shape and size of the defects) localize brain lesions.

Finally, the movements of the eyeballs must be accurately coordinated. Each eyeball is moved by a complex of six external *ocular muscles* supplied by nerves arising in the brainstem. Interference with the central mechanism of coordination, with the nerves, or with the muscles themselves, can result in DOUBLE VISION.

vitamins

A group of natural substances needed by the body for growth, health, and life. With few exceptions, vitamins cannot be synthesized by the body and therefore must be gotten from the diet.

Vitamins are generally divided into two broad groups—fat-soluble (A, D, E, K) and water-soluble (B complex, C).

Vitamin A is needed for the growth of the skeleton, for maintaining mucous membranes, and for keen vision. It is found in leafy green vegetables, yellow fruits and vegetables, fish-liver oils, milk, cheese, butter, and eggyolk. Vitamin-A deficiency leads to NIGHT BLINDNESS, eye changes, and thickening of the cells that cover internal and body surfaces such as the skin and the lining of the gastrointestinal and urinary tracts. Hypervitaminosis A (too much vitamin A) can cause irritability, fatigue, lethargy, stomach pain, joint pain, severe headache, insomnia, night sweats, loss of body hair, and brittle nails.

The vitamin-B complex consists of the following: thiamine (B_1), which is essential for the maintenance of normal digestion and appetite and for the functioning of nervous tissue; riboflavin (B_2), which is important for normal growth and in the formation of certain enzymes; niacin, or nicotinic acid (B_3), which prevents pellagra; and cyanocobalamin (B_{12}), which is needed for the development of red blood cells. All of the B vitamins are found in large amounts in liver and yeast. Heat and prolonged cooking, especially in water, can destroy B vitamins.

Vitamin C, ascorbic acid, is found in citrus foods and green vegetables. A deficiency causes scurvy.

Vitamin D is needed for the normal growth of bones and teeth and for absorbing calcium and phosphorus from the intestines. The vitamin is present in natural foods in small amounts. The needed amounts usually are obtained from supplements added to various foods, especially milk and dairy products, and from exposure to sunlight. Natural foods containing vitamin D include saltwater fish, organ meats, eggyolk, and fish-liver oils. Deficiency of vitamin D results in RICKETS or OSTEOMALACIA, while hypervitaminosis D causes loss of appetite, nausea, vomiting, thirst, excessive urination, nervousness, itch, impaired kidney function, and calcification of tissue.

A lack of vitamin E causes muscle damage, blood disorders (ANEMIA), liver and kidney damage, and infertility. The richest dietary sources of vitamin E are wheat germ, soybeans, eggs, raw seeds and nuts, peanuts, cottonseed and corn oils, liver, and sweet potatoes. Because it is stored in the body for long periods of time, a severe lack is rare.

Vitamin K is needed to help the liver function and to help the blood clot. This vitamin is in many foods, especially leafy green vegetables, yogurt, egg yolk, fish-liver oils, kelp, alfalfa, and blackstrap molasses, and is made by bacteria in the intestines. A lack of this vitamin is marked by blood disorders.

For an extended discussion see *The Wellness Diet* in the section on **Wellness**.

vitiligo

A condition in which light-colored blotchy patches appear on the skin as a result of a localized absence of melanin, the pigment responsible for skin color. The cause is not known but approximately one third of the cases are found to run in families.

Most commonly, the condition affects palms, soles, knees, elbows, armpits, genitalia, and areas around the mouth and eyes. Occasionally, the vitiligo is so widespread that nearly all the skin may become white.

Although persons with vitiligo are generally healthy, there may be an increase in thyroid disease (especially in those over aged 50), DIABETES MELLITUS, and ANEMIA.

About one third of the cases will regress spontaneously, especially in that part of the skin that gets sun exposure. There has been some success noted when these persons are treated over a long period of time, under close medical supervision, with ultraviolet light. (All persons need to guard against sun exposure with the use of sunscreen creams or lotions.)

vomiting

The forcible ejection through the mouth of the contents of the stomach, brought about by a complicated reflex controlled by a vomiting center in the brain. Retching, also known as "dry heaves," is the act of vomiting without the production of stomach contents.

The vomiting reflex can be set in motion by many different stimuli. Direct stimulation of the vomiting center occurs in MENINGITIS, MIGRAINE, and in the state of increased pressure within the skull caused by tumors or hemorrhage. This type of vomiting is not accompanied by nausea; it may also be caused by various drugs.

Many people vomit as the result of emotional shock—for example, at the sight of a bad road accident, or the perception of a disgusting smell; others vomit when unduly excited or anxious.

Travel sickness is a problem for a number of people, particularly the young. It is caused by stimulation of the vomiting center by impulses arising in the inner ear.

The most common cause of vomiting is intestinal disturbance, when irritation brought about by overdistension or inflammation sets up the reflex through the vagus nerve—which serves both to carry stimuli to the vomiting center and to transmit the outgoing nerve impulses necessary for the accomplishment of the act.

The vomiting that often occurs during pregnancy (see MORNING SICKNESS) may be due to changes in hormone balance, but the cause is not definitely known; in many cases it is accompanied by anxiety or other emotional disturbances.

Vomiting in children may herald the onset of an infectious FEVER; in babies it is often the result of injudicious feeding or the swallowing of too much air.

So many disturbances cause vomiting that it is not possible to generalize about the most effective treatment, which must depend on treating the underlying condition. One danger of vomiting to excess, particularly in young children, is loss of water and salts from the body with consequent DEHYDRATION and imbalance of electrolytes. A more immediate danger is inhalation of vomit, which may occur in unconscious or semiconscious persons, and which could cut off the flow of oxygen to the lungs.

von Recklinghausen's disease

A hereditary condition, also known as *neurofibromatosis*, in which numerous bumps (*neurofibromas*) are found all over the body. This disease gained widespread public attention through the film *The Elephant Man*, although few cases are ever as severe as the true case depicted in the film.

Neurofibromas are benign tumors that grow from the skin or in the fibrous tissue surrounding the nerves. When superficial these may be seen as nodules under the skin; if they develop around deeper nerves, they might not be noticed until they have grown large enough to cause symptoms by pressing on surrounding structures.

The symptoms of the disease depend on the severity of nerve involvement. When only peripheral nerves are affected, there may be no symptoms except for a feeling of pressure where they press on nerves. However, when the cranial nerves or the roots of the spinal nerves are involved, serious disability may result. Depending on the nerves involved, deafness, blindness, and numerous other disabilities can occur. Rarely do neurofibromas degenerate into cancerous tissue or do areas affected by them become malignant.

The only treatment for von Recklinghausen's disease is surgical removal of the neurofibromas, where possible. The disease affects one in 3,000 live births. The first symptoms of café-au-lait spots and neurofibromas begin to appear around age 3, although it is not until the first or second decade that the more full-blown disease may develop.

vulvitis

Inflammation of the vulva, the female external sexual organs excluding the vagina. The vulva consists of the labia majora, labia minora, clitoris, urethral meatus, and various glands. Inflammation can be the result of many types of skin disorders.

Infecting organisms that may be involved include the HERPES SIMPLEX virus and the parasitic protozoon, *Trichomonas vaginalis.* Infections by fungus and yeast organisms often are associated with pregnancy, DIABETES MELLITUS, and the use of birth control pills, antibiotics, and other medications that can change the environment of the vagina. This last type of vulvitis (CANDIDIASIS) is characterized by its curdy white appearance and severe itching and usually can be controlled quickly by local applications of an antifungal medication.

In general, dermatological problems such as PSORIASIS, seborrheic dermatitis, and FOLLICULITIS can involve the vulva. Friction, allergies, or irritation can led to "eczematoid dermatitis," which responds well to local medications. It is not uncommon for vulvitis to be initiated by vaginitis spreading to the vulva via an extensive discharge, with resultant severe vulvar edema and itching. Treatment is directed at the underlying cause.

warts

Small solid benign tumors that arise from the surface of the skin as a result of a virus infection.

Warts (or *verrucas*) are extremely common and in the vast majority of cases are completely harmless, although they may be unsightly and irritating. A wart appears when the activity of the virus causes hypertrophy of the papillae of the skin.

This results in the growth of a bundle of fibers from the skin's surface, capped by the horny cells that cover the cuticle. The mass of the wart is surrounded by a ring of thickened cuticle and the fibers can be seen particularly well when the wart has been growing for some time and has become abraded. The color of the wart is usually darker than the color of the background skin, but this is merely because dirt becomes lodged in the minute crevices between the fibers.

Warts are common in children, probably because of a lack of immunity to the causative virus. They often appear more thickly on areas such as the knuckles, the insides of the knees, and the face—where the skin is more likely to be irritated. Adolescents and young adults often suffer from epidemics in schools and other institutions, such as military camps, where physical education and swimming may be conducted in bare feet. The wart transmitted in these cases, the PLANTAR WART on the soles, can be painful because the pressure of the body's weight forces the wart into the skin of the sole. Older people suffer from *senile warts,* and there is a type of *soft wart* on the eyelids, ears, and neck that can occur among people who work with hydrocarbons.

Venereal warts (condylomata acuminata) are spread through sexual contact and appear in the genital areas. (See CONDYLOMA.)

Treatment of warts usually is accomplished successfully, where it is thought necessary, by the simple expedient of removing them by application of a freezing agent such as liquid nitrogen or carbon dioxide snow. Plantar warts unsuitable for this treatment may need surgical excision. Chemical agents for the removal of warts now are little used; their effects are slow and repeated applications are necessary.

wheeze

A noise produced in respiratory diseases and caused by narrowing or obstruction of the larger airways. It is often worse in the morning, during and after exercise, and following a chest infection. A high-pitched wheezing is characteristic of acute ASTHMA.

whiplash injury

When an automobile is hit suddenly from behind, the head and neck of a person sitting inside the struck vehicle move violently backward and forward like the lash of a whip. The movement can damage the neck or—in violent accidents—the spinal cord and even the brain.

A very common complaint even after minor collisions is stiffness of the neck. This usually wears off, but the injury can be severe enough to require the wearing of a collar to limit movement of the cervical spine until recovery is complete. The effects of whiplash injury may take a long time to show themselves, and the development of a "cervical disk syndrome" sometimes can be traced back to an accident that occurred some years before.

Headrests (or more properly, head restraints) fitted to car seats protect against these injuries by preventing the backward whiplash movement of the neck.

whooping cough

An infectious disease of the mucous membranes lining the air passages; also called *pertussis.* It is caused by a coccobacillus called *Bordetella pertussis.* It is mainly a disease of children, who achieve lifelong immunity after infection. Thanks to improved health care and vaccination programs, it is no longer the menace that it once was in heavily populated countries.

Whooping cough gets its popular name from the fact that the irritation of the upper respiratory tract causes convulsive bouts of coughing, followed by a peculiarly noisy crowing indrawing of the breath. Children, particularly those under the age of 1 year, were once greatly at risk from whooping cough. Since the discovery of a vaccine, whooping cough has become a comparatively rare disease.

In cases where vaccination has not been performed, three stages of the disease may be expected to occur. The initial "catarrhal" stage is followed by the "spasmodic" stage, in which all the classical signs appear, and this is followed by the stage of decline. During the spasmodic stage the bouts of coughing and "whooping" last about thirty to forty-five seconds and can be extremely distressing to a child.

The spasmodic stage may last four to seven weeks and in rare cases may leave behind side effects such as EMPHYSEMA or a liability to attacks of ASTHMA. Whooping cough is highly contagious. When a case occurs it is wise to isolate the sufferer from other children, and even from adults who have not had the disease previously or been vaccinated against it. The victim should be kept warm and restricted to bed until the symptoms abate. Spasms of coughing may be relieved by the administration of drugs.

xeroderma

A disorder in which the skin is very rough and dry. The most common form is known also as *ichthyosis simplex,* in which large corrugated papery scales form on the skin (which is deficient in sebaceous glands and sometimes also in sweat glands).

Xeroderma pigmentosum is a rare disease, usually appearing in childhood, in which the skin atrophies (wastes away) and wrinkles. There is a familial tendency. Sufferers have PHOTOPHOBIA (abnormal sensitivity of the eyes to light), and the warty and "keratolytic" lesions of the disease quickly become malignant if exposed to sunlight. Sufferers must be protected from the sun. The skin has the appearance of very old skin even in young people.

yellow fever

An acute viral infection of the liver, kidneys, and heart muscle transmitted by a female mosquito of the genus *Aedes.* It occurs in tropical Africa and parts of the Western Hemisphere lying between Brazil and the southern United States.

In the last century yellow fever killed so many workers engaged in building the Panama Canal that the French Panama Canal Company went bankrupt. During the Spanish-American War in 1900 a team of Army doctors—including Walter Reed—showed that the disease was transmitted by a species of mosquito known as *Aedes aegypti.* An efficient vaccine eventually was produced, giving protection for up to ten years.

There is no known specific treatment for yellow fever. From about three to fourteen days after being bitten by an infected mosquito the person develops a headache, fever, and pains in the muscles. In a severe attack the temperatures rises, the face becomes flushed, and the person becomes confused. After one or two days the fever stops and the person is no longer confused. In severe infection, however, the delirium and fever return, the pulse becomes slow and weak, blood is vomited, there is a great deal of protein in the urine

(PROTEINURIA), and the person becomes yellow from JAUNDICE. Many attacks of yellow fever are mild or subclinical. About 10 to 20 percent of those infected die.

Treatment involves bed rest, fluid maintenance, anticoagulant therapy, and blood transfusions.

The control of yellow fever depends on strict control of the *Aedes aegypti*, which is a domestic mosquito breeding in pools of stagnant water and in water left in the bottoms of old pots and pans and oil drums.

All travelers to places where the disease exists must be immunized at least ten days before they travel.

zoonosis

Any disease shared by man and other vertebrate animals.

More than 150 zoonoses, carried by a variety of animals, are known; but modern medicine and veterinary science have been able to control many of them, or to ameliorate their effects. Even so, some still present a very real threat to human and animal life.

Examples of zoonoses are ANTHRAX, BRUCELLOSIS, PSITTACOSIS, and RABIES.

4

PROVIDERS

allergist/immunologist

The allergist is a specially trained physician concerned with the diagnosis and treatment of all forms of allergy and allergic disease.

An estimated 15 to 25 percent of Americans suffer from some form of allergy. Some allergies, if untreated, can become serious lifelong illnesses, often starting in infancy and early childhood. Clinical allergy and hypersensitivity embrace a wide range of disease states, including asthma, allergic rhinitis (hay fever), eczema, contact dermatitis, urticaria ("hives"), and angioedema (wheals and swelling of skin tissue), drug reactions, insect allergy, and food hypersensitivity.

Allergy and immunology go hand-in-hand. In fact, allergy has been defined accurately as "untoward physiological events caused by a variety of immunologic reactions." Any organ of the body can be involved, but the most common "shock organs" are the nose, skin, and lungs. In most cases, immunologic mechanisms are protective and act as the body's natural defense against infections, ridding it of potentially dangerous substances that may disturb its normal internal environment. Such substances may be introduced from outside the body or generated from within. Allergy is the effect that results when the immunologic mechanisms "backfire" to produce unwanted results.

To diagnose a specific allergy, the allergist must do three things: identify the causal agent, demonstrate that it produces clinical signs and symptoms, and identify the immunologic mechanisms that are causing the problem. This is often difficult to do because there are certain diseases that mimic allergic states but actually are caused by other mechanisms.

The allergist-immunologist is qualified by many years of training. Following graduation from medical school, he must complete a full three years of residency training in either internal medicine or pediatrics. He may then be certified in the one he has chosen by passing the examinations given by that examining board. Following this, he must then complete a full two-year in-hospital fellowship in clinical allergy and immunology, which qualifies him to take the examinations (oral and written) given by the American Board of Allergy and Immunology. In addition, most states require continuing education as a requirement for relicensure.

Most patients today are referred to the allergist by their family doctors.

anesthesiologist

Anesthesiology, which was recognized as a distinct medical specialty in 1937, is concerned with the

351

administration of local and general anesthesia and with monitoring surgical patients safely through the period of unconsciousness to consciousness.

The anesthesiologist (also called *anesthetist*) is a physician well trained in general medicine and surgery who spends an additional four to five years in postgraduate clinical training. During this period he becomes proficient in all areas of anesthesiology, including the techniques of resuscitation, which may be required for surgical patients who develop life-threatening complications while under deep anesthesia.

Owing to well-trained anesthesiologists and the various techniques and support systems available to them, many high-risk patients who only a short time ago would not have been recommended for surgery are now routinely and safely operated on—even in long procedures.

Today's anesthesiologist has a variety of anesthetic agents from which to choose, both for local and general anesthesia. In *general anesthesia*, which causes loss of consciousness, the patient inhales carefully controlled amounts of vapor or gas such as nitrous oxide, halothane, cyclopropane, or trichloroethylene. For *local anesthesia*, during which the patient remains fully conscious, he receives an injection around a nerve trunk to deaden all feeling in the area it serves. In *caudal block* a needle is inserted into the sacrococcygeal notch (area between the sacrum and coccyx) into the epidural space (just outside the spinal cord), killing all sensation in the area below the blockage.

In the recovery room careful monitoring of all vital signs is continued until the patient passes safely from unconsciousness to consciousness. If you become a surgical patient, your anesthesiologist, perhaps never seen in an emergency situation and only briefly in any event, will be one of your most important doctors. He is well worth his fee, which today is billed directly and not included in the patient's hospital charges, as was once a common practice.

cardiologist

A physician who specializes in the diagnosis and treatment of diseases and disorders of the heart and its associated blood vessels. These disorders include coronary heart disease, hypertensive heart disease, rheumatic heart disease, infectious heart disease, and heart defects present at birth.

To become a cardiologist, one must graduate from medical school and then spend at least three years of residency training in internal medicine at an accredited teaching hospital. Following this, there must be additional time spent in residency training in cardiology. The physician can then take an exam to become board-certified in cardiology as a specialty.

Most of the patients the cardiologist sees are referred from general practitioners or other specialists. After the cardiologist has completed his examination and tests to evaluate the extent of the disease and the specific structures involved, he most often refers the patient back to the patient's regular doctor, with a complete report of his findings and his recommendations for continuing treatment. If surgery is indicated, he will work with the regular physician in preparing the patient for such treatment.

During a heart checkup, the cardiologist first will obtain a patient history, asking questions about the patient's age, family medical history, past illnesses, and current symptoms. Even if you have already answered these questions for your regular physician, it is important to cooperate with the cardiologist. Typical complaints of cardiology patients include shortness of breath, chest pain, palpitations, bluish skin color, fainting, and swelling of the feet or ankles.

The cardiologist next performs a complete physical examination, at which time he checks heart and breathing rates, pulse, and blood pressure. He also listens to your chest with a stethoscope to determine if your lungs are congested, if there is fluid in your lungs, and if there is any irregularity in the rhythm of your heartbeat and the sounds made by the opening and closing of the heart valves. He makes chest X-ray studies to determine shape, size, and general condition of the heart and lungs.

The cardiologist then performs a variety of specialized tests, as indicated by your particular signs and symptoms. These tests may include an electrocardiogram (EKG)—probably performed while you are exercising on a treadmill or bicycle—phonocardiography, echocardiography, and, if necessary, cardiac catheterization and cardiac angiography. Once all necessary tests are completed, the cardiologist will arrive at a diagnosis and a decision on the best course of treatment.

cardiovascular surgeon

The cardiovascular surgeon (or "open-heart" surgeon)—with his large team of physicians and specially trained nurses and technicians—may be better known to laymen than any other surgical specialist. This is due largely to the publicity given in the press and on national television to the drama associated with early heart transplant operations, the replacement of diseased or damaged heart valves, and the implantation of artificial pacemakers to govern the rhythmic beating of the heart.

Being able to stop the heart so that it can undergo surgical repair is one of the great achievements of modern medicine. It was made possible by the development of the heart-lung machine, a device that temporarily takes over the function of the heart in maintaining the oxygenation and circulation of the blood to all the organs and their tissues. What is more important than the rare cases of total heart transplantation is the ability of open-heart surgeons to repair congenital or acquired heart defects in children and adults who only a short time ago faced early death or lives of invalidism. A short time after corrective surgery, a child who was once blue-lipped and grossly handicapped can romp and play as normally as other children. This is but one of the many contributions of cardiovascular surgery.

After medical school, a cardiovascular surgeon must undergo seven years of postgraduate training before he is eligible for certification (more training than is required of any other physician). First, he must undergo five years of residency training in general surgery and become certified by the American Board of Surgery by passing oral and written exams. Then, he must take a two-year residency program in cardiovascular surgery.

chiropractor

Chiropractors base their practice on the belief that mechanical disorders of the joints, especially of the spine, have an effect on the nervous system and that interference with this system impairs normal functions and lowers resistance to disease. Such beliefs place chiropractors outside of the mainstream medical community. Chiropractors take patient histories, conduct physical examinations, and give treatments for illness and injury. However, unlike M.D.s, they treat patients primarily by manual manipulation (adjustments) of parts of the body, especially the spinal column.

In addition to straightforward manipulation, chiropractors employ such orthopedic techniques as immobilization and traction. They also use a wide range of special devices for the therapeutic application of ultrasound, vibration, and electric current.

Laws vary from state to state as to whether chiropractors can treat only musculoskeletal problems or whether they can provide a full range of primary care. They do not prescribe drugs or perform surgery.

To become a chiropractor, one must meet educational requirements required by the state and pass a state board examination. The type of practice permitted and the educational requirements for a license vary considerably from one state to another, but, in general, state licensing boards require successful completion of a four-year chiropractic course following at least two years of college. After training, the candidate must pass the test of the National Board of Chiropractic Examiners.

dental hygienist

Dental hygienists, working under the direction of a dentist, provide direct patient care: They remove deposits and stains from patients' teeth, expose and develop dental X-ray films, and perform various other preventive and therapeutic services. Helping the public develop and maintain good oral health is another important aspect of the job: Hygienists may instruct patients in the proper selection and use of toothbrushes and other devices, for example, or explain the relationship between diet or smoking and oral health.

As allowed or not by state law, hygienists may remove deposits from teeth; apply topical fluoride to prevent tooth decay; take medical and dental histories; take X-ray films; make impressions of teeth for study models; and prepare other diagnostic aids. In a few states, dental hygienists may perform pain control and restorative procedures.

Dental hygienists must be licensed. To obtain a license, a candidate must graduate from an accredited dental hygiene school and pass both a written and a clinical examination. For the clinical examination, the applicant is required to perform dental hygiene procedures, such as removing deposits and stains from a patient's teeth.

The curriculum in a dental hygiene program

consists of courses in the basic sciences, dental sciences, anatomy, physiology, and periodontology (study of gums).

dentist

Dentists examine teeth and tissues of the mouth to diagnose and treat diseases or abnormalities.

They take X-ray studies, place protective plastic shields on children's teeth, fill cavities, straighten teeth, repair fractured teeth, and treat gum disease. Dentists extract teeth when necessary and may provide dentures. They also perform correc-

DENTISTRY

PERMANENT TEETH OF RIGHT SIDE OF JAW

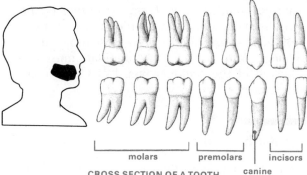

molars   premolars   incisors
canine

CROSS SECTION OF A TOOTH

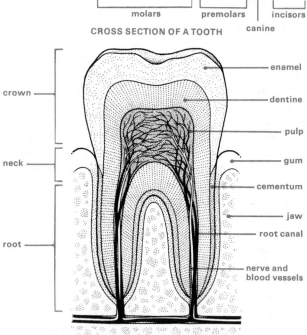

The root of every tooth is securely fixed into a bony socket, and the blood vessels and nerve enter at this site. Enamel, the hardest substance in the body, covers each crown and allows it to endure years of biting, chewing and grinding of foodstuffs.

tive surgery of the gums and supporting bones. In addition, they clean teeth and provide other preventive services.

Most dentists are general practitioners who provide many types of dental care; about 20 percent practice in one of the eight specialty areas recognized by the American Dental Association (ADA). The largest group of specialists are *orthodontists*, who straighten teeth. The next largest group, *oral* and *maxillofacial surgeons*, operate on the mouth and jaws. The remainder specialize in *pedodontics* (dentistry for children); *periodontics* (treating the gums); *prosthodontics* (making artificial teeth or dentures); *endodontics* (root-canal therapy); *public health dentistry*, or *oral pathology* (diseases of the mouth).

To qualify for a license to practice dentistry, a candidate must graduate from a dental school approved by the Commission on Dental Accreditation and pass written and practical examinations. Dental schools generally require four years of undergraduate work. Studies begin with classroom instruction and laboratory work in basic sciences including anatomy, microbiology, biochemistry, and physiology. Courses in preclinical technique and beginning courses in clinical sciences also are provided at this time. During the last two years of training, the student treats patients chiefly in dental clinics.

Most dental colleges award the degree of Doctor of Dental Surgery (D.D.S.). An equivalent degree, Doctor of Dental Medicine (D.M.D.), is conferred by some schools.

dermatologist

A specialist in diseases of skin, hair, and nails. The dermatologist must also have a wide knowledge of the many diseases that, while affecting other systems of the body, also produce changes in the skin.

In skin cancers (see basal cell carcinoma *and* squamous cell carcinoma, *illustrated right) the malignant growth disrupts the tissues and the cells escape from their normal anatomical boundaries. By contrast,* psoriasis *and the* common wart *(see illustration) are not malignant conditions, and the abnormalities of cell growth cause only a thickening or outgrowth of the skin.*

STRUCTURE OF NORMAL SKIN

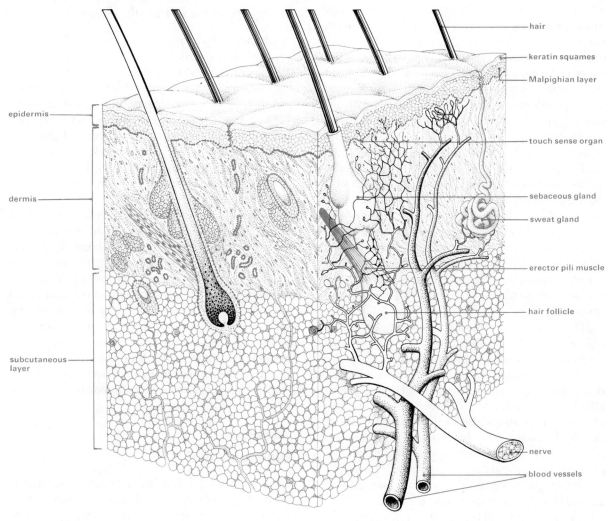

hair

keratin squames

Malpighian layer

epidermis

touch sense organ

dermis

sebaceous gland

sweat gland

erector pili muscle

hair follicle

subcutaneous layer

nerve

blood vessels

SKIN DISEASES

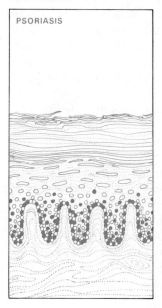

PSORIASIS

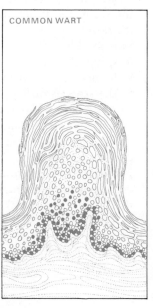

COMMON WART

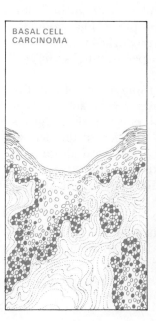

BASAL CELL CARCINOMA

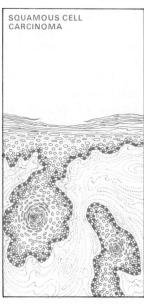

SQUAMOUS CELL CARCINOMA

Skin diseases are very common, representing about 15 percent of all illnesses. Many, especially those caused by infection, are of brief duration and easily controlled, but there are also many that persist throughout life and for which there appears to be no cure. Like other specialties, however, dermatology is advancing rapidly, and these major problems are gradually yielding before advancing knowledge of immunology, virology, molecular biology, and genetics.

The day-to-day work of the dermatologist includes the management of dermatitis caused by a wide range of allergens; other allergic conditions like hives (*urticaria*); fungal infections of the skin such as athlete's foot, jock itch, or scalp ringworm; acne, especially in adolescents; warts (*verrucae*) of all kinds, including plantar warts; herpes simplex infections of the face or genitalia; boils and pustules; psoriasis; the damaging effects of prolonged exposure to sunlight; and cases of possible skin cancer.

When you consult a dermatologist, he or she will be interested in the whole of your previous medical history and family medical history and will want a detailed account of your present skin complaint. Then he or she will closely inspect the affected area, and probably the whole of the rest of your skin, perhaps using a magnifier for a more detailed examination. In some cases, the diagnosis will be immediately apparent and an appropriate treatment can be prescribed. In others, there may be some doubt, and further investigation may be necessary. Skin scrapings may be taken, or even a small biopsy removed under local anesthesia, and these will be sent to the histopathology laboratory for processing, examination, and diagnosis. Bacteriological swabs may be taken for culture, and suspected fungus sampled for microscopy.

Dermatologists have a wide range of effective medications and other treatments, and the repertoire of valuable and effective drugs grows steadily. One important function of the dermatologist, however, is to deal with those skin disorders actually caused by injudicious medication—which, like the effects of sunlight, poses a growing problem.

After graduation from medical school, the prospective dermatologist must complete at least four years of accredited residency training, three of which are in dermatology. He or she is then eligible to take certifying examinations given by the American Board of Dermatology.

emergency-medicine physician

A physician specially trained in treating emergency situations such as accidents or strokes.

It is one of the newest specialties (the American Board of Emergency Medicine was established in 1979) and one of the fastest growing. To become a physician of emergency medicine, residents must have thirty-six months of graduate training in emergency medicine following graduation from medical school. They then must pass oral and written exams given by the American Board of Emergency Medicine.

Most emergency-medicine physicians work in the setting of the emergency room of a hospital; some work in clinics. They see the broadest spectrum of problems of anyone in the health care system. These range from minor complaints or injuries, such as the flu or a small cut that needs one or two stitches, to critical illnesses or injuries, such as a heart attack, that need immediate care by a trained specialist. The emergency-medicine physician must be able to decide which patients are in a life-threatening situation needing immediate care and which patients can safely wait their turn for treatment.

endocrinologist

Special problems that relate to hormone imbalance or growth and development often are referred to an expert for precise diagnosis and treatment. The endocrinologist is concerned with the study and function, in health and disease, of the dozens of different hormones secreted directly into the bloodstream by the endocrine, or ductless, glands. These substances exert a powerful influence on the way we act, think, and respond to the stresses of life.

The major endocrine glands include the *pituitary gland* (traditionally known as the "master gland" because of its great influence on the other endocrine glands), *parathyroid glands, thyroid gland, adrenal glands, islets of Langerhans* (specialized groups of cells in the pancreas that secrete the hormone insulin), *ovaries*, and *testes*.

The body has two complex control systems that make it possible for an individual to respond quickly and efficiently to changes in the environment: the nervous system and the endocrine (or hormonal) system. Ordinarily hormones are re-

THE PITUITARY GLAND – effects of the hormones it secretes into the bloodstream

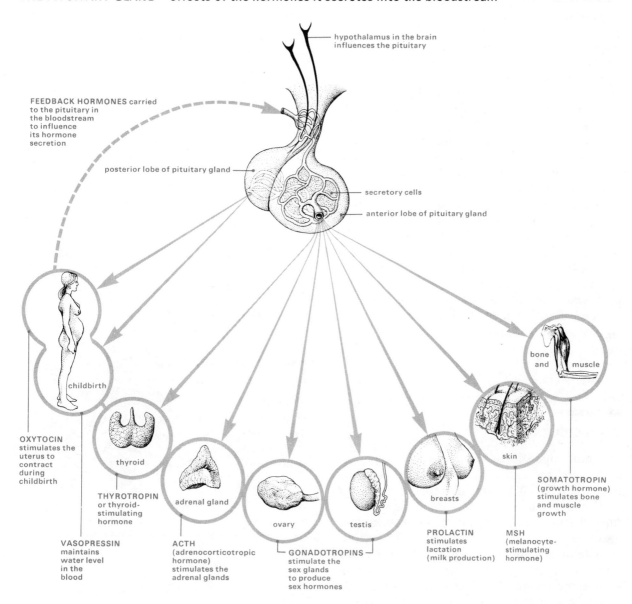

hypothalamus in the brain influences the pituitary

FEEDBACK HORMONES carried to the pituitary in the bloodstream to influence its hormone secretion

posterior lobe of pituitary gland

secretory cells

anterior lobe of pituitary gland

childbirth

bone and muscle

OXYTOCIN stimulates the uterus to contract during childbirth

thyroid

skin

SOMATOTROPIN (growth hormone) stimulates bone and muscle growth

THYROTROPIN or thyroid-stimulating hormone

adrenal gland

ovary

testis

breasts

PROLACTIN stimulates lactation (milk production)

MSH (melanocyte-stimulating hormone)

VASOPRESSIN maintains water level in the blood

ACTH (adrenocorticotropic hormone) stimulates the adrenal glands

GONADOTROPINS stimulate the sex glands to produce sex hormones

leased into the bloodstream following a specific stimulus of an endocrine gland—such as a nerve impulse or a change in the concentration of a specific substance carried to the gland in the blood. In a normal, healthy person the activity of the hormonal system is kept in delicate balance, but sometimes things can go wrong. This is where the endocrinologist comes in.

The endocrinologist deals with diseases that are caused by hormone imbalance. Thus, you are not likely to see an endocrinologist if you have a "garden variety" type of ailment such as a cold, sore throat, or strained back. You may need this specialist, however, if you have a goiter that won't

The pituitary is the "master gland" of the body's hormonal system and influences the activities of the other endocrine glands. It is about the size of a pea and is attached to the base of the brain by a slender stalklike process. This illustration indicates the names and actions of the various hormones the pituitary gland releases into the bloodstream.

regress, or if your physician suspects a problem in your pituitary function.

Certified endocrinologists have graduated from medical school, completed a 3-year residency internal medicine as well as a 2-year fellowship in endocrinology, and passed certifying examinations.

ephebiatrician

A specialist in adolescent medicine. The specialty began to develop in the early 1970s as physicians realized that teenagers have unique needs. They may have outgrown their pediatrician but still have medical needs that are different from those of adults.

Currently there are about one thousand ephebiatricians, according to the Society for Adolescent Medicine. To become an ephebiatrician, one must graduate from medical school and fulfill an internship and residency, usually in pediatrics, family medicine, obstetrics and gynecology, or psychiatry. The physician then spends one to two years in a fellowship in adolescent medicine. A test for board certification is not as yet required.

Ephebiatricians address and treat all medical problems, particularly those of concern to the adolescent, such as menstrual cramps, acne, birth control issues, and sports injuries.

gastroenterologist

The gastroenterologist specializes in the digestive system and the wide range of disorders and diseases that effect it. He or she is concerned with a body system extending a distance of some 30 feet from the mouth to the end of the rectum, and which includes the mouth, throat, gullet (esophagus), stomach, duodenum, pancreas, liver, small intestine (jejunum and ileum), large intestine (colon and rectum), and anal canal.

The gastroenterologist must have an extensive knowledge of internal medicine as well as of the basic sciences underlying the digestion, assimilation, and excretion functions.

Among the many common conditions a gastroenterologist investigates and treats are pharyngeal pouch, swallowing difficulties, narrowing of the esophagus, varicose veins of the esophagus, hiatus hernia, ulcers of the stomach and duodenum, cancer of the stomach, cancer of the pancreas, disorders of the liver and gallbladder, diverticulitis, polyps, ulcerative colitis, irritable bowel syndrome; cancer of the colon, and hemorrhoids.

"Steerable," flexible fiber optic endoscopes have revolutionized the examination of the

THE DIGESTIVE SYSTEM

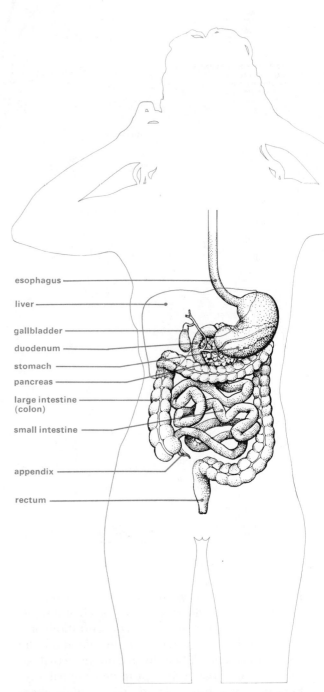

esophagus

liver

gallbladder

duodenum

stomach

pancreas

large intestine (colon)

small intestine

appendix

rectum

The digestive tract is basically a hollow tube which extends from the mouth to the rectum, at the end of the large intestine. Inside this tube, nutrients are digested and assimilated into the body and waste products are formed into a semisolid mass for elimination from the body. Usually nothing serious happens to the automatic working of this complex system. When it does, your physician may refer you to a gastroenterologist.

esophagus, stomach, duodenum, and first part of the small intestine, and have made accessible, for direct vision examination, the rectum and about five feet of the colon. These are the parts of the digestive tract most commonly affected by disease. Now the disease process can often be observed directly, can be photographed in color, and samples (*biopsies*) taken for microscopic confirmation.

The noninvasive methods of CAT and MRI scanning have also greatly increased the diagnostic scope and reliability of the gastroenterologist, enabling him or her to perform, if necessary, a scan of the whole abdomen, so that no important site of disease need be missed. In addition to these methods, ultrasound scanning can be especially useful for liver disease, showing up gallstones, tumors, abscesses, and cysts. In some cases where the exact nature of liver disease is uncertain, the gastroenterologist will take an actual sample of liver (a liver biopsy) through a broadbore needle and send the core of tissue for detailed examination.

Many new and valuable drugs have become available in recent years for gastroenterologic treatment.

The gastroenterologic must work in close association with a surgeon, for many of the diseases he or she is concerned with can be effectively managed only by operative intervention. This applies especially to cancer.

After graduating from medical school, the budding gastroenterologist must undertake a three-year residency in internal medicine and then a two-year fellowship in gastroenterology so as to complete the formal period of training required for certification.

hematologist

The hematologist specializes in disorders of the blood and, to some extent, those affecting the closely associated lymphatic system. A physician trained in the pathological and clinical aspects of blood disorders, this specialist is concerned also with the provision of blood for transfusion and of blood products for the treatment of a variety of disorders.

To become a hematologist, one must graduate from medical school and complete a three-year residency in internal medicine. Once certified in internal medicine, a doctor then fulfills a minimum two-year fellowship required for certification in hematology; many hematologists do an additional fellowship in oncology. The hematologist has undergone a transformation from an expert who spent much of his time in a laboratory producing data for others to use, to a skilled clinician who not only supervises his laboratory but comes more and more into direct contact with patients who are suffering from primary blood diseases; he carries out his own diagnostic procedures and, when a diagnosis is reached, personally supervises the increasingly complex treatments now available.

The hematologist takes a careful history from the patient. Then he examines the patient, paying particular attention to symptoms such as pallor, bruising or bleeding, and enlargement of the lymph nodes in the neck, armpits, or groin. His abdominal examination may detect enlargement of the spleen (under the margin of the left rib) or the liver (similarly placed on the right side). He looks carefully at the mouth and throat for evidence of infection or hemorrhage in the lips, gums, or throat. Blood samples are then taken, upon which a selection of tests from the wide range possible, is carried out.

Once the diagnosis is established, the hematologist often takes personal charge of the treatment. This may be as simple as a course of iron tablets, followed by another blood count to ensure than an anemia has been fully corrected. The condition may, however, be complex—as in acute leukemia—requiring admission to the hospital, the provision of blood platelets for transfusion, the administration of antibiotics for control of infection, and, under blood count surveillance, specific therapy for the leukemia itself.

In many cases, once the diagnosis has been established and the appropriate treatment has been approved, the family physician will resume full responsibility for the patient's medical care and periodic evaluation.

infectious-disease specialist

A patient may be referred to an infectious-disease specialist under a number of circumstances. The typical patient may have a life-threatening infectious illness or an illness that appears to be infectious but in which the cause is not readily apparent; or he may be infected with an organism that requires the use of very potent antibiotics.

Specialists in infectious diseases encounter a great variety of clinical syndromes. Such physicians must be capable of using a number of sophisticated procedures, must be intimately familiar with the large number of antimicrobial drugs available, must be able to select the optimal drug for the specific organism involved, must decide the duration of therapy, and must try to anticipate and prevent potential side effects of any drugs used.

Most experts in this field are concentrated at referral hospitals, the majority being in university hospitals. Usually they are not involved in primary patient care but serve as consultants. Typically, an infectious-disease specialist, after completing medical school, serves an internship and two years of residency training in internal medicine. This is followed by two more years of subspecialty training in infectious diseases. Trainees in the subspecialty gain clinical experience and learn to perform and interpret laboratory procedures to aid in the diagnosis and treatment of infectious diseases. Following this training, they are eligible for board certification in both internal medicine and the treatment of infectious diseases.

Because the subspecialty is a very rapidly changing one—as a consequence of the ongoing development of new pharmacological agents, the identification of previously unknown pathogenic microbes, and the refinement of diagnostic procedures—the specialist must keep abreast of these changes. Several continuing-education activities are offered throughout the year and most subspecialists in this field attend meetings sponsored by the American Academy of Microbiology and the Infectious Diseases Society of America.

internist/general practitioner

A physician trained to provide comprehensive health care for adults, diagnosing and treating physical and mental disorders. In general, he or she does not perform surgery.

Internists' postgraduate training places emphasis on the various organs and organ systems and the diseases that can affect them, such as disorders of the heart and lungs or of the gastrointestinal tract. Most internists then choose to specialize in one of these systems, and as a result true general practitioners are hard to find. However, even the internist who "specializes" in one system, such as the gastrointestinal tract, should be able to provide solid basic care. (See PRIMARY-CARE PHYSICIAN.)

laboratory personnel

Laboratory tests, which detect changes in the body fluids and tissues, play an essential part in the diagnosis and treatment of disease.

Although physicians use the results of laboratory evaluation and diagnosis, they do not perform the tests themselves. Instead, the tests are done by clinical laboratory personnel, who may be either medical technologists or medical technicians.

Medical laboratory technologists have a bachelor's degree in science, as a rule. They perform complicated chemical, hematological, microscopic, and bacteriological tests. These may include chemical tests to determine the blood cholesterol level, for example, or microscopic examination of the blood to detect the presence of disease. Technologists microscopically examine other body fluids; make cultures of body fluids or tissue samples to determine the presence of bacteria, viruses, or other microorganisms; and analyze the samples for chemical content or reaction. They also type and cross-match blood samples for transfusions.

Medical laboratory technicians generally have an associate degree or a diploma or certificate from a private postsecondary school. They are midlevel laboratory workers who function under the supervision of a medical technologist or laboratory supervisor. They perform a wide range of routine tests and laboratory procedures that do not require the analytical knowledge of medical technologists. Like technologists, they may work in several areas or specialize in one field.

licensed practical nurse (LPN)

Nurses who are trained and licensed to provide basic care, such as taking temperatures, giving injections, and changing wound dressings, under the supervision of a registered nurse. They attend a one-year program in practical nursing.

midwife

Midwives manage uncomplicated pregnancies, deliver babies, and give postpartum and gynecological care. Certified nurse-midwives are registered nurses who have received advanced education in midwifery and are certified by the

American College of Nurse-Midwives. They work in clinical collaboration with physicians. They may also direct classes in nutrition, in the techniques of relaxation, in special exercises for pregnant women, and in care of the baby once it is born. Laypeople and other nurses also may practice midwifery in accordance with state laws.

Long accepted in Europe, midwives are becoming more popular in the United States; most work in hospitals.

naturopath

Naturopathy is a system of health care based on the belief that disease is provoked by violation of "nature's laws" and that the reparation of physical or psychological disorder depends entirely on the use of diet, massage, or special bathing procedures. The naturopath believes, not incorrectly, that health is the normal state of the human being, and, quite incorrectly, that it can invariably be maintained by "natural" foods alone.

Although naturopathy may seem a reasonable philosophy for someone in good health, for someone in ill health it may be dangerous. Few naturopaths have formal medical skills and thus they may fail to recognize life-threatening but curable disorders such as tuberculosis. There is no scientific basis for the claims of naturopaths in healing.

neurologist

A neurologist is a specially trained physician who treats diseases and disorders of the nervous system. He sees patients who have symptoms such as headaches, back pain, dizziness, muscular weakness, poor balance, impaired sensation, poor memory, lapses of consciousness, and convulsive seizures. Like other doctors, he tries to diagnose the cause of such complaints by examining the patient, asking questions, and performing or requesting various laboratory tests. Compared with other specialists, however, the neurologist is at some disadvantage because he cannot see, feel, hear, or sample the body parts that concern him; and a neurologist must diagnose disorders in nerve tissue encased by the bones of the skull and spine or concealed deep within the trunk or limbs.

Thus the neurologist must resort to an indirect method of examining the nervous system by observing the way it performs its various functions. He takes advantage of the highly specialized way

the nervous system acts and the location of certain functions in particular parts of the system. For example, a person may have trouble moving the right side of his face and hand. The neurologist knows that impulses for such movements originate in the left side of the brain. He also knows that impulses to the right leg originate near the top of the left side of the brain and that impulses to the face and hand originate next to each other near the bottom of the left side of the brain. His knowledge of nervous-system structures and functions allows him to deduce that this particular patient has a disorder of the lower part of the left half of the brain. In daily practice, he deals with many more complicated problems in pinpointing a neurological disorder, but the principle is always the same. He pieces together changes in the patient's thinking, vision, strength, coordination, sensation, and reflexes and determines where the disorder might lie.

Once a tentative diagnosis has been made, the neurologist may then turn to the wide range of available imaging techniques for confirmation. These include X-ray, CAT or MRI scanning, standard angiography, digital subtraction angiography, air encephalography, and isotope scanning. In some cases, electroencephalography may help. (See specific tests in **Tests**.) These tests also help in discovering the disorder that is causing the problem, such as tumor, injury, ischemia, demyelinization, or inflammation.

The neurologist is a consultant who works best in cooperation with other doctors. He pinpoints neurological problems for primary-care physicians and supplies suggestions for treatment. He refers patients who need surgical treatment to a neurosurgeon. He may himself become the primary-care doctor for patients with chronic neurological illnesses (seizures, multiple sclerosis, Parkinson's disease), but he still remembers to coordinate his care with a general doctor and with specialists in rehabilitation and urology.

Before a neurologist can apply for board certification by the American Board of Psychiatry and Neurology, he must have completed at least four years of postgraduate training and experience; then, to be certified, he must pass the board's extensive written and oral examinations.

neurosurgeon

Neurosurgery is the medical specialty that consists of the evaluation, diagnosis, and surgical treat-

THE HUMAN NERVOUS SYSTEM

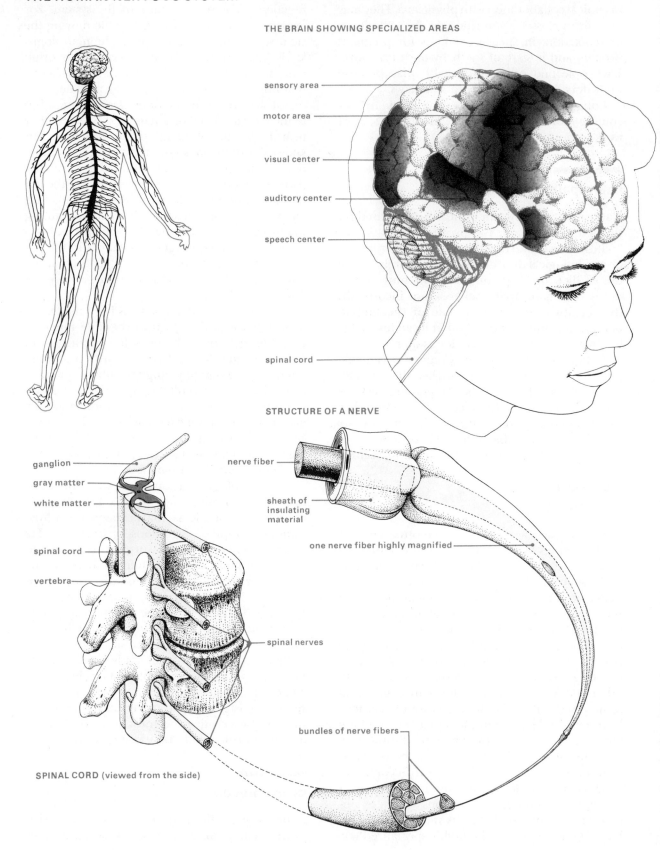

THE BRAIN SHOWING SPECIALIZED AREAS

sensory area

motor area

visual center

auditory center

speech center

spinal cord

STRUCTURE OF A NERVE

nerve fiber

sheath of insulating material

one nerve fiber highly magnified

ganglion

gray matter

white matter

spinal cord

vertebra

spinal nerves

bundles of nerve fibers

SPINAL CORD (viewed from the side)

ment of diseases involving the nervous system (brain, spinal cord, and nerves).

Because of the highly specialized nature of this field, the neurosurgeon generally sees patients on a consultation basis. That is, most of his patients are referred to him by other physicians who suspect their patients may have a disorder of the nervous system that will be amenable to surgical treatment. Because the evaluation of such disorders is a highly intricate and sophisticated process, very often a definitive diagnosis is not made until *after* this consultation. Therefore, the neurosurgeon must also be completely trained as a neurological diagnostician.

Like the sleuth of detective fiction, the neurosurgeon listens, looks, and investigates for clues in order to make a diagnosis. The "history-taking," in which he discusses the symptoms and complaints with the patient, is of utmost importance in providing details as to what the patient actually is experiencing and what the pattern of symptoms has been. This information is pivotal in making the diagnosis, since many disorders of the nervous system follow a special pattern in terms of timing, progress, and anatomical distribution. Therefore, the more accurate the information given by the patient, the more accurate the diagnosis.

The neurological examination that follows is designed to test and evaluate those bodily functions that are related to the activity of the nerves, spinal cord, and brain. These include movement and strength of all extremities, reflex activity, sensation in all extremities and on the face and trunk, balance and coordination, thinking ability, speech, and the special senses of sight, smell, and hearing. Full use is then made of all available imaging techniques, especially CAT and MRI SCAN-

The human nervous system (shown left) can be broadly divided into two parts: the central nervous system (the brain and spinal cord) and the peripheral nervous system (the branching network that supplies our skin, muscles, and internal organs). The brain acts as the controlling center, interpreting all incoming information from the senses and adapting our behavior accordingly. Specific areas on its surface are responsible for the special senses and for generating speech and movement. All the signals between the brain and the body flow up and down pathways in the spinal cord, and this vital structure is well protected by the bony vertebrae. Pairs of spinal nerves attach to the spinal cord at regular intervals and they contain motor and sensory fibers which supply muscles and skin, respectively.

NING and ANGIOGRAPHY (see under *Tests*). Correlating this information with that obtained during the history-taking, the physician arrives at the diagnostic possibilities that confirm his impressions and provide the basis for a specialized plan of treatment.

All of the accredited training programs for neurosurgeons in the United States are geared toward providing these skills. To enter such a program, one must be a graduate of an accredited medical school and have completed at least one year of formal training in general surgery. The actual residency program in neurological surgery is a minimum of four years, but may be as many as seven, depending upon the institution chosen. During the latter part of his residency, the individual may take the written examination given by the American Board of Neurological Surgeons. However, the final examination cannot be taken until the candidate has successfully completed his formal training program and has been in practice for two years in one location. At that time he must submit the case histories and records of all the patients he cared for in those two years as well as recommendations by his colleagues and training institution. He must then successfully complete an oral examination by the American Board of Neurological Surgeons before it will award him a diploma of certification.

This rigorous process is designed to provide the public with the best possible care in a highly specialized field of surgery. A neurosurgeon who is "board certified" has gone through the process and has accomplished all of these objectives. A "board eligible" neurosurgeon is one who has fulfilled all the basic requirements but has not yet completed the oral examination.

nutritionist/dietician

Health professional trained and licensed to apply knowledge of proper dietary principles in the maintenance of good health. He or she also can treat certain diseases caused by nutritional deficiencies.

A bachelor's degree with a major in foods and nutrition or institution management is the basic educational requirement for this field. To qualify for professional credentials as a Registered Dietician (R.D.), the American Dietetic Association (ADA) recommends completion of a coordinated undergraduate program that includes an internship; completion of a bachelor's degree plus an approved dietetic internship or three years of approved qualified experience; or six months of approved qualified experience plus an advanced degree. The internship lasts six to twelve months and combines clinical experience under a qualified dietician and some classroom work.

obstetrician/gynecologist

The obstetrician/gynecologist specializes in treating all the disorders that affect a woman, particularly those involving the sexual organs. The obstetrician usually cares for a woman before, during, and after pregnancy; the gynecologist's care is more general.

Women see a gynecologist in order to find out about their health, sexuality, and fertility. A gynecologist also can help a woman decide what method of contraception is best. It is now well established that women should go to a gynecologist for regular breast exams and cervical smears, particularly women who are in a high-risk group. Some symptoms suggestive of a gynecological disorder are vaginal discharge, abnormal bleeding, low back pain and pelvic pressure, and irritation of the genitalia.

Any woman who is planning to have a baby or who is already pregnant should consult an obstetrician immediately. The obstetrician can guide her throughout pregnancy, conducting routine prenatal exams to ensure both her health and that of the fetus. Study upon study has shown that routine prenatal care begun in the first trimester decreases the chance of complications. The obstetrician delivers the baby and provides care for the newborn.

Approved residency programs for "ob-gyn" candidates run for four years following graduation from medical school. They include broad experience in internal medicine, pediatrics, anesthesiology, urology, and nephrology, as well as in obstetrics and gynecology—including gynecological surgery. At the conclusion of a year in practice, the candidate can take the written and oral examinations given by the American Board of Obstetrics and Gynecology. When he successfully passes such examinations he becomes a "diplomate" of the board, certified as competent in all areas of his specialty. He may then choose to practice as a general ob-gyn specialist, or may continue an extra two years of fellowship training to qualify in one of the subspecialties.

occupational therapist

Occupational therapists treat people of all ages who are mentally, developmentally, or emotionally disabled. Therapists provide their patients with specialized activities that aid them in mastering the skills necessary to perform daily tasks at home, at work, at school, and in the community. For those with a disability, being able to perform a daily activity such as getting dressed without assistance is an important step toward an independent, productive, and satisfying life.

Like other health professionals, occupational therapists usually work as a member of a team that may include a physician, nurse, physical therapist, psychologist, rehabilitation counselor, and social worker. Team members evaluate the patient in terms of their individual specialties and consult with each other to arrive at an overall assessment of the patient's capacities, skills, and abilities. Together they develop goals that meet the patient's needs and decide what treatment methods to use.

Various activities are used as therapy tools. They are designed to prepare patients to return to work, develop or restore basic functions, and aid in adjustment to disabilities. When working with children, occupational therapists often use toys and games to teach a variety of skills. With other patients, occupational therapists use activities of daily living such as meal preparation, bathing, and dressing, which patients practice in clinic areas set up as kitchens and bathrooms. Woodworking, leatherwork or other therapeutic activities are used to increase motor skills, strength, endurance, concentration, and motivation as preparation for applying these skills to the tasks of daily life.

Occupational therapists often work with patients who have lost basic functional skills such as unaided movement of their limbs. Loss of motor skills and coordination may result from spinal cord injury, for example, or be associated with a chronic disease such as muscular dystrophy. Therapists provide individuals with adaptive equipment such as wheelchairs, splints, and aids for eating and dressing. They may design and make special equipment for disabled patients and recommend changes in the home or work environment to facilitate functioning.

Preparation for this field requires a bachelor's degree in occupational therapy. Most states require a license to practice occupational therapy. Applicants for a license must have a degree or certificate from an accredited educational program and pass the American Occupational Therapy Association's certification examination, which awards the title of Registered Occupational Therapist (O.T.R.) to qualified applicants.

Coursework in occupational therapy programs includes physical, biological, and behavioral sciences and the application of occupational therapy theory and skills. These programs also require students to work for six to nine months in hospitals, health agencies, or schools to gain experience in clinical practice.

oncologist

A specialist in the diagnosis and treatment of tumors, both benign and malignant. The oncologist seeks to determine the cause and pattern of abnormal new growth of cells or tissues associated with tumors, malignant or not.

There is much to be discovered about how and why tumors develop, but essentially the process is one in which cells (or a cell) within a group at a particular time in life begin to multiply and either produce an enlarged mass of the original tissue (a benign tumor) or lose their differentiation and grow continuously (a malignant tumor), possibly invading adjacent structures or throwing off cells to form colonies elsewhere in the body (known as secondaries, or metastases). What causes this change is not completely known for each tumor, but several cancer-causing stimuli (carcinogens) are known to provoke the change.

Often the clue to the disease is given in a patient's history. For example, marked weight loss, decreased appetite, blood in the sputum, localized back pain all suggest a lung tumor (and many benign conditions too). It is essential to establish the correct diagnosis before the often tragic news is imparted and before the correct treatment can be commenced.

A wide range of methods of investigation is available. These include X rays, endoscopy, CAT and MRI scanning, biopsy, thermography, radioisotope scanning, angiography, and exploratory operations (see under *Tests*). Having established the presence of a tumor, the oncologist will attempt to discover if it has invaded elsewhere and perhaps spread through the body. If a tumor is cancerous, the oncologist can allot it to a particular stage of development. International medical agreement regarding staging allows the effectiveness of treatments to be compared in cancer centers throughout the world.

Oncologists usually qualify as specialists in internal medicine, then undergo an additional fellowship of clinical training in oncology, which includes radiation therapy, chemotherapy, and hematology. Working usually in a medical center, the oncologist also coordinates the other specialists involved in the management of cancer, such as the surgeons, gynecologists, and radiologists. He may well further specialize to become expert in a subdivision such as colorectal, gynecological, or head and neck tumors; others become involved in research, publicity, and prevention programs.

ophthalmologist

The ophthalmologist's role is to diagnose and treat abnormalities of the eye, both medically and surgically. He should not be confused with the *optometrist*, who is licensed (in many states) only to examine the eyes and prescribe corrective lenses; the optometrist's training and experience may qualify him to recognize evidence of serious disease, in which case he should make a referral to a qualified medical doctor, usually an ophthalmologist. The *optician* is a highly skilled technician who is qualified to fill lens prescriptions. The *orthoptist* and *ophthalmic assistant*, seen in many ophthalmologists' offices, are specially trained persons who are qualified to relieve the ophthalmologist of many routine and time-consuming duties. Such personnel must work under the ophthalmologist's direct supervision; they may apply eyedrops required for special tests and may conduct vision testing using standard eye charts. Orthoptists also assist the ophthalmologist in the management of STABISMUS (squint) and AMBLYOPIA.

The qualified ophthalmologist must have a broad knowledge of general medicine and also years of rigorous clinical training and experience in the diagnosis and treatment, both medical and surgical, of the diseases and injuries that affect vision. After receiving the M.D. degree from an accredited medical school, he must complete four years of postgraduate clinical training. He spends the first year as an intern in general medicine and surgery and the following three years in residency training in an approved program, usually at an eye facility within a medical center or teaching hospital. Here he will gain experience in diag-

THE EYE

The eye is actually a direct extension of the brain. The retina, the light-sensitive structure at the back of the eye, contains millions of rods and cones—specialized nerve endings which convert light into electrical impulses. These impulses are then conveyed by the optic nerve to the visual center at the back of the brain, where the individual interprets them as specific images.

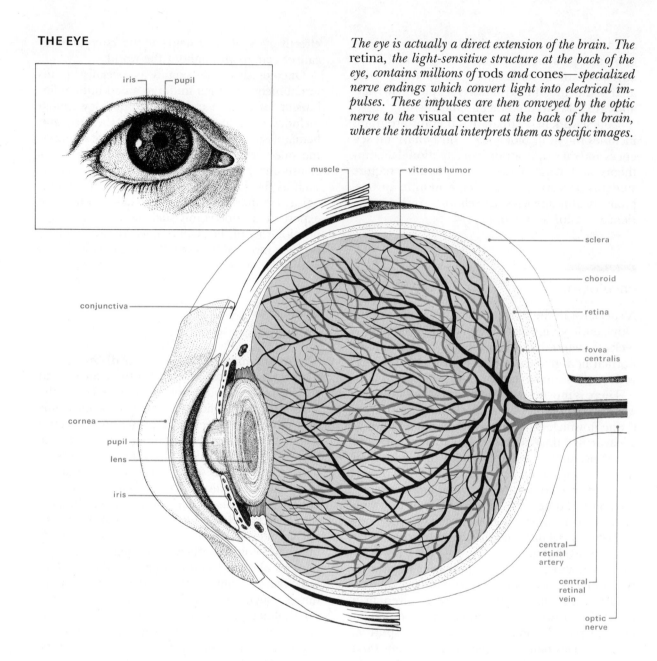

nosing and treating all types of eye disorders, using medical and surgical techniques as needed. After completing residency training, he must practice his specialty for at least one year to be eligible to take the written and oral examinations necessary for certification by the American Board of Ophthalmology. If he should choose to specialize in one specific area of ophthalmology, he may devote an additional year or two after residency to fellowship training in the subspecialty of his choice.

A substantial number of the ophthalmologist's patients seek him out only after their vision has been impaired significantly or when their eyes hurt severely. Very serious damage may have taken place by then. Thus, it pays to heed early warning signs and to seek out expert advice promptly. Some of these signs are: fuzzy vision; double vision; halos; crossed eyes; "cobwebs," "floaters," and flashes of light; sensitivity to light; inflamed eyes; white pupil; and "cat's-eye" pupil (a slit-like, elongated pupil).

It is advisable for adults past the age of 40 to have periodic checkups for glaucoma and, in later years, checkups for cataracts every two years. Patients who have sickle-cell anemia or diabetes should have their eyes examined at six-month intervals.

optometrists

Half the people in the United States wear glasses or contact lenses. Optometrists (*doctors of optometry*) provide much of the vision care these people need.

Optometrists should not be confused with either ophthalmologists or dispensing opticians. *Ophthalmologists* are physicians (doctors of medicine) who specialize in medical eye care, eye diseases, and eye injuries; perform eye surgery; and prescribe drugs or other eye treatment, as well as lenses. Dispensing *opticians* fit and adjust eyeglasses and contact lenses according to prescriptions written by the ophthalmologist or optometrist; they do not examine eyes or prescribe treatment.

Optometrists examine people's eyes to diagnose vision problems and detect signs of disease and other abnormal conditions. They also test to ensure that the patient has proper depth and color perception and the ability to focus and coordinate the eyes. When necessary, they prescribe lenses and other treatment. When optometrists diagnose diseases requiring treatment beyond the optometric scope of practice, they arrange for consultation with the appropriate health care practitioners. Most optometrists supply the prescribed eyeglasses or contact lenses and also prescribe vision therapy or other treatment that does not require surgery. In most states, they cannot prescribe drugs.

Optometrists must be licensed. Applicants for a license must have a Doctor of Optometry degree from an accredited optometric school or college and pass a state board examination or the test of the National Board of Examiners in Optometry. In most states, optometrists must earn continuing-education credits in optometry to renew their licenses.

The Doctor of Optometry degree requires a minimum of six or seven years of higher education consisting of a four-year professional degree program preceded by at least two or three years of preoptometric study at an accredited university, college, or junior college. Most optometry students enter with at least a bachelor's degree.

Optometrists wishing to advance in a specialized field may study for a master's or Ph.D. degree in visual science, physiological optics, neurophysiology, public health, health administration, health information and communication, or health education.

orthopedist

The modern orthopedist is concerned primarily with the diagnosis and treatment of injuries and diseases that affect the bones and joints and with correcting skeletal deformities. His tasks range from the resetting of a dislocated shoulder (which any physician can do) to the highly skilled surgical replacement of a diseased hip joint with an artificial ball-and-socket joint or even surgical repair of a herniated spinal disk (an ability he shares with the neurosurgeon).

How do you choose an orthopedist and how can you know that he is competent? Most often you will be referred to one by your personal physician, who may be able to judge which orthopedist is best qualified to deal with you as a patient and to treat your particular problem. You might also meet an orthopedist for the first time if you are an accident victim and are brought to the emergency room of a hospital, or you might seek one out on the recommendation of a friend who has a similar problem.

The certified orthopedist qualifies by graduation from medical school, followed by five years of postgraduate clinical training and experience. The first year may be a revolving internship in general medicine, or it can, by choice, be entirely in surgery; the second year will be in surgery (such as plastic surgery, neurosurgery, or general surgery); the last three years will be devoted entirely to gaining knowledge and experience in all areas of orthopedics and orthopedic surgery, including pediatric, hand, total joint replacement, and all forms of reconstructive surgery. He or she must then practice for at least three years before seeking membership in the American Academy of Orthopedic Surgery, a society devoted to the continuing education of its members, the encouragement of orthopedic research, and the maintenance of a standard of excellence in orthopedic practice.

The orthopedist works in close cooperation with family doctors, rheumatologists, and other specialists who refer patients to him. When he has made his examination and diagnosis and decided on what treatments are indicated, he will discuss his findings with the referring physician.

As in other specialties, some orthopedists limit their practice to specific surgical procedures and treatments. Thus, if one orthopedist should refer you to another, you may accept his recommendation as being in your best interest. Such re-

THE SKELETON

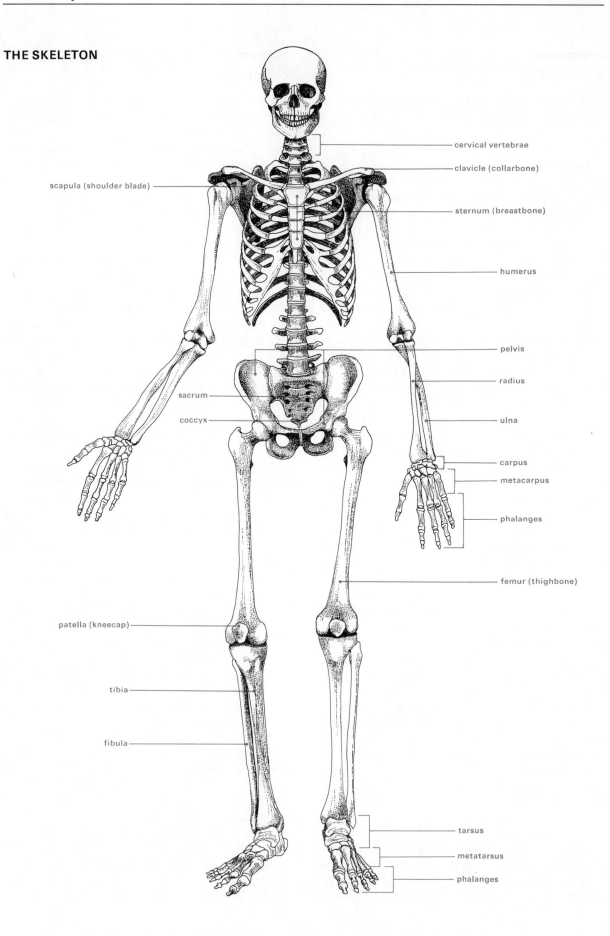

cervical vertebrae

clavicle (collarbone)

scapula (shoulder blade)

sternum (breastbone)

humerus

pelvis

radius

sacrum

ulna

coccyx

carpus

metacarpus

phalanges

femur (thighbone)

patella (kneecap)

tibia

fibula

tarsus

metatarsus

phalanges

ferrals often are made in certain diseases and high-risk surgical cases that the general orthopedist may see only two or three times a year; he knows that the patient will be served better by an orthopedist who deals with such patients regularly.

Recovery from almost any orthopedic problem requires time. Patients should remember that it takes a considerable time to heal a fractured femur (thigh bone) or to recover from a severe back injury. Most of the serious diseases and disorders treated by orthopedists require rehabilitation counseling and treatment. A patient who has just received a new hip or knee joint or a prosthetic leg needs instruction and encouragement to help him become proficient in its use. In order to obtain the best possible results, orthopedists treat the patient with understanding, compassion, and psychological support during the period of readjustment and recovery.

osteopath

Doctors of osteopathy (D.O.s) are similar to medical doctors in their training, licensure, and practice. Their training includes four years of college, four years of osteopathy school, and a residency; whereas M.D.s have twenty-three specialties to choose from, D.O.s have about fifteen.

Osteopaths and M.D.s differ mainly in their philosophy of medicine. Osteopaths believe that the body has a natural ability to defend itself against disease and thus they place great emphasis on preventive care, including diet and fitness. In addition, they are trained to perform osteopathic manipulative therapy, which they use to treat disorders through manipulation of the spine.

otolaryngologist

A specialist in diseases of the ear, nose, and throat, the otolaryngologist must be proficient in the detailed examination of certain very inaccessible

The bones of the skeleton (shown left) are living tissues, quite unlike the brittle and bleached collection of bones seen wired together in museums or biology classes. The skeleton is composed of 50 percent water and 50 percent inorganic salts (mainly calcium and phosphorus) and begins to form in the fetus during the second month of pregnancy. It is the supporting and protective framework of the body and provides points of attachment for the muscles.

areas, such as the recesses of the nasal cavities, the depths of the middle ear, and the vocal cords. He or she is a surgeon who must be a master of microsurgery of extreme delicacy, and yet must be prepared to carry out relatively crude operations on the bones of the nasal sinuses.

Formerly known as oto*rhino*laryngology (-*rhino* refers to the nose), the title of this specialty was shortened, some years ago, for convenience. The otolaryngologist must treat nasal obstruction, severe nosebleeds, deviated septum, allergic rhinitis, nasal polyps, adenoids, Eustachian tube obstruction, and all the common inflammatory problems of the para-nasal sinuses that drain into the nose. The treatment of persistent sinusitis often involves surgical opening, through bone, so that proper drainage of sinuses can be restored. Many otolaryngologists are equipped, both by training and experience, to perform rhinoplasty (cosmetic nose surgery).

The otolaryngologist treats many patients with throat problems, the most common of these being infections of the tonsils and surrounding tissues. Sometimes he has to deal with a *quinsy*—a serious abscess beneath a tonsil—calling for surgical incision. Other diseases include those of the larynx, especially laryngitis, laryngeal paralysis, singer's nodes on the vocal cords, and cancer.

In his management of ear problems, the otolaryngologist commonly treats middle ear infections (otitis media), particularly in children who develop chronic serious effusion so that the mechanism of the middle ear becomes glued up and inefficient.

Working with an operating microscope, under incredibly confined conditions, the otolaryngologist is able to treat the disease of otosclerosis, which cause deafness by leading to a bony fixation of the footplate of the inner of the three ossicles.

The otolaryngologist is also an expert in the diagnosis and assessment of the different forms of hearing loss, using refined instruments to perform various kinds of audiometric examination that can measure hearing loss at different frequencies and intensities and help to determine the cause and the best methods of treatment. He is able to advise on whether a hearing aid will help, in any particular case, and, if so, what kind is likely to be most suitable.

The qualified otolaryngologist is certified by the American Board of Otolaryngology after graduating from medical school, completing five years of residency training, and passing certifying examinations.

THE EAR

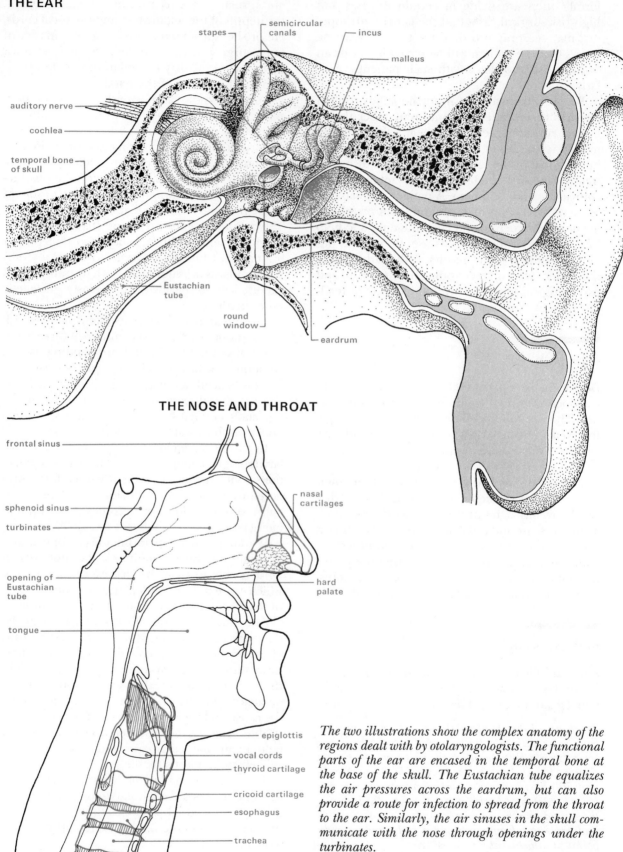

- stapes
- semicircular canals
- incus
- malleus
- auditory nerve
- cochlea
- temporal bone of skull
- Eustachian tube
- round window
- eardrum

THE NOSE AND THROAT

- frontal sinus
- sphenoid sinus
- turbinates
- opening of Eustachian tube
- tongue
- nasal cartilages
- hard palate
- epiglottis
- vocal cords
- thyroid cartilage
- cricoid cartilage
- esophagus
- trachea

The two illustrations show the complex anatomy of the regions dealt with by otolaryngologists. The functional parts of the ear are encased in the temporal bone at the base of the skull. The Eustachian tube equalizes the air pressures across the eardrum, but can also provide a route for infection to spread from the throat to the ear. Similarly, the air sinuses in the skull communicate with the nose through openings under the turbinates.

pathologist

A physician who specializes in the study of the origin, development, causes, and effects of disease.

In most hospitals, there are three types of pathologists: the clinical pathologist, the surgical pathologist, and the autopsy pathologist.

The *clinical pathologist* receives samples of patients' body fluids, tissues, or stool which he examines for the clear presence or the signs of disease. The clinical pathologist performs blood counts and tests to determine the coagulation time and hemoglobin content of the blood. He also takes smears and cultures of suspect materials from patients to isolate and identify viral or bacterial infectious organisms. He also studies patients' urine and stool, and even their stomach contents, to determine their composition, the presence of abnormal elements, and the presence of disease-causing factors. Once the pathologist completes his work, he sends the results back to the patient's physician who ordered them. That physician then uses the results in making a diagnosis and explains it to the patient.

The *surgical pathologist* is usually present at any operation in which tissue is removed from a patient. He may examine tissue while the surgery is in progress to determine if the operation should be modified. For example, an operation will proceed quite differently if a tumor removed is benign rather than malignant. When examining the tissue for a correct diagnosis, the pathologist usually uses a small portion of tissue. This is referred to as a *biopsy.*

The *autopsy pathologist* examines the body after death. An autopsy involves both the inspection of the entire body with organs and tissues intact and the microscopic examination of small samples of tissue. The autopsy is important for several reasons: It can confirm whether the diagnosis in a spent patient was correct; it can determine conditions which may be hereditary and therefore are of importance to surviving relatives; and it can result in the discovery of rare or new diseases. Results of an autopsy should always be explained to family members in an understanding and caring manner.

The pathologist first studies in all areas of general medicine, then spends a minimum of four years in residency training to be eligible for certification in his specialty. He may choose to practice in one of the divisions of pathology explained above, or in all three of them. If a pathologist is interested in a particular organ system, he may limit his practice to that subspecialty—such as hematologic pathology or neuropathology. Pathologists may work in hospitals or maintain private laboratories to which doctors send specimens for study.

pediatrician

Pediatricians are physicians who have acquired a special interest in and knowledge of the health needs of infants, children, and adolescents by virtue of an extensive training in these areas after completion of formal medical education. They have graduated from medical school and fulfilled a three-year residency in general pediatrics, and as well may have completed an additional two- to three-year fellowship in a pediatric subspecialty. Pediatricians are certified by the American Board of Pediatrics. These physicians provide the bulk of primary medical care for children today.

Ideally, first-time parents should choose a pediatrician a short time before the actual birth of the child. The pediatrician frequently is someone recommended by another physician, such as the mother's obstetrician, or by friends or relatives. A meeting prior to the baby's birth allows the parents to assess the physician's attitude without any urgency imposed by the infant's immediate medical needs. It is assumed that the physician has been educated and trained in the health requirements of children, that he therefore has a sincere interest in children and is a personal advocate for them, and that he is comfortable in the management of their illnesses.

The prospective parents need to evaluate how this physician relates to them. Usually it is advisible for both parents to meet the physician at this initial visit, unless circumstances make this impossible. Questions relating to scheduling of visits, office practice, and fees are appropriate to this discussion. In addition, parents need to know when it is best to telephone with routine questions, what the procedure is for obtaining aid in an emergency, and who will cover for the pediatrician when he is away or otherwise unavailable. Many physicians have a routine "telephone hour" to answer necessary but nonemergency questions. Some physicians include nurse practitioners as part of the expanded health team. The parent should ask about and understand the role of these "health care extenders."

Similarly, parents of older children who relocate in a new community should meet the new pediatrician prior to the acute illness of any one child. This again allows for a nonharried interview and assessment of the relationship between the health provider and the family—both parents and children. Ideally, the relationship between the child and the physician—as well as between the parents and physician—should be one of mutual respect and affection.

pharmacist

There are thousands of drugs on the market, and their complexity and potential side effects have caused health professionals and the public alike to rely increasingly on the special knowledge of *pharmacists.* In addition to providing information about drugs and drug treatments, pharmacists dispense drugs and medicines as prescribed by physicians, podiatrists, and dentists. Pharmacists must understand the use, composition, and effects of drugs and how they are tested for purity and strength. They may maintain patient medication profiles and advise physicians on the proper selection and use of medicines. Compounding— the actual mixing of ingredients to form powders, tablets, capsules, ointments, and solutions—is now only a small (but important) part of a pharmacist's practice, since most medicines are produced by manufacturers in the dosages and forms used by patients.

Pharmacists in hospitals and clinics dispense inpatient and outpatient prescription medications and advise the medical staff on the selection and effects of drugs. They may make sterile solutions, buy medical supplies, teach in schools for health professionals, and perform administrative duties. They also may be involved in patient education, monitoring of drug regimens, and drug-use review. In addition, pharmacists work as consultants to the medical team on drug therapy and patient care in hospitals, nursing homes, and other health care facilities. Their role is crucial to safe, efficient, and proper therapeutic care.

Some pharmacists prepare and dispense radioactive pharmaceuticals. Called *radiopharmacists* or *nuclear pharmacists,* they apply the principles and practices of pharmacy and radiochemistry to produce radioactive drugs that are used for patient diagnosis and therapy.

A license to practice pharmacy is required in all states. To obtain a license, one must graduate from an accredited pharmacy program, pass a state board examination, and have a specified amount of practical experience or serve an internship under the supervision of a licensed pharmacist. Internships generally are served in a community or hospital pharmacy.

At least five years of study beyond high school is required to graduate from programs accredited by the American Council on Pharmaceutical Education in the seventy-two colleges of pharmacy. Five years are needed to obtain a Bachelor of Science (B.S.) or a Bachelor of Pharmacy (B. Pharm.) degree, the degrees received by most graduates. A Doctor of Pharmacy (Pharm.D.) degree normally requires six years.

physical therapist

Physical therapists plan, organize, and administer treatment to restore functional mobility, relieve pain, and prevent or limit permanent disability for those suffering from a disabling injury or disease. Their patients include accident victims, handicapped children, and stroke victims. Physical therapy also is used in the treatment of multiple sclerosis, cerebral palsy, nerve injuries, amputations, fractures, arthritis, heart disease, and other conditions.

Therapists may treat patients with a wide variety of problems, or they may specialize in pediatrics, geriatrics, orthopedics, sports medicine, neurology, or cardiopulmonary diseases.

Initially, physical therapists review and evaluate the patient's condition and medical records, perform tests or measurements, and interpret the findings. Then they develop a treatment plan in cooperation with the patient's physician. The goal is to help patients attain maximum functional independence, muscle strength, and physical skills and, at the same time, adapt to what may be a drastic change in physical abilities. Patients often are suffering emotional as well as physical stress, and treatment requires sensitivity in addition to technical proficiency on the part of the therapist.

Therapeutic procedures include exercise for increasing strength, endurance, coordination, and range of motion; electrical stimulation to activate paralyzed muscles; instruction in carrying out everyday activities and in the use of assistive devices; and the application of massage, heat, cold, light, water, electricity, or ultrasound to relieve pain or improve the condition of muscles and skin. To carry out these procedures, therapists must have detailed knowledge of human anatomy and physiology and know what steps to take to treat the effects of disease and injury.

All states require a license to practice physical therapy. Applicants must have a degree or certificate from an accredited physical therapy educational program prior to taking the licensure examination.

Three different types of programs provide educational preparation for entry-level jobs in this field: bachelor's-degree programs in physical therapy; certificate (or second bachelor's-degree) programs for those who already hold a bachelor's in another field, such as biology; and entry-level master's-degree programs in physical therapy. Efforts are under way to raise entry-level educational requirements from the bachelor's- to the master's-degree level.

The physical therapy curriculum includes science courses such as anatomy, physiology, neuroanatomy, and neurophysiology; it also includes specialized courses such as biomechanics, human growth and development, manifestations of disease and trauma, and courses in specific therapeutic procedures. Besides receiving classroom instruction, students get supervised clinical experience in administering physical therapy to patients in hospitals and other treatment centers.

physician assistant

The occupation of physician assistant (P.A.) came into being during the 1960s, when physicians were in short supply. Additional education enabled medical corpsmen trained during the Vietnam conflict, as well as some nurses and others with experience in patient care, to relieve physicians of many essential but time-consuming tasks. P.A.s interview patients, take medical histories, perform physical examinations, order laboratory tests, make tentative diagnoses, and prescribe appropriate treatments. Studies show they have the ability to care for eight out of ten people who visit a family practitioner's office in any one day. P.A.s always work under the direction of a licensed "supervising physician," however. Alternative titles sometimes used by these workers are "Medex" and "physician associate."

About half of all P.A.s assist physicians in such specialty areas as pediatrics and surgery. They perform routine procedures such as physical examinations, provide postoperative care, and assist during complicated medical procedures such as cardiac catheterizations. These specialist P.A.s include child health associates, orthopedic physician assistants, urologic physician assistants, surgeon assistants, and emergency-room physician assistants.

In the early years of the occupation, informal training was not uncommon, but today, nearly all states require that new P.A.s complete a program approved by the Committee on Allied Health Education and Accreditation (CAHEA) of the American Medical Association.

Educational programs generally are two years in length, although some are longer and a few are shorter. Most P.A. programs are located in medical schools, schools of allied health, or four-year colleges; a few are located in community colleges or are hospital-based.

P.A. education begins with a classroom phase that lasts from six to twenty-four months. Classroom instruction includes human anatomy, physiology, microbiology, clinical pharmacology, applied psychology, clinical medicine, and medical ethics. During the program's last nine to fifteen months, students do supervised clinical work designed to develop practitioners' skills. Clinical training begins with a series of clinical practice assignments or rotations that include family practice, inpatient and ambulatory medicine, general surgery, obstetrics and gynecology, emergency medicine, internal medicine, psychiatry, and pediatrics. Sometimes, one or more of the rotations are served under the supervision of a physician who is seeking to hire a P.A.

Postgraduate education for P.A.s is a recent development. Residency programs, as yet unaccredited, are available in emergency medicine, general surgery, neonatology, and occupational medicine.

State laws and regulations govern the use of the title "physician assistant" and the scope of the P.A. practice. Most states require that P.A.s be certified by the National Commission on Certification of Physician Assistants (NCCPA).

physician of nuclear medicine

A specialist who uses radioactive substances in the diagnosis and treatment of disease. For example, he may perform a brain scan to determine if the brain is anatomically and biochemically normal, or he may perform a bone scan to get a picture of the bones.

Nuclear scanning usually reveals abnormalities

that can't be seen on normal X-ray films. Chemicals that contain minute traces of radiation are injected into the body. The chemical is chosen because of its affinity for a particular body part; once injected, it travels there. The radiation emanating from the body is measured; abnormalities are determined by identifying increased or decreased amounts of radiation.

Physicians of nuclear medicine have graduated from medical school and completed a residency in internal medicine, radiology, or pathology, and they have fulfilled an additional fellowship requirement in nuclear medicine. They are certified by the American Board of Nuclear Medicine.

plastic surgeon

When we think of plastic surgery, many of us think immediately of cosmetic surgery, performed to enhance one's appearance. Today, more and more people of average means are turning to plastic surgery in order to improve their looks. While cosmetic surgery cannot produce miracles, it can produce significant improvements in appearance. Some of the more common procedures are: *dermabrasion* to remove acne scars or other superficial disfigurements; eyelid surgery (*blepharoplasty*) to remove extra skin on the upper lids or bags below the eyes; facelifts; and *breast augmentation* or *reduction.* In addition, plastic surgeons often perform *hair transplantations.* The most frequently performed cosmetic procedure is the "nose job," or *rhinoplasty.*

The plastic surgeon is not, however, primarily concerned with cosmetic work; he is essentially a reparative surgeon, dealing with the restoration of function and, when possible, appearance following tissue loss and damage by injury or disease—especially burns, cancer, and automobile accidents. Most cosmetic plastic surgery carried out today is performed on accident victims, young and old, who may need a new ear, nose, or chin or the removal of disfiguring scar tissue. One of the plastic surgeon's most important contributions is in the treatment and rehabilitation of burn victims.

The plastic surgeon must undergo one of the longest periods of training of all physicians and surgeons before he can be certified in his specialty by the American Board of Plastic Surgery. Following graduation from medical school, he will serve a one-year internship, followed by three years of residency training in general surgery and an additional two years of residency in plastic surgery.

It is critical to ensure that you choose a qualified and competent plastic surgeon. To find one in your area who is certified, contact the American Board of Plastic Surgery.

podiatrist

A growing number of foot-ailment sufferers visit a *doctor of podiatric medicine,* or podiatrist, for relief. Podiatrists diagnose and treat diseases and disorders of the foot.

Much of their practice is devoted to treating soft-tissue complaints such as corns, bunions, calluses, ingrown toenails, and skin and nail diseases. To help in diagnosis, podiatrists take X-ray films and order laboratory tests. Depending on the condition, they may fit corrective devices, prescribe drugs, order physical therapy, or recommend proper shoes. Surgery, performed in hospitals, outpatient surgery centers, clinics, or podiatrists' offices, is an increasingly important part of podiatric practice.

Podiatrists are trained to identify systemic diseases such as arthritis, diabetes mellitus, and heart disease. If they find symptoms of a systemic disorder, they refer the patient to a medical doctor while continuing to treat the foot problem.

Most podiatrists provide all types of foot care. After completing additional training, however, some specialize in podiatric surgery, orthopedics (bone, muscle, and joint disorders), podopediatrics (children's foot ailments), or podogeriatrics (foot problems of the elderly).

A license is required for the practice of podiatric medicine. To qualify for a license, an applicant must graduate from an accredited college of podiatric medicine and pass a written and oral examination, or the examination of the National Board of Podiatric Examiners.

Of the four years in podiatry school, the first two are spent in classroom and laboratory work in anatomy, bacteriology, chemistry, pathology, physiology, pharmacology, and other basic sciences. During the final two years, students gain clinical experience while continuing their academic studies. Graduates are awarded the degree of Doctor of Podiatric Medicine (D.P.M.).

Additional education and experience are necessary to practice in a specialty. Board certification is offered in two specialties: podiatric orthopedics and podiatric surgery.

primary-care physician

This is a general term applying to any type of physician who is capable of diagnosing and treating a majority of a person's and family's medical problems. Primary-care physicians are licensed as general practitioners, family practitioners, internists, or pediatricians.

The primary-care physician is trained in his specialty to provide total medical care, being personally able to treat all general diseases and injuries within his competence. But he will refer patients to the proper specialists when their particular knowledge and skills are required; he will resume the medical management of his patients when the specialist no longer is needed. The primary-care physician is concerned with individual needs and with a family's special needs, and is the counselor and friend who is concerned with preventive medicine as well as with the treatment of disease. He not only lances boils, excises splinters, sets simple fractures, treats sore throats, hemorrhoids, childhood diseases, and special complaints of the aged, but he also provides prenatal care, delivers babies (if an obstetrician is not consulted), treats diabetes and heart problems, and, if needed, lends an ear to let a parent talk about the problems of a nonconforming child who is not doing well at home or in school. He takes steps to see that proper vaccinations and booster shots are given, sets dates for physical checkups, and is available by telephone if any special problems arise. In brief, he exemplifies all of the virtues and skills that most of us associate with the revered "old family doctor."

To become a primary-care physician, one must qualify for a license. On a nationwide basis, the minimal requirements for the practice of medicine include graduation from an approved medical school, one year of postgraduate clinical training, and the passing of a state licensing examination. (Graduates of foreign medical schools are required to pass a special additional test that is standard across the country.) Most states will accept in place of their own examination the successful completion of the uniform examination administered by the National Board of Medical Examiners.

psychiatrist

Psychiatry is concerned with the emotional and mental disorders that afflict mankind, with their diagnosis and treatment, and with research to find better ways to prevent, control, or cure them.

A psychiatrist is a physician who, after completing medical school, has had at least a year of internship and three years of psychiatric residency training. During this period of clinical training he has studied and diagnosed a wide range of psychiatric, neurologic, and medical problems. He has learned to recognize and treat mental handicap, personality disorders such as psychopathy and paranoia, psychoses such as dementia and schizophrenia, mood disorders such as depression and the manic-depressive psychosis, and neurotic disturbances such as anxiety, obsession, and hysteria. After completing his clinical training and two years of experience in psychiatric practice, he is eligible to take the comprehensive examinations given by the American Board of Psychiatry and Neurology. Certification of competency in psychiatry is given by the board to those who successfully complete the extensive written and oral examinations.

Patients and doctors are learning that mental illness must be recognized and dealt with much like any other illness. The most important factors for successful treatment are early recognition and professional evaluation of a developing illness, followed by appropriate therapy. Today such treatment is provided largely in outpatient settings—private psychiatrists' offices, community mental health centers, or psychiatric clinics in general hospitals. Inpatient treatment is used only for the most acutely ill, when there is a true emergency and the patient is a threat to himself or others, or is unable to care for himself.

psychologist

Psychologists study human behavior and mental processes in order to understand and explain people's actions. Some research psychologists investigate the physical, emotional, or social aspects of human behavior. Other psychologists in applied fields counsel and conduct training programs; do market research; or provide health services in hospitals or clinics.

Clinical psychologists generally work in hospitals

or clinics, or maintain their own practices. They help persons who are mentally or emotionally disturbed adjust to life. They interview patients; give diagnostic tests; provide individual, family, and group psychotherapy; and design and carry through behavior modification programs. Clinical psychologists may collaborate with physicians and other specialists in developing treatment programs. Some clinical psychologists work in universities where they train graduate students in the delivery of mental health services. Others administer community mental health programs. *Counseling psychologists* use several techniques, including interviewing and testing, to advise people on how to deal with problems of everyday living—personal, social, educational, and vocational. *Educational psychologists* design, develop and evaluate educational programs. *School psychologists* work with teachers and parents to evaluate and resolve students' learning and behavior problems. *Health psychologists* counsel the public in health maintenance to help people avoid serious emotional or physical illness. Other areas of specialization include *environmental* psychology, *population* psychology, *psychopharmacology*, and *rehabilitation psychology*.

A doctoral degree often is required for employment as a psychologist. This qualifies one for a wide range of responsible research, clinical practice, and counseling positions in universities, private industry, and government.

People with a master's degree in psychology can administer and interpret tests as psychological assistants. Under the supervision of psychologists, they can conduct research in laboratories, counsel patients, or perform administrative duties. They teach in two-year colleges, or work as school psychologists or counselors.

People with a bachelor's degree in psychology are qualified to assist psychologists and other professionals in community mental health centers, vocational rehabilitation offices, and correctional programs, and to work as research or administrative assistants.

At least one year of full-time graduate study is needed to earn a master's degree in psychology.

Three to five years of graduate work usually are required for a doctoral degree. The Ph.D. degree culminates in a dissertation based on original research.

Most states require that licensed or certified psychologists limit their practice to those areas in which they have developed professional competence through training and experience.

The American Board of Professional Psychology recognizes professional achievement by awarding diplomas primarily in clinical, counseling, forensic, industrial and organizational, and school psychology. Candidates need a doctorate in psychology, five years of experience, and professional endorsements; they also must pass an examination.

radiologist

The most common medical procedure done today, along with the blood count and urinalysis, is the X-ray examination. Although many X-ray films are taken by highly trained technicians, they are always seen and their meanings interpreted by the radiologist, who sends his reports to the doctors who ordered them. Thus, the radiologist is for the most part a "doctor's doctor." Few physicians will undertake treatment of serious disease or recommend surgery without his consultation. The modern radiologist can explore visually every nook and cranny in every organ system of the body. He may work within the hospital, serving its staff and patients, or he may have an office practice to which patients are sent by their physicians for required examinations or treatments.

The radiologist is not only a master diagnostician but is also a radiotherapist who uses radiant energy to irradiate malignant tumors and treat other conditions. He is first trained in general medicine and surgery, then spends a minimum of four years in postgraduate training to become proficient in all areas of radiology, including those that require invasion of the body to introduce dyes, air, and other contrast materials that are X-rayed as they pass through blood vessels and the organs they serve. In recent years the scope of radiology has been greatly extended by the development of the CAT scanner and the MRI scanner and by the use of digital imaging and intensifying techniques.

Radiology has its own examining board responsible for the educational and clinical training programs of future radiologists, as well as their examination for competence and certification.

Radiology is one of the most important specialties in medicine and is highly safe and effective, both for diagnosis and therapy. Its practitioners are responsible for much of the progress that has been made in recent years in detecting and controlling many of the diseases that afflict us.

recreational therapist

Recreational therapists provide services to people who are mentally, physically, or emotionally disabled. These workers are known also as "therapeutic recreation specialists," a job title that draws attention to the fact that theirs is a health profession.

Recreational therapists employ recreational and leisure activities as a form of treatment—much as other practitioners use surgery, drugs, nutrition, exercise, or psychotherapy. Therapists strive to minimize patients' symptoms and to improve their physical, mental, and emotional well-being. Enhancing the patient's ability to function in everyday life is the primary goal of recreational therapy; enjoyable and rewarding activities provide the means for working toward that goal.

Activities employed by recreational therapists are as varied as the interests and abilities of the people they serve. For example, they might organize athletic events, dances, arts-and-crafts or musical activities, attendance at movies, field trips, or poetry readings. Apart from sheer enjoyment, activities such as these provide opportunities for exercise and social participation. Other goals that the therapist might have in mind when planning an activity include relieving anxiety, building confidence, or promoting independence.

Recreational therapists are found in a variety of settings, including mental hospitals, psychiatric "day hospitals," community mental health centers, nursing homes, adult day-care programs, residential facilities for the mentally retarded, school systems, and prisons. Often they are located in the activities department or therapy department of an organization.

A degree in therapeutic recreation, or in recreation with an emphasis on therapeutic recreation, is the usual requirement for professional positions in this field. An associate degree satisfies hiring requirements in many nursing homes, while a bachelor's degree ordinarily is necessary in community and clinical settings.

Certification is available (but not required) through the National Council for Therapeutic Recreation Certification (NCTRC), which awards credentials for therapeutic recreation specialists and therapeutic recreation assistants.

registered nurse

Registered nurses (R.N.s) handle a variety of tasks related to both health and illness. Typically concerned with the "whole person," registered nurses deal with patients' mental and emotional functioning as well as their physical needs. They observe, assess, and record symptoms, reactions, and progress; administer medications; assist in convalescence and rehabilitation; instruct patients and their families in proper care; and help individuals and groups take steps to improve or maintain their health. The work setting determines the scope of the nurse's responsibilities.

Hospital nurses constitute by far the largest group of nurses. Most are staff nurses who provide skilled bedside nursing care and carry out the medical regimen prescribed by physicians. They also may supervise licensed practical nurses, aides, and orderlies. Hospital nurses usually work with groups of patients who require similar nursing care. For instance, some nurses work with patients who have had surgery; others care for children, the elderly, or the mentally ill.

Registered nurses working in *nursing homes* provide bedside nursing care to patients convalescing from surgery or an illness and to those suffering from chronic illnesses and disabilities. They also supervise licensed practical nurses and nursing aides.

Private-duty nurses give individual care to patients who need constant attention. They may work in a home, a hospital, or a nursing home or rehabilitation center.

Community health nurses care for patients in clinics, schools, retirement and life-care communities, and other community settings. A growing number provide home health care. They may instruct community groups in proper nutrition and exercise and arrange for immunizations, blood-pressure testing, and other health screening measures.

Office nurses assist physicians, dental surgeons, and, occasionally, dentists in private practice, clinics, and health maintenance organizations. Sometimes they perform routine laboratory and office work in addition to their nursing duties.

Occupational health nurses and *industrial nurses* provide nursing care to employees in industry and government and, together with physicians, promote employee health. As prescribed by a doctor, they treat minor injuries and illnesses at work, provide needed nursing care, arrange for further medical care if necessary, and offer health counseling. They also may assist with health examinations and inoculations.

Nurse practitioners are registered nurses who specialize in providing services such as preventive care, physical exams, and counseling under the supervision of a physician.

To obtain the R.N. license that is required by all states, nurses must graduate from an approved school of nursing and pass a national examination administered by the state.

Nursing training programs vary in length from two to five years after graduation from high school, depending on the nature of the program. Programs offered by community and junior colleges take about two years and lead to an associate degree; hospital-based programs last three years and lead to a diploma; college and university programs require four or five years and lead to a baccalaureate degree.

All nursing training programs include classroom instruction and supervised nursing practice in hospitals and other health facilities. Students take courses in anatomy, physiology, microbiology, nutrition, psychology, and nursing. Increasingly, nursing students learn the latest clinical and administrative uses of computers in medicine. In hospitals, for example, nurses routinely use computers to enter and retrieve information about patients, such as their X-ray studies, laboratory test results, or medication orders.

For nurses who prefer close contact with patients, career advancement may mean becoming a *clinical nurse specialist, nurse practitioner, nurse clinician,* or *nurse anesthetist.* Graduate-level preparation is necessary to reach these positions.

respiratory therapist

Respiratory therapists treat patients who have cardiopulmonary (heart/lung) problems that interfere with breathing. Treatment may range from giving temporary relief to patients with chronic asthma or emphysema to emergency care for heart failure, stroke, drowning, or shock. Respiratory therapists are among the first specialists called for emergency treatment of acute respiratory conditions arising from head injury or drug poisoning. Their role is a highly responsible one because a patient who stops breathing for longer than three to five minutes has little chance of recovery without serious brain damage. If oxygen

is cut off for more than nine minutes, death results.

Respiratory care usually involves one or more of the four major kinds of treatment: (1) administering oxygen and oxygen mixtures; (2) using humidity and aerosol mists to keep the respiratory tract moist or to deliver medication; (3) administering chest physical therapy, which includes exercises to reduce the effort of breathing, as well as tapping and coughing procedures to help clear the lungs; and (4) operating mechanical ventilators that replace or assist natural breathing. Mechanical ventilators help sustain life when a patient is unable to breathe spontaneously. This may happen due to a number of causes: coma; paralysis of the respiratory muscles; severe lung, head, or chest injury; or damage from smoke inhalation.

Respiratory-care equipment has become more complex in recent years, and formal training is increasingly important. Voluntary certification is available through the National Board for Respiratory Care.

Formal training programs vary in length and in the credential or degree awarded. Some lead to a bachelor's degree; most of the others are somewhat briefer and lead to an associate degree. Areas of study include human anatomy and physiology, chemistry, physics, microbiology, and mathematics. Technical courses deal with procedures, equipment, and clinical tests.

rheumatologist

Rheumatology is that subspecialty of internal medicine concerned with the body's bones, joints, and muscles and with the diseases that afflict them. The rheumatologist is concerned not only with diagnosis, treatment, and research, but also with public education to help people recognize the symptoms and dangers of diseases, such as rheumatoid and other forms of arthritis, that now afflict millions of Americans.

Few die as a result of rheumatic disease, but without early and adequate treatment, many face a lifetime of pain and increasing disability as well as emotional and economic disaster.

Most certified rheumatologists practicing in the United States serve in teaching hospitals and medical centers or as members of a group practice. Some rheumatologists may practice both internal medicine and rheumatology.

The rheumatologist qualifies for certification

in his specialty by four years of medical college, three years of residency training in internal medicine, followed by an additional two years or more of clinical training and experience in all areas of rheumatology.

The major goals of therapy are to cure when possible, to induce and maintain remissions, and to maintain maximum treatment during acute periods in order to avoid deformities and crippling.

speech pathologist and audiologist

Almost one American in 10 is unable to speak or hear clearly. Speech pathologists and audiologists assist such people by evaluating their speech, language, and hearing abilities and providing treatment. *Speech pathologists* work with those who have communicative disorders resulting from total or partial hearing loss, brain injury, cleft palate, voice pathology, learning disabilities, mental retardation, emotional problems, foreign dialect, or other causes. *Audiologists* assess and treat hearing problems, sometimes by fitting and dispensing hearing aids. Speech and hearing are so interrelated, however, that to be competent in one of these fields, one must be familiar with both.

A master's degree in speech-language pathology or audiology is the standard credential in this field. Payment under Medicaid requires that the practitioner have a master's degree and completion or participation in three hundred hours of supervised clinical experience.

Although licensure requirements vary somewhat, all states require graduation from a master's-degree program in speech-language pathology or audiology, three hundred hours of supervised clinical experience, and an examination.

surgeon

A physician who employs operative procedures to preserve or restore function and/or to cure disease.

One can choose to be a general surgeon or to practice a surgical specialty. The *neurosurgeon* surgically treats diseases of the brain and nervous system. The *orthopedic* surgeon uses surgical methods to correct deformities, diseases, and injuries to the skeletal system. The *pulmonary surgeon* deals with diseases of the lung, and the *cardiovascular surgeon*, with heart problems. The *colon and rectal surgeon* diagnoses and surgically treats disorders of the colon, rectum, and anal canal.

The number of years of training to fulfill the educational requirements for certification as a surgeon (except the orthopedic surgeon) is greater than for nonsurgeon physicians. After graduating from medical school, the orthopedic surgeon must complete four years of formal training before he can enter practice. A five-year residency program is required for the specialist in general surgery or neurosurgery. At this point, he then must pass oral and written examinations given by the American Board of Surgery or the American Board of Neurological Surgery (which also requires two years of practice as a condition for certification). Before taking a two-year residency in cardiovascular surgery, the candidate must already have received certification from the American Board of Surgery. Thus a cardiovascular surgeon spends seven years in postgraduate work before he is eligible for certification.

There is a wide range of societies that the surgeon may join. Regardless of specialty, he may seek membership in the American College of Surgeons. The specialist may then want to join the society concerned with his specialty, such as the American Academy of Orthopaedic Surgeons or the American Association of Cosmetic Surgeons. There also are societies such as the American Society of Transplant Surgeons, to which many different types of specialists belong.

When choosing a surgeon, you should look for one with many years of experience in the procedure you are to undergo. It has been shown that mortality rates are lower in hospitals where experienced surgeons perform a particular procedure frequently than in hospitals where the operation rarely is done. You can check the surgeon's experience, hospital affiliations, and board certification in medical directories available at the library. In addition, you can contact the American Board of Surgery directly.

Whenever surgery is proposed, you should get a second opinion. Over 75 percent of operations in this country are elective surgery, that is, nonemergency procedures. All carry some risk, and you will want to weigh these risks carefully against the benefits. A good surgeon will give you the name of a second surgeon if you ask. If he is unwilling, however, contact the appropriate department at a large teaching hospital or medical center in your area. They will usually supply the names of about three surgeons appropriate to consult for a second opinion.

urologist

The urologist is a physician trained in the disorders of the urinary bladder, the urethra, and the male sexual organs.

URINARY SYSTEM

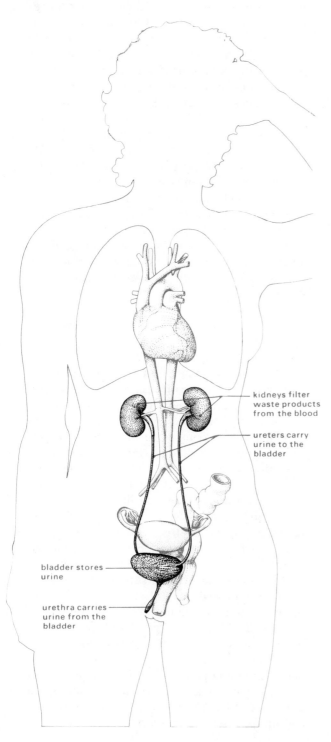

kidneys filter waste products from the blood

ureters carry urine to the bladder

bladder stores urine

urethra carries urine from the bladder

A substantial proportion of the urologist's female patients have symptoms relating to the urinary bladder. These symptoms include a constant sense of pressure in the pelvis, a burning sensation on urination, frequency, urgency, stress incontinence, and backache. In many cases there may be mild to severe infection (*cystitis*) but in many, nothing abnormal is to be found on examination.

The urologist's male patients frequently complain of bladder-emptying difficulties, and this can usually be traced to enlargement of the prostate gland that surrounds the urethra as it leaves the bladder on the underside. Benign enlargement of the prostate is very common in elderly men who may find it increasingly difficult to void urine. The result is that urine accumulates in the bladder, leading to a shorter and shorter interval between experiencing the sense of fullness. Sleep is disturbed and there are frequent nighttime visits to the toilet.

The treatment of benign prostatic hypertrophy is surgical, and the excess tissue can be removed through the urethra itself (transurethral resection of the prostate), through the bladder, via an incision above the pubic bone, or directly by way of an incision through the skin behind the scro-

The urinary tract consists of the kidneys, ureters, bladder, and urethra. In the male, the urethra also has a sexual function since sperm and seminal fluid are propelled along it. The urinary tract is subject to infection, trauma, stone formation, and cancer.

URINARY AND GENITAL TRACT
male

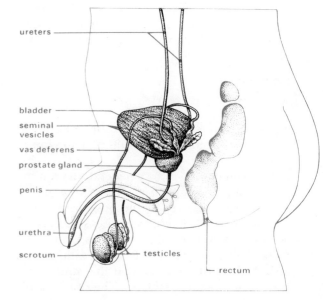

ureters

bladder

seminal vesicles

vas deferens

prostate gland

penis

urethra

scrotum

testicles

rectum

tum (perineal). The same range of choices is available to the urologist treating cancer of the prostate, but in this case, the concern also will be to remove any tumor as completely as possible, and to determine the possibility that the cancer has spread to other parts of the body. Prostate cancers are hormone dependent and when they have spread, removal of the source of male sex hormone, the testicles (*orchiectomy*), will often produce years of remission.

The bladder itself can be the site of many diseases and some of these, such as cancer of the bladder, or certain types of kidney stones may be revealed by the presence of blood in the urine.

Such a sign will prompt the urologist to perform *cystoscopy*—the inside of the bladder is illuminated and inspected through a narrow, straight optical instrument passed into the bladder through the urethra. Cystoscopy is performed under general anesthesia and is an indispensable way of observing the disease process directly and, if necessary, in obtaining a sample (*biopsy*) for examination.

Urologists must graduate from medical school, fulfill a two-year residency program in general surgery, and then an additional three- or four-year residency in urology. They are then eligible to take certifying examinations given by the American Board of Urology.

TESTS

5

acid phosphatase (ACP)

Acid phosphatase is an enzyme found in many tissues throughout the body, but particularly in the prostate gland. When cancer of the prostate is present, the level of ACP in the blood is elevated. Thus, a laboratory test that measures the level of ACP in the blood usually is performed to determine the possible presence and extent of prostate cancer.

The test may be performed also in a woman if rape is suspected. The finding of ACP in the vaginal fluid is an indication that sexual intercourse has taken place.

Although many physicians agree that this is the best lab test for detection of early prostate disease, a high ACP reading can be caused by other conditions such as diabetes mellitus and kidney disease. Therefore, if your ACP level is elevated, your physician will probably order a thorough rectal examination and other tests before making a diagnosis.

As with all blood tests, discomfort and risk are minimal.

acquired immune deficiency syndrome—human immunodeficiency virus (AIDS-HIV) testing

A blood test to determine if a patient has antibodies against the human immunodeficiency virus (HIV), which is thought to cause acquired immune deficiency syndrome (AIDS). A positive result means only that a person has been exposed to the AIDS virus in the past, not that he or she has or will ever get AIDS.

The test is given to all people who are going to donate blood to ensure that their blood is not tainted. Many doctors also advise persons in high-risk groups for AIDS, such as homosexuals, hemophiliacs, and people who have had sexual relations with a known victim, to undergo the test. Various kinds of HIV antibody tests exist, but the test most widely used at present is the ELISA (Enzyme Linked Immuno-Sorbent Assay) test. This is a good screening test and, if positive, the diagnosis should be confirmed with another test, such as the Western Blot test.

As with all blood tests, discomfort and risk are minimal. Results usually are available within a few hours.

383

agglutination

The clumping or sticking together of numbers of small particles in a fluid. Particles or cells (for example, red blood cells or bacteria) demonstrate this phenomenon when they are exposed to an antibody that reacts with an antigen they contain.

This phenomenon is of particular importance in medical diagnosis, as it is the basis for many laboratory tests. For instance, if bacteria of unknown identity are obtained from a patient, they can be mixed with antibodies from laboratory animals. These antibodies are specific to a particular bacterium; if the bacteria taken from the patient agglutinate (clump) on contact with them, they can be identified positively as being the same organism and the appropriate antibiotic can be prescribed.

Another variety of the agglutination test uses the same principle in reverse. Serum (the amber fluid remaining after blood has clotted) of a patient who is suspected of having a particular infection is mixed with fluid containing bacteria that are known to cause that infection. If the bacteria agglutinate, this indicates the patient has antibodies against them.

In practice, this does not mean that a patient currently has a disease, only that he has had it sometime in the past. Often it is necessary to repeat the test after a period of time to see if the patient's titer of antibodies has risen. (The agglutination titer is the highest dilution of a serum that will cause clumping of the bacteria being tested.) If this has gone up, the infection is probably a recent one.

The test usually is performed when the doctor suspects an infection but does not know its cause. Some infections for which there are specific agglutination tests are German measles, tapeworms, and typhoid fever.

Agglutination is also the basis for determining what type of blood you have: A, B, AB, or O. Blood-typing is always performed before a transfusion to ensure that the donor's and the recipient's blood types are compatible. The blood type is determined by noting the type of blood with which a person's serum agglutinates. As an extra precaution, the blood is "cross-matched," that is, a sample of the recipient's serum is mixed with the donor's red blood cells to check that they do *not* agglutinate.

As with all blood tests, discomfort and risk are minimal.

amniocentesis

A diagnostic test carried out in the first half of pregnancy involving the removal of a small amount of amniotic fluid from the womb. It is done usually on an outpatient basis between the sixteenth and twentieth week of pregnancy.

Using ultrasound scanning, the doctor learns the position of the fetus and the location of the placenta. An area of skin on your stomach is cleansed with antiseptic, and a local anesthesia is given; you will remain awake during the procedure. A needle attached to a syringe is inserted through the abdominal and uterine walls where there is the least chance of touching either the placenta or the fetus. Less than 1 ounce of amniotic fluid is withdrawn. Tests on the fluid and cells can detect birth defects such as Down's syndrome, spina bifida, some forms of muscular dystrophy, as well as some blood and brain disorders. The sex of the fetus can also be learned.

Amniocentesis carries a 1 in 200 risk of losing the baby and should only be done for good reason. Infection in the mother or fetus occasionally occurs but is rare.

AMNIOCENTESIS

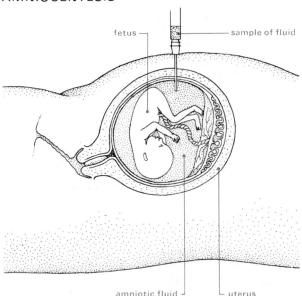

fetus —   — sample of fluid

amniotic fluid —   — uterus

Amniocentesis is a technique for removing a small sample of amniotic fluid from the uterus of a pregnant woman. Analysis of the fluid can show whether the fetus is affected by certain serious disorders such as Down's syndrome and spina bifida. In these cases the mother can be offered a therapeutic abortion; where the result of amniocentesis is normal, she is reassured.

amylase

Amylase, which is an enzyme needed for the digestion of starches, is produced in the pancreas, salivary glands, and liver. The doctor performs a test that measures the level of amylase in a patient's blood if he suspects a disorder of the aforementioned organs or glands.

High blood levels of amylase are indicative of pancreatitis, pancreatic duct obstruction, or other disorders of the pancreas. Low levels may indicate liver damage.

Be sure to tell your doctor if you are taking any drugs when he administers the test; codeine, thiazide diuretics, large amounts of alcohol, and certain other drugs elevate blood levels of amylase.

The test is about 85 percent accurate. As with all blood tests, discomfort and risk are minimal.

angiography

Radiological investigation in which a substance opaque to X rays (radiopaque material) is injected into blood vessels to make them visible on the X-ray plate or viewing screen. The process of outlining arteries is called *arteriography*; that of outlining veins is known as *phlebography* or *venography*. The technique is used not only in demonstrating abnormalities or disease of the blood vessels but also in diagnosing tumors, particularly in the brain. Lymph vessels also can be outlined; the technique is then known as *lymphangiography*. An angiogram of the heart's arteries is termed a *coronary angiogram*.

Before the procedure starts you will probably be given a sedative and asked to urinate. You will lie on your back for the procedure. A local anesthetic is given and the radiopaque material is introduced into the artery through a needle or catheter. A series of X-ray pictures is then taken.

Having an angiogram causes some discomfort; when the radiopaque material is injected, you will feel a momentary sensation of heat. After the anesthesia wears off you may have some pain and swelling at the site of the injection. The procedure lasts from one to four hours, so you will probably be a little stiff from lying on the hard table. After the test you will be required to stay in bed for at least eight hours. Digital Intravenous Subtraction Angiography is a more recent method that is much quicker and involves less discomfort.

CEREBRAL ANGIOGRAM

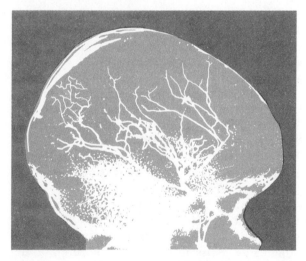

Cerebral angiography is an X-ray technique for displaying the arteries that supply the brain. The normal pattern can be altered by a congenital malformation of the vessels, an aneurysm, blockage with a blood clot, or a brain tumor. The neurosurgeon needs precise information about the location of these abnormalities if he or she is to operate.

auscultation

Process of listening to sounds produced within the body, with the aid of a stethoscope. Auscultation gives information about abnormal body conditions, thus it is a very important part of the physician's examination routine. Stethoscopes are used to listen to the sounds produced by the heart, lungs, major blood vessels, and intestines. Abnormal heart sounds could be caused by faulty heart valves or other conditions. Abnormal lung sounds can be caused by the accumulation of fluid in the lungs or by diseased or obstructed airways. Abnormal bowel sounds can be indicators of serious intestinal blockages.

When used in conjunction with other elements of a physical exam, auscultation is an important means for the health care professional to assess a person's health.

See also STETHOSCOPE in **Medical A–Z**.

barium meal/barium enema

A *barium meal* is used in an X-ray study of the esophagus. Before the X-ray pictures are taken, you will be asked to swallow a cup of barium sulfate, a thick, chalky liquid. Although it is rather unpleasant-tasting, you will not feel any pain. While you are swallowing your "barium milk-shake," a radiologist watches the barium going down the esophagus, as shown on a video screen, and X-ray pictures are taken. In some cases, X-ray pictures are taken while you lie on a table that tilts your head lower than your feet. The whole procedure takes thirty minutes or less.

A *barium enema* is used in an X-ray study of the lower gastrointestinal tract. The same chalky liquid, barium sulfate, is introduced into the rectum through a tube under gentle pressure while you lie on your side. As with all enemas, you will have a feeling of fullness and an urge to defecate; you may also experience some cramps. X-ray pictures are taken both while you hold the barium and when you expel it.

X rays do not pass through barium sulfate, so the substance shows up as an opaque mass on the X-ray film. And, like any liquid, barium sulfate conforms to the shape of its container; thus a clear outline of the gastrointestinal tract can be obtained as the barium passes through.

BARIUM MEAL/ENEMA

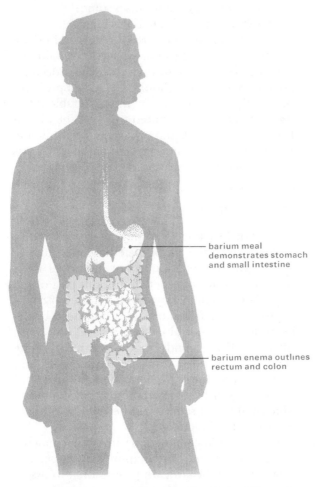

barium meal demonstrates stomach and small intestine

barium enema outlines rectum and colon

Barium sulfate is a radiopaque liquid (one through which X rays cannot pass). It is used extensively in radiology exams to outline the digestive tract. The barium is either swallowed as a meal or injected through the anus as an enema. Using these techniques the radiologist can diagnose peptic ulcers, cancers, pockets in the bowel wall, and other diseases of the bowel.

basal metabolic rate (BMR)

The basal metabolism is the minimum energy used to maintain body functions, including temperature, blood circulation, heartbeat, and breathing. Measuring the metabolic rate is an indirect test of thyroid function. It has, however, been superseded by more direct tests of thyroid function, from which much more information can be obtained.

See also THYROID-FUNCTION TESTS.

bilirubin

A simple blood test for measuring the bile pigment, bilirubin. It is given routinely as part of a complete physical examination, or when liver or pancreatic disease or a disorder of the bile ducts is suspected.

To perform the test, a physician, nurse, or laboratory technician will take a small blood sample. Be sure to tell your doctor if you are taking any medication, since drugs such as thorazine, male hormones, and some antibiotics can increase the level of bilirubin in the blood. Fasting or dieting also can affect bilirubin levels.

An elevated bilirubin level is a fair indicator that something is wrong with the liver, pancreas, or bile ducts. Hepatitis A and hepatitis B invariably cause a rise in the serum bilirubin. Your physician will have to perform further diagnostic tests, such as LIVER-FUNCTION TESTS, to determine exactly what is wrong.

In persons with high bilirubin levels the skin and eyes often become jaundiced, or yellow in color.

See also HEPATITIS TESTING.

biopsy

Removal of a small specimen of tissue from the living body for diagnostic purposes. Diagnosis is made by examining thin slices of the tissue under a microscope. Since only very small pieces are required, tissues can be obtained from within the body by means of special instruments without a major surgical operation. To obtain tissue from the bronchi, intestines, or bladder (all of which have natural openings onto the body surface), doctors use slender illuminated instruments known as *fiberoptic endoscopes.* These include bronchoscopes, gastroscopes, and cystoscopes for viewing the bronchi, stomach, and bladder, respectively. They are flexible tubes with special attachments that can be introduced into the appropriate body opening to the point at which a tissue specimen is to be taken. A gastroscope, for example, is passed via the mouth and esophagus into the stomach where the gastric lining can be viewed and a biopsy taken.

Biopsies of internal organs such as the liver and kidney are performed by means of a long hollow needle that is passed through the skin and into the organ concerned. Skin biopsies are taken directly, under local anesthia.

Most biopsies are sent to the laboratory for processing before being examined under the microscope. This may take a day or two. But sometimes a biopsy is taken during an operation when an immediate result is required for the surgeon to decide how to proceed. In such cases a "frozen-section biopsy" is performed. This is a quick but less satisfactory means of processing the tissue by freezing it before slices are made.

A diagnosis made on biopsy findings is generally a firm one. However, a disease may affect organs in a patchy manner, and, since only extremely tiny pieces are removed, these bits may not have come from the affected parts. Where possible, several "bites" are taken at biopsy in order to reduce the chance of missing affected parts.

blood pressure

This test measures the pressure, or tension, of the blood as it presses against the arteries. There are two pressures to determine: the *systolic* pressure, when the heart muscle contracts, and the *diastolic,* when the heart relaxes.

Blood-pressure testing is part of almost any physical exam and is extremely important. High blood pressure, or hypertension, is a known risk factor for heart disease and stroke, and may be raised years before any other symptoms, such as palpitations, appear.

To measure blood pressure, a device called a *sphygmomanometer* is used. This instrument has an inflatable cuff designed to be wrapped around the patient's arm. Inflation of the cuff by compression of a rubber bulb applies pressure to the arm; this pressure is measured by a mercury-filled air-pressure gauge that is attached to the cuff.

To take your blood pressure, the doctor or nurse will wrap the inflatable cuff around your upper arm while you are sitting or lying down. A stethoscope is placed on the arm, just below the cuff, and air is pumped into it until the pressure in the cuff is greater than the pressure inside the artery. When the pressure is sufficient, it will temporarily cause the artery to collapse and circulation to stop. As the physician listens through the stethoscope, he will slowly lessen the pressure within the cuff by letting air out through a valve. As the blood is forced through the artery, a pulsing sound is heard; the value that appears on the mercury gauge at this point is the systolic blood pressure. As more air is let out of the valve, the pulsing will eventually stop because the pressures outside and inside the artery are equal; this is the diastolic pressure.

The blood pressure reading is recorded in millimeters of mercury pressure and expressed as a ratio, such as 120/70 ("120 over 70"). The top number is the systolic pressure; the bottom, the diastolic. Debate continues over what constitutes a high blood pressure reading, but it usually is agreed that the diastolic pressure is more important in this regard. Generally, it is thought that a diastolic value of 90 to 115 constitutes moderate hypertension, and 115 or above, severe hypertension. If your values are elevated, your doctor will repeat the test several times to ensure the reading is accurate: Many factors such as stress can cause a temporary rise in blood pressure.

See also BLOOD PRESSURE, SPHYGMOMANOMETER in Medical A–Z.

blood testing

Many of the tests described in this section are blood tests. There are two main methods of performing blood tests: venipuncture and the fingerstick method.

In venipuncture, a tourniquet is tied around the arm, just above the elbow, to prevent blood from flowing in the veins in the lower arm. These veins are then more visible to the nurse or doctor. After cleansing the area around one vein with antiseptic solution, the nurse or doctor inserts into the vein a needle connected to a syringe, pulls the plunger, and withdraws a sample of blood. The needle is removed and an adhesive dressing is put on the insertion site. This method has no risk, although the area may become bruised if there was trouble locating a vein. Some people say they feel weak or faint after the blood is drawn, but this is really a psychosomatic reaction; in truth, not enough blood is drawn to make a person weak.

If only a few drops of blood are needed for testing, or if the person is afraid of venipuncture, the fingerstick method may be used. The fingertip is simply cleansed with alcohol and pricked with an instrument called a lancet. The finger is squeezed, causing blood to flow from the insertion site, and a glass tube (pipette) is used to draw up the blood. Again, there is no risk associated with this method, though your finger may feel a bit sore for a while.

See also COMPLETE BLOOD CELL COUNT.

blood urea nitrogen (BUN)

The nitrogen waste product of protein metabolism is called *urea*, and normally it is eliminated by the kidneys. A laboratory test that measures the level of urea nitrogen in the blood is the most common test for kidney disease: When kidneys are not functioning properly, the blood urea level will be higher than normal; a low value may be an indicator of liver disease.

If values are abnormal, your physician will order further tests of renal function before arriving at a diagnosis.

bone marrow aspiration

A test in which a sample of bone marrow is aspirated (withdrawn) for analysis. Such analysis will reveal the number, size, and shape of red blood cells, white blood cells, and platelets, all of which are produced in the bone marrow.

The test is performed when certain conditions are suspected: tumors or cancers that may have spread to the bone, or blood disorders such as anemia and hemolysis (self-destruction of red blood cells).

The test may be performed either in the doctor's office or the hospital. A sedative usually is given before the test. Usually, the sample is taken from the sternum (breastbone) or from the crest of the hipbone. The site is sterilized and a needle is inserted into the outer layer of bone to anesthetize the area. Then a special needle containing a stylus is inserted through the skin to penetrate the bone. Once the needle penetrates to the marrow cavity, the stylus is removed and replaced with a syringe; about a teaspoon of marrow is suctioned out. The specimen is sent to a laboratory for analysis. After the needle and marrow are withdrawn, the physician puts pressure on the site for several minutes to prevent bleeding. You will need to rest for at least half a day. Results will be available later or the next day.

Although there is little risk of complications, there is pain associated with this procedure. The tenderness and pain should subside, however, within a few minutes after the needle is withdrawn. There may be bruising at the insertion site that lasts for about a week, and a local anesthetic may be prescribed.

cardiac catheterization

A test involving the passing of a catheter (a long, flexible tube) into one or more of the heart's chambers. It is done for various reasons, including the collection of blood samples, the detection of abnormalities, and the determination of blood pressure within the heart itself.

On the night before the test, you will begin fasting. On the morning of the test, after receiving a sedative, you will be taken into a special lab. Because you will be awake during the test, you will probably be strapped to an X-ray table to prevent any sudden movements. Your heart rate and rhythm must be monitored throughout the procedure, so EKG leads will be connected to your body.

The catheter usually is inserted through a vein or artery in the groin. After the area is numbed by an anesthetizing agent, the catheter is inserted and guided toward your heart. To aid your doctor in directing the catheter correctly, X-ray pictures are shown constantly on a monitor. The movement of the catheter should feel strange, but not particularly painful. Once the catheter is in the heart, blood samples are taken. Do not feel alarmed if your heart seems to be beating abnormally at this point. Pressure readings from the chambers are taken by a special instrument called a *transducer* that is attached to the catheter.

If your doctor is trying to determine the extent of coronary artery disease, he will move the catheter to the opening of a coronary artery with the help of the TV monitor. A substance that is opaque to X rays is released into the artery to make it visible on the X-ray plate or viewing screen. The doctor probably will repeat the procedure on another coronary artery. This procedure is rather uncomfortable: You will experience a metallic taste in your mouth and feel flushed. The unpleasantness should last about only a minute, however.

The catheter is removed and pressure put on the insertion site for about half an hour. You will have to rest in bed for at least five hours, and in the hospital for at least a day. The procedure itself takes up to three hours and is somewhat exhausting, so you will probably welcome the period of rest. You also will be told to drink plenty of fluids and may even be given fluids intravenously.

Since there is some risk involved with this procedure, you should speak with your doctor before undergoing the procedure to get a clear understanding of the risk. Also, by having the test done at a hospital where many cardiac catheterizations are done, you can minimize your chances of complications.

cervical smear

A test in which cells on the surface of the neck of the womb (*cervix*) are gently removed and examined microscopically. It was pioneered by Dr. George Papanicolaou (1883–1962) and is sometimes called a "Pap smear" or "Pap test."

The smear test was aimed originally at early identification of cancer of the cervix and this is still the main use of the technique. But its value has spread to include assessment of hormone imbalance in menstrual and menopausal disorders, infections, and nonmalignant changes in the tissues.

The technique is simple and painless and can be performed quickly without sedation or anesthesia. The tissue may be sucked into a glass pipette or scraped away with a small wooden spatula or cotton swab. The latter method is more likely to detect abnormal cells, but is less useful for hormone studies.

The material collected from the cervix is placed on a microscope slide and examined under the microscope. In this way, abnormal cells, precancerous cell changes, and cancerous cells can be identified. The examination also may identify signs of inflammation, infection, and cervical warts.

Prior to the development of this test in the 1940s, hundreds of thousands of women died from cervical cancer. Routine testing is now available but approximately eleven thousand women a year still die from this disease. Much publicity has informed the general public of the importance of monthly self-examination of the breasts. Pap smears, on a yearly basis, are also vitally important for women of childbearing age, including sexually active teenagers.

If you are no longer of childbearing age, you should follow the advice of your physician on the frequency of pelvic examinations, but it should be done at least every three years. The absence of symptoms does not mean that all is well.

Cervical cancer is one of the most easily curable cancers when caught in its early stages. It should also be noted that women who begin sexual activity at an early age and women with multiple sexual partners have a higher rate of cervical cancer. However, even women who have never been sexually active can develop this form of cancer.

cholesterol testing

Physicians routinely perform this test to determine the amount of cholesterol in the blood, because it has been proved that high levels of blood cholesterol increase the risk of developing atherosclerosis (hardening and partial obstruction of the arteries), which leads to increased risk of heart attack.

The test usually measures total cholesterol and two lipoproteins called low-density lipoprotein (LDL) and high-density lipoprotein (HDL). HDL is called the "good" cholesterol because it is thought to retrieve cholesterol from cells, while LDL is known as the "bad" cholesterol for its role in depositing cholesterol in the arteries where it builds up and constricts blood flow.

You will be told to fast for twelve to fourteen hours before the test; water is allowed. If possible, avoid thyroid medicines and oral contraceptives for two weeks before testing since they can interfere with results.

Serum cholesterol is measured in milligrams per deciliter. A normal cholesterol reading is usually 180 to 200 milligrams per deciliter of blood; moderate–high, 200 to 240; and severely high, over 240.

As with all blood tests, discomfort and risk are minimal.

chromosomal analysis (chromatin)

Testing to determine an individual's chromosome pattern. Usually it is performed if sexual development seems abnormal, if there is evidence of mental or physiologic disability in a sibling, or if there is a question about an individual's gender.

The physician scrapes a cell sample from the inside of the cheek, treats it so that the cells divide, and stains it. The chromosomes are then visible under the microscope and are photographed and carefully counted.

Normally, human cells contain forty-six chromosomes, twenty-three being inherited from each parent. Abnormalities are detected by checking the patient's sample against the norm; for instance, Down's syndrome results from a person having an extra chromosome number 21, giving him forty-seven in all. A missing or extra chromosome number 23 indicates a sexual abnormality.

The testing is 98 percent accurate and causes no pain or discomfort.

cognitive-capacity screening

A test used to determine if mental disease is due to organic or to psychological problems.

A patient is given about twenty-five simple problems—for example, to add 30 and 20, and then 20 again. If the patient gives more than fifteen correct answers, organic disease is considered unlikely.

The test is extremely controversial, its accuracy never having been completely proved to the satisfaction of many health professionals. More comprehensive analysis by a qualified clinical psychologist will usually make the distinction clear.

complete blood cell count (CBC)

This is actually a collection of several tests performed simultaneously, including red blood cell count, WHITE BLOOD CELL COUNT, HEMOGLOBIN, HEMATOCRIT, and platelet count. CBC is performed routinely as part of a physical exam or when a person enters a hospital for any reason. The test is useful in screening for anemia, in which the number of red blood cells is too low; for infection, in which the number of white blood cells is too high; and for a number of other disorders.

Once a blood sample is taken (see BLOOD TESTING), an automatic instrument is often used to separate the blood into its various components and measure them.

The individual tests are:

■ *Red blood cell count*

The number of red blood cells varies according to sex and age; therefore, after the number of red blood cells in one cubic milliliter of blood is measured, the value is compared with the normal range for one's sex and age.

Although a high number of red blood cells (polycythemia) is not always indicative of disease, it can be a sign of certain serious disorders, such as emphysema.

Low red blood cell levels most often point to anemia. However, levels may also be decreased by severe infections, some cancers, and malaria.

■ *Hematocrit*

This test determines the percentage of your entire blood that is made up of red blood cells. To determine a hematocrit level, a blood sample is spun in a centrifuge. The red blood cells will remain at the bottom and a clarified fluid consisting of white blood cells, platelets, and plasma rises to the top.

Abnormal values usually are indicative of the same problems as are associated with abnormal hemoglobin values; however, this test is slightly more useful in distinguishing between different types of anemia. As with the hemoglobin count, the red blood cell value is often raised in chronic lung disease.

■ *Hemoglobin*

Since hemoglobin is the major component of red blood cells, abnormal hemoglobin values usually indicate the same problems that are associated with abnormal red blood cell values. However, if the red blood cell level is normal but the hemoglobin count is low, iron deficiency anemia is probably present. This condition easily can be treated by diet and iron supplements.

Heavy smoking lowers the hemoglobin count

by converting up to 8 percent to the nonfunctional carboxy-hemoglobin.

■ White blood cell count (total and differential)

White blood cells protect against infection and disease, and a white blood cell count will be performed whenever your doctor suspects an infection.

A total white blood cell count is useful in too many diseases to name; however, an elevated count is usually indicative of a bacterial infection. Appendicitis, leukemia, anxiety, stress, trauma, and pregnancy can also raise the count. A drug overdose, poisoning, or chemotherapy can lower it.

There are many types of white blood cells. If the total white blood cell count is raised, your physician will order a differential count to measure the relative amount of each type in the blood.

To perform this part of the test, a drop of blood is smeared on a slide and examined under a microscope. In this manner the doctor can determine which type of white blood cell is responsible for the overall elevation and better diagnose exactly what type of infection or blood disorder you have.

computerized axial tomography (CAT)

A sophisticated X-ray technique used to detect abnormalities in the head or body. The CAT scanner uses a computer to assemble, from a large number of separate narrow beam X-rays, a highly detailed, cross-sectional picture of the body. The CAT scanner can differentiate between small changes in tissue density, making it helpful in diagnosing head injuries and brain disease.

Your doctor may order a CAT scan for a variety of reasons, including a suspicion of brain tumor, aneurysm, or major artery disease.

There is absolutely nothing to fear in this procedure: There is no pain associated with a CAT scan and the amount of radiation exposure is less than with a normal X-ray exam. Further, the procedure can be done on an outpatient basis.

The machine, which has a cylindrical chamber, comes in two main sizes: one that will allow a view of the whole body and one to view the head alone.

There is very little preparation necessary, although a contrast dye may have to be administered before the test in order to make the soft tissues more visible. Some people may feel flushed or nauseated from the contrast material. Clothed in a hospital gown, you will be asked to lie on a table with either your head or body inside the cylinder chamber. Just as with X-ray exams, it is important to lie perfectly still and, if instructed, to hold your breath. While the scanner is in operation, you will hear the same clicks as during an X-ray exam.

The whole procedure takes about forty-five minutes. Afterward normal activities can be resumed. Results usually are available the same day. Also called *computed tomography* or *CT scan.*

dilatation and curettage (D & C)

A gynecological procedure performed to obtain tissue for examination, to determine the causes of menstrual pain or excessive bleeding from the uterus, or to evaluate the reasons that a woman cannot conceive. After a miscarriage, it may be performed to ensure that the uterus is clean of any remnants of placenta and to halt any associated bleeding. In addition, D & C is the most common means of voluntary abortion in the United States.

A D & C may be performed on an inpatient or outpatient basis, under either local or general anesthesia. About a half hour before the procedure, you will be given a sedative. A transfusion may be given if you have lost a lot of blood due to excessive bleeding. (The D & C itself, however, should not cause you to lose enough blood to require a transfusion.)

During the procedure, you will lie on your back with your knees bent. A series of gradually widening dilators (metal rods of increasing diameter) are passed into the vagina to dilate the cervix. When it is sufficiently dilated, a curette—a rod with a sharp-edged loop at one end—is passed into the uterine cavity. The physician uses the curette to scrape the lining of the womb (endometrium). A sample of the endometrium is sent to the pathology lab for examination.

The entire procedure takes about fifteen minutes. Afterward, you will have to rest in the recovery room for about forty-five minutes—longer if you received general anesthesia. If the D & C was done on an outpatient basis, you can go home the same day; inpatients must stay overnight. Activities that are not strenuous can be resumed when you feel ready; however, strenuous activity, sexual intercourse, and the use of tampons usually

DILATATION AND CURETTAGE (D & C)

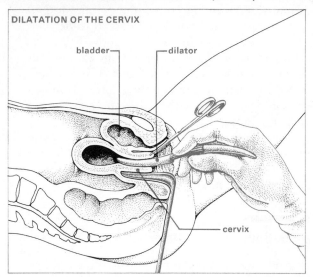

DILATATION OF THE CERVIX

bladder — dilator

cervix

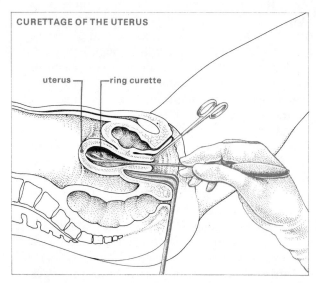

CURETTAGE OF THE UTERUS

uterus — ring curette

A dilatation and curettage (D & C) is the most commonly performed gynecological operation. It is used both for diagnosis (in cases of abnormal bleeding from the uterus) and treatment (for example, after abortions). Progressively larger dilators are used to open the cervix, and then the lining of the uterus is scraped with a ring curette.

are prohibited for about two weeks. You will have to use sanitary napkins for several hours or days, since there is some post-op bleeding.

In most cases, your doctor will prescribe antibiotics to prevent infection, as well as painkillers.

In rare instances, the curette perforates the uterine wall. In this event your doctor may have to perform an emergency hysterectomy.

echocardiography

A safe and painless ultrasound procedure in which high-frequency waves from an emitting source are aimed at the heart in order to gain information about its inner workings. It is useful in detecting fluid between the heart and its lining sac (the pericardium); in determining the size of the heart's chambers; and in viewing the functioning of the heart's valves. The test is more accurate than a chest X ray and shows the actual movement of the chambers and valves.

An echocardiogram usually is ordered if an electrocardiogram (EKG) is abnormal or if a heart murmur is detected through the stethoscope.

To perform the test, the doctor uses a small instrument called a *transducer*, which resembles a microphone, to send high-frequency pressure waves to the heart. The waves that are reflected back from the heart to the transducer are transformed into electrical signals. The EKG machine translates the signals into an image—either a graph or a picture—that can be viewed on a special monitor.

The test, which can be performed in a doctor's office or hospital, is completely painless. Risks are minimal: Unlike the X-ray procedure, no radiation is involved. Usually, an electrocardiogram is performed at the same time; together the two tests take about twenty-five to thirty-five minutes.

If the test shows abnormalities of the heart, a cardiac catheterization study may be ordered.

electrocardiogram (ECG or EKG)

A tracing that represents the electrical activity of the heart. The tracing is an electrocardio*gram*; the instrument used is an electrocardio*graph*. (Both abbreviations are correct; medical personnel commonly prefer "EKG" since it is more distinct when spoken from "EEG"— electroencephalogram.)

The EKG can alert physicians to a wide range of abnormalities: changes in chamber size, heart attack, arrhythmias, pericarditis, and many other conditions that alter the wave patterns of the electrical activity of the heart. An EKG may show changes that are perfectly normal in some individuals but not in others.

The EKG can be traced either on paper or shown on the screen of an oscilloscope. The latter technique is an essential part of intensive care

ELECTROCARDIOGRAM (ECG)

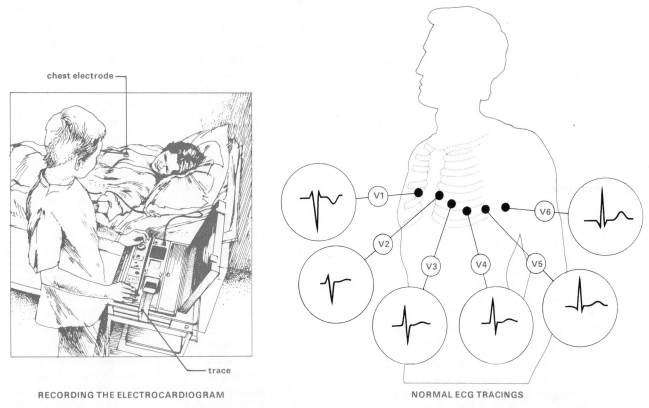

chest electrode —

— trace

RECORDING THE ELECTROCARDIOGRAM

NORMAL ECG TRACINGS

Electrocardiogram (ECG) recordings of the electrical activity of the heart are made from standard points (V1 to V6) on the chest wall. The tracing from each point is different, but should conform to a normal pattern. Abnormalities in the tracing can indicate a variety of heart diseases.

and major surgery, where doctors must constantly assess the state of the patient's heart. Some oscilloscopes sound an automatic early-warning bell if there is any variation in the wave pattern, in order to alert the medical and nursing staffs.

Fetal electrocardiography can be used before and during the induction of labor to assess the state of the baby's heart and to give warning of FETAL DISTRESS. It is achieved by attaching electrodes across the mother's abdomen.

electroencephalogram (EEG)

A test in which a tracing of the brain's electrical activity is obtained by applying very sensitive electrodes to the skull. The instrument used is called an electroencephalo*graph*; the tracing is an electroencephalo*gram*.

All brain functions involve electrical activity

that is detectable through the skull in the same way that heart muscle activity is detectable by an electrocardiogram (EKG) through the chest wall. The tracing of an EEG is very complicated and requires skilled interpretation. Changes from the normal can aid in the diagnosis of such conditions as brain tumors, brain injury, and epilepsy.

Brain-wave patterns of patients with seizures can indicate the type of seizures (petit mal or grand mal) by detecting the buildup of electrical discharge even when the patient has no symptoms.

Usually, a laboratory technician will perform the test in a hospital; it can be done on an inpatient or outpatient basis. About twenty-five electrodes will be placed on your scalp; your head need not be shaved. Although you can eat what you like before the test, no stimulants such as coffee or depressants such as alcohol should be consumed for at least twenty-four hours before.

During the test, you will be told to lie on your back as still as possible with your eyes closed (to avoid stimulation); however, the machine will be stopped periodically so that you can change position.

There is no pain or risk involved. The test usually takes one to two hours, with the machine almost constantly recording electrical waves from the brain. The results, which will probably be interpreted by a neurologist, usually are available the next day. After the test, you will feel perfectly normal.

erythrocyte sedimentation rate

If a sample of blood (treated with an anticoagulant to prevent clotting) is placed in a tall narrow tube, the red cells slowly settle toward the bottom of the tube. In a normal person who is in good health, the process of sedimentation is slow; by the end of an hour the top of the red-cell column will have dropped only 5 to 10 millimeters.

In many diseases in which the blood proteins are abnormal, the sedimentation rate is increased—with figures as high as 100 to 150 millimeters per hour. This constitutes a simple but useful test for the presence of various organic diseases. However, since it provides little information about the type of disease present, it is quite nonspecific.

fibrinogen uptake test

A noninvasive test to identify blood clot (thrombus) formation. Fibrinogen, a protein manufactured by the liver, allows the blood to clot; at an area where a clot is forming, the level of fibrinogen will be abnormally high.

The test usually is performed in the nuclear medicine department of a hospital. You will be given an intravenous injection of radioactive fibrinogen; twenty-four hours later the doctor will record the amount of radioactive fibrinogen detected by a Geiger counter–like device at different sites in the body. If the amount at a particular site is abnormally high, a blood clot is forming at that site.

The test takes about forty-five minutes and causes no pain or discomfort other than the injections of fibrinogen into the vein.

fundoscopy

Examination of the *fundus*, which is the central part of the retina at the back of the eye, using a *fundoscope*, or *ophthalmoloscope*, an instrument with an adjustable lens and a small light at the tip. The fundus is the only area of the body where veins and arteries can be observed directly. During the exam, the optic disk, the place at which the optic nerve enters the brain from the eye, also is observed.

Fundoscopy is a routine part of any physical exam as well as of any eye exam by an ophthalmologist. Properly performed, it is one of the most important tests you can undergo, because clues in the fundus often reveal the first signs of heart and blood-vessel disease, including high blood pressure and hardening of the arteries, diabetes, brain disorders, and eye diseases such as glaucoma. In a person who has had a stroke, little blood clots may be seen.

Adequate fundoscopy involves dilatation of the pupils with mydriatic drops and should be conducted in the dark. The procedure is painless. While you stare ahead, a beam of light is projected through the pupil, and onto the back of the eye. The examination cannot cause harm to the eye.

genetic counseling

Advice to parents about inheritable diseases, especially concerning the likelihood of a disease being passed on to their children.

Counseling is important when there is a history of a hereditary disorder in the family of either parent. If conducted carefully, by a knowledgeable person, counseling can produce a realistic assessment of the risk of passing on the inherited disease to the couple's offspring.

glucose tolerance (blood fasting)

A test to determine the body's ability to stabilize the blood-sugar level after taking a quantity of glucose. It is the most reliable means of diagnosing diabetes mellitus and can also aid in the diagnosis of malabsorption syndromes.

For three days before the test, a diet high in complex carbohydrates or starches should be consumed. At midnight the night before the test, you will begin fasting. At the start of the test, your doctor will obtain both blood and urine samples and then give you a premeasured amount of glucose to drink or eat. Blood and urine samples are obtained and glucose levels measured at thirty minutes, one hour, two hours, three hours, and five hours after you consume the glucose. You will be confined to the doctor's office during this time. You may drink water; food and exercise must be avoided, however, as they affect blood sugar levels.

The test is painless, although it may cause some discomfort because of the confinement and the number of blood samples taken. Results usually are available that day or the next day.

hepatitis testing

Hepatitis means inflammation of the liver. Unless further qualified (such as alcohol- or drug-induced hepatitis), the term usually is taken to refer to a viral infection that causes liver inflammation. Hepatitis testing refers to testing for one of the two main types of viral hepatitis: hepatitis A, or infectious hepatitis; or hepatitis B, serum hepatitis. The doctor will perform such testing if you have been in close contact with someone who has the disease, have eaten a food known to be infected with the virus, or have symptoms of liver disease such as jaundice, lack of appetite, nausea, and muscle aches.

Blood testing, to reveal the presence of antibodies against the viruses, is the most common means of determining if you are infected with one of the two hepatitis viruses.

If results are positive, other liver tests may be ordered. The doctor probably will repeat the hepatitis test in the future, since some persons who recover or are otherwise symptomless carry the hepatitis virus around for years, still posing a health threat by their ability to transmit the disease to others.

intelligence testing (IQ)

A presumed measure of the intelligence of an individual as compared with the intelligence level of the total population. The IQ of a person is obtained by means of a series of tests to calculate his or her mental age, which is then divided by the person's chronological age and multiplied by 100 (to remove the decimal point). The result is the person's "intelligence quotient," or IQ. Thus, a person whose mental age is 12 at a chronological age of 10 will be deemed to have an IQ of 120. Thus, 100 is taken to be the IQ of a person of "normal" intelligence; about half of the population score below 100 and the other half above.

Intelligence tests attempt to establish the mental ability of the subject in a number of different fields. Such matters as vocabulary, arithmetic, ability to reason, general knowledge, and (somewhat less successfully) creativity are tested by the application of a battery of tests worked out by psychologists.

Critics have challenged the fairness of the IQ allocations. They question whether the tests adequately measure the intelligence of children from sectors of the community other than the literate middle class. In the most modern tests, attempts are made to correct imbalances due to language barriers, reading disabilities, or cultural differences.

Ishihara color test

A test devised by a Japanese ophthalmologist, S. Ishihara (1879–1963), to detect color blindness.

The subject is asked to examine a set of cards on which are printed round dots of various sizes, colors, and combinations. On each card the dots of one color (or several shades of one color) form a number or letter, while other colors form the background. The numbers or letters can be read easily by those with normal color perception. Those who are color-blind cannot see them and may in fact detect other patterns that are built into the design.

The tests may be particularly useful in deciding whether a slightly color-blind person can safely be employed in a job where distinguishing between different colors is essential—such as driving a locomotive or connecting color-coded wires in electronic components.

isotopes

These are widely used radioactive chemicals. They are employed in the nuclear medicine department of most hospitals, both in diagnostic tests and in the treatment of certain diseases. After a tiny dose of an isotope is given either by mouth or injection, the isotope's fate in the body can be determined by a device similar to a Geiger counter. Valuable information about the ability of certain organs to concentrate the element concerned can be obtained by analyzing the date generated by this technique. Overactivity of the thyroid gland, for example, can be measured by using a radioactive isotope of iodine.

laparoscopy

Examination of the contents of the abdominal cavity with an instrument known as a *laparoscope.*

You will probably be given general anesthesia for the examination. First, gas (usually carbon dioxide) is introduced into your abdomen through a needle to distend the abdominal cavity and provide room for the instrument to maneuver. A small incision is then made through the abdominal wall below the navel and the laparoscope is inserted through it.

Laparoscopy was first used widely by gynecologists to examine the ovaries, Fallopian tubes, and uterus. A good view of these organs can be obtained, often avoiding the need for exploratory surgery. Minor operations can be performed through the laparoscope with special instruments. Female sterilization by cautery of the Fallopian tubes often is achieved in this way.

The laparoscope can be used to examine other abdominal organs—such as the liver, gallbladder, and appendix—but the views obtained are often less complete than those of the reproductive organs.

Laparoscopy is relatively safe and has few complications. The minor wound heals rapidly, although the necessary introduction of gas may cause you discomfort for a day or two.

liver-function tests

A variety of tests ordered when liver disease is suspected. If bilirubin is elevated, these tests will be performed to confirm and identify liver damage.

In particular, blood levels of four enzymes are determined: AST (aspartate aminotransferase), ALT (alanine aminotransferase), LDH (lactic dehydrogenase), and alkaline phosphatase. If the liver is diseased, these enzymes are released into the bloodstream.

If levels of these enzymes in your blood are elevated, your doctor will probably also measure prothrombin time to determine if blood-clotting mechanisms (controlled, in part, by the liver) are functioning normally. As with all blood tests, the risk and discomfort are minimal.

lumbar puncture (spinal tap)

A test in which cerebrospinal fluid (CSF) is withdrawn and analyzed. Usually it is performed if there is suspicion of an infectious disease of the brain or nervous system such as encephalitis or meningitis. In addition, the pressure of the cerebrospinal fluid before and after removal of the sample is helpful in diagnosing brain tumor or infection. In certain disorders, the introduction

LUMBAR PUNCTURE

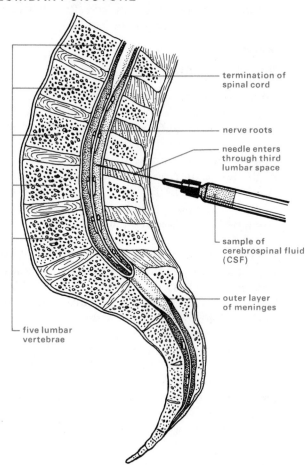

termination of spinal cord

nerve roots

needle enters through third lumbar space

sample of cerebrospinal fluid (CSF)

outer layer of meninges

five lumbar vertebrae

Lumbar punctures are performed by neurologists and other specialists in order to obtain samples of cerebrospinal fluid (CSF). This fluid bathes the brain and spinal cord and is contained between two layers of their enveloping membranes, the meninges. The appearance and chemical composition of CSF changes in diseases such as meningitis, cerebral hemorrhage, and multiple sclerosis; it is therefore an important aid to diagnosis. The lumbar puncture needle is introduced between the third and fourth lumbar vertebrae to avoid damaging the spinal cord.

of air into the space filled by cerebrospinal fluid provides further diagnostic information.

In a spinal tap, a small needle is introduced into the space between the spinal cord and its innermost covering membrane (the subarachnoid space). In most cases the site chosen for insertion is in the lower part of the back, after the area has been infiltrated with a local anesthesia. The tap is performed as you lie on a hospital bed in the fetal position. Once the anesthesia numbs the area, you will feel no pain, only a sense of pressure as the needle penetrates the innermost membrane. Because the penetration is in the lower part of the back, there is very little risk of permanent nerve damage.

After the fluid has been withdrawn and a pressure reading taken with an instrument called a *manometer*, the needle is withdrawn. An adhesive dressing is all that is needed to cover the puncture site.

Your CSF sample is sent to the lab for analysis. You will be asked to lie on your back for the rest of the day and drink plenty of fluids. Some people develop a headache that lasts up to three days after the procedure.

magnetic resonance imaging (MRI)

Like a CAT scan, MRI takes cross-sectional pictures of the body, from which clear, detailed images of the organs can be obtained. The images are even clearer and more detailed than those obtained with CAT scans, however, and MRI also permits biochemical processes within the body to be viewed. Often, tumors too small to be seen with a CAT scan can be found with MRI. No radiation or contrast dyes are used in this process.

The MRI scanner looks something like a large doughnut in a cylinder into which the person's entire body (or part of the body) can be placed. The inside of the scanner contains a powerful electromagnet—so powerful it can stop a wristwatch or erase the magnetically encoded information strips on the back of a credit card. MRI makes use of the tendency of the nuclei of atoms of an element (such as hydrogen or oxygen) placed in such a strong magnetic field to become aligned with the field.

To better understand this, consider that the human body is 90 percent water and that each molecule of water contains hydrogen atoms. Usually, these hydrogen atoms spin back and forth randomly, generating small magnetic fields in different directions. However, when subjected to the strong magnetic field of the MRI scanner, the nuclei of the hydrogen atoms all line up in the same direction. If the nuclei are now exposed to weak radio waves, they will flip; when the radio waves are turned off, the nuclei flip back. This process creates radio signals that are detected by a special receiving instrument and then translated and enhanced by a computer into an image that provides detailed structural and biochemical information.

MRI provides useful information for the diagnosis of numerous diseases, including brain disorders such as multiple sclerosis, brain tumors, and kidney, heart, and lung diseases.

No special preparations are necessary for this procedure, which is done in a special room in the hospital. Wearing a hospital gown, you lie on an examining table and are placed within the doughnut hole of the scanner. Since there is no radiation, risks are minimal; likewise, there are no known complications. After the images are taken by the scanner, they must be interpreted by your physician; results usually are available the next day. The main drawback is the cost: Because the scanner itself is expensive, the cost to the patient also is high. New and more efficient superconductivity materials (which produce the strong magnetic field necessary) are, however, being developed, so MRI scanners may be expected to become smaller and less costly.

mammography

X-ray examination of the breast in the diagnosis of the cause of breast lumps; it is used as a screening test for breast cancer.

A picture is obtained of the soft tissues of the breast in which any potentially cancerous areas may be seen. Mammography can detect tumors in the breast tissue while they are still too small to be palpated readily by a nurse or physician, thus it provides a means for the detection of early cancer.

Tumors detected by mammography may be either benign or cancerous; further tests and often removal of the tumor may be needed before a firm diagnosis can be made.

When having a mammogram, you will be asked to remove all clothing above the waist. You will sit on a stool, stand, or lie down, depending on the type of machine being used. The technician adjusts the machine so that it touches your breast on two sides. An X-ray beam is then passed over it. You will not feel anything except a slight squeezing by the machine. The whole procedure takes twenty to thirty minutes.

Mantoux test

A test to show that you possess at least some degree of immunity to tuberculosis. It consists of the injection of tuberculin, a protein derived from the tubercle bacillus, or a purified protein derivative of tuberculin, PPD. If you are or have been infected with tuberculosis, a positive reaction will occur at the site of the injection within forty-eight to seventy-two hours.

The tuberculin is recognized as a "foreign protein" by your immune system if you have had tuberculosis. The immune system response is a raised, red, itchy, and hardened swelling.

The reaction may also be positive if you have never been infected with TB but have previously been immunized against the disease by an injection of bacillus Calmette-Guérin (BCG) vaccine. A positive reaction is probably due to a symptomless infection in the past. But a negative response is close to certain proof that you have not had the very common primary complex and have no immunity. Negative reactors should consider having BCG.

See also BACILLUS CALMETTE-GUÉRIN, TUBERCULOSIS, in Medical A–Z.

positron emission transaxial tomography (PETT)

A diagnostic technique that allows observation of the biochemical reactions taking place within the brain and other organs in the body. While CAT scans reveal anatomical portraits of each organ, PETT scans give biochemical and metabolic pictures, showing the rate at which different biochemicals are metabolized by body tissues. To accomplish this, the PETT scanner traces positron-emitting isotopes of natural body substances, such as glucose, which are injected into the body; depending on the distribution pattern of the radioactive isotopes, a special computer translates the information into a portrait of the organ being tested. The isotopes to be injected into the body are made by a cyclotron; since the radioactivity can deteriorate within minutes, the cyclotron is located adjacent to the PETT scanner.

Once the cyclotron makes the radioactive isotopes, a small amount is injected into or inhaled by the patient as he lies with his head or body in the PETT scanner, which is a large, hollow cylinder. When the radioactive material travels to the brain, its distribution pattern is recorded and translated by the computer into an image of the tissue being scanned. Comparison of a series of such images affords the physician the chance to observe biochemical changes in brain tissue.

Since abnormal and normal tissues absorb radiation differently, these comparisons allow the doctor to determine if there is dead tissue or a tumor growing in the brain. For example, if a patient who has suffered a stroke inhales radioactive oxygen, a light-colored area will appear on part of the PETT image. This area indicates the part of the brain where tissue death has occurred.

PETT scanning is both painless and safe (one is exposed to less radiation than with conventional X rays). Its main drawback is cost: Very few medical institutions can afford to own the equipment.

plantar reflex/Babinski's reflex

A reflex elicited on stroking the sole of the foot.

Josef Babinski (1857–1932) was a French neurologist. The sign most commonly referred to as Babinski's reflex (or Babinski's sign) is an abnormal reflex (except during infancy) diagnostic of some neurological disorder of the central nervous system. When the sole of the foot of a healthy person is firmly stroked upward, the toes turn downward. When a certain neurological disorder exists, however, the stroking elicits Babinski's reflex: The big toe turns upward instead.

In children under the age of about 2 years, an upward movement of the toes is perfectly normal. But soon after the child learns to walk, a downward movement becomes the norm.

proctosigmoidoscopy

An important method of examination allowing detailed inspection of the inner surface of the rectum and the lower part of the colon. The instruments used range from a simple metal tube to a very sophisticated, steerable endoscope, with fiber optic illumination and viewing channels as well as facilities for taking biopsies. Proctosigmoidoscopy is valuable in cases of suspected cancer, polyposis, diverticulitis, amoebic dysentery, or megacolon.

PLANTAR REFLEX/BABINSKI'S REFLEX

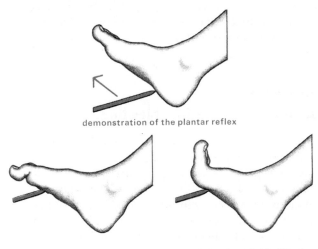

demonstration of the plantar reflex

normal reaction   abnormal reaction   Babinski's sign

If the sole of the foot is stroked firmly with a sharp pointer in the direction shown in the upper diagram, a plantar reflex will be seen, with the toes curling down. Babinski's sign, where the toes curl up, is an indication of disease in either the brain or spinal cord. A positive Babinski's sign is normal in children under 2 years of age because the central nervous system is still maturing.

pulmonary function tests

A series of simple tests that allow the physician to evaluate such lung functions as breathing ability and vital capacity (maximum air volume in one breath).

The tests are performed in the hospital or in the doctor's office. The patient inhales deeply and then exhales forcefully into a tube that is attached to a *spirometer*, a machine that records the total volume of air exhaled as well as the rate at which the air has been exhaled. The values then are compared with normal values, which are dependent on age, height, and sex; deviations from these normal values are suggestive of specific lung diseases.

Usually these tests are performed if you suffer from shortness of breath, wheezing, coughing, or breathing difficulty. They are done also before a chest operation and after bronchodilator therapy to see how the patient is responding.

You should not take any bronchodilator drugs or smoke for five hours before the test. It lasts about twenty minutes; there is no discomfort for most patients, although persons with advanced lung disease may be exhausted afterwards.

The most common tests performed are:
Forced vital capacity (FVC): the maximum volume of air that can be exhaled after maximal inspiration.

Forced expiratory volume in one second (FEV_1): the amount of air expelled during the first second of exhalation. This test is important in the diagnosis of obstructive lung diseases such as emphysema, since the total amount of air exhaled may be almost normal, but the amount exhaled in the first second will be lower than normal due to obstructed airways.

Maximal midexpiratory flow (MMEF): the rate at which air flows during exhalation.

pulse

In everyday usage, "pulse" is taken to be the number of times your heart beats per minute. In more formal medical terms, it is the palpable and sometimes visible change in arterial pressure caused by the pumping action of the heart.

When the heart contracts, blood is pumped through the arteries, causing them to expand slightly. You can feel this pressure at a number of places on the body; usually, one takes the pulse at the radial artery in the wrist. In aerobics classes, the instructor often asks pupils to take their pulse on the right side of the neck directly below the jawline.

The pulse is a useful indicator of health; a slow rate is generally an indication of cardiac efficiency, while an irregular beat may be a first sign of heart or circulatory disorders. The "normal" pulse rate is said to be about 72 beats per minute, but an athlete at rest may have a pulse rate as low as 45. A rate, at rest, as high as 95 is not necessarily abnormal. During strenuous exercise or stress, the pulse rate can go above 200 without harm.

The pulse rate is quicker in children than in adults and slows down progressively throughout life. When a patient is suffering from a fever, the pulse rate usually is elevated. The absence of perceptible pulse is not a definite sign of death; a person suffering from disease or injury may exhibit no pulse even though his heart is still beating.

reflex

A reflex is an involuntary action or movement that occurs in response to a stimulus. Many reflexes may be tested during a general medical examination.

When an appropriate stimulus is provided by the doctor, the reflex response is involuntary; any disturbance in the expected reflex thus affords an objective sign of disturbed neural function. One common test is the "kneejerk" reflex: The doctor firmly taps the tendon just below the kneecap with a rubber-headed mallet; the normal response is for the lower leg to jerk outward suddenly and then return to its former position. The reflex contraction of the pupil to bright light is an important test of the integrity of certain nerve pathways in the brain.

No discomfort or risk is associated with reflex testing.

skin patch

A test to determine the cause of a contact dermatitis (skin inflammation) or other sensitivity reaction.

Since sensitivity reactions can be caused by one or more of a large number of substances to which your body may be allergic, avoidance may be impossible unless the cause is known. To find out the cause, the doctor will apply a small square of gauze to the skin, usually on the upper part of the back. The gauze is impregnated with a pu-

PATCH TEST

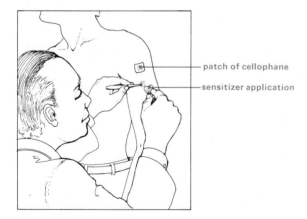
patch of cellophane
sensitizer application

Patch tests are performed in an attempt to identify the cause of allergic contact dermatitis. Possible sensitizers are made up in special creams, and each substance in turn is applied to an area of unaffected skin (usually on the arm). The area is then covered by a patch of impermeable material (cellophane) and left for 48 hours. A positive result, where the skin becomes inflamed, indicates the substance responsible for the dermatitis.

rified extract of the suspected substance or substances. If, after about forty-eight hours, there is an allergic reaction to the substance(s) under test, it can be assumed that the cause of sensitivity has been identified.

stool test for intestinal bleeding

A test to determine if occult (hidden) blood is in your stool. Usually the test is ordered if you have such symptoms as stomach pains, weakness, or altered bowel habits. Occult blood can be a sign of many disorders, including ulcers, hemorrhoids, and bowel inflammation. It is also one of the first signs of bowel cancer. If caught early, bowel cancer need not be fatal.

The test has no risks or complications; the biggest problem for the patient often is embarrassment. If you are in the hospital, your doctor may ask you to try to provide him with a stool sample. If you are coming in for a checkup, he will ask you to bring a sample with you. You can also perform the test at home using a special kit; simply smear a stool sample on the slide provided and mail it in for analysis.

The main problem with the results of stool tests is that many everyday activities—from brushing your teeth vigorously to eating turnips and radishes to taking aspirin, iron tablets, or large doses of vitamin C—can cause false positives. Therefore, your doctor will want to perform the test several times; if all stool samples indicate that occult blood is present, the doctor will order further tests such as a BARIUM ENEMA.

Stool tests may also be taken to detect other abnormalities including bacteria, stool fat, parasites, and worm ova.

stress testing (exercise tolerance test)

Testing to determine if the circulatory system—in particular, the coronary arteries—can meet the heart's increased demand for oxygenated blood during exercise. Narrowed or blocked coronary arteries may meet their function while a person is at rest but they cannot adequately meet the heart's demand while he or she is exercising.

Most modern exercise testing employs a treadmill or a stationary bicycle. Just as if you were going to a gym to work out, dress in comfortable clothes and sneakers. Eat lightly and avoid alcohol, caffeine, and drugs on the day of the test. Do not smoke.

Before you begin exercising, your electrocardiogram (EKG), heart rate, and blood pressure will be taken. While you exercise, you will continue to be monitored. Since the purpose of the test is to determine what level of stress causes symptoms of heart disease, the speed of the treadmill or bike is progressively increased for a set period of time, usually about twenty-five minutes. However, if you develop any signs of distress—such as irregular heartbeat or shortness of breath—during that period, the test will be stopped.

Since the test is performed under the close supervision of a doctor, there is little risk of having a heart attack due to exertion. Since you are the best judge of how you feel, be sure to tell the physician if you feel any discomfort so that the test can be stopped.

thermography

A test that uses infrared heat sensors to measure slight variations in tissue temperatures. It is used to diagnose tumors and blood clots, particularly of the leg, and to determine if impotence is due to organic reasons. While originally hailed in the 1970s as the best tool for diagnosing breast cancer, many medical organizations now maintain that it is not accurate enough to be used in the primary diagnosis of this disease.

The test is extremely safe since it exposes the person to no X rays or radiation. Whatever part of the body the doctor wishes to test is undressed or exposed and put in front of a scanner that looks like a video camera. Depending on how much heat, or infrared energy, is being given off by tissues within the body part, signals are sent to a computer, which takes all the signals and converts them into what looks like a topographic map. Different amounts of emitted heat show up as different colors; abnormalities in the body look like "hot" colors.

The whole procedure, which is risk-free, takes about two minutes; usually it is repeated several times to ensure accuracy.

thyroid-function tests

A battery of tests used to determine if the thyroid gland is functioning normally.

The thyroid regulates metabolism—the rate at which bodily processes occur—by releasing into the bloodstream hormones that travel to organs throughout the body. The most important of these hormones are triiodothyronine (T3) and thyroxine (T4).

The thyroid's function is governed, in turn, by the pituitary gland, which is located at the base of the brain. If your level of thyroid hormones falls too low, the pituitary gland produces thyroid-stimulating hormone (TSH). In response to TSH, a healthy thyroid works harder to push the level of thyroid hormones back to normal.

Thyroid testing centers on measuring the levels of TSH, T3, T4, and two other less important thyroid hormones in your blood. The tests usually are ordered if you suffer from symptoms of either an overactive thyroid, such as rapid heartbeats, palpitations, and unexplained weight-loss, or of an underactive thyroid, with symptoms such as lethargy and weight gain. If the levels of these hormones are found to be abnormal, a special diet and thyroid medication will be prescribed.

As with all blood tests, discomfort and risk are minimal.

ultrasound

A valuable technique for visualizing internal organs, using ultrasonic pressure waves of a frequency as high as 10 million cycles per second. These waves can be formed, like light, into a beam that will reflect from various "interfaces" in the body between structures having different acoustic properties. The technique (also called *ultrasonography*) can be used to inspect organs or structures that will not show up on an X-ray photograph—for example, blood vessels, or gallstones in position in the gallbladder. It has the added advantage over X rays of producing no radiation hazards and is therefore extremely useful for monitoring the developing fetus in pregnancy.

A small percentage of the results are misleading, but the technique is very valuable because it does not disturb the person and can be repeated frequently. In pregnancy the size and shape of the developing fetus can be estimated; moreover, the beating of the fetal heart can be detected from about the twelfth week and the pulse rate counted.

For the procedure you must lie completely still, face up or face down, depending on the organ to be studied. A lubricant is smoothed over the body

ULTRASOUND SCANNING

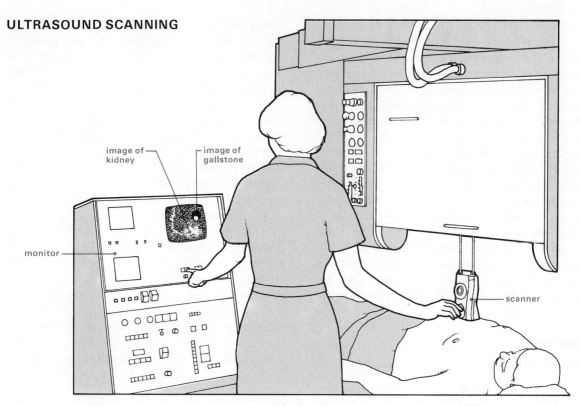

Ultrasound scanning is a technique that measures the reflections of low-intensity, high-frequency pressure waves by the soft tissues of the body. Unlike X rays, ultrasound is not dangerous and can be used in pregnancy. It has also proved valuable in gastroenterology, where it can display the abdominal organs and reveal abnormalities such as gallstones.

area under study, and the transducer—a device that looks something like a microphone—is pressed back and forth over the area. The technician watches the image on a monitor and takes photographs at specific intervals. The procedure is completely painless and lasts fifteen minutes to an hour.

venogram

The veins, like most of their surrounding tissues, are readily penetrated by X rays and therefore do not show up on an X-ray film. To make them visible they must be injected with material that stops the passage of X rays (a *radiopaque contrast medium*). This causes the veins to show up as light areas on the film. Many such materials are available, most of them containing the radiopaque element iodine.

In the venogram procedure, liquids containing iodine dyes are injected into a vein and a series of X-ray pictures is taken as the radiopaque material moves through the vein in the bloodstream.

If the dye's passage is blocked, the blood's passage also is blocked.

The technique is particularly useful in the diagnosis of thrombosis of the leg veins. If you are allergic to iodine or shellfish, make sure that your physician is informed of this before you undergo a venogram.

X rays

X rays, discovered in 1895 by the German physicist Wilhelm Konrad Roentgen (1845–1923), have become one of the best-known aids to both diagnosis and treatment.

A standard radiograph (or "X-ray picture") is produced by placing a body part—the hand, for example—before a sheet of X-ray film enclosed in a light proof envelope and exposing the hand to radiation from an X-ray tube. The bones, being resistant to the passage of X rays (radiopaque), will appear on the film as white unexposed areas, while the soft tissues, being nonresistant (radiolucent), will allow the film behind them to be exposed and blackened by the rays. The result, in photographic terms, is a "negative" picture of the bones of the hand.

Since most soft tissues are radiolucent, their visualization requires special radiographic techniques. (An exception is the lungs: Being air-filled, they are much *more* radiolucent than other tissues and can be studied easily on a simple chest X-ray picture.) A technique with wide applications is to inject or give by mouth or otherwise introduce into the body a fluid contrast material that is opaque to X rays. For example, the upper part of the intestinal tract can be visualized by X rays if the patient first swallows a liquid suspension of barium sulfate (BARIUM MEAL). To visualize the large intestine on an X-ray film, a similar suspension can be given as an enema (BARIUM ENEMA).

Certain iodine-containing compounds can be injected into a blood vessel to allow X-ray visualization of the heart, arteries and veins (arteriogram, VENOGRAM). Similar material, on injection into the circulation, is excreted rapidly by the kidneys, allowing the kidneys to be visualized (*intravenous pyelogram*—IVP). Injection of iodine-containing material into the cerebrospinal fluid (around the brain and spinal cord) allows these structures to be seen on an X-ray picture (myelogram).

A technique for soft-tissue visualization is *tomography*. Movement of the X-ray tube during the exposure allows a plane of tissues to be examined in more detail, since there is no interference by tissues that lie above or beneath. This technique will reveal soft-tissue structures not identifiable on a standard X-ray picture. A more recent development is COMPUTERIZED AXIAL TOMOGRAPHY (CAT). Here multiple tissue planes are viewed by tomography, and the results are analyzed by an attached computer to build up a detailed picture of the soft-tissue structures. This technique is applicable in the diagnosis of tumors and other lesions within the brain, liver, and other organs not easily visualized on X-ray film by other means.

6

PROCEDURES

abortion

A spontaneous or deliberate ending of pregnancy prior to the time the fetus can be expected to live outside the uterus, which is about 20 weeks after conception. Medically the terms *abortion* and *miscarriage* are generally synonymous, but in recent years there has been an increasing tendency for laypersons to use the word *abortion* to mean deliberate termination of a pregnancy; *miscarriage* implies that the ending of a pregnancy has been accidental or spontaneous.

Deliberate abortion has been practiced for thousands of years, but was a quite dangerous procedure until recently. Criminal or "back-street" abortions are still dangerous and may result in death or serious injury.

Legal abortion (carried out by trained medical practitioners, surgeons, or gynecologists) is a relatively safe procedure, especially if performed very early in the pregnancy. The Supreme Court decision of January 1973 made first-trimester (first three months) abortions legal in any setting, including doctors' offices and medical centers.

The technique of an early abortion usually involves aspirating the contents of the womb with a suction catheter. Later abortions (when pregnancy is advanced beyond 12 weeks) may involve more complex techniques and carry a much higher risk of side effects.

For an extended discussion see *Family Planning* in the **Family Medicine and Health** section.

acupuncture

The technique of attempting to produce anesthesia or treat disease by inserting the tips of long needles into the skin at certain points. The needles then are rotated by hand or charged with a weak electric current for five minutes or so.

Acupuncture has been known in China for thousands of years, but until recently it generally has been regarded by Western physicians as a form of "quack" medicine. This view was also taken by orthodox (that is, Western-style) physicians in China itself until well into the 1950s.

However, Mao Tse-tung's instruction to the medical profession in China to "investigate the great treasure house of ancient Chinese medicine" led to a reappraisal of acupuncture. Chinese anesthesiologists were surprised to find that the technique sometimes could induce absence of pain during certain surgical operations.

In the 1960s some Western physicians investigated "acupuncture anesthesia" and found that some patients failed to respond to this method

ACUPUNCTURE

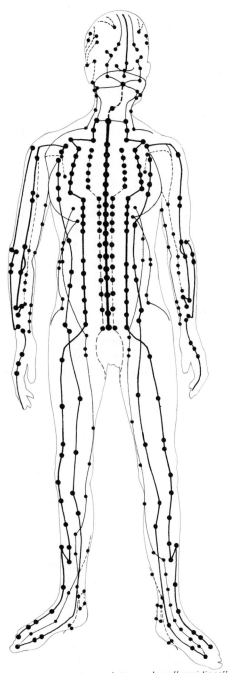

acupuncture points run along "meridians"

This is an acupuncturist's map of the body and shows the various points at which needles can be inserted through the skin—purportedly producing areas of anesthesia in other parts of the body. Many acupuncturists also claim that internal diseases can be cured by their skills. Many conventional doctors are skeptical about its effectiveness.

and continued to feel pain. It was found, however, to have some value in the treatment of chronic pain.

The value of acupuncture in treating disease is dubious, although many Chinese doctors now accept the traditional oriental teaching that acupuncture can be used to treat a wide range of diseases. However, many American physicians point out that the technique has no basis in scientific medicine.

The value of acupuncture in anesthesiology is documented, but its effectiveness as a form of treatment is still under investigation.

Why should it work at all? No Western or Chinese doctor has come up with a truly satisfactory explanation, although some have suggested that the insertion and stimulation of the needles may in some way stimulate the release of endorphins, natural pain-killers present in the body.

amputation

The removal of any part of the body, especially a limb or part of a limb.

Amputation may occur accidentally, as in automobile accidents or war injuries, or it may have to be performed surgically because of severe injury or disease.

Accidental amputation of toes, fingers, legs, and arms is fairly common, particularly in traffic accidents. Other cases occur at home through mishaps with knives, fans, air-conditioning equipment, lawn mowers, blenders, and garbage disposal units. Many amputations occur among workers who fail to observe safety precautions while operating machinery.

In all these cases, immediate surgical treatment is required to alleviate shock, arrest bleeding, and remove the damaged tissues at the edges of the wound. The surgeon will suture (stitch up) and dress the wound and take precautions to ensure that tetanus (lockjaw) and other infections do not develop. In a few cases, it is possible by very skilled surgery to reattach the amputated part—provided it is not too damaged and there has been little delay; it is always prudent to pack the amputated part in ice and bring it with the victim to the hospital.

Deliberate surgical amputation is one of the oldest operations. It is performed in cases of great trauma where a part of the body has been damaged beyond saving, in cases of malignancy where a cancer—most frequently of bone—has developed in a limb, and in cases of gangrene due to trauma, exposure to cold, or vascular disease.

Before the development of anesthesia, amputation was a very rapid and crude procedure; the surgeon's main intention was to remove the limb or other part in a matter of seconds in order to spare the unanesthetized person pain. In the last 130 years, however, since the introduction of anesthesia, techniques of amputation have become much more delicate, so that a reasonably good appearance is obtained after healing. After a limb amputation, an artificial limb usually can be fitted; the psychological adjustment required after amputation may be more difficult than the physical adjustment.

anesthesia

A term generally applied to the deliberate induction of insensibility (either general or local) to make it possible to perform surgical operations.

Before you are administered anesthesia, you will be asked about any drug allergies you may have. In some cases, the choice of whether to receive either a local or a general anesthesia will be yours; the doctor will explain the advantages and disadvantages of each. While general anesthesia may seem preferable because it renders the patient unconscious, local anesthesia without loss of consciousness carries less risk of complications and is associated with a shorter recovery time. If you are given general anesthesia you will have to be taken to a recovery room for at least an hour after the operation so that your vital signs can be monitored.

Complications are rare, but general anesthesia can increase lung secretions, making one prone to pneumonia. If your lungs seem congested, the nurse or doctor will turn you frequently and tell you to breathe deeply and cough to clear the lungs.

One type of local anesthesia, called spinal anesthesia, works by blocking transmission in the spinal nerves. To avoid postoperative headaches that can result from loss of spinal fluid, you may be told to lie on your back for up to a day after the operation.

appendectomy

Surgical removal of the appendix, a small struc-

ture about the size and shape of an earthworm, that is attached to the blind end of the larger intestine (the cecum). Appendectomy is performed whenever the appendix is infected or inflamed (appendicitis).

The operation is usually a simple one, lasting about an hour and performed under general anesthesia. The surgeon makes an incision on the lower right side of the abdomen deep enough to reveal the cecum. After the small intestine is moved aside, the appendix is freed from other structures and tissues, tied off, and removed. Sutures or tiny staples are used to close the incision. A small scar will remain.

Recovery is generally quick. You will remain in the recovery room about forty-five minutes and be up and walking in the room in about five hours. You will probably be able to leave the hospital within two days, drive within seven days, and exercise in two to three weeks. Your doctor will prescribe oral drugs to control postoperative pain.

Complications are rare, particularly if the operation is performed within twenty-four hours of first symptoms. However, if the symptoms go unrecognized, the appendix can become gangrenous and burst, producing peritonitis. Although this infection was once almost always fatal, it can now be treated successfully with antibiotics given intravenously.

See APPENDICITIS/APPENDECTOMY in **Medical A–Z**.

arthroplasty

An operation to rebuild a damaged joint. Damage can occur because of rheumatoid arthritis or osteoarthritis; if it is severe enough to cause chronic pain or disability, arthroplasty may be performed.

Before the operation, you will undergo standard tests including a complete blood count and electrocardiogram (EKG). About an hour before, you will be given a sedative and an IV will be started. The operation usually is performed under general anesthesia.

Knees are a common site for this type of surgery. For total knee arthroplasty an incision is made from the shinbone to the kneecap. A prosthesis is fitted between the shinbone and thighbone while the knee is flexed. The knee is then straightened and the opening sutured.

The operation takes about two and a half hours; you will have to rest in the recovery room for about two hours. The day after the operation you will begin a rehabilitation program with special ex-

ARTIFICIAL JOINTS

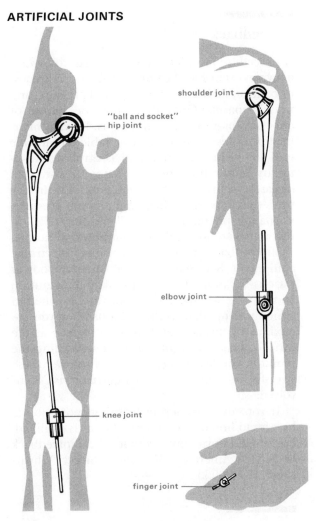

shoulder joint

"ball and socket"
hip joint

elbow joint

knee joint

finger joint

Artificial joints are used to replace joints which have been severely damaged by arthritis. The most successful and widely performed replacement operations are to implant artificial hip joints. The ball and socket is made up of a metal strut and a metal or plastic cup.

ercises for your knee. You will need a walker or cane at first, and your knee will be heavily bandaged. Pain-killers will be prescribed and, possibly, antibiotics as well. A scar will remain from the shinbone to the knee.

See also HIP REPLACEMENT.

arthroscopy

A procedure performed to diagnose joint disorders. It also can be used in performing surgery on a joint.

Arthroscopy can be done on an inpatient or outpatient basis; it takes about one hour. You will probably be asked to fast on the day of the operation. Usually, your doctor will apply a tourniquet or wrap the joint (particularly if it is the knee) in an elastic bandage in order to stop the flow of blood to the joint. After a local anesthetic is injected, a small incision will be made through which an endoscope (arthroscope) can be passed. This allows the physician to observe the joint directly.

During the procedure, the joint may be moved to various positions of extension and flexion. Attachments may be connected to the endoscope so that the joint can be irrigated or a specimen taken for biopsy. Finally the incision will be stitched and bandaged. You can walk the same day, but you should avoid excessive use of the joint for about a week.

During the procedure, the tourniquet may cause some pressure or discomfort. Complications are rare, however.

autopsy

Examination of a body by dissection to determine the cause of death. Conducted by a pathologist, an autopsy (also known as a *necropsy* or *postmortem* examination) may be undertaken with the permission of the nearest relative if death has occurred in a hospital; but if violence or neglect is the suspected cause of death, or if the cause is not precisely known, an autopsy usually will be conducted with or without the relative's permission, according to the laws of the state where the death occurred.

First the pathologist (or the local Medical Examiner) examines the external surface of the body and its orifices (natural openings) and notes any distinguishing marks, wounds, or evidence of disease. Then the abdomen, chest, neck, and skull are opened and all the individual organs removed and examined. Specimens of tissue are taken for microscopic examination. The major blood vessels are opened to assess the state of the inner walls, and in particular the pathologist examines the arteries supplying the heart muscle (coronary arteries) and the arteries of the brain. The stomach and intestinal contents may be kept for analysis as well as specimens of blood and urine.

Where death has been caused by violence, identification of the precise cause is of the utmost importance, since a criminal prosecution may rest on the proof established at autopsy. Wounds, injuries, and poisons all leave particular signs that can be identified, and forensic scientists can nearly always determine with accuracy the cause of death, even in bodies discovered long after death has occurred.

When a death has been investigated fully, the Medical Examiner will inform the appropriate authorities, who will issue a certificate for burial. If the cause is in doubt, or if there is any dispute, the body will not be available for disposal until an inquest has been held.

After the autopsy the body is prepared for burial, with the organs returned to their cavities and the incisions closed.

balloon angioplasty

Also called *percutaneous transluminal coronary angioplasty* or simply *coronary angioplasty*, this is a procedure for widening coronary arteries that have become narrowed due to a buildup of fatty tissue plaque. It is an alternative to heart bypass surgery.

Although introduced only in the last decade, angioplasty has been performed in thousands of patients.

Under local anesthesia, a thin tube or catheter with a small balloon on its end is passed into the clogged artery. Once inside the artery, the balloon is inflated, thus pushing the plaque of fatty tissue against the artery wall and opening up the constricted vessel. The procedure can be performed on more than one artery.

Angioplasty is most successful in opening short segments of diseased vessel; the longer a segment is, the less amenable it is to balloon angioplasty. It is best to have the procedure done at a medical center where it is performed frequently; at such institutions, success rates are 85 percent to 90 percent.

Pain and discomfort are the same as with cardiac catheterization. The procedure is not risk-free: An artery to the heart can tear open, or blood clots can form in the area of the balloon. For this reason, angioplasty is performed with a surgical team and an operating room immediately available.

The main problem with balloon angioplasty is that arteries that have been opened tend to close again within a year in about 25 percent of patients. It is then necessary to repeat the procedure of angioplasty or to perform bypass surgery.

biofeedback

A procedure in which a patient learns to control activities over which he normally has no awareness or control, such as heart rate, blood pressure, and muscle spasms. Once thought to be a form of quackery, biofeedback is now considered by many health professionals to be a valuable therapeutic tool for reducing stress and controlling involuntary body functions. Among stress-related diseases being treated successfully with the procedure are migraine, high blood pressure, Raynaud's phenomenon (or "cold fingers"), severe muscle spasms, and irritable bowel syndrome.

Biofeedback relies on sensitive electronic equipment. Sensors are placed on your body at various locations to measure skin temperature and muscle activity. The sensors are attached to a monitor that detects fluctuations when you are anxious or aroused and displays signals in the form of beeps or light flashes. By watching the monitor, you learn to exercise control over these stressful responses. No discomfort or risk is involved.

If you are considering learning biofeedback, be sure to find out if the practitioner is qualified. For more information, contact the Biofeedback Society of America, 4301 Owen Street, Wheatridge, CO 80033.

blood transfusion

The transfusion of blood from one person to another is now a safe and routine part of medical care. Blood is drawn from donors into sterile bottles or plastic bags containing chemicals to prevent clotting (anticoagulants). Refrigerated donor blood has a storage life of three weeks.

Blood is administered from a plastic bag through a tube (drip set) connected to a needle inserted in a vein in the arm. The rate of administration varies with the needs of the recipient, but in routine cases one unit will be given over two to three hours.

All blood for transfusion is carefully typed for ABO and Rh groups. Except in grave emergencies, only blood of the person's own ABO and Rh type is used and direct compatibility tests are performed between the blood of the donor and that of the recipient.

Whole blood consists of a number of components including plasma (the liquid part), red

BLOOD TRANSFUSION

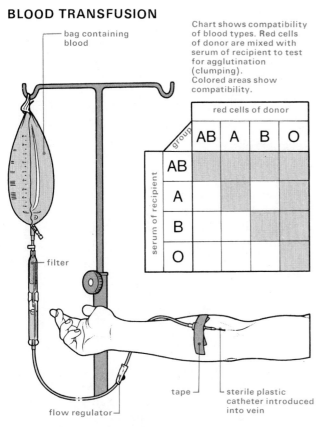

bag containing blood

Chart shows compatibility of blood types. Red cells of donor are mixed with serum of recipient to test for agglutination (clumping). Colored areas show compatibility.

filter

tape — sterile plastic catheter introduced into vein

flow regulator

Blood transfusion can be lifesaving, but stringent checks are necessary before it is performed. The first step is to determine the patient's major blood group (AB, A, B, or O) and Rh (Rhesus) type so that possible donor blood can be selected. Before every transfusion, the blood is "cross matched" as an extra precaution— a sample of the recipient's serum is mixed with the donor's red blood cells to check that they do not agglutinate.

blood cells, white blood cells, platelets, and clotting factors. Usually, each of these components is separated in the blood bank and packaged individually. Component transfusion is now the rule in hospitals. For example, severely anemic individuals receive red blood cells; persons deficient in platelets receive platelets; persons lacking one or more clotting factors receive concentrates of clotting factors.

All blood for transfusion is tested for the viruses that can cause hepatitis and AIDS. Blood that tests positive is discarded. As the result of this screening process, blood-component transfusion remains one of the safest and most important therapeutic tools used in the hospital.

See also BLOOD TYPES in **Medical A–Z.**

bypass

A shunt; a means of circumvention. Specifically, a surgical procedure to create a diversionary channel through which blood or other fluid can circulate around an obstruction.

When an artery becomes narrowed as a result of atherosclerosis or other disease that causes hardening of the arteries, there may be harmful effects on the organ or tissue supplied by the vessel. In addition, a narrowed vessel is likely to become the site of a blood clot that could stop the flow of blood.

Narrowing of the coronary arteries (which nourish the heart muscle) may lead to angina pectoris or to myocardial infarction ("heart attack"). In the limbs, a narrowed artery may produce intermittent claudication with pain developing in the limb on exercise.

In certain sites the problem may now be overcome by the use of grafts to replace the narrowed portion of the vessel or to bypass it. In the heart, narrowed coronary arteries producing angina pectoris can be bypassed by inserting a graft taken from a leg vein or an arterial graft from inside the chest wall (internal mammary graft). Once the graft has "taken," the vein soon assumes the structure of the artery it replaces. In the leg and in the major blood vessels at the lower end of the abdominal aorta (the main artery from the heart carrying blood to the lower part of the body), narrowed or obstructed vessels may be replaced with a variety of plastic grafts. All these procedures demand a high level of surgical skill, but the results can be extremely successful.

After a bypass operation you will remain in the hospital for about two weeks; full recovery usually takes about three months. Once you are home, your doctor may put you on a restricted diet and on a carefully controlled exercise program.

See also CORONARY ARTERY BYPASS SURGERY.

cardiac massage

A technique used in the attempt to restore function to a heart that has stopped beating.

Direct cardiac massage is massage of the heart itself through an opening in the chest; it is performed only by doctors, usually after heart surgery.

External cardiac massage, or *compression,* is performed by means of pressure applied over the sternum (breastbone); this technique combined with resuscitation is called CPR (cardiopulmonary resuscitation) and can save life when performed correctly by a trained person.

cataract removal

An elective surgical procedure to remove a cataract from the eye, often followed by implantation of an acrylic lens. A cataract occurs when the lens of the eye becomes so opaque that it causes defective vision. Surgery is the only effective treatment for a cataract.

Cataract removal may be performed under local or general anesthesia. While the eyelid is held open by a light wire retainer, an incision is made around the margin of the cornea. The lens is removed through the widely dilated pupil and is replaced with an acrylic lens of the correct prescription for your eyesight. Sutures used to close the incision are so fine that they will not have to be removed afterward; no visible scar will remain.

After the operation, which lasts about an hour, you will rest in the ward or in an outpatient recovery room for up to ten hours before going home. Strenuous exercise and bright sunlight should be avoided for two to three weeks. Dark glasses may help. You also will have to clean your eye several times a day and instill eyedrops.

Complications include lens dislocation (in which case your doctor will reposition the lens) and infection, which can be treated with antibiotics. See also CATARACT in **Medical A–Z**.

caudal anesthesia

The use of an anesthetic drug injected into the lower part of the spinal canal to numb the senses in the lower back. It is used during labor and childbirth.

Sometimes the injection is given near the beginning of labor at the stage when contractions are becoming very painful. The woman usually lies on her side with her knees drawn up to her chin. The injection may be given by an anesthesiologist or by the obstetrician. With great care he inserts a needle between two vertebrae into the epidural space. He then pushes a fine tube, or catheter, through the needle into the space and withdraws the needle. The anesthesia is injected through the tube. Its effect lasts for about two hours, and may be reinjected if necessary.

Sensory nerves carrying pain impulses run from the uterus, vagina, and perineal area (between the vagina and anus) to the spinal cord. These nerves are much more sensitive to local anesthetic drugs than are the motor nerves, which control movement in the same area. It is therefore possible to deaden the pain of childbirth while allowing muscle contraction and movement.

cautery

The use of an agent to burn or destroy tissue. The term may also refer to the agent used.

The main use of cautery is to prevent unwanted bleeding during surgical operations. Bleeding from small cut vessels usually can be stopped by cautery, thus eliminating the need to tie off many vessels (which would prolong the operation).

The most simple form of cautery is heat applied by a piece of hot metal, but this seldom is used in modern medicine. In surgery, cautery usually is achieved by a high frequency electric current that heats the tissues and produces hemostasis (localized arrest of blood flow). This is called surgical diathermy, a common technique in which an electrode-heated pair of forceps or a blade is used to cut tissue, ensuring hemostasis as it cuts.

Extreme cold is the agent in *cryocautery*. Gas-cooled probes routinely are used in various operations to destroy tissue by freezing. Cryocautery also may be achieved by the use of liquid nitrogen or solid carbon dioxide, as in the destruction of skin warts.

Chemocautery involves the use of caustic chemicals and is another technique used to destroy skin lesions.

cesarean section

A procedure that allows delivery of a child through an incision in the mother's abdomen. It is named after Julius Caesar, who is thought to have been born in this manner. The obstetrician will advise delivery by cesarean section if he feels it is dangerous—for either mother or child—for the baby to be born through the natural birth passages. It is the method of choice when there are signs of fetal distress necessitating a quick delivery.

In the procedure, an incision is made through the lower part of the abdomen and the lower part of the uterus, through which the child is delivered. The incision may be an up-and-down midline cut

CHOLECYSTOMY

Cholecystectomy, removal of the gallbladder, is usually performed because of gallstones. The surgeon first divides the cystic artery and then ties off the cystic duct (1). The cystic duct is cut and the gallbladder removed (2). Any bleeding vessels are coagulated using a diathermy probe (3).

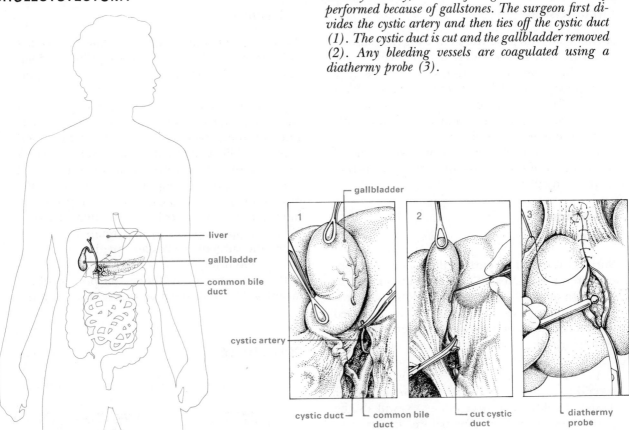

or a crosswise "bikini" incision. It can be done under regional or general anesthesia. A scar will remain where the incision was made. For this reason, most women prefer the low traverse, or crosswise, incision, which, as its nickname implies, can be hidden by a bikini.

See also extended discussion under *Childbirth Options* in the section on **Family Medicine and Health.**

cholecystectomy

Surgical removal of the gallbladder. Usually it is performed if the gallbladder is severely inflamed (cholecysitis) or if there are gallstones (cholelithiasis). While gallstones are fairly common and usually cause no symptoms, they sometimes cause infection, pain, or jaundice.

Before the operation, your doctor will order several tests, such as abdominal ultrasound, to help him observe the gallbladder. A few hours before the operation you will be given a sedative.

In most cases, the procedure is performed under general anesthesia.

An incision is made through the abdominal wall to expose the gallbladder and the bile duct running to the small intestine, is cut off. The gallbladder is removed and the cut in the abdominal wall is sutured, one layer (tissue, muscle, and skin) at a time.

The operation takes one and a half to two and a half hours; afterward, you will rest in the recovery room about two hours. In about two days, you can walk around; strenuous activity should not be resumed for about three weeks. Pain-killers will be prescribed.

While not a high-risk procedure, cholecystectomy does carry the risk of paralytic ileus. In this condition, peristalsis, the normal movement of the small intestine, is interrupted and bloating results. The condition usually corrects itself; if it does not, medication will be given to stimulate the bowels.

A scar will remain on the right side of the abdomen.

circumcision

A minor surgical procedure involving the removal of all or part of the foreskin (prepuce) of the penis. In some ethnic groups, circumcision is performed as a traditional religious rite. Other reasons for circumcision include an abnormal tightness of the foreskin (phimosis) and the belief that it premotes cleanliness.

Circumcision in women involves the removal of the hood of the clitoris; the procedure is rare in Western cultures.

colectomy

Surgical removal of part of the colon. The operation is sometimes called for if a lesion such as a benign or malignant tumor develops in the colon. In many cases, the lesion can be removed without necessitating removal of a length of the colon; however, if recurrent bleeding or infection occurs, a colectomy is needed.

Before the operation, your doctor will perform several tests including a *barium enema* (see under **Tests**). A colonoscopy (see ENDOSCOPY) will also be performed. About an hour before surgery, you will be given a sedative. The operation is performed under general anesthesia.

An incision is made through the abdomen. Once the bowel is freed from surrounding tissue, the segment with the lesion is cut out and removed. The cut ends of the remaining bowel are sewn together so that bowel function will be normal. However, if it cannot be reconnected or if the bowel has been obstructed by the lesion, a temporary COLOSTOMY will be performed. The wound is closed in layers; a long vertical scar just to the left or right of the middle of the abdomen will remain.

The entire operation lasts about two and a half hours; you will remain in the recovery room about the same amount of time. Sedatives and painkillers will be prescribed to ease the soreness of the abdomen. Antibiotics also will be given to prevent infection. Gradually, you can resume nonstrenuous activity; by the second day after the operation, you can walk around. Strenuous activities should be avoided for about a month. If you have a colostomy, you will have to wear a bag to collect fecal waste as it leaves the body. A special diet that prohibits gas-causing foods must be followed.

colostomy

An artificial opening in the large intestine so that it can discharge its contents through the abdominal wall. Colostomies can be temporary or permanent.

A *temporary colostomy* may be performed when cancer has attacked the bottom end of the intestine and the surgeon wishes to divert the bowel contents to facilitate treatment. Persons suffering from severe inflammation of the intestinal wall also may require a temporary colostomy. If the disease is so severe that the rectum must be removed, a permanent colostomy is unavoidable.

In the operation to form a temporary colostomy, the surgeon makes an opening in the abdomen and brings to the surface the tip of a loop of the transverse colon (the middle portion of the large bowel). Once the disease responsible for the

COLOSTOMY

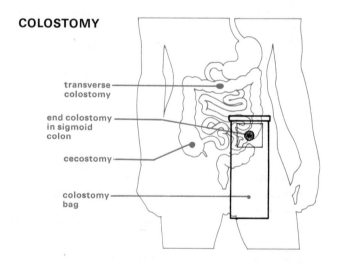

transverse colostomy

end colostomy in sigmoid colon

cecostomy

colostomy bag

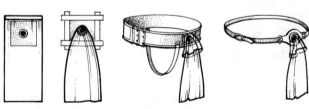

colostomy bags can be held in place by magnets, adhesive tapes or belts

A colostomy is an opening (stoma) made into the large intestine in order to relieve an obstruction. It may be either temporary or permanent, depending on the site. Cecostomies and transverse colostomies are both temporary diversions. End colostomies are permanent openings in the sigmoid colon.

temporary colostomy has been successfully treated, the opening is closed. Usually about three months elapse before closure is possible.

In a *permanent colostomy* the lowest section of healthy intestine is fastened to the skin of the abdomen. The opening, or stoma, is positioned to one side of the midline so that the colostomy appliance (collection bag) will be in a comfortable site.

In the first few days after the operation, the discharge is fluid and collects in a transparent disposable bag attached to the stoma by an adhesive seal. The bag must be changed at least once daily. Later, when the feces become more solid, you may want to switch to bags attached by a plastic flange. These need to be changed less often and are less likely to cause skin irritation. Cosmetic factors are of great importance, and "stoma therapists" can advise you on the use of aids to improve security of adhesion and reduce odor.

Once the immediate postoperative period is over, you may find that your colostomy empties only two or three times a day. Often the timing is so regular that the bag can be emptied before you leave for work in the morning. By paying careful attention to your diet, problems with excess gas production or diarrhea can be minimized.

A permanent colostomy need hardly restrict your normal physical and social activities.

contraception

Any of various techniques for preventing pregnancy. This may be accomplished by a drug, device, or surgical intervention to block the process of fertilization. Contraception permits sexual intercourse without pregnancy resulting. Methods of contraception range from the very unreliable to the almost totally reliable. These methods include coitus interruptus (the act of premature withdrawal of the penis from the vagina before ejaculation); chemical methods such as foams and jellies and the birth-control pill; barrier methods, which are physical devices such as condoms, diaphragms, contraceptive sponges, and cervical caps; and intrauterine devices, or IUDs. (Since 1986 the only IUD available in the United States has been Progestasert; this product contains the hormone progestin, which is slowly released for added protection. This IUD must be replaced yearly as compared with the copper IUDs, which needed replacement every three years. The copper IUDs were withdrawn from the U.S. market be-

CONTRACEPTION

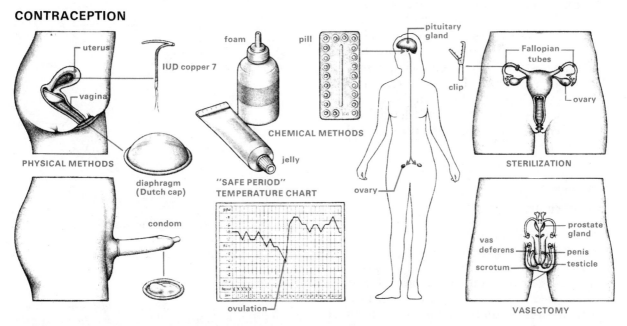

Most contraceptives are either physical devices such as the condom and diaphragm, which act as barriers to the sperm, or chemical methods that either kill the sperm (foam or jelly) or prevent ovulation (the Pill). The intrauterine device (IUD) occupies an intermediate position in that it works by causing local inflammation, and so preventing implantation of a fertilized egg in the womb. Sterilization by closing the Fallopian tubes, or a vasectomy, in which the vasa deferentia are cut, provides permanent contraception.

cause of liability and insurance problems, although they are available in Canada and other parts of the world.)

Another contraceptive option is surgery, either vasectomy for men or tubal ligation for women.

See also "Contraception" in **Family Medicine and Health**.

corneal grafting

Transplanting corneal tissue from one human eye to another. This transplant technique is used to preserve the sight of people who are threatened with blindness when the cornea (the transparent area on the front of the eyeball) turns opaque (cloudy).

There are two main types of corneal grafts: partial- or full-thickness grafts. Full-thickness grafts are better optically than partial grafts; still, in certain circumstances, some surgeons prefer to replace only the outer layers of the recipient's cornea that have turned opaque.

About three quarters of corneal transplants are successful, but the failure of one operation does not necessarily doom the person to blindness. In a few cases it has taken as many as six operations to restore vision.

It can take a month or so for a transplanted graft to "knit" naturally, during which time it is held in place by sutures. These have to withstand considerable pressure, since the pressure behind the cornea exceeds that of the atmosphere.

A major reason for the high success rate of corneal grafting is that the cornea contains no blood vessels; therefore the body's defense system of antibodies cannot attack the corneal transplant to reject it.

coronary artery bypass surgery

An operation in which a portion of a leg vein is used to create a bypass around a clogged artery or arteries. Its purpose is to keep a continuous flow of oxygenated blood to the heart. Usually it is performed if a patient has a severely blocked left main coronary artery or if three or more major arteries are diseased due to arteriosclerosis. Controversy exists as to whether the surgery should be performed in other cases, but it may be recommended to a patient who has angina and is not responding to drug therapy.

Before the operation, you will be given a series of tests such as an electrocardiogram (EKG) and cardiac catheterization to determine if you are strong enough to undergo the surgery and if it will help you. The physician will take an angiogram (see under **Tests**) to determine where any fatty plaques are located. If your doctor decides to go ahead with the operation, you will be prepared for it with a sedative about sixty minutes before, and the nurse will insert a needle so that fluids can be given intravenously. The procedure is performed under general anesthesia.

CORONARY BYPASS

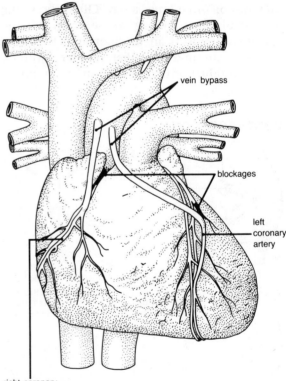

vein bypass

blockages

left coronary artery

right coronary artery and vein

In principle, the coronary bypass operation is simple and involves bypassing the blocked section of the coronary artery with a length of vein taken from the person's leg or a length of artery from inside the chest wall (internal mammary artery bypass graft). In practice, however, the operation calls for a formidable surgical team and expensive equipment.

The operation begins with the removal of a portion of a vein from your leg. Then you will be connected to a heart-lung machine that will bypass your heart during surgery. The chest wall is opened to expose the heart, and a potassium solution is injected to paralyze the heart temporarily. The heart temperature is reduced to 15°C. An opening is made below each of the clogged arteries and vein grafts are connected between this point and the aorta (main artery of the body). Once the grafts are done, the heart-lung machine is stopped and the normal pumping of the heart is resumed.

The operation can take up to six hours; you will then have to rest in the recovery room for at least three hours. Afterward, you will remain in the intensive care unit for about three days while your heart action is being monitored. By three days post-op, your doctor will encourage you to walk around your room; other activities should be resumed slowly, as you feel fit. Pain-killers will be prescribed. Two scars will remain: one where the vein was removed and one from the lower ribs to the breastbone.

Complications sometimes occur, but they can be controlled. Treatment with antibiotics may be necessary if the wound becomes infected. Cardiac rhythm may be disturbed temporarily; this can be treated effectively with drugs.

cryotherapy

A procedure in which tissue is frozen; it is used in the treatment of various disorders, ranging from skin cancer and warts to cervical cancer.

Cryosurgery is carried out with a *cryoprobe*, an instrument containing a freezing agent such as liquid nitrogen. As a treatment for skin cancer, the liquid nitrogen is applied to the malignant tissue to lower the temperature and, in effect, freeze the malignancy to death. The physician must be very careful: If the temperature is not low enough, the malignancy may return; if the temperature is lowered too much, adjacent healthy tissue may be damaged. After cryosurgery, some swelling and oozing may develop at the site.

As a treatment for warts, cryosurgery requires no anesthesia. Liquid nitrogen freezes and destroys the growth; you may be left with a light spot at the site, since the process removes pigment permanently from the area.

debridement

The removal of foreign material, dead tissue, and other debris from a wound. By keeping the wound as clean as possible, infection is discouraged and prompt healing is enhanced. Debridement is commonly used on bedsores and burns.

defibrillation

The use of electrical energy to stop arrhythmias (irregular rhythms) of the heart, particularly ventricular fibrillation.

The ventricles are the two chambers that pump blood out of the heart into the arteries. In a normal heart the ventricles are controlled by the sinus pacemaker, a bundle of fibers in the right atrium that sends out electrical impulses to control the rate of heartbeat.

Ventricular fibrillation usually is a complication of coronary heart disease and, if untreated, causes death within minutes. Treatment of this condition is to stop the fibrillation and resume the heart's normal rhythm.

Defibrillation is performed by applying electrodes to the chest and then passing a pulse of electric current through the chest wall to the heart.

The defibrillator is a machine that gathers electrical charge in capacitors and then discharges it in a fraction of a second. The energy level is usually about 200 to 400 watts per second, which is sufficient to stop the heart quivering and give it a chance to resume its normal rhythm under the control of the sinus pacemaker.

See also ARRYTHMIAS in **Medical A–Z**.

dermabrasion

A technique to scrape away areas of the skin.

Dermabrasion is used mostly to remove the pitted scars of acne from the face. Sandpaper was the first abrasive used, but it has been replaced by special high-speed rotary steel brushes.

The aim of the treatment is to plane down the epidermis (the outer layer of skin) in the scarred area. As long as the glands in the underlying dermis are not damaged, the epidermis will soon grow again.

Local anesthesia is achieved by spraying the skin with a "freezing" fluid. Skin abrasion then takes only a few minutes, although it is followed by superficial bleeding for fifteen to twenty minutes. A dry dressing will be applied for the first day but then the wound will be left open to allow dry crusts to form; these peel off after about ten days. For the first month after the procedure, you should not expose the treated skin to sunlight or cosmetics.

Dermabrasion also has been used to remove facial tattoos and some types of birthmarks.

dialysis

A technique to remove waste products from the blood when the kidneys are unable to perform this task (also called *hemodialysis*).

The most important functions of the kidneys are to excrete the waste products of the body's metabolism and to maintain the correct electrolyte balance of the blood. When both kidneys are failing, these functions have to be maintained artificially.

Dialysis is based on the simple principle of osmosis: Many chemical substances will diffuse through a membrane from a strong to a weak solution.

Blood from a patient in renal failure contains high concentrations of urea and other toxic substances and low concentrations of essential electrolytes such as sodium. During dialysis the patient's blood and the dialyzing fluid (containing the correct concentrations of electrolytes) flow in opposite directions on either side of a membrane. The blood cells are too large to cross the membrane, but the toxic substances diffuse into the dialyzing fluid, while electrolytes pass from the fluid into the blood.

In the familiar kidney machine (hemodialyzer) the membrane is made of a synthetic substance such as cellophane. In peritoneal dialysis the dialyzing fluid is introduced into the patient's peritoneal cavity where the peritoneal membrane serves as the barrier. It is used only in cases where the renal failure is expected to reverse quickly or as a holding operation until a kidney machine becomes available.

Although a kidney machine can maintain life for many years, it is not a perfect replacement for the natural kidney. A patient on long-term hemodialysis tends to develop associated medical problems and to experience severe psychological stress. Successful kidney transplantation is the best treatment of chronic renal failure; most patients are maintained on dialysis only until a suitable donor kidney becomes available. In the event of transplantation failure, the patient can return to dialysis.

The treatment of chronic renal failure is governed by its enormous cost; unfortunately, the majority of patients die without being offered dialysis or transplantation. In an effort to reduce the expense, patients are now encouraged to dialyze at home with standard dialyzing equipment rather than in the hospital. In addition, being at home means the patient can dialyze at convenient times; most choose to do so three nights a week during their sleep.

electroconvulsive therapy (ECT)

A method of psychiatric treatment in which a seizure is caused by passing an electric current through the brain; used in the treatment of some severe mental disorders, especially in cases where medication has not helped. ECT (also called *electric shock therapy*) can impair memory and concentration, and dull both imagination and perception, but sometimes is very effective. It is seldom used nowadays, and when it is, general anesthesia is used to mitigate the unpleasantness.

endarterectomy

The surgical removal of part of the inner layers of an artery together with anything that is impairing the blood flow—such as a clot or fatty deposits (atheromas) on the arterial walls. Also called *thromboendarterectomy*.

The surgeon uses a "coring out" process that leaves behind the smooth inner lining of the arterial wall to act as the new channel for the blood circulation.

It was first performed in 1957 by American cardiac surgeons on the coronary arteries of the heart, in an attempt to increase blood flow to the heart muscle. But in persons with ATHEROSCLEROSIS the entire length of the coronary artery usually is affected and it is technically difficult to remove all the lining of long, convoluted, and tiny blood vessels. So endarterectomy did not prove successful for every person with coronary artery disease. The technique is more successful with the larger arteries, such as those of the limbs.

It was not until bypass operations on the coronary arteries became possible in the late 1960s that surgery for coronary atherosclerosis came into general favor. Since then a number of techniques have been combined: joining together blood vessels from inside the chest wall, bypass, and endarterectomy.

Carotid endarterectomy, to improve the blood flow to the brain by "coring out" the carotid arteries in the neck, has proved successful in most cases.

endoscopy

Examination of the interior of the body through optical instruments inserted into the interior of hollow organs by way of natural passages or, in some cases, through special incisions.

Through endoscopes it is possible to inspect the esophagus (the tube connecting the mouth to the stomach), stomach, large intestine, bladder, air passages of the lungs (bronchi), abdominal cavity, interior of joints, and even the ventricles of the brain (cavities containing cerebrospinal fluid).

The basic technique was invented in the nineteenth century, but instruments were relatively clumsy because they depended on a straight optical pathway; an early endoscope was basically a rigid shaft bearing an inspection lens and a light at the end. With the invention of fibers capable of conducting light (fiberoptics), the shaft of the endoscope no longer had to be rigid. Because of this flexibility, modern instruments make it possible to inspect structures that were formerly inaccessible. Photographs can be taken through the endoscope, and in many cases a fragment of suspected abnormal tissue can be removed through the endoscope for microscopic examination (biopsy).

You will probably be given a sedative to help you relax during the procedure, which consists of passing a flexible tube through your mouth, urethra, or anus to the area under examination. Although the procedure is somewhat uncomfortable, endoscopy usually is not painful or dangerous when performed by a specially trained physician. It can be done on an outpatient basis.

epidural anesthesia

A form of local anesthesia achieved by injecting the anesthetic agent between the spines of the vertebrae into the space (extradural space) just outside the outermost covering membrane (dura mater) of the spinal cord. Also called *peridural anesthesia.*

episiotomy

A small surgical incision made in the vaginal orifice, on one side, to facilitate childbirth and prevent unwanted tearing of tissues.

FIBEROPTIC ENDOSCOPE

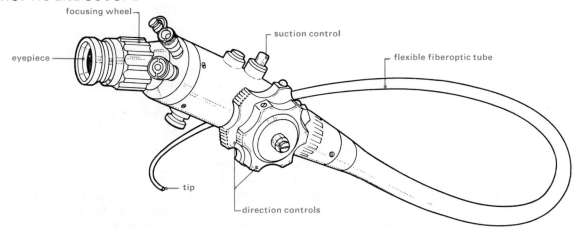

The fiberoptic endoscope shown here permits direct visual examination of the esophagus, stomach, and duodenum. It is a quick and safe procedure in experienced hands and the patient requires only mild sedation beforehand. The long tube, which is swallowed, contains thousands of fibers that project light and also act as a telescope.

EPISIOTOMY

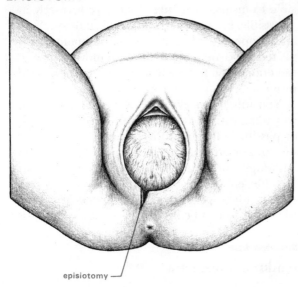

episiotomy —

An episiotomy is a small cut made at the bottom of the vagina at the moment of delivery of the baby's head. It is performed where there is a risk that the baby's head will tear the mother's perineal tissues. The cut is placed to avoid vital structures such as the anus and the supports of the uterus.

During delivery the perineal skin becomes very stretched, particularly if the baby's head is large; as a result, jagged tears of skin and muscles may occur. Many gynecologists believe it is better to prevent this tearing by making a small incision to enlarge the entrance to the vagina just before delivery.

You will feel little or no pain because of the previously administered anesthesia. The surgical wound is stitched up following delivery. It heals rapidly, often with very little discomfort.

gastrectomy

Surgical removal of all or part of the stomach. The extent of the operation depends on the condition for which it is being performed.

Gastrectomy may be indicated in cases of ulceration of the stomach or duodenum that have not responded to medical treatment, in cases of uncontrollable bleeding from ulcers, in the treatment of cancer of the stomach, and for the relief of obstruction to the emptying of the stomach caused by old ulceration near the pylorus, the outlet of the stomach (where scarring has narrowed the passage from the stomach to the duo-

denum, the first part of the small intestine).

Sometime before surgery a nasogastric tube will be inserted through your nose and passed down the esophagus into your stomach to empty it. Although not painful, the tube will be uncomfortable.

During the operation the surgeon makes an incision in the upper part of your abdomen just below the rib cage. A part of the stomach or all of it is removed and the gastrointestinal tract is reconnected. The operation takes two to two and a half hours. As with all major surgery you will have postoperative pain but medication will be given; ask for it if it is not. You will have to remain in the hospital for ten to fourteen days.

After the removal of the stomach or part of it, there may be unwanted aftereffects such as weight loss, anemia, recurrent ulcers, or the *dumping syndrome*. In the last-named, the person either becomes faint and pale about five minutes after a meal and suffers from abdominal rumbling and distention with vomiting and diarrhea, or feels these symptoms coming on about half an hour after a meal. In the first case, symptoms are due to the rapid passage of food into the small intestine; in the latter case, which is far less common, the quick passage of food produces a sharp rise in blood sugar followed by an outpouring of insulin, which leads to an abnormally low bloodsugar level (hypoglycemia). Relief may be obtained by taking small meals, lying down after meals, and learning to take appropriate doses of glucose at the right time.

hemorrhoidectomy

Elective surgery to remove hemorrhoids, a condition in which the veins around the anus or in the anal canal are abnormally dilated. It is done when there is pain, bleeding, large piles, or constant discomfort.

The operation usually is performed in the hospital and lasts about an hour. Before surgery, you will be given a sedative and either a local or general anesthetic. The anal area is cleansed and shaved. One of two surgical procedures is then performed: The hemorrhoids may be tied off and allowed to shrink, or carefully cut away and the wounds sutured. No visible scars will exist.

After the operation, you will remain in the recovery room for about two hours where you will be observed for any signs of bleeding. The next day you will be able to sit up and walk about. You should avoid strenuous exercise and lifting for about three weeks, however.

Although the operation is generally safe, many patients are uncomfortable afterward. Oral drugs will be given for postoperative pain, and laxatives and rectal creams given to ease discomfort during bowel movements.

There is some chance of postoperative bleeding, in which case the blood vessel is sutured. If the wound becomes infected, antibiotics will be administered.

herniorrhaphy

An operation to repair an abdominal hernia, which is the protrusion of a loop of bowel through a defect in the wall of the abdominal cavity. In some cases it is elective surgery performed because the hernia is merely uncomfortable rather than life-threatening. In other instances, it must be performed because the contents of the hernia have become trapped in the muscle wall; without surgery, they can become strangulated or swell and become gangrenous.

The operation usually is performed in the hospital. After you are given either a local or general anesthetic, the surgeon will make an incision just above the groin and cut through muscle and tissues to locate the hernial sac. Its contents—usually part of the small intestine—are returned to the normal position. The surgeon ties off the sac itself and removes it. The incisions in the muscle, tissue, and skin are closed; a small scar will be left just above the groin.

The operation lasts up to two hours; afterward you will remain in the recovery room for up to two hours more. Although you will be able to walk the same day, running or strenuous activity should not be attempted for at least a month. Heavy lifting should be avoided for two months. Most people can resume sexual activity in three weeks.

Several complications are possible. In men, the testes can become irritated or inflamed; this will be treated with application of cold packs to the scrotum, antibiotics, anti-inflammatory drugs, and bed rest. In elderly men, the prostate gland also can become irritated or inflamed, causing urinary retention, which may necessitate catheterization for relief.

Oral medication will be prescribed for any postoperative pain.

See also HERNIA in **Medical A–Z.**

hip replacement

Osteoarthritis of the hip is a very common cause of severe disability, particularly in the elderly. Mostly it is caused by wear and tear, but any injury or disease that damages the joint surfaces tends to accelerate the development of osteoarthritis. Where the cartilage wears away there is considerable pain, which is made worse by walking, and increased stiffness develops in the joint. For mild cases, medication and physical therapy may make life tolerable, but a worn-out joint cannot be regrown. However, there are two main types of operations for the surgical replacement of an artificial joint.

In *cup arthroplasty* the joint socket (acetabulum) on the pelvis is smoothed out and a highly polished metal cup (often of titanium) is placed over the head of the thighbone (femur) to serve as a replacement lining for the joint.

In *total replacement* the head of the femur is removed and replaced with a metal prosthesis permanently embedded in the shaft of the bone. The socket is deepened and a rigid plastic cup is cemented to the bone with an acrylic compound. The operation lasts two to three hours. Afterward, a tube attached to a suctioning device may be put in place at the incision site to draw out blood and fluid in order to hasten healing.

This operation has few complications and brings immediate pain relief and a dramatic improvement in movement range.

A physical therapist will take you through some exercises, which may hurt at first. A special triangular bar above your bed will help you move in bed, where you will be required to stay for four to five days. After that you will be able to move to a chair and to a walker. Your stay in the hospital will be from two to three weeks. Once home you may need to use a cane for a few weeks.

The duration of the new joint's activity is known to be at least a decade.

Replacement of other joints—such as the knee, shoulder, wrist, ankle, and elbow—also has been done but is not yet as widely employed as hip replacement.

hypophysectomy

Surgical removal of the hypophysis, better known as the *pituitary gland.*

About the size of a pea, the pituitary gland is situated beneath the brain behind the eyes. It acts as an intermediary between the brain and the major endocrine glands, controlling the secretion of sex hormones, thyroid hormone, and the adrenal corticosteroids. The pituitary also secretes growth hormone and hormones controlling lactation.

The pituitary may be removed surgically if a tumor forms in the gland—although treatment by radiation therapy often is preferred. It is also removed in some cases of advanced breast cancer when the tumor has been shown to be hormone-dependent. Whatever the cause, after removal of the pituitary, the normal hormone balance of your body needs to be maintained by replacement therapy with synthetic hormones.

hysterectomy

Surgical removal of the uterus or womb. Indications for the operation include cancer of the womb, fibroid tumors, pelvic infections, endometriosis, and excessive uterine hemorrhage. The operation is usually elective.

Various procedures are covered under the term *hysterectomy*. The most radical operation, carried out for overgrowth of fibroids and for cancer of the womb, involves removal not only of the uterus, but also of the Fallopian tubes, the ovaries, and—in the case of cancer—the lymphatic glands that drain the area of malignancy. In this case, an incision usually is made through the lower part of the abdomen. However, if only the cervix or the uterus need to be removed, a vaginal approach may be used, in which an incision is made around and above the cervix. Either procedure is performed under general anesthesia in the hospital. While the vaginal incision will leave no visible scar, the abdominal cut will leave a low, transverse "bikini" scar.

The operation lasts from one to three hours, after which you will remain in the recovery room for about the same amount of time. You will be able to walk around your room the next day; however, most strenuous activities, as well as sexual intercourse, will have to be avoided for about two months. In some cases, if your health is good and you experience minimal vaginal pain or discomfort after the operation, these activities can be resumed sooner.

Contrary to the old wives' tale, sexual desire is not lost after a hysterectomy. However, removal of the uterus means you will be sterile and will no longer menstruate.

Any pain you experience after the operation should be controlled by oral drugs which your doctor will prescribe. There is a chance of complications, including pelvic abscess, inflammation, and hematoma. All are treatable by your physician.

ileostomy

The surgical formation of an opening through the abdominal wall into the ileum (the lower part of the small intestine). The operation is performed whenever the colon has to be removed; the opening then acts as an artificial anus through which the contents of the small intestine are discharged instead of passing through the colon to the natural anus.

The opening does not have muscles like the opening of the natural anus, so if you have an ileostomy you will have to wear a bag continually to collect the fecal matter. This sounds unwieldy, but in fact an ileostomy is perfectly compatible with a normal life.

The colon (large intestine) absorbs water from the intestinal contents. But the waste products discharged through an ileostomy have not passed along the colon; thus they are watery, especially for a time just after the colon has been removed. Later your body will adapt and the fecal matter will gradually become more formed although never completely solid.

ILEOSTOMY

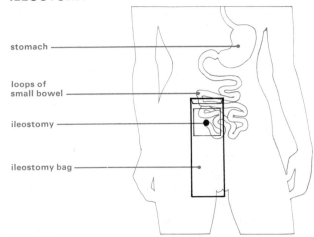

stomach

loops of small bowel

ileostomy

ileostomy bag

An ileostomy is an opening made in the ileum (the last part of the small bowel) to divert fecal material to the exterior, where it is collected in a bag. Ileostomies are necessary when the colon and rectum have been removed.

You may have to make some minor changes in your diet to alter the consistency of the stools or to reduce odor.

You will learn how to look after your ileostomy at the hospital where the operation is performed. Additional help may be obtained from the United Ostomy Association or its chapters, which exist in all fifty states.

See also COLOSTOMY.

immunization

The process by which resistance to infection is artificially induced.

Normally the body resists infection by producing substances called antibodies, which act against infectious organisms. Each infectious organism has on its body surface a substance called an antigen, which the body recognizes as "foreign." Whenever an infectious agent invades the body, the body starts to produce antibodies against this type of organism. The antibodies produced are released into the blood circulation so that they can reach the site of infection.

Each type of organism has its own particular type of antigen, and antibodies produced in response to infection by one type are specific only against that type of antigen.

Usually, after recovery from an infection, sufficient antibody remains in the circulation to protect against further infection by the same organism. This type of resistance is known as *naturally acquired immunity*.

Artificial immunization can be produced in two ways, active and passive. In *active immunization* the antibodies are produced in response to antigens deliberately introduced into the body, usually by injecting the body with the antigens, but sometimes by having them swallowed. These antigens may come in the form of dead organisms, or organisms so weakened (by laboratory methods) that they cannot cause disease but can stimulate antibody production. Increasingly, vaccines are being produced using organisms modified by genetic engineering so as to be safe while remaining strongly antigenic.

If the disease is caused by toxins (poisons) produced by infectious organisms, *antitoxin* production may be stimulated artificially by injecting chemically modified toxins, or *toxoid*.

In *passive immunization*, readymade antibodies against a particular organism are injected. These antibodies may have come from the blood of someone who previously has been infected or immunized, or from animals that have been immunized deliberately so that their antibodies can be harvested for use in passive immunization. Passive immunization provides quicker but only temporary immunity. Active immunization may require a few weeks before antibodies are produced, but the effect is longer-lasting, the degree and duration of immunity varying with different diseases. Sometimes the antigen has to be given in two or three doses to ensure the production of a reasonable quantity of antibody.

Immunization may sometimes produce unpleasant reactions, but this varies with the type of immunization. People who have allergies are more likely to suffer from adverse reactions.

Immunization against several specific diseases of childhood is advisable; not only does this protect the individual child, but it protects the whole community, because if a large proportion of the susceptible population is immune to a disease an epidemic cannot get under way—thus even those who are not, or cannot be, immunized are to some extent protected.

The age at which a child gives the best response to a vaccine varies with the type of immunization.

Most pediatricians follow a plan of immunization that has been approved by the American Academy of Pediatricians. Most school systems mandate that a child must have completed his or her course of immunizations before being allowed to attend school.

induction of childbirth

The use of artificial means to start the process of childbirth, or labor. Sometimes this is carried out when it appears safer for the fetus or mother that the pregnancy be terminated as soon as possible. The timing should be such that the fetus is mature enough to have at least as good a chance of survival outside the uterus (even if in an incubator) as inside.

Sometimes labor is induced not for obstetric problems, but so that it can take place at a convenient time for both mother and doctor.

Labor can be induced in two basic ways. One is the use of drugs, given intravenously, to stimulate the uterus to contract. The other is artificial rupture of the membranes surrounding the fetus. The release of fluid produced by rupture of the membranes sets off uterine contractions. Sometimes artificial rupture of membranes is used in conjunction with induction by drugs.

Induction of labor carries some risk. The uterus may respond to induction by contracting too violently (in which case the uterus may even rupture), or it may not respond sufficiently. The fetus may turn out to be too premature, or it may not withstand the process of childbirth and show signs of fetal distress. If the membranes have been ruptured, there is also a risk of infection. Thus, very careful observation of mother and fetus has to take place throughout an induced labor and, if necessary, a cesarean section may have to be carried out.

Medical indications for induction of childbirth include severe maternal diabetes and severe preeclampsia.

intubation

The introduction of a tube into a body orifice. The term usually is used to mean the introduction of a tube through the mouth or nose into the windpipe in order to maintain an adequate air passage into the lungs. It is carried out in general anesthesia, in cases of unconsciousness due to other causes, and in cases where the breathing is obstructed.

Gastric intubation, the passage of a tube into the stomach through the esophagus, is necessary in some cases of obstruction to the esophagus and in some cases of paralysis of the swallowing mechanism. It is used in cases of intestinal obstruction so that the contents of the stomach can be aspirated. It is also used to wash the stomach out in cases of poisoning.

iridectomy

Surgical removal of a portion of the iris of the eye.

The function of the iris is to let in a controlled amount of light to the retina. It acts much the same as the adjustable lens opening of a camera, which controls the amount of light that hits the film. A portion of iris is removed to improve sight when for some reason the pupil becomes obscured, or when there is another disease that the procedure may improve.

Iridectomy may be *peripheral,* in which a small portion of iris is removed from the base, or *broad,* in which a large area of the iris, including the edge of the pupil, is excised, leaving a keyhole

type of appearance. Peripheral iridectomy is usually curative in subacute glaucoma, and broad iridectomy is often needed in congestive glaucoma. *Optical* iridectomy is used to shape a new pupil and improve vision in cases of central opacities of the cornea or lens; and, finally, *therapeutic* iridectomy may be performed to prevent recurrence of iritis (inflammation of the iris). Peripheral iridectomy is now usually done by laser.

laparotomy

Any surgical operation in which an incision is made into the abdominal cavity.

Laparotomy may be performed in order to expose for surgery any of the organs within the abdomen (such as the stomach, gallbladder, or colon) or for inspection of the abdominal contents. The latter operation, called an exploratory laparotomy, sometimes is required to determine the nature of lumps felt in the abdomen, to inspect a tumor and assess whether or not it is operable, and occasionally to seek the cause of an unexplained fever. Modern diagnostic techniques have made exploratory laparotomy a less common procedure than it was in the past.

laryngectomy

Surgical removal of the larynx, performed especially in cases of advanced cancer.

The larynx ("voice-box") is situated in the throat between the pharynx and the trachea. Laryngectomy destroys the power of normal speech; however, following this procedure, many patients can be taught "esophageal speech." The person swallows air and then belches it up from the esophagus, moving his lips and tongue at the same time to form words. Artificial "voice-boxes," implanted in place of the removed larynx, have also been fairly successful in restoring speech.

laser surgery

Procedures in which a laser is utilized to perform surgery; often used in the prevention of detached retinas and for removal of tumors, growths, and "port wine" birthmarks.

Laser stands for "light amplification by the stimulated emission of radiation." The laser instrument used for surgery is usually a glass rod

LASER SURGERY

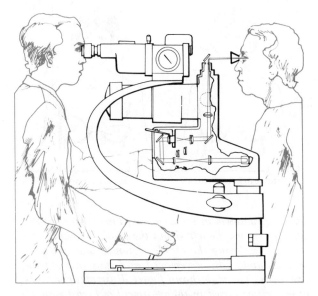

The first surgical use of lasers was in treating certain types of eye disorders, particularly the repair of a detached retina. The intense beam of light is directed into a pinpoint and focused for a split second on the detached part of the retina, producing an inflammation reaction that causes the tissues to fuse together.

filled with a gas such as carbon dioxide. When electrons in the gas are excited, energy is given off in the form of light. The light is amplified and a laser—a narrow, very concentrated beam—is created.

The first surgical use of lasers was in treating certain types of eye disorders, particularly the sealing of retinal holes or areas of degeneration, threatening to cause detached retina. The intense beam of light is directed into a pinpoint and focused for a split second on the damaged part of the retina, producing an inflammation reaction that causes the tissues to fuse together. The laser is now used much more often to treat the disorder of retinal blood vessels, which commonly complicates diabetes.

Laser surgery also shows great promise in removing growths and tumors; it is so precise that doctors can remove tiny areas of tissue leaving healthy adjacent tissue undamaged. The beams cauterize (seal the blood vessels) as they remove unwanted tissue, thus minimizing bleeding and swelling.

lithotomy

The removal of a stone, usually a bladder stone, through an operative incision. Stones may form in the bladder or may enlarge there after being passed from the kidney. The main symptoms are pain, frequent urination, and blood in the urine. An X-ray study usually reveals the presence of the stone. It is removed by the introduction of a crushing instrument via the urethra or, if the stone is too large and hard, by lithotomy—surgical incision into the bladder above the pubis.

Today, stones are removed more frequently by a method called extracorporeal shockwave lithotripsy, which, in effect, disintegrates the stones.

The term also describes a position—the *lithotomy position*—used in the early days of surgery in the operation of "cutting for the stone." The patient lies on the back with the thighs raised and the knees supported and held apart. The position is employed during childbirth, for gynecological procedures, and in operations on the rectum or anus.

lobotomy

Brain surgery in which nerve fibers in the frontal lobe of the brain are cut. Overwhelming depression, incapacitating anxiety, and extreme pain are among the reasons for considering this operation. It is rarely performed now because of its many unpredictable and undesirable side effects, and because of major improvements in drug therapy.

mammoplasty

A cosmetic operation to enlarge or reduce the size of the breast or to restore its shape after a cancer operation.

Reduction mammoplasty is the removal of tissue from the breasts when they are too large or heavy, followed by their cosmetic "reconstruction."

Augmentation mammoplasty is the opposite: enlargement of the breasts. Surgeons currently prefer to implant a sealed bag containing silicone. The implant is placed into a pocket cut into the underside of the breast. There is a *small* long-term risk of scarring and distortion of the shape of the breast, especially if the silicone leaks out of the implant.

Mammoplasty is being used increasingly to restore the breast contours after surgical removal of a breast tumor by partial MASTECTOMY. The volume of the breast may be restored to normal either with a silicone implant or with a graft of fat or muscle taken from another part of the body. With such restorative surgery no form of artificial breast or padding is needed, and the fact that surgery has been performed may be unnoticeable even when the patient wears a bikini.

mastectomy

Surgical removal of breast tissue in the treatment of cancer.

Radical mastectomy was the most commonly employed technique until recently. In this operation the breast, both underlying pectoral (chest) muscles, and the lymph nodes in the corresponding armpit were removed en bloc. Many women found this to be a mutilating operation; in addition, it produced problems of arm swelling and shoulder immobility. Nevertheless, radical mastectomy is unsurpassed in terms of the number of women with early breast cancer who survive for five years or more after operation, and it has been the mainstay of operative treatment for seventy-five years.

Radical mastectomy, however, is no longer standard therapy. A *modified radical mastectomy*— in which the breast, one of the pectoral muscles beneath it, and the auxiliary lymph nodes under the arm are removed—is now probably the most common operation used in the United States.

Some surgeons advocate the use of *simple mastectomy*—removal of the breast only. An even less extensive operation that is being used in selected cases is the *lumpectomy*, in which only the cancerous lump and surrounding tissue are removed. These simpler and less disfiguring procedures have been made possible by improvements in imaging techniques and in the effectiveness of radiation and chemotherapy.

If you have a mastectomy, you will have a bulky dressing on your chest. The arm on the side of your operation will be raised above your shoulder to prevent swelling. You may need medication for pain; and although your arm may hurt, you will be encouraged to use it.

You will remain in the hospital for a week to ten days (for a lumpectomy the hospital stay is a day or two). Before you leave you will be given exercises for the shoulder, arms, and chest muscles to help you regain strength and mobility.

If the breast cancer has already formed distant metastases or large lymph-node deposits, mastectomy alone is ineffective, and your physician will

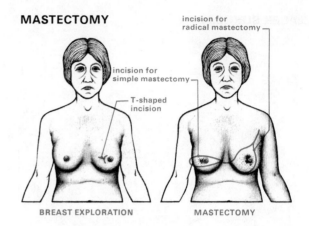

MASTECTOMY

incision for radical mastectomy

incision for simple mastectomy

T-shaped incision

BREAST EXPLORATION   MASTECTOMY

There are many techniques employed in breast surgery. The picture on the left shows the small T-shaped cut used for exploring the nipple region so that any suspicious lumps can be removed and examined microscopically. The right-hand figure illustrates two types of mastectomy used in the treatment of breast cancer.

add various combinations of hormones, drugs, and radiation therapy to your treatment regimen.

meniscectomy

In the knee joint, the medial and lateral cartilages (the *menisci*) are two crescent-shaped wedges of fibrocartilage interposed between the femur and tibia (the thighbone and shinbone, respectively). These menisci compensate for the incongruities in the shapes of the two bones and facilitate smooth movement at the joint. If one or the other meniscus should be torn and displaced by injury, or if it is distorted by a cyst, then it is usually removed surgically (a procedure known as meniscectomy).

Although the knee is principally a hinge joint, once the knee has been flexed it is possible for the tibia to be rotated or twisted. When the leg is bearing weight and the flexed knee is violently twisted, the meniscus can be torn. The torn and displaced fragment of cartilage can jam between the femur and tibia, "locking" the knee so that the leg cannot be straightened. Two thirds of these cases involve the medial meniscus only. Such injuries often are incurred in sports, particularly football.

Initial treatment following injury may be nonsurgical and involve merely splinting the affected joint. A true tear does not heal satisfactorily, however, because the cartilage has virtually no blood

MENISCECTOMY

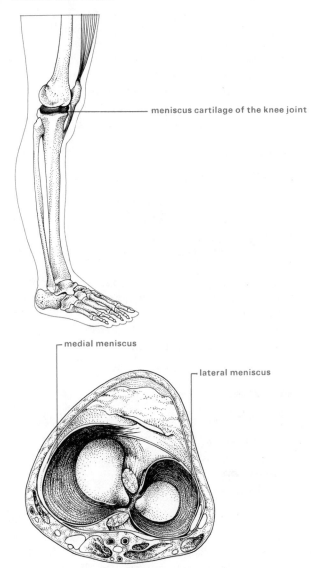

meniscus cartilage of the knee joint

medial meniscus

lateral meniscus

A CROSS SECTION OF THE RIGHT KNEE SEEN FROM ABOVE

The two meniscus cartilages in the knee transmit weight from the thigh to the lower leg. Cartilage injuries result from violent twisting of the knee; torn cartilages do not heal and meniscectomy must be performed.

supply. Therefore, if the symptoms of pain and knee-locking persist, meniscectomy is indicated. With appropriate physical therapy, approximately 75 percent of persons regain complete functional efficiency of the knee joint (a "rim" of fibrocartilage regenerates from the margin of the excised meniscus). In cases where the diagnosis is not clear or where symptoms persist postoperatively, arthroscopy—in which a special optical instru-

ment (arthroscope) is inserted into the joint cavity to permit direct inspection of the damage—can be performed.

oophorectomy

Surgical removal of one or both ovaries.

The operation is carried out mainly (1) on ovaries that are involved in malignant disease, usually with removal of the Fallopian tubes and uterus as well; (2) on ovaries involved in a widespread chronic inflammatory process; and (3) on ovaries that are almost completely destroyed by a large benign tumor. Usually in the case of a benign tumor every effort is made to preserve whatever functioning ovarian tissue is left in order to retain hormonal balance.

Some malignant tumors of the breast are hormone-dependent, and it may be useful in the management of such a cancer to remove both ovaries. About 30 percent of women, particularly those before the menopause, show a degree of remission following oophorectomy.

Removal of both ovaries may be performed in severe cases of endometriosis and is usually accompanied by removal of the uterus and as much of the abnormal endometrial tissue as possible. The operation induces an abrupt menopause, which is the desired effect in endometriosis and in cancer of the breast. However, in cases where this effect is unwelcome, women can be given the ovarian hormone estrogen to help offset the menopausal changes.

Removal of the ovaries, or of the ovaries, uterus, and tubes, is accomplished through an abdominal incision. The operation takes from one to two hours, and you will need to remain in the hospital for seven to ten days. The day after the operation you will be encouraged to get up and walk around. About a week later your stitches will be removed (there is no pain in this). Full recovery takes about six weeks.

orchiopexy

A surgical procedure to move an undescended testicle into the scrotum and attach it so that it will not move back up into the intestinal area. The operation generally is performed by the time the child is 5 years old, but the earlier it is done the better. A testis that is not in the scrotum by the time a child is 6 is unlikely ever to produce sperm. If only one testis is undescended, the other should be able to produce enough sperm to maintain fertility. If a testis remains undescended, an inguinal hernia is more likely to develop; there is a thirty-fold increase in the risk of cancer in that testis; and the testis is more likely to be injured or to undergo torsion (in which it twists on its stalk and cuts off its own blood supply).

pacemaker implantation

A pacemaker is a device that controls heart rate by the rhythmic discharge of electrical impulses.

A small electrical generator is implanted under the skin and an electrode leading from the generator is introduced into the heart itself. Most frequently, pacemaker implantation is performed as emergency surgery when heart rhythm disturbances occur that threaten life. A pacemaker can be implanted temporarily or permanently.

The procedure can be performed on an inpatient or outpatient basis; permanent implantation is almost always done on an inpatient basis in the hospital. Before the implantation, patients usually are prepared with a sedative and a local anesthetic. In more than 75 percent of cases, the surgeon uses the vein-through, or transvenous approach, here described.

The surgeon makes an incision to expose and open the vein in the right outer chest wall. Through this opening, an electrode is passed and led into the right ventricle of the heart. The surgeon also creates a pocket under the skin into which the generator will be placed.

Using fluoroscopy, the electrode is guided into the heart. By coughing and breathing deeply, you will help the surgeon to position and stabilize it. Once it has reached the correct location, the electrode's lead is attached securely to heart muscle with sutures. The lead is connected to the generator (placed in the pocket as described above). The incision is closed; a scar from the collarbone to the side of the shoulder will remain.

The entire operation lasts up to two hours; you will have to be in the recovery room connected to a cardiac monitor for about the same amount of time. For at least forty-eight hours after the operation, electrocardiograms (EKGs) will be taken periodically. You can walk for short distances during this time; other activities should be resumed as your physician advises.

Most new models of pacemakers are powered by lithium batteries with a life of seven to ten years, after which the generator may have to be replaced (electrodes are permanent). Medication will control any postoperative pain, which is usually minimal. There are several devices that need to be avoided, such as microwave ovens, since their electrical fields can disturb heart rates. Complications, which are rare, include malfunctioning of the pacemaker and wound infection.

See also PACEMAKER in **Medical A–Z**.

pancreatectomy

Surgical removal of the pancreas.

This is a major operation with considerable risk, and it is appropriate only for carefully selected persons. The reason for the operation is the presence of pancreatic cancer.

In some cases of cancer a preferred operation is one in which only the head of the pancreas is removed, together with a segment of the duodenum (pancreaticoduodenectomy). In most persons the tumor is too far advanced for simple removal.

phlebotomy

See VENESECTION.

plasmapheresis

A procedure in which blood is removed from the body, separated into components that are then cleansed of toxic or unwanted elements involved in disease, and then returned to the body. It is used in the treatment of various diseases for which no cure is available—including myasthenia gravis, immune complex disorders, Goodpastures syndrome, and thrombocytopenic purpura. For the procedure to be effective, a substantial quantity of blood must be removed; this is done in small quantities over a period of time.

To perform plasmapheresis, the doctor withdraws blood through a needle or catheter. The blood is mixed with an anticoagulant to prevent clotting and spun in a centrifuge to separate its components (red blood cells, white blood cells, platelets, and plasma). The component thought to be responsible for your disease is removed and the rest of the blood is returned to your body. If plasma is removed, it is replaced with a mixture of albumin (a major plasma protein) and saline.

(If any other component is removed, it will be replaced naturally by the body's own processes.)

During the procedure, you may feel chills, dizziness, headache, or ringing in the ears. Usually, these symptoms will go away by themselves, although your doctor may give injections of calcium to help resolve them. In rare instances, a fast pulse or abnormal heart rhythm may develop.

Plasmapheresis is considered safe; a major study of three hundred patients who underwent it found only one major complication—a heart attack in an elderly person. However, since it is a fairly new procedure, other complications may be seen in the future.

A major drawback is its cost: $500 to $2,000 for a single session, with most conditions requiring anywhere from three to twenty-five sessions.

prostatectomy

See TRANSURETHRAL RESECTION OF THE PROSTATE.

rhinoplasty

An operation for the reconstruction of the nose. Generally, it is elective surgery, performed for cosmetic reasons (a "nose job"); however, it may be necessary owing to an accident, fracture, or a deviated septum that is causing breathing difficulties.

If you are choosing to have rhinoplasty for cosmetic reasons, your doctor (most often a plastic surgeon) will photograph your face from various angles and try to show you how the surgery will change your looks. Computer profiles may also be used. Your expectations will be discussed; if you have what the surgeon considers to be unrealistic expectations, you may not be accepted for surgery.

The procedure can be done on an inpatient or outpatient basis. Before the operation you will be given a sedative and an intravenous local anesthesia. Most likely, you will be conscious during the procedure.

During the one- to four-hour operation, the nasal cartilages are reshaped and sometimes the nasal bone is shaved. No external incisions are used.

After surgery, expect to remain in the recovery room for up to two hours with an ice bag on your face to prevent swelling. You will be released either the same day or the next morning.

Even with the use of ice packs, some swelling or discoloration of the face may develop. It can be hidden to some degree with makeup and should disappear in about two weeks. There will be no scar. Oral drugs will be given for postoperative pain. Some risk of postoperative bleeding exists, but this usually can be controlled with ice packs.

sigmoidectomy

Surgical removal of the final descending part of the large intestine (colon), which is joined to the rectum. Usually it is performed because of cancer (sometimes because of ulcerative colitis) in that part of the colon.

After removal of the affected portion, the intestine will be reconnected to the rectum. A temporary COLOSTOMY may be done to allow the intestine to heal. If reconnection is not possible for some reason, a permanent colostomy will be done. The operation last two to four hours and you will remain in the hospital for ten to fourteen days.

slipped disk

Surgery to excise part or all of a herniated disk is called *laminectomy*. Injection of a drug into a disk in order to dissolve it is called *chemonucleolysis*.

The intervertebral disks—which act as "shock absorbers" between the vertebrae and convey flexibility of the spine—may rupture, or "slip," forward or sideways as the result of trauma, weakness of the retaining ligaments, or changes in the fibrous consistency of the disk's outer wall. This condition, known as *herniated disk*, *ruptured disk*, or *prolapsed disk*, is treated first with bed rest, then with physical therapy. If these measures fail to control the pain or if the slipped disk causes so much pressure on the roots of the sciatic nerve that the muscles are unable to perform their function, surgery may be needed.

In deciding whether to operate, the physician will perform various tests, including X rays and a CAT scan (see COMPUTERIZED AXIAL TOMOGRAPHY under Tests). Before the operation, you will be given a sedative and a general anesthesia. An incision is made lengthwise down the affected vertebrae, and the herniated disk is removed. Any remaining disk particles are removed through suction, and the opening is closed in layers.

The operation takes up to four or five hours; you will then rest in the recovery room for about three hours. You may be encouraged to walk around the next day, but you should not lift or run for about a month. About two weeks after the operation, you will begin rehabilitation exercises to help your back and stomach muscles regain strength. Pain-killers will be prescibed.

If any wound infections develop, they will be treated with antibiotics. There is also some chance that urinary retention may occur; a catheter will then be inserted to allow normal urination until the condition corrects itself. A back scar will remain.

Another possible surgical option is to fuse two adjacent vertebrae using a bone graft. This is called *spinal fusion.*

Chemonucleolysis is a nonsurgical means of treating slipped disks. In this procedure, the doctor injects a solution of a drug called chymopapain into the soft central part of the herniated disk. This portion of the disk dissolves and pressure on the sciatic nerve is reduced, thus alleviating pain. While chemonucleolysis offers the advantage of eliminating the need for hospitalization, there is some controversy as to its success rate and its use is not routine in the United States, although it is very popular in Canada and Europe.

splenectomy

An operation to remove the spleen.

The spleen is an organ that lies next to the stomach. One of its functions is to remove worn-out blood cells and foreign particles from circulation; with the lymph nodes, it plays a part in the formation of antibodies. If the spleen is lacerated or ruptured, excessive, uncontrollable hemorrhaging occurs, and the spleen must be removed. Other conditions indicating splenectomy are cancer of the lymph nodes and certain blood disorders. Removal of the spleen does not lead to any permanent disabilities in an adult.

Before the operation, a number of tests including a complete blood count, chest X ray, and electrocardiogram (EKG) will be performed. Several units of compatible blood will be reserved for a transfusion. An intravenous needle will be inserted into one arm so that fluids can be given to prevent dehydration. One inserted in the other arm will be used for the blood transfusion, if it

is needed. You will be given a sedative and a general anesthetic.

After the abdomen is sterilized, an incision will be made through the skin, tissue, and muscle so that the liver, gallbladder, and spleen can be examined. The spleen is separated from surrounding tissues and removed. A portion of the omentum, a fold in the abdominal lining, is sutured over the space, and the incision is closed.

The entire operation takes four to five hours; afterward, you will rest in the recovery room for about the same amount of time. You should try to walk around your room the next day; however, strenuous activities should be avoided for about a month. Pain-killers will be prescribed. You will also receive a vaccine against pneumonia, since resistance to infection is lowered in persons after splenectomy.

If a wound infection should develop, it will be treated with antibiotics. A scar will be left across the abdomen.

stapedectomy

A surgical procedure involving the drilling of the footplate of the stapes and the insertion of a plastic or stainless-steel piston to restore hearing in the treatment of otosclerosis.

sterilization

Any process or act that makes a man or woman infertile while leaving sexual desire and capacity unaffected. Sterilization is being used increasingly as an alternative to contraception by couples who have completed their families or do not want to have children.

Sterilization can be accomplished through surgery, vasectomy (for men), or tubal ligation (for women). HYSTERECTOMY also causes sterilization.

sympathectomy

Surgical removal of the sympathetic nerve supply to an artery. The procedure allows the vessel to relax and expand, so that a greater volume of blood can pass through it.

thoractomy

The surgical opening of the chest cavity (thorax) necessary for access to the heart and lungs.

thyroidectomy

Surgical removal of the whole thyroid gland or part of it.

The main indication for this operation is in cases of *thyrotoxicosis,* where medical treatment with antithyroid drugs has failed, particularly in persons under the age of 40. It is also indicated in the treatment of large goiters. About nine-tenths of the gland is removed in operations for thyrotoxicosis, leaving in place the part of the gland that is in close relation to the parathyroid glands. The operation is a common one but is sometimes followed by complications ranging from damage to the "recurrent laryngeal nerve," which causes postoperative hoarseness, to tetany due to inadvertent removal of parathyroid glands. Tetany is a condition of muscle cramps, numbness, and tingling of the hands and feet associated with insufficient parathyroid secretion.

SYMPATHECTOMY

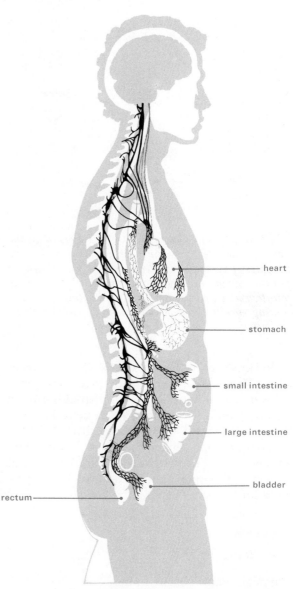

THE AUTONOMIC NERVOUS SYSTEM

The autonomic nerveous system has two components— the sympathetic (black) and parasympathetic (gray)— both of which supply the internal organs. Sympathectomy is an operation, usually performed in the neck or the low back, to improve the blood flow to the arms or legs by cutting the sympathetic nerves to the arteries.

STAPEDECTOMY

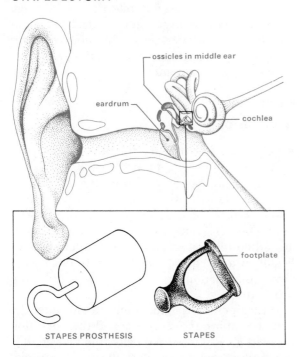

Hearing depends on the sound-transmitting function of the ossicles (little bones) of the middle ear. Occasionally, in a disease called otosclerosis, the footplate of the stapes becomes fused to the cochlea. The resulting deafness can be cured by a stapedectomy, an operation in which the stapes is replaced with a tiny stainless-steel piston.

THYROID AND PARATHYROID

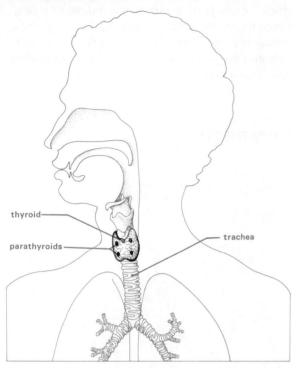

The thyroid gland lies in front of the trachea in the neck and secretes thyroxine, a hormone that controls the rates of many bodily activities. The four pea-sized parathyroid glands embedded within the thyroid secrete parathormone, a hormone that is essential for maintaining correct levels of calcium and phosphorus in the blood.

Recurrence of thyrotoxicosis may occur in about 10 percent of cases; the occurrence of symptoms due to an insufficiency of thyroid hormone (hypothyroidism) is under 10 percent. Periodic medical checks are required after thyroidectomy.

The operation also is indicated in the treatment of cancer of the thyroid, but because of the radical nature of the operation the occurrence of complications may be higher.

tonsillectomy

Surgical removal of the tonsils.

The indications for the operation have changed in recent years. Most surgeons are unwilling to operate because difficulties with the tonsils usually resolve themselves with puberty—in girls rather later than in boys; they prefer to operate only in cases of recurrent severe infection with ear complications, or in obvious cases of chronic

TONSILLECTOMY

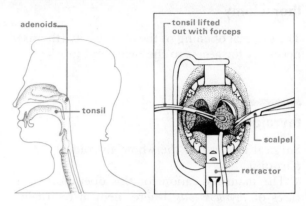

Tonsillectomy is carried out most often on children who have frequent attacks of acute tonsillitis. The tonsils are removed under general anesthesia by cutting them off the side wall of the throat with a scalpel and lifting them out with forceps. Very often, the adenoids are removed at the same time.

infections that do not respond to medication.

In adults it may be necessary to remove the tonsils when they are the seat of a new growth (tumor). The operation usually is performed under general anesthesia for children up to the age of about 12; for teenagers and adults the surgeon may prefer local anesthesia. The most common complication is postoperative bleeding, which requires urgent treatment.

tracheostomy

An operation in which the trachea ("windpipe") is opened from the front of the neck and a tube inserted to allow air to reach the lungs. It becomes necessary when the windpipe is obstructed or narrowed as the result of an illness such as diphtheria or angioedema. Tracheostomy may be necessary also when respiration has to be maintained artificially by a mechanical ventilator. In emergency airway obstruction, tracheostomy is a lifesaving procedure.

If the opening is made immediately under the chin and above the thyroid gland the operation is called *high tracheostomy;* below the thyroid, it is *low tracheostomy.* In practice the operation frequently involves cutting through the center of the thyroid gland.

The entry into the windpipe is made by cutting a vertical slit through the skin and fatty tissues of the neck, and then through the front wall of the trachea. Tracheostomy tubes then are inserted:

TRACHEOSTOMY

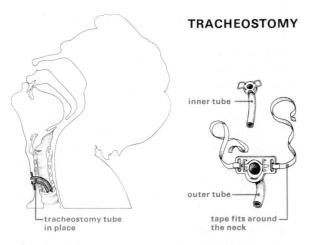

A tracheostomy is an opening made in the trachea ("windpipe") through which a tube is inserted to create an emergency airway. The main indications for a tracheostomy are (1) an obstruction in the larynx or upper respiratory tract, and (2) an unconscious patient who needs to be attached to an artificial respirator for a considerable period.

an outer tube first, which remains in position, and an inner tube, which may be removed or coughed out if, for example, it becomes blocked with mucus. The tubes are made of hard rubber or metal and a dressing is inserted between the outer tube and the wound. The entrance to the inner tube is protected by medicated gauze to act as an air filter. If a mucus buildup occurs, suctioning the tube clears it.

When there is a permanent obstruction the tubes must be left in place. In other instances, such as diphtheria, the tubes are left in for three or four days and then removed, after which the wound heals.

If you have a tracheostomy that is to remain in place indefinitely, you will be taught how to clean and suction it yourself at home. People with a permanent tracheostomy can learn to speak again by regurgitating air from the esophagus (esophageal speech).

transurethral resection of the prostate (TURP)

An operation in which a portion of the prostate gland is removed. The prostate gland lies around the urethra, just under the bladder in men. With age, the prostate frequently becomes enlarged and may obstruct the urine flow. This, in turn, can cause bladder and kidney infection. TURP

PROSTATE GLAND

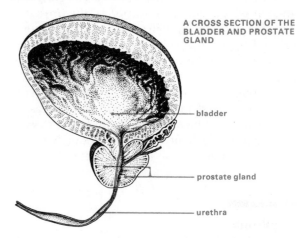

A CROSS SECTION OF THE BLADDER AND PROSTATE GLAND

bladder

prostate gland

urethra

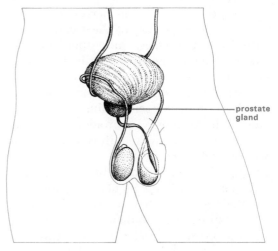

prostate gland

The prostate sits at the base of the bladder and secretes fluid into the urethra during sexual excitement. Most prostates enlarge after middle age and may cause urinary symptoms. Partial or total removal of the gland (prostatectomy) may then be necessary. The two methods most widely used are to remove the gland through a small abdominal incision or to extract the core of the gland through the urethra—a techique known as transurethral resection.

will then be performed. If, however, the prostate is extremely enlarged or if cancer is suspected, a more radical procedure may be needed.

Before the operation, you will be given a number of tests including urine culture and complete blood count. About an hour before, you will be given a sedative and an intravenous needle will be inserted so fluids can be given later. A regional nerve block is the usual anesthesia.

During the operation, the doctor will insert a resectoscope into the urethra to observe directly the prostate gland and bladder. He will then insert a cutting instrument through the resectoscope and cut off the enlarged portion of the prostate. A urinary catheter is put in after surgery to remove urine. The entire operation takes about an hour; you will rest in the recovery room for about two hours.

Although you can walk the day after surgery, you should avoid strenuous activity for at least a month. You will be prescribed pain-killers as well as antibiotics to fight infection. About 5 to 15 percent of men become impotent after TURP.

vagotomy

The cutting of the two vagus nerves. It is performed sometimes as part of the treatment of uncontrolled peptic ulcer, since stimulation by the vagus nerves is one of the main factors in secretion of the digestive juices (hydrochloric acid and pepsin) by the stomach. Persons with duodenal ulcers commonly secrete abnormally large amounts of hydrochloric acid; vagotomy results in a lower acid output and thus reduces the chances of further ulceration.

The vagus nerves begin in the brainstem, travel down the neck close to the jugular vein, and then pass to the abdomen where branches serve the various digestive organs. In their course the vagus nerves also provide branches to the heart and lungs.

Vagotomy may be *complete* or *selective*; in the latter case only some of the branches are cut, thereby reducing the likelihood of unwanted side effects such as diarrhea.

Before surgery a nasogastric tube will be passed through your nose and down the esophagus into your stomach to suction out fluid and gas. Although not painful, the tube will be uncomfortable. As with all major surgery you will experience pain afterward but pain-relieving medication will be available. You will have to remain in the hospital for ten to fourteen days.

valvotomy

Literally, "cutting a valve." The valves of the heart normally consist of two or three separate flaps (cusps) that are free to move as the valve opens and closes. As a result of disease (rheumatic fever, for example), the valve becomes inflamed and the cusps may become damaged or scarred, causing them to stick together. The valve becomes narrowed and no longer functions normally, presenting a considerable obstacle to the free flow of blood. This condition is called *stenosis* of the valve—*mitral stenosis* or *aortic stenosis*, for example, depending on which valve is affected.

To overcome the obstruction of the stenosed valve, the valve cusps are opened surgically (valvotomy) to allow free movement and an unobstructed flow of blood. In many cases it is thought wise for the diseased valve to be removed and replaced with an artificial valve (prosthetic valve). The choice of operation depends on the severity of the damage to the valve cusps—although valvotomy is a technically simpler procedure than valve replacement.

Before the procedure your lungs will be checked (to prevent respiratory complications), and cardiac catheterization will be performed. The operation lasts anywhere from one to four hours, and you will remain in the hospital for about two weeks. Full recovery may take a few months, as with any cardiac surgery. If the valve is replaced rather than repaired, you may receive anticoagulant drugs afterward to prevent clot formation, and you will periodically need to have blood tests.

vasectomy

A surgical procedure that makes a man sterile by cutting out sections of the vasa deferentia (the tubes that carry sperm) and tying the ends, thereby interrupting the route that sperm must travel to be ejaculated and cause conception.

A man will not be considered sterile until all live sperm left in the tubes beyond the cut sections are ejaculated. This may take several months, during which time another form of birth control is required. At the end of this period consecutive sperm counts are made; two or three negative results are needed before the operation can be considered successful. The person himself will not notice any difference in his sexual activity, since most of the fluid ejaculated at orgasm comes from the prostate gland and seminal vesicles, which are untouched; the secretion of male hormone from the testicles continues without interruption, so that virility and sexual arousal and desire are not affected.

See also STERILIZATION.

VASECTOMY

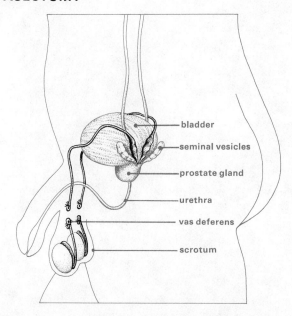

Vasectomy is a method of male sterilization carried out through a small incision in the scrotum. The vasa deferentia are cut and tied back, as pictured above, so that sperm can no longer pass from the testes to the urethra. Only rarely can a vasectomy be reversed successfully.

venepuncture

The puncture of a vein with a hollow needle, most commonly performed for the removal of blood samples for laboratory testing, but also for the injection or transfusion of drug solutions, blood, or other fluids.

The most accessible veins for these purposes are those on the inner side of the elbow (antecubital fossa), although veins on the hand, wrist, and (in small infants) the scalp and neck may be used.

Blood commonly is drawn with a plastic syringe attached to the needle.

venesection

The "letting of blood" as a therapeutic medical procedure. Also known as *phlebotomy.* It was widely practiced in earlier centuries, but the indications for its use were far from clearly established. Usually it was carried out by cutting an arm vein and allowing the blood to run into a basin ("venesection" literally means the cutting of a vein). Today the procedure is the same as giving a pint of blood at your local hospital.

In modern medicine it is used only rarely. In polycythemia there is an overproduction of red blood cells. The simplest method of reducing the red blood cell count is to remove blood, usually 500 cubic centimeters at a time, using a needle and a length of plastic tubing. In hemochromatosis, excessive amounts of iron accumulate in the body and, since iron can be removed from the body only in the form of the hemoglobin pigment in the red blood cells, venesection is the treatment of choice.

FAMILY MEDICINE AND HEALTH

As health-care costs have spiraled, so has consumer awareness of the importance of adequate, economical health care. At the same time, the number of options available to individuals seeking competent medical care has grown enormously. The concept of the "second opinion" in medical diagnosis, the realization that some medical-surgical procedures are not always necessary, and the necessity of justifying expensive treatments to insurance companies have made family health care a much more complex, confusing subject.

It makes sense, then, for families to know and learn as much as possible about what is and is not normal in behavior, development, growth, and aging. Adult heads of families need to know when professional guidance is indicated, when a health-care practitioner is providing adequate care, and what their options are. The purpose of this chapter is to introduce families to the major health issues they will encounter as the family evolves. These include the kinds of biological pressures women sometimes feel as their lives unfold; how couples can plan and control their reproduction; the changes and challenges of pregnancy and labor; the choices couples have in determining the environment, management, and quality of labor and childbirth; and the pros and cons of breastfeeding versus bottle feeding. The reader will also find sections on necessary immunizations and preventive practices to keep children healthy and happy; childhood illness and disease, both simple and complex; the care and feeding of teenagers; and sources of help when the family is in crisis.

7

THE CYCLE OF WOMANHOOD

The past fifty years have brought sweeping changes in the way society views women. The feminist movement, societal pressures, scientific advances, and demographic and economic changes have created a sometimes confusing picture of woman's role as mother, sex object, nurturer, mate, career person, breadwinner, and political being. One of the results of these changes is that many women now believe they can and—must—"have it all": family, career, love, marriage, good health, a physically fit body, and the continuing opportunity to evolve and grow emotionally.

At the same time that the media and society urge women to aim higher and work harder, there is a growing trend among American parents to have children at a later age than their ancestors did. This is due in part to the goals of career, identity, and self-fulfillment that motivate women during their 20s and early 30s especially. This trend poses a challenge both for families and for practitioners of family medicine.

At opposite sides of the age spectrum, adolescent girls and older women face societal pressures that may affect their self-esteem and emotional maturity. Little girls approaching puberty may find themselves confused by the conflicting messages they see and hear regarding growing up, independence, responsibility, and the desirability of loving and being loved. Women approaching menopause can at times experience severe emotional distress over what they perceive as a loss of "womanliness." For the aging woman there is the constant sense—perpetuated by television, cinema, and advertising—that growing older is somehow unnatural and unattractive. Hundreds of beautiful, vital older women continue to disprove this notion, but the message is still there.

Woman's biology, meanwhile, remains basically unchanged. While modern obstetrics can implant a fertilized egg in a woman who in an earlier era would have been considered barren, the basic facts of puberty, childbearing, and change of life persist, despite our efforts to grow up too fast, work too hard, achieve the impossible, and stay young forever.

Normal Developmental Events in the Female

■ *Puberty*

Puberty is defined as the time in which the *secondary sex characteristics* begin to develop and the

437

individual becomes, for the first time, capable of reproducing. Secondary sex characteristics are those features, such as breasts and body shape, that distinguish males and females from one another but are not directly involved with reproduction. Adolescence, on the other hand, is less precisely fixed in time and refers to the whole set of emotional, physical, psychological, social, and maturational changes an individual goes through during and after puberty.

For girls, puberty is characterized by a widening of the hips, the appearance of breasts, the development of pubic hair, and the onset of menstruation (*menarche*). The normal age range of menarche for girls in North America is 10 to 15 years; the average age is $12\frac{1}{2}$. For boys, puberty is marked by a broadening of the shoulders, deepening of the voice, and the appearance of pubic and facial hair; it occurs usually between the ages of $12\frac{1}{2}$ to $16\frac{1}{2}$, with a mean age of 14.

■ *Physical and Physiological Changes of Puberty*

The "growth spurt" peculiar to adolescence begins, for girls, between ages 10 and 14; this is somewhat earlier than the age range for boys. On average, the adolescent girl will gain 2 to 8 inches in height and 15 to 55 pounds in weight. This period of growth usually ends at 16 or 17 years of age.

It is no coincidence that many adolescents appear "leggy" and awkward; the extremities actually do grow first and may therefore appear larger than normal for a time, before the rest of the body "catches up." The face, also, grows disproportionately, with the forehead and nose enlarging first, then the mouth and lips, and finally the jaw.

Teenage boys and girls differ in their patterns of fat distribution. In girls fatty tissue is deposited more heavily over the thighs, hips, buttocks, and breasts, which accounts for the rounder, more "womanly" appearance of the older adolescent girl.

The secretion of estrogen, the female sex hormone, causes the pubescent girl's skin to soften and thicken. Sebaceous, or oil-secreting, glands are more active during puberty, particularly in the genital areas and on the face, neck, shoulders, and upper chest. This accounts, in part, for a common complaint of adolescence: acne. (See *Common Health Problems in the Adolescent* later in this section.)

Sweat glands also become more active during puberty, while body hair becomes more prominent. Pubic and axillary (armpit) hair appears in both girls and boys and may take up to four years to reach full development.

The physical and physiological events of puberty are under the control of the *pituitary gland* in both boys and girls. Situated at the base of the brain, the pituitary releases hormones that in turn stimulate the sex organs to produce *gametes*, or sex cells—ova (eggs) and the sex hormones estrogen and progesterone from the teenage girl's ovaries.

One or two years before menarche the prepubescent girl begins to secrete estrogen in a cyclic pattern. Menarche usually occurs about two years after the changes of puberty first appear. During the first few years after the first menstrual period, menstrual bleeding is often irregular and scanty and may not occur in conjunction with ovulation. The onset of menstruation is believed to be dependent upon attainment of body weight of at least 106 pounds (48 kilograms), but this can vary according to race and other factors.

■ *Psychological and Emotional Changes of Puberty*

The physical changes of puberty occur so rapidly that the adolescent girl may have difficulty adjusting to them. Her body image alters radically, while her peer group attaches enormous significance to the development of breasts, pubic hair, and "curves." For both boys and girls, adolescence is a time of extreme self-awareness, self-consciousness, introversion, and rebelliousness. Awakening sexual feelings, the guilt such feelings bring, and the combination of confusion and alienation brought about by a changing body image can make the teenage girl an extremely difficult person to live with at times. (See *Psychosocial Problems in the Adolescent* later in this section.)

■ *Sexuality in the Adolescent Girl*

Strong sexual feelings are a normal part of a healthy adolescent girl's development. Whereas teenage boys' sexual feelings tend to be centered in the genitals, with girls sexuality tends to be more generalized, less well defined, and more closely linked to their total personality.

Recent studies suggest that at least 40 percent

of girls and 80 to 95 percent of boys experience sexual intercourse by the end of adolescence. At the same time, research indicates that, in general, casual sexual relationships usually are not acceptable among teenagers; there appears to be some sense of a need for strong commitment before sex is considered an acceptable activity. In recent years there has been a trend in our society toward more permissive attitudes regarding teenagers' sexual behavior. This trend poses a challenge for families, sex educators, and health professionals who treat families and teenagers. More important, it places still greater responsibility on the adolescent girl, who may or may not be emotionally capable of dealing with the consequences of her actions.

Fertility is, strictly speaking, the physical capacity to conceive. Since ovulation occurs at the menarche, teenage girls must be considered to be fertile from the time of the first menstrual period.

Adolescent pregnancy is one of the major health problems in the United States today, with more than a million teenagers becoming pregnant each year; 600,000 births occur from these teenage pregnancies every year. According to recent statistics, the United States has the highest birth rate among 15- to 19-year-olds in the Western Hemisphere. Clearly, adolescent sexuality is a major issue for American families, legislators, and health professionals.

■ The Childbearing Years

The childbearing years actually begin with the onset of fertility and end with menopause (the end of menstruation). Although motherhood has always been viewed by society as a special, almost sacred, institution, our concept of motherhood is ever changing. This change is due to political, social, economic, and demographic factors as well as to scientific advances in contraception and fertility that make it possible for women to have more control over family planning.

The decision to have children may be influenced by many factors, some of them relatively new and some as old as motherhood itself. For some women, though, there is a sense of biological and societal pressure—a desire to be like one's contemporaries, to "nest," to reproduce oneself while there is still time. Women who do choose to establish themselves in a career sometimes find that they feel "rushed" to have a baby as soon as their professional identity is firmly founded.

The national tendency of families to bear children later in life has both advantages and drawbacks. In an ideal world, a woman would not conceive until she was emotionally, physically, and socially mature and capable of taking on responsibility for another's life. It may be that women who bear children at a later age bring to motherhood an added maturity and sense of self-fulfillment that enable them to contribute even more to their children's development.

The age at which women usually become first-time mothers now ranges between 24 and 39. During the first half of this decade, in fact, the only age group that experienced an increase in fertility were women between 30 and 34 years old, whose rate of births per 1,000 women rose to 72.2 from 60.0 four years earlier.

Statistically speaking, with older mothers there is a slightly increased risk of some anomalies in the fetus, including Down's syndrome (mongolism) and other, rarer disorders. Although the American College of Obstetrics and Gynecology has said that for the majority of healthy women over the age of 35, there is no likelihood of major problems with the pregnancy or the baby, nevertheless there are certain risks. During their pregnancy women over 35 have a slightly higher risk of developing hypertension (preeclampsia) or diabetes (refer to *Pregnancy and Childbirth* later in this section for details on these disorders); they are also somewhat more at risk for miscarriage and stillbirth. At the same time, older women are more likely than younger women to have certain underlying health problems, such as chronic hypertension or diabetes, which may influence the outcome of a pregnancy. Finally, the ability to become pregnant does appear to decrease with age, so that women over 35 may have a harder time becoming pregnant.

It is important to bear in mind, however, that there is no "ideal" age at which to have a baby. A healthy, successful pregnancy depends on a number of factors ranging from proper nutrition and prenatal care to the mother's emotional well-being and maturity. A woman at any age who takes care of herself and gets adequate medical care during her pregnancy is a better candidate to have a baby than one who is young and ignorant of her body's functions, and who does not take responsible care of herself and her unborn baby from the moment she knows she is pregnant.

There are numerous tests to diagnose chromosomal and other abnormalities of the fetus before the pregnancy is too far advanced. These offer the option of abortion if a severe defect is found (see *Pregnancy and Childbirth* later in this section).

■ *Menopause*

The word *menopause* means, simply, the end of menstruation, or the time when a woman stops having monthly periods. The end of the menstrual period is one part of a larger event, commonly called the "change of life," which has to do with the body slowing down its production of estrogen. Health professionals refer to the whole time period around the menopause as the *climacteric.*

Menopause normally occurs in one's 40s or 50s. The average age overall is 51 years. Menopause occurring before age 35 is called "premature" menopause; if it occurs after age 58 it is considered "delayed" menopause.

Contrary to popular notions, menopause does not make women fat, masculinized, emotionally unstable, or sexless. It is a natural process, just like the first menstrual period of puberty, through which all women must pass.

One of the first signs that menopause is approaching is a change in the menstrual cycle, such as a missed period, heavier or lighter flow, shorter or longer flow periods, or spotting between periods. The change can appear also as several missed periods in a row until finally there are no periods at all. Differences in the menstrual pattern can go on for several years, depending on the amount of estrogen circulating in the bloodstream. Irregularities with the period can sometimes be a sign of something more complicated, however, and should always be reported to your gynecologist or family doctor. In particular, bleeding from the vagina that happens after a long absence of periods (six months or more) can be an early sign of serious problems. Women in the menopausal age group should be aware of changes in the pattern of their periods and should report such changes to their doctor.

A common sign of menopause is the *hot flash* or *hot flush,* which is a transient flushing of the skin that starts in the face and neck and sometimes spreads to the back or chest. Other possible symptoms of menopause include changes in the way the skin feels, extreme changes in mood, difficulty sleeping, abnormal discharge from the vagina, pain in the back and joints, and vaginal pain with or without intercourse. Not every woman will experience these problems. When they do occur, these symptoms are caused by a decrease in the amount of estrogen circulating in the body, and although all women experience a drop in estrogen with menopause, some women have fewer "side effects" from this decrease than others.

The menopause can be a difficult time for women emotionally as well as physically. Such things as changes in the family structure, the illness or death of one's parents, the stress of becoming a grandparent, or a spouse's difficulty—or one's own—in adjusting to retirement can create barriers to communication between family members and cause tension. The media's messages about growing older, especially for women, are often unfair and misleading, suggesting that women in middle age are less attractive, less energetic, and even less emotionally stable than their younger counterparts.

If you are a woman in this age group, it is helpful to be aware of new stresses in your life and to try to examine your life-style and habits to see what can be done to reduce the effects of stress on your emotional and physical life. A reliable and trusted family physician or internist can sometimes help to point out stressful situations that can be controlled and suggest ways of coping.

Severe symptoms of stress, such as fatigue or insomnia, should always be reported to your physician. Some of the more severe symptoms of estrogen loss associated with the menopause may mimic symptoms of severe stress, and some of these can be controlled with simple measures. Other problems of menopause—such as hot flashes, sleep disturbance, nervousness, dizziness, palpitations, mood swings, vaginal pain, and joint pain—may be alleviated by hormone-replacement therapy. This therapy, which involves giving estrogen pills, usually in conjunction with progesterone, another female hormone, is not a cure-all and should be discussed at length before it is prescribed. It is now believed that estrogen replacement carries few risks, providing the woman is free of certain preexisting medical conditions.

Advances in health care have increased the life expectancy of American women significantly, so that a woman in her 40s or 50s today can expect to live well into her 70s. This means that at menopause, nearly a third of your life remains ahead of you. The enjoyment of that all-important third depends upon good health, a little bit of luck, and the right attitude.

PREGNANCY AND CHILDBIRTH

8

Perhaps no event in a family's life affords such wide-ranging changes—or so much excitement—as the natural processes of pregnancy and childbirth. Pregnancy and birth are unique situations in which an essentially healthy family seeks the regular intervention of trained health care professionals. Even though pregnancy and childbirth are "natural" occurrences, regular prenatal care by a qualified professional is essential to detect any disease processes or other problems that may be occurring without causing symptoms. It is important for the childbearing family to have contact with an obstetrician/gynecologist or certified nurse-midwife whose competence, qualifications, and judgment they trust. Equally important is the family's active participation in the whole process. The best obstetrical patients are a woman and family who are interested in and knowledgeable about the pregnancy and impending birth. By understanding what pregnancy and childbirth mean, both in a medical sense and in terms of the way they affect family dynamics, a family is better able to cope with the changes—and occasional discomforts—that take place and better prepared to face the responsibilities of parenthood.

Ovulation

The regular production of a single, ripe egg from the woman's ovaries is called *ovulation*. Normally it occurs fourteen days before the next menstrual period, *not* necessarily fourteen days after the previous period. This means that you can know when ovulation occurred only in retrospect; you can't know exactly when it *will* occur. If, however, a woman's cycle is fairly regular and conforms to the normal twenty-eight-day cycle of most women, it means that ovulation occurs approximately between days 13 to 15 of the cycle, if the first day of the menstrual period is considered to be day 1. The ovum, once shed from the ovary, lives for about eighteen hours.

Fertilization

The joining of the ovum with a sperm from the male is called *fertilization*. Although as many as 500 million sperm may be contained in one ejaculation, only one sperm actually fertilizes the ovum. About a million sperm ejaculated from the penis will arrive at the uterus and Fallopian tubes,

FEMALE REPRODUCTIVE ORGANS

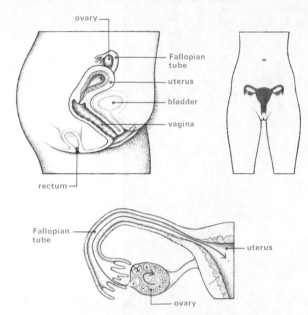

The reproductive system of the female, unlike that of the male, undergoes regular cyclic changes which revolve around ovulation—the release of an egg from the ovary. The egg passes along the Fallopian tube into the cavity of the uterus. If it has been fertilized, the egg embeds itself in the lining of the uterus; if not, the egg and the lining of the uterus are shed at menstruation.

and they can live in the female reproductive tract for up to seventy-two hours.

Given the eighteen-hour life of an ovum and the seventy-two-hour life of a sperm, it follows that unprotected sex occurring between days 11 and 15 in a regular twenty-eight-day cycle can produce a pregnancy.

Implantation

Implantation usually occurs at the beginning of the first week after fertilization, that is, between days 7 and 9 after the ovum joins with the sperm. The fertilized ovum moves slowly down the Fallopian tube toward the uterus, doubling and quadrupling in size by simple multiplication of its cells as it travels. After some basic cellular development has taken place, the *conceptus*, or product of conception, embeds itself completely in the lining of the uterus, or *endometrium*, burrowing in with the help of projections, called *chorionic villi*, that develop on its outer surface. Once im-

planted, the conceptus will be nourished through the uterus until it is fully developed and ready to be born.

Duration of Pregnancy

Normal pregnancy lasts, on average, 266 days from the date of fertilization, or 280 days (forty weeks or nine calendar months) from the first day of the last menstrual period. Obstetricians and midwives may calculate the gestational age of the unborn baby based on ten "lunar months," or twenty-eight-day months that correspond to the phases of the moon. The simple way to calculate your own due date is to take the first day of your last menstrual period, subtract three months and add seven days. If, for example, your last period started on December 12, your due date would be determined as follows:

	December 12
minus	3 months
=	September 12
plus	7 days
=	September 19 due date

A normal pregnancy is considered to last forty weeks plus or minus two weeks. The due-date calculation described above is accurate only for a regular, twenty-eight-day cycle. If your cycle is shorter than twenty-eight days, your due date would be slightly earlier than this calculated date because ovulation would have occurred earlier in the cycle; if your cycle usually lasts longer than twenty-eight days, you would ovulate somewhat later in the cycle and thus would be due a little bit later than the due date shown above. If your cycles are irregular, the best you can do is to estimate your due date, accurate to within a week or two.

This forty-week gestation is the same for all women regardless of age, race, or geographic location. Multiple gestations, however (such as twins, triplets), tend not to last the full forty weeks.

■ *Boy or Girl?*

All cells in human beings contain forty-six chromosomes, or twenty-three pairs of chromosomes, including one pair of sex chromosomes. The pair of sex chromosomes consists of two X chromosomes in a female and one X and one Y chromosome in a male. The other twenty-two pairs

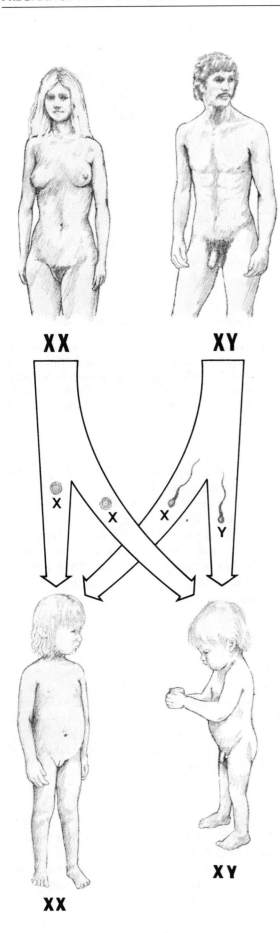

are responsible for all hereditary characteristics other than sex.

The ovum donated to the fetus by the mother contains twenty-two chromosomes plus one sex chromosome which is always an X since it comes from the female. In other words, the ovum contains only half the full complement of chromosomes that a cell should contain, because it will eventually merge with a sperm containing the other half. The sperm possesses twenty-two chromosomes plus one sex chromosome which may be either X or Y, since the male cells contain both. If the sperm that fertilizes the ovum contains an X chromosome, then the fertilized ovum will have the sex chromosome combination XX and will become a girl. If a sperm containing a Y chromosome reaches the ovum and fertilizes it, then the resulting fetus will be male, with XY sex chromosomes.

Thus the baby's sex is determined by the contribution of the male partner. Some scientists are now exploring theories about various ways in which a couple might influence the sex determination of their child during conception, but for now it appears to be entirely up to chance.

Early Signs of Pregnancy

Even before you take a pregnancy test that proves positive, you may suspect you are pregnant. There are numerous signs and symptoms of pregnancy, some merely suspicious and some definitely diagnostic.

Among the symptoms of pregnancy are fatigue, nausea and vomiting, and breast tenderness. Some women report a change in the way certain foods taste, or a continuous, unpleasant metallic taste in the mouth, altering their subjective experience of certain foods, alcohol, or tobacco. These changes may be caused by other factors, and therefore none of these is considered to be diagnostic of pregnancy.

Objective signs of pregnancy are those that are observed by another, trained, individual. These include amenorrhea (absence of a menstrual period), constipation, weight gain, vomiting, breast

From each parent a baby inherits 22 "body" chromosomes plus one sex chromosome (46 in all). The sex chromosome carried in the ovum is always X, that in the sperm either X or Y. The combination of these determines the baby's sex: XX chromosomes result in a female child, XY in a male.

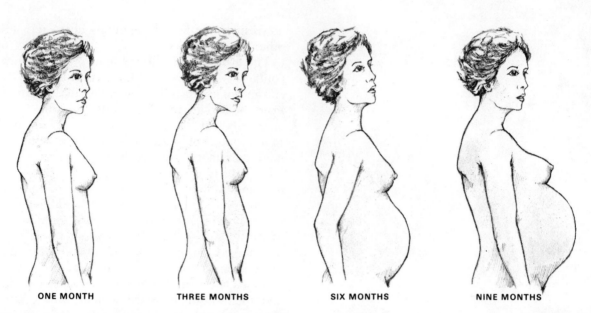

ONE MONTH   THREE MONTHS   SIX MONTHS   NINE MONTHS

The first signs of pregnancy are the absence of periods, morning nausea, and water retention. Breasts usually enlarge slightly and become tender, the skin becomes warm, and the mother enjoys a "glow" caused by increased hormone levels. Her girth will not increase before three or four months. The middle of pregnancy sees rapid fetal growth with corresponding maternal enlargement. Fetal movements are usually felt at around the fifth month. The mother's circulation and pulse rate increase. Toward the ninth month the enormous womb may make breathing shallow and large meals uncomfortable.

swelling, and increased frequency of urination. Also included are changes in the appearance of pelvic organs such as the vagina and uterus; changes in skin tone and pigmentation; the palpable outline of the fetal body along the abdomen (this does not occur until after the midpoint of the pregnancy); increased height of the uterus in the abdomen; the *uterine souffle,* a soft blowing or swishing sound heard in the pelvis with a stethoscope, caused by blood pulsating through the placenta; and positive results of pregnancy tests. Commonly used pregnancy tests today look for the hormone *chorionic gonadotropin,* which is present and detectable in the urine of pregnant women about a week after the missed period. The tests are accurate in about 98 percent of cases.

Embryonic Development

After the union of sperm and ovum, the conceptus consists of one cell. As the conceptus moves along the Fallopian tube toward the uterus, it divides to form two cells, then four, then eight, and sixteen. By the time implantation occurs, about a week later, the conceptus consists of a group of cells around a small bag of fluid which in turn

contains a number of cells that are in the process of differentiating into the fetus. The cells that surround the sac of fluid, called *chorionic cells,* are equipped to help the conceptus penetrate and embed itself within the uterine lining. They also secrete chorionic gonadotropin, a hormone that is involved in maintaining the pregnancy in conjunction with other hormones from the pituitary gland and the ovaries.

■ 4th Week

By the end of the fourth week after the first day of the last menstrual period, the embryo is about two weeks old and is just big enough to be seen without a microscope, were it outside the womb. It is about 2 millimeters (0.08 inches) long from crown to rump, and its heart and kidneys are about to be formed.

■ 5th Week

At the end of the fifth week after the last period, or three weeks' gestation, the spine and central nervous system are beginning to develop. The liver is actually beginning to function, and blood is starting to circulate.

■ 6th Week

At the sixth week after the last menstrual period, the embryo is four weeks old and 4 mm. (0.16 in.) long from crown to rump. The brain is forming, there are visible "limb buds" that will develop into arms and legs, and the digestive tract also is forming.

■ 7th Week

The embryo's developing muscles are being activated by nerves by the seventh week, and the atria of the heart have divided into two separate chambers. The length of the embryo is about 1.3 centimeters (0.50 in.).

■ 8th Week

The beginnings of the bones are present as the primitive shape of the skeleton begins to form. The embryo's mouth, nose, and upper lip form during this period. Sex glands are beginning to appear, and the beginnings of the lungs are in evidence.

■ 12th Week

The baby-to-be has fingers and toes now, although they still may be somewhat fused. Movement of the embryo's small parts is possible at this stage. The facial features are recognizable, and all of the vital organs have been formed. The external genital organs are forming, although the distinction between male and female genitalia is difficult to discern at this point. The embryo is about 6 cm. (2.34 in.) long and weighs from 14 to 18 grams (0.49 to 0.63 ounces).

■ 18th Week

By the end of the eighteenth week, the fetus is moving vigorously; occasionally, the mother can detect these movements. The fetus has fingernails and toenails; its facial characteristics have developed further and are more recognizable and individualized. *Meconium,* or fetal stool, is beginning to form in the intestines; *lanugo,* a fine downy hair, covers the entire body. Scalp hair is beginning to grow, and the sex of the fetus is more easily determined by the appearance of the external genitals. The fetus is now 15 to 16 cm. (6 in.) long and weighs around 200 g. (7 oz.).

■ 20th Week

This period marks the halfway point in a pregnancy. Tooth buds are forming, and the fetal heart sounds can be heard with a fetuscope (a specially shaped stethoscope). The fetus at twenty weeks is by no means viable, but it is fast approaching the time when its vital organs will be mature enough for it to survive outside the womb.

■ 24th to 26th Week

By now the embryo is actively swallowing amniotic fluid, and *peristalsis* (the rhythmic movements of the intestines that allow digested material to pass through) has begun. Respiratory movements may occur during this period, although the lungs are not sufficiently mature to allow independent life outside the womb, except in rare instances. All the organs are well formed now, and for the rest of the pregnancy the fetus will simply grow and mature. The fetus's length is approximately 33 cm. (13 in.). It weighs 0.675 to 0.79 kilograms (1.5 to 1.75 pounds).

■ 30th to 32nd Week

The fetus is six calendar months old by the date of the last menstrual period. Its skin is wrinkled and covered with a white, cheesy protective substance called *vernix caseosa.* This period is considered to be the earliest time of viability outside the womb, although fetuses have survived delivery at an earlier age. The lungs are still immature at this stage, and a baby born thirty to thirty-two weeks after the last menstrual period would require aggressive intervention to survive. The fetus, if born now, would weigh approximately 1.35 to 1.58 kg. (3 to 3.5 lb) and would be about 40 cm. (16 in.) long.

■ 36th Week

The baby is almost completely mature at this point. Vernix still covers most of the skin, lanugo is starting to fade away, and the fingernails are almost to the fingertips. By now, the baby has assumed the position in the abdomen that it will have until delivery.

■ 40th Week

Length of the full-term fetus ranges from 47 to 52 cm. (19 to 21 in.); weight may be from 3 to

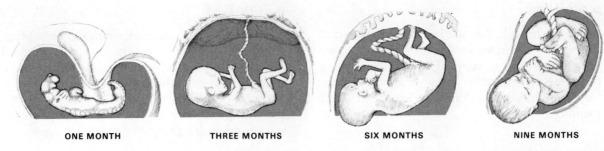

ONE MONTH   THREE MONTHS   SIX MONTHS   NINE MONTHS

The fetus grows from a single cell, increasing its weight about 6 billion times. At two months, the baby's heart is beating and its limbs and some of its bones have formed. At about three months, the placenta has developed and the fetus weighs 1 ounce. At seven months it weighs $2\frac{1}{4}$ pounds, and during the last two months it trebles in size.

3.6 kg. (6 lb. 10 oz. to 7 lb. 15 oz.). Some variation on those parameters may occur, depending on maternal and fetal characteristics, but these are the average dimensions. The baby's skin is pink and shiny, with little lanugo remaining and little vernix except in the folds of skin of the armpits and groin. The breasts protrude somewhat in both boys and girls.

The Products of Conception

Besides the developing fetus, the "products of conception" consist of the placenta, the umbilical cord, the membranes, and the amniotic fluid. These four parts comprise the unborn baby's entire world.

The *placenta*, or "afterbirth," is the means by which the growing fetus exchanges oxygen, nourishment, and wastes with the mother. Unlike other embryonic parts, the placenta does not begin to develop until the third week after fertilization. Before that, the conceptus is nourished by a primitive *yolk sac* such as that formed in chicken eggs. The placenta is formed from the original group of chorionic cells surrounding the fluid sac at the time of implantation. The placenta resembles a flat disk covered with blood vessels; the umbilical cord emerges from its center. At forty weeks, or the birth time of a full-term fetus, the average placenta is about 17.5 centimeters (7 inches) in diameter and 3.75 cm. (1.5 in.) thick. It weighs about 6.75 kilograms (1.5 pounds), or about one sixth of the full-term baby's weight.

The placenta has two portions. The *maternal side* is the side attached to the uterine wall; its surface is red, fleshy, and rough-looking. The *fetal side* faces the interior of the womb; it is covered by a membrane called the *amnion* that gives the

fetal side of the placenta its gray, shiny appearance. The umbilical cord attaches to the center of the placenta on the fetal side.

The maternal and fetal circulations are completely independent of one another. The fetal blood circulates from the developing fetus to the placenta and returns to the baby through the placenta. The mother's blood nourishes the placenta by means of the uterine artery and leaves the uterus by the uterine veins. The blood of mother and baby never mix, except for the occasional escape of a few fetal blood cells into the maternal circulation. This is normal and may occur throughout the pregnancy. At the time of delivery even more fetal blood cells may get into the mother's circulatory system; it is these cells that are responsible for *Rh (Rhesus) factor* sensitization in mothers with Rh negative blood. Most drugs, including alcohol, caffeine, and nicotine, are capable of crossing the placenta into fetal circulation; these substances may cause harm to developing fetal organs or the fetal nervous system. Viruses and some bacteria also are able to cross the placenta and infect the fetus in the womb. Antibodies, including Rhesus antibodies, can pass to the fetus.

The *umbilical cord* carries fresh, oxygen-rich blood from the placenta to the fetus by means of the umbilical vein, and it carries waste products from the fetus back to the placenta by means of two umbilical arteries. At the time of delivery, the average umbilical cord usually measures 50 to 55 cm. (20 to 22 in.) in length and about 2 cm. (0.75 in.) in diameter. It attaches to the fetus at the *umbilicus*.

The *membranes* are two thin structures called the *amnion* and the *chorion*. They lie within the uterus and form the "bag of waters" or *amniotic sac* filled with *amniotic fluid* in which the developing fetus lives. The major function of the membranes is to maintain the amniotic fluid within the sac throughout pregnancy. If the sac is ruptured, the fluid drains out through the vagina, eventually causing uterine contractions and termination of the pregnancy. Sometimes the sac does not rupture until delivery; at other times the bag breaks during the powerful contractions of active labor. Still other labors are brought on by the deliberate rupture of the sac at term. Occasionally, the sac breaks without causing subsequent contractions and labor. When this happens, if the pregnancy is at term, it may be desirable to induce labor with medications to avoid infection of the uterus. Once the protection afforded by the intact bag of waters is gone, the mother is vulnerable to infections ascending from the vagina. Such infections, once they reach the uterus, are very risky for the baby. Thus, labor may be induced to prevent possible risks of infection to the fetus.

Sometimes the amniotic sac may rupture before a baby is ready to be born. If the fetus is not mature, it may be possible to maintain the pregnancy a while longer by preventing uterine contractions with medications. These medications, which may be given orally or intravenously, relax the smooth muscle of the uterus to prevent or postpone labor.

Amniotic fluid is formed in the early stages of embryonic development. Early in pregnancy there is more fluid volume than fetal body size, so the young fetus has ample room to move about vigorously within the sac. At about the thirtieth week of pregnancy, the baby has grown larger, tending to become more fixed within the sac, usually in a longitudinal position. At thirty-six weeks the amniotic sac contains, on average, about 1 liter, or 2 pints, of fluid. This amount gradually decreases until the expected date of delivery. After the fortieth week, the fluid may diminish more rapidly, so that at forty-two weeks there may be only 100 to 200 milliliters (3.3 to 6.6 ounces) of fluid remaining.

Amniotic fluid is made up of protein, water, urea (and other waste products from the fetal blood), fat, sugars, skin and tissue cells, white blood cells, enzymes, and lanugo hair. The fluid provides a soft, safe liquid environment in which the fetus can grow and move with freedom. It protects the fetus from pressure and trauma, acting as a "shock absorber" against maternal injury to the abdomen. The fetus also swallows some amniotic fluid during development, which enhances development of its digestive and respiratory mechanisms.

Because amniotic fluid represents the fetus's *internal* as well as external environment, its contents can provide an accurate picture of fetal development, well-being, and abnormalities. *Amniocentesis*—a medical procedure that involves obtaining a sample of amniotic fluid from the sac—can be a valuable diagnostic tool when fetal immaturity, growth retardation, disease, or deformity is suspected.

The procedure is relatively simple and does not require general anesthesia. A long needle is passed through the abdominal wall, after the position and location of the placenta and fetus have been determined by ultrasound scanning. A sample of amniotic fluid is drawn up into a hypodermic needle and later analyzed in a laboratory. Complete results of the analysis can take up to three or four weeks.

Amniocentesis usually is done between the fourteenth and sixteenth week of gestation if abnormalities such as Down's syndrome (mongolism) or spina bifida are suspected. This is early enough that if these or other serious anomalies are diagnosed, the mother can safely undergo a therapeutic abortion before the fetus is considered viable and probably before the mother has felt fetal movement.

Later in the pregnancy, amniocentesis can be done to determine fetal lung maturity in the case of premature labor, or fetal well-being if other, simpler tests have suspicious results.

Amniocentesis often is performed on pregnant women 35 years old and older because of a statistically increased risk of fetal anomalies associated with increased maternal age. It should be noted, however, that amniocentesis is an invasive procedure that carries a definite, if slight, risk of premature labor, miscarriage, or damage to the fetus or placenta (this last possibility is very rare). Other, less invasive tests are available for diagnosing specific anomalies or disease (see *Diagnostic Tests of Pregnancy* later in this section); amniocentesis is not performed routinely or for such nonmedical reasons as determining the sex of the unborn fetus.

Discomforts of Pregnancy

There are as many different physical experiences of pregnancy as there are labor and delivery stories. Some women look and feel wonderful throughout pregnancy. Others experience nausea, swollen feet, constipation, and heartburn from the moment they miss a period until they give birth. Fortunately, most of the discomforts that pregnancy causes have simple solutions, and many diminish as pregnancy advances.

■ Nausea and Vomiting

Nausea, a strong feeling that you are about to vomit, may be the first sign of pregnancy that you experience. It is believed to be due to the sudden presence of the hormone chorionic gonadotropin and to changes in the way your body metabolizes carbohydrates. It is often more severe early in the day, hence the term "morning sickness." It is very common during the first trimester of pregnancy.

Nausea often is brought on by the odors of certain foods or cigarette smoke. One obvious way to prevent it is to avoid those smells that provoke it, although this often is not possible. It is also frequently relieved by raising the body's level of glucose in the bloodstream. This is best done not by eating a large amount of simple carbohydrate, such as a candy bar—this may actually worsen the sensation—but by taking several small meals a day. Foods to be avoided are greasy or spicy preparations, and meals should be as plain as possible, such as dry toast or a few crackers. If you are particularly prone to nausea upon arising, it can be beneficial to eat something dry, such as plain toast, before getting out of bed. Try also to get up slowly.

Vomiting in the first trimester of pregnancy often accompanies nausea; it may also occur without warning. It is more common early in the day but can occur at any time. Severe, frequent vomiting, known as *hyperemesis gravidarum*, may require hospitalization for a short period of time. It is not harmful to the mother or fetus as long as it is treated properly. Any pregnant woman who vomits more than three or four times a day should consult her doctor.

The interventions described above to relieve nausea may also be helpful in preventing vomiting. Both nausea and vomiting generally diminish by the end of the tenth week of pregnancy and should end entirely by the thirteenth or fourteenth week.

■ Urinary Frequency and Urinary Tract Infection

Along with nausea, one of the first things that can signal pregnancy is an increase in the frequency of urination. This is particularly noticeable at night and is due to the increasing pressure on the bladder by the growing uterus. This should not be associated with any discomfort. There is not much that can be done about urinary frequency, except to maintain good muscle tone in the pelvic area by doing frequent "Kegel's exercises." These exercises involve a rhythmic, repetitive tightening and loosening of the pelvic floor muscles, a feeling of "raising" the pelvic floor as though it were an elevator. Such exercises, diligently maintained throughout pregnancy, not only help to prevent involuntary leakage of urine as the uterus grows in size, but also may be of benefit during labor, especially in the "pushing" stage.

Even if you experience severe urinary frequency, you should *never* decrease your fluid intake. Pregnancy represents a great demand on your body's blood and fluid volume, and decreasing your oral fluid intake can cause problems with your health as well as with fetal development. If, however, urinary frequency is associated with pain, burning, a sense of urgency, and/or the release of only a small amount of urine each time, you may have a *urinary tract infection*. Such infections are common in pregnancy because of mechanical pressures and changes in the chemistry of the urinary and reproductive tracts.

Normal urinary frequency that is not associated with infection will subside after about the twelfth week of pregnancy, only to return in the third trimester as the weight and size of the uterus once again put pressure on the bladder. Urinary tract infection (UTI), however, may recur throughout pregnancy and can cause premature labor if untreated.

If you suspect that you have a UTI, you should notify your obstetrician or midwife as soon as possible. He or she may take a "clean-catch" specimen of your urine (one that is obtained after first cleansing the perineum and urethral opening) to send to a laboratory for analysis. If bacteria are found in your urine, you will most likely be treated with oral antibiotics for a week to ten days.

Although you are more prone to develop UTIs during pregnancy, there are ways to prevent their occurrence. These measures—which should be practiced even in nonpregnancy—include drinking four to six glasses of water a day, always wiping or cleaning the perineum from the front to the back, and urinating both before and after intercourse, so that the bladder is kept empty.

■ *Constipation*

Constipation is an unpleasant, common "side effect" of pregnancy related to an increase in the circulating levels of the hormone progesterone, which reduces the motility of the intestines. Later in pregnancy, the growing fetus may displace the intestines, further worsening the condition. In addition, iron supplements commonly given to pregnant women can contribute to constipation.

If constipation is severe, you can ask your doctor or midwife for a prescription for stool softeners. Constipation is best treated, however, by increasing your intake of fluids and roughage (dietary fiber), and by maintaining a reasonable level of daily exercise.

■ *Changes in Taste*

Changes in the way foods taste are among the earliest symptoms of pregnancy and vary according to individual women. The new taste may be described as metallic or bitter and is often associated with unpleasant smells or with foods that bring on nausea, particularly cigarette smoke, alcohol, and fatty foods. A simple way to cope with this problem is to use a strong mouthwash and to carry gum, mints, or hard candies with you.

Although it is a cliché repeated over and over again in television situation comedies, some pregnant women do indeed experience strong cravings for certain types of foods. There is no harm in indulging such cravings, providing the foods desired are somewhat nutritious and do not take the place of other nutritionally sound food items. Cravings for inedible items such as dirt, clay, or household starch sometimes occur during pregnancy. such cravings, known collectively as *pica*, should be reported to your obstetrician.

■ *Heartburn*

Heartburn, also known as *pyrosis*, is not the same as simple indigestion. It is a painful, burning sensation in the lower part of the chest, usually accompanied by the regurgitation of a small amount of acidic fluid from the stomach. It is caused by the displacement of the stomach as the fetus grows.

Simple ways to prevent heartburn include taking small, frequent, dry meals; avoiding overeating; avoiding fatty, fried, or overly spicy foods; and avoiding lying down right after meals. Heartburn that occurs at night when you are lying flat in bed may be remedied by elevating your head and upper back with several pillows.

Severe heartburn that is not remedied easily should be reported to your physician or midwife. There are many antacid preparations that are safe to take in pregnancy, particularly those containing aluminum and magnesium, but you should not take any preparation, including sodium bicarbonate ("baking soda") without first consulting your obstetrician. Such preparations can cause severe temporary imbalances in your body's electrolytes.

■ *Hemorrhoids*

Hemorrhoids, which are really varicose veins of the anus, are another common discomfort in pregnancy related to both constipation and increased pressure on veins in the perineal area. You can help to avoid hemorrhoids by avoiding constipation and straining at bowel movements, but if you develop severe hemorrhoids, topical ointments, suppositories, warm soaks, or ice packs may provide some relief.

■ *Skin changes*

Skin changes usually do not occur early in pregnancy, but some women complain of dry skin or spots on the face. The spots usually disappear around the end of the thirteenth week, but the dry skin may persist owing to hormonal changes. Other skin changes that occur later in pregnancy have to do with pigmentation. *Chloasma*, or "the mask of pregnancy," is a darkening of the skin over the forehead and eyes that may occur to a greater or lesser degree after week 16; it is worsened by exposure to the sun. Chloasma is caused by hormonal changes and usually disappears after pregnancy.

Striae gravidarum, or silvery stripes along the abdomen and buttocks (popularly known as "stretch" marks), may occur in mid- to late pregnancy and fade after the birth of the baby. Darkening of the nipples and areolae occurs commonly in dark-haired women or women in their first pregnancy. The *linea nigra*, a dark line along the midline of the abdomen, occurs in about half of all pregnant women and fades after the pregnancy is terminated.

■ *Breast Swelling and Discomfort*

The breast swelling and tenderness that normally

occur in many women premenstrually continue as the period is missed; within a very short time the swelling and soreness are even more obvious. The nipples may be particularly sensitive to touch, and the breasts may have a tingling sensation. These changes are related to increased levels of estrogen and progesterone. After the sixth week or so, there is an appreciable change in breast size, and there may be an accompanying increase in the number and size of superficial veins over the breast, as well as an increase in nipple size. The only intervention to reduce breast tenderness and discomfort is to wear a supportive, well-fitting bra and to avoid trauma or stimulation of the breasts and nipples.

■ Nasal Stuffiness and Nosebleeds

Increased levels of circulating estrogen in pregnancy can cause swelling of the lining of the nostrils, which can lead to nasal stuffiness and nosebleeds (also called *epistaxis*). The use of a cool-air vaporizer can alleviate some nasal congestion and irritation. Nasal sprays, nose drops, and decongestants are to be avoided unless recommended by your doctor.

■ Backache

As the weight and size of your lower abdomen increases, your center of gravity moves forward. At the same time, because of hormonal changes there is a relaxation of pelvic and pubic joints, resulting in a "waddling" gait. These changes in posture and walk can result in low backache, especially in the latter half of pregnancy.

There are numerous exercises to relieve low backache, including "tailor-sitting" (sitting cross-legged with the ribcage lifted), pelvic tilt movements, and back-strengthening exercises. Consult your doctor or midwife for a list of good back exercises. In addition, sensible shoes are a must during late pregnancy, and proper body mechanics need to be applied when lifting, twisting, or moving from a sitting to a standing position.

■ Leg Pain and Cramps

In the last month or so of pregnancy, as the fetal head moves down into position in the pelvis, you may experience shooting pains in the low back and down the thighs. These pains are the result of pressure on the sciatic nerve and may be quite disconcerting. Finding positions that relieve the pressure on the nerves is up to the individual woman. It may help to avoid walking for long distances, but lying completely supine is not recommended. Not only does lying flat on your back do little to relieve the pain, but late in pregnancy it can also temporarily reduce the flow of blood from the placenta to the fetus. Lying on your side, particularly the left side, or elevating the legs may prove helpful in relieving leg pain.

Cramps in the lower legs are particularly bothersome to some women during late pregnancy. Although the exact cause has not been determined, leg cramps in pregnancy are believed to be partly due to an imbalance in your body's ratio of calcium to phosphorus, which is due, in part, to an increase in the consumption of dairy products during pregnancy. You should consult your doctor if you suffer from severe leg cramps. Some people recommend reducing your intake of dairy products and taking oral calcium supplements to correct the imbalance, but this should be discussed with your doctor first. While a painful cramp is occurring, it may be helpful to flex the foot upward at the ankle while maintaining the leg in a straightened-out position; this will stretch the calf muscle.

■ Vaginal Discharge

You may notice an increase in the amount of normal vaginal discharge throughout the pregnancy. This is the result of an increase in the blood supply to the vagina and cervix and is quite normal. If, however, you notice a change in the normal color of the discharge or an offensive odor, you should report this to your doctor immediately. Just as you are more prone to develop urinary tract infections in pregnancy, the slight alteration in your body's acid-base balance means you are also more likely to get candidiasis or other vaginal infections. Other symptoms of vaginal infection might include itching or irritation of the labia or the vagina.

A yeast or bacterial infection of the vagina is treated with fungicidal or bactericidal cream or other preparations. In addition, good hygiene measures such as wiping the perineum from front to back, taking frequent showers, avoiding douching, and using a cornstarch-based or other nonperfumed powder can help prevent vaginal infections. It helps, too, to wear cotton rather than nylon panties and to avoid wearing tight trousers or constricting pantyhose.

■ *Swollen Ankles*

Edema (swelling) of the feet and ankles is fairly common in mid- to late pregnancy, especially after you have been standing or sitting for long periods. This is due to an increase in your body's fluid volume, and it may be relieved by elevating the legs.

Severe edema can cause discomfort in the feet and ankles. Although even severe swelling is usually normal, it can be associated with a rise in blood pressure and other symptoms of a potentially dangerous condition known as *preeclampsia* (see under *Problems in Pregnancy* later in this section). As such, swelling needs to be reported to your obstetrician or midwife, and sudden increases in the amount of fluid retained, or the sudden appearance of swollen hands and swelling of the face, require evaluation. In some instances, swelling can be treated with dietary modifications and diuretic preparations. Reducing your intake of salt and cutting down on spicy foods, which may cause you to drink more fluids and retain more water, are two simple treatments for excessive fluid retention.

■ *Varicose Veins*

Discoloration and prominence of superficial veins in the legs may cause discomfort and distress during the second and third trimesters of pregnancy, as the growing fetus exerts downward pressure on the organs and inhibits good return of blood from circulation in the lower extremities. Discomfort from varicose veins can be minimized by frequently elevating the legs, avoiding long periods of sitting or sitting with the legs crossed, and wearing support pantyhose or elastic stockings.

■ *Faintness*

The changes in a pregnant woman's blood volume and the tendency of circulating blood to "pool" in the leg veins can contribute to a feeling of faintness or dizziness, both in early pregnancy and in the second and third trimesters. This condition may be aggravated by standing in warm, crowded places and by arising rapidly from a lying or sitting posture to a standing position.

If you experience faintness, you should not try to fight the feeling, but should lower yourself to a sitting position as quickly as possible, with your head held low. In general, it is best for the pregnant woman to avoid standing up suddenly or standing for long periods of time. Sometimes gently flexing and moving the feet and legs while standing or sitting can prevent "pooling" of blood.

■ *Shortness of Breath*

As the top of the uterus rises into the upper abdomen during the latter half of pregnancy, it may exert pressure on the diaphragm. This can cause a feeling of shortness of breath and actually can reduce the "vital capacity" of the lungs—the maximum amount of air that can be inhaled and then exhaled. Sitting up straight in a tall chair and elevating the upper back on several pillows while lying down usually relieves this condition somewhat.

■ *Braxton-Hicks Contractions*

Irregular, painless contractions of the uterus that occur throughout pregnancy and are not associated with labor are called *Braxton-Hicks contractions*. They generally increase in frequency and intensity as the pregnancy progresses and may become more regular as labor approaches. True Braxton-Hicks contractions are normal and represent no cause for alarm. Contractions that occur well before the due date, however, and are regular and cause a noticeable tightening of the uterine muscle require evaluation. (See discussion of premature labor under *Disorders in Pregnancy* later in this section.)

■ *Fetal Movement*

Fetal movement ("quickening") actually begins around the twelfth week of pregnancy. The mother does not begin to become aware of the baby's movements, however, until around the eighteenth to twentieth week. Quickening may first be experienced as a fluttering sensation that gradually increases in intensity and frequency. As your pregnancy progresses, you may find that your baby has a definite sleep-wake cycle. Many fetuses, in fact, seem to prefer being active while the mother is trying to sleep! Regular fetal movement is one of the simplest ways to determine fetal well-being. Any long period—such as forty-eight hours—during which the baby stops moving, although it is probably normal, should be reported. In the view of some obstetricians, anything less than two fetal movements an hour warrants investigation.

■ *Rib and Ligament Pain*

Toward the end of pregnancy you may experience pain at the costal margin, the place where the ribcage ends at the lower end of the chest. In some women the pain is stronger or felt only on the right side. It is caused by the growing uterus exerting pressure on the lower ribs. It may be felt as more severe when sitting. Unfortunately, nothing can be done to relieve it except to avoid postures that aggravate it, such as slumping or slouching. Delivery of the baby alleviates the problem.

Between weeks 16 and 20, you may experience a sensation like a dragging, continuous, aching pain in the lower abdomen, usually on the right side. It is caused by stretching of the ligaments that support the uterus and usually is exacerbated on standing up after sitting for long periods. Like rib pain, nothing specific can be done to relieve ligament pain, but it is harmless and usually passes after about eight weeks.

■ *Emotional Changes*

Pregnancy being one of the major events in the life of a family, it is understandable that the pregnant woman as well as the father-to-be and siblings-to-be go through many emotional changes with regard to the eventual birth of the new baby. A certain amount of jealousy on the part of the baby's future brothers and sisters and the father-to-be is to be expected. It is likewise quite normal for the mother-to-be to experience *ambivalence*, or mixed feelings, about the change in her life the pregnancy represents. At some point, however, a feeling of acceptance of the pregnancy occurs, along with, at times, *introversion*, or a turning-inward of one's feelings about oneself and the pregnancy.

Mood swings similar to those sometimes experienced premenstrually are not uncommon throughout pregnancy and are due partly to hormonal changes and partly to the emotional stress and physical discomforts of pregnancy. An understanding family can be a big help to a pregnant woman who sometimes feels emotionally overwhelmed by the changes taking place in her body and her body image.

Prenatal Care

Nowhere in health care is there a better example of preventive medicine than the regular prenatal (or antenatal) care sought by healthy families who are expecting a baby. The only way problems can be recognized, treated, or simply avoided is with regular visits to a private obstetrician, an obstetrical clinic, or a nurse-midwife *starting as soon as you suspect you are pregnant*. Part of the reason for the continuing high infant mortality rate in the United States, compared with the rates in other major industrialized nations, is the absence of good prenatal care among many lower socioeconomic groups.

■ *Rest and Sleep*

It is normal to feel unusually fatigued in early pregnancy. You should not try to fight this, but acknowledge your body's requirement for extra rest if possible. The amount of extra rest and sleep you need is a highly individual matter; a total of ten hours of rest a day is considered ideal. At the very least, you should make a point not to get *less* rest than you did before the pregnancy, even if you do not feel particularly tired.

Fatigue may result in sound, blissful sleep, but sometimes anxiety or other problems may cause restlessness and insomnia. You should always discuss these kinds of problems with your doctor or midwife during your prenatal visits if they are not easily resolved by tried-and-true methods of relaxation and sleep inducement. It is generally agreed, however, that sleep medications are to be avoided during pregnancy.

■ *Exercise*

Most obstetrical experts now agree that exercise during pregnancy has many benefits. "Exercise" in this context, however, does not mean physical exertion beyond normal daily activity, but the maintenance of reasonable physical activity that does not cause pain or undue exertion. Pregnancy is certainly not the time to try to go beyond your normal, prepregnant capacity for exercise or to take up any new forms of exercise. Nor is it the time for exercise that involves a physical danger, such as skiing or jumping horses. Activities such as swimming, golfing, playing tennis, running, or bicycling may be continued safely during pregnancy, as long as you stop before you feel really tired. Many obstetricians feel that aerobic exercise is unwise during pregnancy, both because of the risk of injury and because of changes in blood flow to the extremities.

■ Diet

A well-balanced diet is essential in pregnancy, and pregnancy is no time to try to cut back on calories. Even if you were overweight before you became pregnant, you should be taking in 300 to 500 extra calories a day beyond your usual intake. You should never consume fewer than 2,220 calories a day, and you should try to increase your protein intake to more than 1 gram of protein per kilogram (2.2 pounds) of body weight. Some experts recommend a daily protein intake of at least 75 grams. Nonmeat sources of protein include cheese and dairy products, peanut butter, and beans. You should also pay attention to your calcium and iron consumption. Your calcium intake during pregnancy should be at least 1.2 grams a day, and you should maintain a daily intake of about 18 milligrams of iron a day throughout the childbearing years. Additionally, a diet high in fiber content may prevent the constipation that is sometimes brought on by pregnancy.

■ Alcohol, Drugs, and Caffeine

There is disagreement among obstetrical health-care providers about whether any amount of alcohol is acceptable on a regular basis during pregnancy. Some feel an occasional glass of wine with dinner cannot cause harm to the fetus; others say up to two drinks per day are acceptable. Still others ban alcohol altogether for the duration of pregnancy.

It is clear that excessive amounts of alcohol consumed by the mother cause injury to the developing fetus; it is probably better to be on the safe side and restrict your intake to no or occasional drinks only.

No drug should be taken in pregnancy, even an over-the-counter preparation such as aspirin or antacid tablets, without first consulting your doctor. Even such seemingly harmless drugs as those that are sold without prescription can cause harm to a developing fetus, and almost all drugs the mother takes cross the placenta into the fetal circulatory system.

Caffeine is one of the most common drugs enjoyed by adults. The amount of caffeine most adults take in on a daily basis, however, is not advisable for a developing fetus. For this reason, many obstetricians recommend cutting out coffee, tea, colas, and chocolate during pregnancy. If you feel you cannot cut out caffeine altogether, it is best to be aware of how much coffee, tea, and cola you are drinking and to limit yourself to one or two servings per day.

■ Travel

As long as you are healthy and your pregnancy is uneventful, you do not need to eliminate travel. However, you should keep your long-distance traveling to a minimum and consult your doctor or midwife before taking a long trip. Many airlines will not accept pregnant passengers after the thirty-fifth week of pregnancy, and it is probably not a good idea to journey too far from home after that time.

■ Dental Care

Good oral hygiene and preventive dentistry are just as important during pregnancy as they are at any other time. X-ray examinations and major dental surgery usually are avoided during pregnancy, but you should not avoid your dentist just because you are pregnant.

■ X-ray Examinations

In general, all X-ray exams are contraindicated during pregnancy because of the possible hazards of radiation to the developing fetus. If, however, an X-ray study is necessary during pregnancy because of an accident or illness, you should inform the doctor or X-ray technician that you are pregnant *before* you undergo the procedure.

■ Smoking

Smoking is discouraged at all times, but especially during pregnancy. Smoking in pregnancy will cause you to give birth to a smaller baby than if you did not smoke at all, and low birth weight is one of the primary contributors to the relatively high infant mortality rate in the United States. Smoking after the sixteenth week of pregnancy can cause both mental and physical retardation of the unborn baby. If you are contemplating becoming pregnant and you smoke, it is best to quit *before* you become pregnant.

■ Sex

Sexual intercourse during pregnancy is normal and healthy and can continue right up until labor starts. As the pregnancy continues, the growing abdomen may make it necessary to modify the positions in which sexual intercourse takes place. Sometimes the woman in advanced pregnancy may be so uncomfortable in general that she does not wish to have sex. This is normal and should not be a matter of great concern.

It is likewise normal for sexual desire to diminish or disappear during pregnancy in some women. This should be treated with understanding by the partner, and the couple should know that normal sexual desire will return once the pregnancy is over. Some women, on the other hand, may feel increased sexual desire during pregnancy and may enjoy heightened sexual response at this time.

There are instances in which sexual intercourse in pregnancy is not advised. A woman who has had one or more miscarriages should consult her doctor on the question of vaginal intercourse during the first trimester of the pregnancy. Any sign of a threatened miscarriage, such as vaginal bleeding or abdominal cramping, should result automatically in cessation of all sexual activity until the doctor has been notified of the situation and says sex can resume.

■ Bathing and Douching

Pregnancy is no reason to alter your habits of hygiene. You should continue to bathe as you always have. Keep in mind, however, that there is an increased tendency to faint in pregnancy and that your center of balance is changed from your nonpregnant state. For this reasons, nonslip bathmats in the shower and tub are essential, and you should avoid taking baths or showers that are too hot or last too long. When getting out of the bathtub, always get up slowly and hold on to guardrails at the sides of the tub.

Douching is not recommended during pregnancy for the same reasons that it is not advised in general: It can destroy the naturally occurring "good" bacteria and other organisms that normally inhabit the vagina, resulting in an upsetting of the normal chemistry of the vagina and in an increased risk of infection. If you feel you must douch, then you should use only plain water or very dilute vinegar.

Danger Signs

Certain symptoms and warning signs that occur in pregnancy deserve immediate attention. Those symptoms that should be reported to your physician or clinic *immediately* are:

■ Vaginal Bleeding

Bleeding from the vagina, even "spotting" or scant amounts of pinkish fluid, before the twenty-eighth week of pregnancy indicates that there is a chance of miscarriage, or *spontaneous abortion*. If you note blood coming from your vagina, you should go to bed and notify your doctor as soon as convenient. If the bleeding appears to be heavy and is accompanied by cramping or pain, notify your doctor at once and go to bed. After the twenty-eighth week of pregnancy, bleeding can signify the beginning of labor. Your physician should be notified as soon as possible.

■ Continuous Abdominal Pain

Severe abdominal pain that is *continuous*, not intermittent or occasional, should be reported to your obstetrician immediately. This can be a sign of partial or complete detachment of the placenta from the uterus, a rare and dangerous condition.

■ Breaking of the "Bag of Waters"

A gush of fluid from the vagina, or even a steady trickle of fluid, can mean that the amniotic sac has ruptured. Labor usually ensues rapidly. It is important to note the color and appearance of the fluid and to notify your physician or midwife to arrange for admission to a hospital.

■ Blurred Vision or "Spots" Before the Eyes

In the second half of pregnancy, misty, blurry vision or spots before the eyes can signal *preeclampsia*, a condition of pregnancy in which the blood pressure rises significantly above baseline values. If you experience any of these symptoms, you should go to bed, remain quiet and calm, and call your doctor at once.

■ Continuous, Severe Headache

A severe headache that does not resolve within several hours, particularly one that is felt in the forehead and front of the head, may also be a sign of preeclampsia. Notify your physician of this symptom if the headache seems unusually severe or does not resolve within a reasonable time period.

■ *Recurring, Steady Contractions Before the Due Date*

Uterine contractions that recur at regular intervals and increase in intensity or frequency well before your due date should be reported immediately to your physician or midwife. If you are experiencing premature labor, you may need to be admitted to the hospital to receive medications to suppress labor until your baby is mature. If you think you are having premature contractions that are more intense or more regular than Braxton-Hicks contractions, go to bed and call your doctor. You may actually be able to feel a tightening at the top of the uterus with each contraction.

Other symptoms that may require attention and should be reported within twenty-four hours are:

■ *Fever*

A rise in temperature to more than 100°F (38°C) usually needs to be treated aggressively and may require brief hospitalization.

■ *Urinary Pain and Frequency*

Some amount of frequency and urgency associated with urination is normal in the first and last trimesters of pregnancy. Pain or burning on urination, however, and urgency or frequency greater than that experienced before can mean that you have a urinary tract infection, a common occurrence in pregnancy because of changes in your body's chemical balance. Because a urinary tract infection can bring on labor before the due date, it needs to be treated as soon as possible.

■ *Swelling of the Face, Hands, and Ankles*

Excessive swelling (edema) of the feet, hands, and face needs to be distinguished from simple *dependent edema* of the feet and ankles that occurs in pregnant and nonpregnant persons after standing or working on one's feet for many hours. Dependent edema usually is relieved by elevating the feet for a period of time. Severe swelling of the feet that is not relieved by elevation, or swelling of the face and hands, such that rings or bracelets have to be removed or become uncomfortable, may be associated with preeclampsia and should be reported as soon as convenient.

■ *Absence of Fetal Movement*

It is normal for a baby to rest or stop moving for rather long periods, and it is fairly common to experience no movement for several days between the twentieth and twenty-fourth weeks of pregnancy, or for the baby to "rest" for up to twenty-four hours toward the end of pregnancy. Absence of movement for forty-eight hours or more should be reported to your physician or clinic.

■ *Severe Vomiting*

It is normal to vomit quite a bit during the first fourteen weeks of pregnancy; however, if it becomes so severe that you cannot retain any solid food or liquids, your physician should be notified. During the last trimester of pregnancy occasional vomiting may occur, but recurrent, excessive vomiting merits medical attention.

Disorders in Pregnancy

■ *Premature Rupture of Membranes (PROM)*

Breaking of the amniotic sac significantly before the due date, as described earlier, may require hospitalization and treatment with medications to postpone labor until the baby is mature enough to survive outside the womb. PROM can occur spontaneously, for no apparent reason, or you can develop a "leak" in the amniotic sac that causes fluid to gush or drip out of the vagina continuously. The loss of amniotic fluid means the uterus loses its protection against the outside world, making the mother more prone to ascending uterine infection. If signs of infection are present, antibiotic therapy may be initiated and the fetus may be delivered, either vaginally or by cesarean section, regardless of its maturity. The reason for this is that maternal uterine infection can be extremely hazardous to the fetus, and delivery is the safer option. If infection is present and labor has not followed PROM, *induction of labor* with the hormone oxytocin may be required.

If there are no signs of maternal infection, and

if gestational age is 34 weeks or more, labor may be induced with oxytocin after waiting twenty-four hours to permit an increase in maternal-fetal levels of corticosteroids in the circulation. These hormones help accelerate the maturation of fetal lungs.

If the gestational age of the baby is less than 34 weeks, labor may be suppressed or prevented temporarily by the use of drugs to allow the fetus more time to mature. A drug called *betamethasone*, a synthetic corticosteroid, may be given to the mother to initiate maturation of the baby's lungs. The mother will be placed on bed rest and monitored closely. After the baby has reached 34 weeks' gestational age, labor may be induced.

■ Premature Labor

Labor that occurs before the thirty-seventh week of pregnancy is called *preterm labor*. If the mother has a condition such as preeclampsia, kidney disease, or cardiovascular disease, so that continuing the pregnancy would jeopardize her well-being, then no effort is made to stop labor. If certain other conditions are present, labor is likewise allowed to progress. These conditions include: active labor with the cervix dilated 4 centimeters (1.6 inches) or more; fetal complications such as anomalies or Rh isoimmunization; ruptured membranes with or without maternal infection; hemorrhage; and fetal death.

In the absence of these conditions, and if fetal lung maturity is doubtful, the woman may be given drugs to suppress labor. The woman who is experiencing preterm labor might be kept in the hospital until she reaches thirty seven weeks of pregnancy. Or, in the hospital, she might be kept on intravenous labor-suppressing drugs until all contractions have ceased, then be sent home on oral *tocolytics* (antilabor drugs); at home, she would be kept on modified bed rest and monitored closely in visits to the obstetrician.

■ Incompetent Cervix

A cervix that thins out ("effaces") and dilates in midpregnancy, significantly before the fetus is capable of survival outside the uterus, will cause miscarriage at around the twentieth week of pregnancy. If cervical dilation—which is painless in this case—can be diagnosed before it progresses too far, or if the woman has a history of miscarriage at around the twentieth week of gestation, the treatment is *cerclage*, or insertion of perma-

nent sutures (stitches) around the cervix to maintain it in a closed state until the pregnancy reaches term. This procedure normally is performed around the fourteenth week of pregnancy. The sutures are removed at term to allow cervical dilation and labor to ensue. The procedure has a success rate greater than 75 percent.

■ Preeclampsia/Eclampsia

A condition that sometimes occurs in late pregnancy is *preeclampsia*, in which two of the following three conditions are present: elevation of blood pressure; edema of the hands, feet, or face; and protein in the urine. No one knows exactly what causes preeclampsia to occur, but it poses risks to the fetus as well as to the mother.

Preeclampsia is treated with bed rest and drugs, although the only real "cure" is delivery of the baby. Once the uterus is emptied, preeclampsia usually resolves fairly quickly. If preeclampsia is not diagnosed and treated, however, it can progress to *eclampsia*, which is an exceedingly dangerous condition. It is usually preceded by a severe headache, visual changes, irritability, and sometimes pain below the heart in the center of the belly. These symptoms lead quickly to convulsions, or "fits," which last a minute or so and are followed by a period of unconsciousness. True eclampsia is relatively rare today because of diligent monitoring of pregnant women for symptoms of preeclampsia during prenatal visits.

■ Hypertension

Hypertension (elevated blood pressure) can occur in pregnancy without preeclampsia, or it can predispose a woman to develop preeclampsia. Because elevated blood pressure involves constriction of many of the blood vessels, it can cause insufficient blood flow to the placenta, resulting in a placenta that is chronically insufficient, or a fetus that is small for gestational age, immature, or compromised.

Hypertension that occurs in pregnancy is treated with bed rest, drugs, and diligent monitoring of fetal well-being.

■ Diabetes

Sometimes a woman who has never had *diabetes mellitus* develops it during pregnancy. Diabetes mellitus is a condition in which the body is unable to manufacture enough *insulin* to metabolize carbohydrates, so that the body cells are forced to break down fat and protein for energy. Diabetes that occurs only during pregnancy usually is detected by the presence of sugar in the urine, an abnormal occurrence. This condition is called "gestational diabetes."

Women who develop gestational diabetes rarely need to take insulin to control their body's sugar imbalance. Usually a restricted-calorie, low-carbohydrate diet is sufficient to control symptoms and maintain blood sugar at normal levels. Such women may require hospitalization, however, for a few days or weeks after the condition is diagnosed, until their blood sugar is brought under control by diet. If you develop gestational diabetes, you may have to be taught to monitor your blood sugar by the use of "finger sticks," puncturing the skin of the finger with a lancet, dropping a small specimen of blood onto a chemically treated strip of paper, and observing color changes on the paper to determine your blood sugar level. Another way to monitor gestational diabetes is by testing voided urine with chemically treated strips of paper and recording the results.

Gestational diabetes poses certain risks to the fetus, thus the mother may require more rigid monitoring during pregnancy than she would if she did not have this condition. Sometimes labor may be induced several weeks before the due date, since babies of all diabetics tend to be larger than normal, and their large size may pose problems for vaginal delivery.

Gestational diabetes usually resolves within twenty-four hours of delivery.

■ Hydramnios

The presence of an excessive volume of amniotic fluid within the amniotic sac is called *hydramnios.* The cause usually is not known, and in most cases the pregnancy is otherwise normal. Some instances of hydramnios, however, are associated with multiple gestation (twins or triplets), diabetes, preeclampsia, and fetal abnormalities. Because the uterus and abdomen are so enlarged, the mother may feel marked discomfort toward the end of pregnancy. Usually the woman with hydramnios is not treated except with monitoring and comfort measures. Her abdomen may be scanned by ultrasound to rule out fetal anomalies.

■ Anemia

In pregnancy, because the volume of circulating blood is so greatly increased, it is normal for the blood to be somewhat diluted. Anemia—a reduction in the blood's *hemoglobin* content—is quite common in pregnancy, however, and can be hazardous. As a result, many women are given iron supplements routinely during pregnancy to prevent anemia.

Symptoms of anemia are subtle and may be confused with other normal symptoms of pregnancy. Usually they are not recognized until the condition has advanced significantly. They include fatigue, lethargy, lack of energy for performing normal daily tasks, and pallor.

■ Hemorrhage

Vaginal bleeding that occurs after the twenty-eighth week of pregnancy is called *antepartum hemorrhage. Incidental hemorrhage* may result from ulcerations or minor injuries to the genital tract, or it may signal the start of labor as the fetal head descends into the pelvis, putting pressure on the small blood vessels of the cervix.

Placenta previa is another possible cause of antepartum hemorrhage and is much more serious. In this condition, the placenta, which normally is attached to the uterine wall high up in the uterus, is instead attached to the lower uterine segment near the cervical opening. Because of the proximity of the placenta to the cervix, bleeding invariably occurs either before the onset of labor or during labor. The amount of bleeding is usually quite heavy and is not associated with any pain. Depending on the location of the placenta, delivery may be vaginal or by cesarean section.

Abruptio placentae is a relatively rare, dangerous condition in which the placenta separates prematurely from the uterine wall, either completely or partially. This may be accompanied by light to heavy bleeding or may occur without any bleeding. The most significant symptom of this condition is continuous, severe abdominal pain. The uterus becomes rigid and board-like, and the fetal heartbeat may not be audible by conventional methods through the uterine wall. This condition requires immediate hospitalization and possible cesarean delivery.

■ Placental Insufficiency

In *placental insufficiency*, for reasons that are not clearly understood, the placenta either develops abnormally or, once developed, fails to function efficiently. As a result, the fetus does not receive sufficient oxygen or nutrients from the placenta. Such a fetus develops very slowly and is at risk because the placenta at some point will no longer be able to provide adequate oxygen to it.

Where placental insufficiency is suspected, diligent, frequent monitoring of fetal well-being by the use of various tests will help to determine when and if the fetus is compromised; rapid delivery by the vaginal or cesarean route may be indicated.

■ Existing Maternal Conditions

A woman who has a chronic medical disorder, such as cardiac disease, diabetes, hypertension, lupus erythematosus, sickle-cell disease, or rheumatoid arthritis, is likely to experience a worsening of that condition if she becomes pregnant. Although pregnancy is a normal, natural state, it represents a stress on a healthy body because of changes in blood volume, hormone balance, mechanical pressures, and other conditions; a woman whose health is already compromised may experience greater difficulty during pregnancy.

Modern obstetrics has made it possible for women to sustain a pregnancy who twenty or thirty years ago might not have been able to bear children. Such a woman, however, is considered a "high-risk" patient, and she requires the intervention of a medical expert. Extreme modifications in life-style may be required during the pregnancy, and delivery may not be possible by "natural" methods.

Diagnostic Tests of Pregnancy

■ Amniocentesis

When fetal anomalies are suspected, amniocentesis (discussed earlier in this chapter under *Products of Conception*) is performed. Later in pregnancy, amniocentesis may be done to determine fetal lung maturity in the case of premature rupture of membranes or preterm labor. Before amniocentesis is performed, the abdomen may be scanned by ultrasound to locate the placenta and the fetus in the uterus.

■ Ultrasound

Ultrasound scanning, or a *sonogram*, may be performed at various points throughout the pregnancy to determine any of the following: gestational age; possible cephalopelvic disproportion (where the fetal head is too large to fit through the pelvis); fetal viability and well-being; fetal presentation (which part of the baby will enter the pelvis first); multiple gestation; hydramnios (an excessive volume of amniotic fluid); fetal anomalies; placental insufficiency; placenta previa; abruptio placentae; spina bifida; fetal position in the abdomen; normal fetal growth and development.

The procedure, described simply, involves projecting pressure pulses of extremely high frequency into the abdomen through a transmitter, or *transducer*. The pulses are reflected, in different ways, off tissues of varying densities, and the returning echoes are transformed into electrical signals displayed on a video screen.

A sonogram is painless, takes twenty to thirty minutes, and may cause discomfort only in that the pregnant woman must lie flat on her back for the entire procedure. If you are to have a sonogram, you may be asked to drink a quart of water two hours before the procedure and not to empty your bladder. This is because the distended bladder is used as a landmark for locating the cervix and uterine segments.

■ Chorionic Villus Sampling

Chorionic villus sampling (CVS) is a relatively new procedure developed to permit early detection of chromosomal abnormalities in the fetus, the most common being Down's syndrome (mongolism). Other, more rare genetic disorders also may be detected through this technique.

The procedure usually is performed between the ninth and eleventh week of the pregnancy. A small plastic catheter is passed into the vagina through the cervix and into the uterus in the vicinity of the chorionic villi, the tiny vessels formed on the embryonic fetal membranes that will develop into the placenta. Samples from the villi are obtained with a syringe attached to the catheter, and the specimens are analyzed in a laboratory.

Complications following the procedure are rare, although not enough is known as yet about the procedure to make accurate assessments of the risks. There is a slight risk of miscarriage from CVS, as well as a slight chance of infection. There is also a small but significant chance of misdiagnosis of a fetal abnormality. Other possible complications are as yet unknown.

■ *Maternal Serum Alphafetoprotein (MSAFP)*

An extremely simple procedure that is becoming more popular as a diagnostic test in pregnancy is the study of maternal levels of a particular type of protein from the fetus in the mother's bloodstream. A small sample of the mother's blood is drawn and analyzed in a laboratory for quantity of *alphafetoprotein*, which normally increases within certain parameters with each week of the pregnancy. Abnormally high or low values can mean such genetic abnormalities as *spina bifida* (a condition in which the spinal column of the fetus is improperly closed), multiple gestation, chromosomal abnormalities, and other, rarer anomalies. The test, which is performed between weeks 16 and 18 of gestation, will also reveal a miscalculation of the due date.

■ *Nonstress Testing/Oxytocin Challenge Test*

A widely accepted, simple test of fetal well-being is *nonstress testing* (NST). It requires the pregnant woman to be monitored externally for fetal heart rate (FHR) for at least thirty to forty minutes, with the mother lying on her back with her head and shoulders slightly elevated and an electronic fetal monitor attached to her abdomen with a belt. *Reactive* NST, which suggests fetal well-being, shows *accelerations* (increases) in the FHR coordinated with movement of the fetus. NST might be required in pregnancies that go significantly beyond the due date, in cases where no fetal movement is felt for several days, or where there is a maternal condition, such as diabetes, that might compromise fetal health.

An *oxytocin challenge test* (OCT), also called a *contraction stress test* (CST), is also used to evaluate fetal well-being and may be ordered if results of NST are suspicious. The FHR is monitored during three uterine contractions within a ten-minute period. The contractions may occur spontaneously or, more commonly, may be induced with a small amount of intravenous oxytocin or by nipple stimulation of the woman, which also releases small amounts of naturally occurring oxytocin. In a healthy fetus, there should be no *deceleration* (slowdown) in the FHR with contractions or just after contractions. Decelerations that occur in the FHR with uterine contractions may mean that the baby is not receiving adequate oxygen during contractions and may be compromised in labor and delivery.

■ *Biophysical Profile*

For routine assessment of fetal well-being, a *biophysical profile* (BPP) may be performed in conjunction with ultrasound scanning. A healthy fetus, as determined by BPP, is one that shows "breathing" movements, body movements, flexed arms and legs, and adequate amounts of fluid in the amniotic sac—all appearing on a sonogram. It also has reactive NST, as defined above.

Normal Variations in the Fetus at Term

■ *Fetal Lie*

In 98 percent of pregnancies, at the time of delivery the baby's body lies parallel to the mother's long axis—a *longitudinal* lie. Either the buttocks present first or the head, known as *breech* or *cephalic presentation*, respectively.

In the remaining 2 percent of pregnancies at term, the fetus lies *obliquely*, with its spine at an oblique angle to the mother's spine, or *transversely*, with its spine at right angles to the mother's. With the baby in an oblique or transverse lie, the shoulder descends into the pelvis first; this sort of presentation cannot be delivered vaginally. Sometimes, an oblique lie converts to a longitudinal lie when labor commences. If, however, the baby remains in a transverse or an oblique lie, delivery will have to be by cesarean section.

■ *Fetal Presentation*

In 96 percent of longitudinal lies, the head is the presenting part ("cephalic" presentation). The remaining 4 percent present bottom first ("breech" presentation). Depending upon whether the baby's feet descend below the pelvic brim, a breech baby may be delivered safely by the vaginal route, or a cesarean delivery may be required. Because the head is the largest diameter of the baby's body to pass through the cervix and pelvis, a head-first presentation is the most natural and safe way for delivery to take place.

A breech baby who does not convert by itself to a head-first presentation by the thirty-third or thirty-fourth week of the pregnancy may sometimes be rotated from the outside of the abdomen

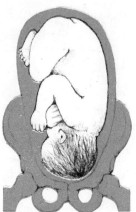
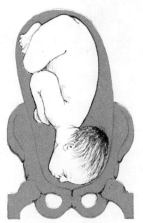
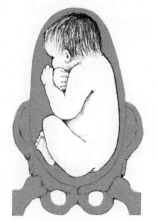
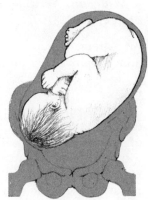

NORMAL (CEPHALIC) PRESENTATION   **BROW OR FACE**   **BREECH**   **OBLIQUE LIE**

The normal presentation, i.e., the baby's position relative to the cervix, is head down with chin on chest. In "brow" (or "face") presentation the baby's neck is extended, and labor may be delayed. Cesarean section may be required; this is also usually the case for breech presentation (bottom first) and sometimes for the oblique lie, although this often corrects itself when labor begins.

by the obstetrician exerting gentle manual pressure on the abdominal wall. This is known as *external cephalic version* and is performed in the labor and delivery suite of the hospital.

Of the possible head-first or cephalic presentations, the *vertex* presentation, in which the neck is bent forward and the baby's chin is on its chest, is the most favorable and also the most common. When the head is partly extended or held straight up-and-down, in a so-called "military" attitude, the brow or face presents into the pelvis first. This can slow labor or cause damage to the baby and thus may require delivery by cesarean section.

Labor

■ Onset of Labor

No one knows exactly what maternal or fetal mechanisms cause labor to start when it does. Among the possible mechanisms involved are increased sensitivity of the uterine muscle to natural levels of oxytocin in the bloodstream; decreasing levels of the hormone progesterone near the delivery date, which may cause the uterus to contract; increasing levels of estrogen, causing the uterus to become more irritable; production by the fetus of a hormone that stimulates labor; the presence of the hormone prostaglandin just prior to labor, causing the uterus to contract; and increased stretching of the uterus by the growing size of the baby, causing the release of substances that stimulate the uterus to contract.

■ Induction of Labor

Labor may be *induced* artificially for various maternal and fetal indications if labor does not occur naturally within a reasonable time period around the due date. Labor may likewise be induced artificially before the due date for various maternal and fetal indications, such as class A diabetes or a series of nonreactive NSTs. Obviously, any condition that has the potential to jeopardize fetal health and well-being necessitates immediate or rapid delivery. If such a delivery can be accomplished vaginally, induction by the use of oxytocin is justified. Such induction is not without risks, however, and is not to be taken lightly.

■ True vs. False Labor

With any pregnancy, you can experience "false alarms" that cause you to go to the hospital, convinced that "this is it," only to have the contractions die down or find that no dilation of the cervix is occurring. No one should ever feel embarrassed about going to the hospital for almost any reason during the latter part of pregnancy, since it is far better to be overcautious than undercautious. Sometimes, however, careful self-monitoring can help distinguish true from false labor.

In true labor contractions are regular when timed. For example, contractions that are almost exactly five minutes apart for an hour or more are likely to be "the real thing," and some midwives and obstetricians use the maxim of one hour of contractions coming five minutes apart as the standard for coming to the hospital.

The contractions of false labor tend to be irregular and do not increase significantly in intensity, duration, or frequency. True labor, on the other hand, tends to bring stronger and longer contractions which gradually become more frequent. False labor tends to be felt only in the front of the abdomen, whereas the contractions of true labor often start in the lower back and radiate to the abdomen. False labor may be alleviated with walking. True labor, on the contrary, may actually worsen with walking, or at least not seem to ease with walking.

Stages of Labor

Labor has three distinct stages. Stage 1 starts with the onset of contractions and ends with full dilation of the cervix to 10 cm. (4 in.). Stage 2 begins with complete dilation and ends with the birth of the baby. Stage 3 begins with the birth of the baby and ends with delivery of the placenta.

■ Stage 1

The first stage of labor is divided into two phases. The *latent* or *prodromal phase* begins with the onset of contractions. The initial contractions may be felt first in the lower back, eventually radiating to the lower abdomen, and may occur irregularly, gradually becoming more regular in the intervals between them. At first they may be as far apart as every twenty or twenty-five minutes, but they will gradually become more frequent. As the frequency increases, the intensity of the discomfort that is felt also increases, so that you may be unable to talk or walk through the contractions.

Initial contractions may last only about thirty seconds; however, as labor intensifies the contractions will be felt for a minute or so; between contractions the uterus relaxes completely. The latent phase is said to end when the cervix is dilated 4 to 5 cm. (1.6 to 2 in.); by this time contractions will probably be five minutes or less apart. Rupture of membranes, or breaking of the "bag of waters," is possible during the latent phase as contractions become more powerful. You may also experience passage of "bloody show," which is a small quantity of blood and/or mucus from the cervix. Bloody show may appear first, before labor starts, and is almost always a sign of impending labor.

In a woman who is having her first baby, the latent phase lasts, on average, 8.6 hours. For a woman who already has had one baby or more, the latent phase averages 5.3 hours. There are many variations in these numbers, but for a woman having her first baby, the latent phase should not last longer than 20 hours; for a woman who already has borne a child, it should not last longer than 14 hours.

The *active phase* begins with cervical dilation of 4 to 5 cm. (1.6 to 2 in.) and ends with full dilation to 10 cm. (4 in.). Some childbirth educators refer to the period just before full cervical dilation as the "transition" phase of labor.

During the active phase, contractions occur approximately every three to five minutes and last forty-five to sixty seconds or more. During the active phase, you may find yourself irritable and restless. You may be afraid of losing control and may feel hopeless from time to time. These feelings are normal and may be alleviated by the active support of the coach and labor nurses. It is quite common to vomit, hiccup, or belch during the active phase. Perspiration and feelings of rectal pressure are also common. If the membranes have not ruptured during the latent phase or have not been artificially ruptured (*amniotomy*) by the obstetrician to enhance labor, they may rupture during the active phase. An increased amount of "show" appears during the active phase.

In all, the first stage of labor usually lasts between four and eighteen hours in a woman having her first baby; if you already have had one or more babies, your first stage may last from half an hour to twelve hours.

■ Stage 2

Very strong sensations of rectal pressure, similar to the feeling you have before you are about to pass a bowel movement, usually signal the onset of the second stage of labor. An examination by the nurse, midwife, or obstetrician will confirm full cervical dilation. You are then instructed to "bear down" strongly or "push" with each contraction. Many women find the second stage an enormous relief, although contractions are just as intense as before, because they can now "do something" about the pain. Pushing can provide a sense of control regained and, perhaps for the first time, a feeling that labor is about to be over.

The baby's head descends into the birth canal with each push, finally emerging beyond the perineum to be delivered. Very quickly afterward the shoulders emerge, then the entire body. The baby's respiratory passages will be suctioned im-

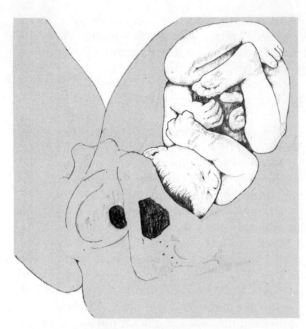

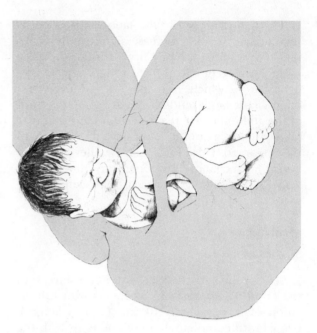

When the cervix is fully dilated, the baby's head passes transversely through the bony arch of the pelvis before turning to face downward. As the nape of the neck passes under the arch the head moves upward and backward (chin moves away from chest).

After the baby's head is born, it turns to the side without assistance (restitution). The upper shoulder dips under the arch, followed by the other shoulder, body and arms, pelvis and legs.

mediately, usually after the head is delivered and before the shoulders emerge. The umbilical cord is clamped and cut, and the baby usually begins to cry shortly afterward. His breathing may sound spluttery and irregular at first.

The second stage averages one hour for the first baby, fifteen minutes for the second and subsequent babies. Many midwives and obstetricians, however, will allow the second stage to go on as long as four hours, providing the baby is not compromised and the mother is able to continue the pushing effort.

■ *Episiotomy*

Occasionally, the obstetrician or midwife may make a small cut in the perineum as the baby's head is about to be delivered. This cut is called an *episiotomy* and is discussed in some detail later in the next chapter under *Special Issues in Labor and Delivery.*

■ *Stage 3*

The third and final stage of labor commences with the delivery of the baby and ends with the spontaneous delivery of the placenta, or afterbirth. The uterus continues to contract rather powerfully after the baby is delivered, and, usually within a few minutes after delivery of the baby, the placenta separates from the uterine wall and a gush of blood may come from the vagina. At the same time, the umbilical cord may lengthen. When these signs are observed, you may be asked to bear down as you did for delivery of your baby. The placenta then is delivered by gentle traction on the umbilical cord, or it falls out without effort. After the placenta is delivered, you may be given an injection of oxytocin either intravenously or intramuscularly to aid the uterus in contracting, thus preventing further blood loss.

9

CHILDBIRTH OPTIONS

M uch has changed since our mothers gave birth to us. Twentieth-century childbirth practices in America have gone from simple home birth to team-attended birth in the hospital delivery rooms. Today's mothers enjoy greater freedom of choice, yet there is often occasional extreme intervention on the part of the obstetrician. Although the general trend has been and continues to be toward more and more sophisticated monitoring and intervention throughout pregnancy, labor, and delivery, nevertheless, as a consequence of feminist politics, enhanced media emphasis on patients' rights, and other factors, women today are capable of exercising more control over their childbirth experiences than would have been available to them twenty or even fifteen years ago.

Many efforts have been made by women and health-care professionals to stress family-centered care of the pregnant woman and her support persons before, during, and after delivery. At the same time, malpractice lawsuits against obstetricians and other childbirth professionals have emphasized the need for strict monitoring of mother and baby during labor and delivery and have put pressure on the medical research community to come up with even more precise, and possibly more invasive, monitoring tools.

It is up to the pregnant woman and her family to learn as much as they can about their options in labor and delivery in order to make intelligent, informed choices. By carefully reviewing the available options; preparing for the childbirth experience, and knowing what to expect, the expectant family can maintain a sense of control over its experience and can avoid misunderstandings and unpleasant surprises.

Choice of Practitioner

■ Certified Nurse-Midwife

A certified nurse-midwife (C.N.M.) is a registered nurse with advanced training in obstetrics who is licensed by the state and recognized by the American College of Nurse-Midwives as qualified to provide health care to mothers and babies during pregnancy, labor, delivery, and the immediate postpartum period, as long as the pregnancy falls within the boundaries considered "normal."

A nurse-midwife's focus may be somewhat different from that of an obstetrician in that she has

463

been trained as a nurse, not as a physician. For that reason, and because she may see fewer patients and only healthy ones, she may have more time to spend with patients and may be more willing to talk about such larger issues as family planning, breast-feeding, fetal development, physical and physiological changes of pregnancy, discomforts of pregnancy and possible treatments, and so on. Because midwives see only normal, healthy patients for the most part, they can sometimes offer their patients fewer invasive measures during pregnancy and labor, such as intermittent rather than continuous monitoring and limited internal examinations, as well as alternative positions for delivery, which will be discussed in greater detail later in this section.

The fees a midwife charges for her services vary from state to state and from birthing center to hospital, but, in general, midwives charge somewhat less than obstetricians do, especially in major urban centers.

Midwives now are licensed to practice in all fifty states. If you are looking for a midwife but don't know how to find one, the American College of Nurse-Midwives has a current registry of midwifery services throughout the United States and can refer you to a qualified midwife in your area. The College's number is 202-347-5445. Most private insurers will now reimburse clients for midwifery services, and midwifery care is covered under Medicaid, but you should check with your private insurer before engaging the services of a midwife for your pregnancy.

The essential limitation of midwifery care is that a nurse-midwife is trained to manage only healthy pregnancies independently. In conjunction with an obstetrician, a midwife may co-manage pregnant patients who have underlying medical problems or problematic pregnancies, but if you are an obstetric risk for any reason, including age in some cases, you may be referred to a "high-risk" specialist obstetrician. Midwives are, however, trained to recognize any subtle changes during the course of a pregnancy that could signal potential problems, and they will immediately refer such a patient for an obstetric consultation.

Obviously, if your labor ends in a cesarean section for any reason, your midwife will not be able to perform the surgery, although she may remain with you throughout the operation. Depending on the hospital or birthing center, if extreme complications ensue during labor, delivery, or the postpartum period, you may have to be hurried to an obstetrician you have never met before, although your midwife may be able to accompany you.

■ Obstetrician

An obstetrician is a medical doctor who specializes in fertility, conception, contraception, gynecology, pregnancy, and childbirth. Obstetrician's fees for management of pregnancy and delivery vary from place to place, ranging as high as several thousand dollars in some cities. Insurance companies routinely reimburse policyholders for "fair and prevailing costs" of obstetric management, which may or may not cover all of your doctor's fees.

■ Family Practitioner

A family practitioner or family physician is an M.D. who specializes in family medicine—pediatrics and adult medicine. Sometimes family physicians also perform gynecological examinations and act as obstetricians.

Choice of Delivery Setting

■ Birthing Center

A birthing center is a place designed to facilitate the process of giving birth. It is not a hospital: It is not usually equipped with an operating room, for example, or with anesthesia equipment. It is not intended for high-risk deliveries, nor is it equipped to handle the special needs of pregnant patients who have medical or physical problems. Usually there are no "delivery rooms"; instead there are rooms that serve as both labor rooms and delivery rooms, with beds and sometimes chairs that can be adjusted to allow for safe, controlled delivery and, when necessary, repair of any trauma to the perineum.

Many women prefer the atmosphere of a birthing center because it has nothing of the sterile, clinical feeling of a hospital. The rooms usually are decorated to look like bedrooms, with curtains and comfortable furniture. Often the woman in labor is free to wander the halls and sometimes even walk outdoors. The emphasis in a birthing center usually is on as little intervention as possible, simply "letting nature take its course," doing little or nothing to induce, augment, or otherwise interfere with the course of labor.

The major drawback of a birthing center is that a woman who develops a medical problem during labor or whose unborn or newborn baby shows signs of compromise must be transported immediately to a hospital. Most if not all qualified birthing centers are affiliated with nearby hospitals and have a team of "back-up" obstetricians ready to handle problem births. Since women who qualify for birthing-center deliveries are essentially healthy women, the chances of having to be transported are low, but there is still the possibility.

To avoid such last-minute, traumatic transfers of patients and babies, birthing centers generally have strict criteria for the patients they will accept. Such factors as underlying health disorders (diabetes, cardiac problems, sickle-cell disease, hypertension, and glandular disorders, for example), previous problem pregnancies, and, in some cases, extremes of maternal age (very young or old) may cause a woman to be declined by a birthing center. Such a patient may still have a "birthing-center experience," however, if she chooses a hospital with flexible policies and an obstetrician or obstetrician-midwife team that is sympathetic to the patient's specific requests.

Most private insurers reimburse policyholders for qualified birthing-center maternity care, as does Medicaid. If you are not sure, always check with your insurance representative first.

■ *Hospital Labor and Delivery Unit*

A labor and delivery unit in a hospital generally is equipped to handle cesarean sections, some minor surgeries related to obstetrics, and anesthesia of all types. The degree of sophistication that a labor and delivery unit possesses, however, can vary from place to place, particularly in nonurban settings. Some hospitals, for example, are classified as high-risk referral centers for large metropolitan areas, so that patients with severe medical disorders during pregnancy and labor may be transferred there from smaller, less "high-tech" medical centers.

Many hospital labor floors have "birthing rooms" equipped with infant warmers, resuscitation equipment, and "birthing beds," so that both labor and delivery take place there. Others provide "delivery rooms" to which the laboring patient is moved (usually by stretcher) when it is time for the baby to be delivered. Depending on the hospital, a labor/delivery unit may look very much like a hospital, with bright lights, bare walls, and an antiseptic smell, or it may be much more home-like and comfortable.

The chief advantage of giving birth in a hospital, as opposed to a birthing center, is that in the event of an emergency all the necessary personnel and equipment to handle the problem are within reach. Many kinds of specialists in both obstetric and newborn care can be called upon to provide quality care at a moment's notice.

Giving birth in a hospital can have drawbacks, however, for a patient who is healthy and wants to control major aspects of her experience. Some hospitals have fairly restrictive policies about what the laboring patient can and cannot do in terms of moving about, having minimal monitoring equipment, eating and drinking during labor, use of intravenous (IV) solutions, and positions for delivery. In such a setting, a woman may be less comfortable than she would like to be and may be frustrated by her relative lack of choices.

Other hospitals are very flexible and will allow a laboring woman as much freedom as she requires. Much depends on the policies of the individual obstetrician or midwife, and a woman choosing a doctor or midwife to manage her pregnancy should find out what the attitude of the childbirth professional is toward such matters as alternative positions for labor and delivery, the use of IVs, continuous versus intermittent fetal monitoring, and so on.

Some of the more old-fashioned aspects of labor and delivery are still in existence at some hospitals, although their necessity is debatable. Some hospitals still routinely "prep and shave" the pubic area and perineum of laboring women when they are admitted; others routinely give an enema to the labor patient on admission. Many hospitals and obstetricians no longer believe in the necessity of the prep, the shave, and the enema and object to the discomfort it causes the patient. If you are concerned about this, you should check with your doctor or midwife, or ask your "tour guide" when you take a tour of the labor and delivery unit prior to giving birth.

In general, it is a good idea for you and your coach, husband, or support person to tour the labor floor before your due date arrives. Most hospitals and birthing centers routinely offer such tours at regularly scheduled dates, and this is an excellent opportunity to ask questions that might not occur to you otherwise. It also gives you an idea of what to expect when you enter the hospital or birthing center to have your baby.

Here are some important questions to ask:

• Are birthing beds available? If there are birthing rooms, are they very popular and will it be difficult to get into one? Are there special requirements for patients using birthing rooms, such as forgoing pain medications or anesthesia?

• Can laboring patients walk around or sit in a chair during labor instead of being confined to bed? Are some patients restricted from walking (for example, if membranes are ruptured)?

• Are IVs routinely inserted in all laboring patients? If so, can the IV be postponed until labor is active, and can an IV pole on wheels be provided so that the patient can walk with the IV in place?

• Can the baby be given to the mother immediately after it is delivered, provided that there are no problems with the baby? Can the baby stay with the mother in the recovery room rather than going to the nursery immediately?

• If a cesarean section is required, can the father or coach accompany the mother in the operating room? (Obviously, if the cesarean is of an urgent or emergency nature, or if general anesthesia is to be administered, there is no compelling reason for a support person to be present.) If not, can the baby be given to the coach/father as soon as possible?

• Are episiotomies (cutting of the perineum to ease the delivery of the baby's head) routinely performed? Are there ways to avoid episiotomy if the perineum appears to have adequate stretching capacity?

■ *Home Birth*

Home births are a controversial issue in America. In Great Britain, which enjoys a relatively low infant mortality rate, home births, especially for the second and subsequent babies, have been routine for many years, although the tide there may be turning in favor of hospital births. In many other industrialized nations, home deliveries are commonplace and America's love of hospital births is considered somewhat odd. Nevertheless, the prevailing attitude in the United States still seems to be against home birth for reasons of safety. Women who genuinely desire to deliver at home, and who have had uneventful pregnancies and, in some cases, a history of previous low-risk de-

liveries, often can succeed in giving birth at home if they are persistent. It may be difficult to find an obstetrician willing to perform a home delivery partly because of insurance problems. A midwife may be a more likely candidate to perform a home delivery, although insurance issues once again can be a sticking point. The American College of Nurse-Midwives may be able to provide referrals of midwives who do home deliveries, or you may be able to persuade your obstetrician either to deliver your baby at home or refer you to someone who will. In various parts of the country, such as California, home births are more usual and less difficult to arrange. Be sure to inquire of your insurance provider, however, about whether home birth is covered under your policy before you undertake the project.

Prepared Childbirth

Since the early decades of this century, it has been known that the pain of childbirth can be caused in part by ignorance, fear, and lack of preparation. A response to this has been the concept of "prepared childbirth," or "psychoprophylaxis." This idea, simply stated, holds that the woman who enters labor fearful and ignorant of what to expect may experience more difficult, and even more painful, childbirth than one who has been educated about the course of labor and whose knowledge gives her some measure of control. There are many sound physiological reasons why this is so, and many millions of women remain thankful to Grantly Dick-Read, Margaret Gamper, Elisabeth Bing, Ferdinand Lamaze, and other pioneers of prepared childbirth.

Almost all major hospitals and birthing centers now provide their own classes or can make referrals to private classes in prepared childbirth. The childbirth educator aims to teach expectant families what labor is, how it progresses, what the various stages will feel like (although this is difficult to do in advance!), and how to cope with the increasing discomfort of labor and delivery. The breathing and relaxation exercises and other points taught in such classes can promote better muscle tone, deeper relaxation, better understanding, more assertiveness, and less fear. Although no amount of preparation can truly afford the patient a precise idea of what to expect the first time around, it appears very clear that the more preparation, the easier, more joyful, and less problematic the childbirth experience is likely to be.

Support Persons in Labor

The labor "coach" may well be the most important figure in a woman's labor and delivery experience. Ideally, this is a close friend, relative, lover, or husband of the laboring woman who has attended childbirth preparation classes with her and is prepared for the experience. The coach's support may take the form of silent hand-holding, vigorous back rubs, foot massages, helping with position changes, and speaking encouraging words. The coach should learn and practice the breathing and relaxation exercises with the woman so that he or she can assist and remind her during labor. Coaches should pack their own "Lamaze bag" when they go into the hospital with the woman, including snacks, books, and other amenities, since the coach can and should expect to stay with the woman throughout the entire labor if possible.

Most hospitals allow a support person to remain with the woman throughout labor and delivery, and some are flexible with regard to numbers, allowing as many as two or three persons in the room. A busy labor and delivery unit, however, is not an appropriate place for a "party," and the laboring woman may find several companions distracting.

A sensitive coach should be constantly attuned to the needs of the woman, knowing when to be silent and supportive and when to be chatty and encouraging. The woman in labor may feel very anxious; she may scream, curse, threaten, and otherwise behave antisocially; this is quite common and should be understood and forgiven by the coach.

A truly prepared and supportive coach is a valuable asset to the obstetric team and to the patient. He or she may feel almost as drained and exhausted as the laboring patient toward the end of the experience, but the outcome—seeing a marvelous, unique creature come into being—is well worth the effort.

Alternative Positions for Labor

Contrary to popular notions put forth by movies and television, labor does not always—and should not always—take place with the woman flat on her back, a prisoner in a hospital bed. Walking during labor, especially in the early phases, is often more comfortable for the woman; it adds the force of gravity to the strength of contractions to help dilate the cervix, and has been shown to be effective in reducing some women's need for pain relief while causing no harm to mother or baby.

Many women find sitting in a chair at the bedside more comfortable than lying in bed, especially if they experience back pain during labor, and again the force of gravity is used to help dilate the cervix.

Many childbirth educators stress the importance of changing positions as much as possible during labor, even if you are confined to a bed for whatever reason. The classic "Lamaze" position, known in hospital terminology as "high Fowler's," has the patient sitting straight up in bed, with pillows behind her back and shoulders for support and pillows under her knees.

Some women seek out more unusual positions between contractions, such as on all fours or squatting, and these positions are fine, provided the woman is comfortable, the fetus shows no signs of distress (as evidenced by changes in the heart rate), and there are no medical contraindications. The patient's comfort and the baby's well-being are the most important considerations when choosing a position for laboring.

If "back labor" is a problem, some women find the side-lying, or "lateral Sims's" position more comfortable. This position makes a great deal of sense physiologically and may in fact be required at times during labor to increase the fetal heart rate. When a woman in labor or late pregnancy lies flat on her back, the baby's weight compresses the mother's vena cava and abdominal aorta, the two largest blood vessels descending from the heart. This compression reduces the amount of blood that flows from the mother to the placenta, thus restricting the amount of blood and oxygen the baby receives. Prolonged compression of these blood vessels can cause the fetal heart rate to drop suddenly or gradually. The first, simplest, and most obvious intervention for a decrease in fetal heart rate is to have the mother lie on her side, usually her left side because of the location of the great blood vessels. In addition to the enhanced blood flow to the fetus, the side-lying position takes weight off the mother's back muscles and allows for continuous massage of the lower back by the coach or nurse.

Alternative Positions for Delivery

■ *Lithotomy*

The classic position of the mother for delivery, and the one most commonly portrayed in books, on television, and in film, is *lithotomy*, with the woman on her back, with or without her head and shoulders slightly elevated, legs and feet spread apart and elevated with the support of "stirrups." This is the position women assume for gynecological exams as well. Lithotomy allows for maximum visualization of the pelvic organs and the position of the emerging baby's head. It also affords the childbirth professional maximum control over the emergence of the baby's head and the subsequent delivery of the shoulders, body, and afterbirth. If an episiotomy is necessary, the lithotomy position makes it easy to infiltrate the perineum quickly with local anesthesia, cut a perfect incision, and repair the episiotomy quickly, thoroughly, and comfortably afterward. For these and other reasons, lithotomy has become the position most preferred by the medical establishment for delivery.

It must be noted, however, that almost all of the advantages of lithotomy have to do with the convenience of the doctor or midwife, and less to do with comfort and control for the laboring woman. If you think that you might prefer another position for delivery, you should discuss this with your obstetrician or midwife in advance and explore all of the possibilities. A flexible and experienced practitioner should be able and willing to deliver a baby in an alternative position.

■ *Side-Lying*

For the reasons discussed earlier, you may find the side-lying position a comfortable one for delivery. This can be accomplished with a coach or assistant supporting the top leg and holding it comfortably away from your body. This is best done on a birthing bed or regular bed and would probably be uncomfortable or unfeasible on a delivery table.

■ *Birthing Chair, Chair or Toilet*

Some hospitals and birthing centers provide "birthing chairs" that can be manipulated to allow the baby to be delivered through an opening in the seat. You may find this especially suitable for the pushing stage of labor, since gravity can help bring the baby's head down and out of the birth canal. The birthing chair may require the practitioner to kneel, squat, or lie on the floor, and so it may not be very popular with the obstetrical staff. It may also provide for less control of the delivery because with the mother in this position the force of gravity brings the baby out more quickly.

A regular chair may be comfortable for laboring and for some pushing, but at the point when the baby's head emerges, it may be difficult for the midwife or doctor to control the delivery without someone lifting the mother up above the seat of the chair. Some birthing centers and hospitals allow patients to push while sitting on a toilet. This makes sense because many patients describe the feeling of having to push as being similar to the feeling of having to pass a bowel movement. Once the baby's head is visible below the perineum, however, it is advisable to get up off the toilet and squat or lie down, which may be difficult to do quickly if the toilet is more than a few feet from the bed.

■ *Supported Squatting/All Fours*

In the "supported squatting" position the woman squats with her knees bent, partially supporting herself with her thigh muscles and partly assisted by another person behind her back holding her under the arms. The woman may lean slightly against the body of the person behind her. This position is very popular at some birthing centers and may be especially useful for the woman who is having her first baby and is unfamiliar with the sensation of pushing or does not feel a strong urge to push. The squatting position requires strong thigh muscles, a strong back, and a strong support person! It may be used for several minutes at a time, with the woman resting on her side or sitting up between pushes.

A woman also may try pushing on all fours in the bed, holding the side rails of the bed for support. This is a variation on the squatting position that does not require a support person behind the woman. Delivery in such a position can be controlled fairly easily, but the woman's legs and back may tire out before the head is delivered.

■ *Underwater Birth*

Giving birth under water has been done to some

extent in Russia and has gained popularity in some parts of the United States, such as California, but it is still fairly unusual. While it does make sense in some respects, some people feel hesitant about the safety of letting a newborn emerge into water, and it would probably be difficult to find a hospital equipped to do underwater deliveries, never mind finding an obstetrician or midwife willing to "take a dip" in order to deliver a baby. The practice may catch on eventually, however.

Pain Relief During Labor

■ *When Is Pain Relief Necessary?*

The question of analgesia and anesthesia for labor and delivery is a controversial one and has as many right answers as there are different experiences of labor. A few women find uterine contractions unbearable and simply lose all control of themselves during labor, making even the simplest interventions difficult. Other women find themselves able to breathe deeply through the contractions as they were instructed to do in their childbirth classes and, though uncomfortable, never feel that the pain is beyond their control. Few women find labor painless, but different women have different pain thresholds, and different cultural backgrounds in some cases dictate a person's experience of and response to pain.

Any woman who expects or thinks she is entitled to a pain-free experience is not only being unrealistic, but she is also likely to sabotage her labor experience. Extreme responses to pain, such as muscular tension, hyperventilation, and terror, cause physiological changes that can slow down cervical dilation, reduce the amount of oxygen the baby receives, and actually make the experience of pain worse.

The decision to take pain medication to enhance relaxation or dull sensation is one the woman, her support person, and the doctor or midwife should make as a team, after discussing all the options, the advantages, and the disadvantages. Sometimes, in extreme cases your physician or midwife may overrule you and insist on persuading you to take some form of pain relief, or he or she may insist that you don't need anything just yet. Obviously, a relationship of trust between patient and childbirth professional is an asset in such cases.

■ *Analgesia*

Pain relief in milder forms is routinely available to labor patients in most hospitals and some birthing centers, providing there are no medical contraindications to taking such medications. *Narcotic analgesics*, such as meperidine, are the most commonly used, and although they do not completely remove pain, they are often valuable in helping the patient to relax and cope better with her contractions. According to *Williams Obstetrics*, the definitive medical textbook for obstetricians, such drugs, administered in appropriate doses once labor progress has been established, have no deleterious effect on labor and, providing the mother and fetus are closely observed following administration, pose little or no threat to mother and fetus. Some women experience little relief from narcotic analgesics in labor, however; the drugs' effectiveness depends on the woman's pain threshold, the amount of pain she is experiencing, and the phase of labor she is in.

Narcotic analgesics are usually given in one of two ways. The drug can be given intravenously so that it goes straight into the bloodstream. In this way, the drug gives rapid pain relief. It also is metabolized quickly by the liver, so that only a small amount of it crosses the placenta to reach the baby. Narcotics may also be given via the intramuscular route, into the buttock or thigh. This method takes longer to provide relief and allows the drug to stay in the system a little longer.

Occasionally, a patient may have a severe response to a narcotic analgesic, such as "flushing," loss of consciousness, or a skin reaction. These side effects are rare, and patients receiving narcotic analgesics should not be concerned if they feel a little dizzy or "high" for the first few minutes after administration. These drugs have the advantage of being relatively short-acting while still allowing greater relaxation; they do not wipe out sensation the way that anesthesia does, and their extreme effects, if experienced, can be reversed quickly with the narcotic antagonist naloxone.

■ *Anesthesia*

There are several types of anesthesia available for pain relief during various stages of labor.

Epidural or regional anesthesia: The epidural has become an extremely popular method of pain relief for the active phase of labor. In this method, a flexible plastic catheter is introduced between vertebrae in the lower back and into the space just outside the outer layer of membranes protecting the spinal cord. Medication (anesthesia) injected through the catheter blocks the conduction of nerve impulses from the extremities and abdomen to the central nervous system.

The epidural procedure may take more than a few minutes, often requires the patient to sit up on the side of the bed, and may be somewhat frightening to some patients. It is not appropriate for patients with chronic lower back pain, spinal structural abnormalities, back injury, or other medical conditions. The catheter is introduced through a large needle that is not felt by the patient because the area has been numbed with local anesthesia. The patient may perceive some sensations of pulling and tugging and may feel a brief sensation of electrical current in her back and legs when the catheter is passed.

The advantages of epidural anesthesia (when done correctly) are as follows: It completely blocks pain sensation in the abdominal area; it seldom produces untoward side effects; if administered while labor is active, it should not slow down the course of labor; the mother remains alert and aware of what is going on around her so that she is able to participate in the childbirth experience. Disadvantages include the fact that even with an experienced anesthesiologist, the epidural may fail or affect only one side of the body; occasionally there can be severe side effects, such as rapid and dramatic lowering of maternal blood pressure, which can in turn reduce the amount of oxygen the baby receives; the woman's sensation from about the navel down is completely removed, thus she no longer feels the urge to void (and must be intermittently catheterized if labor takes a long time) and may be unable to feel the urge to push when the second stage of labor arrives.

If the catheter is not placed correctly it may inject a major blood vessel. If this happens and a large amount of anesthesia is administered, the woman can have a severe toxic or systemic reaction, which can include mental disorientation, nausea, unconsciousness, skin rash, and changes in blood pressure and respiration. If the catheter is placed into the spinal column itself and anesthesia is administered, there is a possibility of severe headache after the catheter is removed. These possibilities are rare, however.

Spinal anesthesia or ''saddle block'': In this method of anesthesia, medication is injected directly into the spinal fluid. Spinal anesthesia is used most often for cesarean section, so that the woman can remain awake during the procedure,

but occasionally it is used for vaginal delivery if complete blockage of sensation is required. The procedure is similar to that for epidural anesthesia, except that the medication is injected directly into the spinal fluid, with no catheter remaining in the back. Spinal anesthesia blocks sensation so that the woman has to be instructed when to push. The most common serious side effect of spinal anesthesia is a rapid reduction in blood pressure, which can adversely affect the fetus. "Spinal headache," which occurs twenty-four hours or so after delivery and can last several days, is more common when larger needles are used: it is treated with bed rest and increased fluid intake.

Both epidural and spinal anesthesia are considered quite safe for the fetus, since little of the anesthetic drug crosses the placenta to the fetus.

Paracervical, pudendal, and local anesthesia: Other types of anesthesia are less commonly used but may be useful for specific phases of labor. The *paracervical block*, which involves the injection of anesthesia into nerve groups on either side of the cervix through the vagina, can be used after active labor is established (cervical dilation of 4 to 5 centimeters/1.6 to 2 inches). It can provide relief from the pain of cervical dilation without anesthetizing the vagina or perineum. It is not as popular as epidural anesthesia today, however, because it carries a greater risk of causing depression of the fetal heart rate and can create trauma in the cervical area.

Pudendal block, which involves numbing the nerves of the perineum through a needle inserted into the vagina, can provide relief from the pain of the last part of labor and the "pushing" stage, but it does not relieve the pain of contractions. It is especially useful if forceps delivery is needed or if episiotomy repair is to be very complicated and protracted. It may reduce the woman's urge to push, but it has little effect on the fetus if properly administered.

Local anesthesia commonly is administered at the time of delivery for both the cutting of an episiotomy and the repair of an episiotomy or lacerations of the perineum or rectum. It is simple, relatively free from complications, and can be done quickly and effectively. Unfortunately, however, large amounts of anesthesia must be used to achieve complete blockage of sensation. It is administered by injection with a small needle into the muscle, subcutaneous fat, and skin of the perineum.

General anesthesia: This is used most commonly

for cesarean section when there is a need for rapid delivery of the baby, or when deep relaxation of uterine muscles is needed (as for a premature delivery or a breech delivery). It is seldom used for vaginal delivery, and the "twilight sleep" experience of many of our mothers or grandmothers is, for the most part, a thing of the past. Babies born to women under general anesthesia can be compromised at first, if large amounts of anesthesia have been used for a long period of time. For the mother, too, general anesthesia remains the riskiest of all anesthesia options.

Special Issues in Labor and Delivery

■ *Episiotomy*

The surgical cutting of the perineum, in a sterile manner, prior to delivery of the baby's head is called *episiotomy*. It is done from the bottom of the vagina usually straight down toward the rectum and then to one side, with the object being to prevent tearing into the anus from too-rapid delivery of the head or delivery of a head too large to be accommodated by the stretching of the perineal tissue. It is done quickly, usually after adminstration of some local anesthesia with a hypodermic needle, but also may be done without anesthesia if the perineum is numb from the constant pressure of the baby's head.

Episiotomy is a controversial issue for many women and health professionals. It is not always necessary, and it takes an experienced and wise practitioner to judge when the perineum will stretch adequately and when it will not. Many obstetricians and some midwives routinely cut episiotomies simply to prevent the possibility of the perineum tearing, and indeed it is far better to have a clean, sterile cut that can be cleanly repaired than a jagged tear.

If you feel strongly about episiotomy, you should discuss it with your doctor or midwife before you go into the hospital to have your baby. You should try to be open-minded about it if your doctor or midwife is willing to be, because there are situations where the perineum simply will not stretch any further. This has to do with the woman's individual anatomy and the size of the baby's head; the need for a last-minute episiotomy does not mean that a natural childbirth experience has "failed."

There are measures that may help in avoiding an episiotomy. These include: "Kegel's exercises" (discussed earlier in this section under *Discomforts of Pregnancy*); perineal massage, which involves you and your partner stretching the skin of the perineum with the use of clean or gloved fingers at regular intervals throughout the latter part of pregnancy and during labor; pushing between contractions instead of with them (the diminished urge to push can result in more controlled pushing); and pushing with contractions in an extremely controlled fashion, using breathing-and-blowing techniques to control the force of the pushes.

■ *Cesarean Section*

Cesarean section, or abdominal delivery of a baby, is major surgery. It is not to be undertaken lightly—not to be done because the patient or physician is feeling impatient or to relieve or avoid the pain of labor. There are specific indications for cesarean section, and many definite risks, as with all major surgery.

The most common indications for cesarean are *cephalopelvic disproportion*, in which the baby's head is simply too large to pass through the maternal pelvis, or the maternal pelvis is too small to accommodate an average-size baby's head; *fetal distress*, where the fetal heart rate shows signs of compromise, suggesting that rapid delivery is the safest option (sometimes, also, the results of various tests performed on the fetus during labor can indicate distress); *arrested labor*, where for unknown reasons labor simply stops and complete cervical dilation cannot be achieved; *arrested second stage*, where the mother's pushing efforts do not achieve delivery of the baby's head; *fetal malpresentation* or *malposition*, such as breech position or transverse lie; and any maternal or fetal condition that would make vaginal delivery difficult or dangerous.

The incision of the skin for a cesarean delivery may be either up-and-down or transverse. The uterine incision is almost always transverse, along the lower segment of the organ. This is done so that subsequent deliveries can be vaginal if possible; because of the musculature of the uterus, a "low-flap" incision, once repaired, can withstand the contractions of labor at a later time without the danger of the old suture line rupturing. The so-called "classical" incision, which is an up-and-down cutting of the middle and upper segments of the uterus, is done only for a few very specific indications and involves the active part of the muscle. After one classical incision, all subsequent deliveries must also be by cesarean and must be scheduled before labor ensues, as vigorous uterine contractions could cause the old suture line to break open.

If you know in advance that you are going to require a cesarean delivery, or if it becomes necessary during labor but is not an emergency, there is no reason why your experience has to be a cold, frightening "surgical" one rather than a quiet, calm, patient-centered experience. If you opt for epidural or spinal anesthesia for your cesarean delivery, you can be fully awake and aware of your baby's birth, and the chances are that your husband or support person can be there with you for the birth.

The risks of cesarean delivery are, primarily, postoperative infection and bleeding, and, during and immediately after surgery, the possibility of anesthesia complications. These risks are minimized by the use of epidural or spinal anesthesia, but there will be cases where general anesthesia is necessary. Many physicians give antibiotics intravenously during cesarean delivery to avoid the possibility of infection, and the chances of postoperative hemorrhage are small. All major surgery, however, has the risk of major complications, and you should discuss these with your physician in advance if it appears that you may require a cesarean delivery.

Full recovery from abdominal surgery takes up to eight weeks. For the first twenty-four hours or so, you will probably experience fairly severe pain from your incision, which can be alleviated by the judicious administration of narcotic analgesics intramuscularly or intravenously. You will probably not be allowed to eat or drink anything for the first twenty-four hours, except perhaps small amounts of ice or water. A catheter will be placed into your bladder before surgery to prevent the bladder from becoming distended and will probably remain in place for the first twenty-four hours or so after surgery.

After the first twelve to twenty-four hours, you will be expected to get out of bed—slowly and with assistance—and sit in a chair and eventually walk around. It is very important in the first twenty-four hours to breathe deeply and cough and to change position frequently so that fluid will not collect in the bottom of your lungs due to shallow or "lazy" breathing. Also, by getting out of bed and moving around, you encourage your bowels to become active again and thus you will be able to resume taking solid food. Until

then, however, your intravenous solution will prevent dehydration; you will not "starve."

Usually, patients remain in the hospital for about five days to a week after cesarean delivery; by the time you go home you will still feel "creaky" and sore but you will be eating and moving well. You may be restricted to bed rest with minimal trips to the bathroom and minimal baby care during your first few weeks at home; if possible, a family member or hired baby nurse/housekeeper should arrange to live in or spend days with you during that time. You may be allowed only one stair-climbing exercise a day at first; if the baby's room is upstairs, you may want to move things to the first floor, or stay on the second floor as much as possible.

Vaginal birth after a cesarean is a very real possibility for most women. Unless the first cesarean delivery is done because of some maternal problem that is not likely to change, a woman who has had one cesarean delivery has a very good chance of having her second baby vaginally. This is something you should discuss with your doctor or midwife at your six-weeks' postpartum checkup or earlier if desired. In general, the more cesareans you have, the greater the likelihood of having another cesarean delivery because of the risk of rupturing the old incision.

■ *Forceps Delivery*

The application of sterile forceps, which look something like large spoons, to the head of the baby to assist with delivery is referred to as a *forceps delivery*. Indications for forceps delivery include any condition that threatens the life of the mother or the fetus. If, for example, the mother has a heart condition or severe preeclampsia that would make vigorous pushing difficult or dangerous, forceps delivery is the preferred mode of delivery. Sometimes the administration of epidural or spinal anesthesia makes vigorous pushing impossible, and forceps might be indicated in this instance. If, on the other hand, the baby's head is on the perineum and there is a sudden episode of fetal distress, forceps represent a quick and safe way to achieve rapid delivery.

There are risks to both mother and fetus in forceps delivery, but a skillled practitioner can minimize or obviate those risks. The possible serious complications include damage to the baby's facial nerves; trauma to the fetal head and face; trauma to the maternal perineum, vagina, and cervix; increased chance of postpartum hemorrhage; and increased chance of neonatal depression.

Ideally, forceps delivery should be accomplished with deep maternal anesthesia, preferably epidural or spinal. Slight bruising of the baby's face is common after forceps delivery and usually disappears within a few days.

■ Postpartum Care

For years the standard postpartum stay for mothers with normal vaginal deliveries was three days or more. Nowadays, it is sometimes possible to stay for a shorter period, providing all is well with mother and baby. The rationale for the longer stay was to ensure that there would be no postpartum hemorrhage or problem with uterine involution (the gradual shrinkage of the uterus back to the nonpregnant size), and to observe the newborn for any signs of neonatal compromise or distress. The advantages of staying for the full three days are, first, that the mother can sometimes get more rest in the hospital than she would at home (although the hospital is not always the most restful place to spend time!), and, second, that instruction to new mothers on bathing babies, general baby care, and breast-feeding is usually available from the postpartum nursing staff. If you think you might want to go home sooner than three days after you deliver, you should discuss this with your doctor or midwife ahead of time. (Many birthing centers send patients home within twenty-four hours of delivery, to be visited at home by a midwife on the second or third postpartum day.)

10 BREAST-FEEDING

Since 1970 the number of women in the United States who choose breast-feeding over bottle-feeding has increased dramatically. According to a 1980 survey conducted by the Federal Centers for Disease Control, 51 percent of white mothers were feeding their children exclusively by breast-feeding compared with just 19 percent in 1969. Among black mothers, 25 percent breast-fed their babies in 1980, up from 9 percent in 1969.

Most physicians applaud this trend. It is known that breast milk gives babies the most complete nutrition possible as well as extra immunity from childhood illnesses. The office of the Surgeon General has urged hospitals and employers to do more to promote breast-feeding in order to help the nation meet the Federal Government's goal of having 75 percent of newborns breast-fed by 1990.

Clearly, breast-feeding has advantages over bottle-feeding, but both methods have pros and cons. Whether to breast-feed or bottle-feed ultimately is the mother's choice and there are many factors to consider in making that decision.

Lactation—How It Works

The female breast consists of a small amount of glandular tissue and a much larger proportion of fat. The size of the breasts is determined largely by the amount of fat, while milk production depends on the glands. Since all women have about the same number of milk glands, breast size has no bearing on a woman's ability to produce ample milk. There may be fewer milk glands in large breasts than in smaller breasts.

Every woman experiences changes in her breasts during pregnancy. The breasts enlarge, the nipples and their surrounding areolas darken, and the woman sometimes feels tingling sensations. During pregnancy the increased levels of the hormones estrogen and progesterone stimulate breast-duct proliferation and prepare the glands to produce milk.

In the weeks prior to giving birth, a woman may notice a sticky discharge from her nipples. This is *colostrom*, which becomes the breast-fed baby's first food during the two to five days it takes for the mother's actual milk to begin flowing.

Colostrom has a high fat, high mineral, and moderate protein content; also, it contains high levels of antibodies that provide the baby with early immunity to diseases that the mother has had. Most important, colostrom gives the baby the fluid it needs in the first few days of life. The presence of colostrom encourages the baby to suck (although it doesn't take long for most babies to discover that sucking is pleasurable in and of itself).

Sucking actually encourages the production of breast milk through the "let-down" reflex. This reflex is initiated by the pituitary gland, which releases the hormone *oxytocin*. This hormone causes the muscle fibers surrounding the milk glands to contract, forcing milk into the ducts behind the nipple. Some women experience a sensation of milk rushing into the breasts; others do not. The let-down reflex can be triggered by emotional as well as physical stimulation. Sometimes just the sound of the baby's cry will stimulate the flow.

Most women experience some pain while breast-feeding in the days immediately following delivery. These "afterpains," which feel like menstrual cramps and can be mild or severe, are caused by the uterus returning to its normal size. Since oxytocin helps the uterus to contract in the days following delivery, breast-feeding prompts the uterus to return to normal more quickly, and the afterpains may be stronger for the breast-feeding woman. Afterpains also are likely to be stronger for a woman who has given birth previously.

Breast or Bottle?

Although breast milk is the "natural" food for babies, breast-feeding is not always easy at the beginning. In fact, most new mothers find it a process that has to be learned. No mother should feel pressured to breast-feed if she would be happier giving the bottle. On the other hand, women who have any inclination at all toward feeding their babies at the breast should be given as much encouragement and support as possible.

■ *Nutrition*

One of the compelling reasons for choosing to breast-feed is that breast milk is better for babies. Quite simply, human milk is the perfect food for human babies. Formula, usually made from cow's milk, is only second best.

Most bottle-fed babies thrive on formula but a few experience digestive problems. *Gastroenteritis,* or stomach upset, occurs more often in bottle-fed infants. To prevent gastroenteritis, bottles, nipples, and containers for formula must be scrupulously sterilized.

Bottle-fed babies can become fat if overfed, and a production of more fat cells in infancy may promote a tendency to obesity later in life. On the other hand, with formula it is easy to count the number of ounces a baby is taking. And although you cannot overfeed with breast milk alone, the only way to know if a breast-fed baby is getting enough nourishment is to see that the baby is gaining weight and growing.

■ *Cost and Convenience*

Breast-feeding is thought to be less costly than bottle-feeding simply because there are no bottles or formula to buy. The breast-feeding mother must maintain a diet rich in fluids, vitamins, and protein. Some women who choose to breast-feed may regain their prepregnancy figures more quickly because babies utilize a supply of calories.

An advantage of bottle-feeding is that it offers the baby nourishing food and suckling comfort, independent of the mother's state of health. Breast-feeding, in contrast, *is* affected by the mother's health. Illness, fatigue, anxiety, and even menstruation can reduce the supply of breast milk.

Mother's milk, sterile and of the perfect temperature, is ready to drink when baby is hungry. Formula requires some preparation, and the bottles must be refrigerated until feeding time. Usually parents or the caretaker prefer to warm the bottles even though the baby does not mind cold formula. Going out even for an afternoon with a bottle-fed baby requires carrying all the necessary paraphernalia. Night feedings for breast-fed infants are usually easier, especially if the infant sleeps near the mother.

■ *Working Mothers*

The father or another person can help in caring for a breast-fed infant but the burden of feeding falls upon the mother. If she works outside the home she may have to miss at least one feeding a day. Somehow, in the confines of the busy workplace, she may have to find time to pump her breasts and perhaps store the milk. It is easy to see how some women become overwhelmed with the task of trying to maintain breast-feeding while holding a job. Some employers are becoming more sensitive to the needs of working parents, but much more progress needs to be made.

■ *Privacy*

Most women enjoy the physical contact of breast-feeding but a few find the idea repugnant. Some are alarmed if they find that breast-feeding awakens sexual sensations. If a woman feels awkward about the physicality of nursing then she and the baby would probably fare better with the bottle. It is most important that the mother be happy with the feeding situation. Sometimes babies must be fed in public; this may be disconcerting for a shy and modest nursing mother. Although the breasts can be bared discreetly (there are even clothes designed specifically for nursing), some mothers may still feel uncomfortable. If the mother cannot relax, then her ability to breast-feed will be hampered. Bottle-feeding can be done anywhere, by anyone, without embarrassment.

Drugs and Breast-feeding

Breast-fed infants usually are not affected by specific foods that their mother consumes in moderation, but any drugs that the mother ingests may cross over in varying amounts to the breast milk. Some of the drugs that a nursing mother should be very cautious in using include the following:

• Oral contraceptives inhibit milk production and should be avoided.

• Over-the-counter medications should be treated like prescription drugs, and a physician should be consulted before any of these medicines are taken.

• Cigarettes are harmful to both mother and child, and recent studies on passive cigarette smoking indicate that children whose parents smoke are more susceptible to respiratory diseases than are the children of nonsmoking parents.

• Alcohol is believed by some physicians to be harmful even if consumption is moderate, and these doctors say that drinking should be avoided until the end of lactation. However, most doctors maintain that moderate drinking by the mother does the baby little harm and may even have an overall positive purpose if an occasional beer, glass of wine, or cocktail helps the nursing mother to relax.

• Marijuana contains an active ingredient that is fat-soluble and therefore appears in breast milk. The drug should be avoided by nursing mothers. (The situation for children born to heroin and cocaine addicts is very grim. These children are born addicted to the drugs, and it goes without saying that any women who abuses these substances should not breast-feed.)

Learning How to Breast-feed

Ninety-five percent of all new mothers are physically capable of breast-feeding if they desire to do so. As previously stated, breast size has no bearing on milk production, and many women have successfully nursed twins.

Even women who adopt a baby have been able to stimulate their breasts to produce enough milk, but this is a difficult process and takes hard work and absolute determination. Advice from a dedicated pediatrician or an organization such as the La Leche League is necessary in these special cases.

In Western society, where breast-feeding is a choice rather than a necessity, many first-time mothers learn how to breast-feed without the benefit of having observed an older generation of women do so. At first, breast-feeding may seem like a lot of trouble, but a little patience usually produces results that satisfy mother and baby.

If a new mother chooses to make a wholehearted try at breast-feeding, then she should keep in mind that she is learning a skill and not get discouraged. Especially at the outset, the baby should be encouraged to nurse as much as possible to stimulate milk production; avoid using a bottle as a substitute until milk production is well established.

The newborn should be put to the breast as soon as possible, even right after birth if both mother and baby are healthy and capable. At first, mother and baby will be practicing and getting to know one another, so the mother should not worry if the feeding situation is not immediately perfect. Breast-fed babies in particular tend to lose weight in the first few days of life; this is normal. Babies sometimes lose as much as half a pound but they usually gain it back in about five days. The new nursing mother should remember also that the newborn is receiving that valuable fluid, colostrom, in the days before her milk starts flowing.

Each baby reacts differently to the first feeding.

Some babies are eager to suck while others need gentle prodding. Sucking is an instinctive response. Most babies will turn toward the breast to nurse after a gentle stroke on the cheek. When the baby feels the nipple on her lips, she usually will grab on and suck.

In order for the baby to get any nourishment, the mother must be sure that the baby takes the entire nipple as well as the surrounding areola into the mouth so that colostrom or milk will be pumped out. If the baby must be taken off the breast, the mother should gently insert a finger between the nipple and the baby's lips to break the suction.

Breast-feeding can help to foster a close physical and emotional bond between mother and baby, but a baby also needs affection and closeness above and beyond the feeding contact. Forcing a sleepy baby to suck at the breast will be frustrating for both mother and infant. It is better for the mother to take her cue from the baby and let the baby suck when interested. A baby who is very upset and screaming should be calmed by holding, rocking, walking, talking, or any other method that works, before being offered the breast. If a baby seems distracted by outside noises or activity, the mother should try to get the baby to focus on her by maintaining eye contact and speaking softly.

■ Positions for Nursing

It is very important that the new mother begin nursing in a comfortable position. Many mothers prefer to sit up while nursing. This requires a chair that supports the back and allows both feet to rest on the floor. Some mothers feel that a rocking chair offers the best comfort. The mother should support the back of her baby's head in the crook of her arm while the baby's body lies across her lap. The baby's mouth should be brought up to the mother's breast, and pillows can be used so the mother can avoid having to bend over for the infant to reach the breast. The baby may enjoy having a hand free to explore the mother's breast.

Some mothers may prefer the "football" position, in which the baby's body lies nearly parallel to the breast, cradled between the mother's arm and rib cage. Other mothers may find it more comfortable to lie on their side while nursing, and this position is especially helpful for mothers who have had a cesarean section. The baby may lie parallel to the mother or "upside down" with feet toward her head. Mother and infant should be well supported by pillows.

During first feedings the breasts may be very full and block the baby's nostrils. Since babies can only breathe through their noses at first, it is important to ensure an adequate airway. This is done easily by gently depressing the breast above the areola so that the baby can breathe freely.

Many hospitals offer instruction in breast-feeding to new mothers, and nurses on the post-partum floor often assist with individual instruction. Childbirth educators sometimes include classes on breast-feeding in their childbirth preparation courses. Midwives and pediatricians also are helpful sources of advice.

■ When and How Often

Initially mothers should nurse their infants as often as possible to stimulate milk production. Early feeding should last long enough to allow the let-down reflex to function. One rule of thumb is to allow the baby five minutes on each breast during feedings on the first day. If the mother's nipples are not too sore, she can increase the feeding time to ten minutes for each breast at every feeding on the second day, gradually increasing to fifteen or twenty minutes as her nipples toughen. Most physicians recommend giving both breasts at a feeding, starting with the breast last used in the previous feeding. In this way each breast gets the maximum stimulation from the baby's eager initial sucking.

As the milk supply becomes established, babies may nurse for as long as thirty minutes at each breast. Since a baby will take most of the milk in the first five to eight minutes, much of this sucking gives the baby pleasure and comfort (though the breasts will always produce a little milk as long as they are stimulated). Newborns may nurse as often as every half hour. Most pediatricians advise feeding "on demand," whenever the baby seems hungry. But parents should be cautioned that crying does not always signal hunger.

It may be easier on the new mother to lengthen the time between feedings to two hours once her milk is established. When a woman becomes experienced with her baby, she should nurse as often and as long as she and the baby require it. As babies grow and can take in more nourishment at a feeding, the time between feedings will increase to three or four hours. Generally, night feedings will be given up sometime between the baby's second and sixth month.

New mothers should not be dismayed at the thin, bluish, and watery appearance of their milk.

Even though it does not look nourishing, breast milk is the "cream of the cream" for babies.

■ *The Baby's Responses*

The individuality of each child can be seen clearly in the early stages of breast-feeding. Certain babies are so eager to nurse and suck so forcefully that they are rough on the mother's breast. If a baby begins to gum or chew on the nipple, the mother should remove the baby from the breast for a few moments.

Babies who are very excitable quickly show frustration if they lose hold of the nipple. Some can become inconsolable. These babies need to be handled quietly and gently and be fed only when calm.

Sometimes babies can be reluctant to take the breast because they are sleepy, uninterested in feeding, or very slow-moving. A sponge dipped in cool water and dabbed on the forehead can gently remind a baby to nurse. Undressing the baby may produce alertness, but some babies are distressed at having their clothes removed. Any attempt to force the child to the breast usually will make the baby very angry.

Possible Problems

There are some inconvenient but temporary problems that may occur with breast-feeding. If these are dealt with quickly and properly, breast-feeding should become a blissful experience for mother and baby. Some women never have any difficulty, while others may experience some of the following complaints:

■ *Inverted Nipples*

The nipples are flat or sunken into the rest of the breast. A woman who intends to breast-feed should toughen her nipples by pulling on them and rolling them between thumb and forefinger. Her husband can help by stimulating the breasts orally during pregnancy. Breast shields, worn for the last three and four months of pregnancy, gently stretch the areola, gradually forcing the nipple through a hole at the center of the shield. The shields may be worn at the beginning of breast-feeding, but in any event they should be worn for no more than two hours at a time as they tend to collect moisture that may irritate the breasts.

The mother can help the baby to grab the areloa on a flatter breast by expressing a small amount of milk and then pulling and gently pinching the areola into an oblong shape that can be put into a hungry baby's mouth.

■ *Engorgement*

When mother's milk arrives suddenly, the breasts can swell and may feel very hard, hot, and painful. Even the areola can become so distended that the baby will not be able to grab on and suck enough to relieve the pressure. To remedy this, the breasts should be bathed in hot water and some milk should be expressed. Breast-feeding mothers should wear a well-fitted nursing bra, which will help to support very full breasts and reduce muscle strain.

If the baby doesn't nurse enough to keep the mother comfortable, cold washcloths or wrapped ice placed on the breasts often provide some relief.

■ *Sore Nipples*

If the nipples become sore, then the baby's time at the breast must be shortened—until the nipples toughen. The mother should not pull the sucking baby off the nipple but instead break the suction with a finger. It's helpful for the nursing mother to keep her nipples dry and exposed to the air as much as possible. If soreness does develop, treat it with one of the special creams or ointments formulated for nursing mothers. Some women find that exposing their breasts near the light of an ordinary bulb helps soothe sore breasts.

■ *Cracked nipples*

A sharp pain that begins and persists as the baby sucks is the sign that the nipple has a small crack. A physician may prescribe a cream, and the affected breast must be rested for a day or two. Milk should be expressed manually from the breast until the baby can suck again.

■ *Plugged Duct*

If a mother feels a small, hard, and painful lump in her breast, it may be a plugged duct; milk pools above the blockage in the duct and cannot flow out. The breast should be bathed in warm water repeatedly and then the baby should nurse. If the lump doesn't then disappear, an abscess could be forming.

■ Breast Abscess

If infection enters a neglected crack in the breast, an abscess may form. An abscess can be very painful and make an area of the breast hard and red. The abscess must be treated immediately by a physician. Usually if it is caught and treated with antibiotics in its early stages, the baby can continue to suckle.

■ Illness in Mother

Usually, by the time a mother shows the symptoms of an ordinary illness, the baby has already been exposed. In such a case, the baby can continue nursing. But if the mother contracts a serious infectious disease, then cessation of nursing might be advisable. The mother should consult a physician if she has any questions.

■ Biting the Nipple

Later on, when the baby begins teething, he or she may bite the breast toward the end of a feeding. This can be very painful for the mother and should not be tolerated. The mother should stop the biting by slipping her finger between the baby's gums and saying "No!" to the baby in a firm tone.

■ Leaking

As the newborn sucks one breast, the other may leak. The mother can wear pads in her bra to catch the flow; these should be changed when they become wet. Sometimes the flow of milk can be halted by firmly pressing the nipple.

■ Preference for One Breast

Occasionally a baby will show a definite preference for one breast over another. Some authorities say that the preference for the right or left breast indicates the dominance of the right or left cerebral hemisphere, while others insist that the preference is due to the position the baby adopted in the womb. It may simply be that the milk flows more readily from the preferred breast.

Whatever the reason, the mother may become lopsided if the baby nurses vigorously at one breast only. Sometimes changing the baby's feeding position and putting the baby to the "neglected" breast first may help. The mother may need to express milk from the less favored breast, but eventually the breast will adjust to the lesser demands.

Expressing Milk

This means simply that the mother herself forces milk from the breast. The mother massages her breast with downward strokes that reach the areola; this should be done all around the breast. The mother then runs her thumb firmly down the breast until it reaches the edge of the areola. As she presses in and up, milk will squirt out. The mother knows that she has finished when the milk comes out in droplets. If the milk is to be used by the baby, it should be expressed into a sterile container. Several models of manual breast pumps are available and electric breast pumps can be rented.

There are many reasons why a mother might express her milk. She may wish to breast-feed an infant from whom she is separated, say, a premature baby who is still hospitalized. The demands of a newborn may vary from one feeding to the next and any milk that is left in the breast should be expressed to promote adequate milk production. Some babies will choke if milk rushes out of the breasts too quickly; by expressing some milk at the beginning, the mother will ensure a comfortable flow for her baby. Mothers who return to the workplace may wish to have their own milk, instead of formula, given at the feedings they miss.

Success with Breast-feeding

One of the important factors influencing a woman to continue with breast-feeding is the support she receives from her closest companion, whether it be husband, lover, family member, or best friend. Many people are jealous of the special unity of mother and child in the breast-feeding situation. Furthermore, it is difficult for mothers to keep their self-confidence if they face a barrage of concerns about their ability to produce enough milk.

A husband may feel especially jealous of the baby's closeness to his wife's breasts, which to him may be objects of physical pleasure. Husbands should take heart in the findings of doctors Masters and Johnson, that nursing mothers are more eager to resume sexual relations after childbirth than are women who do not breast-feed. It is important that husband and wife communicate with each other about all aspects of the baby's care. The husband can help with feeding by burping the baby and by giving an occasional relief bottle or bottle of water.

A few women hesitate to breast-feed if they have other children, fearing that it will create too much jealousy. These mothers should realize that siblings will be jealous of a new baby no matter how that baby is fed. Breast-feeding may even give the mother a free hand to play with an older child. The mother should take some reassurance from the fact that she is giving her baby something special, even though it means she will need to spend more time with the older children.

■ *Ensuring the Milk Supply*

The nursing mother should get plenty of rest, avoid stress and tension as much as possible, eat a healthy diet, and drink plenty of fluids. Depending on the amount of milk a woman produces, she needs anywhere from 500 to 1,200 calories beyond a normal prepregnancy diet. The nursing mother needs a well-balanced diet rich in protein and dairy products and including grains, fruits, and vegetables. If the mother eats a poor diet she will not shortchange the baby, but she will deplete her own physical resources and therefore diminish her milk supply.

The mother must drink plenty of fluids or her body will become dehydrated and her milk production will decline. To avoid this she should drink at least three quarts of fluid a day, including one quart of milk (low-fat or skim if fat consumption is a problem). Most obstetricians continue to prescribe the multivitamin and mineral supplements given in pregnancy for the mother as long as she breast-feeds.

The nursing mother may find her breast milk diminishing as the demands of daily living encroach upon her. It is important that the mother remember to relax and take care of herself to ensure breast milk for her baby.

Breast-feeding as Contraceptive

In the United States breast-feeding is *not* a reliable form of contraception. In some societies—certain African tribes, for instance—where mothers carry their children constantly and nurse them frequently, breast-feeding does seem to offer a reliable form of contraception and family planning. The contraceptive effect appears to be linked to round-the-clock breast-feeding. In most modern societies, women who breast-feed work toward giving up night feedings as soon as possible and limiting the number of feedings a baby takes per day.

Some women never menstruate while they continue to nurse. For other women menstruation can be regular or irregular. Some babies seem to be cranky during their mother's menstruation. In a study of twenty-seven Scottish women who were lactating, menstruation resumed at an average of thirty-three weeks after delivery, but ovulation did not occur until thirty-six weeks postpartum. No women ovulated who were breast-feeding six or more times a day.

If a woman becomes pregnant while still breast-feeding, she may continue to nurse if she desires, but she should, of course, consult her obstetrician or midwife.

Weaning

In the strictest sense of the word, weaning begins when the baby is introduced to other foods in addition to breast milk, but, practically speaking, weaning means giving up the breast. Each mother must decide what is easiest for her, keeping in mind that breast-feeding—even if practiced for only a few weeks or months—has many benefits.

Many babies will be weaned to a bottle before six months or before solid foods are started. If a mother intends to follow this course, she should begin giving an occasional bottle before the baby is two months old, or it may become increasingly difficult to get the child to accept a new food source.

Some breast-fed babies can be weaned directly to a cup, but usually this means still offering one breast-feeding a day until the baby is a year old. It is very important to remember that although a baby younger than one year old can get adequate nourishment from solid foods and whatever formula he or she can drink from a cup, sucking is still a comfort that the infant badly needs.

Gradual weaning is best for mother and baby. The mother should give up one feeding at a time. Generally speaking, it is easiest to start with the feeding the baby is least interested in, usually the noontime feeding. Often the evening feeding will be the last to go. Mothers should be open-minded about how long weaning will take and should keep in mind that babies are hesitant to give up breast-feeding if they are feeling ill.

With gradual weaning, a mother's breasts will not usually feel uncomfortable. If they do feel too full the mother should nurse the baby for fifteen to thirty seconds on each breast to relieve the pressure. A word of caution: Nursing for as long as five minutes would stimulate the breasts too much. Some mothers will feel relieved about giving up breast-feeding. Others should be prepared to feel sad about the loss of this special bond between mother and child.

Some babies begin to show a lack of interest in breast-feeding as early as four or five months, when there is a developmental spurt. Others seem happy to nurse for as long as the breast is offered. There is currently a debate about how long a child should be nursed. Advocates of extended breast-feeding say that nursing into the child's second or third year fosters a stronger, more loving bond between the mother and her child, who benefits also from being allowed to grow up at a more leisurely pace.

Critics respond that mothers who nurse their children until the child is 2 or 3 years old have difficulty letting their children grow up. There is almost no clinical evidence on the effects on the child of long-term breast-feeding. However, mothers who intend to nurse their children for longer than eighteen months should be aware that it is difficult to wean a 2-year-old and that they will probably face criticism from others. The ultimate decision about how long to breast-feed, however, must be the mother's and her family's. The happiness of mother and child should be the deciding factor.

Bottle-feeding

Many babies are fed successfully on bottles of commercially prepared formula. One advantage of bottle-feeding is that others beside the mother can feed the baby. Bottles need some preparation, but parents can share in the responsibility of feeding so that the new mother can get more rest.

Obstetricians formerly prescribed drugs to suppress lactation in the mother but this is no longer considered necessary. Without stimulation from a suckling infant, lactation ceases. If breasts become uncomfortably full in the days following the baby's birth, ice packs may alleviate some of the tenderness; analgesics also may help. Mothers should wear a well-fitting bra and avoid any stimulation of her breasts, including direct spray from a shower. Heat, such as that from a sauna, steam bath, or bath, should be avoided. Lactation usually is suppressed between forty-eight and seventy-two hours after delivery.

■ *Formula*

Most formulas are cow's milk that has been modified to be more like human milk. These formulas are not the same as human milk but they are good for babies. Formula made from soy protein is available for babies who are found to be allergic to cow's milk. There are several brands of formula that come with or without iron. The baby's doctor will determine if formula with iron is needed. Many mothers choose a particular brand of formula because they are given free samples of it before leaving the hospital. If it seems to agree with the baby, then the mother should stick with the brand she originally tried. Formula comes in four different ways:

- Powdered formula is the most economical. It is light to carry and easy to store. But it must be accurately mixed with boiled water.
- Liquid concentrate needs measuring, mixing, and refrigeration after being made.
- Quart cans of ready-to-feed formula are heavy to carry but easy to use.
- Ready-mixed formula in presterilized bottles is easy to use but very expensive.

■ *Equipment and Sterilization*

Glass or plastic baby bottles are available as well as a variety of nipples for bottles. Some latex and silicon nipples are claimed to be orthodontically better for babies, more like a mother's nipple. What is most important about a nipple is that its opening should be large enough to satisfy the baby's sucking but not so large as to let the milk flow too quickly. The way to test a nipple is to turn a bottle upside down and be sure that the milk only drips out. Whatever type of nipple or bottle is used, what matters most is that everything connected with the preparation of formula be kept clean and sterile. There are plastic bottle liners that come on a roll and are presterilized. These can be placed in a bottle or holder and filled with formula. Even though the nipples must still be sterilized, these liners offer great convenience to some families.

For the first three to four months of a baby's life, bottle-feeding equipment must be sterilized because of the risk of gastroenteritis. When you prepare formula, remember that *handwashing* is important to reduce the number of germs that come into contact with the bottles and formula. In addition, everything used to make up the bottles—measuring cups, storage containers, spoons, nipples, nipple covers, and the bottles themselves—*must be sterilized.*

There are two methods of sterilization. *Terminal sterilization* involves filling the bottles with formula, putting the nipple in the bottle upside down with the cover on loosely, and boiling the bottles in a large pot or sterilizer in about 2 inches of water for twenty-five minutes. With the *aseptic method* of sterilization, all equipment is placed in a couple of inches of water and vigorously boiled for five minutes. Tongs and a pouring cup, both sterilized, should be used to bottle the formula. Powdered or liquid concentrate formula should be mixed with water that has been boiled for five minutes. One other method of preparing a bottle calls for putting the formula in a sterile jar, washing a bottle and nipple well, and putting the formula in the bottle right before it is given to a baby. This is less work but it means last-minute preparation, which could frustrate a very hungry baby. Whatever method you use, as soon as the bottles are completed they should be placed in the refrigerator. The baby doesn't care if the formula is warm or cold as long as it is about the same temperature at each feeding. Any formula that the baby doesn't drink at a feeding should be thrown away.

■ *Feeding*

Just as with breast-fed babies, bottle-fed babies should be fed on demand. A newborn's needs will come at irregular intervals, but as the baby grows older a pattern will be established. A baby should not be forced to take more than he wants from a bottle, because his needs will vary from feeding to feeding. Bottle-fed babies may want additional water separately, but their formula should be prepared exactly according to the manufacturer's directions.

Babies should be held close when feeding on the bottle. The nipple should be well back in the baby's mouth and the bottle should be tilted so that the nipple is always full of milk. Propping the bottle not only denies the baby closeness to her caretakers, but it also carries the risk of the baby choking and can cause ear infections (if milk runs into the Eustachian tubes). Bottle-fed babies need comfort as well as nourishment. They may need to be burped more often during a feeding than breast-fed babies, but it is best to watch the baby for any discomfort before arbitrarily burping in the middle of a feeding.

■ *Weaning*

If the baby is to be weaned to a cup sometime at the end of the first year, then she should be introduced to one at about 4 or 5 months of age. Babies should take their bottles sitting on someone's lap; even though bottles in bed may make going to sleep easier, this may cause tooth decay or choking and make a child fiercely attached to the bottle. Weaning a toddler is difficult, and many children will not give up their bottles until well into their third year. It is most important that the family take an accepting attitude to the older child who still wants a bottle. Eventually the child will outgrow the bottle.

11

NORMAL INFANT DEVELOPMENT

B abies change rapidly in their first year of life. Watching a baby grow from a tiny, squirming newborn to a busy little person can be an amazing experience. A baby's growth pattern during the first year can be an important indicator of the baby's health and well-being. However, since each infant is unique, the rate of development varies between individuals, and can be affected by the baby's gestational age at birth (amount of time spent *in utero*), by the baby's condition at birth, and by the birth experience itself. Although all parents like to compare their child's appearance and achievements with other children's, this is not considered a meaningful indicator of future size, strength, looks, or intelligence. Babies who are premature and small for their gestational age generally "catch up" quickly, usually by the first birthday or earlier. Any questions or doubts should always be referred to a qualified professional.

A baby's growth and development can be measured or gauged in terms of average standards that allow for individual variation. Four aspects used to evaluate normal growth and development are physical characteristics such as height and weight, motor ability (gross and fine coordination), language, and social skills.

■ *The First Month*

At birth a baby is small. Its average weight is 6 to 9 pounds (2.7 to 4 kilograms), its average length 18 to 21 inches (45 to 53 centimeters). Initially the baby may be quite funny-looking: the head is too big for the body and it may be misshapen, swollen, or bruised by a vaginal delivery (a baby delivered by cesarean section doesn't usually get pushed, pulled, or squeezed as much). There are two soft spots, or *fontanelles*, on the top of a baby's head: one diamond-shaped in the front, and a smaller, triangular one in the back. These close as the baby's skull bones grow together (at 6 to 18 months and 8 to 12 weeks, respectively). Reddish areas on the face, head, and neck are very common in fair-skinned infants at birth. These "stork bites," as they are called, generally fade in a few weeks. A baby's nose may look flattened, and there may be small white dots on the nose, cheeks, or forehead. The dots, called *milia*, also disappear within a few weeks.

A newborn's skin is loose, wrinkled, and pink,

483

and it may be mottled in places or bluish around the mouth, hands, or feet. A yellow tint to the skin can be caused by newborn, or "physiologic," jaundice. This occurs in about 50 percent of all babies on the second or third day and disappears in one to four weeks. At birth, a baby's body is covered by a white, cheesy substance called *vernix*. It is also not uncommon for a baby to have a soft, thin layer of hair on its body. This body hair, called *lanugo*, will fall out within a few weeks. The baby may have a lot of hair on her head, or she may be completely bald. The baby may lose her first head of hair in a few months, and the hair may grow back a completely different color. The eye and skin color also may change. Permanent eye color usually is established by age 6 to 12 months. The color of the tops of a baby's ears is frequently a good predictor of future skin color.

A newborn baby can breathe only through his nose, not its mouth, so it is important to keep the nostrils clear and clean. A baby's tear ducts usually do not function until age 1 to 3 months, so when a newborn cries, he probably won't shed any tears. The baby's belly usually protrudes due to its undeveloped abdominal muscles. The umbilical cord dries up and falls off in one to two weeks.

The practice of circumcision (the surgical removal of the foreskin from the glans penis, usually done before the baby goes home from the hospital) is no longer routine; indeed, it has become a controversial issue. It should be done only as a conscious and informed choice made by the parents. The American Academy of Pediatrics maintains that there are no valid medical reasons for circumcision. Possible complications of circumcision include hemorrhage, infection, loss of penile skin, injury or laceration to the glans penis or scrotum, urethral fistula, and strictures.

An infant generally maintains a flexed position, with her arms and legs bent and close to the body and her fists closed (not unlike the "fetal" position it occupied in the womb). A newborn will move her arms and legs vigorously, turn her head from side to side, and as she gets older will try to lift her head up. Though her hands are closed most of the time, she will grasp on to objects; in fact, babies seem to hold on instinctively to fingers. Babies also have a tendency to reach their hands toward their own mouth.

The normal temperature for infants is somewhat higher than that for older children, usually ranging between 99.4°F (37.4°C) and 99.7°F (37.6°C). The average heart rate in a newborn is 120, and newborns, on average, breathe about 35 times per minute. A newborn normally has several neurological reflexes that disappear as he grows and develops. "Rooting," in which the newborn turns his head instinctively toward the side on which his cheek is stroked, helps the baby prepare for nursing. As any breast-feeding mother knows, the sucking reflex is strong in babies almost as soon as they are born. Newborns also startle easily as part of a reflex response that involves jerking the legs and arms up violently.

Preferred positions for sleeping include prone (lying flat on the belly) with the head to one side, and side-lying, propped against the side of the crib or warmer. These positions help prevent aspiration of stomach contents (sucking them down the windpipe) if the baby spits up. Newborns sleep a great deal at first, but when awake they display varying degrees of alertness. Crying, the most extreme alert state, serves many purposes. It distracts the baby from unpleasant stimuli such as hunger or pain; it allows the baby to expend energy; and it almost always elicits a satisfying response from parents. Some infants cry more than others, and, provided hunger, pain, wet/dirty diapers, and illness are not present, parents should not be unduly distressed by their infant's crying from time to time.

A newborn's language skills are primitive but effective. Babies cry to show discomfort or displeasure. Most have different, distinct cries to signify pain, hunger, and distress, and they quickly develop "happy" sounds as well. While eating or looking at a familiar face, the infant may make small, throaty sounds of pleasure. During the first month, a baby sees between 8 and 10 inches in front of her and can fixate upon objects or parents' faces when she is 2 to 4 weeks old. Babies love to be touched, stroked, spoken to, and smiled at: A baby often will quiet down or smile in response to these stimuli. Indeed, early stimulation and socialization are an important part of a baby's healthy development.

■ *1 to 3 Months*

In the first few months of life physical growth is extremely rapid. On the average, babies gain 5 to 7 ounces (141 to 198 grams) a week and increase their length by 1 inch (2.5 centimeters) every month during the first six months. A baby's head also grows rapidly (as measured by an average increase in circumference of 0.6 inch/1.5 centimeters monthly for the first six months). This reflects the ongoing development of the brain and nervous system, which continues after birth. Neurological development is evidenced by improvements in visual acuity. Visual range extends to several feet and peripheral vision expands so the baby can follow objects in a range of 180 degrees. Hearing also becomes more specific as the baby learns to locate sounds by turning his head and looking in the same direction. Tear glands begin to function, the posterior fontanelle closes, and motor control increases.

Between the ages of 1 and 3 months a baby gains the strength and control to lift his head and uses his arms for support. At 3 months most babies can sit momentarily (when positioned) with their head steady or may begin to be able to roll over. They hold their hands open now most of the time, and enjoy sucking on their own fingers; they frequently clasp their hands together or clutch at blankets or clothing. At 3 months a baby may hold a rattle or toy but probably will not reach for it yet.

A baby's vocabulary increases as well; his cries become more differentiated and new sounds emerge. A baby will coo, squeal, or laugh at the sound of a familiar voice, as if he were trying to "talk back" to you. A baby begins to take more interest in his surroundings, starts to recognize faces and familiar objects (such as a bottle), and smiles spontaneously as well as responsively. At this age a baby is less apt to cry while he's awake and may begin to sleep through the night, with naps taken during the day.

■ 4 to 6 months

Growth continues at the same rapid rate until age 6 months, by which time birth weight is usually doubled. Thereafter, weight gain slows to 3 to 5 ounces (85 to 141 g.) per week and increases in height decline to about a half inch (1.27 cm.) per month. At 5 months old a baby is able to breathe through her mouth as well as her nose. Drooling generally begins around the fourth month, followed by teething, which starts at approximately 6 months. Signs of teething include increases in drooling and finger-sucking, and biting on toys or hard objects. A baby's gums can be sore and inflamed, so some babies may be irritable or have difficulty eating or sleeping. (A doctor should be consulted in the event of serious problems.) At about 6 months, the first teeth erupt. One or two central lower incisors are usually the first to break through. Six months is also usually the recom-

mended age at which to add new, solid food to the baby's diet. (Cereal and strained or pureed fruits and vegetables are introduced, one kind at a time.) Any questions concerning a baby's diet, eating habits, or weight gain should be discussed with a pediatrician, nutritionist, or pediatric nurse.

Baby will seem much steadier and her movements more purposeful as her coordination develops and her motor control increases. A baby can now sit erect (when propped up or in a chair) with her head steady and her back fairly straight. Sitting up in a baby seat, or propped with pillows, allows the baby a vertical perspective on the world, rather than the horizontal or sideways view she gets while lying down. When lying on her stomach, a baby can use her arms to raise her head and chest up to a 90-degree angle. When lying on her back, she often will put her feet to her mouth. Now she can roll over in almost any direction, front to back and vice versa. With assistance, baby can stand and bear most of her own weight. She enjoys more physical activity, and loves to be held or bounced on your lap.

At this age babies are becoming more alert, and they interact more with their environment. Toys and games are fun as the baby develops eye-hand coordination. Brightly colored toys such as balls, blocks, or mobiles can encourage a baby's ability to look for, reach out for, hold on to, and transfer objects from one hand to the other. Once a baby gets hold of a favorite thing, she will begin to resist attempts to pull it away.

Babies also grow more talkative. The use of both vowel and consonant sounds allows "baby-talk" to imitate real word sounds. Most of these word sounds consist of one syllable and may be the precursors of real words—"ma" or "da," for example. These little chatterboxes now start to acquire conversational skills; they answer when spoken to and seem to expect a response to their vocalization. Such "conversations" often are punctuated by baby's laughs, squeals, and shrieks.

The unique aspects of a baby's personality become more apparent as the baby grows. Some babies are very active and noisy; others are more calm and peaceful. Many babies don't speak much until they are a year or older, but they nevertheless make their needs and wishes known. Baby is becoming a more active participant in family life; she fusses to be picked up and to get attention, and she recognizes the difference between family members. She also prefers some special toys over others. She likes familiar people and surroundings and may even show some fear of strangers at this age.

■ *7 to 9 months*

Babies follow the same basic pattern of growth, but at an individualized pace. Some will be bigger than average; some may have no teeth or hair but be very verbal; others may be small and quiet but very active. Each baby is unique. Regular visits to a doctor or nurse-practitioner are important to monitor baby's growth and development. Early recognition of physical or developmental delays allows for early intervention and treatment, thereby increasing the chances of a better outcome.

Between 7 and 9 months of age, baby's lower teeth may have already poked through, and the upper teeth may be coming in. He will also be growing stronger and more active. Most babies start to sit up by themselves, maintaining the position without support for an increasingly long period of time. A baby may begin to crawl by wriggling on his stomach and pushing with his arms. (He may go backwards at first!) Some babies use the sides of the crib, or furniture, to pull themselves up on their feet and may even attempt to walk while holding on.

At about this age, babies get very busy with their hands; they like to make messes and they like to make noise. At mealtimes they may begin to try to feed themselves (using their fingers) and may like to bang a cup or utensil on the table. A baby of this age will reach out and grab at toys, food, or familiar faces. His little hands display more dexterity as he develops a *pincer grasp* (thumb against the fingers). With increased use, one hand usually begins to emerge as the dominant one, that is, the stronger one he reaches out with first. More babies are right-handed than are left-handed, but dominance of one side or the other has not been proved to be a valid indicator of future aptitude or ability.

A baby's powers of observation become sharper as he watches people's facial expressions and their mouths as they speak. Babies appear to be instinctively drawn to human faces. Making funny faces at your baby, calling him by name, speaking to him clearly and frequently, and repeating words will help him to learn by imitation. He may practice talking to himself and may like to play with his own reflection in a mirror. Speech development varies greatly from child to child, so although a baby may have a wide range of facial expressions and vocal sounds, he may not say anything resembling real words for several more months. Some babies will be using simple sounds like "baba" or "googoo" and may say "mama" or "dada," but not specifically in response to their parents. However, most babies will vocalize generally (laugh, cry, hoot, or babble) in response to familiar faces, toys, or activities. A baby should learn to react to simple commands, especially "no-no!" (This is an important word for him to learn early, but it should be used only when necessary.)

As a baby develops stronger bonds to his mother (or primary caretaker), he may cling to her and show fear and anxiety if he is separated from her. This is commonly called *separation anxiety.* A baby also may show dependence on or strong preference for a certain toy or blanket, deriving comfort from its presence and experiencing distress when separated from it. This display of separation anxiety is related to stranger-anxiety; the baby may act shy initially and fret or cry in the presence of unfamiliar people, especially if his mother leaves. Since this is a stressful experience for the baby, he needs to be comforted and reassured that his mother will return.

Just as he makes clear his preferences for people or toys, baby demonstrates his likes and dislikes for certain foods. He may clamp his mouth shut and refuse to eat something, or immediately spit it out if he doesn't like it. At this age also a careful observer might notice some regularity in a baby's bowel and bladder function, but it will be many months more before he is ready to begin toilet training.

By age 7 months, baby should enjoy playing quietly alone in his playpen. He should be provided with a variety of interesting things to play with and he probably will be fascinated by his own body parts. (This type of play is normal and you should encourage it by touching and naming parts of his body for him.) Babies enjoy interacting with their environment. Squeak toys or toys that move or come apart can be particularly exciting. Games like pat-a-cake or peek-a-boo and play with hand puppets, which encourage parent-child interaction, also can be stimulating for a baby at this age. A routine activity like bath time can be enhanced by floating toys.

As a baby becomes more mobile, more adept with his hands, and more curious about his environment, parental awareness and protection of his safety become more essential. Accident prevention is very important for infants and young children since they are at high risk for injury from poisoning, burns, falls, suffocation, and aspiration (inhalation of small objects or food pieces which lodge in the windpipe and cause the baby to choke). (See the section on **Wellness**, under *Safety First*, for ways to prevent accidents inside and outside the home.)

■ *10 to 12 Months*

In the first year of life a baby grows and changes considerably. Her birth weight triples and she increases her original length by 50 percent. At 12 months she resembles a small person more closely than she did as a tiny newborn. Although still a bit large for her body, her head appears to be in better proportion, with the head circumference almost equal to the chest circumference. She still has a "potbelly" and her legs look "bowed" and too short for her body. (As she grows and begins to bear weight while walking, these will straighten out.) Baby has six to eight *deciduous* (primary or baby) teeth, and the soft spot over her forehead (the anterior fontanelle) is almost closed (it will close completely by age 18 months).

Her control over her body has improved dramatically. She lies down now only to sleep or nap and, when awake, prefers a more upright position. She sits up easily, without difficulty or assistance, and she gets around well, crawling on her hands and knees with her belly off the ground. She may even try to crawl up or down stairs. (A child gate should be placed in front of staircases to prevent accidents.) She stands and walks while holding onto someone's hands or the furniture. At 12 months she may stand or even walk for a moment without assistance, and she can sit herself down without falling.

Baby's improved fine motor control and coordination are demonstrated by her more precise pincer grasp and use of her thumb. At mealtime she is able to pick up small pieces of food—a raisin or a crumb, for instance. Baby is able to feed herself with her fingers. By using both hands she can hold her bottle, and she may try to use a spoon or cup, even though she spills a lot. During playtime she is able to put things into a container and take them out again. In this way she begins to understand the concepts of size and space. She likes to drop or throw things deliberately to have them picked up. She may search for a fallen or hidden toy, showing a primitive understanding of *object permanence* (an object still exists even if out of sight). She can also grip a crayon and make marks on a piece of paper. Her little hands can turn pages in a book (usually many pages at a time) and she begins to notice and appreciate the pictures. Her index finger is used to point out or poke at things.

Comprehension of language precedes ability to speak. By 12 months a baby should understand the meaning of "no!" (A parent may begin to set limits on inappropriate behavior and to teach the child a few simple rules.) At this age a baby usually will respond if her name is called. She also may know how to wave "bye-bye." She may follow other simple commands such as "bring it to me" and may be able to hand you specific objects when named. Her vocabulary may include three or more words in addition to "mama" and dada," which she now uses appropriately to refer to her parents. She may recognize the names of other people, animals, and objects. The simple words that a child of this age uses generally refer to all the related things in a group, rather than to one thing in particular. For instance "daw" (or dog) may signify all animals.

Baby is becoming a very social creature. She loves to be the center of attention and will put on quite a show for an audience. She likes to be involved in daily routines, go on errands, and "help" with household chores. If she feels left out, baby usually will protest loudly, and she now reveals a more complex variety of emotions, including happiness, affection, sympathy, fear, anger, and jealousy. In seeking affection, she may climb up on laps or reach out her arms to be picked up and held. When asked, she may even give kisses or hugs. Baby may tire easily, since at this age she is very active and is learning all the time. When tired or frustrated she may throw a temper tantrum, and will need to rest and be comforted.

A child develops both cognitive and physical skills through play. Push-pull toys, wheeled walkers, swinging chairs, and jumping all encourage walking and the use of baby's legs. Rolling a ball back and forth with baby promotes interactive and cooperative play and the idea of taking turns. Clapping and games like pat-a-cake stimulate coordination. Toys that come apart, fit together, make sounds, or stack teach her object relations and cause-and-effect and improve manual dexterity. Stimulating the senses is another way to help a baby learn: she loves music (repetitive, rhythmic sounds), colors, and flashing lights, and the feel of different textures and temperatures also heightens her awareness of herself and her environment. Since they enjoy being touched and tickled, babies love exercises like "this little piggy" and "Simon says." Reading simple stories and nursery rhymes and looking at the illustrations with baby reinforces her language skills and can be a very pleasurable experience.

■ *The Second Year*

By the time he reaches the age of 2 years, baby has become a toddler. The last of his baby teeth are coming in (he usually has between sixteen and twenty—twenty make a full set). He has also grown a full head of hair (this is usually the time for his first haircut). He is three to four times bigger now than he was at birth, but his rate of growth slows down significantly from now until adolescence. Between the second and the ninth or tenth year, he will gain an average of 4 to 6 pounds (1.8 to 2.7 kg.) per year and grow at an average rate of only 3 inches (7.6 cm.) per year. The legs grow more, and faster, than the trunk, making the child's appearance better proportioned as he matures. He may still look bowlegged, and his potbelly is even more pronounced due to the lumbar curve (or swayback) in the small of his back, which develops as he learns to walk, but this will disappear as his muscles develop. A child grows in spurts, with sudden increases interspersed with periods of relatively little change. In general, mature, adult height can be predicted by doubling a child's height at the age of 2 years. By the end of his second year, a child's neurological system is almost mature, and his brain development is 75 percent complete. He has all his brain cells, but they are still growing. The areas governing speech, vision, cognition, and concentration still are developing.

By his second birthday, a child is quite surefooted. He can run as well as walk, go up and down stairs, and climb on the furniture (which he likes to do). He may still be a bit clumsy getting up, bending over, or sitting down, but he very seldom falls. His posture is still immature; he holds his elbows and knees slightly bent and he may lean forward and hunch his shoulders as he walks or runs. His balance is improving, and he can stand on one foot for a moment or jump in place. He is very ambitious and likes to test his physical abilities.

A 2-year-old uses his hands now better than ever before. At this age one hand clearly seems dominant over the other: He will be either left-or right-handed. His fine motor coordination has improved, so that now he can turn the pages of a book one at a time, pick up and put down tiny objects with ease, unwrap a candy, untie his shoes, or undo a button. He struggles to be more independent and is able to undress himself, wash and dry his hands, feed himself with a spoon, and drink from a cup. He may also put his toys away. His ability to open things (doorknobs, cabinets, faucets, and the tops of boxes or bottles) can get him into trouble. Since most 2-year-olds are totally oblivious to danger, all of his new powers, combined with his curiosity, can seriously threaten his safety.

Language skills improve dramatically between the ages of 2 and 3. A child's vocabulary can be anywhere from six to one thousand words, with the average being around fifty words. A toddler begins to formulate simple sentences by combining these words, two or three at a time. He uses basic grammar, which is often incorrect, although he may begin to use plurals. He knows his own name and calls himself by it, and he talks to himself almost continuously. He is very curious and wants to know the names of people and things around him. His fondness for imitation, repetition, and rhyming words persists, and he will enjoy singing songs and nursery rhymes and making all sorts of animal or machine noises ("Old MacDonald" and the "ABC" song are classic examples).

During the second year, a child begins to experience conflicts between his own needs for independence and self-gratification and his desire to please his parents and conform to their desires. His dependence upon and fear of separation from his mother interfere with his desire to explore his world and act independently. This may be evidenced by the toddler playing away from his mother, yet running back and clinging to her periodically. The tantrums a child throws now may be caused not only by fatigue or frustration, but also by his stubborn resistance to authority. He may try to assert his own will at mealtime, in refusing to eat certain foods, or at bed or nap time. Bedtime often represents separation from his mother as well as exclusion from adult activities.

The issue of toilet training also involves this basic conflict: A child's natural desire to let go and relieve himself at will versus the desire to hold back and go only when his parent permits. A child is usually physically and emotionally ready to begin this stressful task between the ages of 2 and

3 years. It takes patience; as with everything else, some children catch on sooner than others—girls usually sooner than boys. Bowel control usually precedes bladder control, but by age 2, most children are capable of holding their urine for up to two hours and usually can tell when they need to go. When reminded, a child at this age usually can stay dry all day, but nighttime control takes longer to achieve. A special potty seat can make the process easier for the child, or he may in fact enjoy flushing the toilet.

A child of this age has not yet learned to play with her peers—she's much too wrapped up in her own world and her relationship with her parents. She is still very demanding of her parents' attention, is quite possessive of her toys, and resents other children's intrusions.

A 2-year-old is characterized also by his activity and curiosity. He is fascinated by adult activities and is a great imitator (he may also like to wear Daddy's shoes). He likes active games like tag, and can throw or kick a ball, build towers with blocks, and draw lines, dots, or circles with a crayon.

12

COMMON CHILDHOOD AILMENTS

C hildren are at high risk for a variety of health problems, both acute and chronic. A child's age and stage of growth and development make him susceptible to several acute health problems: infectious and contagious diseases, allergic reactions, dental disease, accidents, and a range of behavioral problems.

Fortunately, many of these can be prevented or ameliorated by early establishment of good health practices. Most important among these are regular checkups, including proper immunizations (see schedules under "Immunizations"), good hygiene and nutrition, adequate rest, and exercise. A child also needs affection and emotional support, and appropriate peer interaction and play activities. All of these can be fostered through "anticipatory guidance" (planning for and being aware of the milestones of a child's development with regard to good health practices) by the child's parent or caretaker.

In addition, many chronic conditions first become apparent in childhood. Congenital anomalies (birth defects) that may require corrective surgery or special equipment, and chemical or metabolic disorders necessitating daily medications or special therapy can have significant long-term effects on a child's life and the lives of those around him.

ACUTE HEALTH PROBLEMS

Characteristically, children become very sick very suddenly and then often recover just as quickly. Common among their acute illnesses are respiratory problems, ear infections, gastroenteritis, fevers, urinary tract infections, and acute kidney disorder.

Upper Respiratory Tract Infections

The most common childhood illnesses are upper respiratory tract infections. Almost everyone is familiar with the congested sinuses, watery eyes, mucus-filled "runny nose," and fatigue that characterize upper respiratory tract infections. Recurrent colds are not unusual in children; preschoolers average six colds a year, decreasing to three per year as children reach their teens. Colds are caused by viruses, which are spread by airborne water droplets (sneezes), by shared objects (toys, cups, and the like), and by bodily contact. Children are particularly good transmitters because they like to touch, explore, and put things into their mouths. Colds and other viruses generally are spread at schools and day-care centers where there are many children coming into contact with each other.

Currently there is no cure for or means of preventing upper respiratory tract infections. The disorder must run its course. Treatment is symptomatic and includes rest, fluids, and acetaminophen (for fever or body aches). Nasal congestion or obstruction severe enough to interfere with eating or sleeping can be a problem, especially for small infants, who are nose-breathers. Cool-mist humidifiers in the room can moisten the air and help loosen secretions, making it easier for the child to breathe. Nasal aspirators (bulb syringes), which directly remove mucus from the outer nasal passages, also can help. Nasal sprays and oral decongestants can also be used for immediate short-term relief; however, extended use is not recommended and may cause dependency or worsening of symptoms when discontinued. Consult your pediatrician before giving any medications.

■ *Pharyngitis (Sore Throat)*

This infection commonly affects the oropharynx, the back of the mouth where it meets the throat. Although 80 to 90 percent of all cases are caused by viruses, they are often mistakenly referred to as "strep throat," a name that refers to the bacterial agent most frequently responsible for this type of throat infection: group A beta-hemolytic *Streptococcus.* (Streptococcal pharyngitis is known also as "tonsillitis.")

These infections, both viral and bacterial, are rare among children less than 1 year old, and most common between the ages of 4 and 7 years. In general, symptoms of viral infection develop more gradually and produce a shorter, less severe illness, with fewer complications than the bacterial infections, in which onset of symptoms is rapid and more severe, with longer duration of symptoms. The symptoms themselves are similar in both types of infection. They include: fever, malaise, sore throat, difficulty swallowing, and decreased appetite. On exam, the child's oropharynx will appear red and swollen (in a bacterial infection, small patches of whitish exudate may be visible at the back of the throat), and the lymph nodes on the sides of the neck may be enlarged and tender. Both bacterial and viral pharyngitis will be treated symptomatically, with rest, pain-killers (acetaminophen), humidified air, and plenty of fluids (to prevent dehydration and help nourish a child who may refuse to eat solid foods). An older child may find saltwater gargles soothing to the throat. Often, antibiotics

(usually penicillin) will be prescribed for at least ten days. Antibiotic therapy is indicated to relieve symptoms but also—and more important—to prevent more serious complications. Streptococcal infections can have severe repercussions, causing and spreading other illnesses such as otitis media, nephritis, rheumatic fever, and lower respiratory tract infections (all of which are discussed below).

■ *Epiglottitis*

The epiglottis is a small flap-like structure that covers the entrance to the larynx ("voice box") when a swallowing motion is made, thereby preventing aspiration of food or fluids into the airway. Epiglottitis is a rapid, progressive bacterial infection of this structure, causing inflammation and swelling that narrows the entrance to the airway; it can be a life-threatening emergency if the airway is completely occluded. Fortunately, it is rare. Respiratory difficulty resulting from this infection most commonly affects children aged 3 to 6 years. Symptoms include fever, difficulty swallowing, drooling, noisy and difficult breathing, and muffled or hoarse voice. Care must be taken during examination and treatment not to irritate the area further and possibly aggravate the child's condition. Immediate medical help should be sought, since hospitalization usually is required to protect the airway and the child's ability to breathe. A seven- to ten-day course of intravenous antibiotic therapy will be initiated to reduce the infection, and an endotracheal tube may be inserted temporarily (for one to three days) to keep the airway open. In some severe, emergency cases a tracheostomy may be performed (a small surgical incision is made in the throat, below the larynx, and tube is placed directly into the trachea to ensure air passage to and from the lungs). Possible complications of epiglottitis include pneumonia, pericarditis, meningitis, and arthritis.

Lower Respiratory Tract Infections

Lower respiratory tract infections involve the larynx ("voice box"), the bronchi (large airways), the bronchioles (small airways), and the alveoli (air sacs). The corresponding inflammations or diseases affecting these structures are known, respectively, as *laryngitis, bronchitis, bronchiolitis,* and *pneumonia.* Symptoms generally include coughing, wheezing, and breathing difficulty, possibly accompanied by fever. Breathing difficulty can be frightening for both the parent and the child. The parent must try to remain calm and reassure the child. If the child can cough or talk, he is also able to breathe and is probably getting enough air. A qualified health professional should be consulted, however, if the difficulty persists or if the child has a history of severe respiratory infections or a chronic heart or lung disease. Coughing is the body's way of expelling mucus and other unhealthy or irritating substances from the respiratory tract and is therefore a necessary and even a healthy response to infection. A very persistent or severe cough, however, can be debilitating as well as distressing and uncomfortable and can interfere with eating and sleeping. In these cases, or in the presence of fever or chest pain, a doctor should be consulted who can prescribe a cough suppressant or other medication if indicated. Home remedies like warm tea with honey and lemon, humidified air, and chest compresses or salves also can be effective.

■ Laryngitis (Laryngotracheobronchitis)

Inflammations of the larynx and the upper trachea ("windpipe") are known commonly as *croup.* Swelling associated with inflammation causes these structures to narrow, allowing less air to pass and making breathing more difficult. Inflammation is caused generally by irritation or infection. Viral infections are most frequently responsible; bacterial causes are less common. Before immunizations were available, and in countries still lacking adequate immunization programs, measles and diphtheria have been common causes.

The incidence of croup increases during the winter and early spring, and the disease usually begins, or worsens, at night. It is more prevalent and more severe in younger children (under three years) and in infants, whose respiratory passages are smaller and more easily compromised by swelling. The tendency to develop croup therefore diminishes as the child grows, although some children are recurrently afflicted with this syndrome as a consequence of upper respiratory tract infections. In approximately 15 percent of all cases, the children are found to have a family history of the disease.

Symptoms include hoarseness; a "barking"

cough; rapid, noisy, high-pitched breathing (called "stridor"); nasal flaring; and noticeable retractions of the neck and rib muscles.

As with all infections, treatment includes rest, which reduces demands on the body. A calm, comfortable environment that decreases anxiety and promotes rest and relaxation can ease difficult breathing. Plenty of fluids prevent dehydration, promote adequate nutrition in the event of diminished appetite, and soothe the irritated, inflamed throat. Humidified air is an important part of treatment. Many types of home vaporizers are available. Cool-mist vaporizers are as effective as those with hot steam, and they are safer: They won't cause burns if accidentally spilled or overturned. If no vaporizer is available, a parent can sit with the child in a closed bathroom with the hot water running. The steam produced can temporarily ease the child's breathing. A child's condition usually will improve in three to seven days. If there is no improvement, if breathing worsens, or if there is severe fever (greater than 103°F/39.4°C) or persistent fever (higher than 101°F/38.3°C for twenty-four hours or above normal for three days), a professional should be consulted.

Complications can involve the spread of infection to other areas, causing otitis media, bronchiolitis, and/or pneumonia (see respective entries below). With extreme swelling of the larynx, complete obstruction can occur. This is an emergency, since the child then can suffocate. Emergency treatment includes maintenance of an open airway by endotracheal intubation or tracheostomy (discussed above under "Epiglottitis").

■ Bronchitis

Caused by inflammation of the middle airways, bronchitis results from invasion by one of several viruses that attack the respiratory tract. As with most respiratory tract infections, bacterial invasion is not as common. Environmental factors such as air pollution and noxious chemicals may contribute to the cause. Inflammation of the bronchi alone (bronchitis), without other respiratory structures being affected, is very rare in children. Bronchial inflammation usually occurs in conjunction with either upper or lower respiratory tract disorders. A dry, "hacking" cough, wheezing, and possibly fever are the characteristic symptoms. Treatment includes fluids, rest, and humidified air.

■ *Bronchiolitis*

This inflammation causes narrowing of the small, lower airways. It results from viral infection, frequently follows upper respiratory tract infections, and occurs most often during the winter. It is common in young infants (90 percent of those affected are less than 1 year old). Although rare after age 2 years, bronchiolitis is the third leading cause of death in the 2- to 12-month age group. Incidence is greater among infants born prematurely. It may begin with cold symptoms (nasal congestion and discharge) and progress to coughing and breathing difficulty. Wheezing may be heard as trapped air tries to escape through the narrowed air passages; nasal flaring and sucking in of the flesh between the ribs also may be evident. As breathing becomes more rapid and labored, the infant may become restless and irritable, unable to sleep, and uninterested in food. (Small, frequent feedings may be better tolerated by the baby.) These more severe cases may require hospitalization for oxygen and transfusion. As with other respiratory infections, treatment is directed at relief of symptoms, therefore home treatment includes humidified air, lots of rest, and plenty of fluids. Antibiotics are not given unless the infection is clearly bacterial or is associated with another bacterial infection (otitis media or pneumonia, for instance). A new antiviral drug, ribavirin, can be given in an aerosol.

■ *Pneumonia (Bronchopneumonia)*

Acute inflammation of a section or sections of the lungs, in which the air sacs are clogged by fluids and cells, is common in early childhood and infancy. Neonatal pneumonias (affecting infants less than 1 month old) are caused predominantly by bacteria. Pneumonias in children 1 month to 5 years old are caused more often by viruses. Pneumonias can also result from fungus infections and inhalation of foreign bodies such as small pieces of food, fluid, vomit, coins, or gum (see below, under *Accidents and Emergencies*). Pneumonias can complicate other illnesses, especially upper respiratory tract infections, measles, or long-term diseases such as asthma or cystic fibrosis. It is not uncommon for a bacterial pneumonia to follow a virus infection.

Diagnosis is made by physical exam, X-ray study, blood analysis, and history or reports of symptoms. Symptoms vary depending on the causative agent and the amount of lung tissue affected. Onset of symptoms can be slow or sudden, usually manifested by fatigue, malaise, and mild or high fever. The cough may be slight or severe and initially may be nonproductive, progressing to a "loose" cough productive of whitish sputum. (Dark yellow or green sputum suggests bacterial infection.) Anxiety and rapid, noisy, or labored breathing or chest pain may also be present.

Treatment is dependent on the specific cause, but it generally includes basic relief of respiratory difficulties: fluids taken orally to loosen secretions (unless the child is too sick to drink), humidified air, a restful environment, and antibiotics if indicated. Most pneumonias can be treated at home, but in severe cases or with very young or debilitated children, hospitalization allows for close observation and monitoring of vital signs, fluid balance, and respiratory state, while also providing oxygen and intravenous therapy and a lifesaving staff and equipment in the event of an emergency.

Otitis Media (Middle-Ear Infection)

Manifested most often as a complication of upper respiratory tract infections, otitis media is a common disease of early childhood. This infection is caused most often by bacterial agents that spread from the upper respiratory tract via the Eustachian tube to the middle ear. The middle ear is a small, air-filled space located behind the tympanic membrane (eardrum) and connected to the nasopharynx (the upper part of the throat where it meets the nasal passages) by the Eustachian tube. Normally these tubes are closed and open only to allow for drainage from the ear into the throat, or to equalize the pressure between the middle ear and the outside air. If the entrance to the tube opens, germs can spread from the throat up to the middle ear, causing infection. In response to this infection, the ear becomes inflamed and fills with fluid and pus. As the fluid and infection in the ear increase, pressure causes pain by pushing on the eardrum.

This process predominantly affects infants and young children because the Eustachian tubes in children are shorter, wider, and straighter than in adults, making it easier for organisms to spread. Young children have large amounts of lymphoid tissue in the pharynx which may obstruct the opening of the Eustachian tube, preventing adequate drainage. Infants and young children also spend more time lying down; thus, greater upward pressure is exerted on the nasopharyngeal entrance to the tube, making it more likely to open inappropriately. When the child is in a horizontal position, normal drainage of secretions away from the ear is impeded due to the lessened force of gravity, with pressure and pain resulting.

As pain and pressure increase in the middle ear, the child becomes irritable and uncomfortable, holding or pulling at his ear, shaking his head, and crying or verbally complaining of pain. One or both ears may be affected. The child with acute infectious otitis may also have a high (104°F/40°C) fever; swollen glands, vomiting, and diarrhea are not uncommon. The child may refuse to eat, since sucking and chewing seem to aggravate the pain. If left untreated, in severe cases the tympanic membrane may rupture as a result of the increased pressure. The child then will experience an immediate relief from pain; the infected fluid may be evident in the outer ear, and the fever will gradually subside. The eardrum will heal, although scarring may occur that can impair hearing.

Medical treatment involves a ten- to fourteen-day course of antibiotics (usually penicillin), in conjunction with acetaminophen to reduce fever and pain. Hot compresses or a hot-water bottle over the ear may ease the pain temporarily. Patients should be reevaluated after antibiotic therapy to make sure the treatment is effective and uncomplicated by other infections. Some difficult or recurrent cases may require surgical drainage of the middle-ear space by placement of tiny tubes inserted through the tympanic membrane (myringotomy). The most common complication of acute infectious otitis media is hearing loss; rarely, mastoiditis (infection of the part of the mastoid bone that is adjacent to the ear) and meningitis (inflammation of the membranes of the spinal cord or brain) have been associated. Serous otitis media, also known as "glue ear," is a noninfectious condition in which uncontaminated mucus or serous fluid accumulates in the middle ear as a result of blocked Eustachian tubes. The condition may occur after antibiotic treatment of acute otitis media, or it may be associated with allergies. Although the condition may resolve spontaneously, if it persists or causes hearing loss, treatment will be necessary. Treatment focuses on reducing hearing loss by removing the blockage (sometimes by surgical excision of lymphoid tissue) or by facilitating drainage by the placement of myringotomy tubes.

Gastroenteritis

Occasional episodes of vomiting, diarrhea, abdominal pain, and irritability occur among children of all ages. The most frequent cause is gastroenteritis, an inflammatory disorder of the stomach and intestines. If severe or prolonged, these attacks of vomiting and diarrhea may produce dehydration, the loss of body fluids and electrolytes (important minerals that help maintain the body's chemical balance). This can be life-threatening, especially in a young child. The younger the child, the more dangerous dehydration is. Gastroenteritis is most common in children living in malnourished or debilitated hot climates (which promote the growth and abundance of infectious organisms), and poor living conditions (lack of sanitation, improper hygiene, and contaminated food or water). Infants who are not breast-fed tend to suffer more from diarrhea.

Acute vomiting, diarrhea, and abdominal pain may be caused by a variety of factors: emotional stress or fatigue, food poisoning, certain medicines (some antibiotics in particular), food allergies or intolerances, and bacterial, viral, or parasitic infections of the gastrointestinal tract. After bacterial infections, viral infections are the second leading cause of vomiting and diarrhea with consequent dehydration. Incidence of both bacterial and viral infections is higher from November to May and rarely occurs from June to October. Gastroenteric symptoms can also be caused by some parasites. In the United States, hookworms, flukes, and protozoan infections like amebiasis and giardiasis can produce abdominal pain and diarrhea.

Vomiting is one of the body's protective mechanisms, ridding the stomach of irritating substances. It can be caused by simple gastric distention from overfeeding or air in the stomach. It is also often one of the first symptoms in a number of common infections (ear, urinary tract, kidney, and upper respiratory tract). Vomiting is usually mild and temporary; however, if severe or prolonged, it may be more serious, causing discomfort as well as dehydration and electrolyte imbalances. A risk of any type of vomiting, especially in young children, is *choking*, or *aspiration* (see below, under *Accidents and Emergencies*).

Diarrhea is an increase in the number or liquidity of a child's stools. When assessing for diarrhea, individual variation of bowel functioning must be considered, but any change from normal should be evaluated for an increase in the number of stools, a noticeable increase in fluid content, or a tendency for stools to be bloody or greenish in color. This information can be helpful to the doctor or nurse practitioner.

Mild or *moderate gastroenteritis* usually resolves in a few hours to a few days. Simple home treatment consists of bed rest, close observation for signs of dehydration (see Table 1, page 497), and replacing solid foods with a clear liquid diet (see Table 2, page 497) until the child's condition improves. Some authorities recommend that milk and other dairy products be decreased during the illness (and for one week after it resolves), since the irritation of the intestine may cause temporary milk intolerance and exacerbation of the diarrhea.

Severe gastroenteritis, which involves prolonged vomiting, bloody stools, and signs of dehydration, with the inability to take fluids by mouth, requires immediate intervention and, most likely, hospitalization. In-hospital treatment of severe gastroenteritis centers around immediate intravenous fluid replacement to restore circulating volume and correct electrolyte imbalances. A hospitalized infant or child with severe gastroenteritis should be isolated from other patients (to prevent possible transmission of the disease). The child will be closely monitored and initially will receive nothing by mouth in order to rest the gastrointestinal tract. Examinations and various tests will be needed to discover the cause of the disease.

Chronic or *recurrent gastroenteritis* requires medical evaluation and treatment. Causes of chronic vomiting or diarrhea can include inherited bowel disorders or congenital obstruction of the digestive tract.

Fevers

A fever is a body temperature above normal (98.6° Fahrenheit/37° Centigrade) and is often the first sign of infection. Fevers can occur from simple overheating, as a reaction to immunizations, milk allergy, or thyroiditis, or as a result of strenuous physical activity. Although the normal body temperature is set at 98.6°, fluctuation is normal, both between different children and in the same child at different times of the day. It is usually slightly lower in the morning and slightly higher in the afternoon, and it lowers again in the evening. The method of taking a child's temperature also will produce varying results. Normal, for temperature under the armpits, is 97.6° (36.4°C), slightly lower than the normal oral temperature of 98.6° (37°C), which in turn is lower than the normal rectal temperature of 99.6° (37.5°C). The rectal temperature is considered more accurate and safer to take than the oral temperature: A very young or very sick child may be unable to keep his mouth closed long enough, and there is greater danger of a thermometer breaking in a child's mouth.

Very high fevers are not unusual in children; however, if accompanied by delirium, unresponsiveness, trembling, or convulsions, or if the child looks very ill, a doctor should be consulted immediately. In general, medical help should be sought if a child has an elevated temperature for more than three days, or a fever greater than 101° (38.3°C) for more than twenty-four hours, or a fever greater than 103° (39.5°C) after taking antipyretics (fever-reducing agents such as acetaminophen). Severe fevers require quick intervention to reduce the child's temperature. The child should be cooled by removing warm clothing or blankets, giving plenty of fluids to prevent dehydration, keeping the room cool (ideally air-conditioned), and bathing in cool water.

Most fevers will resolve and the child will be back to normal in a few days: the source of the fever should be considered, however, since fever is an important indicator of many illnesses that may require treatment.

Perhaps the most frightening event associated with fevers is a *febrile convulsion* or *seizure*. These are among the most common pediatric neurologic disorders, affecting 3 to 5 percent of all children. Occurring most frequently in children between 6 months and 3 years of age, the highest incidence is found in children less than 8 months old. Boys are twice as likely as girls to be affected. The exact cause of these seizures is uncertain. Treatment consists of quickly lowering the child's temperature and preventing very high fevers in the future by close attention to even slight fevers. Although seizures usually pass quickly and may not recur or have lasting effects, it is important for the child to be fully evaluated to rule out serious infections of the nervous system (meningitis or encephalitis, for example) or a neurologic disorder such as epilepsy. (See discussion of Seizure Disorders below, under *Chronic Health Problems.*) Repeated febrile convulsions can lead to epilepsy.

Unusually high fevers have been associated also with a recently identified encephalopathy (brain disorder) known as *Reye's syndrome*. It affects children from 2 months old to adolescence, with the highest incidence between 6 and 11 years. This condition is believed to be a sequel of viral infections (most often the respiratory type); the child may seem to recover, but then he suddenly develops a high fever with vomiting and may appear lethargic or delirious. A relationship between this syndrome and large doses of aspirin has been suggested but not proved. Aspirin manufacturers are required by law to carry the following warning on packages: "Children and teenagers should not use this medication for chicken pox or flu symptoms before a doctor is consulted about Reye's syndrome, a rare but serious illness. Keep this and all drugs out of the reach of children. In case of accidental overdose, seek professional assistance or contact a poison control center immediately. As with any drug, if you are pregnant or nursing a baby, seek the advice of a health professional before using this product."

Urinary Tract Infections/Acute Kidney Dysfunction

Infections of the urinary tract are an extremely common and significant childhood health problem. All ages are affected, with the peak incidence between 2 to 6 years. Females are ten to thirty times more likely to develop these infections. A simple urinary tract infection (UTI) is characterized by bacteria in the urine; normal urine is uncontaminated, or sterile, before it leaves the body. Bacterial infections (most commonly caused by *Escherichia coli* organisms) travel up the urethra, causing inflammation. A child may or may not be symptomatic. Symptoms of infection in the lower urinary tract include frequency and urgency of urination, straining or burning on urination, an abnormal stream, and cloudy or foul-smelling urine. In more severe infections abdominal pain may be present and vomiting may occur.

Many factors have been associated with urinary tract infections. The female anatomy, with a shorter urethra and the urethral opening closer to the anus (a site that favors bacteria), accounts for the higher incidence among girls. Poor hygiene such as unchanged diapers and infrequent washing allows for the accumulation of bacteria at the urethral entrance. "Holding" the urine without voiding for long periods of time allows any bacteria in the urine more time to grow, spread, and cause inflammation. Chronic constipation can block the urine from emptying out of the bladder. Vaginitis, pinworm, diaper rash, or any infection in the area can spread to the inner urinary tract structures.

Although urinary tract infections are troublesome—they can make a child very uncomfortable, are likely to recur, and can lead to serious kidney problems—prevention and treatment are relatively simple. To prevent the contamination of the urethra, little girls should be taught to wipe themselves *from front to back*. Good hygiene should be encouraged in small children, with frequent diaper checks for babies. Although regular washing is important, tub baths (especially with oils) are to be avoided since the water can carry bacteria into the lower urinary tract. Clothes and diapers should not be tight or constricting. Drinking lots of fluids helps to flush out the whole urinary tract. Juices such as unsweetened cranberry or apple juice help to acidify the urine, which discourages bacterial growth. Prevention is, of course, the best treatment; however, antibiotic therapy is often important to eliminate the infection.

Bacterial infections that invade the lower urinary tract (the urethra and bladder) can spread to the upper urinary tract, the ureters (which connect the bladder to the kidneys) and the kidneys themselves—causing *pyelonephritis* (acute inflammation of the kidneys). This acute, upper UTI is characterized by more severe symptoms (fever, chills, vomiting, flank pain, and tenderness over the kidneys) as well as by lower UTI symptoms. Chronic or recurrent inflammation can cause scarring and permanent damage. Treatment involves antibiotics, fluids, bed rest, antipyretics, and comfort measures. Hospitalization may be necessary.

Acute glomerular nephritis (or *glomerulonephritis*) is one of the more common kidney disorders of childhood. It is a noninfectious, inflammatory process that attacks the kidneys as a reaction to certain strains of streptococcal infection. It develops ten to fourteen days after some, but not all, streptococcal infections. This disease affects children between the ages of 2 and 12 years. Peak occurrence is at 6 years, and it is rare in children younger than 2. Boys are affected twice as often as girls.

Initial signs of glomerular nephritis include swelling of the eyes and face and the passage of small amounts of dark-colored urine. The child's abdomen also may be swollen and tender and vomiting may occur. The child may be pale, irritable, lethargic, may refuse to eat and complain of headache. Complaints of headache may reflect an increase in blood pressure, which is a common finding.

There is no real treatment for acute nephritis. Usually the child recovers completely in one to three weeks. Bed rest and a low-salt diet are encouraged. Medical evaluation is important to guard against possible complications. These are rare but include encephalopathy (due to increased blood pressure) and acute kidney failure.

SIGNS AND SYMPTOMS OF DEHYDRATION

PHYSICAL

SKIN:
  dry and parched
  pale or mottled
MUCOUS MEMBRANES:
  dry and pale
SUNKEN FONTANELLES (in infants)
SUNKEN EYES
BODY FLUIDS:
  decreased tears
  decreased saliva
  decreased urine output
LOSS OF BODY WEIGHT
RAPID PULSE AND RESPIRATION

BEHAVIORAL

EXTREME LISTLESSNESS

Table 1

SUGGESTED DIET FOR GASTROENTERITIS

FIRST 24 HOURS

water
uncarbonated cola or ginger ale
tea
Jell-O
apple juice
Gatorade

DAY 2 (after diarrhea/vomiting stops)

crackers
rice, rice cereals
mashed potatoes
applesauce
bananas

DAY 3

regular diet with limited milk and other dairy products

Table 2

Dental Problems

Tooth decay, in the form of cavities (*caries*), is a prevalent and serious ailment that affects almost all children of all age groups. The ages between 4 and 8 and again between 12 and 18 years are perhaps the most vulnerable times, when new teeth are forming.

Good dental care should begin with the first tooth. By age 3, when all the "baby teeth" are in, the child should be having regular dental checkups. Parents should help with and encourage plaque removal by regular brushing and flossing. Fluoride protection can assist in the prevention of tooth decay. Whether or not there is fluoride in your water supply, you can boost protection by using a commercial fluoride mouthwash or toothpaste, or both. It is also important to avoid excessive consumption of cariogenic foods—foods that contribute to cavity formation, like candy and soda.

Malocclusion (crooked, crowded, and uneven teeth) and dental trauma also are serious threats to the health of a child's teeth. Orthodontic treatment (braces) to correct malocclusion problems is most effective when started between ages 10 and 13, after the second or permanent set of teeth comes in. During the active and sometimes reckless years of childhood, dental damage and injuries are not uncommon; boys, as a group, generally sustain more injuries than girls. If a tooth gets broken or knocked loose, it should be preserved in a saline (saltwater) solution and be taken with the child immediately to the dentist for reimplantation.

Allergies and Food Intolerances

It is likely that nearly one in 5 Americans suffers from some type of allergy. Allergies affect various parts of the body, most frequently the skin and the respiratory and gastrointestinal systems. Allergies have a strong genetic component: They tend to run in families. An individual's age and environment also affect the development of certain allergies.

Allergies are a hypersensitivity, or adverse reaction, to specific substances (usually protein), which then trigger the allergic response (a rash, sneezing and wheezing, or diarrhea, for example). These allergy-causing substances enter the body as the child eats, breathes, touches, or otherwise comes into contact with dust, pets, plant pollen, soaps, food additives, medications, and the like.

Food allergy is the most common type during the first year, as the child is exposed to new foods. Children tend to become less allergic to foods as they grow older, however. Cow's milk, eggwhite, and wheat are some of the most allergy-inducing foods for infants. These should be avoided or substituted for (with soy milk, for example), although by 2 years of age most milk-sensitive children can tolerate it in increasing amounts. Skin problems such as infantile eczema and atopic dermatitis can be precipitated by milk or eggs. Whereas most younger children manifest allergic reactions as gastrointestinal upsets, older children tend to react with respiratory (asthmatic) symptoms. Although asthma often has no allergic components, it may be associated with allergic rhinitis (hay fever), allergic conjunctivitis (red, watery, or swollen eyes), and atopic dermatitis. (See discussion of Asthma below, under *Chronic Health Problems*.)

Diagnosis of allergy usually is based on the history of precipitating factors, physical exam, and skin testing. Treatment consists of removing (or limiting) the offending agent, following a special diet, and eliminating dust, mold, pollen, and pets from the environment. A physician or allergy specialist can prescribe oral antihistamine medication, nasal decongestants, or steroid creams for relief of symptoms. Comfort measures, good hygiene, and rest also are important to prevent infectious complications.

Some food intolerances can be confused with food allergies; however, food intolerances like phenylketonuria (PKU), galactosemia, and lactose intolerance are more severe, chronic conditions caused by genetic metabolic defects in which certain essential enzymes are missing. Most state laws require testing for *phenylketonuria* at birth. This disease can be treated by careful diet control, but if undiagnosed and untreated, PKU can cause central nervous system damage and retardation. *Galactosemia* can cause severe liver damage, cataracts, and mental retardation due to the body's inability to process galactose, which comes from milk. Treatment is a diet that excludes milk or products containing galactose and lactose. *Lactose intolerance* is less severe, involving a decreased ability to digest milk lactose; symptoms include severe diarrhea and possible dehydration. Lactose intolerance is a rare but lifelong condition, most commonly affecting Asians, blacks, and American Indians.

Accidents and Emergencies

Accidents are the number 1 cause of death in all children between the ages of 1 and 14 years. Early childhood is a time of increased activity, curiosity, and mobility, and these traits, combined with a child's unawareness of danger, make accidents particularly common. Death and disability from injury are unfortunately very real threats to a child's health. Motor vehicle accidents are the most frequent cause of accidental injury; other injuries include falls, drowning, burns, cuts, poisoning, choking, and electric shock. Accidents are more frequent in summer than in winter, and statistically they affect more boys than girls. Most accidents occur in and around the home. Parents need to be aware of the safety threats in a child's environment and "childproof" their home as much as possible.

Auto accidents are a constant threat to drivers, passengers, and pedestrians of all ages. Small children should be placed in specially designed car seats secured to the back seat of the car. Larger children should use a seat belt—as should adults. From a very young age children should be taught that streets are not play areas but dangerous places where the rule is to look both ways before crossing.

A child's age and stage of development affect the types of accidents that are most likely to befall him. Small infants are most likely to sustain injury in falls from a bed or table. As a child learns to crawl and climb, falls continue to be a threat. The child becomes more independent and preoccupied with play activities and is often unaware of the hazards of high places, traffic, or deep water. Young children like to put things in their mouths, hence the risk of poisoning, choking, and burns from hot drinks or electric cords.

Accidental *poisoning* is a very real threat to children under 5 years. Poisoning can occur by swallowing, inhaling, or splashing toxic materials in or on the mouth, nose, eyes, or skin. However, accidental ingestion of, or exposure to, hazardous substances can be prevented. *Prevention means keeping all chemicals, medicines, cleaning solutions, and pesticides out of sight and reach of children.* Keep safety caps on bottles securely closed, and keep poisons in their original containers clearly labeled. Never call medicine "candy." If the child does swallow a harmful substance, check with the poison control center or local emergency room before inducing vomiting. Splashes to the skin or eyes should be flushed with running water. In addition, all children between 9 months and 6 years of age should be routinely screened for lead poisoning.

Corrosive chemicals and cleaning products can cause *chemical burns*. Children may also burn themselves on hot water, a stove, heater, or fire; these are called *thermal burns* Clothing should be removed from the affected area and all burns should immediately be flushed with running water. All but very small, minor burns should be evaluated by a doctor at once, since infections can be a serious complication of burns.

Electrical appliances, wires, and outlets can cause burns and electric shocks. *Electrical burns* may not appear severe at first, but they can be very destructive; medical attention is imperative. In the event of electrical shock, the source should be disconnected immediately, before you touch the child. If the child is not breathing, call the rescue squad. Or, if a qualified person is available, start cardiopulmonary resuscitation immediately.

Choking, or foreign-body aspiration, is the accidental inhalation of small objects, food, or fluids into the airway. This is a leading cause of death among toddlers, since obstruction of the airway can cause difficulty breathing and, in severe cases, suffocation. (Turning the child over, mouth down, and delivering several sharp blows between the shoulder blades is the best method of dislodging the object.) If the object or material is small enough it may be inhaled all the way into the lungs, causing a pneumonia. Children sometimes swallow strange objects or put them into their ears, eyes, nose, or other orifices. A doctor should be consulted; the parent should not attempt removal, since this could cause further injury. (A foreign body in the eye may be flushed out gently with clean water.)

Sometimes children's play and sports can get rough or out of control, causing *sprains* or *fractured limbs*. Ice should be applied, the limb elevated, and the child taken to the hospital for X-ray evaluation. All children bump and bruise themselves. Most such events are minor and quickly forgotten; however, any severe head injury, especially one that involves a loss of consciousness or blackout, or is followed by confusion, lethargy, severe headache or vomiting, requires immediate neurological evaluation by a doctor.

Cuts or *lacerations* to the face or scalp tend to bleed profusely, often appearing much worse than they actually are. As with any cut, the wound should be rinsed with cool water and covered with a clean cloth. Steady pressure over the site should stop the bleeding. Any cut larger than a few centimeters or one that doesn't stop bleeding should be surgically cleansed and sutured by a professional. Immunization against tetanus should be kept up to date (see *Immunizations*); dirty cuts and insect or animal bites may require a booster shot. All cuts and bites should be cleansed thoroughly to prevent infection; in some cases antibiotics may be prescribed. (For more on accident prevention, see *Safety First* in the section on Wellness.)

Communicable and Infectious Diseases

Throughout childhood, every child is exposed to a variety of disease-causing agents—most frequently bacteria and viruses. Infectious diseases spread quickly through schools, playgrounds, and day-care centers. Because of their close physical contact and unlearned habits of hygiene, children cannot help but infect each other and those around them. Most of these diseases can be prevented. The most important form of protection is, of course, proper immunization. Immunizations currently are available against most contagious diseases (see *Immunizations*).

Problems Requiring Surgery

Hospital admission for any reason can be a traumatic experience for both the child and his family. If possible, a child should be well prepared for such an important event. Some hospitals have preadmission tours of the facilities, with opportunities for the child to ask questions and find out what to expect. There are also many books available for children that describe the hospital environment. Many hospitals can now accommodate parents of young children so that they may stay with the child overnight. Emergency admissions may be especially distressing. The stress imposed by the hospital atmosphere and the fear of body-altering surgery may be intensified if the child is in pain or feels sick and uncomfortable. Many necessary tests and procedures associated with surgery are painful as well as frightening. Regression to an earlier stage of development is very common. Even older children may display

COMMUNICABLE DISEASES

Name	Cause & Transmission	Signs & Symptoms	Treatment	Vaccine	Complications
CHICKEN POX	Virus, spread by skin contact, respiratory secretions, shared objects. Contagious for approximately 1 week after rash is first seen. Incubation: 1–2 weeks	Fever, malaise; itchy red blistering rash erupts that forms crusts on face, trunk, arms, and legs.	Prevent itching; give cool baths; cut fingernails; keep skin clean and dry; apply baking-soda paste.	No	Bacterial infection of skin rash can occur; pneumonia, encephalitis, and Reye's syndrome are possible, but rare.
DIPHTHERIA	Bacterium, spread by skin contact (rash), respiratory secretions, shared objects. Contagious for 2–4 weeks. Incubation: 1–2 weeks	Variable. Similar to upper respiratory infection: fever, nasal discharge, sore throat, cough, hoarse voice, severe breathing difficulty.	Bed rest, antibiotics, antitoxin	Yes	Inflammation of the heart muscle, or a nerve (or nerves); occurs rarely. Asphyxia
PERTUSSIS ("Whooping cough")	Bacterium spread by respiratory secretions, shared (contaminated) objects. Contagious from prodromal through acute phase. Incubation: 5–21 days	PRODROMAL: nasal drip, watery eyes, sneezing, cough, low fever (lasts 1–2 weeks). ACUTE: cough, high-pitched crowing sound on inspiration (whooping), thick expectoration, mucus plug; may vomit.	Antibiotics, immunoglobulin, bed rest, humidified air, fluids	Yes	Pneumonia, lung-tissue damage, otitis media, weight loss, dehydration, convulsions, hernia
MEASLES (rubeola)	Virus, spread by respiratory secretions and other body fluids. Contagious for 4 days before to 5 days after rash. Incubation: 10–20 days	PRODROMAL: fever, aches, nasal drip, red and white spots in mouth; in 3–4 days, rash appears on face and spreads downward; 3–4 days later rash turns brownish.	Bed rest, vaporizer, antipyretics, fluids, cool baths; keep skin clean and dry.	Yes	Otitis media, pneumonia, bronchitis, obstructed airway, conjunctivitis, encephalitis
MUMPS	Virus, spread by saliva. Contagious directly before and after swelling. Incubation: 14–21 days	PRODROMAL: fever, headache, malaise; in 3 days earache (worsens when chewing), painful swelling of cheeks (parotid glands).	Bed rest, pain relievers, fluids, hot or cold compresses	Yes	Deafness, encephalitis, cardiac problems, arthritis, hepatitis, male sterility following orchitis.
RUBELLA (German measles)	Virus, spread by respiratory secretions and other body fluids, and by feces and contaminated objects. Contagious 7 days before to 5 days after rash. Incubation: 14–21 days	Low fever, headache, malaise, rash on face spreads down body. Rash is pinkish red, raised, gone by third day.	Comfort measures, rest, antipyretics if feverish. Keep child away from pregnant women.	Yes	Rare (arthritis, encephalitis). Can cause fetal defects in pregnant women.

COMMUNICABLE DISEASES

Name	Cause & Transmission	Signs & Symptoms	Treatment	Vaccine	Complications
ROSEOLA	Probably a virus. Manner of transmission and incubation period are unknown. Limited to children 6 months to 2 years.	High fever; in 3–4 days fever drops and rash appears (pink bumps on trunk). Rash spreads to face and limbs; lasts 1–2 days.	Antipyretics (aspirin, acetaminophen)	No	Febrile seizures
SCARLET FEVER	Bacterium, spread by respiratory secretions and by contaminated objects, food, or milk. Contagious during incubation and approximately 10 days beyond. Incubation: 2–4 days	High fever, vomiting, headache, chills, abdominal pain. Then sore, swollen, red throat and rash (small, red dots on body). Face is flushed without rash.	Antibiotics, bed rest, fluids	No	Otitis media, peritonsillar abscess, sinusitis, rheumatic fever, glomerulonephritis
TUBERCULOSIS	Bacterium, spread by respiratory secretions. Active disease is always contagious. Infection can be detected in 2–10 weeks by test.	Variable: fever, malaise, weight loss, cough. Site of infection varies, but most common in lungs. Can be asymptomatic.	Bed rest, antitubercular drugs for 18 months	Yes	Pulmonary tuberculosis can spread and cause infection in most parts of the body, but most often in the bones.
POLIOMYELITIS	Virus, spread by oral-fecal routes and by direct contact. Contagious for 1–6 weeks. Incubation: usually 7–14 days	Three forms— ABORTIVE: fever, sore throat, headache, vomiting, abdominal pain. NONPARALYTIC: same as abortive form, with pain and stiffness in neck, back, and legs. PARALYTIC: same as above, with recovery, then signs of paralysis.	Bed rest, physical therapy, respiratory assistance (if needed)	Yes	Respiratory arrest, permanent paralysis, muscle weakness
TETANUS ("lockjaw")	Bacterium (tetanus spores) enter into damaged tissue from contaminated soil or object. Incubation: 1–54 days, but usually less than 14 days	LOCAL TETANUS: muscle rigidity near infected site may persist or resolve spontaneously. GENERALIZED TETANUS: stiff neck, jaw, mouth; facial muscle spasms; rigid trunk and limb muscles; difficulty swallowing; slight stimuli cause convulsions.	Tetanus immuno globulin, hospitalization	Yes	Respiratory difficulty; 30 percent mortality. Survival past fourth day allows good prognosis. Recovery takes weeks.

SKIN INFECTIONS

Name	Cause	Description	Treatment	Comments & Complications
IMPETIGO	Bacteria	Fluid-filled bumps erupt to form itchy crust.	Antimicrobial cream; remove crusts, wash.	Usually heals without scarring.
TINEA CAPITA (ringworm)	Fungus	Itchy, scaly patches on scalp, neck	Antifungal pills or ointment; clip hair, shampoo often.	Person-to-person or animal-to-person transmission
TINEA CORPORIS	Fungus	Round, red, scaly patch; may appear ring-shaped (clear in center); itchy.	Antifungal pills or ointment	Animal (pet)-to-person contact
TINEA CRURIS ("jock itch")	Fungus	Round, red, scaly patches on thighs (groin area); itchy	Apply imidazole cream; wash frequently.	Rare in preadolescent children. Teach good hygiene.
TINEA PEDIS ("athlete's foot")	Fungus	Scaly patches between toes, soles of feet	Antifungal pills, liquids, or powders	Rare in children; rarely contagious.
CONJUNCTIVITIS ("pink eye")	Bacteria	Red, swollen eye; yellow, crusty drainage	Antibacterial drops, ointment	If vision is affected, treatment by a specialist is urgently required.
	Virus	Red, swollen eyes	Time, self-resolving	
WARTS	Virus	Small, firm bumps on exposed areas, hands, and feet	Caustic agents, surgical removal	Common in children; may disappear spontaneously.
INSECT BITES:				
Mosquitos, fleas	Foreign protein	Itchy, red bumps	medicated cream, cool baths, antihistamines	May infect and cause scarring.
Bees, wasps, ants	Stinger; foreign protein	Itchy, red bumps; pain, swelling; possibly vomiting	Remove stinger; cleanse, apply cold compresses.	May cause anaphylactic reaction in sensitive individuals.
HEAD LICE	Saliva of louse; poor hygiene	Itching scalp; small, white bugs, eggs	Apply medicated cream; shampoo (gamma benzene).	Skin irritation may become infected.
BODY LICE	Lice bites; poor hygiene	Itchy, red bumps	Wash body (gamma benzene) and clothing.	
SCABIES	Skin-to-skin contact	Very itchy linear bumps. Black specks on wrists.	Wash body (gamma benzene); wash clothing in hot water.	Wash all family members at once.

unusually dependent or childish behavior. Children of different ages and personalities have varying abilities to understand the principles or aspects of a surgical procedure. The discussion of the surgery should be done in as clear, direct, and honest a way as possible.

A variety of conditions exist that require *surgery*: a life-threatening emergency, correction of a structural abnormality, removal or repair of a malfunctioning organ, or alteration of a pathological condition. A common reason for emergency surgery is major injury resulting from a severe accident. Less acute surgical conditions include complete intestinal obstruction, hernia, acute appendicitis, and tonsillectomy. Correction of congenital structural abnormalities may be

done at birth and may require a series of operations as the child grows.

Emergency operations are those that are required immediately to preserve life. The major indication is *excessive bleeding*. Bleeding into the brain or lungs or excessive blood loss in itself can cause sudden death or permanent disability. Emergency surgery often can prevent or correct these conditions.

Symptoms of *intestinal obstruction* or blockage are usually rapidly progressive. Abdominal pain and distention, nausea and vomiting, and possibly fever are common signs. The child may have no bowel movement or in some cases may pass a bloody mucoid stool or may even have diarrhea or constipation. The dangers of this situation if left untreated include intestinal rupture and peritonitis, or severe dehydration and shock. Treatment may consist initially of an attempt to release pressure by passing a tube into the stomach through the mouth or nose; this may relieve the pressure and may "unplug" the intestine. A barium meal may be used both to help diagnose and visualize the obstruction on an X-ray film, as well as to help push the obstruction through. Surgical intervention involves manually correcting the problem. Sometimes, if there is damage to the intestine itself, a temporary colostomy will be performed to allow the intestine to rest. (The end of the intestine will be brought out of a small incision on the side of the abdomen; bowel contents then empty out into a bag.) This type of alteration in body image can obviously be very distressing to a child and her family.

A *hernia* is the protrusion or bulging of a structure through an abnormal opening. Surgical repair of these defects is extremely common during infancy and early childhood. Surgical intervention often is required to prevent functional disorders or constriction and decreased circulation to the affected part. Herniations can occur through the abdominal wall, or the inguinal canal. An *umbilical hernia* is usually evidenced by an abnormal swelling or bulge, which enlarges as the child cries. Most common hernias are seen near the navel, or in the inguinal canal of the testes. A *hiatal hernia* causes feeding problems and regurgitation, as part of the stomach protrudes through the diaphragm. Surgical repair consists of tightening the diaphragmatic opening and securing the stomach inside the abdominal cavity. Some other types of hernias are noticed and repaired within a few weeks of birth. Recovery usually is uncomplicated.

Acute appendicitis is the most common reason for abdominal surgery during childhood. It is rare in children less than 2 years old. The appendix is a small structure at the end of the cecum, the pouch where the large intestine begins. In appendicitis this structure becomes inflamed and swells; if undiagnosed and untreated the condition can progress to perforation and peritonitis. The inflammation usually is caused by obstruction of the appendix. Dietary and bowel habits may be contributing factors. The symptoms of appendicitis are abdominal pain, tenderness in the right lower quadrant, vomiting, and fever. These symptoms can vary and may resemble other types of illness. Treatment consists of surgical removal of the appendix (appendectomy). Recovery from an uncomplicated appendectomy is usually uneventful and involves a hospital stay of about four days. Recovery from a perforated appendix may take up to two weeks in the hospital and involves intravenous antibiotic therapy.

Tonsillitis usually occurs as a result of bacterial pharyngitis (see Pharyngitis). Enlargement of the adenoids and lymphatic tissue surrounding the pharynx makes it difficult for the child to breathe. Although most cases of tonsillitis are treated conservatively with antibiotics, tonsillectomy is perhaps the most frequently performed pediatric surgery—although it is performed less routinely now than in the past. Tonsillectomy refers to the removal of the palatine tonsils, and is indicated for patients with chronic, persistent sore throats or who have a related significant respiratory problem. The term *adenoidectomy* refers to the surgical removal of the adenoids. Usually this is performed in conjunction with a tonsillectomy, when breathing is impaired or when the child suffers from recurrent otitis media (see Otitis Media). Generally, tonsillectomy is done in children over 3 or 4 years old. The most significant complications are excessive bleeding and regrowth or hypertrophy (overgrowth) of the lymphatic tissue.

Significant *structural anomalies* often require some type of medical or surgical correction to maintain or improve a child's ability to function. The most severe deformities, such as cardiac defects, necessitate immediate surgical correction. Some anomalies become apparent only as a child grows and develops, certain urinary tract anomalies, for example. Treatment of conditions like "clubfoot" may initially involve special legs braces as well as surgery in more severe cases. The problem of *hydrocephalus* (excessive accumulation of cerebrospinal fluid) demands an initial surgery to insert a shunt (a specialized drain) and periodic surgeries as the child grows in order to refit the device.

CHRONIC HEALTH PROBLEMS

Children with chronic physical conditions are challenged by more than the average childhood tasks of growth and development. These children require regular medical supervision and special adjustments that may include daily medications, a modified diet, and extra protection. Chronic ailments that have no cure—like diabetes mellitus, asthma, sickle-cell disease, and seizure disorders—can have profound effects on a child's development as well as serious implications for career and life-style choices, related health problems, and even life expectancy.

Diabetes Mellitus

This disease is the most frequent endocrine disorder affecting school-aged children. It results from the absence or inadequate production of the hormone *insulin*, which is made in the pancreas and is essential to carbohydrate metabolism. Insulin is responsible for moving glucose (simple sugar) out of the bloodstream and into the cells where it can be used as energy. Diabetes is influenced by both genetic and environmental factors and can occur at any age. The likelihood of developing diabetes increases with age.

Currently several types of diabetes have been identified and classified:

Insulin-dependent diabetes mellitus (IDDM) is perhaps better known as "juvenile-onset," or type I, diabetes. The person requires daily insulin and must take care to avoid ketoacidotic coma, which can have severe consequences.

Non-insulin-dependent diabetes mellitus (NIDDM), or "adult-onset diabetes," can occur at any time and is more common among obese people. This is controlled by diet or by drugs taken orally.

Gestational diabetes is caused by the metabolic and hormonal changes of pregnancy. Pregnancy may aggravate preexisting disease.

Impaired glucose tolerance is the term for nonsymptomatic or borderline diabetes.

Signs and symptoms of uncontrolled type I diabetes (*hyperglycemia*) include increased thirst, hunger, and frequent and copious urination. Abdominal discomfort, nausea and vomiting, dry skin, and blurred vision occasionally occur. Behavioral symptoms include regression (bed-wetting is common), irritability, and constant fatigue. In contrast, symptoms of *hypoglycemia* (too little sugar, usually as a result of too much insulin) are sweating, shaking, weakness, confusion, headache, and coma. Treatment is by insulin injecttion. With patience and persistence and through the use of play therapy, most children can learn to draw up and inject their own insulin, make appropriate diet choices and exchanges, and monitor their glucose levels by simple blood and urine analyses.

Asthma

Asthma is the third leading cause of children's hospitalizations. The incidence seems to be increasing in the population and there is a strong tendency for the disease to run in families; Hispanic children seem to be more predisposed. Asthma attacks are frequently exacerbated by upper respiratory tract infections, allergies, and stress; they occur more often at night. Difficulty breathing and talking, wheezing, and mucus-producing cough are common symptoms. Although many kids outgrow asthma, many need consistent medication to remain symptom-free. Routine maintenance medications include theophylline (as pills, sprinkles, or elixir) in combination with an aerosol pump containing a bronchodilator. In acute attacks, the child should be taken to the hospital where she may receive epinephrine injections, as well as intravenous theophylline and possibly steroids.

Sickle-Cell Disease (Sickle-Cell Anemia)

This is an inherited disease that is most frequently found in black people. During a crisis, or acute attack, the red blood cells become sickle shaped when they are deprived of oxygen, under stress, or dehydrated (as may occur during periods of overexertion). The sickled cells impair circulation, causing pain, most commonly in the abdomen and joints. Related symptoms include weakness, loss of appetite, and fever. Long-term effects are manifested by growth retardation and delayed sexual maturity, bone deformities, and increased risk of infection. Treatment is aimed at relief of symptoms with rest, warmth, plenty of fluids, supplemental oxygen, and analgesics and antipyretics for pain and fever. Blood transfusions may be needed.

Seizure Disorder (Epilepsy, Convulsions)

This is a disorder of the brain. Seizures can be acute, nonrecurring events, most commonly caused by high fever (see above, *Fevers*). Seizure disorders also can be chronic. Chronic seizure disorders may be inherited or the result of permanent brain damage, most commonly head trauma.

Mental ability usually is not affected or related

to the two most common forms of seizure activity. These are tonic/clonic seizures (grand mal) and absence seizures (petit mal). *Grand mal seizures* are the more severe type. The seizing child actually loses consciousness and the muscles alternately relax and contract; there may be an excessive amount of saliva in the mouth. The child can quite possibly sustain serious injury from falling or choking. Parents should provide a relatively safe environment and nonstressful activities for a child with this condition. The seizures last only a few seconds, but are usually followed by a period of lethargy and confusion.

Petit mal or *absence seizures* are much less dramatic and less dangerous. These are characterized by a brief lack of attention, possibly accompanied by eye-blinking or twitching. Attacks may occur several times in a day. Often the child is unaware that anything has happened; however, if frequent, these events can disrupt learning and concentration. These are most common between the ages of 4 and 12, and the child may possibly outgrow them. Both grand mal and petit mal seizures can be controlled effectively by medications.

Behavioral Problems

Growing up can be an emotionally confusing, frustrating, and sometimes frightening experience. Children are struggling constantly to please their parents and later on their friends; at the same time they seek to satisfy their own needs and desires. Conflicts are unavoidable. A child's ways of dealing with these conflicts are often annoying or disappointing to the parents. It takes many years and a lot of patience on both the child's and the parents' parts for the child to learn to behave in a socially acceptable manner; some children never learn.

Different children have different ways of expressing their emotions. In general, *a parent should pay close attention to behavior that is persistent, uncharacteristic, or unusual for a particular child.* Crying, apathy, speech or learning disabilities, hyperactivity, sleepwalking, bed-wetting, thumb-sucking, masturbation, temper tantrums, and lying can be annoying, but they may be appropriate at a certain age or stage of development. Such behavior should be closely observed and investigated, however, as possible clues to more complex physical, emotional, or social problems.

Discipline is important for children. It provides them with consistent standards of behavior, en-courages self-control, and helps them develop a sense of responsibility. Parents' goals and expectations should be reasonable, however, taking into consideration a child's stage of development and individual personality. Excessive or inconsistent discipline may confuse a child and lead to rebellion, depression, or other personality disorders. Since children learn from example, parental behavior strongly influences a child's psychosocial development.

Young children cry a lot, especially before they are able to communicate verbally. Crying is their most effective way of expressing their needs, frustrations, or fears. Uncontrollable, unrelieved, prolonged crying is not healthy, however, and should be interpreted as a warning of physical pain, rather than as a behavioral problem. The same is true for extreme apathy or lethargy. With the exception of frequent rest periods, healthy children normally are very active and interested in their surroundings. If organic or physical disease has been ruled out, and if the child continues to appear withdrawn or depressed, the child may have a real emotional problem.

Children who don't begin speaking as early as their peers, who stutter or stumble over their words, or who are slow to learn, may worry their parents. These children should have their hearing carefully tested. Late or garbled speech may resolve spontaneously as the child improves her verbal abilities and becomes more self-confident. If problems persist, specialized help should be sought, since many of these problems can be corrected. Emotional tension and excessive attention to the problem may make it worse.

Healthy children are very active; however, a condition of *hyperactivity* can exist. Hyperactivity may be a sign of an attention-deficit disorder. This condition is characterized by disorganized, nonproductive, inappropriate behavior, unusual sleeping patterns, and/or over-reaction to stimuli. It usually manifests before age 7 and, paradoxically, it may be treated with amphetamines, often in conjunction with behavior modification therapy. Many children will outgrow their need for medication. In recent years some health-care professionals have advanced the notion that food additives and other dietary factors may play a part in hyperactivity.

Sleep disorders are not uncommon. Approximately 15 percent of all children have walked in their sleep. Most sleepwalkers start before the age of 10 and discontinue the behavior by age 15. The child will not recall the episode. Saftey precautions are important to prevent accidents and a regular sleep schedule or reduction of stress may help resolve the disorders. Sleep terrors and nightmares often occur. Shortly after sleep begins, the child may awaken with a scream and appear panicstricken. These events usually resolve themselves and the child remembers little about them.

Enuresis, or bed-wetting, may accompany these events or may be a separate phenomenon. This problem is more common in males and may be associated with a family history of the disorder. Although most children have achieved daytime dryness by age 5, and some will also be dry at night, 90 percent of children do not attain complete nighttime dryness until the age of 12. Reminding the child to void and decreasing fluid intake just before bedtime will encourage dryness. A child's bladder control and capacity may prevent total control until neuromuscular development is complete. A child who is normally dry, and completely toilet trained, may regress to wetting during periods of severe stress, although physical reasons also must be looked for.

Thumb-sucking, self-rocking, and *masturbation* are common and normal behaviors for a young child and may increase when the child is sleepy or upset. Essentially they are comforting actions that the child can provide for himself. The child normally outgrows behaviors like thumb-sucking and rocking as he finds other interests and methods of gratification. The precious thumb usually is given up by the age of 5 or 6, although regression under stress is not unlikely. Depending upon the parents' attitudes and beliefs, masturbation is either discouraged or accepted, but as a private act.

A *security blanket* or favorite pet may be a source of controversy if the child refuses to give it up. But if parents avoid drawing attention to the treasured object, most children eventually will lose interest in it.

As a response to *frustration*, a young child will express herself by acting out or throwing a temper tantrum. It takes time and experience before children learn self-control. Between the ages of 2 and 4, children do not tolerate frustration well; they are seeking to gain more control over themselves and their actions. They express themselves through physical and verbal aggression and demonstrations of will. Screaming, kicking, and name-calling are not unusual. A child in this condition is best left alone to sort things out for herself. Punishment is rarely appropriate. The exception is potentially harmful aggression or extremely destructive or violent behavior, which should not be tolerated. Displays of temper gradually disappear or subside as the child's personal style of coping evolves.

Social and *moral development* is a lengthy and highly individualized process. As children grow, their personalities change and develop in response to new situations and circumstances. For instance, a normally outgoing child may be shy on the first day of school. Repeated refusals to go to school may be part of a more pervasive social withdrawal. Negative aspects of school should be minimized and the process made as pleasant and as easy as possible; the child should be encouraged to accept going to school.

Young children have very active imaginations; fantasy and games of pretend are important to their normal development. *Lying*, in the form of "pretend" or exaggeration, is common, as are lies told to conceal wrongdoing. A child should be reassured of her own real worth and of her parents' unconditional love for her. Because young children are not capable of abstract thought, it is difficult for them to understand the concepts of stealing or cheating. Even very young children can, however, clearly understand firm prohibition. As the child grows, such behavior may be tried as a result of peer pressure. If allowed to persist beyond the realm of innocence, however, a seriously maladaptive pattern may develop. Other types of maladaptive behaviors may also begin as a result of innocence, curiosity, or peer pressure. Exposure to and experimentation with drugs, alcohol, and cigarettes are now so widespread as to be almost unavoidable. Parental attitudes and example, as well as a child's self-esteem, general state of emotional stability, and sense of well-being, play significant roles in determining a child's choice of abstinence, or substance abuse.

Preventive Practices and Anticipatory Guidance

Childhood is a vulnerable time, fraught with many changes and challenges. By being aware of possible threats to a child's safety parents can anticipate and prevent situations that may be particularly harmful to a child at various developmental stages.

Complete, balanced nutrition helps a child maintain a healthy body. Children need adequate protein for normal growth. Carbohydrates, fats, and sugars supply energy. Vitamins and minerals ensure maintenance of all body systems. Good hygienic practices will diminish the risk of infections, parasites, and vermin infestation. Ensuring that a child receives the routine schedule of immunizations is essential to supplement the body's own immune system and protect against infectious disease.

All children should be observed regularly by a physician who can advise on nutrition and immunization and detect early signs of disease or developmental delay. Health care should always include regular dental check-ups.

The number of accidental deaths and injuries in childhood demonstrates the crucial need for implementation of effective safety measures. The home of a young child should be "childproofed." Measures include: guards on high windows and stairs; foolproof storage of poisons, caustic substances, sharp objects, and plastic bags; maintenance of safe electrical outlets and appliances; and cautious use of stoves and open flames. Every home has its own unique hazards and should be evaluated carefully. As the child grows older, the parent should remain aware of potential dangers in the home.

Education of preschool, school-age, and adolescent children by both teachers and parents should include recognition and prevention of sex-ual abuse. The child's age, mental ability, and emotional development must be weighed carefully so that he or she is not overwhelmed, frightened, or confused by too much information. Emphasis can be on such notions as, "No one has the right to touch the private parts of your body," and "Just because someone acts nice to you doesn't mean that he/she is incapable of doing mean things." Most important, open communication between parent and child should be encouraged, and parents should be alert to possible signs of sexual abuse, such as changes in behavior, appetite, and school performance, or regressive behavior such as bed-wetting, tantrums, and anxiety toward strangers.

Accident prevention outside the home can be promoted through education. The child should be taught the dangers of traffic, water play, and recklessness in climbing. Teaching the child to swim and to behave appropriately in swimming areas will diminish risks.

Awareness of the normal development stages, behavior, activities, and patterns of peer interaction can prepare parents to respond helpfully. Familiarity with the parameters of normal growth and development enables parents to recognize abnormalities that need professional attention. Health care providers should be consulted in the event of any doubts or insecurities.

13

IMMUNIZATIONS

The goal of immunization is to put an end to disease. This has been achieved, for example, in the case of the deadly disease smallpox: Through successsful global vaccination, smallpox was declared eradicated in 1980 by the World Health Organization. WHO's current goal is to reduce deaths and illnesses from diphtheria, pertussis (whooping cough), tetanus, measles, polio, and tuberculosis through immunization of every child, worldwide, by 1990. Effective immunization currently is available for these diseases and many others, including mumps, rubella (German measles), typhoid, yellow fever, hepatitis B, pneumococcal and meningococcal infections, influenza, and cholera. Recent advances in biomedical research and technology are making new vaccines safer, less expensive, and more effective.

The importance of routine immunization in the prevention and eradication of infectious disease cannot be overemphasized. This is true on a global as well as an individual level. Within the first two years of life all children should be vaccinated against diphtheria, pertussis, and tetanus (collectively called the DPT vaccination); against measles, mumps, and rubella (collectively called

the MMR vaccination); and against polio. All children should also be tested for tuberculosis at the age of 12 months or at 15 months, before the MMR vaccine is given.

The terms *immunization* and *vaccination* commonly are used interchangeably. "Immunization," which is the more inclusive term, describes the process by which an individual is protected against or made resistant to a disease. "Vaccination," in current usage, has come to mean the actual inoculation with a vaccine to establish resistance to a specific infectious agent. The word *vaccine* is derived from "vaccinia," the name of the "cowpox" virus that was used formerly to immunize people against smallpox.

The U.S. Department of Health and Human Services defines a vaccine as "a suspension of attenuated live or killed microorganisms (bacterium, virus, or rickettsia) or fractions thereof administered to induce immunity and thereby prevent infectious disease." A vaccine can make a person immune to a disease in much the same way that actually contracting the disease can prevent a future recurrence of the disease: by the process of *immunization*. A substance that is foreign to the body (bacterium or virus) is called an *antigen*. Immunization occurs when the body reacts to an antigen by developing antibodies that are "specific" for it—that is, they are designed for fighting that particular virus or bacterium and, if the person is exposed to it again, they will "remember" it and inactivate it, thus preventing the disease that it causes from taking hold.

The products used for immunization, called "immunobiologics," include vaccines, toxoids, and antisera from human or animal donors. They are given most commonly by intramuscular (IM) or subcutaneous (SC) injection, usually into the upper arm, buttock, or thigh. Some vaccines, such as the Sabin oral polio vaccine, can be taken by mouth.

There are two basic kinds of immunization: active and passive. *Active immunization* occurs when the body responds to an antigen and actively produces specific antibodies that render a person immune. This can happen either by receiving a vaccine or by exposure to the disease itself. *Passive immunization* occurs when the body acquires ready-made antibodies without exposure to the antigen. Passive immunization can occur in the fetus in blood received through the placenta, during infancy through the mother's breast milk, or by direct injection of antibodies, such as gamma globulin injections once a person is exposed. Passive immunity is only temporary, however, because once the "borrowed" antibodies are used up, the body does not produce more; the body has never been exposed to the disease itself and so cannot "remember" what the antigen (disease-causing organism) "looks like" to make antibodies against it. Thus the person is once again susceptible to infection by the particular disease-causing antigen.

Active immunization is the method used for the routine schedule of immunizations that all children should receive in the first few years of life (see Table 1 for recommended schedule of active immunization for normal infants and children). This means that the child receives a vaccine containing all or part of a disease-causing microorganism or a product of that microorganism. This process provides the antigen that stimulates the recipient's immune system to produce antibodies.

The infectious microorganism in the vaccine may exist in one of several forms. It may be alive ("attenuated") or killed ("inactivated"). Most vaccines against viral infections contain the attenuated form. In such cases, the organism is alive, but it has been aged and altered in such a way that it does not cause disease. The live attenuated vaccines include the combined measles, mumps, and rubella vaccine; the Sabin oral polio vaccine; and the tuberculosis, or BCG, vaccine. These live attenuated vaccines provide immunity that lasts a lifetime, while the inactivated-virus vaccines usually require a sequence of several immunizations or periodic "booster shots."

Most of the inactivated vaccines against bacteria (such as the cholera, typhoid, and plague vaccines) and some viral inactivated vaccines (such as the hepatitis B and influenza vaccines and the injectable polio vaccine) produce a less complete immunologic response than that produced by some live attenuated preparations; protection is short-lived and should only be used when live attenuated forms cannot be used. This is why repeat doses of inactivated vaccines are necessary to provide complete protection, although even partial protection will generally decrease the severity of the disease if it *is* contracted.

In addition to attenuated and inactivated types of vaccines, there are vaccines containing *toxoids.* Toxoids contain a modified bacterial toxin that has been made nontoxic but is still able to stimulate antitoxin production by the body. Diphtheria and tetanus toxoids given in the DPT injection are common examples of this.

The terms *multivalent* and *polyvalent* refer to a vaccine containing several strains of the same species of bacterium or virus. The pneumococcus vaccine, for example, is effective against the twenty-three most prevalent types of pneumococci.

Passive immunization is induced by the transfer of preformed concentrated antibodies contained in fractions of blood—either human immune globulin, human plasma, or animal serum. Human immune globulin consists of the "gamma globulin" fraction as well as other blood proteins obtained from blood products donated by adults who have antibodies against the particular disease. This solution is sterilized and modified so that it cannot transmit such diseases as hepatitis or AIDS. However, because it is so highly concentrated, injections of the solution can sometimes be painful; in some individuals it can cause severe *anaphylactic* (allergic) shock or other systemic reactions, although this is rare. In addition to these drawbacks, passive immunization by vaccination is, as already mentioned, short-lived, usually lasting only a few months. Passive injection of preformed antibodies can, however, be very important in certain circumstances:

• for individuals whose immune systems are de-

RECOMMENDED SCHEDULE FOR ACTIVE IMMUNIZATION
OF NORMAL INFANTS AND CHILDREN

Recommended Age	Vaccine/Disease	Comments
2 months	DPT, Oral Polio Vaccine (OPV)	
4 months	DPT, OPV	
6 months	DPT (OPV)	OPV optional
12 months	Tb test	May be given simultaneously with MMR at 15 months
15 months	MMR	
18 months	DPT, OPV	
4–6 years	DPT, OPV	
14–16 years	Td	Should be repeated every 10 years for the duration of life

SOURCE: Adapted from the American Academy of Pediatrics' Report on Infectious Diseases

Table 1

ficient and who are therefore unable to make their own antibodies

- when there is no vaccine available to stimulate active immunization against a disease, as in the case of hepatitis A
- when exposure to infection occurs in a susceptible (nonimmunized) person and there isn't enough time for the body to actively produce its own antibodies, a process that normally takes about fourteen days
- when an infectious disease is already present and giving antibodies can lessen the severity of symptoms (as with diphtheria or tetanus) or actually decrease the effect of the toxin (as with botulism)

Passive immunization through injection of specific immune globulin is available for many diseases, including measles, hepatitis A and B, varicella zoster (chickenpox), rubella, rabies, and tetanus. Distribution of the mumps and pertussis immune globulin preparations was discontinued in the United States in 1980 because neither was very effective and because active immunization against both by means of the MMR and DPT vaccines had become widespread.

Since immunization is important in protecting the health of individuals and in preventing the spread of disease, public health laws requiring children to receive routine immunizations before entering school exist in all states and in many countries outside the United States. These requirements may vary from state to state, but generally they mandate three DPT injections, three polio vaccinations, and one MMR injection before enrolling in school (see Tables 1 and 2). The

American Academy of Pediatrics' Committee on the Control of Infectious Disease strongly urges that every parent keep a record of all immunizations received. The Academy considers this record a vital document as important as a birth certificate or passport. The prescribing physician should maintain a complete record, but given our highly mobile society, it also makes sense for every parent to request a copy, including all the following information:

- date of administration
- age of recipient
- immunobiologic administered
- manufacturer, lot number, expiration date of substance
- site, route, and amount given
- any reaction or contraindications to the substance

This record can be very useful as proof of immunization for school, travel, or military or other institutions, or if future medical conditions arise that may involve the original inoculation.

There are only two recognized exceptions from most public health requirements governing immunization. These are a physician's certificate stating the medical reasons for withholding the vaccine, or a document stating that the child's parents follow a religion that does not permit immunization.

There are several medical conditions in which vaccines should not be administered. There are, of course, exceptions, but general contraindications to vaccination include serious chronic illness, seizure or neurological disorder, fever, leukemia, immune system disorders, steroid ther-

RECOMMENDED IMMUNIZATION SCHEDULES FOR CHILDREN AND ADULTS NOT INITIALLY IMMUNIZED IN EARLY INFANCY

Time	Younger than 7 years	Older than 7 years
1st visit	DPT, OPV, Tb test	Td, OPV (no OPV if older than 18 years)
1 month later	MMR	MMR
2 months later	DPT, OPV	Td, OPV
4 months later	DPT, (OPV)	——
8–14 months later	——	Td, OPV
10–16 months later	DPT, OPV	——
Age 14–16 years	Td	Td
Boosters	Td every 10 years	Td every 10 years

SOURCE: *Immunization in Clinical Practice*, Vincent A. Fulginiti (Philadelphia: J. B. Lippincott & Co., 1982).

Table 2

apy (cortisone or prednisone, for example), radiation therapy, or gamma globulin received in the previous three months.

The measles, mumps, and rubella combined vaccine (MMR) should not be given to persons who are allergic to eggs, chicken, rabbit, or duck, or to the antibiotic neomycin. Nor should it be given to pregnant women. (In general, unless urgently needed, all drugs should be avoided during pregnancy.) The vaccine against pertussis is not normally given to children older than 7 years, since at that age the risks of the vaccine begin to outweigh its benefits (because the disease is less dangerous and less likely to occur in an older individual). A physician should be consulted if there is any doubt about any vaccine.

Vaccines provide one of the safest, most reliable and most effective methods modern medicine has of controlling the death and illness caused by infectious disease. In most cases, the benefits yielded by the process of immunization far outweigh the possible risks or side effects. Most side effects of vaccination are mild and temporary, lasting only a few days and causing only slight discomfort. It is important, however, to distinguish between a predictable "normal" reaction and signs of a more severe reaction.

There are two basic ways the body can respond to an immunobiologic: either *locally*, at the site in which the solution has been injected, or *systemically*, with the whole body or a body system being affected. Local reactions are quite common and usually are not serious. Some swelling, redness, and soreness at the site may occur in the first day or two. A mild systemic reaction is also a fairly common response. It can be manifested as a low-grade fever or a mild rash. Serious systemic reactions, which are much less frequent, include hypersensitivity, anaphylaxis, shock, and nerve or brain damage. A brief summary of reported reactions to specific immunobiologics follows:

Measles vaccine: No more than 15 percent of children will have a slight rash or fever for a few days, starting five to twelve days after receiving the vaccine. Rarely (one case in 1 million doses) a central-nervous-system (CNS) disorder may occur, such as encephalitis (inflammation of the brain) or encephalopathy (a degenerative disease of the brain).

Mumps vaccine: Very infrequently, after receiving a mumps vaccine, mild mumps-like symptoms may occur, involving a low fever and swelling of some of the salivary glands. Inconclusive connections exist between this vaccine and CNS disease; however, even if they do exist, they are extremely rare.

Rubella vaccine: Mild rash, swollen lymph nodes, and fever may occur following vaccination but should resolve within a few days. Joint pain may occur within three to ten weeks and is more common in females and adults. The chance of developing arthritis is quite unlikely (less than 1 percent). Pain, numbness, and tingling of the hands and feet also have been reported. All women of childbearing age should receive this vaccine, since the disease can cause severe birth defects if contracted during pregnancy. Women should wait at least three months after vaccination before getting pregnant, however, and of course pregnant women should not be vaccinated.

Diphtheria toxoid: Since this usually is given in solution with either pertussis or tetanus toxoid or both, it has been difficult to determine possible reactions. Most acute reactions usually are attributed to the pertussis element. Side effects to DT (the vaccine without pertussis) are uncommon but usually are more severe in adults than in children. Therefore, in persons older than 7 years of age, tetanus-diphtheria (Td) toxoids, which contain a lower dose of the diphtheria toxoid, are given. Side effects of Td have been predominantly local and mild, including soreness, swelling, and itching.

Tetanus toxoid: This substance rarely is given without the diphtheria element, and for the first four doses it usually is given in the DPT form. When given as a booster (recommended every ten years), it is given either alone or in the Td form discussed above. Reactions to the tetanus toxoid are generally local (pain, swelling, redness at the injection site). Rarely, anaphylactic reactions (facial and neck swelling, itching, flushing, and breathing difficulty) may develop.

Pertussis vaccine: Reactions associated with this inactivated bacterial suspension seem to be more frequent and more varied. Therefore, a child with a fever or a neurological disorder (especially seizures or a family history of seizure disorder), or any child older than 7 years probably should receive the DT or Td without the pertussis element. Less severe, typical side effects that may develop shortly after receiving the injection (and subsiding within twenty-four hours) include irritability, fever, and loss of appetite. Local irritation and, rarely, abscesses or infection at the site also may occur. Much less common are serious systemic reactions such as anaphylaxis, shock, sudden infant death, excessive fever, and cardiorespiratory arrest.

Polio vaccine: The oral live polio vaccine rarely has side effects. There is, however, a very slight incidence (one in 4 million) of a person recently vaccinated, or someone in close contact with such a person, becoming permanently crippled or even dying. The risk of this happening increases with age above 18 years and in individuals who have other diseases or are receiving treatment (steroids, chemotherapy, or radiation) that lowers the body's resistance to infection. The injectable killed polio vaccine is recommended for these individuals. The injectable inactivated polio vaccine has no known risks, but it is generally considered to give less effective protection against polio.

Influenza vaccine: This vaccine has no known major adverse effects; however, it is not given to persons with severe hypersensitivity to eggs, allergy to the mercury derivative thimerosal, or a history of Guillain-Barré syndrome, a rare neurological disorder. It is especially recommended for health care workers and those persons at risk for serious complications from influenza. This population includes those with heart or lung disease, kidney problems, severe anemias, diabetes mellitus, impaired immune systems, and healthy individuals older than 65 years.

The vaccines described below, although considered safe and effective, are not routinely given to healthy children or adults. They may be indicated for persons with certain physical conditions or occupations or for those who travel to foreign countries where there is some likelihood of exposure to the disease. The need for, risks, and benefits of specific vaccinations should be discussed with your physician.

Hepatitis B vaccine: This inactivated virus vaccine generally is reserved for people at greater risk because of occupational, social, environmental, or familial factors. It is given in three doses over a period of six months. Side effects are rare but have been neurologic when they have occurred. Since hepatitis B (once known as "serum hepatitis") is a known precursor of liver cancer, the value of this vaccine for those who need it outweighs most other considerations.

Meningococcus vaccine: Available in one subcutaneous dose, this vaccine is given to control specific outbreaks of illness from an isolated organism, and for travel to countries where outbreaks are common. It is generally not given to pregnant women, and there are no known side effects.

Pneumococcus vaccine: Also given in a single subcutaneous dose, this vaccine is administered to individuals at increased risk (persons with a dysfunctional or missing spleen; chronic heart/lung, kidney, or liver disease; diabetes mellitus; or cerebrospinal fluid leaks) and to healthy individuals older than 65.

14

ADOLESCENT GROWTH AND DEVELOPMENT

Adolescence is the period of great transition from childhood to mature adulthood. During this time, the child changes physically, mentally, emotionally, and socially. The adolescent strives to integrate the parts of the personality developed during childhood and to achieve a unique sense of self. As the child undergoes these radical changes, she forms a mature identity in preparation for living as an independent adult.

The changes during adolescence encompass all areas of the person. Physically, children reach sexual maturity and the capability to reproduce. They attain full body height and weight, and develop an "adult" appearance due to secondary sex characteristics. Emotionally, they begin to separate from their parents and to see themselves no longer as children but as unique and independent people. Through emotional separation, they begin forming attachments to people outside their family. Intellectually, adolescents move from the concrete methods of childhood reasoning to more abstract adult thinking.

Though the changes of adolescence are normal and absolutely necessary in each person's life, they cause an upheaval in the child's life and in the lives of those around her. These changes, and the varying degrees of disturbance, often characterize adolescence as a period to be suffered through. The psychologist Anna Freud saw the conflict and strife experienced during adolescence as essential to growth and maturation. As the child adjusts to personal changes, there must be a clear upset in the former equilibrium in order to ensure proper growth and development.

The concept of adolescence varies from culture to culture. In less complex and less industrialized societies, adolescence may be a short, circumscribed period or ritual marking the passage of the child into the adult world. In our complex Western society, adolescence has been infiltrated with increasing influences and aspects that must be coped with and integrated into a meaningful sense of self and society. Often to young adults and their parents, the phase of adolescence seems to last well into the mid-20s.

While the child is going through the tumultuous period of adolescence, parents too are experiencing profound changes in their roles and in their sense of self. Parenthood becomes an even greater challenge. Before, the parents were responsible for providing food, clothing, shelter, and medical care. Now, in addition, they must act as teachers, advice-givers, and role models. And often the child responds to their best efforts with anger, hostility, and depression. Is it any wonder that parents often share their adolescent's confusion?

As adolescence progresses there is the excitement of watching the adult emerge out of the child. Yet the transformation evokes ambivalent feelings in the parents as they see their child growing increasingly free and independent of them. Sometimes parents feel hurt because their child seems to withdraw and distance herself from them. They must try to remember that this is a necessary process whereby the child is forming her identity and achieving autonomy.

The teenage years are usually synonymous with adolescence, and adolescence is divided into three stages within this period. Early adolescence (10 to 14 years) is associated with great physical change as the child enters puberty and becomes capable of reproduction. As the physical changes slow down, the person enters middle adolescence (15 to 17 years), in which the bulk of mental maturation occurs. Late adolescence (17 years and up) focuses on psychosocial development, emotional maturation, and the refining of social interactions. It is normal for young people to mature at different rates; development is often seen to start earlier in girls than in boys. For each person, the interpretation of growth and development must be unique.

Physical Changes of Adolescence

Although the terms *puberty* and *adolescence* are often used interchangeably, they are not synonymous. As discussed previously, *adolescence* refers to the entire process of transition from child to adult, encompassing all aspects of the person. *Puberty*, on the other hand, is the much shorter period of physical change when the child's body matures and becomes capable of reproduction. Puberty usually marks the onset of adolescense.

■ Onset of Puberty—External Development and Secondary Sex Characteristics

Puberty in both boys and girls is marked by the appearance of secondary sexual characteristics and the development of external genitalia. *Primary* and *secondary sexual characteristics* are terms used to differentiate between the body parts directly related to reproduction (primary) and those that distinguish the sexes (secondary). Primary characteristics include the ovaries, uterus, and testicles. Secondary characteristics include breasts, pubic hair, facial hair, and axillary (underarm) hair.

Females generally reach puberty one and a half to two years before males, between the ages of 10 and 14 years. Onset of puberty in males usually is seen from 12 to 16 years of age. Once puberty begins it is usually complete within three years.

Onset of puberty is under hormonal control. The role of hormones in the maturation process involves a highly complex and sensitive interaction between parts in the brain and the reproductive organs. From an early age in the child (about 6 years), levels of the sex hormones gradually increase until a feedback system is triggered and puberty is initiated.

The hypothalamus in the brain begins producing follicle-stimulating-hormone-releasing factor (FSHRF) and luteinizing-hormone-releasing factor (LHRF). These substances travel within the brain to the anterior pituitary gland and cause the production of follicle-stimulating hormone (FSH) and luteinizing hormone (LH). In the female, FSH controls ovulation (release of the mature ovum, or egg) and production of one of the female sex hormones, progesterone. LH controls the maturation of the ova and production of estrogen, another of the female sex hormones. In the male, FSH controls spermatogenesis (production of sperm). LH causes testicular maturation and the production of testosterone, a male sex hormone. As the child enters puberty the ovaries or testicles become the primary site of sex hormone production. In the prepubescent child small amounts of sex hormones are produced from the adrenal glands, located above each kidney. The adrenal synthesis of sex hormones continues throughout adult life, providing small amounts of both female and male sex hormones in all men and women.

As the child begins to experience hormonal shifts, she may also experience behavioral changes. The varying levels of sex hormones may bring on moodiness or depression. As secondary sex characteristics begin to develop at this time, the child may feel ambivalent as her familiar child's body begins to transform into an adult body. Periods of moodiness in the pubescent person are normal and should be treated as such.

The development of breasts, pubic hair, and

MALE AND FEMALE SEX HORMONES

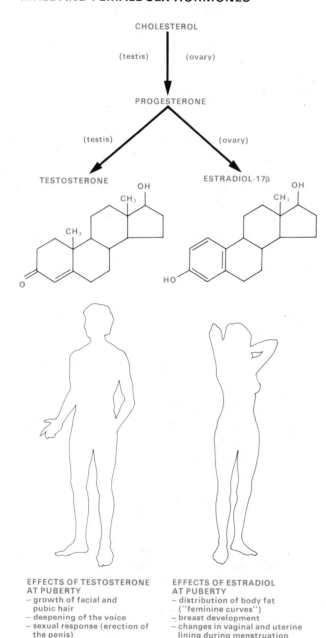

CHOLESTEROL

(testis)   (ovary)

PROGESTERONE

(testis)   (ovary)

TESTOSTERONE   ESTRADIOL-17β

EFFECTS OF TESTOSTERONE AT PUBERTY
- growth of facial and pubic hair
- deepening of the voice
- sexual response (erection of the penis)
- muscular development

EFFECTS OF ESTRADIOL AT PUBERTY
- distribution of body fat ("feminine curves")
- breast development
- changes in vaginal and uterine lining during menstruation
- distribution of body hair

Testosterone is the male sex hormone and estradiol and estrone are the two major female sex hormones (estrogens); they play important roles in the development and function of the adult. Both testosterone and estradiol are manufactured by the body from cholesterol, and as the illustration shows, the molecular structure of these hormones is remarkably similar. Both the male and female sex hormones—testosterone and estrogens—can be prepared synthetically for therapeutic use.

external genitalia progresses in well-ordered stages corresponding to the maturation of internal organs. J. M. Tanner, a psychologist and writer on adolescent development, has described the external development process in five stages. Pubic-hair development in both males and females starts at stage 1 with no hair growth. Stage 2 is the first appearance of pubic hair, which is sparse, light in pigmentation, and fairly straight. In males, hair growth begins at the base of the penis; in females hair growth is seen first along the labia majora (the outside lips of the vulva). In stages 3 and 4, the pubic hair becomes coarser, darker, curlier, and spreads to cover the area surrounding the penis or the vulva completely. Stage 5 signifies mature adult distribution and hair characteristics. Pubic hair may spread to the inner thigh and abdomen in most men and some women, depending on their genetic makeup.

Male genital growth is outlined similarly in five stages. Stage 1 is prepubescence, when the penis and testicles are childlike in size and texture. In stage 2, the testicles enlarge and the scrotal skin begins to darken and roughen. There is only slight penile enlargement at this stage. At stages 3 and 4, growth of both testicles and penis continues. The development of the glans penis (head of the penis) occurs in stage 4, along with further darkening of the scrotal skin. As in pubic-hair growth, stage 5 brings full maturation and growth of penis and testicles.

Stage 1 of female breast development is the childlike flat areola (the darker skin surrounding the papilla or nipple). The breast bud forms in stage 2 as hormonal activity increases. A small bump is formed as the areola and papilla elevate. The diameter of the areola increases. Further elevation of breast bud and papilla occurs in stage 3, with continued enlargement of the areola. In stage 4 a second mound is formed as the areola and papilla enlarge and separate from the shape of the breast. Again stage 5 represents full breast growth. The areola falls back into a continuous line with the breast shape, while the papilla continues to project. Adolescent boys may experience some breast tenderness and swelling during puberty. This is confusing and worrisome to young men, but it is a normal consequence of hormonal activity and will eventually subside.

Spontaneous erections are a common and embarrassing experience of adolescent boys. The new high levels of testosterone can cause erections to occur with no perceived stimulation. This can happen sometimes several times a day and in inconvenient situations. The erection will subside by itself, and the incidence of spontaneous erections will decrease as the boy gets older. In the meantime, assuring the boy of his normalcy and understanding the embarrassment that he may feel can help him cope with the situation.

As the adolescent begins to develop mature breasts or testicles, it is wise to teach regular testicular and breast examination. Though the incidence of abnormal growth in the breasts or testicles is very low during adolescence, regular self-examination will set a precedent for the future; it helps the adolescent become familiar with his or her own unique structure, and aids in the early detection of any abnormal growth. The uncircumcised male should clean any smegma (normal white, cheesy secretion) that collects under the foreskin.

In addition to pubic-hair growth, the adolescent experiences increased body hair in the axilla, legs, and—in the male—the face and chest. Male facial hair usually appears between ages 14 and 16, varying widely from boy to boy. Shaving traditionally has been a significant step for males, but it can often be just as meaningful to girls. Having "too little" or "too much" hair is often distressing for both sexes.

■ Onset of Reproductive Capability— Menses

Menarche (first menstrual period) traditionally marks the beginning of "womanhood," though it is viewed differently among different individuals and cultures. Some young women find it a positive experience, while other young women find it extremely upsetting. Most young women fall somewhere in between.

As with all new experiences, it helps to be prepared and to have even a small idea of what is to be expected. Sometimes girls start menstruating much earlier than their parents expect, taking both generations by surprise. In North American populations, improved nutritional status and general state of health have lowered the average age of the menarche. There is no absolute normal age for a girl to start menstruating; it usually occurs between age 10 and 15 years. Often young girls feel very self-conscious about menstruating much sooner or much later than their friends. It is important to help the young girl at this time to recognize that each person is unique, and that each matures and develops at her own rate.

Menstruation is controlled by the body's levels

of estrogen and progesterone in relation to the levels of FSH and LH. The menstrual period encompasses the entire cycle. For simplicity's sake, this cycle is most often described as a period of twenty-eight days, but a normal period can range anywhere from twenty-one to forty days. The menstrual cycle is a process that includes maturation and release of the ovum, changes in the uterus to prepare for possible conception, and discarding of the ovum and uterine lining when conception does not occur.

Every woman is born with all the ova she will ever produce in her two ovaries. The ova lie in their immature state until the hormonal system initiates maturation, and the woman begins to go through a monthly cycle.

Under the control of FSH and LH, each month an ovum matures and separates from one ovary or the other. FSH controls the growth of the follicle in the ovary, while LH controls actual ovulation. At ovulation, the mature ovum moves from the ovary into the adjacent Fallopian tube, where fertilization of the ovum occurs if sperm are present at this time. The ovum moves through the Fallopian tube, taking 5 to 6 days to reach the uterus; if it is unfertilized it dies within 24 hours and is discarded with the menstrual fluid. Spermatazoa can survive in the Fallopian tube for 24 hours or longer.

Ovulation usually occurs about midcycle. The ovum is able to be fertilized only in the Fallopian tube. Conception cannot occur once the ovum has left it. It is important to emphasize to the adolescent that ovulation is very hard to predict, and that prediction cannot be used as a method of birth control. (See discussion of ovulation earlier in this section, under *Pregnancy and Childbirth*)

Estrogen and progesterone cause the vaginal and uterine environment to go through many changes throughout the menstrual cycle in preparation for possible conception.

The length and characteristics of the menstrual flow vary from woman to woman. A typical flow lasts two to eight days. Daily average blood loss is from 30 to 100 milliliters, and daily average iron loss is from 0.5 to 1.0 milligrams. Adolescent menstrual cycles tend to be irregular for several years. The cycle may vary widely in length, sometimes skipping one to several periods in a row. Often the menstrual cycles are *anovulatory* (ovulation does not occur) for the first few years after menarche. Again, however, this is not true in all women and cannot be counted upon as protection for sexually active adolescents.

Cramping during the menstrual periods is usually associated with contractions of the uterus as it expels the menstrual fluid. These cramps are experienced in the pelvic, abdominal, and lower back regions. Though it is not the norm, some women experience extreme *dysmenorrhea* (painful menstruation). Dysmenorrhea will be discussed below in "Common Health Problems of Adolescents." (For more information about the female reproductive cycle, see above, "Pregnancy and Childbirth," and "Family Planning" later in this section.)

■ *Spermatogenesis*

Onset of reproductive capability in males is less discussed than the menarche. As stated previously, women are born with all the ova they will ever produce. The male, on the other hand, does not begin to make sperm (*spermatogenesis*) until after puberty is initiated, and then he continues to synthesize new sperm throughout his adult life.

Sperm production occurs in the testicles, protected by the scrotal sac located at the base of the penis. The testicles are located outside the body to ensure the optimal temperature for sperm production, which is a few degrees lower than normal body temperature. The scrotal sac has the ability to contract and bring the testicles closer to the body in cold temperatures, and to relax in order to keep the testicles farther away from the body when internal or external temperature increases.

Puberty and reproductive maturity in the male are initiated and controlled by some of the same hormones as in the female. Luteinizing hormone (LH) controls the secretion of the primary male sex hormone, testosterone, an androgen produced in the testicles. Follicle-stimulating hormone (FSH) in conjunction with testosterone is responsible for spermatogenesis. Testosterone also controls the normal growth and development of the testicles and penis and the secondary sexual characteristics.

Reproductive capability is marked by the boy's ability to ejaculate. This may happen first with masturbation, partnered sexual activity, or, very commonly, *nocturnal emission* ("wet dreams"). As with menarche, the normal age range of first ejaculation varies widely. Twelve to 16 years are common parameters for onset of puberty; spermatogenesis usually occurs one to two years later.

Nocturnal emission is caused by a buildup of seminal fluid in the seminal vesicles. It is an involuntary release during sleep often accompanied by dreams of a sexual nature. Nocturnal emissions persist into adulthood. Early discussion and preparation makes this important development easier for the adolescent boy to understand.

■ *Growth Spurt and Voice Changes*

As in toddlerhood, the child experiences a large growth spurt during adolescence. In females the growth spurt usually begins in stage 2 of puberty, and 90 to 95 percent of full height is reached by stage 5. Males usually begin the growth spurt at stage 3 and may reach complete height at stage 5, but they often continue to grow for the next five years. Males also experience an increase in muscle mass at stage 4. At this time the *epiphyses* (ends of the long bones in the arms and legs) fuse, thus limiting overall height. Adipose (fat) tissue takes on an adult distribution that is particularly noticeable in females. A huge increase in appetite may accompany the growth spurt.

During puberty the child will begin to experience skin changes. The *sebaceous glands* of the skin begin to manufacture more sebum (the normal lubricating substance of the skin), often leading to the common dilemma of excessively oily skin and acne. The *apocrine* sweat glands, located in the axillary (armpit) and genital regions, begin functioning. The apocrine glands produce more sweat than the *eccrine glands* located over the rest of the body. As adolescents begin to get oilier skin and an increased perspiration production, they will naturally become more interested in good hygiene, but may often need gentle reminding to ensure regular hygienic practice during the early years of adolescence.

Changes in the larynx bring *voice changes* to both the male and female, though much more noticeably in the male. As the vocal cords grow, the boy will often experience drastic changes in voice pitch, which often is manifested by embarrassing squeaking and cracking accompanied by periods of a surprisingly deep voice. These gradually modify to the deeper voice of the mature male. The female also experiences changes that cause her voice to become slightly deeper and fuller, though this occurs without disruption of voice sounds.

Psychosocial Changes in the Adolescent

Along with the major physical changes experienced in adolescence, the child goes through profound changes emotionally and mentally as she grows toward mature adulthood. After a period of relative order in her life as a child, adolescence brings upheaval. Order is disrupted, and the person begins to reevaluate herself in relation to her family, peers, and society as a whole. She needs to struggle to see herself as a separate human being, not just an extension of her family. Any period of great change can cause high levels of stress. The child is often confused, feeling sometimes all child, sometimes all adult, and usually a nonintegrated mix of the two.

Adolescence is similar in some ways to toddlerhood. As a toddler, the child learns to walk, speak coherently, feed herself, and control bladder and bowel elimination among other milestones. All these events work to bring the child a sense of autonomy and separateness from her primary caregiver. The adolescent, too, goes through great physical changes. The child leaves childhood, where most of her needs have been met by her parents, and enters adolescence, where she realizes that there is a vast world outside her familiar childhood environment.

Adolescence is a period of endless possibilities and choices. It is a time of discovery about oneself, one's parents and friends, about sexual relationships, and about the world as a whole. It is also a time of *ambivalence*: The child wants to grow up, yet wants to remain safe and secure as a child. She desperately needs to confirm her separateness and unique identity. She is easily frustrated by limits on her control. She may often become hostile and angry in response to perceived threats to her fledgling sense of independence.

Psychologically the adolescent has many tasks to complete in the change from childhood to adulthood. The developmental psychologist Erik Erikson has described each stage of the life cycle in terms of universal "tasks" that each person must successfully complete in her own way. He has described the adolescent period as one of "identity versus role confusion." He sees the formation of "identity" as an ongoing process throughout the stages of life. The adolescent incorporates the parts of herself developed as a child into a more unified and unique sense of identity. This is achieved through successful completion of infant and childhood tasks and the development of what is called "abstract thought."

Robert Havighurst, a human developmental specialist, has established several developmental tasks appropriate for assessing the adolescent's development. These include sexual identification and preparation for adulthood in terms of financial security, occupation, and intimate relationships. The adolescent must also develop an *ideology*, a set of ethics and values that will act as a guide. The development of an ideology helps the adolescent to become established as an independently thinking adult. She may often reassess the values she was raised with, and either reject them, modify them, or make them a part of her own personal values.

Erikson describes "role confusion" as the opposite of successful identity integration. With too many sudden changes and not enough support, the adolescent may experience feelings of self-doubt and insecurity. She may "over-identify" with certain life-styles or peer groups in trying to define her role and reestablish a feeling of order in her life.

This sense of confusion is normal to some degree in adolescents, as it is with persons of any age going through many changes. Confusion does not necessarily indicate abnormality. The adolescent is getting mixed messages. She is treated like a child but expected to act like an adult, and vice versa.

An important part of the adolescent period is the increase in understanding of the world. The Swiss psychologist Jean Piaget has published much work concerning the cognitive characteristics of each stage as the child grows toward adulthood. In the prepubescent school-age years, the child engages in what is called "concrete thought." Concrete thought allows the child to grasp the concepts of reversibility and the concreteness of objects and events. In adolescence, the person begins to develop "formal abstract" cognitive patterns.

The adolescent becomes able to think in terms of abstraction and hypothesis, to move beyond the realm of immediate experience and use reasoning to begin to understand other aspects of life. The development of abstract thinking makes the child more inclined to think about morals, values, and ethics. This aids significantly in the shaping of a well-formed identity.

Typical adolescent *rebelliousness* comes from a need to separate and control. The adolescent must assert independence and grasp control wherever possible. Parents often get the brunt of adolescent hostility and anger. The parent reminds the adolescent of the old child-parent dependent relationship, and when she feels threatened in her new role, she fights to make sure she does not lose it. The adolescent cannot always see that it is unnecessary to discard everything from her childhood in order to establish independence. With enough parental support and understanding during this time, the adolescent eventually is able to settle into a more comfortable adult parent-child relationship.

Adolescents use many things as a focus of their rebellion. Some may seem trivial, others may be very hurtful. Parents' unrelenting opposition to the adolescent's rebellion often causes the child to go to extremes. It is important to set limits on the child's behavior, however. The limits should be set for safety reasons, out of respect for others' feelings, and for the sake of the parents' sanity. The adolescent is often testing her parents to see how far she can go without creating an actual permanent break. A situation without any rules or limits is frightening; the adolescent needs room for rebellion and control, but she is still a growing child, without the experience or developmental maturity she needs to guide her through many situations.

Parents who are feeling helpless and desperate in the presence of a wayward teenager need to know that for the child the myriad physical, physiological, and hormonal changes of puberty are creating emotional turmoil. As part of normal, healthy development, the adolescent's self-awareness is at a peak, and her concerns are mainly directed inward. Change in body image can lead to a temporary loss of security, which may manifest itself in blatant hostility toward parents. Sexual arousal may be causing the adolescent to feel bewildered and without identity for a time.

It has been observed that some elements of "normal" teenage behavior, such as mood swings, depression, and regressive and antisocial behavior are quite similar to pathologic behaviors in adulthood characteristic of mental illness. Parents may find some relief by joining parental support groups, trying to maintain some line of communication with teenage children, and giving their adolescent rebels a little room to breathe and to grow.

The absence of blatant rebellion during adolescence does not necessarily prevent one from accomplishing the developmental tasks and attaining normal maturity. Adolescents have numerous ways of coping and creating a separate identity. It is important to note, however, that a continued dependent role with little or no development of independent thinking may be just as worrisome as a blatant challenge to authority. As described above, there are varying degrees of

adolescent behavior that may all be considered normal.

To promote full adolescent growth, the parent needs to recognize the changing relationship between the parent and the child, and listen to what the adolescent is communicating (verbally and nonverbally). It helps to use flexibility in the relationship and be prepared for what may seem to be the withdrawal of their child's love. This withdrawing behavior may flip back and forth as the adolescent attempts to define the separation and distancing. Parents should never forget that they also have rights during the adolescent years.

Some degree of depression is normal in the adolescent. This is often caused by the adolescent's confrontation with irrevocable changes as she grows from child to adult. The ordered, familiar world of childhood loses its security, and the adolescent faces fear of what may turn out to be unmanageable situations. Depression may center around sexual feelings and changing body image, worries about peer acceptance, doubts about achievements, and decisions about the future. Sometimes separation and loss of the child-parent relationship simply evokes feelings of sadness.

Adolescents are not immune from maladaptive, or *constitutional*, depression. Constitutional depression is that which is elicited by seemingly inconsequential circumstances, and is chronic in nature. Constitutional depression is often seen to run in families and is considered a pathological condition requiring professional treatment.

Suicidal ideation (expression of suicidal feelings or intent) and *gestures* are very common among adolescents. Suicide has become the third leading cause of death in the 15- to 24-year age group. Suicidal feelings and gestures are often an outcome of feelings of depression. The adolescent may be expressing an impulsive anger, a wish to hurt someone with her death. She may be acting out a plea for help in what she feels as unmanageable situations and feelings, or she may be truly self-destructive. Any suicidal ideation or gesture *must* be taken seriously.

Sometimes the adolescent is not expressing an actual desire to die but is making a statement that something in her life or feelings is not right. The adolescent should be questioned about her suicidal ideation. This can be frightening for the person who is presented with the situation, but it is often exactly what the adolescent is looking for. The degree of suicidal intention can be screened by questioning the person as to her actual plan of action; a well-thought-out, realistic plan suggests a more serious death intention. The adolescent's access to the means of death should be explored.

Any suicidal gesture calls for professional help. The adolescent may be acting impulsively, and the underlying emotional disturbances must be investigated. Suicidal ideation should be carefully evaluated for the degree of imminent danger. A third party, such as a physician, is often necessary for effective management of the situation.

Included in the emotional development of the adolescent are changes in social orientation. Usually, as a child the person spends a great deal of time with the family, associating to lesser degree with the peer group. As the child moves into adolescence and begins to separate from her family, her peer group becomes increasingly important. This change is often frustrating to the parents, when it seems as though the child is never at home anymore.

The peer group plays a major role in the stages of adolescent development. The peer group becomes a secure atmosphere as the adolescent distances herself from the family. Among her peers, the adolescent feels more comfortable expressing her feelings and exploring changes experienced in common. The peer group acts as a standard for what is normal and deviant, especially in terms of physical changes as the adolescent develops a heightened sense of her body image. Within the peer group, the adolescent begins to form close heterosexual and homosexual friendships, which act as a start for experiencing adult intimate relationships.

A healthy sense of competitiveness is developed as the adolescent refines her skills and achievements in comparison with what others are doing. Issues about life-style, career, and further education are explored and defined through the ideas of contemporaries. The peer group socializes and teaches the adolescent adult interaction, independent of the adolescent's role in the family. In the peer group, she is not viewed as part of her family, but as an equal and a participant.

As essential as the peer group is in adolescent development, it is often a source of distress. Cliques are common among adolescents and are exclusive by definition, leaving out those who do not fit the standard. Some adolescents have a few close friends but long to be included in a more "popular" group. The feelings of isolation and exclusion can be very painful at any point in life, but especially so during adolescence. Some people find other activities, which they may use to compensate for a lack they see in their social lives. Others react more maladaptively. Parents cannot plan or fix their children's social lives, but they can offer support and understanding in the inevitable painful periods of peer interaction.

Common Health Problems in the Adolescent

The great physical and psychological changes characteristic of adolescence cause many health problems. As adolescents mature, good health becomes crucial to ensure normal growth and development, both emotionally and physically. It is important during these years to build a strong foundation for optimal health through adulthood.

The adolescent may, through normal rebelliousness, ignore or blatantly refuse sound health care advice. The parent does not have the same degree of control of the child's health care as before. Often the adolescent does not share her health concerns with her parents or others out of a sense of shame, a need for privacy, or ignorance.

It is important for parents to become familiar with the common health problems of the adolescent and thus be able to anticipate and detect problems. Encouraging the adolescent to take responsibility for her own health care will facilitate the treatment of existing problems and promote a sense of responsibility in future health maintenance. The health problems discussed in this section do not belong exclusively to the adolescent period; nor do they include all the health problems that may be encountered in adolescence.

■ Acne

Acne is one of the most distressing and common problems of adolescence. As adolescents become acutely aware of their body image, blemishes on the face, chest, or back can be devastating to self-image and esteem.

Acne vulgaris is seen most commonly on the face, neck, shoulders, and back, since these are the areas with highest sebaceous gland activity. The sebacous glands produce sebum, which gives the skin an oily quality. Sebum is a normal and necessary skin product, which acts as both a natural moisturizer and a surface antimicrobial agent. At puberty, there is an increase in sebaceous gland activity, which makes the adolescent more prone to acne. Increased levels of androgens contribute to the incidence of acne. More boys than girls suffer with acne, but 80 percent of all adolescent girls develop it to some degree.

Sebum, keratin, and microbes commonly found on the skin contribute to the formation of the characteristic lesions of acne. A plug of matter forms that blocks a follicle duct in the skin. These impactions are referred to as *comedones* (blackheads). Due to the blockage, the duct becomes distended, causing local irritation to the tissue. If the lesion ruptures, infection may start, causing an inflammatory response. Acne vulgaris is usually described as either *noninflammatory* or *inflammatory*. Inflammatory acne generally is considered more severe, with larger, reddened, often pus-filled lesions that commonly leave scars on healing.

Acne often occurs in midadolescence and ranges from an occasional pimple to severely inflamed lesions. There is no clear evidence that acne is caused or exacerbated by any specific foods. It often continues into adulthood, though usually to a lesser extent.

There is no definitive cure for acne. Treatment usually is aimed at prevention of infection and permanent scarring and at improvement in appearance. For simple, noninflamed acne, the focus of treatment is frequent cleansing with mild astringents. Care should be taken to avoid excessive drying of the skin; it is wise to consult a dermatologist as to the most suitable products. Frequent washing of the affected area helps to remove the excess sebum and keratin, and works to prevent the formation of impactions. In all cases, squeezing the lesions should be avoided. This will only cause increased tissue damaged.

In more severe cases of acne, peeling agents are sometimes effective in reducing the lesions and preventing further formation. Peeling agents include astringents, creams, lotions, and ultraviolet light. They all cause a drying and increased sloughing of the skin. In severe inflammatory acne, antibiotic therapy is used in conjunction with topical medication.

■ Infectious Mononucleosis

Infectious mononucleosis is caused by a virus of the herpes family, and most often in the 12- to 25-year age group. It has been referred to as the "kissing disease," since it is commonly transmitted through intimate contact. The main route of transmission is by close salivary contact. Mononucleosis usually presents with vague symptoms, is self-limiting, and rarely causes serious complications. The disease has an incubation period of one to two months. The acute phase of the illness occurs at this point and lasts two to four weeks. During this period, the person generally complains of sore throat, mild fever, and enlarged lymph nodes, most often seen in the neck and groin areas. The symptoms may be accompanied by nausea, diarrhea, weight loss, chills, sensitivity to light, muscle and joint pain, and enlarged liver and spleen. Some jaundice may occur secondary to liver enlargement. After the acute period subsides, the person may experience an extended period of mild to severe fatigue lasting from a few weeks to months.

Treatment of mononucleosis is aimed at relieving the symptoms, since the disease itself resolves spontaneously. Aspirin or acetaminophen usually is given to relieve headaches, fever, chills, and any aches and pains. Bed rest is recommended, depending on the person's energy level. As long as there is evidence of an enlarged spleen, physical activities that risk blows to the abdomen or chest are discouraged in order to prevent rupture of the spleen.

Mononucleosis is rarely long-lasting and debilitating. Many mild cases go completely undetected. Serious complications such as forms of anemia, rupture of the spleen, or neurological problems are extremely rare.

■ Amenorrhea

Amenorrhea refers to the absence of menstrual flow. Amenorrhea is divided into two types, *primary* and *secondary*. *Primary amenorrhea* refers to delayed menarche, when menstruation is still not initiated by the age of 17. *Secondary amenorrhea* is the cessation of menstrual flow after the establishment of regular menstrual periods. Amenorrhea has several possible causes: hormonal dysfunction, anatomic abnormality, pyschological problems, and pregnancy.

Primary amenorrhea must be evaluated in relation to the stage of puberty. Even though puberty generally begins by 12 years, it is not initiated in some people until much later. Late onset of puberty may warrant further evaluation to rule out hormonal disturbances.

When puberty is under way and amenorrhea exists, the adolescent should be evaluated for anatomic defect, such as absence or malformation of the reproductive organs, the organs' inability to respond to hormonal stimulation, or anatomic obstruction to flow. Obstruction may be caused by an imperforate hymen or abnormal vaginal structure. These are usually correctable by surgical procedures.

Emotional problems may cause a delay in menarche. The adolescent may be experiencing great stress, often unconsciously, due to mixed feelings about growing up and becoming reproductively mature.

Secondary amenorrhea is often caused by hormonal changes, which may arise from severe emotional stress or sudden environmental change. Physical stress such as strenuous athletic training or extreme weight gain or loss may affect hormonal activity. Girls suffering from anorexia nervosa often experience amenorrhea.

Pregnancy is the most common cause of secondary amenorrhea, and this must always be checked, even if the girl denies sexual activity. The adolescent may have a strong sense of guilt and ambivalence about sexual feelings and activity, and may use denial to cope with these feelings. If incest or rape has occurred, the adolescent may also be afraid of actual or imagined retaliation.

Chronic illness can sometimes cause either primary or secondary amenorrhea. These illnesses include thyroid dysfunction, adrenal dysfunction, diabetes mellitus, and cardiac and kidney problems.

■ Dysmenorrhea

Dysmenorrhea refers to painful menstrual periods. A great many young women experience some degree of painful cramping during the menstrual flow; some experience severe cramping that becomes incapacitating. School and job absences in the female population are most commonly due to menstrual discomfort.

Dysmenorrhea is described as *primary* or *secondary*. Primary dysmenorrhea is most common. It is related to the release of normal body substances, *prostaglandins*. Prostaglandins increase contractions of the uterus in its effort to expel the menstrual fluid, and irritate the nerve endings in the uterine lining. Primary dysmenorrhea occurs only in ovulatory menstrual cycles, and is therefore less common in early adolescence.

Secondary dysmenorrhea is caused by anatomic defects, dysfunction of the uterine lining,

and adhesions related to infections. Secondary dysmenorrhea usually is not seen in adolescents.

The amount of menstrual discomfort, of course, varies from woman to woman, as does the perception of the cause of pain and the response to the pain. Menstrual pain should not be dismissed as an hysterical response to hormonal changes, or viewed as part of "being a woman." Significant pain indicates the need for effective treatment. Aspirin, acetaminophen, and ibuprofen are all effective menstrual pain-relievers. In some cases, the adolescent will need more aggressive treatment to alleviate the discomfort. Emotional aspects of the pain should be investigated when the situation indicates a need.

■ Dental Caries

Adolescents have a high incidence of dental caries (cavities), which are caused by inadequate dental hygiene, often compounded by inadequate hygiene as a child. Large quantities of "junk food" and candy contribute to the problem. As in other areas of health care, it is important that the adolescent practice regular dental care, including frequent dental checkups, to help prevent serious disease in the future.

Early adolescents may have the added responsibility of wearing corrective *orthodontic devices.* This is usually a cause of embarrassment to the child, who should be encouraged to practice very careful hygiene at this time and should be reminded of the benefits of the device.

■ Scoliosis

Scoliosis is a deformity of the spine involving some degree of curvature to one side. It can occur anytime throughout childhood. Causes of the spinal curvature can be congenital, traumatic, or compensatory for other structural defects. *Idiopathic* or *genetic scoliosis* often is seen in the adolescent as she begins the growth spurt toward skeletal maturity. Though it does occur in both males and females, adolescent girls are affected about eight times more often than adolescent boys. It may be suspected if one shoulder seems higher than the other.

Early diagnosis is extremely important for optimal recovery. The child should be evaluated for scoliosis from about 10 years of age until skeletal maturity. In mild to moderate scoliosis, there is rarely any discomfort or blatant disfigurement. If the curvature becomes more severe, the child will suffer from respiratory problems, cardiac problems, and pain related to nerve compression.

Screening for scoliosis can be done by observation. As the curve becomes greater, there will be noticeable asymmetry in the shoulders, pelvis, and hips. A screening involves having the undressed child bend over from the hips, and observing for any spinal deviation from the midline.

Treatment depends on the degree of curvature. If detected, very mild curvature can be treated with exercises, but it is difficult to detect visually.

Moderate curvature usually is treated with the external *Milwaukee brace*. The brace is made of plastic with steel parts and leather straps. It is worn from the neck, extending to the pelvic area, covering most of the buttocks in the back. The brace is not removed except for perhaps an hour a day, and daily exercises are necessary to ensure normal spinal and abdominal muscle maintenance. Usually the brace is needed for one to two years. Readjustment should be done every three months during this time. When skeletal maturity is reached, the brace is worn for gradually shorter periods, usually only at night, until bone maturity is absolutely certain.

In the case of more severe curvature, surgical correction is needed. Surgery involves fusing the spine and the internal placement of a rod to stabilize the spine. After surgery a jacket-like cast will be applied to the upper body to ensure optimal correction. The cast remains in place for six months.

The incidence of scoliosis is generally very traumatic for the adolescent. It is usually detected and treated just at the time when body image and peer-group participation are of extreme importance. Correction with the external brace can extend over years. Normal adolescent rebelliousness, combined with the child's desire to be "normal" and accepted by her peer group, often makes compliance with the corrective regime difficult. The brace does not limit movement, but it does limit types of clothing and certain activities, and it may elicit unfavorable reactions in people who view handicaps as a stigma. The adolescent will have to cope with these feelings.

With either method of correction, the adolescent needs much sympathy and understanding in order to maintain a positive self-image. Encouraging her to verbalize her feelings of frustration and anger is particularly important. Allowing her as much control and independence as possible will help to further her compliance with the corrective regime.

■ *Eating Disorders—Anorexia Nervosa, Bulimia, Obesity*

Sound nutrition in the adolescent is extremely important in order to ensure attainment of full height during the period of rapid growth and to lay the foundation of good health as an adult. But how to achieve this—especially as the adolescent begins to spend more and more time away from home?

Adolescents are notoriously prone to bizarre eating habits—ranging from unusual but healthful to unusual and life-threatening. In response to societal and peer pressure and to their own perception of their body image, adolescents (especially if female) may continually try new, fad diets. Snacking, especially on junk food, may deprive the child of needed vitamins, minerals, and protein. Forcing a proper diet may provoke further rebellion.

Allowing the adolescent to take more responsibility for good nutrition may be a more successful approach. Classes in school or informal discussions with professionals can help the adolescent learn sound nutritional principles, their own individual needs, and pleasant ways to meet them. Most adolescents are more concerned about their nutritional status than their parents are led to believe from their eating habits.

As annoying as some adolescent eating habits may be, medical intervention rarely is needed, except in cases of actual eating disorders such as anorexia nervosa, bulimia, and obesity.

Anorexia nervosa is a condition of extreme self-imposed limitations on nutritional intake resulting in severe weight loss to the point of starvation. The weight loss usually is very rapid. Females are affected ten times more often than males. Though it is most common among adolescents, anorexia nervosa may also be seen in children and adults.

There are many theories about the causes of anorexia nervosa. Most attention has been given to the psychodynamics of the disease, but there may be some evidence of hypothalamic malfunction in the brain as a factor also. Psychodynamically, the victim often manifests problems in asserting independence and control. She may have deep ambivalent feelings about growing up and about sexuality. Dynamics within the family structure may be strongly involved.

The victim is usually of normal weight or slightly overweight. A distorted body image may cause her to see herself as fat, even as she becomes dangerously underweight. Often an obsession with food is noticed; she may spend much time preparing food that she does not eat. As well as extreme dieting, the victim may engage in strenuous physical exercise, self-induced vomiting, and laxative abuse.

The victim may have other physical signs related to extreme weight loss. Amenorrhea is very common, as is a growth of fine downy hair (lanugo) on the body.

Treatment is aimed at correcting the malnourished state and treating the underlying emotional disturbances in the victim and family. The victim may need hospitalization with forced feeding and behavior modification. Psychotherapy is used in conjunction with the medical regime to explore the cause.

It is important to develop the victim's sense of responsibility toward her health and eating habits. This can help the adolescent use her desire for control and independence in constructive ways. It is important to remember that parents and other family members need a great deal of support during this time; they should not hesitate to seek counseling for themselves individually and as a family unit (see below, *Family Therapy*).

Bulimia often is associated with anorexia nervosa. Bulimia is defined as binge eating followed by self-induced vomiting. There often is no significant weight loss, and the condition may not come to medical attention until the victim seeks help.

Due to underlying emotional disturbances, the victim will compulsively overeat, then vomit. This purging is associated with feelings of guilt and fears of weight gain. Treatment is almost always on an outpatient basis. It is focused on weight gain if indicated, and on dealing with the underlying emotional distress. If bulimia goes untreated, the victim will often suffer from erosion of tooth enamel and esophageal lining from repeated contact with the acidic gastric contents. Loss of potassium through frequent vomiting may cause a chemical imbalance in the system, in severe cases leading to death from heart irregularities. Psychiatric treatment may also be necessary.

Obesity is a problem in all stages of life, but it is especially stressful in adolescents as they become more conscious of body image and sexuality, and seek both peer and societal approval. The majority of obese adolescents were obese as children, and the high percentage who remain obese as adults demonstrates the difficulty of successful treatment. As well as emotional problems, obesity increases the risks of many diseases and the dangers of any surgical procedure, and it can have detrimental effects on normal growth in the child and early adolescent.

Obesity is defined as an excess of 20 percent above ideal body weight for the person's height and build. Weight by itself is not always an accurate indication of true obesity. A person's skeletal frame and muscle mass must be taken into consideration to determine how much of the weight is fat deposits. Genetics appears to play a large part in childhood obesity. Though causes of obesity have been found in endocrine or metabolic malfunction, the number of these cases is minimal. Obesity due to overeating and lower activity levels is by far the rule.

Obese adolescents usually eat more and exercise less than normal-weight adolescents. They eat more at one time and eat more rapidly, often without hunger or the sense of satiation. Night eating is common. Sometimes obesity has more to do with lower activity levels than with the consumption of increased daily calories, but the prime cause is excessive intake.

The adolescent who is obese from childhood usually suffers early devaluation in a society that is extremely fitness oriented, and this can lead to low self-esteem. In adolescence, with its heightened sense of body image, obesity can mean a loss of self-worth. As the person experiences emotional distress from personal interactions with the peer group and society as a whole, she may resort to food as a gratification and comfort. Self-deprivation (dieting) fails because the emotional need for food is overwhelming. The continued obesity may begin to serve as an excuse for noninvolvement in deeper personal interactions, thus shielding her from the repetition of painful experiences.

To treat obesity successfully, all aspects must be taken into consideration. Since the early adolescent years are a period of rapid growth, adequate nutritional intake is essential. No one should follow a weight reduction plan that deprives the body of necessary nutrients, because the detrimental effects may be greater than the benefits of weight loss. Since this is especially true in adolescents, it is advisable to seek professional guidance in the development of a weight reduction plan. As the person goes through a tremendous growth spurt in puberty, *weight maintenance* diets rather than reducing diets are often used as a means of control. As the adolescent's height increases, the weight will be more evenly distributed over the frame.

Behavior modification techniques are widely used in weight loss treatment. It is important to help the person realize what the parameters of hunger and satiation are, learn to eat more slowly, and recognize the times of emotional stress that lead to seeking comfort in food. It is especially important to follow an exercise program together with calorie reduction. Exercise promotes appetite reduction and development of muscle and acts as diversion. Physical activity also can help the adolescent develop a sense of accomplishment in an area often avoided.

The adolescent needs great support in any weight reduction plan. She must find other ways to satisfy emotional needs besides food. To develop a necessary sense of motivation, it is helpful to use realistic and tangible benefits as incentives. The importance of food cannot be eradicated, and it is therefore necessary to provide the adolescent with low-calorie alternatives to high-calorie choices. Helping the adolescent participate in food preparation may aid in developing a sense of responsibility and control over her intake. Small changes are much easier to implement than drastic overhauls. Any goals and changes must be made with the adolescent's full participation, based on what she feels she can realistically accomplish.

Family support is essential for any plan. Parents and, if possible, siblings are encouraged to change eating habits at home. If the adolescent feels that she alone is being deprived, treatment rarely will be successful. Support groups can provide the adolescent with a place to feel accepted, a feeling often missed in peer interaction. Groups can promote weight loss through the use of normal adolescent competitiveness. The sense of isolation is diminished as the adolescent realizes she is not the only person attempting to lose weight.

The treatment of obesity can be difficult, slow, and frustrating. Though the problem often seems overwhelming to the adolescent, her family, and even professionals, the benefits of weight loss, both emotional and physical, are such that every effort should be made to assist the adolescent in a safe, effective reduction plan.

■ Substance Abuse

The use of drugs and alcohol is becoming an increasingly recognized problem among all adolescents. Adolescents may experiment with these in an exploratory manner, as a social activity, or as a means of escape from internal or external stressors. Substance use often is learned from adult role models, either in the immediate environment or through the media. It can be adopted as a means of demonstrating a level of sophistication. It can also be a way of displaying rebellion, or a means of forming a separation from the perceived oppressive adult standard of behavior.

The fear of drug and alcohol abuse can be overwhelming for parents of adolescents. These fears often lead parents to lecture incessantly or become excessively suspicious of "strange" behavior and social events. Though these fears are understandable, this kind of reaction can cause more harm than good. It is important for the parent to realize the prevalence of such use, while keeping in mind the importance of social interaction in adolescent development. It is most helpful to establish open communication with the adolescent about the subject of drug and alcohol use and abuse. In these discussions, the parent should try to avoid moralizing or directing blame at peers or at the adolescent herself. This may only cause alienation of the adolescent, with feelings of anger and increased confusion, and may further the possibility of substance misuse. Rather, in open, nonjudgmental discussions, the parent can help the adolescent learn and understand the nature of commonly abused substances, and the dangers of their use and abuse. Adolescents may be experiencing concerns about their own or their friends' habits, and may welcome a chance to express these concerns and to ask questions on the subject.

In speaking of drugs and alcohol, it is helpful to differentiate between commonly used terms. *Abuse* implies use of a substance for reasons other than medical, in a way that results in detrimental effects physically, psychologically, or socially. *Misuse* is used to describe the overuse of a substance, or bad judgment in its use. *Addiction* or *dependence* is the state of a physical or psychological need for the substance in order to function. The physical dependence is accompanied by a psychological dependence on the psychic effects of the substance.

There are many dangers involved. Impaired judgment due to alcohol or drugs can result in inappropriate social behavior, accidents (especially associated with cars), and incidences of violence. Physical damage is possible, such as alcohol-induced liver damage, coma from accidental overdose, or cognitive dysfunction due to organic damage to the brain. Substances abused often are illegal, which adds the danger of trouble with the law.

In adolescents drug abuse presents a high risk of developmental delay, which can result in maladaptive behavior into adulthood with an inability to use appropriate coping mechanisms.

If substance misuse or abuse is suspected, the parent should attempt frank confrontation and discussion. When this is not possible, a third party should be sought to explore the possibility with the adolescent. In any case of substance abuse, professional help is mandatory.

■ Accidents and Injuries

Accidents account for most of the adolescent deaths in this country. Common accidents involve automobiles, drowning, falls, and firearms. Most of these accidents are made more tragic by their preventability.

Accidents and injuries often are caused by reckless, impulsive behavior. This kind of behavior may be due to an overabundance of energy which adolescents dispel by pushing themselves to the limit—at high speeds in cars, in daring competitions, or by straining their physical capabilities.

Sports injuries are especially common among adolescents, due partly to their fierce sense of competitiveness. Another factor is the mismatching of children in different stages of physical maturity in sports activities.

Prevention of accidents and injuries is difficult. Parents, teachers, and health providers should work together to supply safe means of physical outlet, while informing adolescents about the vulnerability of the human body.

Adolescent Sexuality

Emerging sexuality is one of the most obvious changes of adolescence. The adolescent grows from a child, who may have minimal interest in sex, to a person who sometimes thinks of nothing else. Adolescents begin to have sexual feelings and physical sexual responses, and through pyschosocial development they begin to see the possibilities of sexual relationships.

Everyone's sexuality develops at its own pace. Some adolescents begin to take a distinct interest in sex in very early adolescence, while others start much later. In American society children are confronted with multitudes of sexual issues from an early age, especially through the media. Adolescents often are led to believe that since "everyone else" is having sex, they should too. As they strive to achieve their identity as adults, adolescents are particularly vulnerable to this kind of influence, which puts them at risk of becoming involved in situations they might not be ready for.

Sexuality is an essential part of every person, and it is important to help adolescents adjust to their emerging sexuality. Parents should be ready to discuss issues of sexuality in general and how they pertain to the adolescent's own life. What are her feelings about her own sexual development? What does she do or want to do in terms of sexual activity?

Sexuality can be very frightening for the parents of adolescents. It seems to be tangible evidence that they are losing the dependent child. The parent may watch the adolescent beginning to explore sexuality and feel overwhelmed by the thought of what lies before the child—all the complications and risks of sexual relationships. The parent may be troubled by moral questions concerning adolescent sexual activity, or premarital sexual activity in general, which the child does not share. These issues rarely are resolved by lecturing or attempting to lay down strict rules, nor are they resolved by ignoring the situation. No one can become instantly comfortable with a situation just because he or she is forced to confront it. Thus it is helpful to the parent as well to discuss with the adolescent her feelings and her related concerns about sexual activity.

Adolescents often experience *guilt feelings* associated with sexual thoughts and activities. These may arise from past associations, from blatant warnings against sexual feelings and activities, or from the natural confusion and ambivalence of adolescence. As the adolescent becomes more comfortable with her sexuality, these feelings usually are resolved, though some experiences may lead to deeper feelings of guilt and indicate a need for professional help.

As adolescents become more aware of their sexual feelings, they commonly spend much of their time daydreaming in sexual fantasy. This provides an opportunity to explore new feelings in a safe and controlled situation. Sexual fantasies help adolescents begin to see themselves as sexual persons, and to adapt to this role.

Masturbation is often rediscovered in adolescence from early childhood when children first discover their genitalia. Masturbation is as individual as any other sexual activity. Some individuals masturbate all through childhood. Others start again in adolescence, while others never feel the need to masturbate. Masturbation is a way for adolescents to further explore their sexual feelings and their unique physical responses. It can help ease the transition into sexual relationships: The young person becomes used to responding sexually and these feelings become less strange and confusing. Familiarity with one's own body is useful in providing effective sexual education, and helps to promote a sense of sexual responsibility.

As adolescents begin to explore sexuality with others, *homosexual issues* may arise. Homosexual feelings and activity are common as the young person struggles with identity formation in conjunction with the arrival of strong sexual feelings. It is not unusual for a child or adolescent to begin to discover sex with a good friend of the same sex. Homosexual feelings and activity may pass as the adolescent begins to feel more comfortable in sexual situations, or these feelings may grow toward a definite homosexual orientation.

With our society's strong bias toward heterosexuality, an adolescent who experiences either passing or permanent homosexual feelings and activity may find this a source of distress. He or she may need support in order to understand these feelings and cope with them.

Sexually transmitted diseases (STDs) are among the risks of sexual activity. The adolescent should have correct information concerning common diseases, methods of transmission, symptoms, treatments, and prevention. STDs carry a strong connotation of shame, which often prevents adolescents from obtaining necessary information and treatment. The adolescent should understand that STDs are very common and should be approached like any other illness. Lack of information and education will lead only to increased numbers of cases of preventable diseases and ineffective treatment of existing cases.

The most common STDs include gonorrhea, herpes, syphilis, non-specific urethritis, venereal warts, and pubic lice. *Gonorrhea* is caused by the transmission of a bacterium from an infected person to another. The bacteria live only in warm, moist, dark places such as the vagina or penis. They soon die on contact with air. Gonorrhea cannot be contracted through inanimate objects (doorknobs, toilets seats) or nonintimate contact. Symptoms in the female include vaginal discharge that is white, yellow, or green in color. Painful urination and lower abdominal pain also may occur. If infection has occurred in the throat or anus, the women will experience a sore throat or anal discharge. Males may exhibit painful urination, with an intermittent or continuous discharge from the penis. Sore throat or anal discharge can occur also. There may be no symptoms at all: 80 percent of all infected women and 10 to 20 percent of men will be asymptomatic.

Gonorrhea is treated with a course of antibiotics. Untreated gonorrhea will not go away by itself. It can cause permanent damage to the reproductive organs, resulting in sterility. Women with untreated gonorrhea who give birth risk passing the infection to the baby's eyes, which, if untreated, could cause blindness. Sexual activity should not be resumed until follow-up tests have shown the infection to be cured. Transmission can be prevented through the use of condoms or discussing with potential partners the possibility of infection.

Herpes is caused by a highly infectious virus passed via close contact. Herpes type I occurs as cold sores in or around the mouth. Cold sores are not usually passed by sexual contact. Herpes type II is usually found in the genital region and is associated with sexual contact. Herpes lesions appear as eruptions or blisters at the area of transmission. They are usually very painful. Once the virus has entered the body, it is there for life. The lesions are not active continuously, but occur in intermittent outbreaks. Transmission occurs through direct contact with a herpes sore, very often from the genitalia of one person to another. Transmission can occur while the sores are present, or up to twenty-four hours before they appear.

After contact, the initial outbreak may appear one to three weeks later, but could occur up to a year later. Before the appearance of the sores, the person experiences a tingling in the affected area. The sores then appear as painful blisters which sometimes ooze fluid. The sores may last up to two weeks, then go away by themselves.

At this time, there is no cure for herpes. A good measure of control is possible with a drug called Acyclovir. Once contracted, the virus remains in the person's peripheral nerves. The number and frequency of subsequent outbreaks is highly individualized. Outbreaks are often precipitated by stress, emotional upset, fatigue, illness, or excessive exposure to sunlight. The subsequent outbreaks are usually less severe than the first. During an outbreak, the person should avoid all sexual contact. He or she must also be careful to prevent spreading the sores from one part of the body to another, especially the eyes, where corneal ulceration could occur. Keeping the sores clean and dry will help healing and prevent bacterial infection.

The best form of prevention is to avoid sexual contact with a person who has active lesions. It helps to ask potential partners if they have herpes; using condoms will add extra protection.

Syphilis is less common than gonorrhea or herpes, which have reached epidemic proportions. But syphilis still exists, and can cause very serious damage if left untreated. Syphilis is caused by a spirochete that enters the body through a mucous membrane. The disease is divided into three separate stages. The first stage is characterized by a painless sore at the point of contact, called a *chancre*. The chancre will disappear in about six weeks, whether the disease is treated or not. The chancre may occur inside the vagina or anus, and since it is not painful, it may go undetected.

The second stage of the illness appears several months after the first. The person may develop a generalized rash with flu-like symptoms. These also will disappear by themselves. If the disease is allowed to go into the third stage, many systems of the body may be affected, possibly leading to death.

Diagnosis of syphilis is made with a blood test, and the disease is then treated with a course of antibiotics. Sexual activity should be avoided until a follow-up test confirms successful treatment. Untreated syphilis can pass from a pregnant woman to the fetus, causing possible problems at birth. Use of condoms and avoidance of promiscuous sexual activity can prevent transmission of this disease.

Venereal warts are wart-like bumps occurring in or around the vagina, anus, penis, or testicles. They are caused by a virus. Usually the warts are painless, but they may become irritated and itchy. Diagnosis is made by direct observation. Treatments include application of an ointment that kills the virus, freezing the warts and removing them, or surgical removal. If the warts are not treated they will become larger and more numerous.

Pubic lice ("crabs") can be transmitted through close contact, or shared clothing or bed linen. They are highly contagious. The first symptom is usually a severe itching in the genital area. The lice are found usually in the pubic hair and can be seen with the naked eye. Pubic lice must be treated with a prescription shampoo. All clothing and bedding should be washed in normal detergent and hot water to kill any lice or eggs.

In the event of an STD, the adolescent needs much support and understanding—especially since she may view her condition as shameful. The widespread incidence of STDs and the need for treatment should be emphasized and information provided so as to prevent future infection.

Sexual transmission is also a means of contracting the deadly disease *AIDS,* or acquired immunodeficiency syndrome, which has grown from a rarity in the early 1980s to an epidemic among certain population groups. AIDS, which is caused by infection with the human immunodeficiency virus (HIV), is spread through unprotected sexual contact with an infected person (as well as through sharing of contaminated needles with an infected drug user, transfusions of contaminated blood products—before blood donations began to be screened for HIV—and across the placenta to the fetus of an infected woman during pregnancy). AIDS destroys the body's immune system, rendering its victims unable to fight off infections that would otherwise do no harm. It is most common among homosexual and bisexual men and intravenous drug users, but it has been found in some preschool, schoolage, and adolescent children.

Adolescent Pregnancy

The increasing number of pregnancies in adolescents points up the great need for effective birth-control counseling. Embarrassment may prevent the adolescent from seeking effective birth control. Often adolescents have received misinformation about contraceptive methods. They may believe that practices such as withdrawal or douching are adequate to prevent pregnancy, or they may be ignorant of the mechanical aspects of effective birth-control methods. Characteristic of the adolescent period, the person may feel ambivalent about her sexuality. She may not want to admit even to herself that she is contemplating or engaging in sexual activity. Obtaining and using birth control adds a tangible aspect to sex, which she may wish to avoid.

Many adolescent boys are not taught that preventing pregnancy is also their responsibility, so they leave it all to their partner. Often adolescents are unable to see the consequences of their actions. They may believe they cannot become pregnant or cause pregnancy because they are "sterile," or because it is "the first time," or because they do not have sex "often" enough. There is no evidence that providing information about such matters will promote sexual activity—as is argued by some opponents of sex education in schools.

Providing birth-control counseling and access to adequate information is paramount in preventing unwanted pregnancies and in teaching adolescents responsibility for their sexual lives. Pregnancy occurring in an adolescent brings with it the possibility of problems in every aspect of the person's life. The girl is at a vulnerable stage physically, emotionally, and socially. Pregnancy at this point can be very detrimental.

Physically, the girl is going through rapid growth. She needs abundant calories and protein to ensure her own normal growth; pregnancy only increases her need for calories and protein. The added burden of pregnancy in the still-growing body puts both the pregnant girl and the fetus at risk for growth impairment and related problems. Because of these factors, adolescent pregnancy is almost always considered high-risk in terms of prenatal care and delivery. Younger adolescents are in much greater danger, since they are usually in the middle of the growth spurt. The risk decreases in middle and late adolescence.

Emotionally, the girl may still be very much a child. She is going through a separation from her family and trying to establish independence. Though many adolescent girls feel that pregnancy will firmly establish their independence and adulthood, it often accomplishes the opposite. Adolescents are rarely able to support themselves financially, much less a baby as well. Financial circumstances alone may throw the adolescent back into a directly dependent role.

An adolescent parent must deal not only with her own psychosocial development, but she becomes responsible for the well-being and normal development of a demanding infant. This is a challenge for the best-equipped adults; for an adolescent who is dealing with rapid change and identity-formation in herself, it can be overwhelming. Ideally, a mother should have the mental development or experience to realize the extent of the responsibility of child-rearing. But the adolescent is still part child. Her visions may be very idealistic, but they have little basis in reality.

As social contacts, peer interaction, and developing relationships take on great significance, the pregnant adolescent often finds herself left out. This is even more likely after the baby is born. The resentment may lead her to ignore her baby's needs rather than isolate herself further from normal adolescent activities.

The pregnant adolescent may believe that the pregnancy will solidify her relationship with the father of the baby. Though many adolescent fathers remain active and supportive in both the baby's and mother's lives, more often the girl finds herself abandoned with the pregnancy and the consequences. The adolescent may not have all the support, resources, and options that an adult would enjoy. A feeling of resentment, coupled with a lack of complete understanding and emotional development, increases the risk of child abuse and neglect. This is not to imply that adolescents cannot be excellent parents, or that parenthood necessarily inhibits their normal development into adults. But the adolescent who decides to continue her pregnancy and to keep the child will require unfailing support and understanding in every aspect of her life in order to make the situation as healthy and successful as possible.

Adolescent fathers are often forgotten in the problem of adolescent pregnancy. They are viewed commonly as the villains who are shirking responsibility. Adolescent fathers are often not given a chance to help in the parenting process or to offer their support. They are as limited in their independence and emotional maturity as the mother. Fear and confusion may prevent them from asserting themselves in the situation. The occurrence of pregnancy can be as devastating for them as it is for the girl, and they are often not given the support they need.

Several options are now available for the pregnant adolescent. Many girls are choosing to terminate the pregnancy with voluntary abortion. In some states abortions can be obtained without parental consent. In the early stages of pregnancy, abortion is a safe, relatively painless, and brief procedure. It is wise for the adolescent choosing abortion to make this decision *early* in the pregnancy, since this eliminates many of the risks of the more complicated abortion procedures performed after twelve weeks of pregnancy.

Deciding to have an abortion is never an easy process. The adolescent may have an especially difficult time in making this decision and in coping with her feelings after the procedure. She needs help and counseling at this time to facilitate the decision-making and to come to the best option for herself and the situation. Though it is important to offer help, it is essential that the adolescent make the decision *herself*. She should never be forced into either having the baby or having an abortion. Options, feelings, and realities must be thoroughly discussed in order to help the girl come to the best decision. She will need further support no matter what the decision is. (See above, *Pregnancy and Childbirth*, and *Family Planning*, in the next chapter.)

Adolescence may seem fraught with danger and pain, but adolescents and their parents should not forget that this is a time of change and growth leading to a desirable outcome. The actual process of change can be a wonderful experience, both stimulating and painful. In the more painful times, the parent and adolescent should try to keep a broad perspective, and remember that anticipation and good preparation help to ease the difficult periods and enhance the joyful ones.

15

FAMILY PLANNING

The decision of whether or not to have children is one that will affect the quality of your life for many years, and it should not be made lightly. Many modern couples weigh the costs and responsibilities of raising children and deliberately and responsibly choose not to make that commitment. Other couples decide to postpone having children until they have attained a particular age, life-style, or career level. In planning their family, they are planning their future.

The term *family planning* is an important one that should be fully understood. Family planning includes not only birth control and contraception but also planned pregnancy, voluntary termination of pregnancy (abortion), voluntary sterilization, and, in some cases, medical investigation of fertility and extreme measures such as *in vitro* fertilization or artificial insemination. In many cases, family planning also includes adoption of children. The quality of family life depends in large part on careful, successful, mutual family planning.

INFERTILITY

The strict medical definition of infertility is the inability of a couple to conceive after at least one year of unprotected, regular sexual intercourse. If the woman is 30 years old or more, she and her partner should probably begin investigation of their fertility problem after six months to avoid losing too many potentially fertile years. "Infertility" can also describe a woman's recurrent inability to maintain a pregnancy to a time when the fetus is viable outside the womb. Having successfully borne children does not preclude the possibility of a couple becoming infertile later.

It is estimated that 10 to 15 percent of all couples in the United States are infertile by the above definition. The inability of a couple to bear children, or to conceive more children after the first one or two, can place a severe strain on their relationship, even leading to the dissolution of the marriage. In dealing with this extremely sensitive issue, the couple should seek the help of a physician who specializes in fertility and conception. The causes of infertility in a particular couple must be clearly understood, and neither partner should be made to carry blame or guilt for the failure to have a child.

Primary fertility exists when a couple has never conceived; *secondary infertility* occurs when a couple has difficulty conceiving or carrying a pregnancy to viability after already successfully giving birth to at least one child. Even if one or both partners have successfully fathered or borne children with other partners, it does not necessarily mean that the present partner is automatically the cause of the infertility. It can seriously hinder the investigation of fertility when one partner refuses to undergo tests on the grounds that he or she has already demonstrated fertility.

The components of fertility are deceptively simple. The man must be able to produce a sufficient number of normal, motile (freely moving) sperm. The male reproductive tract must have passages that are open to allow the sperm to pass through, and the ejaculation must be sufficient to deposit the sperm near the woman's cervix. The sperm must be able to ascend through the cervix, despite thick cervical secretions, move up through the uterus, and reach the Fallopian tubes. All of this must take place at or around the time of ovulation, since the life of a sperm is no longer than seventy-two hours.

In the woman, each reproductive cycle must result in a normal, fertilizable ovum (egg) that moves from an ovary into the Fallopian tube. Once united with the sperm, the fertilized ovum must continue down the Fallopian tube into the uterus, where it meets a receptive endometrium (uterine lining) that allows it to implant, grow, and develop into a healthy fetus. The products of conception (placenta, amniotic sac and fluid) and the ovarian hormones must nourish and maintain the pregnancy to a time when the fetus can survive outside the womb.

■ *Variations in "Normal Fertility"*

It generally takes five to six months of unprotected intercourse for pregnancy to occur. In 20 percent of cases, conception occurs within the first month. A great many couples, however, require as much time as two to five years or more before they have their first baby, despite an absence of factors causing infertility. Besides this normal variation in the ability of couples to conceive, a person's fertility varies throughout his or her reproductive life. A woman's fertility generally decreases somewhat as she approaches menopause; in men the pattern is not so clearly understood.

It would appear that something like "luck" or chance is involved in the ability to conceive; clearly, it is more than just physical and physiological ability. It is known, for example, that psychological factors are important in a couple's ability to conceive. Emotional difficulty can undermine a woman's fertility, and in extreme cases it can produce amenorrhea (absence of menstrua-

tion). Any woman who has stopped having periods temporarily because of a geographical move, an extreme change in life-style, or an emotional trauma can testify to this. In a more practical sense, marital difficulty can sometimes delay conception by perhaps reducing the frequency of sexual intercourse. All of these factors, plus the unknown—the "luck factor"—can play a part in family planning.

Examination and Assessment

Before a couple seek medical intervention for their apparent "failure" to conceive, they should consider a number of factors. If they are 25 or younger, many physicians might advise them to "keep trying" for another year or so after the traditional medical definition of infertility has been met before undergoing a complete infertility workup. The couple at any age should consider the frequency and timing of their intercourse and look for obvious problems—for example, a partner who is constantly traveling for business purposes. A "fertility problem" can result if one partner works nights while the other works during the day; each partner is tired out at a time when the other is most interested in having sex.

It is important to remember, too, that despite the strict medical definition of infertility, it is entirely possible for a couple to miss conceiving at the crucial midcycle time in the woman's fertility cycle every single month for a year without actually being infertile. For this reason, many physicians are reluctant to undertake a fertility workup until the couple has tried to conceive for at least two years. If the woman is over 30 years old, the workup might be hastened, as mentioned earlier.

If you do feel you meet the criteria for a potential fertility problem and you decide to seek medical help, it is useful to have an idea of what to expect.

■ *Medical History*

The physician will ask both of you about any prior pregnancies and their outcome (with other partners as well as together), any spontaneous abortions (miscarriages) or voluntary abortions, cesarean sections, pelvic or abdominal operations, and diseases of the endocrine, circulatory, and digestive systems (such as hypothyroidism, diabetes, and ulcerative colitis, all of which can affect fertility indirectly or directly). The physician will want to know the woman's menstrual history: whether or not she has always had regular menstrual periods, at what age she experienced menarche, whether she experiences dysmenorrhea (painful periods), and any signs or symptoms she might have that would suggest ovulation (changes in vaginal discharge, abdominal pain occurring midway between menstrual periods, and changes in basal body temperature).

A thorough sexual history will be taken, including questions about the number and frequency of previous relationships, use of contraceptives of all types, the fertility of former partners, how long the current relationship has lasted, and any previous fertility evaluations. There is known to be a positive relationship between the number of sexual partners and the incidence of pelvic inflammatory disease (PID) and subsequent infertility. You will be asked about frequency and regularity of current sexual intercourse, different positions used for intercourse, and use of lubricants and douches (many vaginal lubricants and douches are spermicidal).

The physician will probably also ask about the results of previous gynecological exams, especially if any abnormalities were noted. He or she will also ask about any gynecological treatments for chronic infection or abnormal Pap tests (which could suggest potential abnormalities of cervical mucus); any history of sexually transmitted disease; all medications used, current and past; and prior use of fertility drugs.

■ Investigation of the Male Partner

Sperm count: Strict numbers of sperm do not necessarily dictate fertility or infertility. In general, if a man's sperm count falls below 60 million per cubic centimeter of ejaculate, he may have difficulty fathering a child, but there are exceptions to this rule. Sperm count will, as a rule, be increased by abstaining from sex for several days; many experts suggest that serious attempts at conception should involve abstinence for two to three days before the twelfth or thirteenth day of the woman's cycle. Additionally, having sex as often as two or three times a day is believed by some fertility specialists to decrease sperm counts to below the optimum level for conception.

Sperm type and quality: To determine that sperm are normal and motile, a large proportion of those viewed under a microscope should be completely motile and have normal shapes.

Causes of low sperm counts include congenital

abnormalities, undescended testis or testes (one testis or both testes remaining in the abdominal cavity in early infancy instead of descending into the scrotal sac), and diseases that affect the testes, such as mumps, gonorrhea, or syphilis. In addition, a sedentary life-style, living in high altitudes for long periods of time, and raising the temperature of the genital area (by too-tight underwear or trousers, too-frequent hot baths, or other factors) have all been shown to contribute to low sperm counts. Some drugs, such as marijuana, alcohol, antidepressants, and antipsychotic agents, have been linked to changes in male hormonal cycles and hence to low sperm counts or other reproductive problems.

Semen analysis involves collecting ejaculate in a sterile container following masturbation or intercourse and examining a specimen under a microscope within a few hours. It is useful to abstain from intercourse for two to three days before the analysis. Normal ejaculate should be alkaline in pH and should contain more than 60 million sperm per cubic centimeter; at least 80 percent should be motile, while fewer than 20 percent should have abnormal (nonoval) forms.

Reproductive-tract patency: Congenital misplacements of the urethral opening to the penis, also called *hypospadia* and *epispadia*, can prevent ejaculation of semen close to the cervix. (This condition can be corrected surgically and usually is detected in infancy.) A more common and less obvious problem is a *varicocele*, a varicosity of veins in the reproductive passages of the male. This can cause low sperm counts, reduced sperm motility, and inadequate development of the testis. In addition, an enlarged prostate gland (*prostatitis*) can exert pressure on surrounding structures, blocking passage of sperm. Prostatitis usually can be treated with medication to permit normal ejaculation and a varicocele can be corrected surgically.

Hormonal disorders: These are less common causes of infertility in men than they are in women, but occasionally thyroid disorders, diabetes, or *hyperprolactinemia* can interfere with fertility in men. In this last condition, the man has abnormally high levels of the hormone prolactin. This can be treated with administration of another hormone.

Other factors: It is estimated that at least 5 percent of all infertility, male and female, is related to psychological and emotional factors. No matter which partner appears to be the infertile one, psychological stress can affect the couple as a unit and can by itself interfere with fertility. Stress can cause hormonal imbalances and behavioral changes and must be regarded as a major factor— or at least "ruled out"—in any infertility investigation.

Premature ejaculation, in which the male partner discharges semen before entering the woman or immediately upon entering her vagina, can result in sperm being placed too far from the cervix to fertilize an ovum. Likewise, the use of just one position for intercourse could play a part in misdepositing the sperm. Suggested positions to enhance the ascendance of sperm to the cervix include elevation of the woman's hips during intercourse and using the male-superior position with the woman remaining on her back for at least one hour afterward.

Male chromosomal or genetic abnormalities can result in infertility that is not treatable. Chromosome damage can be caused by chemical and radiation exposure, resulting in low sperm count and large numbers of abnormal sperm. This damage is usually permanent and, even if conception is successful, might result in a chromosomally abnormal offspring. On the other hand, men who have undergone chemotherapy or radiation therapy for cancer often have lowered sperm counts and abnormal sperm cells as a temporary condition (up to five years after treatment is discontinued). There is a possibility, however, of potential birth defects from conception that occurs after chemotherapy or radiation treatment. One alternative is to have the husband donate sperm to a sperm bank before cancer treatment is undertaken, so that the wife may later be artificially inseminated with her husband's normal sperm.

■ *Investigation of the Female Partner*

Anovulation (*absence of ovulation*): Approximately 10 to 15 percent of infertility is caused by abnormalities of ovulation; either pregnancy or the surgical recovery of ova from the woman is the only absolute proof that ovulation exists. It is possible for a woman with normal menstrual cycles to fail to produce an ovum with each cycle. Nevertheless, even a woman who ovulates only three or four times a year may have no difficulty conceiving.

Anovulation is one of the first things that must be ruled out in the investigation of the woman. Certain factors in the woman's history are strongly suggestive of normal ovulation: for example, a history of regular menstruation, changes in mucus discharges from the vagina, changes in libido, midcycle spotting, breast tissue changes, and lower abdominal discomfort at midcycle. If you are a woman with lengthened menstrual cycles, infrequent periods, or cycles longer than thirty-five days or shorter than twenty-one days, you are more likely to have some sort of ovulatory dysfunction than a woman who has normal, twenty-eight day cycles.

After the ovum is released from the ovary, the uterine lining increases in thickness and produces secretions to aid in implantation of a fertilized ovum. At the same time, the woman's basal body temperature (BBT) rises approximately 0.5° to 1° Fahrenheit (0.5° Centigrade), and remains a little higher in the second half of the menstrual cycle if ovulation has occurred. In addition, the ovary produces greater quantities of the hormone progesterone during the second half of the cycle in preparation for the nurturing of a fetus; this higher level of progesterone can be detected with a blood test.

A simple way to determine if ovulation is occurring is the BBT chart. If ovulation occurs, the BBT reaches its low point near the time of ovulation, then rises. A BBT chart is made by the woman taking her temperature at the same time every day (in the morning before arising) and plotting the values on a graph. This should be done for at least a few months if not longer to determine whether regular ovulation occurs. Another test of ovulation is the obtaining of progesterone levels in blood at significant times in the menstrual cycle. At the same time, cervical mucus changes can be observed by the woman on a daily basis and noted in a diary; moreover, specimens can be analyzed by the physician. Normally, just prior to ovulation, the cervix produces more mucus, and the mucus becomes more stretchable, forming a characteristic pattern on a microscope slide.

Still another way to determine if ovulation is occurring is home prediction tests, which use artificially manufactured antibodies to measure levels of *luteinizing hormone*. LH levels normally rise twenty-four to twenty-six hours before ovulation. Pap smears taken in a series during the cycle can document maturation of vaginal cells under the influence of estrogen, suggesting normal hormonal variations. *Endometrial biopsy*, which involves taking a very small sample of the uterine lining and examining the cells, is a very accurate way to determine if ovulation is taking place. Usually it is performed in a doctor's office with very little discomfort to the patient. This test, however, would be used only if simpler tests, such as the BBT chart, were inconclusive or yielded suspicious results. Finally, ultrasound scanning is being used increasingly to demonstrate development of *ovarian follicles*, the immature ova cells, and ovulation.

Anatomical abnormalities: In rare cases the uterus, ovaries, or both may have congenital abnormalities that have prevented their development. This usually results in absence of menstruation. More commonly, Fallopian tubes are blocked by scar tissue or congenital obstruction, preventing passage of sperm to the ovum or movement of the fertilized ovum down into the uterine lining. Scar tissue may be formed without the woman knowing it from a bout of pelvic inflammatory disease (PID), gonorrhea, or chlamydial infection. Use of an intrauterine device (IUD) can cause a low-grade inflammatory condition of the uterus that can create scar tissue. Additionally, having an *ectopic pregnancy* (implantation of fertilized ovum *outside* the uterus), especially in the Fallopian tube, can cause a serious medical condition, especially if the pregnancy goes undetected until the conceptus ruptures. Rupture of an ectopic pregnancy results in bleeding into the pelvic cavity and often in damage to the reproductive structures near the site.

Anatomical abnormalities such as a *septate uterus* (a uterus divided into two parts by a thin wall of tissue) or incompetent cervix (a cervix that effaces and dilates before fetal viability is assured) can cause recurrent miscarriage, an infertility problem in which conception occurs but the woman is unable to carry the pregnancy to term. Less common anatomical defects that may prevent the normal maintenance of pregnancy are problems with the endometrium, or uterine lining, a weak uterine muscle wall that cannot tolerate the expansion that occurs with pregnancy, or uterine tumors (*fibroids*).

Adhesions (joining of two surfaces that are normally separate) of both the Fallopian tubes and the uterus can interfere with the transportation of the fertilized ovum and with passage of sperm to the waiting ovum. *Polycystic ovarian disease*, or Stein-Leventhal syndrome, in which the ovaries are enlarged and contain many fluid-filled sacs, is also a contributor to infertility.

Anatomical defects as causes of infertility are probably the easiest to diagnose. Blocked tubes or uterine obstruction can be observed with a procedure called a *hysterosalpingogram*, where a radiopaque fluid is flushed through the uterus and its passage through the tubes is confirmed. Common side effects of the procedure, which is usually performed in a hospital without anesthesia, are cramping and tubal spasm, but these effects are short-lived.

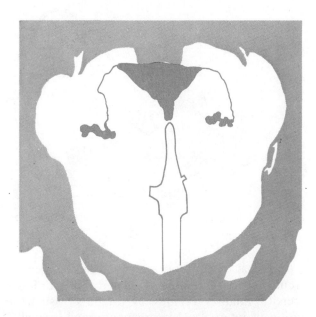

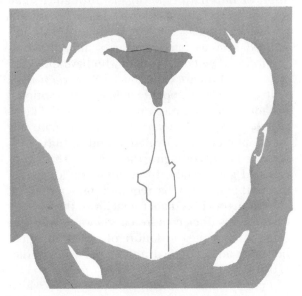

To obtain a hysterosalpingogram a radiopaque liquid is injected through the cervix; obstructions in the uterus and the Fallopian tubes can thus be detected on moving X-ray film. In the top example the uterus is normal and the Fallopian tubes are open—there is some spillage of the fluid at the ends of the tubes around the ovaries. In the bottom picture, however, both Fallopian tubes are shown to be blocked close to the uterus.

*Laparoscopy is a technique for direct visual exami-
nation of the pelvic organs. The abdominal cavity is
first inflated with gas passed through a hollow neddle
and the patient is tilted so that the intestines move
away from the pelvic organs (below); the laparoscope
is then inserted, allowing the doctor to inspect the
uterus, ovaries, and Fallopian tubes (right).*

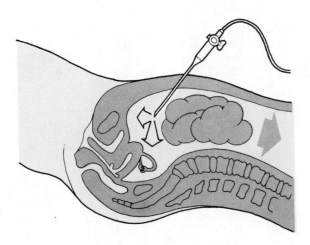
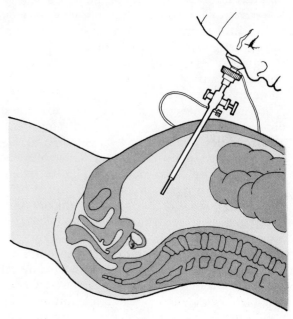

Cervical incompetence is evidenced by recurrent miscarriage that is associated with painless
cervical dilation. *Laparoscopy,* the direct visualization of internal pelvic organs through a small
incision in the abdomen, can diagnose many anatomical problems that might otherwise go unnoticed, such as defective ovaries and adhesions.

Medical conditions: Woman who have dieted to
excess or who have experienced *anorexia nervosa*
(extreme loss of appetite related to emotional
instability) may have a complete cessation of menstrual periods (*amenorrhea*), which naturally
would intefere with ovulation and fertility. This
is treated by encouraging the woman to eat properly and gain weight. In severe cases, long-term
psychotherapy may be required. Other medical
conditions such as diabetes mellitus, thyroid disease, or insufficient adrenal gland activity can
cause amenorrhea or failure of ovulation. Alcoholism or addiction to drugs can decrease ovarian
activity as well.

Endometriosis, a painful condition in which
uterine tissue is deposited elsewhere in the pelvic
cavity, has a positive association with infertility in
women. It is diagnosed by laparoscopy or ultrasound and can be treated with various drugs,
including oral contraceptives, synthetic male hormone, and synthetic hormone-releasing factor.

Other factors: Inflammation of the uterine lining, called *endometritis,* can be caused by various

infectious diseases, rendering the tissue unfavorable for implantation of a conceptus. The presence in either the man or the woman of *antisperm
antibodies,* immunological cells that fight off
sperm as though it were a hostile invading organism, have been found in some infertile couples. This condition can be detected through
laboratory analysis of both the male partner's semen and the female partner's cervical mucus. *Hostile cervical mucus* that is unreceptive to sperm for
reasons other than antisperm antibodies also can
be detected through laboratory analysis of semen
and mucus obtained from the cervix after intercourse (*postcoital test*).

Some hormonal defects, such as excessive prolactin secretion by the pituitary gland, inadequate
progesterone production after the ovulatory
phase of the cycle, and high levels of male hormones produced in the woman, also can interfere
with ovulation and, hence, fertility. These various
disorders are diagnosed through both medical
and surgical analyses.

Treatment of Infertility

■ *Drugs*

Anovulation usually is treated with administration
of several drugs. Clomiphene is a popular fertility

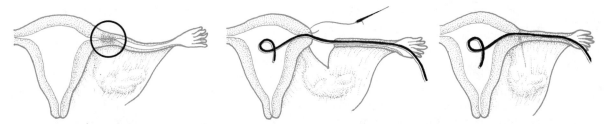

A blocked Fallopian tube can sometimes be corrected surgically, especially if the blockage is close to the uterus, as shown above. The blocked section (left) is removed and a tubal splint (fine nylon catheter) is passed through the tube into the uterus (center) before the shortened tube is sutured onto the uterus (right). The tubal splint maintains the normal tubal canal and can be removed easily through the cervix (neck of the womb) once the healing process is complete.

drug that has been used successfully in hundreds of thousands of women. It is given in tablet form on certain days of the cycle to enhance ovulation. The most common side effect, and a very serious one, is multiple pregnancy resulting from fertilization of more than one ovum. Other drugs that stimulate ovulation include human menopausal gonadotropin, bromocriptine, and gonadotropin-releasing factor. Other complications besides multiple pregnancy include cyst formation and a condition called "hyperstimulation syndrome," which causes the ovaries to enlarge.

Many anatomical abnormalities can be corrected surgically. Incompetent cervix, for example, often is treated very successfully by *cervical cerclage,* or encircling of the cervical opening with a ring or loop of suture during the first trimester of pregnancy. The suture is removed when the fetus reaches term. Other, rarer anatomical defects can be repaired through new microsurgical procedures utilizing lasers and other techniques. Tubal adhesions, strictures, or scar tissue can sometimes be reversed surgically, although even the latest techniques are not always successful. In general, the more severe the scarring, the more difficult it is to correct the problem surgically. Sometimes the surgery itself can cause irritation to pelvic structures, creating more adhesions or leading to the reformation of adhesions. Surgical intervention for polycystic ovaries has met with some success, although the ovaries will sometimes produce ripe ova in response to a fertility drug, without the need for surgery.

Hormonal disorders, depending on the gland affected, may be reversed by administration of other hormones. The existence of hostile cervical mucus does not yet have a clearly proven treatment; artificial insemination is an obvious way to allow conception to occur in cases where the antibodies originate with the male partner. Occa-

sionally, when the antibodies are the woman's, allowing the woman's immune system to remain free from exposure to sperm for a prolonged period can lower her antibody levels. This is accomplished through use of a condom for at least six months to prevent contact between her partner's sperm and her body. At the end of the waiting period, unprotected intercourse is carefully timed to coincide with the woman's most fertile time, so that conception may take place before the woman's antibodies begin to build up again. This method of combating the problem has met with only partial success, however, and at the present time there is no proven treatment for immunological infertility.

■ Artificial Insemination

This procedure is indicated in cases where the fertility problem is primarily that of the male partner. Semen from an unknown donor is introduced into the woman's vagina during her most fertile period, and the procedure is repeated two or three times each menstrual cycle until conception occurs. Donor insemination is successful 50 percent of the time within the first two months and 90 percent of the time within the first six months. In these cases the baby will have the genetic contributions of the wife and of the donor. Artificial insemination using the husband's sperm is indicated only in specific situations, such as severe, uncorrected premature ejaculation, failure of erection, anatomic defects that prevent satisfactory placement of semen within the woman's reproductive tract, low semen volume per ejaculation with normal concentrations of normal sperm, and, in some cases, low sperm counts. The husband's sperm may be "banked" in several deposits and concentrated by mechanical means to enhance sperm count and motility or, as mentioned previously, in cases where the husband must undergo chemo- or radiotherapy for cancer.

■ *Adoption*

Adoption of an infant or young child is still a popular way to solve the problem of childlessness. Parents of adopted children as well as the children themselves are living testimony to the fact that a child does not have to be related by blood to truly belong to a family. Adoption of healthy white infants has become increasingly difficult, however, as growing numbers of childless white couples seek such babies. Alternatives include adoption of Asian babies and babies from Central and South America (although immigration procedures can take years), and adoption of black, Hispanic, or handicapped infants and older children. Most cities or counties have readily available information about adoption through the local government children's welfare agency.

■ *Laboratory Techniques*

Newer procedures available to a limited number of infertile couples, depending on the nature of the fertility problem, include *in vitro* and *in vivo* fertilization techniques. In vitro fertilization, first successfully done in 1978 in Britain, involves the surgical removal of a ripe ovum from the woman's ovary, fertilization of the ovum with the husband's sperm in a culture medium outside the womb, and implantation of the ovum in the mother's womb after a few days of growing and enlarging. The birth of the world's first "test-tube baby" was met with great joy and hopefulness by many couples who were childless because the wife's tubes were permanently blocked, preventing passage of the fertilized ovum to the uterus. The procedure is expensive, however (prices range from $4,000 to $6,000 per procedure), and usually is not covered by insurance. Further, the technique may require three or four attempts and has a success rate of only about 20 percent at the best hospital facilities. Also, very few hospitals are offering the procedure.

In vivo ovum transfer involves the surgical transfer of an ovum fertilized by the husband's sperm in a female donor to the uterus of the infertile partner. In such cases the baby will not have the genetic contribution of the wife, but the wife will nurture the fetus and give birth to it. In vivo techniques are far less common than in vitro procedures and are at least as expensive.

Couples having difficulty conceiving should always first undergo a thorough fertility workup, starting with the least invasive, most common-sense investigation and proceeding to the more complicated ones, before seeking such heroic techniques as in vitro fertilization. A fertility workup by a reliable expert can cost several thousands of dollars exclusive of any corrective treatment and the amount covered by insurance policies varies from state to state. For more information about infertility, treatments, and insurance coverage, couples can write to the American Fertility Society, 2131 Magnolia Avenue, Suite 201, Birmingham, Alabama 35256. Telephone: 205-251-9764.

■ *Surrogate Motherhood*

Surrogacy, in which a donor mother becomes pregnant by artificial insemination with the sperm of the fertile partner, carries the baby to term, and then gives the baby up for adoption by the childless couple, is becoming a source of public controversy, as well as an option that is growing in popularity. Several would-be surrogate mothers have gained notoriety by changing their minds about giving up the baby after its birth and have challenged the adoptive parents' rights in court. As a result, media coverage of such court cases has turned what should be a sensitive, private issue into national news. Until the issue of the adoptive parents' versus the surrogate parents' rights is resolved—if it ever is—couples considering such a solution would do well to tread carefully and have trustworthy legal counsel at every step.

CONTRACEPTION

The term *contraception* refers to the prevention of conception or impregnation. Although several relatively easy methods of contraception are readily available in Western countries, the number of unplanned and unwanted pregnancies that either end in abortion or go to term for adoption is still considerable. Numerous studies have been done on why some women take risks with their fertility and sometimes end up with an unwanted pregnancy; it is clear that denial—the notion that "this is not happening to me" or "this cannot happen to me"—plays a part.

An unwanted pregnancy can place severe strains on a relationship; indeed, it may well be the cause of a breakup. For a single woman, an unplanned pregnancy can wreak great havoc. Although many single women in modern society have consciously chosen to bear children alone, so that single motherhood is no longer the social stigma it once was, it is nevertheless extremely difficult for many women to carry the responsibility for a child singlehandedly. Not just the financial burden, but the emotional price of raising a child alone can create a stressful atmosphere for the single-parent family.

In an ideal world, responsibility for contraception would be shared equally between male and female partners; in reality, the sole burden is often on the woman. Because women pay the price of failed contraception, all too often they are held responsible for ensuring that contraception is used; in any case, it is the woman who cannot afford to "take a chance" in a relationship where the foundations are not secure. Safe, early abortion is still a legal, available option for women who can afford the procedure, but there is always a very slight risk of complications from any invasive procedure, and there are often psychological problems that arise from abortion, especially when the woman is ambivalent about the pregnancy. For these reasons, abortion should never be thought of as a last-ditch attempt at contraception. Abortion is an option that women should resort to only when contraception has failed.

As our society has become better nourished and healthier, the age at which women become fertile (that is, the onset of menstruation) has gradually become younger and younger, with most girls in industrialized Western nations reaching puberty around age 13. At the same time, as the average life span in industrialized countries increases, so does the age at which menopause usually occurs. Thus, a woman's reproductive life in Western countries lasts almost forty years in some cases; in developing countries this span is much shorter. It is logical, then, but unfortunate that most girls become capable of reproducing before they are ready—emotionally, financially, and socially—to support and nurture a child.

This tragic fact is borne out by the phenomenal rate of teenage pregnancy in the United States. Pregnancies among teenage girls in this country now number more than a million annually, with 600,000 of these pregnancies resulting in births each year. The future for the majority of these child-mothers is exceedingly dim. Yet birth control is available for most of those who seek it. The problem with many teenagers appears to be a combination of immaturity and misinformation. Many misleading ideas are passed among teenage girls, such as the notion that "you can't get pregnant the first time you have sex." Some researchers believe that teenagers are psychologically and emotionally incapable of seeing the future consequences of their actions, so that seeking birth control is beyond their decision-making capability. Other studies have shown that some teenage girls associate the deliberate use of contraceptive devices with guilt about premeditated sex; in other words, they feel all right about having unprotected intercourse if they are "taken by surprise" or "swept off their feet" with passion, but they feel guilty about obtaining contraception in advance, since this implies a conscious plan to have sex.

While many parents and fundamentalist church groups object to explicit sex education in public schools, recent research has shown that thorough sex education is the best defense against unwanted pregnancies. Far from encouraging promiscuous behavior, which is the common argument against public-school sex education, teaching teenaged girls and boys about responsible sexual behavior is likely to reduce significantly the staggering number of unwanted adolescent pregnancies in the United States, while also cutting down on the number of abortions performed each year.

There are many methods of contraception currently available in the United States. Each method has its drawbacks and advantages, and couples seeking a new method of family planning should be aware of the drawbacks, pitfalls, and good points of each before making a decision that could affect the quality of their relationship. For Roman Catholics and other religious groups who maintain that "artificial" methods of contraception are sinful, "natural" methods such as the "rhythm" system or the "fertility awareness" methods, or a combination of these methods, may be acceptable alternatives to barrier methods or the Pill.

Types of Contraceptives

■ Rhythm System

This method involves abstaining from intercourse during a woman's midcycle time, that is, between days 10 and 18 of her menstrual cycle (with the first day of the menstrual period counted as day 1). This method is popular among Roman Catholic populations, where artificial methods are prohibited by canon law. Unfortunately, this contraceptive method has a high failure rate, especially among women who do not ovulate at exactly the same time each cycle, or who have irregular periods.

■ *Fertility Awareness Methods*

In women who have subjective evidence of ovulation, such as midcycle pelvic pain (*Mittelschmerz*), spotting, and changes in vaginal discharge, it is possible to chart "fertile" times each cycle and exercise abstinence from intercourse at "unsafe" times. Even if your cycles are irregular, as long as you have symptoms of ovulation, it is possible to avoid unsafe times with some degree of accuracy; however, ovulation may precede symptoms by several hours or a day.

Changes in basal body temperature (BBT) are a more precise, scientific way to predict ovulation, although, like other fertility awareness methods, this system works best in retrospect. In other words, it is much easier to know exactly when you *began ovulating*, rather than when you *will begin*. A person's BBT fluctuates both daily and cyclically; a woman's BBT rises and falls throughout the day, being its lowest just before rising from sleep. At the same time, on a cyclical basis a woman's BBT reaches its low point near the time of ovulation. After the ovum is released from the ovary, the BBT rises by about 0.5° to 1°F (0.5°C) and maintains this slightly higher temperature during the second half of the menstrual cycle if ovulation has occurred. You can use this physiological curiosity to your advantage by taking your temperature orally each day just prior to getting out of bed in the morning. By plotting the values on a chart, you should be able to observe a trend in your BBT—providing you ovulate regularly—that enables you to predict your fertile times with some accuracy. This method, like the others described above, is problematic for women whose periods are irregular or those who do not ovulate on a regular basis.

Other predictors of ovulation include the symptoms mentioned previously, such as pelvic discomfort, midcycle spotting, and changes in cervical mucus. At ovulation, the cervical mucus discharged from the vagina is more copious, clearer, and more stretchable. Awareness of these signs combined with BBT charting and keeping track of your cyclical "calendar" can enhance the accuracy of these methods.

"Natural" contraceptive methods have several advantages: compatibility with religious beliefs in cases where canon law prohibits artificial means of pregnancy prevention; avoidance of the medical risks of certain birth control methods, such as the Pill; and enjoyment of sex that is unaffected by the occasional discomforts or reduced sensation that occurs as a result of some of the barrier methods, such as the diaphragm or condom. Disadvantages include the fact that none of the systems mentioned is very accurate (the suggested failure rate is 20 to 30 percent) and that partners must abstain from intercourse for fairly long periods of time during the possibly fertile phase of the woman's cycle.

■ *Withdrawal Method*

The "withdrawal" method of pregnancy prevention requires that the man remove his penis from the woman's vagina prior to ejaculation. This is also known as *coitus interruptus*. This method is not considered to be very reliable, because some semen may be released into the vagina prior to ejaculation. In addition, some men may find it very difficult to hold back from ejaculating until they have withdrawn from the woman's vagina. A great deal of self-control and perfect timing are required. This method puts the burden of responsibility entirely on the male partner. Withdrawal is better than no method at all, but it has a high failure rate, and many couples are left feeling frustrated and unsatisfied with sex when this method is employed.

■ *Barrier Methods*

Condoms: The condom, "rubber," or "sheath" is one of the most popular contraceptive methods worldwide. The condom is a latex rubber or animal-skin sheath that is unrolled onto the erect penis before intercourse takes place. The ejaculate, including the sperm, is held within the condom; no direct contact takes place between semen and vagina. To work properly in preventing contact of sperm with vaginal tissue, the condom must be removed carefully after the penis is withdrawn from the vagina, *while the penis is still partially erect.* While withdrawing the penis from the vagina and removing the condom from the penis, great care must be taken to avoid spilling the contents of the condom into or near the vaginal opening.

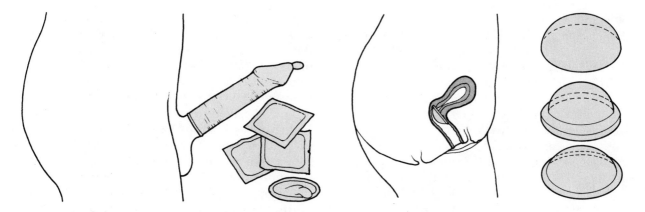

The condom consists of a thin latex rubber sheath drawn over the erect penis before intercourse. The seminal fluid is retained in the reservoir at the end.

The diaphragm or Dutch cap is always used in conjunction with a spermicidal cream; it must be correctly inserted into the vagina before intercourse to cover the cervix and left in position for 6 hours afterward.

Causes of failure with condom use are due mainly to improper use: not putting the condom on until some genital contact has already taken place; leaving the condom in place—and the penis in the vagina—until the penis becomes flaccid, which makes safe removal of the condom from the vagina difficult; and accidental slippage of the condom from the penis after ejaculation. In addition, reusing condoms is absolutely unacceptable—they are for single use only; use of very old condoms that have been stored, say, in a wallet or jacket pocket for years is foolish; use of petroleum-jelly-containing vaginal lubricants can sometimes eat away at synthetic-rubber condoms, leaving holes or destroying the integrity of the sheath. (Use a water-soluble lubricant, such as K-Y Jelly, or a spermicide instead.) Finally, the condom is a highly effective method if *used*; that is, if the condom is opened, unrolled, and put on the penis before intercourse takes place, *not* if the condom sits on the dresser top in its foil packet. Using a spermicidal foam or cream as a vaginal lubricant in addition to the condom enhances the condom's effectiveness.

Condoms come in many shapes, brands, textures, and even colors; they are available in prelubricated and nonlubricated forms in all drugstores. They can also be purchased at most family planning clinics, some discount stores, and even in vending machines in gas stations and public restrooms. The advantages of condoms are many: They are relatively inexpensive and are easily available without a prescription; no medical exam is necessary before their use is undertaken; they are

lightweight and easy to carry; there are no known side effects or health hazards associated with condom use. Perhaps most important, condoms provide effective protection against the transmission of sexually transmitted diseases such as herpes, syphilis, gonorrhea, chlamydia, and AIDS.

Disadvantages of condoms are few, but some couples find them sufficient to shun condom use. Some men and women report decreased sexual sensation when condoms are used. The responsibility for contraception is borne exclusively by the man when condoms are the sole method of birth control, although the woman partner may purchase, store, and carry condoms and spermicide with her. Some spontaneity in sexual play may be lost by the man having to stop while he unwraps and puts on the condom, although the couple may incorporate putting on the condom into foreplay.

The Diaphragm: The diaphragm is a domeshaped, soft rubber device about 3 inches in diameter that is inserted into the vagina before intercourse and used in conjunction with spermicidal cream or jelly. Inserted properly, the diaphragm covers the woman's cervix, effectively barring contact of semen (and hence, sperm) with ovum.

Diaphragms come in various sizes; a gynecologist, nurse practitioner, or nurse-midwife prescribes a particular size and/or style based on a fitting which is done in conjunction with a pelvic exam. The diaphragm is inserted up to four hours ahead of time and must remain in place for at least six hours after intercourse has occurred; if intercourse takes place again within six to eight hours after the first contact, additional spermicidal cream or jelly must be inserted into the vagina with an applicator, taking care not to disturb the placement of the diaphragm.

A diaphragm should be washed thoroughly with mild soap and warm water after it is removed, allowed to dry, and then stored in an appropriate container (one is included in the package when a diaphragm is prescribed). It should be inspected periodically by being held up in the air against a bright light (not touching the light source but placed in the line of vision before a bright light); the woman should examine it carefully for minute pinholes, tears, or other signs of loss of integrity that could allow sperm to penetrate through to the cervix.

Diaphragms are obtained by prescription and only after a physical exam of the pelvis and a "fitting"; they are relatively inexpensive. Many brands of spermicidal foams, jellies, and creams are available over-the-counter at all drugstores; these vary in price and must be used each time the diaphragm is used. The spermicide is smeared on both sides of the diaphragm (about a teaspoon is sufficient) before insertion. The diaphragm is inserted by folding it in half, pushing it deeply into the vagina with one or two fingers, and then checking its placement with a finger inserted into the vagina. When properly placed, the diaphragm should completely cover the cervix.

Advantages of the diaphragm include its high effectiveness rate when used properly (estimated at 97 to 98 percent), the lack of life-threatening risks or health hazards associated with its use, the partial protection it provides against vaginal or cervical infections (enhanced by the use of spermicides containing the ingredient nonoxynol-9), and the ease with which diaphragm use can be discontinued when a couple wishes to start a family.

There are various disadvantages to the diaphragm, which must be weighed by prospective users against the relatively low-risk, effective contraception it offers. Use of the diaphragm requires a medical examination, a prescription, and a fitting. Diaphragms must be refitted or rechecked for correct size after childbirth and following a weight loss or gain of 20 pounds or more; spermicidal jelly or cream can be expensive and has a slight allergenic potential; both the spermicide ingredients and the latex contained in the diaphragm itself may cause allergic reactions in a small number of women or their partners. Women who find touching their genitalia aesthetically or morally offensive will not be able to undertake the self-examination and genital manipulation required for insertion and inspection of the diaphragm. In addition, it has been suggested that the slight pressure the diaphragm can exert against the bladder may be responsible for a higher rate of cystitis (bladder infection) or urethritis (inflammation of the lower urinary tract). Thus, women with chronic bladder or urethral infections may wish to avoid this potential additional trauma. Some couples report discomfort during intercourse related to diaphragm use; this usually can be alleviated by a refitting and examination of insertion methods to ensure proper, nontraumatic placement. The major disadvantage of the diaphragm is the amount of planning and caretaking that goes into its use. Some couples feel that the necessity of inserting it before intercourse interferes with spontaneity; indeed, proper placement may take a few minutes at first, but the man can actively participate in the insertion and placement of the diaphragm as a part of foreplay. In this way, too, the man can take on some of the "work" of maintaining adequate contraception.

The cervical cap: The cervical cap is a small, thimble-shaped device that fits over the cervix; it is used in conjunction with vaginal spermicides and stays in place via suction. Although the cervical cap is widely used in Europe, its use in the United States is considered investigative, and it is not yet easy to obtain. If you are interested, you can get information about the cervical cap, and the cap itself, at some women's health centers, college health services, medical/gynecological clinics, and private physicians' offices. There are limited numbers of facilities offering the cap, however. The best results with the cervical cap come from custom-fitted devices; the degree of suction between cap and cervix depends on how good the fit is. It can remain in place for twenty-four hours or more.

The advantages of the cap are similar to those of the diaphragm. Disadvantages include the cap's limited availability, greater difficulty with insertion than with the diaphragm, and difficulty with removal. There is some question of an association between the cervical cap and toxic shock syndrome (TSS) and also between the cap and cervical dysplasia. Any cervical anatomical abnormalities, such as cysts, erosion, or an unusually long or short cervix would probably preclude use of the cap.

Vaginal sponge: The vaginal sponge, introduced in 1983, is a soft, pliable, disk-shaped sponge with a cup-shaped indentation in one side. It is preimpregnated with an effective, well-known spermicide and is inserted easily into the vagina much in the manner of a diaphragm; it is removed by means of a cloth loop attached to its back side. The sponge is available without a prescription and is readily available in most drug and discount stores. Like the diaphragm, the sponge combines the use of a barrier with a spermicide to prevent pregnancy. The manufacturer's recommendations say that the sponge can be left in place for twenty-four hours and will remain effective for that length of time. That means that the sponge can be inserted nearly twenty-four hours before intercourse takes place, which theoretically enhances sexual spontaneity.

The advantages of the sponge, in addition to those discussed above, are its ease of insertion and its disease-preventing potential. Disadvantages include its cost, which can be prohibitive in some cases (most drugstores charge approximately $1 per sponge), and its failure rate, which at the present time reportedly ranges from 30 percent to less than 5 percent. There is also a slight risk of vaginal-cervical irritability from the sponge, and there is still some lingering concern about toxic shock syndrome. Some reported side effects include an offensive discharge and increased absorption of vaginal secretions, resulting in a dry vagina.

Spermicides used alone: When used in conjunction with condoms, diaphragms, or the cervical cap, spermicides enhance contraception; indeed, the diaphragm is not an effective method without spermicide use. Spermicides used alone, in the form of vaginal suppositories, tablets, foams, jellies, creams, and prefilled applicators must be inserted usually not more than an hour before intercourse takes place; some require at least fifteen minutes to dissolve. The effectiveness of spermicides alone lasts for no more than an hour. They are easily available in drugstores and other retail stores and are easily inserted into the vagina. Their effectiveness rate, however, is reported to vary from 70 to 90 percent, depending upon how much of the product is used, the timing of insertion, and repeated intercourse after the one-hour time limit without reinserting more spermicide. Obviously, this method is better than no method at all, but spermicidal effectiveness is greatly increased by combining its use with one of the barrier methods available.

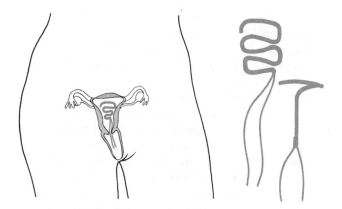

The IUD or coil is available in a variety of shapes; once correctly inserted into the uterus, it can usually be left in position for several years. The nylon string protruding through the cervix is to aid removal and to check for its presence.

■ *Intrauterine Devices (IUDs)*

Because of increasing concern about its safety, the intrauterine device is no longer widely available in the United States. The way in which the IUD works is still not entirely clear, although it is believed to create a low-grade inflammation of the uterus, effectively preventing implantation of a fertilized ovum.

The IUD, which sits permanently in the uterus just above the cervical opening, is meant to be checked periodically by a physician and replaced every few years (removal is achieved by means of a string that hangs through the cervical opening). Women having IUDs inserted are also instructed to check placement of the device from time to time by feeling the string at her cervix with a finger.

Although the IUD had a high effectiveness rate (estimated between 96 and 99 percent), common side effects included severe menstrual cramps, increased menstrual flow, and midcycle spotting. An association has been made between IUDs and increased incidence of pelvic inflammatory disease (PID), a painful infection of the pelvic organs that can affect fertility, among other dangerous conditions.

■ *Oral Contraceptives*

"The Pill" is available in many brands, dosages, and formulations. It works by modifying natural hormone "feedback" systems. Present-day pills contain estrogen and/or synthetic progesterone, which works to prevent conception in many ways.

Estrogen inhibits the secretion of *follicle-stimulating hormone* (FSH), thereby preventing ovulation. Estrogen in the dosage found in the Pill also prevents implantation of a fertilized ovum, and progesterone in birth-control pills maintains the cervical mucus in a thick form hostile to sperm.

The Pill has been in use since the early 1960s, but it has gone through cycles of popularity and unpopularity. Medical technology has improved the safety and effectiveness of oral contraceptives such that today, except for women who smoke, are over age 40, or have specific medical conditions, the Pill is an excellent, easy form of contraception that actually may have some health benefits beyond pregnancy prevention. The possible side effects, however, are many, and some women may find them sufficient to make this form of contraception unacceptable.

Minor side effects include breast tenderness, weight gain, nausea, acne or other skin changes, change in libido (increased or decreased), bleeding in midcycle ("breakthrough bleeding"), emotional changes, fatigue, missed periods, and increased incidence of vaginal infection. All of these may be temporary or mild, and changing the type of pill may alleviate the particular symptom. There are other, potentially serious side effects that have been documented in various long-term studies. These include thromboembolism (blood clot formation), myocardial infarction (heart attack), stroke, high blood pressure, liver disease, and migraine headaches. Women with cardiovascular problems, liver problems, or a history of headache or migraine should avoid taking the Pill. No link has been found between the Pill and cancer, despite early fears about an increased risk of cancer from oral contraceptives.

The Pill is available in two basic forms, the combined estrogen-progesterone pill and the "mini-pill," which contains progesterone alone. Women who desire to take the Pill must first see a physician or qualified nurse-practitioner for a history and physical exam; the Pill is obtained by prescription and refills usually are given only after a second examination has taken place. Especially for women just starting a regimen of oral contraceptives, such parameters as blood pressure and weight gain must be assessed regularly by the prescribing physician.

The birth-control pill in the combined form is taken at the same time each day for twenty-one days and then stopped for seven days. Within a few days after the last pill of the cycle is taken,

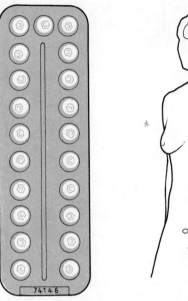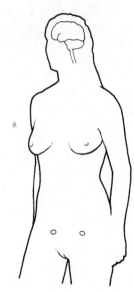

The combined estrogen-progesterone contraceptive pill inhibits the release of hormones from the pituitary gland in the brain. These are necessary to encourage maturation of the ovum in the ovary.

estrogen-progesterone levels in the blood fall and "withdrawal bleeding"—a false period—occurs. Some manufacturers provide seven "blank" pills dyed a different color to be taken during the "off" week; this removes the danger of women forgetting to take their pills again after the seven days off. Some combined pills—known as *triphasics*—alter the proportions and dosages of estrogen and progesterone at various times in the pill cycle to more closely mimic the body's own estrogen-progesterone secretion cycle. The "mini-pill," which is prescribed less often than the combined pill, is taken every day with no off time. Some women find the absence of a nominal "period" with this method disturbing, but the progesterone-only pill may be indicated for some women who cannot take estrogen for various medical reasons.

The Pill is widely available through private physicians, medical clinics, college health services, Planned Parenthood, and women's clinics. Its many advantages have already been discussed. Additional disadvantages to those described above include the expense, which can be considerable for those on a fixed or limited income, and the necessity of getting more frequent gynecological examinations than would normally be required. To put things in perspective, however, truly "long-term" studies of the health risks of oral contraceptives have yet to be seen, because the method

TIPS FOR THOSE TAKING ORAL CONTRACEPTIVES

- Start the first round of birth-control pills with the next menstrual period after you have filled the prescription. The exact starting day depends on the manufacturer's instructions; some say to start on the first day of the next period, others on the first Sunday after the period begins, and so on. Consult the package insert or your physician if instructions are not clear.

- Take one pill at the same time each day for 21 days, then take no pill (or the "blank" reminder pills) for the following week. Try to take the pill as part of a daily ritual, such as flossing your teeth in the morning or doing sit-ups; this will help you to remember.

- Menstruation will occur a few days after you stop the hormone-containing pills. On the eighth day after taking the last hormone pill, start a new package of pills.

- If you miss one pill, take it as soon as you remember. If it is already the next day, take it together with your pill for that day. Use a backup contraceptive until the pill cycle is complete.

- If you miss two pills, take the two as soon as you remember and then take two the next day. Continue to take one pill each day until the package is gone. Be sure to use backup contraception, such as condoms.

- If you miss three pills or more, start another method of contraception immediately; don't bother to take the pills left in the pack. Wait for your next menstrual period, then start a new pack according to the instructions, as though you were starting the pills all over again.

- Whenever you have missed one or more pills, schedule a pregnancy test if no withdrawal bleeding occurs at the end of the pill cycle.

- Don't worry if you miss a period after a cycle in which you have missed no pills. Continue the pill cycle as usual. If you miss two periods in a row, consult your physician for an exam and pregnancy test.

- If you experience "breakthrough" bleeding or spotting during the 21 days of hormone pills, keep taking the pills and consult your physician if it continues. If you experience severe cramping or excessive bleeding, call your health care provider as soon as possible.

- If you experience any of the following symptoms, report them *immediately* to your health care provider: severe headache, difficult or blurred vision or visual disturbance, chest pain, abdominal pain, severe leg pain, or numbness/tingling of the extremities.

SOURCE: Adapted from Janet Griffith-Kenney, *Contemporary Women's Health: A Nursing Advocacy Approach*, (Menlo Park, Calif: Addison-Wesley Publishing Company, 1986), chap. 24.

---

has only been in existence for less than three decades.

Contraindications to taking the Pill, besides those already mentioned, include pregnancy, diabetes mellitus, breast or uterine cancer, liver disease, history of blood-clotting disorders, hypertension, uterine bleeding, and lack of regular menstrual cycles for one year or more in adolescents. Also, women with the following conditions who are taking oral contraceptives should be checked at least every three months by a physician: migraine headache, seizure disorder, depression, and menstrual irregularities.

When discontinuing the Pill, ovulatory cycles usually return shortly after the last round of pills; however, it is not uncommon for a few months to pass before a normal menstrual cycle resumes. If you have stopped the Pill in order to become pregnant, it is advisable to wait a few months, using another method of contraception, before having unprotected intercourse. The calculation of the actual due date of the pregnancy will be more accurate if at least two normal periods have occurred before conception; otherwise, there will be a larger margin of error in due-date calculation.

See box for instructions on the use of oral contraceptives.

■ *Other Contraceptive Methods*

The "morning-after pill" is given in a series of tablets containing high doses of synthetic estrogens or progesterone or both. It must be started within twenty-four hours or so after intercourse in order to be effective. Side effects are similar to those of oral contraceptives, with occasional severe nausea and vomiting reported. If pregnancy occurs in spite of this method, there is a possibility of birth defects related to the high levels of hormones contained in the pills.

VOLUNTARY STERILIZATION

Voluntary sterilization is an excellent means of pregnancy prevention. It is accomplished in a man by the operation known as *vasectomy*, and in a woman by means of *tubal ligation* ("tying the tubes"). The main problem with both methods is their permanence. Many couples, even though they do not wish to have more children, find the idea of permanent contraception frightening and disturbing. They may have the idea in the back of their minds that life can sometimes "throw a curve" and that one day, for reasons not now apparent, one or the other of them may wish to have more children. Indeed, if there are any such doubts among people seeking permanent contraception—even the slightest degree of doubt—sterilization is not advisable.

At present there exists no form of effective sterilization for either a woman or a man that can be reversed easily. Although some success has been reported with reversals of both tubal ligations and vasectomies, these are isolated cases, and both procedures are performed with the understanding that they are irreversible.

Voluntary operative sterilization should be undertaken, then, under specific conditions. Even going beyond the couple's desire to prevent any further pregnancies, the man or the woman undergoing the procedure should be convinced that, no matter what happens to the existing children or the relationship, he or she desires no more children.

Voluntary sterilization offers many benefits to the individual or couple who seek it. It means that the rest of one's life can include sexual intercourse free of the mechanical barriers and the occasional psychological barriers posed by certain forms of contraception. Some couples may find that their sex life takes on new meaning and excitement once the fear of accidental pregnancy is removed.

The choice of whether the man or the woman should be the one to undergo the operation is a difficult one. In general, the male operation is simpler and carries fewer risks. Tubal ligation, however, is also a relatively simple procedure with minimal health hazards. A couple that is uncertain about who should have the sterilization procedure would do best to discuss the issue with a trusted physician and arrive at an informed decision after discussion of the benefits and disadvantages of both operations.

Many states have laws requiring that informed consent for either tubal ligation or vasectomy or both be signed and witnessed a considerable length of time (a month, for example) before the actual surgery can be performed. This waiting time, it is hoped, reduces the number of operations performed on patients who are ambivalent about being sterilized. Also, there are circumstances in which a patient may not be exercising full powers of judgment in the matter, for example, a man or woman just out of surgery, a woman in labor or immediately postpartum, or a patient with a psychiatric history.

Vasectomy

Male sterilization is achieved by interrupting the tubes that carry sperm from the testes to the penis. These tubes are called the *vasa deferentia* (singular: *vas deferens*), hence, the name of the operation is *vasectomy*. It is a minor procedure that normally takes about twenty minutes or so. It is usually done under local anesthesia. A 2–3 cm. incision is made over the vas deferens on either side of the scrotum; the tubes are isolated and cut; the cut ends usually are looped back on themselves and secured with clips or plastic tubing; or the tubes are coagulated to prevent spontaneous rejoining of the ducts. The skin is repaired with absorbable stitches, and the man is instructed to apply ice to the scrotum if swelling or pain occurs and to wear a scrotal support for a week or so. Perhaps the most important thing a man should know about vasectomy is that *it can take up to six weeks to clear residual sperm from the vasa*, so the couple should use a reliable form of birth control for that time period following the procedure.

There are no effects on the man's sexual per-

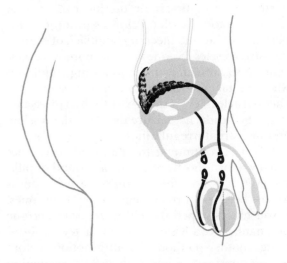

Vasectomy is a minor operation done to cut and tie off the vasa deferentia—the tubes that conduct sperm from the testes to the uretha. This is done through a small incision close to the top of the scrotum

formance from the surgery; the volume of ejaculate remains about the same, the ability to get and maintain an erection is unaltered, and the ejaculate appears the same as before. The man should bring in semen samples at the end of the six-week waiting period for a sperm count to determine the effectiveness of the procedure, and he should be rechecked at six months and one year to ensure that the ducts have not rejoined.

Reversal of a vasectomy, as mentioned above, is still relatively rare. Depending on the method used to occlude the tubes, there is a 14 to 55 percent success rate in reestablishing fertility after vasectomy. Possible side effects of the operation include the formation of *hematomas*, which are collections of clotted blood in local tissue, the formation of *sperm granulomas*, which are tumor-like nodules formed around remaining sperm, and spontaneous reconnection of the vasa, mentioned earlier.

Tubal Ligation

Female sterilization is accomplished commonly by tubal ligation. It is also a secondary effect of *hysterectomy* (removal of the uterus, Fallopian tubes, and sometimes the ovaries) performed for more complex medical indications. Tubal ligation usually involves making a small incision just below the navel, isolating the tubes one at a time, and then occluding them by one of various possible means. Clips, electrical cauterization, or permanent sutures are the usual ways of assuring that the tubes remain closed.

The tubal ligation procedure can be done through the abdomen, as described above, under local, regional, or general anesthesia, or through the vagina by means of a *laparoscope*. The procedure usually takes about fifteen minutes and requires a short stay in the hospital (two to three days). If a woman desires tubal ligation during her stay in the hospital following delivery of her baby, the surgery usually is done on the first to third day postpartum.

Complications of tubal ligation include damage to nearby loops of bowel, infection, bleeding, and the possible hazards of general or regional anesthesia. There is, as with all surgery, a small failure rate, so that occasionally a woman finds herself pregnant after undergoing tubal sterilization.

Reversal of tubal sterilization, like vasectomy reversal, has been accomplished successfully in some cases, but it is still not routine. Depending on the portion of the tube occluded, the surgical technique, and the length of tube remaining, there can be a success rate as high as 70 percent, "success" being defined as pregnancy ensuing.

In a few cases, sterilization affects a woman's attitude about herself and her sexuality. Similarly, sometimes after a vasectomy a man might find himself struggling with sexual potency for psychological reasons. Such problems might best be dealt with by a sex therapist, professional counselor, or gynecologist specializing in sex problems. In the majority of cases, the couple find the burden of contraception lifted and actually enjoy sex more as a result.

It should be emphasized that, although tubal ligation and vasectomy are excellent, safe methods of permanent birth control, they are certainly

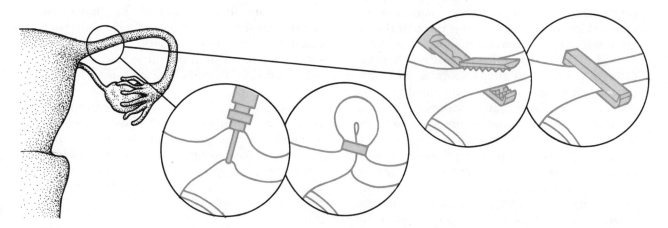

The most modern methods of female sterilization consist of blocking off the Fallopian tubes by the application of rings or clips. This can be performed through a very small abdominal incision using a laparoscope and a special attachment.

not right for everybody. Because they involve "going under the knife," the use of anesthesia, and sometimes a stay in the hospital, they should be carefully weighed against other available contraceptive options before any decision is reached.

ABORTION

The issue of voluntary abortion (also called "elective," "therapeutic," or "induced" abortion) is a highly controversial one in the United States. Religious, ethical, political, feminist, and legislative leaders have all expressed opinions publicly about whether a woman's right to govern her own body outweighs the possible moral consequences of deliberately terminating a pregnancy. More recently, members of the antiabortion movement in the United States have made their feelings known by bombing abortion clinics around the country. The issue may never be resolved legislatively, and it will certainly never be resolved in terms of its moral correctness or incorrectness. Nevertheless, safe, legal abortion remains an important option for millions of American women each year.

Considering the fact that illegal abortions were once the single largest cause of maternal deaths in the United States, the 1973 Supreme Court decision legalizing abortion—and thus putting abortion in the hands of only skilled physicians with adequate facilities to perform the procedure—was a giant step toward improving the health status of American women.

Voluntary or elective abortion must be distinguished from *spontaneous abortion*, or miscarriage, in which the uterus contracts spontaneously, the cervix dilates, and the products of conception are expelled from the woman's body through the vagina. Spontaneous abortion is known to occur in a large proportion of all pregnancies, often because the embryo has gross abnormalities. Spontaneous abortion may be accompanied by relief on the part of the woman experiencing it if the pregnancy was not desired in the first place, disappointment if the pregnancy was desired; if it occurs early enough, it may go undetected as anything more than "menstrual" bleeding or "spotting" and cramping. If you do experience a miscarriage, it is important to remember that miscarriage is very probably the body's system of "quality control," reducing the possibility of carrying to term a baby that is abnormal. The system is, of course, not foolproof, as evidenced by the occasional baby that is born full-term with deformities ranging from mild to life-threatening in nature.

Voluntary or induced abortion, on the other hand, is a procedure the pregnant woman must consciously choose, ideally before the pregnancy has progressed very far.

Indications for Induced Abortion

■ *Medical Reasons*

Occasionally, the pregnant woman may have a severe underlying illness that may be exacerbated by the pregnancy to such a degree that her life or health are threatened. Examples include severe cardiac disease, tuberculosis, severe diabetes, kidney disease or psychiatric illness of an extreme nature. Other chronic conditions may in some instances provide a medical indication for induced abortion, although medicine and obstetrics have progressed to a point of such advanced diagnostic and monitoring capability that many women today are sustaining healthy pregnancies who would never have been able to do so ten or twenty years ago.

If a pregnant woman has never had *rubella* (German measles) and has never been vaccinated against it, she must be extremely careful to avoid exposure to the disease, especially during the first trimester of pregnancy, when the fetus is most at risk for developing congenital anomalies. Exposure to rubella at any time in the pregnancy is still considered dangerous, although perhaps less so in the latter two trimesters. Definite exposure to rubella is a strong indication for abortion, since babies born with congenital rubella often are severely retarded. In addition, exposure to other diseases, such as *cytomegalovirus* or *toxoplasmosis*, can cause severe retardation in the fetus and would provide a compelling reason to seek an induced abortion.

Abortion may also be advised in cases where genetic or chromosomal or other congenital anomalies are diagnosed in the fetus during pregnancy. Such conditions as *Down's syndrome* (mongolism) or *spina bifida* may be indicated by diagnostic tests such as amniocentesis or chorionic villus sampling.

■ *Nonmedical Reasons*

Among the many nonmedical reasons for seeking

abortion are a woman's recognition that having a baby at this particular time in her life might damage her physical or emotional well-being, jeopardize the relationship she is in now, or adversely affect the well-being of existing children. Some women seek it because they already have all the children they want, others because they have decided for some reason not to have any children.

Sometimes having a child is not financially feasible for a woman, perhaps because she is unmarried or already has several children. A child that is conceived in rape, in coerced sex, or in a relationship that has been or continues to be traumatic for the woman is likely to be an unwanted child. Some women may feel they are too young or too old to have a child; others may want children very much but want them when they plan for them, not before. Whatever the reasons, once a woman has made the decision to have an abortion, she deserves adequate counseling both before and after the procedure, as well as treatment that is compassionate and respectful.

How Safe Is Legal Abortion?

Medical and historical documents from earlier in this century describe the horrific illness and death that occurred in many women as a result of "backstreet" or "septic" abortions. Death could result from excessive bleeding, severe infection, a systemic reaction to toxic substances ingested into the body, or combinations of the above. The uterus, once invaded by an unsterile instrument, provides an excellent medium for rapid bacterial growth. An unskilled abortion may not empty the uterus completely of all the products of conception, causing the uterus to contract ineffectively. The bleeding that occurs normally after the uterus is emptied is thus prolonged, and a woman in such circumstances can bleed to death very rapidly. Additionally, some of the toxic substances eaten by or introduced into the uterus by a woman desperate to terminate a pregnancy could produce severe, often fatal poisoning.

Therapeutic abortion as it is performed today involves all the principles of surgical asepsis, so that anything entering the uterine cavity has been sterilized beforehand. No excessive bleeding takes place, and women are monitored carefully after the procedure to ascertain that all the products of conception have been expelled. Nevertheless, even when performed legally by a skilled practitioner, abortion may involve risks to the patient's health and well-being. These will be discussed below. The risk of death from abortion, however, is considerably less than that accompanying a pregnancy that is carried to term. The most important factor in determining the amount of health risk from abortion is the duration of pregnancy—the later in the pregnancy the abortion is performed, the greater the risk to the woman. The estimated death rate for abortions performed at sixteen weeks or later in the gestation is far greater than for those performed at eight weeks or less.

Abortion Procedures

■ *Early Abortion*

Abortion performed up to twelve weeks' gestation is termed "early" abortion, or "first-trimester" abortion.

"Morning-after pill": With this method, relatively high doses of synthetic estrogen are given for the three days following possible conception. The drug causes the uterine lining to shed, the way it sheds with the menstrual period. Nausea and vomiting are common side effects with this procedure.

Menstrual regulation/miniabortion: Very early in the suspected pregnancy (often before conventional pregnancy tests will be accurate), from about five to seven weeks' gestation, the procedure known as menstrual regulation or "miniabortion" may be performed. This consists of introducing a small piece of suction tubing into the uterus and gently sucking out the contents. This is performed without general anesthesia, usually in a doctor's office or clinic, and causes minimal discomfort.

Vacuum aspiration: A pregnancy of no more than eleven or twelve weeks' gestation often is terminated by this method. The cervix may be dilated by means of cones made of dried seaweed (*laminaria*). The cones are introduced into the cervical opening where they swell slightly, slowly dilating the cervix. An alternative method is the introduction of increasingly larger instruments called *sounds*. A small plastic tube is then introduced into the uterus, and a suction device is hooked up to the tubing to remove the products of conception.

The vacuum-aspiration procedure may be performed with premedication, such as analgesics or sedatives, and/or with general anesthesia or regional anesthesia. It can be done in a doctor's office, a clinic, or a hospital. The woman is in the lithotomy position for the procedure (the supine position, with feet in stirrups, as used for a pelvic exam). The perineal area is "prepped" with an antiseptic solution before the tubing is introduced into the uterus. The entire procedure usually takes less than five minutes, and the patient usually goes home within a few hours. If you are undergoing a vacuum-aspiration abortion, you may experience cramping and discomfort during the suctioning; afterwards you should experience little or no discomfort and only slight bleeding from the vagina.

After the procedure you will probably have a slight menstrual-like flow for a few days. You will be instructed to watch for unusual bleeding, high temperature, foul-smelling discharge from the vagina, abdominal or pelvic pain, or general ill feeling, all of which could signal an infection or retained products of conception. You will be given an appointment for a checkup a week or so after the abortion.

Dilatation and curettage (D & C): In this procedure, the patient is prepared in a way similar to that described above for the vacuum aspiration. General or regional anesthesia may be used; the cervix is dilated with sounds as for vacuum aspiration, and a *curette*, a small, spoon-shaped instrument, is introduced into the uterus to scrape the products of conception from the endometrium. After the procedure, you may be given a synthetic oxytocin hormone preparation to assist the uterus in contracting. You can expect to experience some cramping during the procedure and afterward, and a small amount of vaginal bleeding is normal. You will probably stay overnight in the hospital and be discharged the following day with instructions to look for signs of excessive bleeding or infection. You should schedule an appointment for a checkup a few weeks later.

■ Late-Abortion Procedures

Abortions that take place after twelve weeks' gestation are termed "late" or "second-trimester" abortions, and, as previously mentioned, they carry a greater health risk to the woman.

From the thirteenth to the fifteenth week, a *prostaglandin suppository* may be introduced into the vagina. Prostaglandins are naturally occurring substances that act somewhat like oxytocin in that they cause the uterus to contract. The products of conception are expelled gradually by the uterine contractions, just as a fetus would eventually be expelled by labor. The average length of time for a prostaglandin abortion ranges from eight to twenty-four hours; therefore, obviously, a hospital stay is required and the pain caused by the contractions is similar to the pain of labor. Other possible side effects include chills, vomiting, diarrhea, and damage to the cervix.

From sixteen to twenty-four weeks' gestation, prostaglandins may be injected into the amniotic sac much in the manner of an amniocentesis. Again, labor is induced to expel the products of conception; this procedure may take even longer because of the advanced age of the fetus. Side effects are the same as those described above, but may be even more severe. In addition, there is the risk of having a retained placenta or placental fragments after the fetus is expelled; the placenta may have to be removed with a curette, much as in a D & C.

For the same gestational period, a woman may receive a *saline injection* into the amniotic sac. Fetal death usually occurs within a short time, and the fetus and placenta are expelled at the end of labor. Labor usually starts within twelve hours after the injection; sometimes oxytocin is given intravenously to speed up labor. Labor often lasts as long as twenty-four hours and is considerably painful, as with prostaglandin procedures. The placenta may occasionally be retained and will need to be removed by D & C in that case. Among the many potential hazards of saline abortion are severe fluid and electrolyte imbalance, shock, hypertension, infection of the pelvic organs, and blood-clotting disorders.

When other late-abortion procedures are not advisable, or when the patient wants a tubal ligation at the same time as the abortion, a *hysterotomy* may be performed. This is a miniature cesarean section, and the fetus may be delivered alive and survive for several hours if gestational age is advanced enough. Risks of this procedure are the same as for any major surgery.

The many hazardous side effects and risks of late abortion procedures have already been mentioned. In addition, it is important to consider the psychological and aesthetic discomfort of actually going through what will probably be a long and painful labor, with the possibility of delivering a live fetus in all but the saline procedure. The woman who undergoes an abortion in the second trimester of pregnancy not only risks her physical health and future reproductive capacity, but is also at greater risk for psychological and emotional strain in the time period around the procedure.

Obviously, there will be many cases where a second-trimester abortion is unavoidable, but as much as possible it is advisable to have an abortion early in the pregnancy.

Counseling for an Abortion

If you think you want to have an abortion, you should talk with your gynecologist or family physician first. He or she will probably ask you about your feelings regarding the pregnancy, your current relationship with the father, and your general health status. It is advisable for you to know as much as possible in advance about the procedure you are going to have, as well as to talk with a trusted friend, family member, or social worker about the decision and your feelings before you undergo it. While many women experience regret, guilt, and grief following an abortion, you are more likely to be able to cope with these feelings if you make a fully informed decision and are aware of your feelings beforehand.

If the abortion was the result of failed or unused contraception, your gynecologist may offer you another method of birth control before you leave the office or the hospital.

Problems Following an Abortion

In addition to the hazardous side effects of specific procedures already mentioned, every invasive procedure carries the risk of infection. In rare cases, such infection can render a woman sterile by causing damage to reproductive organs. Most infections that occur after an abortion are accompanied by obvious symptoms, such as fever, muscular ache, foul-smelling vaginal discharge, and pelvic/abdominal pain.

In rare cases during a D & C the uterine wall may be punctured, resulting in severe bleeding. In such a case, the abdominal wall would be opened with an incision and the damage sutured. In addition, any procedure performed under general anesthesia has risks from the anesthesia itself, such as pneumonia from aspiration of stomach contents, severe systemic reactions, coma, and death. Fortunately, these risks are quite low.

Psychological problems following an abortion are common. Guilt feelings may last for a considerable time, and it is not uncommon to go through a "grief period," such as that following the death of a loved one, lasting several months. Depression can occasionally accompany the feelings of guilt and loss. Such negative effects may be heightened by pressure from religious beliefs, family members, or antiabortion literature. Counseling before the final decision to have the abortion, with a complete description of the procedure including physical and emotional feelings the woman is likely to have, can help to minimize the negative psychological after effects. Support and understanding from the doctor who performs the procedure, his staff, and family members and friends are of great value. Whatever an individual's feelings about abortion, as long as it remains legal in the United States, a woman's decision to have an abortion is a very private one, and her right to compassionate, respectful treatment must not be denied.

16

FAMILY THERAPY

T he family is the critical link between the internal forces of personality and the wider forces of society and culture," wrote the late Nathan W. Ackerman, a pioneer in the development of pyschotherapy for the whole family group.

Family therapy focuses on the entire family rather than on the individual who may be experiencing a particular problem. It is based on the concept that all family members are interdependent, directly or indirectly affecting each other's emotional well-being.

In 1984, over 1 million American families sought family therapy or counseling. These families sought therapy for many reasons: specific mental illness of a family member; suicide or attempted suicide; chronic or catastrophic physical illness; anorexia nervosa; marital stress or infidelity; child abuse; sexual dysfunction; remarriage; birth or death of a family member; school failure or difficulty; the stress of children leaving home. In short, any factor that affects the family's sense of stability and well-being may become the catalyst for the family seeking help.

The problems of families are ever-changing and often are shaped by society at large. For in-stance, many families now seek help in treating alcoholism and drug abuse and in coping with AIDS (acquired immune deficiency syndrome).

The professionals who offer treatment to families come from many disciplines. Psychiatrists, psychologists, social workers, nurses, and marital and pastoral counselors all offer some form of therapy. Many have earned specialized degrees in family therapy. There are more than two dozen family therapy journals and more than three-hundred specialized family therapy institutes in the United States. Many therapists do both family and individual therapy. The practice of family therapy, which not long ago was still a new concept, today has become a mainstream treatment of choice.

Historical Perspective

Family therapy is a relatively young field in comparison to individual psychotherapy. In the 1950s a number of therapists throughout the country began to note that schizophrenics who had been helped by psychotherapy in the hospital often would relapse upon returning to their families. Sometimes even a visit to the hospitalized patient by a family member would trigger psychotic behavior. The pioneers of family therapy began to ignore a basic psychoanalytic principle, which holds that having other family members present during the therapy session "contaminates" the therapeutic relationship. The context in which a person lives, especially his relations with the immediate family, was found to have a direct impact on a patient's emotional well-being.

Another revolutionary practice in family therapy involved its use of the one-way window, tape-recording, and videotaping. These devices revealed subtle interactions among family members. In addition, for the first time, senior therapists could observe their students at work, and therapists in training could watch their teachers—and themselves—on videotape. Psychiatry had always insisted on the patient's right to privacy and confidentiality, but family therapists insist that videotaping is not only a valuable teaching tool, but that it also provides a valuable check on the therapist. The fact that others will review the session, say family practitioners, makes the therapist more attentive to his own critical role and less likely to act on impulse or against the interests of the group.

Types of Family Therapy

Family therapy is characterized by a direct approach on the part of the therapist which invites the family members to participate in the process of trying to communicate—with and about themselves and with one another. Treatment of the family may be short- or long-term depending on the complexity of the problem. Short-term therapy usually involves a specific goal or is oriented toward solving a crisis, usually over a period of from six to eight weeks. It helps if family members keep an open mind about the length of time the process of treatment will take.

■ Individual Family Therapy

In this approach, each family member has a single therapist. Occasionally the family as a whole may meet together with the therapists to take stock of the family situation and work out specific issues that have been explored in the individual sessions. This works well when family members need to establish their individuality, with the family serving as a reference point. There can be drawbacks to this type of therapy if the therapists are in disagreement; family conflicts may be heightened

in response to the therapists' reactions. Also, the therapists are unable to form a complete picture of each family member, as they would if the entire family were present at therapy sessions (conjoint therapy).

■ Conjoint Therapy

In conjoint family therapy, *the family unit works together in the same room, with the same therapist at the same time.* The family is viewed as a system that has processes that transcend the characteristics of any or all of the individual members. This is the most common type of family therapy.

■ Combined Therapy

While the family unit is being seen in conjoint therapy, one or more family members also may be seen individually. This is *combined therapy.* Sometimes various combinations of family members are seen, for example, just parents together or just children together.

■ Multiple-Family Group Therapy

Here, four or five different families meet weekly because of common problems or issues. Working with several therapists, family members learn to form relationships outside their family unit; the acquisition of social skills helps them to become more adaptable and better able to cope with problems thrown in their path. Group members form a valuable support group even after the formal therapy sessions have ended.

■ Multiple-Impact Therapy

In multiple-impact therapy, as in multiple-family group therapy, several families are brought together, but this is done intensively, with therapists and families staying together for a three-day weekend or week-long encounter. With this intense and time-limited approach families learn to work together in a community of families. Multiple-impact-therapy groups work toward solving a definite problem. Because of the intense nature of this therapy, it should not be used with families that have a psychotic member.

■ Network Intervention

Here, the family unit meets not only with a team of therapists but also with as many as forty friends, relatives, neighbors, and perhaps other interested parties, such as physicians or police officers, who come to the family's home in order to help that family solve its problems. Providing a network that is larger than an immediate family is thought to help the family explore new forms of communication and become "unlocked" from destructive family patterns. Network intervention usually lasts for only a few sessions. It is an intense and exhausting approach carried out in the hope that a lasting support group will emerge.

The Use of the Genogram in Family Therapy

Family therapy's strength lies in its responsive techniques and practical problem-solving, with less emphasis placed upon theory. The *generational approach* is the most highly developed in family therapy to date. In this approach, the therapist uses special symbols on a family tree to note events that are psychologically important (such as separations and divorces). This is called a genogram; the symbols enable the therapist and the family to track patterns of behavior from generation to generation. Destructive patterns that have passed on from one generation to the next can be avoided in the future if a family's behavior and self-image can be altered. Genograms are most useful in extended families where several generations are represented. For a family that has little or no awareness or contact with an earlier generation, a family therapist probably would not use the genogram.

Concepts of Family Functioning

In 1981 the family therapists Green and Franco identified twelve major concepts of family functioning from the literature written by family theorists to date. These are areas that a family therapist will explore as he or she assesses the ways to help a family in need.

Concept 1: The family as an open system

Family members function both inside and outside the family and influence one another. Family members are interdependent, and if one family member's behavior is disturbing it will be returned in kind (reciprocated) by another family member.

Concept 2: Family stability and change

Families tend to function as if governed by a set of rules but will be able to change over time. Family members will react to restore stability that has been threatened by the behavior of another member. Family units will adjust their codes of behavior to accommodate life-cycle or other changes in a family member, but families in trouble lack the flexibility needed to accomplish this.

Concept 3: Family and social organization

The therapist must understand the relationships between the family unit and other systems, such as the extended family, school, workplace, and ethnic and religious affiliations. This is the context within which the family functions, and the therapist must know which systems have the greatest impact on the family. In turn, the family itself provides the context for the relationships between individual members: between spouses, between siblings, and between parent and child.

Concept 4: Family communication disorder

All behavior in social situations involves some sort of communication. All communication has a content (what is said) and a relationship (how it is presented). If these two facets of communication are usually contradictory—as, for example, when a mother tells a child she loves him but pushes him away—then family members will feel confused, and disturbed behavior may result.

Concept 5: Individuality and family conflict

Each family member has individual perceptions, needs, and beliefs that may place him or her in disagreement with the family as a whole. Each family develops a way of managing conflict. In some families, members are willing to compromise and work out solutions together. Other families avoid conflict altogether, ignoring the needs of individual members. In some families there is a competitive approach to conflicts, with individuals unwilling to compromise.

Concept 6: Marital conflict and the parental alliance in well-functioning families

In a family that is functioning well, spouses manage conflict by maintaining a strong alliance that is the product of accepting each other's differences and working to satisfy each other's needs. Even if parents disagree they usually support each other in front of the children. The child is not allowed to enter into husband-wife conflicts as "judge" or "umpire."

*Concept 7: Dysfunction and unresolved
marital conflict*

Failure to resolve marital conflict because of constant competitive bickering or avoidance of confrontation may precipitate involvement of third parties in the marital problems. The presence in the conflict of others such as lovers, policemen, mental health professionals, or children will intensify old problems and cause new problems to emerge.

*Concept 8: The "triangled" child and
the breaching of generational boundaries*

It is inappropriate for a child to become involved in a marital conflict. If a child becomes referee, decoy, ally, or even surrogate spouse or parent, then he forms a "triangle" with his parents. The child's ability to become independent is threatened if he becomes too involved in the problems of either parent, and a greater distance may be created between the parents. Overprotection, scapegoating, and interparent competition may occur when roles are altered.

Concept 9: Transference and projection

Spouses sometimes choose each other in a conscious or unconscious effort to avoid or replicate patterns of behavior experienced in childhood with their own parents. The way that one spouse responds to the desires of the other brings the feared or desired behavior into play.

*Concept 10: Parent involvement with
family of origin*

Spouses owe their prime loyalty to their new family. A policy of give-and-take in dealings with one's spouse's family of origin should minimize the chances of divided loyalties.

Concept 11: Affective expression

Rigid family rules can restrict the expression and possibly the experience of feelings and thereby cause disturbed behavior.

Concept 12: Incomplete mourning

A code of conduct that blocks family members from showing and sharing grief about death and other losses may make it difficult for a family member, especially a child, to separate from the family and find an individual identity. The family member will be locked into "anxious attachment."

Therapy with the whole family will work if *permanent* changes in the structures of communication and behavior are made. The challenge faced by family therapists is to offer families the kind of help that eventually lets them function well on their own.

Where to Get Help

In larger cities in this country there are many institutes devoted to family therapy. One of the foundation establishments is the Ackerman Institute, 149 East 78th Street, New York, New York 10021. Phone: 212-879-4900.

In smaller communities, you may find local clinics, physicians, hospitals, and some churches that are able to recommend appropriate family therapists. Listings in the phonebook yellow pages usually indicate whether or not a professional therapist specializes in treating families. Clients should be sure that any therapist they choose has proper training. Libraries will have the *National Register of Health Service Providers.* Psychologists are listed under their area of specialization and credentials are given. The guides published by the American Psychological Association and American Psychiatric Association also list specialists in the field of family therapy.

The American Family Therapy Association in Washington, D.C., has a nationwide membership. Its telephone number is 202-659-7666.

SECTION THREE

WELLNESS

W hat is health? Many people—and even many physicians—would define health as being "not sick." "I'm healthy when my nose isn't running." "I'm healthy when my arthritis isn't acting up." "I'm healthy as long as I don't have cancer."But is that really *health*? What about the sedentary, obese individual who loves hamburgers and french fries? Is this individual healthy?

Many of us think about our health only when illness occurs. And much of our health care system focuses on heroic efforts to cure the ill individual. But consider the case of the two lifeguards at the beach on a rough, stormy day. One lifeguard sees a man in distress, rushes into the surf, and performs a heroic rescue and resuscitation. He sees a woman screaming for help, rushes in once more, performing another heroic effort. The other lifeguard, observing the dangerous conditions, gets out his bullhorn and warns people away, meanwhile walking back and forth on the beach to prevent any more individuals from entering the water.

Heroic efforts to cure illness are both needed and welcomed. But equally important are the less glamorous and more mundane preventive efforts to maintain a state of "health" or "wellness."

The majority of us must rely, for the most part, on hospitals, physicians, and other health care providers for treatment when illness occurs. But for preventive efforts, we can, to a large extent, rely on ourselves. There are certain life-style choices we can make to prevent illness, to prolong life, and even to "feel" good. For instance, we can modify our diet to reduce the risk of heart disease or cancer; we can stop smoking; we can avoid the sun; we can drink moderately and never when we drive; we can keep trim and exercise regularly; we

can avoid illicit drugs; and we can have regular physical examinations by a physician.

This chapter will be devoted to "wellness"—to explaining how the individual can maintain an optimum state of health.

What is a realistic ideal of wellness? Is the attractive, thin, and limber aerobics instructor the ideal of wellness? Could Winston Churchill, who ate, drank, and smoked cigars until the age of 87, also be categorized as "well"? What about the occasional athlete or runner who dies suddenly of a heart attack?

Even as we pursue health and fitness, factors like age and heredity exert a strong influence on how long we will live and on whether we will develop major, life-threatening disease. And "luck" comes into play as well, as when a fit man in his early 50s—with both his parents in their 90s and still active—is killed in a freak accident as a car in the opposite lane spins out of control.

True, such events sometimes *do* happen. But much more often it is *we* who decide our fate. To a substantial extent we can be our own lifeguards.

The Scientific Method

Many claims have been made that a variety of regimens, both dietary and otherwise, will promote "health" and "wellness." The recommendations for a healthy life-style that appear in this chapter are those that have been accepted by the scientific and medical communities.

The rationale for the actions of the scientific and medical communities is based largely on what is known as the "scientific method." Essentially, the scientific method begins with observation and proceeds to the formation of a hypothesis. The hypothesis is tested in experiments, after which a conclusion is reached. When repeated experiments consistently come up with similar findings, and there are few studies that contradict these findings, it is likely that the hypothesis is valid.

For instance, it was observed during World War II that the strict rationing of high-fat foods necessitated by wartime constraints had an unexpected benefit: a reduction in heart-attack fatalities. That observation, combined with a number of others, led to a hypothesis: High-fat diets contribute to heart disease. Numerous studies and experiments were performed with animals and with groups of people, and over a period of years evidence began to accumulate that high-fat (and high-cholesterol) diets did indeed contribute to the development of heart disease. By the mid-1980s the medical and scientific communities were in agreement: High-fat diets promote heart disease.

A similar kind of rationale has gone into the recommendations of medical experts on methods of preventing heart disease and cancer and on the ways in which we can prolong life.

Although the average individual may not feel qualified to evaluate the scientific and medical literature—nor may he or she have the time or inclination—an understanding of how and why the medical community has come to a given conclusion will give the individual greater confidence in its recommendations.

In This Chapter . . .

Here you'll find·what the medical and scientific communities currently believe are the best methods of preventing disease and promoting health.

We'll begin with a discussion of heart disease and cancer: In developed countries, these diseases account for the greatest number of deaths. To a large extent, cancer and heart disease can be controlled by life-style modifications with regard to diet, exercise, smoking, and certain other factors. We'll come to understand what these diseases are, how the risk factors contribute to their development, and how we can modify these factors to reduce our risk.

A separate discussion on nutrition is also included, since nutritional practices are important in preventing heart disease, in reducing the risk of cancer, and in promoting overall "health." Likewise, there is a discussion of exercise and its benefits (most agree these are significant), as well as its potential risks.

We'll also discuss how to maintain a "safe" lifestyle. Accidents are the number 4 killer (after heart attack, cancer, and stroke) in the United States. A discussion of how to avoid motor vehicle collisions, falls, fires, and other accidents is included in this chapter. Another important component of a safe life-style is avoidance of drug and alcohol abuse, and this too is discussed.

There is a final caution: In no way should the recommendations in this chapter be substituted for the advice of your physician. The recommendations given here are valid for the average individual and for the population as a whole. If you are a "healthy" individual with no visible illness, the guidelines given here will probably be in substantial agreement with your physician's advice. But only your physician knows you, your history, your combination of risk factors, and your state of overall health. The chapter is designed as an adjunct to your physician's advice. It is not intended to substitute for it. Consult your physician if you have any questions as to what's right for you.

17

THE HEALTHY HEART

Shortly after World War II, officials of the United States Public Health Service, alarmed at what seemed to be an epidemic of heart deaths in the United States, began a major effort to understand and combat heart disease. They decided to study a typical sample of Americans over the space of a generation. As their headquarters they chose a white frame house in Framingham, Massachusetts, a small town some thirty miles southwest of Boston.

The data provided by the study were designed to include an analysis of each participant's heredity, life-style, and medical history. The data, they hoped, would yield the answer to the question uppermost in their minds: Why do some individuals develop heart disease while others do not?

In 1949, more than two thirds of the town's residents between the ages of 30 and 62 agreed to enter the Framingham Heart Study, committing themselves to return at periodic intervals to the study headquarters. When the study began, 5,127 of the 5,209 people involved in the study had no heart disease, and all but 2 percent of those who entered the study stayed with it. Almost four decades after the study began about half of the participants were still alive, with the oldest well into his 90s and the youngest in his 60s.

The Framingham study was especially important in that it was a large *prospective* study. That

is, it took a group of individuals and followed them over a period of time to determine how they fared. It is far easier to undertake what is known as a *retrospective* study, in which individuals already ill from a disease are analyzed as to what vulnerabilities they have in common. But the data from a retrospective study, although valuable, are far more open to question than those of a prospective study like Framingham.

The Framingham findings were:

• Smoking, high blood pressure, and high cholesterol levels are strongly linked to heart disease.

• Other important risk factors are gender (men are more likely to develop heart disease than are women), obesity, "Type A" personality, family history of heart disease, and low activity level.*

Individuals with one or more of these "risk factors" are more likely to develop heart disease. These factors are not, of themselves, a "death sentence," but they do render the individual more likely to die of cardiovascular causes. There are, though, some simple steps we can take to reduce our risks of developing heart disease.

Age, sex, and heredity are immutable; they cannot be altered. But other important risk fac-

---

* The Framingham data on activity level and personality type are not entirely conclusive, but other studies confirm a link between these factors and heart disease.

tors *can* be managed by the individual. Evidence continues to accumulate—not only from Framingham but from numerous other studies as well—that by lowering cholesterol levels, stopping the use of tobacco, and controlling high blood pressure we can reduce the risk of developing cardiovascular problems. It's probably prudent as well to increase one's activity level—many doctors recommend regular exercise—and to reduce levels of stress, when possible.

Conclusion: All of us do have some degree of control. By *adding* risk factors, we tip the scales on the side of disease. By *removing* risk factors we help our heart to function in maintaining life.

Major risk factors:

- Smoking
- High Blood Pressure
- High Cholesterol
- Male Gender
- Obesity
- Family History of Heart Disease
- Low Exercise Level
- "Type A" Personality
- High Stress

The Powerful Pump

The heart is a muscular organ about the size of a large pear. It has four chambers, two on the right and two on the left. The upper chambers are called the *atria*, while the lower chambers are called the *ventricles*. Connected to the heart are the major blood vessels, which divide and subdivide throughout the body into smaller and smaller vessels that supply the tissues.

Fired by electrical impulses, the heart contracts and relaxes, or "beats," some 100,000 times each day, receiving blood through the veins and sending it out again through the arteries to supply the cells of the body with oxygen and nutrients. The heart pumps about 1,500 to 3,000 gallons of blood each day.

Like all the other tissues of the body, heart tissue also requires oxygen and nutrients in order to function. The blood that the heart pumps also supplies the heart muscle, which has its own system of vessels—the coronary arteries (see illustration)—that supply it with oxygenated blood. Conditions that affect these arteries will affect the functioning of the heart.

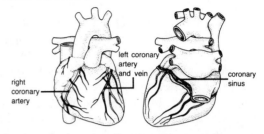

CORONARY ARTERIES

FRONT SURFACE OF HEART   BACK SURFACE OF HEART

The heart muscle receives its oxygen supply from the right and left coronary arteries. If either of these vessels becomes blocked, a "heart attack" occurs—with muscle damage, chest pain, and possibly death. The coronary veins drain into the right atrium via the coronary sinus.

When Things Go Wrong

Of the current United States population of about 245 million, over 64 million individuals have some form of *cardiovascular disease.* That term usually brings to mind the so-called "heart attack." But cardiovascular problems include also such disorders as stroke, angina, arrhythmia, and congestive heart failure.

Although cardiovascular disease usually doesn't show up until the later years (usually in the 50s and 60s), it begins with processes that start in childhood. The predominant forms of cardiovascular disease involve atherosclerosis, or "hardening of the arteries."

The earliest change in the vessels consists of a fatty streak, rich in lipids and white cells. As the child enters adulthood and then middle age, the typical fatty streak turns into the fibrous (atherosclerotic) *plaque*, composed of blood-vessel tissue, white cells, fat droplets, scar tissue, cellular debris, cholesterol, and calcium.

About one-half of all Americans have significant atherosclerosis at the time of death. And, although most people think of atherosclerosis as a disease of aging, the ravages of the disease can begin in the early 20s. Autopsy studies of young soldiers killed in Vietnam and Korea showed that substantial numbers had atherosclerotic plaques.

As the atherosclerotic plaques build up on blood vessel walls, the vessels of the heart become constricted, choking off the heart's blood supply. The heart muscle, lacking oxygen and suffocating in its own waste, gives out a cry of pain. In medical terms this type of chest pain is known as *angina pectoris.*

As vessels continue to narrow, it becomes easier for a clot to form. The consequence is a *heart attack*, which results from total blockage of the coronary arteries. A heart attack, also known as a *myocardial infarction,* is characterized by death of a part of the heart muscle.

Angina pectoris differs from heart attack in that the blood circulation is not completely cut off. Often, the heart's supply of blood is enough for normal needs but proves insufficient when the heart comes under strain. For instance, running for a train might trigger an anginal attack, but walking might not.

Strokes can occur when atherosclerosis develops in the vessels of the brain. This type of stroke is known as a *cerebral thrombosis.* Strokes can also be the consequence of a wandering clot, or embolus, that moves along in the bloodstream until it becomes stuck in one of the arteries of the brain. Stroke may also be caused by bursting of a defective artery in the brain.

Arrhythmias often result from atherosclerosis. These abnormal rhythms result from disturbances of the network of electrical-conducting tissue that regulates the pumping of the heart. Arrhythmias are particularly common following a heart attack, because the death of heart muscle also damages the heart's electrical tissue. The result is a malfunctioning heart and consequent disability.

Congestive heart failure is *not* the same as a heart attack. It occurs as a result of damage to the heart muscle or valves; the damage may be the consequence of heart attack, atherosclerosis, high blood pressure, or other condition. The injured heart muscle is unable to pump sufficient blood into the tissues, causing blood to back up behind the heart. As a result, fluid accumulates in the lungs or in the tissues.

Typical symptoms of congestive heart failure include swelling of the legs or difficulty in breathing. Treatment usually is directed at the cause. For example, high blood pressure should be treated with medication and diet.

Intermittent claudication may occur when atherosclerotic disease begins to affect the blood vessels of the extremities, particularly those of the leg. The key symptoms are pains, aches, or cramps in the leg (most often the calf) that occur on walking.

• • •

Heart transplants may catch the headlines, but they are only a small part of the fight against heart disease. In the 1970s and 1980s, death rates from heart disease, which rose throughout the 1960s, have declined at a rate of 2 percent per year. In part, the decrease can be attributed to improved medical care, better coronary-care units, and training in the techniques of cardiopulmonary resuscitation (CPR).

But there are other factors that help to explain the declining death rates. Prevention has been equally important. Many individuals have stopped smoking; numerous Americans have cut down on their consumption of cholesterol and fats; many more persons with hypertension are controlling their condition with medication and/or life-style changes; and great numbers of men and women are dedicated to running, cycling, swimming, and other forms of exercise.

Heart Attacks: The Symptoms Spell Emergency

A heart attack is a medical emergency. If you or anyone you are with begins to show the symptoms of a heart attack, get help immediately.

The warning signals are these:

- Uncomfortable pressure, fullness, squeezing, or pain in the center of the chest lasting 2 minutes or longer.
- Pain spreading to the shoulders, neck, or arms.
- Severe pain, dizziness, fainting, sweating, nausea, or shortness of breath.

  Not all of these warning signals occur in every heart attack. If even some begin to occur, don't wait. Call for medical attention.

Know what to do if heart attack strikes:

- Find out which nearby hospital has 24-hour emergency cardiac care, and tell your family and friends to call this facility in an emergency.
- Keep a list of emergency rescue service numbers next to your telephone and in your pocket, wallet, or purse.
- If you detect the warning signs of a heart attack, call the Emergency Medical Service or town rescue squad.
- If you can get to a hospital faster without waiting for the ambulance, have someone drive you.

If you are with someone who is showing the signs of a heart attack:

- Act immediately, even if the person denies that he or she is having a heart attack.
- Call the Emergency Medical Service or get to the nearest hospital emergency room that offers 24-hour emergency cardiac care.
- If you are trained, give CPR (cardiopulmonary resuscitation) when it becomes necessary.

Adapted from *1988 Heart Facts,* American Heart Association

To sum up, the recent decline in cardiovascular fatalities has been attributed—probably rightly so—to the progress that has been made in controlling the major risk factors for heart disease with medication, diet, and life-style changes.

The Role of Hypertension

Contributing to the development of heart and blood vessel disease is *hypertension*, or high blood pressure. Blood pressure is the force the blood exerts against the blood vessel walls. An individual with high blood pressure has a pressure level that exceeds optimum levels.

Blood pressure is defined in terms of the *systolic* (upper) reading, which is the pressure at the moment of the heart's contraction, and the *diastolic* (lower) reading, which is the pressure when the heart is relaxed. Normal blood pressure hovers around 125 systolic, and 80 diastolic. High blood pressure is defined generally as a reading above 140 systolic and 90 diastolic.

Hypertension causes injury to the blood vessels, making it easier for atherosclerosis to develop. It is also the major factor in the development of stroke. In addition, hypertension makes the heart work harder, resulting in an enlarged heart, poorer function, and congestive heart failure. Hypertension can result in damage to the eyes and kidneys as well.

In the majority of individuals with high blood pressure, the precise cause cannot be determined. This type of hypertension, known as "primary" or "essential" hypertension, accounts for about 90 percent of all cases. In the 10 percent of individuals with hypertension for which a cause can be discerned and corrected, it may be due to a narrowing of blood vessels that has existed from birth, to a kidney that produces a blood-pressure-provoking enzyme, renin (renovascular hypertension), or to a tumor that causes overproduction of epinephrine (pheochromocytoma).

In many cases, hypertensive persons have no symptoms. Their condition is discovered only in the course of a screening exam or annual physical. In other persons, the condition may produce symptoms such as morning headache.

For the individual with essential hypertension—the type for which a precise cause cannot be determined—treatment modalities include drugs and life-style modifications. A number of powerful and potent drugs are available for treating hypertension: These include: *diuretics*, drugs that increase the excretion of salt and water from/by the body; *Beta-blockers*, drugs that act to ease the heart's pumping action; *Vasodilators*, drugs that act directly on blood vessels to expand them; *Sympathetic nerve inhibitors*, drugs that prevent the sympathetic nerves from narrowing blood vessels; and *ACE inhibitors*, a relatively new class of drugs that interferes with the body's production of angiotensen, a chemical that causes the arteries to constrict.

Equally as important are life-style changes: reduction in salt intake and intake of dietary fats, exercise, weight reduction, and various approaches to stress reduction such as relaxation therapy and biofeedback. These life-style modifications, basic to a well-designed hypertension treatment program, are also helpful in reducing the risk of heart disease for an individual who is not suffering from hypertension.

Salt intake. A reduction in *sodium intake* is particularly important for persons with hypertension. They should limit their dietary intake of salt to 2 grams of sodium per day. This goal can be achieved by avoiding table salt, withdrawing salted foods from the diet, and substituting herbs and spices for salt in cooking.

Convenience foods, processed foods, dairy products, and "fast foods" are particularly high in sodium. Note that it is actually sodium intake, not merely salt intake, that must be reduced. Salt is sodium chloride, but substances commonly used in food processing—monosodium glutamate (MSG), for example—also contain sodium. Hypertensives need to watch their intake of these substances too. *Read labels carefully.*

Life-style. Other important measures to take include weight reduction and exercise. A number of studies have shown that regular exercise reduces blood pressure (regular exercise, of course, also helps in weight reduction). In addition, overweight individuals are far more likely than normal-weight individuals to suffer from hypertension, and weight reduction often brings down blood pressure. In addition to its effect on blood pressure, obesity also exerts an independent adverse effect on cardiovascular health.

Reduction in fat intake, while not directly contributing to the control of hypertension, is believed to slow the development of atherosclerosis and to reduce cardiovascular risk. For the individual with hypertension, who is already at increased risk of heart attack or stroke, these additional life-style changes are critically important.

Stress. The treatment plan for an individual who

A SHORT GUIDE TO SODIUM CONTENT OF FOODS

Foods	Approximate Sodium Content (in milligrams)
BREADS, CEREALS, AND GRAIN PRODUCTS	
Cooked cereal, pasta, rice (unsalted)	Less than 5 per $\frac{1}{2}$ cup
Ready-to-eat cereal	100-360 per oz.
Bread, whole-grain or enriched	110-175 per slice
Biscuits and muffins	170-390 each
VEGETABLES	
Fresh or frozen vegetables (cooked without added salt)	Less than 70 per $\frac{1}{2}$ cup
Vegetables, canned or frozen with sauce	140-460 per $\frac{1}{2}$ cup
FRUIT	
Fruits (fresh, frozen, or canned)	Less than 10 per $\frac{1}{2}$ cup
MILK, CHEESE, AND YOGURT	
Milk and yogurt	120-160 per cup
Buttermilk (salt added)	260 per cup
Natural cheeses	110-450 per $1\frac{1}{2}$-oz. serving
Cottage cheese (regular and lowfat)	450 per $\frac{1}{2}$ cup
Process cheese and cheese spreads	700-900 per 2-oz. serving
MEAT, POULTRY, AND FISH	
Fresh meat, poultry, finfish	Less than 90 per 3-oz. serving
Cured ham, sausages, luncheon meat, frankfurters, canned meats	750-1,350 per 3-oz. serving
FATS AND DRESSINGS	
Oil	None
Vinegar	Less than 6 per tbsp.
Prepared salad dressings	80-250 per tbsp.
Unsalted butter or margarine	1 per tsp.
Salted butter or margarine	45 per tsp.
Salt pork, cooked	360 per oz.
CONDIMENTS	
Catsup, mustard, chili sauce, tartar sauce, steak sauce	125-275 per tbsp.
Soy sauce	1,000 per tbsp.
Salt	2,000 per tsp.
SNACK AND CONVENIENCE FOODS	
Canned and dehydrated soups	630-1,300 per cup
Canned and frozen main dishes	800-1,400 per 8-oz, serving
Unsalted nuts and popcorn	Less than 5 per oz.
Salted nuts, potato chips, corn chips	150-300 per oz.
Deep-fried pork rind	750 per oz.

SOURCE: U.S. Department of Agriculture, *Dietary Guidelines for Americans.*

has hypertension may also include various relaxation and biofeedback therapies. Biofeedback therapies involve giving patients immediate indications of their blood pressure levels, eventually allowing them to control their blood pressure. While not effective in every hypertensive individual, these therapies have been shown to lower blood pressure in a significant number of individuals. More on the relaxation therapies can be found below, under *The Role of Stress.* See also BIOFEEDBACK under **Procedures** and RELAXATION THERAPY in **Medical A–Z.**

For a precise treatment program, consult a physician. A family physician who knows you and your medical history can design an effective plan of therapy. Improvement can be expected, provided you follow the plan wholeheartedly and without fail.

The Role of Cholesterol

The medical community has come to a firm consensus that persons with hypertension need to keep their blood pressure under control. Cholesterol and saturated fats, however, are more recent suspects in the disease process; indeed, they may be the major villains in the piece.

Cholesterol, a soft, fat-like substance found in all cells of the body, is used to form cell membranes and certain hormones as well as other necessary chemicals. It is essential—in small quantities. There is now a substantial body of evidence demonstrating that high blood cholesterol plays a major role in the development of heart disease.

Blood cholesterol levels are determined in part by heredity and in part by diet. Diets high in saturated fats and cholesterol tend to raise blood cholesterol levels, thereby (it is believed) increasing the risk of death from heart disease.

The case against cholesterol consists of several kinds of evidence: evidence that high levels of blood cholesterol are associated with heart-death risk, evidence that certain kinds of diets increase heart-disease risk, and evidence that lowering blood cholesterol may be beneficial.

The evidence has been accumulating since World War II, when food rationing in Europe was associated with lowered heart-attack rates. With the end of the war came a renewed affluence and cardiovascular deaths climbed, perhaps because Europeans once more began to consume meat, butter, and eggs—foods high in saturated fats.

By the 1960s and late 1970s, evidence linking diet, cholesterol, and coronary heart disease continued to mount. For instance, cholesterol and related substances are found in atherosclerotic deposits, suggesting a possible role. Further, cholesterol consumed in the diet often ends up in those atherosclerotic plaques, suggesting but not proving a link.

Animal experiments demonstrate that monkeys fed a typical American diet develop atherosclerosis. When the monkeys are introduced to a low-fat diet, their atherosclerotic lesions ultimately regress and disappear.

Such experiments are impractical in humans, and the evidence linking cholesterol and heart disease must be sought from the epidemiologist and the clinician, who study existing groups and populations. The Framingham study, for instance, pointed to elevated blood cholesterol levels as a major risk factor for coronary heart disease.

Other epidemiological reports make cross-cultural comparisons. For instance, the so-called Ni-Hon-San study investigated coronary deaths among populations of Japanese living in Japan, Hawaii, and San Francisco. The study showed that as the Japanese migrated to the United States and began to adopt a diet high in saturated fats and cholesterol, coronary deaths likewise rose. Compared to Japan, death rates were higher in Hawaii and even higher in San Francisco.

Ideally, evidence for the role of diet would come from a major study of large numbers of patients over a long period of time. Unfortunately, such a study would require at least 60,000 participants and would take a decade to complete. It would be difficult to motivate, would be difficult to conduct with control groups (could a high-fat diet for the controls be justified?), and, finally, it would have a prohibitive price tag.

■ What the Experts Recommend

A 1985 consensus conference report from the National Institute of Health represented a jelling of opinion among heart disease experts that diet, cholesterol levels, and heart disease were inextricably linked.

Two years later, in October of 1987, the National Cholesterol Education Program released an updated report calling on physicians to monitor every American adult's blood cholesterol level and to prescribe diets (and in some instances medication) for those found to be at risk.

The Good and The Bad

In the story of cholesterol, there are villains and there are heroes. Cholesterol, which can't dissolve in the blood, is circulated in the body by the aid of a protein that can associate with fats. These lipoproteins are of several types, the "good" and the "bad." Low-density lipoprotein, or LDL, is the "bad guy": It favors deposition of cholesterol in tissues. High-density lipoprotein, or HDL, comes to the rescue: it is the "good guy," serving as a magnet to keep cholesterol from invading arterial walls. There is also another protein, known as very-low-density lipoprotein (VLDL), which carry another type of fat known as triglyceride.

The total cholesterol in the blood is that contained in all types of carriers—the HDL, the LDL, and, in small amounts, in the VLDL. Levels of these lipoproteins are determined by genetic tendencies, by diet, and by activity levels. Vigorous exercise, for instance, raises blood levels of HDL.

A desirable level of the LDL "bad guy" is 130 mg/dl, while LDL levels between 130 and 160 are considered borderline-risky. Patients with LDL levels above 160 are considered at high risk.

The 1987 report included these recommendations:

• All Americans should have their blood cholesterol tested once every five years.

• A single set of desirable cholesterol levels for all age groups is now available (previously, desirable cholesterol levels varied according to age):

Below 200 mg/dl: low risk

Between 200 and 240 mg/dl: borderline-high risk

Over 240 mg/dl: high risk

• Low-fat diets are indicated for patients deemed to be at risk.

• When fat-restricted diets fail to lower blood cholesterol, drug therapy may be necessary.

Drug therapy cannot be universally recommended because evidence for the long-term safety of cholesterol-reducing medications is not yet in.

Useful drugs include cholestyramine, colestipol, and nicotinic acid. Another cholesterol-lowering drug, lovastatin, came on the market in 1987.

Experts estimate that at least one quarter of all Americans will be found in need of either drug or dietary therapy to bring their blood cholesterol levels down to desirable levels.

Talk of milligrams of cholesterol, saturates and polyunsaturates, percentages and poundages can be confusing. We need to translate what we know about the benefits of low-fat, low-cholesterol diets into action at the grocery counter and refrigerator.

The arithmetic of cholesterol-counting is simple if we follow a chart like the one here, "A Primer on Fat, Saturated Fatty Acids, and Cholesterol in Foods." For example, it shows that a breakfast of two eggs and waffles would provide more than

---

PRIMER ON FAT, SATURATED FATTY ACIDS, AND CHOLESTEROL IN FOODS

MEAT/POULTRY/FISH/ALTERNATES

You can trim off most visible fat. But cholesterol is found in both lean and fat. Dry beans and peas (often used in place of meat) contain no cholesterol and most contain very little fat.

		Total fat grams	Saturated fatty acids grams	Cholesterol milligrams
Beef arm, roasted:				
Lean and fat	3 ounces	16	8	80
Lean only	3 ounces	6	3	77
Ground beef, cooked:				
Regular	3-ounce patty	17	7	77
Lean	3-ounce patty	15	6	80
Pork rib, roasted:				
Lean and fat	3 ounces	20	7	69
Lean only	3 ounces	12	4	67
Beef liver, fried	3 ounces	9	2	372
Chicken, light and dark meat, roasted:				
With skin	3 ounces	12	3	75
Without skin	3 ounces	6	2	76
Halibut fillets, broiled, with margarine	3 ounces	6	1	48
Tuna salad	½ cup	10	2	40
Crabs, hardshell, steamed	2 medium	2	0	96
Dry beans, cooked	½ cup	1	trace	0
Peanut butter	2 tablespoons	16	2	0
Egg, large, cooked	1 yolk	6	2	274
	1 white	trace	0	0

BREADS/CEREALS/OTHER GRAIN PRODUCTS

Grains are naturally low in fat and cholesterol, but ingredients used in preparation of bread and cereal products may contain considerable amounts. Some spreads also add fat, saturated fatty acids, and cholesterol.

		Total fat grams	Saturated fatty acids grams	Cholesterol milligrams
Bread:				
White	1 slice	1	trace	0
Whole-wheat	1 slice	1	trace	0
Bagel, plain	1 bagel	2	trace	0
Biscuit	1 biscuit	5	1	trace
Roll, dinner	1 roll	2	1	trace
Coffee cake	1 piece	7	2	47
Danish pastry	1 piece	12	4	49
Doughnut, yeast	1 doughnut	13	5	21
Muffin, blueberry	1 muffin	5	2	19
Pancake	1 pancake	2	1	16
Waffle	1 waffle	8	3	59
Oatmeal, cooked	½ cup	1	trace	0
Shredded wheat	1 biscuit	trace	0	0
Granola	⅓ cup	5	3	0
Rice, white, cooked	½ cup	trace	trace	0
Fried rice	½ cup	6	1	51
Cookie, oatmeal	1 cookie	2	1	1

MILK/CHEESE/YOGURT

Low-fat milk provides about the same nutrients as whole milk but less fat, saturated fatty acids, and cholesterol.

		Total fat grams	Saturated fatty acids grams	Cholesterol milligrams
Milk:				
Whole	1 cup	8	5	33
2% fat	1 cup	5	3	18
Skim	1 cup	1	trace	5
Buttermilk	1 cup	2	1	9
Yogurt:				
Low-fat plain	8-ounce carton	4	2	14
Low-fat fruit-flavored	8-ounce carton	2	2	10
Cottage cheese:				
Creamed	1 cup	9	6	31
Low-fat	1 cup	4	3	19
Cheese:				
Natural Cheddar	1 ounce	9	6	30
Mozzarella, part skim milk	1 ounce	5	3	15
Process American	1 ounce	9	6	27
Macaroni and cheese	$\frac{3}{4}$ cup	17	7	32
Vanilla ice cream	$\frac{1}{2}$ cup	7	4	30
Vanilla ice milk	$\frac{1}{2}$ cup	3	2	9

Source: U.S. Department of Agriculture, *Dietary Guidelines for Americans.*

VEGETABLES

Served plain, vegetables are low in fat and none of them contain cholesterol. But added ingredients and extras such as sauces can change the picture.

		Total fat grams	Saturated fatty acids grams	Cholesterol milligrams
Potatoes:				
Baked	1 medium	trace	trace	0
French fries	10 strips	8	3	0
Chips	10 chips	7	2	0
Au gratin	$\frac{1}{2}$ cup	19	12	56
Cabbage:				
Cooked	$\frac{1}{2}$ cup	trace	trace	0
Coleslaw	$\frac{1}{2}$ cup	2	trace	5
Stir-fried vegetables	$\frac{1}{2}$ cup	3	trace	0

FRUITS

Fruits add interesting colors, textures, and flavors to meals and snacks. Most are very low in fat and none contain cholesterol.

		Total fat grams	Saturated fatty acids grams	Cholesterol milligrams
Apple	1 medium	trace	trace	0
Avocado	$\frac{1}{2}$ medium	15	2	0
Banana	1 medium	1	trace	0
Olive, green	5 large	3	trace	0
Olive, ripe	5 large	5	1	0
Orange	1 medium	trace	trace	0
Peach	1 medium	trace	trace	0
Strawberries	5 berries	trace	trace	0
Mixed fruit with cream dressing	$\frac{1}{2}$ cup	10	3	18

FATS/SWEETS

Fat can add up from the "extras" you add and the desserts you eat.

		Total fat grams	Saturated fatty acids grams	Cholesterol milligrams
Butter	1 tablespoon	11	7	31
Margarine:				
Soft	1 tablespoon	11	2	0
Stick	1 tablespoon	11	2	0
Vegetable oil (corn)	1 tablespoon	14	2	0
Salad dressing:				
Mayonnaise	1 tablespoon	11	2	8
Mayonnaise-type	1 tablespoon	5	1	4
Italian, low-calorie	1 tablespoon	trace	trace	0
Italian	1 tablespoon	9	1	0
Cream:				
Sour	1 tablespoon	3	2	5
Light (table)	1 tablespoon	3	2	10
Nondairy, frozen	1 tablespoon	2	1	0
Cream cheese	1 ounce (2 tablespoons)	10	6	31
Cake, frosted, devil's food	$\frac{1}{12}$ 8"-layer	11	5	50
Brownie	1 brownie	6	1	18
Pie, apple	$\frac{1}{6}$ pie	18	5	2

700 milligrams of cholesterol. In contrast, a breakfast of toast, peanut butter, and a dish of fruit—say, sliced banana with a little cream—would contain less than 50 milligrams of cholesterol.

How fats affect our cholesterol levels is somewhat more complicated. Intake of certain types of fats raises blood cholesterol levels. Other types of fats, however, cause a lowering of blood cholesterol.

Fats are classified in three types: saturated, monounsaturated, and polyunsaturated fats.

Of the three types of fats—saturated, monounsaturated, and polyunsaturated—the saturated fats are the undesirables. *Saturated fats*, which are generally of the kind that *remain hard at room temperature*, like lard and butter, tend to raise blood cholesterol. Foods of animal origin tend to be high in saturated fats and cholesterol; for example, fatty cuts of beef, pork, and lamb; butter, cream, and whole milk; hard cheeses made from cream and whole milk. Vegetable products high in saturated fats include certain types of shortening such as coconut oil and palm oil. These two oils are commonly used in commercially prepared cookies, pies, and nondairy creamers.

Polyunsaturated fats, when substituted for saturated fats, will lower the level of cholesterol in the blood. They are found typically in vegetable oils that *remain liquid at room temperature*, such as corn oil, safflower oil, cottonseed oil, sesame seed oil, soybean oil, and sunflower seed oil.

Monounsaturated fats are found in foods like peanuts and peanut oil, olives and olive oil, and avocadoes.

Although not yet incorporated into most current recommendations, studies currently indicate that monounsaturated fats are at least as effective as polyunsaturates in lowering blood cholesterol. Diets high in monounsaturates are typical fare in Greece and Italy, where life expectancies are as high as, if not higher than, those in the United States.

There is no reason that a low-fat diet cannot be nutritionally adequate. The American Heart Association points out that in Japan, where fat intake is only 10 to 15 percent of total calories, life expectancy is higher than in the United States.

To replace the saturated fats in our diet, the AHA recommends that Americans adopt a diet high in carbohydrates. Reducing the fat intake to 30 percent of total calories is probably a realistic goal (typical American meals add up to a fat intake of 40 percent of total calories). Often, reducing fat intake can be accomplished in a relatively painless fashion by replacing high-fat, high-cholesterol red meat and pork with fruits, vegetables, pasta, low-fat dairy products, fish, and poultry.

At the supermarket and at restaurants, we should be alert for "hidden fat." Saturated fats form part of the marbling in meat and exist in large amounts in hard cheeses and cream cheese, in deep-fried foods, in cream soups, ice cream, and chocolate. Many commercially prepared baked goods like cakes, pies, and cookies, as well as processed meats like frankfurters and bolognas, are high in saturated fats. Coffee creamers and granolas likewise are high in saturated fats.

Restaurant meals also may contain substantial amounts of fats. Dishes steamed, stewed in broth or their own juices, poached, roasted, or stir-fried are better choices than dishes described on the menu as creamed, fried, buttery, *au gratin*.

What about proteins? Proteins are essential but many high-protein foods are also high in fat. Many of us consume far more protein than we

---

A Fish Story

Another dietary fat has been catching the headlines: fish oil. This "fish story" began in the early 1970s, with a study of Greenland Eskimos. The research showed that although 40 percent of the calories in the Eskimo diet come from animal fat, heart attacks are relatively uncommon. The logical explanation—that the Eskimos are genetically resistant to heart disease—did not seem to explain the findings, since Eskimos who move to Denmark seem to be as prone to heart disease as the ordinary Dane.

The answer seemed to be in the diets these Eskimos consumed: diets high in fat from marine sources—fish, seal, walrus, and whale. A recent study from the Netherlands suggests that eating fish several times a week reduces the risk of heart attack.

The mechanism of action seems to be related to the effect of fish oil on blood platelets, which are small corpuscles that form clots. Although platelets and their clot-forming action are essential in repairing wounds, platelets also form an important part of the atherosclerotic plaque. Fish oils provide another material, known as eicosapentaenoic acid, or EPA, which interferes with the chemicals that enhance platelet action.

Foods highest in EPA include salmon, mackerel, bluefish, and herring. Fish oil or its extracts cannot yet be recommended for general use, although at some later point recommendations may change. Still, having several fish meals a week makes sense as part of a healthy diet.

Recommended Foods

- Eat fruit, vegetables, cereals, pasta, low-fat dairy products, fish, poultry, and lean meats.
- Reduce the intake of high-fat, high-cholesterol foods like pork, bacon, red meat, frankfurters, bologna, butter, cream, hard cheese, whole milk, and eggyolk.
- Ignore the salt shaker and minimize the amount of highly salted foods.
- Know that processed foods may contain hidden quantities of saturated fats, cholesterol, and salt.

---

need. We could reduce our protein intake without harmful effect and get the benefit of less fats in our diet. Beans, which contain substantial amounts of protein, can replace animal foods in many instances. Bread and pasta, once thought of as villains, are now vindicated. We can use them in place of some of our animal protein calories. (See the discussion of proteins later in the section, under *The Wellness Diet.*)

Do we need fat at all? The answer is yes— though in smaller quantities than previously believed. One teaspoon of polyunsaturated oil each day provides all the fat we really need. Most of us eat far more fat than we require.

The Role of Stress

Most physicians, and indeed much of the general public, have an intuitive sense of the potential link between stress and heart disease. Solid data are hard to come by, however, since stress is an intangible and cannot readily be measured.

Among the best known of the postulated correlations between stress and heart disease is the relationship between what has been termed *Type A* behavior pattern and heart disease.

The story began when an upholsterer was called in to fix the chairs in the waiting room of two San Francisco cardiologists, Drs. Meyer Friedman and Stanley Rosenman. The upholsterer commented on the peculiar pattern of wear on the chair seats: The front edges were worn but the backs were as new as the day the chairs were bought. The observation meant little then, but it came to mean more as other observations, including a study of 3,500 subjects with coronary artery disease, demonstrated that patients with certain types of behavior patterns were more likely to suffer from coronary artery disease.

A number of other reports confirmed these results, including studies at Columbia University, where cardiologists found narrowed arteries in 32 percent of the type A patients. Still, probably because psychosocial factors are difficult to document, a role for the type A pattern has been hard to prove.

Drs. Friedman and Rosenman, in the best-selling book, *Type A Behavior and Your Heart,* define this behavior pattern as "an action-emotion complex that can be observed in any person who is aggressively involved in a chronic, incessant struggle to achieve more and more in less time." According to Drs. Friedman and Rosenman, typical type A persons cannot wait on lines. They suffer from constant "hurry sickness" and are obsessed with finishing. Type A's also have an obsession with numbers, attempting to acquire more and more (usually money) as representative of their achievements. Status is particularly important to the type A. Finally, and possibly most importantly, the type A is intensely aggressive, with a free-floating hostility that is triggered readily, often by apparently minor events.

This portrait of the typical type A is a stereotype. Few individuals are all type A; indeed, most people have some type-A characteristics, but some have them to a greater extent. The degree to which the individual can limit the expression of his or her type-A characteristics, the more likely it is that the risk of heart disease will be minimized.

Drs. Friedman and Rosenman suggest ridding yourself of "hurry sickness" by scheduling fewer appointments in a day and allowing yourself to answer only absolutely essential calls immediately. Listen more, talk less. Try to find some time for yourself. Try to curb your hostility, both by having a sense of humor and by using your reasoning powers. Finally, enjoy life: Have friends, develop hobbies, look at a tree or flower and savor its beauty.

Another important tool for reducing stress has found its way from the temples of the Orient to the cardiologists' laboratory. Various forms of *meditation* have been shown both to lower blood pressure and to reduce stress.

The techniques used in the relaxation therapies are those employed for centuries in Eastern religious rituals. Modified for Westerners, the techniques rely on quiet surroundings, sitting still, and some repetitive mental pattern such as counting

---

* Meyer Friedman, M. D., and Ray H. Rosenman, M. D., *Type A Behavior and Your Heart* (New York: Fawcett, 1987).

one's breaths or repeating a word or phrase.

Meditation techniques appear to evoke an actual physical response: a reduction in blood pressure by altering the activity of the sympathetic nervous system, which controls the body's involuntary functions. Studies performed by Western clinical researchers confirm the positive effects of meditation. For instance, one study reported that patients doing meditation reduced their blood pressure by 10 to 15mm. Confirmation of the positive effects of the meditation therapies led to endorsement by the National Institutes of Health in the 1984 Joint Commission report on hypertension.

Meditation techniques probably do help lower blood pressure. Advocates also claim that meditation allows individuals to deal better with other stresses in their lives. For religious individuals, praying may evoke deep relaxation. For modern skeptics, simple breathing exercises, done once or twice a day, may be all that are needed.

Another nonpharmacologic treatment of hypertension is *biofeedback*. Biofeedback techniques for lowering blood pressure use instruments to inform patients immediately about the effect of their efforts on their vital signs. One technique involves an automated blood-pressure measuring device with a standard blood-pressure cuff and a small microphone or light system. The sound or sight is a signal that registers changes in your blood pressure level and encourages you to control the level yourself.

Some limited studies indicate that biofeedback may be effective in lowering blood pressure, and, like the meditation therapies, biofeedback has been endorsed in the 1984 Report of the Joint Committee on Hypertension.

The Role of Smoking

Cigarette smoking is the single most important and most preventable cause of illness and death in the United States today. More than 320,000 deaths annually can be attributed to cigarette smoking, more than the total number of American soldiers killed in World War I, Korea, and Vietnam combined.

Although the correlation between cigarette smoking and lung cancer is better known, equally as important is the link between tobacco and heart disease. Smokers have two to four times the risk for sudden cardiac death than non-smokers.

At least ten major studies, from Framingham

onward, have indicated that cigarette smoking is a major risk factor for heart disease. (Pipe smokers and cigar smokers are also at risk, but to a lesser extent than cigarette smokers.)

People who stop smoking decrease their risk of heart disease (as well as the other ills associated with smoking). The risk of heart disease attributable to smoking drops by about 50 percent one year after the person quits. If your're a smoker, you can't say to yourself, "What's the use, I'm already going to die." If you stop smoking today, you'll still be reducing your risk.

For an extended discussion of smoking and its risks, as well as on ways to quit, see *What Is Cancer?* Meanwhile, keep in mind that heart disease and cigarette smoking are inextricably linked, and that cigarette smoking is one of the most important risk factors. For a healthy heart, stay away from cigarettes.

Exercise Level

Each day millions of Americans put on exercise clothes and sneakers and take to the roads and pathways, running, jogging, cycling their way to what they hope will be better health. Are they pursuing a nirvana that they never can achieve? Perhaps. Exercise cannot guarantee health. Still, regular exercise can tilt the odds, reducing the risks of heart disease (and of adult-onset diabetes and osteoporosis as well).

One of the earliest studies on the effects of exercise was a comparison of the incidence of heart disease in drivers and conductors of double-decker buses in London. This 1953 study, although somewhat primitive in its methods, showed that the conductors, who presumably had to go up and down the stairways all day, had less heart disease than the drivers, who stayed behind the wheel all day.

The positive effects of exercise on the heart have been confirmed by numerous studies. For example, studies involving 17,000 Harvard alumni show that as little as 2,000 calories' worth of exercise weekly can reduce the risk of heart disease by up to one third.

Exercise seems to affect factors like blood pressure, cholesterol, blood sugar, body fat, and ability to handle stress, thereby reducing the incidence of heart disease. For example, regular exercise lowers blood pressure and has a positive effect on blood cholesterol levels. Mild hypertension, for instance, can sometimes be treated with exercise alone. Exercise also affects blood cholesterol. Sometimes total cholesterol goes down in individuals who exercise, but even when that does not occur, exercise is likely to increase the amount of the "good cholesterol"—high-density lipoprotein, or HDL—in the blood.

Exercise is a natural "high," causing the body to release beta-endorphin, a chemical with effects similar to those of morphine. Release of beta-endorphins is believed to be responsible for the so-called "runner's high" and for the "top of the world" feeling experienced by many who exercise. Exercise seems to help in stress control, although the data are not conclusive. (Whether stress control through exercise helps reduce heart disease is uncertain.)

Exercise also helps control weight. The calories we consume in food must be expended in daily activities and maintaining body functions, or the result will be deposition of additional fat. Exercise promotes consumption of those calories.

Other effects of exercise are even more potent. Low-calorie diets tend to cause the body to reduce its metabolic rate and its consumption of calories, resulting in loss of muscle tissue, feelings of deprivation, and sometimes even in nutritional deficiencies. Exercise, on the other hand, raises the metabolic rate, not only during exercise but for hours afterward. As a result, exercise increases the total number of calories used at rest. Further, exercise increases the amount of muscle, or lean body mass. Since obesity is an important risk factor for heart disease, both independently and in combination with hypertension, exercise plays an important part in the lower heart-death rates seen in active, fit individuals.

Exercise also seems to help control blood sugar. In individuals with mild, adult-onset diabetes, exercise helps increase sensitivity to insulin, the hormone that controls blood sugar levels. While this effect may not be important in the majority of Americans, for the several million individuals with mild adult-onset diabetes, and in those with latent, undetected adult-onset diabetes, it may be significant. (Diabetics are generally at higher risk of cardiovascular death.) Exercise also helps in controlling the overweight that seems to be related to the genesis of adult-onset diabetes.

■ The Right Exercise for You

The type of exercise that builds cardiovascular endurance is known as aerobic exercise. These activities include running, swimming, aerobic dance, cycling, and even brisk walking. Continuous exercise for twenty to thirty minutes three to four times a week, not including warm-ups and cool-downs, is needed to reach and maintain cardiovascular fitness.

The standard recommendation is to exercise vigorously enough to increase your pulse rate to 75 percent of maximal. The maximal pulse rate can be estimated as a figure equivalent to 220 minus one's age (for an individual 50 years old, 75 percent of maximal pulse rate would be 170). This figure, by the way, is something to be worked toward gradually, especially if exercise is a change from a sedentary life-style. One need not be a fanatic about exercise to achieve protective levels of cardiac fitness.

For older individuals, age need not be a barrier to an appropriate exercise program if a doctor's examination fails to show reason for concern. However, exercises that put less strain on the joints'—like walking, exercise bicycling, and swimming—may be better for older individuals.

■ The Risks?

Many of us may remember the sudden death of James Fixx, the runner-writer whose books helped spread the fad for jogging. Fixx had a history of heart disease but ignored repeated warning signs. Incidents like this are relatively uncommon, but to prevent them, an exercise program needs to be carried out in an informed way.

For individuals under 50 who have a family history of sudden death, or personal problems with fainting, chest pain, shortness of breath, or cardiac irregularities, a medical examination is essential. If you have been fairly sedentary for years and are over 35 or have a family history of heart disease, you too should consult a physician before taking up an exercise program. In some instances the physician may wish to perform a stress test, an examination in which the patient exercises while an electrocardiogram or other cardiac monitor records the activity of the heart. (Although stress testing has come under criticism as an inadequate predictor, a better, noninvasive, essentially painless screening test for heart-disease risk during exercise has yet to be developed.)

Cardiac problems do not rule out exercise, however, and even individuals who have suffered heart attacks can undertake medically supervised fitness programs.

Other risks of exercise—besides cardiovascular risks—include effects on menstrual periods in women and injuries to bone, ligaments, and tendons of the knees, hips, and ankles.

See also the extended discussion of fitness later in this section, under *The Wellness Diet.*

■ *The Message*

Although critics of the fitness boom continue to carp, the majority of workers in the health field agree that continuous, aerobic exercise is, on balance, beneficial to the heart. Many attribute at least part of the recent drop in cardiovascular death rates to increased fitness, although other factors have probably played a role as well. The message: Regular exercise is part of a healthy lifestyle.

Overweight

Obesity—defined as weighing 20 percent or more over one's ideal weight—significantly increases the risk of developing cardiovascular disease. Numerous epidemiological studies, from Framingham onward, have shown that obesity puts the individual at increased risk of heart disease. It's a logical association: as the body puts on fat, so do the linings of the blood vessels.

Weight reduction can reduce blood pressure, which in turn reduces cardiovascular risk. And even independently of its effect on blood pressure, weight reduction can reduce the risk of heart disease.

There is some controversy, however, as to when the risk begins. Some studies show that while extremely overweight individuals are at increased risk, so are those who are underweight. Although some researchers say that the excess risk associated with underweight is because the persons in question are also cigarette smokers, this explanation has left many unsatisfied. To compound the confusion, the 1959 Metropolitan Life Height and Weight Tables, the previous standard of "ideal weight," have been revised upward to take more recent findings into account. And while some heart experts and fitness advocates exhort all individuals to keep their weight within 5 pounds of ideal, others point out the dangers,

both physiological and psychological, of excessive dieting. The many Americans who are between 5 to 15 pounds over their ideal weight are left to wonder whether or not they are at risk.

It's clear that those who are truly obese—20 percent heavier than the ideal weight for their gender, height, and body build—need to control their weight. For the rest of us, the verdict is not yet in. Consult your doctor if you're concerned.

See also the extended discussion of obesity later in this section, under *The Wellness Diet.*

Steps to a Healthier Heart

A healthier heart depends on *you.* To keep your heart healthy:

• Have your blood pressure checked. If you find out you have hypertension, follow the prescribed treatment program, which may include medication. If your doctor prescribes medication, take your pills, even though you may not feel sick.

• Know your cholesterol levels. This is particularly important if you have a family history of heart disease. A restricted diet may be necessary if cholesterol levels are excessively high. Medication also may be required.

• Follow a diet that is low in cholestrol and saturated fats. For the majority of Americans, fats should comprise no more than 30 percent of total intake of calories. Include fiber in your diet.

• Reduce your salt intake. This is particularly important for individuals with high blood pressure. A high intake of sodium-containing foods can worsen high blood pressure.

• Control your weight. Obesity has been linked to the development of hypertension and to an increased cardiovascular risk.

• Do not smoke. Smoking has no place in a healthy life-style.

• Exercise regularly. Regular, moderate exercise reduces cardiovascular risk.

• Know what to watch for. If you begin to suffer from chest pain, palpitations, or shortness of breath, see your doctor.

Additional information can be obtained from the National Center of the American Heart Association or from your local affiliate.

American Heart Association
National Center
7320 Greenville Avenue
Dallas, Texas 75231
(214) 373-6300

18

WHAT
IS
CANCER?

C ancer—much dreaded but often little understood—is not a simple disease. *Cancer* is not one disease but many: It is a general term for more than a hundred different disorders, including lung cancer, breast cancer, and colon cancer, among the most frequent forms.

Cancer is a disease that affects the cells of the human body. Cells are the subunits of the body—each individual is made up of billions of cells. So that body tissues can grow and repair themselves, cells ordinarily reproduce by dividing in two. Usually, because these processes are under the control of the cell's genetic material, cell reproduction and division occurs in an orderly way so that the body's shape and form is retained.

Sometimes things go wrong, however, and cells begin dividing too rapidly, with no order whatsoever. The result is a tumor. Tumors are sometimes *benign*, meaning that they are confined to the part of the body where they occurred. Benign tumors usually can be removed and will not come back.

But some tumors are *malignant.* Malignant tumors, or cancers, begin to invade surrounding tissues as they grow. Cells sometimes break off and spread through the bloodstream to other parts of the body, forming new tumors, or *metas-*

tases. Unfortunately, even after removal of a malignant tumor, cancer may come back if the cells have already spread sufficiently.

Cancer arises when certain agents—viruses, chemicals, or radiation—attack the genetic material of the cell. This genetic material, or DNA, controls the form and nature of the human body—from the intelligence in our brain to the shape of our foot. Cancer-causing agents disturb the cellular machinery, and in some way the cells are no longer under the controlling influence of their genetic material. (One recent theory indicates that normally "quiet" genes are triggered by these agents.) The result: uncontrolled growth, or cancer.

According to cancer researchers, science in recent years has come to a far clearer understanding of the causes of cancer. The centerpiece has been the discovery of the *oncogene.* Oncogenes are the cancer-causing genes; they produce hormones that stimulate cell growth and division. Under normal circumstances, the oncogenes function in cell growth and division. When cells have ceased to grow, oncogenes are "turned off." When cancer occurs, these genes are "turned on" and uncontrolled cellular growth is the consequence. With the discovery of the oncogene has come an understanding of how these genes are "turned on," "turned off," or lost, either by action on those genes themselves or by action on *promotor* genes or *suppressor* genes. For oncologists this era is tremendously exciting—the discovery of the oncogene has been a quantum leap forward. Some predict that our improved understanding of what happens at the oncogene level will lead to improved treatment and prevention and fewer cancer deaths.

Risk Factors

Although heart disease is the number 1 killer in the United States, cancer runs a close number 2. The symptoms and signs of the two diseases are quite different, but the possibility that a given individual will develop either disease is assessed in much the same way. Cigarette smoking, high-fat diets, and obesity strongly influence the vulnerability of the individual to develop either disease. (Another risk factor for skin cancer is excessive exposure to sun.) By themselves, however, risk factors are not necessarily a "death sentence."

A report on the avoidable risks of cancer concluded that the factors determining whether an individual will develop cancer fall into three categories: nature, nurture, and luck.

Nature relates to the individual's genetic make-up at the time of birth. Certainly, this can affect an individual's risk of cancer. For example, exposure to the sun is more likely to cause skin cancer in a fair-skinned Northern type than in an olive-skinned Mediterranean type. Certain rare cancers appear to be clearly dependent on genetic make-up. They include retinoblastoma (a cancer of the eyes), as well as ataxia-telangiectasia, an inherited immune deficiency that makes persons more likely to develop lymphoma, leukemia, and stomach cancer. Other inherited conditions appear to predispose individuals to skin cancer and colon cancer.

Some cancers seem to "run in families." Familial factors seem to be at work in breast, colon, and brain cancer. Certain types of leukemia (a cancer of the immune cells of the blood) are rare among Asians, and another type of cancer, Ewing's sarcoma, is uncommon in blacks.

Still, it is often difficult to separate genetic influences from those of the environment. Families often share the same dietary habits, the same cultural influences, and the same geographic origin.

But even when a person has a genetic predisposition, that individual can take measures to minimize his or her risk. For example, individuals who know that a particular type of cancer "runs in the family" might take particular care to have regular screening exams—stool blood test for colon cancer or breast exams for breast cancer. And sometimes removal of a precancerous mole may prevent malignant melanoma, while removal of a precancerous polyp may prevent colon cancer.

A factor even more important than nature is *nurture*—what people do or have done to them, from the cradle to the grave. Unlike nature, nurture—the extrinsic or environmental factors that affect our risk of developing cancer—is largely under our control; it can be modified by the choices we make.

Another factor bearing on the cancer risk in any given individual is *luck*. In the case of cancer, it may operate by determining the ways in which particular changes occur in particular cells at a particular time. In the same way that luck may involve some but not others of us in traffic accidents, luck is a factor in the chances that any given individual will develop cancer. But in a large group, good and bad luck will tend to cancel each other out, meaning that for the population as a whole, luck is a minor factor.

(Note also that age is a factor: Cancer is a disease primarily of older and middle-aged individuals, and the older a person becomes, the greater his chances of developing cancer.)

Of the three major determining factors, only one is under our control: "nurture," meaning those environmental, extrinsic, cultural, and societal factors that we can modify by personal, political, or corporate choice.

Risks We Can Control

In 1964, a committee operating under the auspices of the World Health Organization recognized the importance of these kinds of outside factors when it stated that "the categories of cancer that are thus influenced, directly or indirectly, by extrinsic factors . . . account for more than three-quarters of human cancers." But the term "extrinsic factors" (or the phrase "environmental factors" which sometimes is substituted for it) has often been interpreted to mean only man-made chemicals, an interpretation inconsistent with the original meaning.

Current thought on this issue suggests that exposure to harmful chemicals or radiations plays a relatively minor role in the cancer risk of the average individual. The majority of cancers are related to smoking, diet, and exposure to sun—factors that we can readily modify through personal choice. The environment is not only what is imposed on us at our jobs, in the air we breathe, in the water we drink, or at our doctors' offices. *It is also our personal environment that we ourselves create.* We have it in our power to tilt these "extrinsic factors" in our favor. And for most individuals, the necessary changes are relatively simple to make. The National Cancer Institute says:

"Reducing the risk of cancer doesn't mean giving up the pleasures of life. It just means adjusting and changing one's tastes a bit."

■ *Smoking and Cancer*

Most reports of a so-called cancer epidemic are, by all accounts, somewhat premature. The incidence of most cancers has failed to increase in the last few decades, while screening and treatment methods have led to improved outcomes. But if there is indeed an epidemic of any type of cancer, it is in the incidence of *lung cancer.*

Figures from the National Center for Health Statistics show that lung cancer is the only major cause of cancer deaths that has been increasing steadily since 1950. And the cause of lung cancer is almost always *cigarette smoking*.

Most estimates indicate that cigarette smoking is responsible for about 85 percent of lung cancer deaths. Tragically, lung cancer is difficult to detect in the early stages, and present methods discloses only 25 percent of lung cancers at a localized stage when they can be cured. Lung cancer is the most common cancer among men and the second most common cancer among women. And with increased numbers of women who smoke has come a concomitant increase in lung cancer cases: Lung cancer is the leading cause of cancer death among women between 55 and 74 years of age.

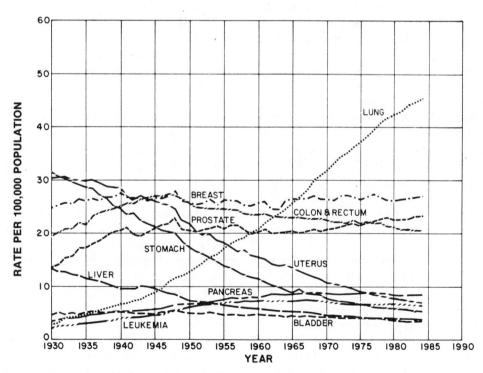

CANCER DEATH RATES* BY SITE, UNITED STATES, 1930-84

* Rate for the population standardized for age on the 1970 U.S. population
Sources of Data: National Center for Health Statistics and Bureau of the Census, United States.

Note: Rates are for both sexes combined except breast and uterus female population only and prostate male population only.
Source: Cancer Facts & Figures—1987, American Cancer Society.

Lung cancer is the only major cause of cancer deaths that has been increasing steadily since 1950. Cigarette smoking is responsible for the majority of lung cancer deaths.

Evidence also indicates that cigarette smoking is associated with a number of other cancers as well. Cigarette smoking has been linked to cancer of the larynx, mouth, esophagus, pharynx, bladder, and pancreas. Overall, smoking is believed to be responsible for about 30 percent of cancer deaths.

Pipe and cigar smokers are less at risk for lung and bladder cancer than cigarette smokers are, but they run similar risks of oral, esophageal, and laryngeal cancer. And their risks are higher than those of nonsmokers. Similarly, smoking low-tar, low-nicotine cigarettes may somewhat reduce the risk of lung cancer, if the smoker does not inhale more deeply, take more puffs, or smoke more cigarettes. But those who smoke low-tar, low nicotine cigarettes run greater risks than if they did not smoke at all.

Nor is smokeless tobacco innocuous. In the last twenty years, while cigarette smoking has waned, smokeless-tobacco consumption has increased. "Smokeless tobacco" includes chewing tobacco and snuff, which is of finer consistency and is held in the mouth without being chewed.

In March 1986 the Surgeon General released a report on the health consequences of smokeless tobacco, warning that it is strongly associated with cancers of the oral cavity and pharynx. Also, because the chemicals contained in smokeless tobacco probably enter the bloodstream, it is likely that the health consequences associated with cigarette smoking—namely, heart disease, hypertension, peptic ulcers, and effects on an unborn child—can be linked to smokeless tobacco as well. Further, the nicotine contained in smokeless tobacco is addictive. This form of tobacco is used heavily by male adolescents and young male adults, and its use is increasing in these groups. According to the Surgeon General, all individuals need to be aware that smokeless tobacco does pose health risks.

In addition to cancer, the risks of smoking include a higher risk of developing the chronic lung diseases, mainly bronchitis and emphysema. These diseases cause about 60,000 deaths each year, and between 80 and 90 percent have been attributed to smoking. The chronic lung diseases have in common symptoms like a mucus-producing cough, wheezing, and shortness of breath. Symptoms develop slowly, often as a result of smoking. Bronchitis and emphysema occur because smoking damages the cilia that cleanse the respiratory tree. Smoking also damages the elastic tissue of the lung, causes the production of destructive enzymes, and blocks the production of inhibitors that protect the lung tissue.

Smokers suffer more from minor respiratory infections, miss more days of work because of respiratory infections, and more often report cough and sputum. The "smoker's cough" is not harmless: It is often an early sign of chronic lung disease.

Smoking has damaging effects on the unborn child. Infants born to women who smoke typically weigh less than those born to nonsmokers. Premature deliveries are common in women who smoke, with an increased risk of infant death as a consequence.

Smokers may also be endangering nearby nonsmokers. Evidence indicating possible adverse effects of so-called passive smoking has begun to mount, causing the Surgeon General to publicize the dangers of such passive exposure. And an increased awareness of the potential dangers of passive smoking has been reflected in a push for restrictions on smoking in public places and in the workplace.

Current evidence indicates that tobacco is also addictive, inducing dependence patterns similar to those of heroin, cocaine, and amphetamines. But while "shooting" heroin is illegal, cigarette smoking is not.

Overall, cigarette smoking is responsible for about 320,000 deaths each year. The economic costs are enormous as well: A study released in September 1985 by the U.S. Congress's Office of Technology Assessment estimated that $12 billion to $35 billion is spent annually to treat smoking-related diseases and another $27 billion to $61 billion is lost in productivity from smoking-related diseases.

For the individual, the costs of a smoking habit are plain: an increased risk of cancer, heart attack, and respiratory disease. More important, the person who stops smoking benefits, even if he or she quits in middle age. For example, the risk of coronary artery disease attributable to smoking declines by about 50 percent one year after quitting. After ten years, the heart-disease risk approaches that of a person who has never smoked. Lung cancer risks likewise decrease. For ex-smokers, lung cancer death rates are only 40 percent of those of smokers after five years of not smoking, while after fifteen years of not smoking, ex-smokers had a mortality rate only slightly greater than that of nonsmokers.

Still, many smokers find it difficult to quit. If you smoke, this short list, adapted from the American Cancer Society's *Quitter's Guide*, may make you more aware of the reasons and provide some alternatives to cigarettes:

Stimulation: Cigarettes seem to give you pep, help you concentrate. You can substitute a brisk walk, exercises, or a cold shower.

Handling: You like the ritual of holding the cigarette, tapping the cigarette on the ashtray. You can find something else to hold in your hands, perhaps a coin, perhaps a pen or pencil.

Relaxation: You seem to get a sense of pleasure out of smoking. But consider the harmful effects: Those may take some of the pleasure away.

Crutch: You may light up when you're angry or depressed, using smoking as a tranquilizer. You have to realize that smoking isn't really helping. Instead, cry on a friend's shoulder. Dealing with stress without smoking may be easier than you think.

Craving: Many smokers perceive a "craving" for cigarettes. Evidence does, in fact, suggest some degree of physical addiction. Although it's often hard to stop, cues can reinforce the individual's determination not to smoke. And once you have stopped, it may be easier to resist the temptation to smoke because it's much too tough to quit again.

Habit: Many individuals smoke without realizing they are smoking. Try to make smoking conscious. Ask: Do I really want this cigarette?

Some smokers just decide to quit. Something pushes them—be it a news report, the warning of a physician, the appearance of a cough, or just a sense that "enough is enough"and they just stop smoking. But for many, Mark Twain's comment about how "easy" it is to quit—"I ought to know because I've done it a thousand times"—is all too true. Strategies include nicotine-containing gums and group support programs. While some quitters do well with group programs, others prefer to go it alone. Choose a strategy that fits your personality and life-style.

Programs available include the following:

Freedom from Smoking, sponsored by the American Lung Association. This is a twenty-day, do-it-yourself program. Local chapters may also have group programs available. Contact your chapter of the American Lung Association.

American Cancer Society–sponsored programs. The fee, if any, is determined by the local chapter. The American Cancer Society also has copies of its *Quitter's Guide* available from local chapters. Con-

tact your local chapter of the American Cancer Society.

Smokenders, a for-profit group, has helped many.

And don't neglect your physician as a resource. He or she can supply information on the health benefits of quitting, on possible quitting strategies, and on pharmacological adjuncts like nicotine-containing gum.

One major deterrent for would-be quitters is the prospect of weight gain. In fact, only one third of smokers gain weight, one third remain the same, and one third, who exercise more and take additional care with their diet, actually lose weight.

Many people do quit smoking. While 37 percent of the U.S. population were smokers in 1976, only 30 percent of the population still smoke. The major declines have been in the numbers of male smokers: 42 percent of U.S. males were smokers in 1976, while 32 percent of U.S. women were smokers. In 1985, 33 percent of males were smokers, while 28 percent of women were smokers. Among high-school and college-aged individuals, more females now smoke than males.

Most smokers tend to start during adolescence and early adulthood. Many smokers admit: *If they knew then what they know now, they would never have started to smoke.*

In truth, smoking has become far less popular. Dating services and personal ads have many calls for "attractive young woman, nonsmoker." And 79 percent of Americans feel that smoking should be restricted in the workplace. A recent editorial in the *Journal of the American Medical Association* states: "only for consenting adults, in private." Major health organizations call for restrictions on cigarette advertising and there is a major public awareness of the deleterious effects of smoking.

Reducing your risk of cancer is largely within your control. Smoking is responsible for more than one third of all cancers. It is, as tobacco companies never hesitate to remind us, a matter of personal choice. You can choose not to smoke. Make that choice: *Don't smoke.*

■ Diet and Cancer

The traditional American fare—steak and french fries, washed down with a can of beer and topped off with a slice of apple pie—is on the way out. Most experts agree: The American diet, high in fats, low in fiber, containing few fruits and vegetables, has a negative impact on our health. Not only is a high-fat diet harmful to our heart, but diets high in fat, low in fiber, containing few vitamin-rich fruits and vegetables, are likely to increase cancer risk as well. Current evidence suggests that up to 35 percent of all cancer deaths may be related to diet.

The evidence—obtained in laboratory studies and in studies of groups or populations of individuals from all over the world—came into focus in the early 1980s, as the National Cancer Institute asked an independent body, the National Academy of Sciences, to report on the evidence linking diet and cancer risk. This independent assessment, published in 1982, indicated that it would be feasible to recommend some dietary modifications. In March 1985, the booklet *Diet, Nutrition, & Cancer Prevention: A Guide to Food Choices* (available by calling 1-800-4-CANCER) was published, under the auspices of the National Cancer Institute and the National Institutes of Health.

What provided the rationale for these recommendations? According to Dr. Peter Greenwald of the National Cancer Institute, it was "that more and more studies done by different investigators, using different methods and different populations all showed consistency: an accumulation of evidence suggesting that individuals could lower their cancer risk by modifying their diet."

■ Foods That Help

The recommendations for a diet that will reduce the risk of developing cancer are these:
• Increase the amount of dietary fiber.
• Reduce your consumption of dietary fat.
• Be sure to include the cruciferous vegetables— brussels sprouts, cabbage, broccoli, cauliflowers, and turnips—in your diet.
• Choose vegetables high in vitamins A and C.
• Take care to preserve freshness when storing nuts, grains, and seeds.
• Drink alcohol only in moderation, if you drink at all.

Fiber. The term *fiber* is used to refer to the food components that are not readily digested by the intestinal tracts. Foods high in fiber include vegetables, fruits, whole-grain breads and cereals, legumes like peas and beans, and brown rice. A possible link between diet and colon cancer was first suggested in 1969 when it was noted that individuals in Africa and India, who consumed relatively large amounts of fiber, were at lower

risk of colon cancer than individuals in the more developed countries, where lesser amounts of fiber were consumed. The precise reason for the protective role of fiber is unclear, although a number of suggestions have been advanced: Fiber speeds the transit time of food through the intestines, decreasing the time that potential food carcinogens remain in contact with the intestinal lining; fiber alters the kinds of bacteria in the colon; or fiber reduces the internal production of potentially carcinogenic chemicals in the intestines.

The exact connection between dietary fiber and cancer is complex and research continues. We do know that individuals who eat substantial amounts of fiber do not become obese, and that their diets are also lower in fat and higher in vegetables that are rich in vitamins A and C. The fiber-containing foods are a wholesome substitute for fatty foods, and fiber-rich fruits and vegetables often contain other important nutrients. Most Americans now consume about 10 to 20 grams of fiber daily. Current National Cancer Institute recommendations state that most individuals ought to consume about 25 to 35 grams of fiber a day.

To put more fiber into your diet, choose fruits, vegetables, peas and beans, and breads and cereals made from whole grains. The skins of fruits and vegetables are high in dietary fiber. So instead of grabbing a croissant for breakfast, choose a bran muffin instead. At lunch and dinner, skip the rolls and have an extra serving of vegetables. Put a bowl of luscious fresh fruit on the dinner table instead of a pastry dessert. Fiber supplements probably aren't a good idea for everyone just yet, since all studies to date relate to the protective effects of fiber-containing *foods.*

• • •

• NCI recommendations on fiber suggest that we should choose these foods *more often*:
• Whole-grain products:
  bakery products like bran muffins; whole-wheat crackers; rye, brown, oatmeal, pumpernickel, bran, and corn breads; whole-wheat English muffins; bagels
  breakfast cereals like bran cereals, shredded wheat, whole-grain or whole-wheat flaked cereals; those listing high dietary fiber content
  other foods made with whole-grain fiber like whole-grain waffles, pancakes, pasta, and taco shells

other whole-grain foods like barley, buckwheat groats, bulgur wheat
- Fruits and vegetables:
  apples, pears, apricots, bananas, berries, cantaloupes, grapefruit, oranges, pineapples, papayas, prunes, raisins
  carrots, broccoli, potatoes, corn, cauliflower, brussels sprouts, cabbage, celery, green beans, summer squash, green peas, parsnips, kale, spinach, other greens, yams, sweet potatoes, turnips
- Dried beans and peas:
  black, kidney, garbanzo, pinto, navy, white, lima beans; lentils, split peas, black-eyed peas

These foods should be chosen *less often*:
- Refined bakery and snack products:
  refined flour breads (white breads), quick breads, biscuits, buns, croissants, snack crackers and chips, cookies, pastries, pies

Fat. High dietary fat intake appears to be linked to an increased risk of cancers of the breast, colon, endometrium (uterus), and prostate gland. This evidence comes from both population (epidemiologic) studies and from animal studies, in which animals ingesting high-fat diets had an increased incidence of breast and colon cancer. Correlations of international incidence and death rates with the components of diet also indicate that colon cancer is linked to total dietary fat intake. Studies of individuals who already have developed colon cancer also suggest a link, although the evidence is not definitive. (Some of the data on fat intake and increased risk of colon cancer are conflicting, but in many instances variable fiber intake may account for the discrepancies.) The precise reason for the role of fat intake in cancer risk is unknown, although some evidence has implicated bile acids and sex hormone production.

The average American consumes about 40 percent of his or her calories from fat. Current recommendations, from the National Academy of Sciences, the National Cancer Institute, and the American Cancer Society, suggest that individuals reduce their fat intake to 30 percent of total calories. Studies have not been able to differentiate between the effects of saturated fats and those of unsaturated fats on cancer risk (although the two do have differing effects on heart-disease risk). This recommendation is, by the way, similar to the recommendations of the NIH Consensus Committee and the American Heart Association for a healthy-heart diet.

• • •

Techniques for cutting down on fat intake include the following:
- Eat more breads, cereals, vegetables, and fruits.
- Choose lean meats and low-fat products.
- Try low-fat meals such as salads, low-fat soups, bean dishes, lean meat or fish, and vegetable mixed dishes.
- Trim all visible fats from meats before and after cooking.
- Remove skin from poultry.
- Broil, poach, or roast meats and drain the fat from the pan.
- Substitute broth for grease in cooking.
- Cut down on the *amounts* of salad dressing, fats, cream, and rich sauces you use.
- Choose *more often* low-fat poultry, fish, and meats like chicken, turkey, and rock cornish hens (without skin); fresh, frozen, water-packed fish and shellfish.
- Choose *less often* higher-fat poultry, fish, and meat such as duck and goose, poultry with skin, frozen fish sticks, tuna packed in oil.
- Choose peas and beans rather than nuts and seeds.
- Choose trimmed beef, lamb, veal, and pork with little marbling or visible fat.
- Choose *more often* low-fat or skim-milk dairy products. These might include low-fat skim milk or buttermilk; low-fat yogurt, skimmed evaporated milk, nonfat dry milk; low-fat cheeses like ricotta, pot, farmer, cottage, mozzarella, or skim-milk cheeses.
- Choose *less often* full-fat dairy products like whole milk, butter, whole-milk yogurt, sweet cream, sour cream, half-and-half, whipped cream, other creamy toppings; also choose less often full-fat soft cheeses like cream cheese, cheese spreads, Camembert, Brie; hard cheeses like Cheddar, Swiss, blue, American, Jack, Parmesan; and coffee creamers (including nondairy), cream sauces, cream soups.
- Choose sherbet, frozen low-fat yogurt, ice milk rather than ice cream.
- Choose *more often* "diet" and low-fat salad dressings, along with low-fat margarines.
- Choose *less often* vegetable and salad oils, shortening, lard, meat fats, salt pork, bacon, mayonnaise, and high-fat salad dressing, margarine, gravies, butter sauces.

• Choose fruits and vegetables and breads and cereals for snacks.

• Choose *less often* snack foods like doughnuts, pies, pastries, cakes, cookies, brownies, potato chips, snack crackers, canned puddings, icings, candies with butter, cream, or chocolate, granola, and croissants.

• Food preparation: Baking, oven-broiling, boiling, stewing, poaching, stir-frying, simmering, steaming are preferable to deep-fat frying and sautéeing.

• Seasoning with herbs, spices, or lemon juice is preferable to fatty gravies, sauces, cream, or butter.

Cruciferous vegetables. Both epidemiologic (population) and animal studies suggest that the cruciferous vegetables—which include cabbage, brussels sprouts, broccoli, kohlrabi, cauliflower, rutabaga, and turnip—may have a protective effect. Epidemiologic studies suggest that diets including these vegetables may reduce the risk of gastrointestinal and lung cancers, while animal studies reveal that these vegetables may be highly effective in preventing chemically induced cancers. Experimental work is being directed currently at identifying which component or components of these vegetables are protective. Current guidelines from the National Cancer Institute suggest choosing several servings of these vegetables each week.

Vitamins and minerals. Evidence suggests that diets rich in vitamins A and C may protect against cancer. This means that each day you should include in your diet several servings of fruits and vegetables rich in vitamins A and C.

Consumption of foods rich in vitamin A has been linked to a reduced incidence of cancers of the oral cavity, pharynx, larynx, and lung. Carotenoids are compounds like beta-carotene that are converted to vitamin A in the body. Carotenoids are found in carrots, sweet potatoes, peaches, apricots, cantaloupes, and other yellow-orange fruits and vegetables like broccoli, kale, and spinach.

Another form of vitamin A called preformed vitamin A occurs only in animal foods like whole milk, cheese, butter, eggyolk, and liver. (A different form of preformed vitamin A—retinyl acetate or retinyl palmitate—is found in multiple-vitamin pills and in some fortified foods.) The protective role of preformed vitamin A has not been determined.

Animal studies show that vitamin C can inhibit the formation of potentially carcinogenic nitro-

samine compounds. Vitamin C may protect against gastric and esophageal cancers. Foods rich in vitamin C include oranges, grapefruits, strawberries, and green and red peppers.

It is best to consume sufficient amounts of vitamin-rich foods rather than relying on vitamin supplements, because the protective effects may not come only from vitamins themselves but perhaps from some other component of vitamin-rich foods as well. Do not use vitamin A supplements (particularly in doses above the recommended daily allowances) because of potentially toxic effects.

■ *The "Enemies List"*

Here are the dietary traps and how to avoid them:

Aflatoxins. Certain molds that occur naturally on nuts, grains, and seeds produce potent carcinogens known as aflatoxins. Aflatoxins produce liver cancer in animals and may be linked to cancer in humans as well. Aflatoxins are not a significant problem in the United States, since commercially sold nuts, grains, and seeds are monitored by the Food and Drug Administration and by industry. However, do take care to store nuts, grains, and seeds in dry, sealed containers. Throw away these foods if they become moldy.

Alcohol. Heavy drinkers, particularly those who smoke, are at increased risk of cancers of the oral cavity, larynx, and esophagus, and the liver. Alcohol also results in cirrhosis of the liver, which increases the likelihood of developing liver cancer. Studies indicate an increased risk of cancer of the mouth, pharynx, and larynx, particularly in individuals who smoke. Studies from all over the world indicate a close link between cancer and alcohol abuse, with French studies indicating that heavy drinking and cigarette smoking together exert a more deleterious effect than either alone. Note, however, that pure ethanol is not carcinogenic: Heavy drinking may promote cancer either by acting in combination with some other compound, like tobacco; by leading to poor nutrition; or by acting through some carcinogenic substance other than ethanol contained in alcoholic beverages.

Current recommendations suggest moderation in the consumption of alcoholic beverages. Individuals should limit their intake to two or fewer drinks per day. It should be noted that scientists at the National Cancer Institute and researchers at other institutions have found evidence suggesting that women who consume three or more drinks *a week* may be somewhat more at risk of developing breast cancer than women who do not drink at all. The evidence, though, is still inconclusive and no public health recommendations have been made.

Obesity. Obese individuals—those 20 percent or more above their ideal weight—are at increased risk of cancer. This increased risk was demonstrated in a massive study performed by the American Cancer Society, which found a markedly increased incidence in cancers of the uterus, gallbladder, kidney, stomach, colon, and breast to be linked to obesity. Women 40 percent or more overweight had a 55 percent greater risk while men had a 33 percent greater risk. Animal experiments also indicate that cancer incidence is reduced by maintaining animals at their ideal weight.

Salt-cured, smoked, and nitrate-cured foods. Conventionally smoked foods—for example, hams, some sausages, and fish—may absorb tars that contain potentially carcinogenic chemicals much like those in cigarette smoke. Since food processors are now using a different smoking process, this risk may apply only to conventionally smoked meats.

Some limited evidence indicates that salt-cured or pickled foods may increase the risk of stomach and esophageal cancer. An increased risk of these cancers is found in Japan and China, where salt-cured and pickled foods are commonly consumed.

Evidence also indicates that nitrates and nitrites, often used in food preservation to prevent botulism and improve color and flavoring, may contribute to the production of *nitrosamines.* Nitrosamines are potent carcinogens in animals and may be carcinogenic in humans as well. Nitrate-containing foods include bacon, frankfurters, and luncheon meats such as bologna and salami. Although the National Cancer Institute has no current recommendations regarding consumption of salt-cured, smoked, or nitrate-cured foods, the American Cancer Society does suggest moderation in intake of these foods. Prudence would suggest that a frankfurter at every meal is neither a balanced nor a cancer-free diet. (As mentioned above, vitamin C acts to inhibit the formation of the nitrosamines.)

The above aren't the only dietary cancer risks you've heard about and these aren't the only cancer-preventive agents you know. What about the others? Dr. Greenwald of the National Cancer Institute indicates that the role of many of the following substances, either for good or bad, has been exaggerated, and that no current recommendations are warranted.

Additives. Dr. Greenwald indicates that food additives do not appear to pose much risk. Population studies, for example, have been unable to identify any positive evidence. There is little evidence on the cancer risk of unintentional additives such as pesticides, Greenwald points out. Some food additives have been found to cause cancer in animals and have been banned. Artificial sweeteners like saccharine (as well as cyclamates) have been shown to cause bladder cancer in rats, but epidemiologic studies show no clearcut evidence of increased risk in moderate users.

Caffeine. Coffee was at first implicated in cancer of the bladder and prostate, but later studies failed to confirm these findings. Most researchers currently find the data on coffee risk unconvincing.

Cholesterol. So far, cholesterol does not appear to be implicated in the genesis of cancer. There is little evidence that a high intake of cholesterol, apart from a high fat intake, is likely to increase the risk of cancer. Late in 1986, however, some studies linked high blood cholesterol levels to colon cancer. Most experts feel that the high blood cholesterol levels are acting as a marker for high fat intake; individuals with high blood cholesterol levels also consume substantial amounts of fat.

Vitamin E. It has been suggested that vitamin E, as well as selenium, which is a trace mineral may act as anticancer agents. Both vitamin E and an enzyme (a substance promoting certain chemical reactions in the body) that depends on selenium act as *antioxidants*, able to block damage to the cellular genetic material (DNA) from some carcinogens. These substances prevent cultured cells pretreated with carcinogenic chemicals from becoming malignant. The potential is that compounds that are antioxidants, such as vitamin E and selenium, prevent the occurrence of alterations in the genetic machinery of the cell that set the stage for the genesis of cancer. Although trials evaluating the effects of these agents are under way, neither the American Cancer Society nor the National Cancer Institute currently offers any recommendations. And both the NCI and the ACS indicate that "megadoses"—doses far above the recommended daily allowances—offer no real benefits. Both selenium and vitamin E can be toxic, and for this reason the medically unsupervised administration of these agents cannot be recommended.

■ *Summing Up*

In short, you can structure your diet to reduce your cancer risk. These actions are critical:
• Avoid obesity
• Cut down on fat intake
• Eat high-fiber foods
• Include foods high in vitamins A and C
• Include cruciferous (cabbage family) vegetables
• Be moderate in the intake of alcoholic beverages
• Avoid aflatoxin exposure
• Be moderate in consumption of salt-cured, smoked, or nitrate-cured foods

Many of these measures also help reduce our risk of heart disease. For instance, by reducing fat intake and avoiding obesity, we reduce our risk of heart disease. Eating plenty of fiber may also have cardiovascular benefits. And vegetables and fruits high in vitamins A and C as well as the cruciferous vegetables are attractive alternatives to the high-fat foods that contribute both to heart attack and cancer risk.

Moderation is the key: A healthful, *varied* diet low in calories and fat, combined with moderate amounts of exercise and keeping trim, will go a long way to reducing cancer risk.

Additional information can be obtained from these organizations:
• The American Cancer Society. Contact your local chapter.
• The Cancer Information Service Office of the National Cancer Institute. In most locations, dial 1-800-4-CANCER. By calling this number, you can obtain a copy of the NIH booklet, *Diet, Nutrition and Cancer Prevention*, as well as other information on cancer and cancer prevention. In Alaska, call 1-800-683-6070; in Hawaii on Oahu, call 524-1234 (collect from neighboring islands).

Spanish-speaking staff members are available in California, Florida, Georgia, Illinois, Northern New Jersey, New York City, and Texas.

You can also obtain a copy of the booklet, *Diet, Nutrition and Cancer Prevention: A Guide to Food Choices*, by writing the National Cancer Institute, Bldg. 31, Room 10A18, Bethesda, MD 20205.

Sun, Skin and Cancer

The fashionable flaunting of a suntan may get you smiles, but it's far from being a badge of health. Exposure to sun is believed to contribute significantly to the development of the more than 500,000 cases of nonmelanoma skin cancer and the more than 27,000 new cases of melanoma that are estimated to occur in 1988.

Nonmelanoma skin cancer, primarily what is known as *basal cell carcinoma* but also *squamous cell carcinoma*, is the most common cancer among whites in the United States. Although this cancer is readily curable, it does result in 2,000 deaths each year. Melanoma, although less common, is far more lethal: Of the estimated more than 27,000 individuals who will be diagnosed in 1988, some 5,800 will not survive.

The role of sun exposure in the development of skin cancer is suggested by several observations:
• The incidence of (nonmelanoma) skin cancer is greater at the lower latitudes, where exposure to sun is greater. A 1977-78 study showed that for white males the incidence in Detroit was 172 per 100,000, but the incidence in Albuquerque was 752 per 100,000.
• Skin cancers tend to occur at sites on the body that are most exposed to sun.
• Skin cancers tend to occur more often in individuals whose occupations expose them to the sun, for example, seamen, farmers, outdoor construction workers, and telephone linemen.

The incidence of nonmelanoma skin cancer is directly proportional to ultraviolet exposure and inversely proportional to skin pigmentation. Nonmelanoma skin cancer tends to occur most often in Caucasians, less often in Asians, and least often among blacks. Individuals are at particular risk if they are fair-skinned or if they have had relatives with skin cancer. Skin cancer tends to be somewhat more common in men.

Sunlight contains *ultraviolet rays*, which are believed to be related to an increased incidence of skin cancer. In a sampling of U.S. cities where skin pigmentation might be expected to be a relative constant, incidence rates for squamous cell carcinoma and basal cell carcinoma are closely linked to exposure to ultraviolet radiation (actually to one type of ultraviolet light—ultraviolet B, or UV-B). For melanoma, the more lethal form of skin cancer, sunlight is a risk factor but apparently a less influential one.

Experts agree: The chief risk factor for nonmelanoma skin cancer is exposure to sun, and the evidence indicates that the risk is greater at higher doses. Avoiding overexposure to sunlight is the chief method for preventing nonmelanoma skin cancer. Nor is *artificial* UV light without risk:

Avoid exposure from sunlamps and tanning booths as well.

Melanoma, the more lethal but less common type of skin cancer, is also linked to sun exposure, but less directly. There is a relatively high incidence of melanoma in white individuals who work indoors and who have been exposed to sun during weekends or winter vacations. Some evidence suggests that intense, intermittent exposure—for instance, travel to resort areas involving short periods of high-level exposure—is a risk factor. Blistering sunburns during childhood and adolescence also appear to increase melanoma risk. Exposure during childhood may be particularly hazardous: An Australian study indicated that migrants arriving in Australia before age 10 had the same risk of native-born Australians, while migrants arriving after age 15 had one-quarter the rate of native-born Australians. (Also playing a role in the development of melanoma are precursor lesions—called *dysplastic nevi*—which develop during adolescence.)

Excessive exposure to sun contributes not only to skin cancer but also to premature aging. Wrinkling of the skin, loss of elasticity, and color change all appear to result from excessive sun exposure.

The sun is the cause of at least 90 percent of all skin cancers. But there is good news: Almost all skin cancers are preventable.

■ Sunscreens

Sometimes it is possible to avoid exposure to sun, but when that is not possible, sunscreen lotions provide protection against exposure to cancer-causing radiations. The choice of a sunscreen is based on your skin type, the length of time you spend in the sun, the intensity of the sun's rays where you live, and the type of formulation you prefer. The Food and Drug Administration designates five degrees of protection according to the products' Sun Protection Factor (SPF):

SPF 2 to 4	Minimal sun protection
SPF 4 to 6	Moderate sun protection
SPF 6 to 8	Extra sun protection
SPF 8 to 15	Maximal sun protection
SPF 15 or greater	Ultra sun protection

Products of SPF 15 or greater provide the greatest amount of protection against sun-induced skin damage and against sun-induced skin cancer. Especially if you're fair-skinned, and even if you're

not, a product with a high SPF is preferable to one with a lower SPF, when available.

Sunscreens contain chemicals that protect against the sun's rays: PABA, or para-aminobenzoic acid, and PABA esters; cinnamates; benzophenones; and anthranilates. PABA was the original compound; it was commonly used in a 5-percent solution in alcohol. More popular today are the PABA esters, compounds like glyceryl, padimate A, and padimate O, which are more popular than the original PABA because they do not stain clothing yellow. The PABA and PABA esters are available in either an alcohol or a cream base. The alcohol base stays on longer but may irritate the skin, while the cream base acts as a moisturizer but washes off more easily. Also available are water-resistant sunscreens that stay on longer. Protection may also be provided by the cinnamates, which wash off more easily than PABA.

PABA, PABA esters, and the cinnamates, while providing excellent protection, do not completely screen out all ultraviolet light. They protect primarily against UV-B, the familiar sunburn- and skin-cancer-causing rays. Less well-understood are the UV-A radiations, which have been suggested as contributing to wrinkling and skin cancer. For this reason, sunscreens often combine PABA, PABA esters, or cinnamates with UV-A screens. These are the benzophenones, effective primarily against UV-A, and the anthranilates, moderately effective at screening both UV-A and UV-B.

Some persons may be allergic to PABA or PABA esters. Non-PABA sunscreens also are available. Individuals may also be allergic to the cinnamates. An allergic reaction might possibly be due to other ingredients in the sunscreen—fragrances or preservatives, for example—and switching to another brand might solve the problem. Consult your physician, dermatologist, or pharmacist to find a sunscreen that suits you.

■ Recommendations

The Skin Cancer Foundation, a nonprofit organization concerned with cancer of the skin, supports research and education programs to help reduce the incidence of skin cancer. To limit the damage done by the rays of the sun, the Skin Cancer Foundation recommends these simple steps:

• Limit your sun exposure during the midday

hours (10 AM to 2 PM, or 11 AM to 3 PM Daylight Saving Time), when the sun is strongest. Plan outdoor activities for the morning or late afternoon or evening.

• Wear protective clothing—a hat, long-sleeved shirt, and long pants.

• Apply a sunscreen before every exposure to the sun, and reapply when necessary, at least every two hours, for as long as you stay in the sun. The sunscreen should be reapplied after you have been swimming or perspiring heavily. Do not forget to cover the ears, lips, nose, hands, and other prominently exposed areas.

• Use a sunscreen in high-altitude activities like mountain-climbing and skiing. At high altitudes the exposure to damaging rays is greater. The sun is also stronger near the equator.

• Use a sunscreen even on overcast days. The sun's rays may still be damaging when filtered through clouds.

• Individuals at high risk (outdoor workers, fair-skinned persons, and persons who already have had skin cancer) should apply sunscreens every day.

• Certain drugs and medications may cause *photosensitivity*, an increased sensitivity to sunburn. If you are using skin medication, you may need to take additional precautions. Consult your doctor.

• If you develop an allergic reaction to your sunscreen, change the product. You should be able to find a sunscreen on the market that you can use.

• Beware of reflective surfaces like sand, snow, concrete, and water. Sitting in the shade may not be protective.

• Sunscreens should be used both winter and summer. Sunscreens are needed in the snow, since sun reflected on snow can produce as much penetration as sun reflected on sand. The wind can thin sunscreens, so reapply often.

• Avoid tanning parlors. The UV light in tanning booths is as risky as that from the sun.

• Keep young infants out of the sun. Begin using sunscreens as early as 6 months of age.

• Teach sun protection early. Children should be taught to protect themselves against the sun, since sun damage accumulates over a lifetime.

Additional information may be obtained from the Skin Cancer Foundation, 245 Fifth Avenue, New York, NY 10016. Telephone: 212-725-5176. Your local chapter of the American Cancer Society can also provide information.

A Few Other Risks

For the majority of individuals, the major risks are those posed by cigarette smoking, diet, and exposure to sun. However, smaller numbers of individuals may be exposed to cancer risks as a result of X-ray, drug, or workplace exposures. Although these risks are less significant in terms of the numbers of individuals affected, efforts should nevertheless be directed at eliminating or controlling them.

■ *X rays*

Ionizing radiation—the type of radiation contained in medical X rays or radioactive fallout—may account for up to 3 percent of human cancers. Because ionizing radiation may affect the molecular structure of the cells, it may damage the cell's genetic material, leading to an increased risk of cancer.

Medical X rays do pose a certain degree of risk. Early radiologists had high rates of leukemia, a blood cancer. But later radiologists—armed with the recognition that excessive X-ray exposure was risky—took precautions, and today their risk is no greater than that of other physicians. Before 1950, too, radiation was used to treat or monitor a number of conditions. Women in whom fluoroscopy, an X-ray technique, was used to monitor treatment of tuberculosis, received relatively high doses of radiation; ten to fifteen years later, they had a higher incidence of breast cancer. Similarly, children once were treated with intense radiation to reduce the size of the thymus gland, a now-outmoded form of treatment that led to an increased risk of thyroid cancer and leukemia. Radiation had also been used to treat scalp ringworm and large tonsils.

The risks of nuclear radiation were seen in atomic bomb survivors in Japan: Increased rates of acute leukemia and cancers of the breast, thyroid, lung, stomach, and other organs were seen. Radioactive fallout, as is produced during atmospheric weapons tests, did seem to increase cancer risk in those accidentally exposed to very high levels; atmospheric weapons tests have since been banned.

Today, measures are taken to reduce the risk of cancers resulting from X rays. But X-ray procedures are often needed, and the benefits frequently outweigh the risks. For example, for a woman at risk of breast cancer, particularly if she is over 50 years of age, the benefits of detecting cancer early outweigh the potential risk of repeated mammograms.

Minimizing excessive exposure to medical X rays may reduce your cancer risk. Sometimes, that chest X ray or dental X ray "just to make sure" isn't needed. But always undergo X rays when they're really needed. Often, as in the case of mammography, the benefits are greater than the risks.

■ Drugs

In the last half-century, "miracle" drugs brought cures for once-fatal illnesses. Still, altering the body's chemistry to treat disease can have unintended effects: Drugs can contribute to the development of other disorders, including cancer. Drugs are believed to account for 2 percent of all cancers. An informed patient and conscientious physician carefully weigh the benefits of a drug against its risks, and make an educated decision on that basis.

Among the drugs that have been linked to cancer have been the *estrogens*, which are hormones, produced mainly by the ovaries, that help regulate menstruation, pregnancy, and female body features. Some middle-aged and older women have been prescribed synthetic "replacement" estrogens to alleviate the symptoms of menopause that may develop when ovarian production of these hormones stops. Replacement therapy, particularly over a prolonged period of time, has been linked to an increased risk of cancer of the lining of the uterus. The role of replacement estrogens in breast cancer is less clear.

If you suffer from menopausal symptoms, discuss the need for estrogens with your physician. While certain risks of estrogen therapy do exist, therapy may be necessary and beneficial. The decision must be made on an individual basis by you and your physician.

Oral contraceptives (most contain estrogens as well as another hormone, progesterone) have been the focus of much medical research. Data are not always consistent. Early studies indicated that certain groups of women who use birth control pills may have an increased risk of breast cancer. The current consensus is that there is little evidence linking oral contraceptives used in the U.S. with an increased risk of breast cancer. Other reports have linked oral contraceptives to a higher risk of cervical cancer, even after taking into account sexual activity and other risk factors. Some reports indicate that women who use the Pill may actually be at a *lower* risk of ovarian and endometrial (uterine) cancers.

However, a different formulation of birth control pill was available at one time and was taken off the market in the late 1970s. These pills, known as "sequential" pills, seemed to result in an increased incidence of endometrial cancer.

Another estrogen-like compound, DES or *diethylstilbestrol*, was prescribed during the 1940s and 1950s to prevent miscarriage. Although studies in the 1930s had indicated that DES could cause cancer in animals, the drug continued to be prescribed until the 1970s, when a rare vaginal and cervical cancer was found in women whose mothers had received DES. Whether these daughters are at increased risk of other types of cancers is unclear. Sons have been reported to have an increased incidence of sperm abnormalities and cancers of the reproductive tract. Probably 4 to 6 million Americans—mothers, daughters, and sons—have been exposed to DES.

If you are a woman whose mother took a drug to prevent miscarriage while pregnant with you, you should go to a doctor for examination of your vagina and cervix. You should probably be examined yearly, with a breast and pelvic exam as well as a Pap test. DES sons should be examined for genital defects such as undescended or underdeveloped testicles, but no increased risks of cancer are known to occur in DES sons.

Male hormones, or androgens ("steroids"), are chemically related to the estrogens. Synthetic androgens are used to treat cancers, genetic disorders, and blood and endocrine disorders. These androgens are the "anabolic steroids" sometimes used by athletes to increase body mass and boost athletic performance. Some evidence indicates that androgen administration may increase the chances of developing liver cancer.

Other drugs also may increase the incidence of human cancers. They include *phenacetin*, once an ingredient of a number of pain-killers; methoxypsoralens, used to treat psoriasis; and chlornaphthazine, a drug used to treat both Hodgkin's disease and the blood disorder polycythemia vera. And paradoxically, some very powerful drugs used in cancer treatment or in organ-transplant recipients may also induce cancer. Still, the benefits of treatment most often outweigh the risks.

■ Cancer at Our Jobs

Investigators attribute 4 percent of cancer deaths

to occupational factors. For the average individual who is not exposed to proven carcinogens, this probably means that occupational factors play a relatively minor role in his or her cancer risk. Occupational cancer tends to be concentrated among relatively small groups of people among whom the increased risk may be quite large. For instance, workers exposed to vinyl chloride are 200 times more likely to develop liver cancer than the average individual. The risks can often be reduced or eliminated once they are identified. Current recommendations to the individual worker for minimizing cancer risks emphasize the importance of following safety measures designed to reduce exposure to hazardous substances. These safety measures have been designed by regulatory agencies, industry, and organized labor.

Workplace cancers have been with us for a long time. Since 1775, when Percival Pott reported on a rare cancer of the scrotum common among London chimneysweeps, a disease then known as the "soot-wart," workers in certain occupations have been known to be at greater risk of certain types of cancer because of their exposure to chemicals, dusts, metals, or radiation.

One classic instance of workplace-related cancer involves those cancers attributed to exposure to asbestos, a name given to a group of minerals that occur naturally as masses of fibers, which can be separated into thin threads and woven. Asbestos has been commonly used in the construction and shipbuilding industries—often for fireproofing and insulating. Reports relating asbestos exposure to lung cancer and to asbestosis, a lung disease, have been appearing since 1935. And since the early 1960s, mesothelioma, a rare cancer affecting the lining of the chest and abdomen, has been linked to asbestos exposure. Mesotheliomas have been reported following asbestos exposures of as little as two months. Most cancer cases have occurred among asbestos workers and miners, but during World War II, numerous workers, particularly in the shipbuilding industry, suffered damage. And cases of lung cancer and mesothelioma have been found among the wives, sons, and daughters of asbestos workers who brought the asbestos fibers into their homes on their clothing. Today, asbestos exposure is regulated by the Occupational Safety and Health Administration (OSHA), which requires protective equipment for workers and regulates the number of fibers in the workplace.

Vinyl chloride made its appearance in the headlines in 1974 when the B. F. Goodrich Com-

pany indicated that three workers in its Louisville, Kentucky, plant had angiosarcoma, a rare form of liver cancer. This announcement caused the NIOSH to initiate studies of workers in the vinyl chloride industry. The studies found that workers who had been working with vinyl chloride for five years or more and whose initial exposure had begun at least ten years earlier had higher than expected rates of liver cancer, as well as cancers in other organs. Vinyl chloride, a colorless gas, is an important ingredient in phonograph records, product packaging, medical tubing, household utensils, and a number of other plastics. Although plastic products were shown to pose no danger to the average individual, workers in vinyl chloride plants are 200 times more at risk from liver cancer.

Other important workplace carcinogens include dyes (which have been reported to induce bladder cancer) and metals such as arsenic, chromium, cadmium, and nickel. An arm of the World Health Organization (a United Nations agency) known as the IARC (International Agency for Research on Cancer) reports on carcinogenic chemicals.

Although the list of cancer-causing chemicals is growing, it is small considering the many chemicals, both manmade and natural, in our workplaces and our environment. Many chemicals do not cause cancer. When used properly, many chemicals have no harmful effects whatsoever.

But if you work in an industry where you are exposed to potential carcinogens, be sure to follow safety rules. Have periodic physical examinations, and, if you are exposed, avoid personal habits that expose you to greater risk. For example, tobacco users who have been exposed to asbestos are at greater risk than they would be if exposed to either agent alone.

■ *Water/Air Pollution*

Although air and water pollution could potentially affect large numbers of individuals, current assessments indicate that pollution seems to play a relatively small role in overall cancer risks.

Lung cancer is higher in cities, but workplace factors and cigarette smoking may be responsible for the difference. As noted above, asbestos is a known carcinogen that once had wide use as a building material. Asbestos is found in the air around the workplaces of certain industries such as shipbuilding, asbestos mining and manufacturing, insulation work in construction and building, and automotive brake repair. The degree of risk to the general public is uncertain but probably small. Health risks usually arise when asbestos fibers are set free during mining, drilling, sawing, or spraying, or when materials with asbestos in them start to decompose. Some concerns have been raised about children's exposure in old school buildings.

Radon, a radioactive material normally present in soil and water, may result in cancer. When it enters a well-insulated home, it may be retained within, precipitating the development of cancer. Some investigators suggest that 10,000 cases of lung cancer will be attributed to radon exposure. However, excessively high indoor levels of radon may be lowered by relatively simple venting systems that cost about $1,000.

Another important "air pollutant" is cigarette smoke. Some studies indicate that cigarette smoke inhaled by nonsmokers may be harmful to them. The extent of the hazard posed by both radon and passive smoking, however, remains unclear.

Current evidence suggests that the drinking water of most communities poses little cancer risk. But concerns have arisen that hazardous waste disposal sites can leak, causing contamination of groundwater and wells. Industrial plants may introduce carcinogenic effluents into drinking water. And the chlorine used to purify water supplies may react with substances in drinking water to form chemicals (these are known as trihalomethanes, or THMs) that may be carcinogenic. U.S. water supplies are monitored by the Environmental Protection Agency and by local and state groups.

But although in isolated cases drinking water may contain excessively high levels of carcinogens, the evidence to date seems to indicate that the drinking water in most communities has little influence on cancer risk.

There is one postulated risk, however, that has proven significant. Since the mid-1970s, scientists have theorized that certain types of chemicals, primarily those known as the chlorofluorocarbons (once used in aerosol propellants, refrigerators, and air conditioners, nonessential uses that have since been banned in the U.S.), which were dispersed into the atmosphere, caused changes in the earth's atmosphere. It was predicted that high levels of these chemicals would destroy the "ozone layer" that protects the earth from ultraviolet rays. (Other risks of ozone depletion include climatic changes, smog, and acid rain.) Despite the U.S. ban, use of chlorofluorocarbons in refrigerants,

electronic solvents, specialty dry cleaning, foam-blowing agents, and other specialty uses have raised global emission rates almost to 1974 levels.

It is particularly worrisome that data are now coming in indicating that ozone depletion has already occurred and is continuing to occur as the global rate at which the chlorofluorocarbons are dispersed into the atmosphere continues to increase. Because the ozone layer filters out ultraviolet rays (ultraviolet rays play a role in the development of skin cancer), depletion of the ozone layer is likely to lead to additional cases of human skin cancer. The extent of this risk, however, is not certain at this time.

Cancer Screening

The *first line of defense* against cancer consists of those actions we ourselves can take to reduce our cancer risk: not smoking, modifying our diet, and avoiding exposure to the sun.

The *second line of defense* consists of cancer screening and detection techniques. Early detection and screening means that cancer can be diagnosed and treated when it is curable. With improved treatment techniques—the last decade has seen significant advances—many cancers are treatable when they are detected at an early stage.

Some of the more common cancers—those of the colon and breast—can be detected readily with currently available screening techniques. Some of the best known techniques are also the most critically important.

Cancer of the breast often can be detected early through breast self-examination, breast examination by a doctor, or mammography, a low-dose X-ray picture of the breasts.

The American Cancer Society recommends that women between the ages of 20 and 40 should do a breast self-examination every month, should have their breasts examined by a physician every three years, and should have at least one baseline X-ray study (mammography) obtained between the ages of 35 and 40. Individuals at particularly high risk of breast cancer are those with a personal or family history of breast cancer, those who have never had children, and those who have had their first child after 30. These individuals should probably be screened more often.

For women over 40 years of age, self-examination is recommended every month, a doctor's exam is recommended every year, and mammog-

BREAST SELF-EXAMINATION (BSE)

Here is how to do BSE: Breast self-examination should be done once a month so you become familiar with the usual appearance and feel of your breasts. Familiarity makes it easier to notice any changes in the breast from one month to another. Early discovery of a change from what is "normal" is the main idea behind BSE.

If you menstruate, the best time to do BSE is 2 or 3 days after your period ends, when your breasts are least likely to be tender or swollen. If you no longer menstruate, pick a day, such as the first day of the month, to remind yourself it is time to do BSE.

1. Stand before a mirror. Inspect both breasts for anything unusual, such as any discharge from the nipples, puckering, dimpling, or scaling of the skin. The next two steps are designed to emphasize any change in the shape or contour of your breasts. As you do them you should be able to feel your chest muscles tighten. **2.** Watching closely in the mirror, clasp hands behind your head and press hands forward. **3.** Next, press hands firmly on hips and bow slightly toward your mirror as you pull your shoulders and elbows forward. Some women do the next part of the exam in the shower. Fingers glide over soapy skin, making it easy to concentrate on the texture underneath.

4. Raise your left arm. Use three or four fingers of your right hand to explore your left breast firmly, carefully, and thoroughly. Beginning at the outer edge, press the flat part of your fingers in small circles, moving the circles slowly around the breast. Gradually work toward the nipple. Be sure to cover the entire breast. Pay special attention to the area between the breast and the armpit, including the armpit itself. Feel for any unusual lump or mass under the skin. **5.** Gently squeeze the nipple and look for a discharge. Repeat the exam on your right breast. **6.** Steps 4 and 5 should be repeated lying down. Lie flat on your back, left arm over your head and a pillow or folded towel under your left shoulder. This position flattens the breast and makes it easier to examine. Use the same circular motion described earlier. Repeat on your right breast.

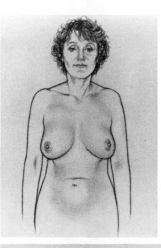

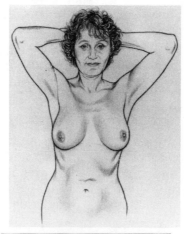

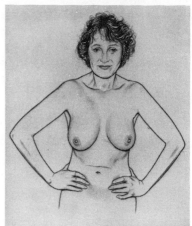

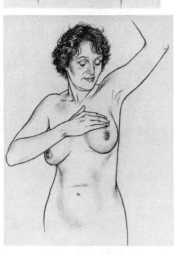

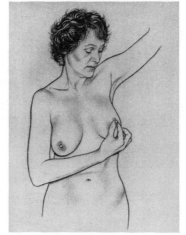

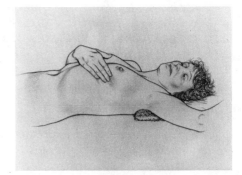

Source: Breast Exams—What You Should Know, National Cancer Institute.

raphy should be done every year after 50. Between the ages of 40 and 49, breast X rays should be performed every one to two years.

Cancer of the colon can likewise be detected early. Individuals aged 40 and over should have their stools tested for occult (hidden) blood. (Colon cancer is more common in older individuals.) Current American Cancer Society recommendations indicate that specimens should be collected each day at home over three days while the individual follows a specific diet. Screening for occult blood is inexpensive.

Individuals over 50 years of age should also have a digital rectal examination performed by a physician each year. In this examination a gloved hand is used to examine the rectum for lumps or masses.

Also recommended for persons over 50 years of age is the proctosigmoidoscopy. This test involves visualization of the intestine through a tube with a light and a magnified viewing system that is much like a telescope. The most recently available sigmoidoscopes are flexible, and allow additional visualization of the colon (they reach much farther into the intestine) while causing much less discomfort than earlier rigid instruments. Although uncomfortable, the test is a highly effective screening tool. For individuals over 50, the American Cancer Society recommends two successive negative proctosigmoidoscopies one year apart, and thereafter the test should be performed every three to five years. Individuals at higher risk—those with a personal or family history of colon cancer, those with a family history of polyps, and those with ulcerative colitis—should be screened more often.

Probably the best-known screening test is the "Pap test," used to screen for cancer of the cervix (the mouth of the womb). When detected before cancer cells have spread beyond the superficial layers, cervical cancer is almost 100 percent curable. The Pap test is reliable, inexpensive, and easy to perform. The physician takes a scraping of cells from the inside of the cervix with a small wooden spatula or Q-Tip, and a pathologist examines the samples for malignant changes. In a joint statement made in January of 1988, the National Cancer Institute, the American Cancer Society, and the American College of Obstetricians and Gynecologists recommended that all women who are or have been sexually active, or have reached age 18 years, have an annual Pap test and pelvic examination. After a woman has had three or more consecutive, satisfactory, normal annual examinations, the Pap test may be performed less frequently, at the discretion of her physician. Women who are at higher risk—those with any abnormal Pap test or those who are sexually active with multiple partners—should be screened at least annually.

Cancer of the endometrium, or the lining of the womb, generally strikes women after menopause. Currently, the pelvic examination is recommended as screening for endometrial cancer. In addition, any woman at increased risk—risks include obesity, infertility, failure to ovulate, abnormal uterine bleeding, and history of estrogen therapy—should undergo some form of endometrial tissue sampling at menopause and thereafter as recommended by her physician. The most accurate procedure for obtaining endometrial tissue is dilatation and curettage (D & C), which is a simple surgical procedure. During the D & C the cervix is opened and dilated, and the inside of the uterus is scraped. Other endometrial sampling techniques, using aspiration and suction (these can be done in the office), appear promising, and these techniques are used by many physicians to screen high-risk women.

The importance of a medical examination during which cancer-related tests (screening tests and physical examinations) are performed also needs to be recognized. The American Cancer Society recommends a cancer-related check-up every three years for individuals between 20 and 40 years of age and yearly for individuals over 40. These physical examinations should include screening tests as well as a physical examination for cancers such as testicular and prostatic in males; breast, ovarian, cervical, and endometrial in females; and cancers in the mouth, neck, skin, thyroid, lymph nodes, and colon for both sexes. At this time, your physician can discuss with you ways in which you can reduce your cancer risk.

A physical examination once every three years before 40 years of age and once a year after age 40 is far less costly than initiating treatment once a cancer has developed.

In short, the recommended screening tests are these:
Pap test—
• (at least every 3 years)
Colorectal tests—
• digital rectal examination by physician every year after 40
• stool blood test yearly after age 50
• Proctosigmoidoscopy every 3 to 5 years after

age 50 following 2 annual exams with negative results

Breast-cancer detection—

• Breast self-examination for all women over 20
• Physician examination at least once every 3 years between ages 20 and 40 and then every year
• Mammogram every year for asymptomatic women age 50 and over, and baseline mammogram between ages 35 and 39. Women 40 to 49 should have mammography every 1 to 2 years, depending on history, X-ray exposure, and physical findings.

It should be stressed that the above recommendations are general guidelines for the average individual who has no symptoms. Ask your physician how these guidelines relate to you. He or she knows you, your family history, and your other risk factors, and will interpret these recommendations in the light of your medical history.

Attention to possible early warning signs of cancer is equally important. For many years, the American Cancer Society has publicized seven early warning signs of cancer.

• Change in bowel and bladder habits
• A sore that does not heal
• Unusual bleeding or discharge
• Thickening or lump in the breast or elsewhere
• Indigestion or difficulty swallowing
• An obvious change in a wart or mole
• A persistent cough or hoarseness

While none of these symptoms is a sure sign of cancer, if any lasts longer than two weeks, be sure to consult your doctor. Do not wait for symptoms to become worse. An examination at this point can enable your physician to catch the disease at an early, curable stage. Denying symptoms may give the disease a chance to spread, reducing the possibility of complete and relatively painless cure.

There are also some preventive actions directed at specific cancers. These are particularly important for individuals at high risk, although they should be of concern to all individuals.*

Cancer of the larynx. Individuals at particularly high risk are those who are heavy drinkers or smokers and those who have had cancer of the oral cavity or lung. This cancer can be detected early. Cutting down on drinking or smoking minimizes the risk. Early warning signs include hoarseness or bleeding from the throat.

* Adapted from Daniel G. Miller, M.D., "Cancer Prevention: Steps You Can Take," in the *American Cancer Society Cancer Book* (New York: Doubleday, 1986).

Cancer of the mouth and throat. Factors increasing the risk of oral cancer include broken teeth that irritate tissues in the mouth; ill-fitting or broken dentures; heavy smoking or drinking; a non-healing sore or white patch. Anyone with a sore that does not heal or bleeding from the throat should consult a physician or dentist. Minimizing consumption of alcohol and eliminating tobacco use will reduce risk.

Cancer of the lung. Cigarette smoking puts you at increased risk. Others at increased risk include those with a history of tuberculosis, those with a chronic cough, and those who have worked in occupations in which they have come into contact with asbestos, nickel, chromates, or radioactive material. Eliminating smoking and minimizing occupational exposure to hazardous substances helps reduce the risk. Unfortunately, this cancer is not often detected at an early, curable stage.

Cancer of the kidney and bladder. Individuals at increased risk include those with congenital abnormalities of the kidney and bladder (your physician will probably have informed you of these); those who have been exposed to chemicals like naphthalines, aniline dyes, or benzidines; those with frequent urinary tract infections; those with a history of schistosomiasis, a parasitic disease seen in the tropics; those who use tobacco. Note that blood in the urine is an important sign that may indicate bladder or kidney cancer. Although not necessarily a sign of cancer (blood in the urine is more commonly found with infection), you should consult your physician. Further, frequent urinary tract infections may be the result of underlying cancer.

Cancer of the prostate. Individuals at increased risk include those with a history of venereal disease and those with a history of prostate infections. Persons over 50 also are at increased risk; they should be aware of the symptoms of prostate cancer and should have the prostate examined regularly by a physician. Early symptoms include interruption of urine flow, frequent urination, inability to urinate, blood in the urine, painful or burning urination, and persistent pain in the back, hips, or pelvis. These symptoms are common also in benign enlargement of the prostate, a common condition in older men, and in bladder or prostatic infections.

Cancer of the testes. Individuals at risk include those with undescended testicles. This cancer is most common in men under 40. Men, like women performing breast self-examination, can perform a testicular self-examination once a month. Each testicle can be examined by rolling it gently between the thumb and fingers. Feel for a firm lump about the size of a pea. Most lumps are noncancerous, but you should consult your physician if you find one.

Cancer of the stomach. Individuals at greater risk of stomach cancer are those with a lack of normal stomach acid, those with pernicious anemia, or those with chronic gastritis or polyps. Ulcers and ulcer symptoms often mimic cancer. If symptoms last more than one month, consult a physician. Also, avoid excessive amounts of salt-cured, smoked, or nitrite-cured foods: There is suggestive evidence that these may be implicated in the development of stomach cancer.

Cancer of the colon. Individuals with a history of polyps or a family history of colon or rectal cancer are at greater risk. Any change in regular bowel habits, including constipation or diarrhea, abdominal pain, weight loss, fatigue, or bleeding into the stool, should be a signal for a visit to a physician. A high-fiber diet seems to reduce the risk of developing cancer of the colon.

Cancer of the cervix. Individuals with more than five completed pregnancies, those who have had intercourse before age 18, and those who have had a history of syphilis or gonorrhea and multiple sexual partners are at greater risk. This cancer is generally slow-growing and can be cured when detected early by a Pap smear. Early symptoms are uncommon, but may include spotting between periods or after intercourse. Adult women should have a Pap smear at least every three years.

Cancer of the endometrium. Women at greater risk are those who have completed the menopause, who have never been pregnant, who have a family history of endometrial cancer, who are obese, or who have diabetes or hypertension. These women should have some form of endometrial sampling (either a D & C or endometrial aspiration) at menopause. Exposure to estrogens may also increase the risk of endometrial cancer. Early symptoms include bleeding or spotting after menopause.

Cancer of the ovary. This type of cancer is detected at the time of a pelvic examination. Early symptoms are rare but may include abnormal menstrual bleeding, pain, or an increase in abdominal size with vague abdominal complaints.

Cancer of the breast. Women at greater risk are those with a family history of breast cancer, those who have never had a baby or who have had a baby after age 30, those who consume a high-fat diet, and those with previous breast cancer. Breast self-examination, examination by a physician, and mammography are recommended as preventive measures, as indicated. This cancer often is curable if identified early.

Skin cancer. Risk factors for skin cancer include very fair skin, history of prolonged exposure to the sun, a history of skin cancer, and moles in areas typically irritated by clothing or shaving. According to the Skin Cancer Foundation, the warning signs of skin cancer are these:

- A skin growth that increases in size and appears pearly, translucent, tan, brown, black, or multicolored.
- A spot or growth that continues to itch, hurt, crust, scab, erode, or bleed.
- An open sore or wound on the skin that does not heal or persists for more than four weeks, or heals and then reopens.

To sum up, individuals at higher than average risk for cancer include:

- Those who have close relatives with cancer of the breast, stomach, colon, prostate, lung, or uterus. Although the risk in this case is higher than average, it is not that much higher. It's not a foregone conclusion that you'll have cancer, even though your relatives have had the disease. But if people in your family have had these cancers, let your doctor know so that he or she can help you watch for signs of the disease.
- Those who have been exposed to cancer-causing agents on the job. Common carcinogens include nickel, chromate, vinyl chloride, and asbestos dust. Health hazards from asbestos have been seen among workers in the shipbuilding trades, asbestos mining and manufacturing, insulation work in building construction, and auto repair (brake linings). If you work in a job at which you may be exposed, follow safety procedures. Consult your doctor if you have been exposed, and if you smoke, stop.
- Those who have had X-ray treatments involving head and neck. Individuals who have received X-ray treatments to the thymus, tonsils, or in the treatment of adenoids, whooping cough, ringworm, and acne may be at increased risk of thyroid cancer. Consult your doctor. Even if thyroid cancer does develop, it can be cured.

Excessive X-ray exposure may increase cancer risk. While most medical X rays today are adjusted to deliver the lowest dose possible without sacrificing image quality, you should check with your physician about the *need* for X rays. You probably could do without that dental X ray "just to make sure." On the other hand, don't avoid needed X-ray exams for fear of cancer: The benefits of detecting disease (for instance, detecting breast cancer by mammography) outweigh the potential risks.

• Women whose mothers took DES (diethylstilbestrol) while pregnant with them.

Estrogens, often given to women at menopause to control symptoms like hot flashes or thinning of the vaginal lining, may be associated with certain risks. Prolonged estrogen treatment has been linked to an increase in the risk of uterine cancer. However, estrogens *can* be given safely. Women need to discuss the risks and benefits of estrogens with their physicians.

Cancer Facts and Figures

• In 1988 it is estimated that close to 500,000 Americans will die of cancer.

• About 985,000 new cases of cancer will be diagnosed in 1988.

• About 30 percent of Americans now living ultimately will develop cancer, according to present rates. Cancer will strike in about 3 of every 4 families.

• Cancer is primarily a disease of older and middle-aged persons. However, it kills more children between ages 3 and 14 than any other disease.

• Lung cancer is the only major cause of cancer death that has been increasing steadily since 1950, an increase attributed to the numbers of smokers entering middle age.

• Lung cancer is the most common cancer among males, followed by colorectal and prostate cancer, in that order.

• Breast cancer is the most common cancer in females, followed by lung and colorectal cancer. While in 1950 colorectal cancer was the second most common malignancy among females, in 1988 lung cancer was the second most common cancer among females. Lung-cancer deaths among women have accelerated sharply, primarily because of the increased number of women smokers entering age groups at risk.

• Stomach-cancer death rates have decreased in the United States, both for men and women.

• The American Cancer Society estimates that of the close to 500,000 cancer deaths, about 175,000 might have been prevented by earlier diagnosis and treatment.

• The National Cancer Institute estimates that at least 80 percent of cancers are caused by factors that are under our control. If we alter our lifestyles— eliminate smoking, modify our diet, avoid excessive exposure to sun—there is evidence that we can reduce our risk of getting cancer.

Cancer Control: In Your Hands

The evidence is accumulating: Much of your cancer risk is in your hands. Scientists now believe that most cancers are related to life-style: what you eat, drink, and/or smoke. To a large extent, you can control your cancer risk by making some simple—and often pleasant—changes in the way you live. Dr. Daniel G. Miller, of the Strang Clinic in New York, estimates that up to 50 percent of cancer deaths could be eliminated by preventive strategies that include life-style modifications.

And should you develop cancer, you can increase your chances of a cure by paying attention to early detection and screening: Be watchful for the warning signs of cancer; see your physician as recommended for checkups; and have yourself screened as appropriate for breast, colon, and cervical cancer.

To reduce cancer risk:

Do not smoke. Smoking is the most important risk factor, causing 30 percent of all cancer deaths. It's responsible for 83 percent of lung-cancer cases. Chewing tobacco ("smokeless tobacco") is harmful as well, posing a risk for mouth and throat cancers.

Modify your diet. Dietary factors may be responsible for as many as 35 percent of all cancers, according to some estimates. For healthy nutrition that reduces cancer risks:
• Eat more cabbage-family vegetables
• Add more high-fiber foods
• Choose foods high in vitamins A and C
• Reduce the amount of fat in your diet
• Avoid salt-cured, smoked, or nitrite-cured foods

Avoid obesity. Obesity is linked to cancers of the uterus, gallbladder, breast, and colon. Exercise and a lower calorie intake may help you avoid weight gain.

Moderate your alcohol intake. Heavy drinking increases the risk of liver cancer. It also increases the risk of cancer of the larynx, throat, mouth, and esophagus, especially for persons who smoke.

Avoid too much sun. Most cases of nonmelanoma skin cancer are sun-related. Try to avoid the midday sun, between 10 AM and 3 PM, and if you must go out then, protect yourself with a strong sunscreen—at least SPF 15—and wear long sleeves and a hat. Don't use indoor sunlamps or tanning parlors.

Cancer: A Curable Disease

A diagnosis of cancer is no longer a death sentence. In the early 1900s, few cancer patients had any hope of survival. Even in the 1930s, only 1 in 5 individuals with cancer was alive 5 years after diagnosis. Today, however, 40 percent of those who get cancer will be alive 5 years after diagnosis.

Actually, survival statistics are even higher, because some deaths in this group are caused by such factors as heart disease, accidents, and other degenerative diseases. The "relative" survival rate of today's cancer patient is actually 49 percent: He or she has a 49 percent chance of surviving diagnosed cancer.

Cancer therapy has made considerable strides in the last decade and a half, with improved management and diagnosis. A number of cancers that once had a very poor prognosis are now being cured: acute lymphocytic leukemia in children, Hodgkin's disease, Burkitt's lymphoma, Ewing's sarcoma, Wilms's tumor, rhabdomyosarcoma, choriocarcinoma, testicular cancer, ovarian cancer, and osteogenic sarcoma.

Much of the progress has been relatively subtle. Developments include better staging (that is, determining how far the disease has spread followed by appropriate treatment for that stage), as well as new and improved combinations of cancer drugs. Well-designed treatment programs often include more than one kind of therapy—radiation, chemotherapy, and surgery—often in combination.

Directions for current and future research:

• *Monoclonal antibodies.* Fusing cancer cells to normal immune cells produces specific antibodies that seek out chosen targets on cancer cells.

• *New drugs.* About 50 drugs have been found effective against certain cancers, and others continue to undergo testing.

• *Immunotherapy.* This holds the hope of harnessing the body's disease-fighting systems.

• *Bone-marrow transplants.* This technique has promise for patients with leukemia.

• *Chemotherapy, radiation therapy, and surgery.* Improvements have made possible more conservative management (for example, fewer permanent colostomies for persons with colon cancer, while many more of those with laryngeal cancer will be able to retain their voice).

• *Improved detection methods.* These include CAT scanning (computerized axial tomography), NMR (nuclear magnetic resonance imaging), thermography (heat patterns), and diaphanoscopy (transillumination with a beam of light).

• *Preventive interventions.* Work is directed toward (1) interrupting the development of cancer; and (2) studying the possibilities of chemoprevention with agents like synthetic retinoids (cousins of vitamin A), betacarotene, folic acid, and certain vitamins and minerals; also studying the effects of dietary intervention in women with breast cancer.

19

THE WELLNESS DIET

Each day we are bombarded with nutritional information—and *misinformation*. New diet books become overnight best sellers. Nationwide health organizations stress the importance of diet. The National Cancer Institute tells us to adopt an anticancer diet. The American Heart Association tells us to reduce our fat and cholesterol. The National Institutes of Health term obesity a "killer disease."

What are the facts? And what are the fallacies?

How can we apply sound, scientific principles to design a diet that is safe, healthy, and nutritionally sound? How can you design the diet that is right for you?

Elements of the Diet

The major building blocks of the diet are the basic substances contained in the foods we eat. We need a certain amount of energy: The energy we use is measured in the form of calories (the "calorie" is the amount of heat needed to raise 1 liter of water by 1 degree Celsius). A given food is said to provide a certain number of these calories. Our need for energy, or calories, varies according to our activity level, height, and body composition.

Some of what goes into our diet is essential: certain minimum quantities of carbohydrates, proteins, vitamins, and minerals. To a large extent, however, we get more than we need of many important components of the diet, especially fats and cholesterol, sugar, salt, and even protein.

■ Fats and Cholesterol

Discussed earlier, in connection with heart disease and cancer, a diet high in fats and cholesterol contributes to the development of these chronic diseases. Fat also promotes weight gain: While 1 gram of protein or starch contains only 4 calories, 1 gram of fat contains 9 calories.

We do need sufficient amounts of one nutrient supplied by fats: *linoleic acid.* Most of us need no more than a teaspoon of fat a day, however, and in adults the body synthesizes all the cholesterol we need. Also, although butter, oils, meat products, cheeses, and whole milk are thought of as typically "fatty foods," even fruits, vegetables, and potatoes have lesser amounts of fats.

An individual who takes care to limit the amount of fat in his or her diet—avoiding red meat, using minimal butter and oil, scorning hard cheeses and whole milk—will still get enough fat as long as he or she is consuming sufficient amounts of other foods.

■ Protein

The word *protein* comes from a Greek word meaning "to come first." Most people think of protein as the most important nutrient, and, in fact, protein is needed on a daily basis for growth and for the function and repair of tissues. Bones, teeth, cartilage, blood and other body fluids, muscles, skin, and organs like the liver, kidney, eyes, and brain all need protein. Protein is essential also for production of antibodies and for the hormones and enzymes that regulate body functions.

Many different types of proteins are found in the human body, but all consist of the amino acids. Over one hundred amino-acid "building blocks" may make up one protein. Of the twenty-two amino acids that exist in nature, all except nine can be made in the human body. These nine amino acids, termed the "essential amino acids," must be supplied in the form of food.

Most Americans consume far more protein than they need. The major sources of protein in the American diet consist of meat and milk products—foods of animal origin. These foods are, to a large extent, also high in fat and cholesterol. About 6 to 7 ounces of protein per day is enough for the average adult.

Vegetable protein—derived from beans, peas, and many vegetables—is a low-fat alternative to meat and meat products. However, while meat and milk proteins (from red meat, milk, fish, poultry, and eggs) supply all nine essential amino acids, most vegetable proteins lack one or more of the essential nine.

Vegetable proteins should be used in combination. For instance, the Mexican tortilla usually is made of corn flour, which is low in the essential amino acid *lysine*. It is eaten along with beans, however, which have enough lysine but are low in *methionine*, another essential amino acid. Substantial amounts of methionine, however, can be gotten from corn. Other similar combinations are rice and beans, cereal and milk, pasta and beans, peanut butter and wheat bread. Nutritionists today call them "complementary" combinations.

To obtain substantial amounts of protein from vegetable sources, be sure to combine a *grain* such as corn, rice, wheat (bread, pasta, cereal), seeds, barley, or oats with a *legume* such as soy products (soybeans, tofu), peanuts, black-eyed peas, lentils,

---

DIET AND CHRONIC DISEASE

Diet is at the center of efforts directed at the prevention of two major chronic diseases: heart disease and cancer. In previous sections, we have discussed how dietary strategies help reduce the risk of heart disease and cancer:

• Reduce intake of fat. This will help prevent both heart disease and cancer. Americans currently get about 40 percent of their calories from fat. Individuals should reduce the number of calories they get from fat to 30 percent.

• Reduce intake of cholesterol and saturated fat to less than 10 percent of total daily calories and cholesterol intake to less than 300 milligrams per day. Polyunsaturated fats should be substituted for saturated fat when possible.

• Maintain desirable weight. Obesity—defined as weighing 20 percent or more above your ideal weight—increases the chances of developing heart disease or cancer.

• Include fiber-containing foods in your diet. The evidence is strong that fiber-containing diets reduce cancer risk. There is also suggestive evidence that fiber may reduce heart-disease risk.

• Include fruits and vegetables containing vitamins A and C in your diet. Foods containing vitamins A and C seem to reduce the risk of cancer. Fruits and vegetables are also good alternatives to fatty foods like meat, pork, cakes, and heavy desserts.

• Cabbage-family (cruciferous) vegetables seem to reduce the risk of cancer. Include vegetables like broccoli, cabbage, and brussels sprouts in your diet.

• Limit salt intake. This recommendation of the American Heart Association is disputed by some experts, who contend that persons with normal or below-normal blood pressure need not limit consumption of salt. All agree, however, that persons with high blood pressure ought to limit the amount of salt they consume.

• Limit intake of nitrite-containing foods. Bacon, frankfurters, sausages, and other processed meats that have nitrite as a preservative may contribute to the development of cancer.

• Moderate alcohol intake. Alcohol abusers are at higher risk of cancer.

These are the guidelines, yet many consumers don't know how to translate them into action at supermarket checkout counters. Also, these guidelines are directed only at the major chronic diseases. There is much more to know in putting together the elements of a healthy, nutritionally sound diet.

lima beans, or chickpeas. Grains and legumes can likewise be combined with smaller amounts of meat or milk products.

In this way, vegetarians can obtain a healthy, nutritious diet. And vegetarians who take care to observe sound nutritional principles may actually prolong life by avoiding artery-clogging cholesterol and fats.

Even athletes don't need "extra protein." The protein requirement for a 200-pound man is readily met by cereal and milk for breakfast, 4 ounces of chicken for lunch, and less than 6 ounces of lean meat for supper. Athletes who are trying to increase weight by increasing muscle mass may need slightly more, but still not more than is supplied in the normal diet.

The average individual aged 19 years and over needs only 0.36 grams of protein per pound of ideal body weight. Thus, a 120-pound woman needs 43 grams of protein, readily supplied by cereal and skim milk for breakfast, $\frac{3}{4}$ of a cup of cooked beans for lunch (be sure to include a grain with this as well), and 4 ounces of chicken for supper.

It is best to consume a variety of foods. This ensures not only that you will obtain sufficient amounts of the essential amino acids but sufficient amounts of the other nutrients as well.

■ *Carbohydrates: Sugar and Starch*

The much-maligned potato is now coming into its own. Foods like potatoes, rice, and pasta—especially when eaten without high-fat butter, oil, or sauce—are not really fattening. They have fewer calories, ounce for ounce, than meat or poultry, and they are lower in artery-clogging fats and cholesterol.

These foods—the so-called starchy foods—are high in carbohydrates, which are the body's main source of energy. Carbohydrates are classed as either simple or complex. *Simple carbohydrates* are contained in table sugar, milk sugar, fruit sugar, and the like. The more complex carbohydrates are made up of many of these simple "sugar" building blocks.

The body breaks the complex carbohydrates down to glucose, which supplies the fuel for the heart, brain, and muscles.

The complex carbohydrates, or the starches, have important assets. They often contain substantial amounts of fiber, which may protect against cancer. They provide bulk in the diet, leading to a feeling of fullness. And they also provide important nutrients: vitamins, minerals, and trace elements.

Refined sugar (table sugar or *sucrose*), on the other hand, supplies calories without giving us any additional vitamins, minerals, trace elements, or proteins. The body does not actually need refined sugar: Sufficient amounts of body fuel can be provided by starches and fruit sugars. And refined sugar is the enemy of the dentist because it promotes tooth decay.

■ *Fiber*

Dietary fiber is the material from plant cells that is not digested or is only partially digestible. Vegetables, fruits, and whole-grain products contain different types of fibers.

High-fiber diets are believed to reduce the risk of some cancers by promoting bowel function and the removal of toxic wastes. A high-fiber diet also increases levels of HDL, the "good" lipoprotein in the blood, suggesting that it may help promote cardiovascular health. Similarly, fiber may also improve the processing of sugar by diabetics. And because fiber creates a feeling of fullness, it may aid in weight control.

Other claims for fiber remain unproved. Similarly, further work has to be done on the relative benefits of vegetable, fruit, and grain fibers.

■ *Salt*

From culture to culture, salt has been used to preserve and season foods. The Japanese consume salt primarily as soy sauce. Americans simply put a saltshaker full of sodium chloride on the table. This need and craving for salt has extended through time and throughout many cultures.

But in our modern society, this craving is essentially maladaptive. Scientists speculate that the herbivorous diet of fruits, nuts, and grains of the tropical savannas, where salt was difficult to obtain, was typical throughout much of human history. Only recently have we abandoned it for the meaty and salty diet of modern times. The result: tastes that are not adapted to our needs.

High blood pressure is pervasive in the United States and the developed countries of Europe. While we do need a certain amount of salt, many Americans may consume five to ten times as much as they actually need. Major health organizations now warn that our salt intake is far too high. Experts agree that hypertensive individuals should reduce their salt intake, and the American Heart Association extends this recommendation to all Americans.

Foods high in salt include not only the perilous pretzel but many processed foods as well, such as dried and canned soups, hard cheeses, pickles, even breakfast-cereals. And it is actually the sodium, not the "salt," that is the villain. Sodium is contained not only in salt but also in food additives like monosodium glutamate (MSG). Processed meats, baked goods, ketsup, and mustard all contain sodium in one form or another. *Read labels.*

See also the extended discussion of dietary salt—and its role in high blood pressure—in the earlier chapter, *The Healthy Heart.*

Vitamins

In the old days of sailing ships, scurvy—a disease marked by bleeding gums, mental disturbances, and ultimately death—disabled many ships and crews before the end of a long voyage. In 1753 a Scottish naval surgeon, James Lind, wrote that he had cured and prevented scurvy by giving citrus juices to sailors while on a ten-week cruise. In 1795 the British navy ordered that a regular supply of lime juice be issued to all ships (thus the name "limeys" for British sailors). Eventually scientists discovered that scurvy was caused by a lack of vitamin C, or ascorbic acid, in the diet.

To prevent deficiency diseases such as scurvy, small amounts of *trace substances* like vitamin C and certain inorganic substances known as *minerals* (which include calcium, magnesium, and potassium) are essential to the diet.

Vitamins are defined as organic (carbon-containing) substances that in small amounts are essential to proper body functioning. There are thirteen known essential vitamins.

Four *fat-soluble* vitamins:

- vitamin A
- vitamin D
- vitamin E
- vitamin K

Nine *water-soluble* vitamins:

- vitamin C
- Eight B-complex vitamins

  thiamine, B_1 cobalamin, B_{12}
  riboflavin, B_2 pantothenic acid
  niacin, B_3 biotin
  pyridoxine, B_6 folic acid

Fat-soluble vitamins dissolve in oil and certain other organic solvents like chloroform; they do not dissolve in water. High doses of fat-soluble vitamins are more likely to produce toxic effects than are high doses of water-soluble vitamins. Still, toxic reactions have been reported following excessively high doses of certain water-soluble vitamins.

The above thirteen vitamins are the only vitamins recognized as *essential* by the scientific community. There is a continuing debate, however, as to what quantities of these vitamins are required. Some experts maintain that we need only enough vitamins and minerals to prevent the deficiency diseases. Others maintain that larger amounts are needed for optimal health.

The debate has become so heated that a 1985 revision of the 1980 Recommended Dietary Allowances (RDAs) by its own appointed committee was rejected by the National Academy of Sciences. As revised, recommended values for vitamins A and C were lowered for both men and women, a guideline that critics said conflicted with the Academy's own recommendations that we should eat sufficient quantities of vitamins A and C to protect against cancer. At stake here: Should the RDAs be set at amounts that merely protect against nutritional deficiencies, or should they be set a bit higher, at amounts that might promote the best possible health?

Some in the nutrition field promote the value of vitamin and mineral supplements in doses far above the 1980 Recommended Dietary Allowances. Physicians and scientists usually contend that these megavitamins and megaminerals are unneeded. Some excesses are positively known to be harmful. Megavitamin and megamineral therapy is not part of the mainstream of medical and scientific thought. The Nobel-prizewinning scientist Linus Pauling took a fringe position when he argued for the benefits of vitamin C.

■ *Vitamin A*

Since ancient times, physicians have known that foods high in vitamin A will cure night blindness. An Egyptian papyrus recommends treating this affliction—one of the first signs of vitamin-A deficiency—with ox liver or the livers of cocks.

The cause of vitamin-A deficiency was first identified by a Danish pediatrician, C. E. Bloch, who noted that between 1910 and 1920, many Danish children suffered from xerophthalmia (a type of eye disorder) and from impaired growth. Suddenly—with the blockade of Danish ports in 1917 by the German Navy—these symptoms

FOOD AND NUTRITION BOARD, NATIONAL ACADEMY OF SCIENCES-NATIONAL RESEARCH COUNCIL
RECOMMENDED DAILY DIETARY ALLOWANCES,[a] Revised 1980

Designed for the maintenance of good nutrition of practically all healthy people in the U.S.A.

Age (years)	Infants 0.0-0.5	0.5-1.0	Children 1-3	4-6	7-10	Males 11-14	15-18	19-22	23-50	51+	Females 11-14	15-18	19-22	23-50	51+	Preg-nant	Lact-ating
Weight (kg)	6	9	13	20	28	45	66	70	70	70	46	55	55	55	55		
(lb)	13	20	29	44	62	99	145	154	154	154	101	120	120	120	120		
Height (cm)	60	71	90	112	132	157	176	177	178	178	157	163	163	163	163		
(in)	24	28	35	44	52	62	69	70	70	70	62	64	64	64	64		
Protein (g)	kg × 2.2	kg × 2.0	23	30	34	45	56	56	56	56	46	46	44	44	44	+30	+20
FAT-SOLUBLE VITAMINS																	
Vitamin A (µg RE)[b]	420	400	400	500	700	1000	1000	1000	1000	1000	800	800	800	800	800	+200	+400
Vitamin D (µg)[c]	10	10	10	10	10	10	10	7.5	5	5	10	10	7.5	5	5	+5	+5
Vitamin E (mg α-TE)[d]	3	4	5	6	7	8	10	10	10	10	8	8	8	8	8	+2	+3
WATER-SOLUBLE VITAMINS																	
Vitamin C (mg)	35	35	45	45	45	50	60	60	60	60	50	60	60	60	60	+20	+40
Thiamin (mg)	0.3	0.5	0.7	0.9	1.2	1.4	1.4	1.5	1.4	1.2	1.1	1.1	1.1	1.0	1.0	+0.4	+0.5
Riboflavin (mg)	0.4	0.6	0.8	1.0	1.4	1.6	1.7	1.7	1.6	1.4	1.3	1.3	1.3	1.2	1.2	+0.3	+0.5
Niacin (mg NE)[e]	6	8	9	11	16	18	18	19	18	16	15	14	14	13	13	+2	+5
Vitamin B-6 (mg)	0.3	0.6	0.9	1.3	1.6	1.8	2.0	2.2	2.2	2.2	1.8	2.0	2.0	2.0	2.0	+0.6	+0.5
Folacin[f] (µg)	30	45	100	200	300	400	400	400	400	400	400	400	400	400	400	+400	+100
Vitamin B-12 (µg)	0.5[g]	1.5	2.0	2.5	3.0	3.0	3.0	3.0	3.0	3.0	3.0	3.0	3.0	3.0	3.0	+1.0	+1.0
MINERALS																	
Calcium (mg)	360	540	800	800	800	1200	1200	800	800	800	1200	1200	800	800	800	+400	+400
Phosphorus (mg)	240	360	800	800	800	1200	1200	800	800	800	1200	1200	800	800	800	+400	+400
Magnesium (mg)	50	70	150	200	250	350	400	350	350	350	300	300	300	300	300	+150	+150
Iron (mg)	10	15	15	10	10	18	18	10	10	10	18	18	18	18	10	h	h
Zinc (mg)	3	5	10	10	10	15	15	15	15	15	15	15	15	15	15	+5	+10
Iodine (µg)	40	50	70	90	120	150	150	150	150	150	150	150	150	150	150	+25	+50

[a] The allowances are intended to provide for individual variations among most normal persons as they live in the United States under usual environmental stresses. Diets should be based on a variety of common foods in order to provide other nutrients for which human requirements have been less well defined. See text for detailed discussion of allowances and of nutrients not tabulated.

[b] Retinol equivalents. 1 retinol equivalent = 1 µg retinol or 6 µg β carotene. See text for calculation of vitamin A activity of diets as retinol equivalents.

[c] As cholecalciferol. 10 µg cholecalciferol = 400 IU of vitamin D.

[d] α-tocopherol equivalents. 1 mg d-α tocopherol = 1 α-TE. See text for variation in allowances and calculation of vitamin E activity of the diet as α-tocopherol equivalents.

[e] 1 NE (niacin equivalent) is equal to 1 mg of niacin or 60 mg of dietary tryptophan.

[f] The folacin allowances refer to dietary sources as determined by *Lactobacillus casei* assay after treatment with enzymes (conjugases) to make polyglutamyl forms of the vitamin available to the test organism.

[g] The recommended dietary allowance for vitamin B-12 in infants is based on average concentration of the vitamin in human milk. The allowances after weaning are based on energy intake (as recommended by the American Academy of Pediatrics) and consideration of other factors, such as intestinal absorption; see text.

[h] The increased requirement during pregnancy cannot be met by the iron content of habitual American diets nor by the existing iron stores of many women; therefore the use of 30–60 mg of supplemental iron is recommended. Iron needs during lactation are not substantially different from those of nonpregnant women, but continued supplementation of the mother for 2–3 months after parturition is advisable in order to replenish stores depleted by pregnancy.

cleared. The explanation: The German blockade made butter—formerly a prized export—readily available to the Danes. Butter, which contains substantial amounts of vitamin A, was consumed in preference to lard or margarine, which contain very little of the vitamin.

Deficiencies of vitamin A can also result in skin problems and breakdown of the linings of the respiratory tract, intestinal tract, and genitourinary tract.

Food sources for vitamin A include foods containing beta-carotene:

- carrots
- peaches
- apricots
- potatoes
- yellow vegetables and fruits
- dark green, leafy vegetables

The body converts beta-carotene to vitamin A within the body. This conversion, however, is relatively inefficient: Only one third to one fourth

ESTIMATED SAFE AND ADEQUATE DAILY DIETARY INTAKES OF SELECTED VITAMINS AND MINERALS[a]

VITAMINS Age (years)	Infants		Children and Adolescents				Adults
	0–0.5	0.5–1	1–3	4–6	7–10	11+	
VITAMINS							
Vitamin K (μg)	12	10–20	15–30	20–40	30–60	50–100	70–140
Biotin (μg)	35	50	65	85	120	100–200	100–200
Pantothenic Acid (mg)	2	3	3	3–4	4–5	4–7	4–7
TRACE ELEMENTS[b]							
Copper (mg)	0.5–0.7	0.7–1.0	1.0–1.5	1.5–2.0	2.0–2.5	2.0–3.0	2.0–3.0
Manganese (mg)	0.5–0.7	0.7–1.0	1.0–1.5	1.5–2.0	2.0–3.0	2.5–5.0	2.5–5.0
Fluoride (mg)	0.1–0.5	0.2–1.0	0.5–1.5	1.0–2.5	1.5–2.5	1.5–2.5	1.5–4.0
Chromium (mg)	0.01–0.04	0.02–0.06	0.02–0.08	0.03–0.12	0.05–0.2	0.05–0.2	0.05–0.2
Selenium (mg)	0.01–0.04	0.02–0.06	0.02–0.08	0.03–0.12	0.05–0.2	0.05–0.2	0.05–0.2
Molybdenum (mg)	0.03–0.06	0.04–0.08	0.05–0.1	0.06–0.15	0.10–0.3	0.15–0.5	0.15–0.5
ELECTROLYTES							
Sodium (mg)	115–350	250–750	325–975	450–1350	600–1800	900–2700	1100–3300
Potassium (mg)	350–925	425–1275	550–1650	775–2325	1000–3000	1525–4575	1875–5625
Chloride (mg)	275–700	400–1200	500–1500	700–2100	925–2775	1400–4200	1700–5100

[a] Because there is less information on which to base allowances, these figures are not given in the main table of RDA and are provided here in the form of ranges of recommended intakes.

[b] Since the toxic levels for many trace elements may be only several times usual intakes, the upper levels for the trace elements given in this table should not be habitually exceeded.

of ingested beta-carotene is converted to vitamin A.

Preformed vitamin A is found in:
- organ meats (kidney and liver)
- eggyolk
- butter
- cream

Too much vitamin A is dangerous. The toxic effects of high doses of vitamin A were responsible for the violent reactions afflicting Arctic explorers who had eaten polar bear liver, which contains huge amounts of vitamin A. Drowsiness, irritability, headache, vomiting, mental disturbances, redness of the hands and feet, as well as peeling skin occurred shortly after they had consumed the liver. For infants under 6 months of age, 18,500 to 25,000 IU can be toxic. Similarly, adults ingesting quantities greater than 25,000 to 100,000 IU per day can likewise suffer toxic effects. The list of symptoms caused by excess vitamin A is long: loss of appetite, weight loss, loss of hearing, anemia, blurred vision, drying of the skin, itching, arm and leg pain, abnormal bone growth, bleeding tendency, irritability, and birth defects. Similarly, excessive ingestion of foods high in carotene—such as green vegetables, carrot juice, tomatoes, citrus fruit, or yellow vegetables—can result in yellowish-orange skin, particularly on the palms, feet, forehead, nose, and groin.

The key, then, is moderation. Too much of vitamin A can be toxic; too little can be equally dangerous. Because all fat-soluble vitamins such as vitamin A accumulate when taken in excess, a vitamin-A intake consistent with the RDA is probably sufficient. This amount is readily obtained from a balanced diet including green and yellow vegetables, dairy products, fruit, and occasional organ meats.

■ Vitamin D

Vitamin D is often called the "sunshine vitamin." Rickets, the disease caused by vitamin D deficiency, results in bone deformity (bowed legs) in children and in osteomalacia (softening of the bones) in adults.

When sunlight is present, vitamin D is produced in our bodies from dehydrocholesterol found under our skin. This vitamin is essential for normal bone growth, development, repair, and maintenance. Along with another hormone (parathyroid hormone), it regulates phosphorus and calcium metabolism and absorption.

Dietary sources of vitamin D include:

- eggs
- milk
- butter
- cod liver oil

Most commercial milk is fortified with vitamin D. If a child whose diet is low in vitamin D does not get enough sun, rickets will develop, and unless the vitamin D deficiency is corrected early, the child will become deformed. Black-skinned people are more susceptible to vitamin D deficiency because sunlight cannot easily penetrate skin pigment.

However, excessive amounts of vitamin D, from vitamin-D supplements, may have toxic effects: in children, growth retardation, weight loss, failure to thrive, and nausea; in adults, kidney malfunction, vomiting, nausea, and high blood pressure. Toxic effects can readily occur with vitamin pill supplements. The toxic dose is unclear, but except when indicated, as in deficiency, prolonged intake above 2,000 IU is probably dangerous.

■ Vitamin E, Tocopherol

Vitamin E is an essential nutrient. It is an *antioxidant*, a chemical that protects against destructive attack by oxygen on cell membranes. Humans really need minimal amounts of vitamin E, however, because it is excreted and used up slowly, because it can be regenerated from vitamin C, and because the human body has other antioxidants available to it.

Vitamin E is present in all foods. Good sources include:

- the vegetable oils (especially good sources)
- olives
- chocolate
- cabbage
- asparagus
- wheat germ
- spinach

Vitamin E deficiency has been reported only in premature infants who cannot get vitamin E from their mothers and in patients who are unable to absorb fats.

In animals, however, vitamin E deficiency has been shown to lead to loss of fertility, leading to claims of vitamin promoters that vitamin E improves sexual performance. This claim is totally fallacious, since the vitamin-E-deficient animals readily engaged in sexual activity. Vitamin E is also said to ease painful calf muscles, prevent heart disease, and increase vigor—all unproved.

Theoretically, the antioxidant qualities of the vitamin might retard aging and prevent cancer. Although there is some suggestive evidence, these properties remain unconfirmed.

■ Vitamin K

Vitamin K is essential to the body's blood clotting mechanism, which prevents us from bleeding to death from cuts and wounds or from internal bleeding.

In humans, vitamin-K deficiency is rare, because the vitamin is found widely in plant and animal foods and because intestinal bacteria usually make over half of what we need. However, vitamin K supplementation may be indicated in certain instances:

- in newborn infants, in whom minimal vitamin K is received from the mother and in whom the gut is almost sterile, containing few bacteria
- in adults consuming diets low in vitamin K who are also receiving antibiotics (which destroy intestinal bacteria)
- in individuals with impaired flow of bile into the intestine resulting in malabsorption of both fat and vitamin K
- diseases such as tropical sprue, which are associated with impaired absorption from the intestine

Vitamin K rarely is recommended in megadoses, and large doses of vitamin K can be toxic. Toxic reactions have been reported following its medical use.

■ Vitamin C

A lack of vitamin C, or ascorbic acid, was responsible for the scurvy noted in sailors on long voyages. Vitamin C deficiency may result in appetite loss, fatigue, irritability, joint pain, and skin lesions, progressing ultimately to bleeding gums and internal hemorrhage.

The foods from which we obtain vitamin C include citrus fruits—although these are not the best sources. Black currants, sweet peppers, broccoli, turnip greens, kale, and brussels sprouts are even higher in the vitamin than are citrus fruits. Cabbage, spinach, watercress, and cauliflower are also high. Tomatoes are the main source of vitamin C in the American diet.

Some evidence suggests that foods high in vitamin C may protect against cancer, and the National Cancer Institute as well as the American Cancer Society recommend a varied diet including sufficient amounts of foods containing vitamin C.

Advocates of megavitamin therapy maintain doses much higher than the RDA are needed for optimum health. In *Vitamin C, the Common Cold,* *and the Flu,** Linus Pauling suggests a minimum intake of 2,300 mg. High doses of vitamin C are commonly suggested in the prevention and treatment of colds. Despite a good deal of study—Pauling's prestige lent credence to the theory—the positive effects of megadoses of vitamin C still remain unproved.

Vitamin C is viewed, overall, as relatively nontoxic. To a large extent, this is correct, because it is a water-soluble vitamin that is largely excreted rather than stored. Megadoses of vitamin C, however, can cause rebound scurvy when intake is stopped. Reported side effects include gastritis as well as formation of kidney stones. Vitamin C also may interfere with the action of anticoagulant drugs.

Healthy individuals probably need no more than 200 mg., which can be obtained readily from a varied diet containing sufficient amounts of fruits and vegetables. And although the risks of megadose vitamin C therapy are probably small for most individuals, the benefits are probably equally elusive.

■ *Vitamin B₁, Thiamine*

Severe deficiency of vitamin B_1 results in beri-beri (literally, "I can't, I can't"), a disorder characterized by extreme weakness. Beri-beri was at one time common among Asians who ate large quantities of polished rice. Thiamine is contained in rice husks, and this nutrient was lost in the polishing process.

Rich natural sources of thiamine include the following:

- yeast
- rice husks
- wheat germ
- soybean flour
- liver
- pork

Lesser amounts are found in lean meats, poultry, eggs, seafoods, as well as in oats, barley, brown rice, nuts, potatoes, asparagus, beans, broccoli, peas, corn, cauliflower, and other fruits and vegetables. Many flours and cereals are now enriched to replace thiamine lost in processing. Thiamine deficiency is rare in the United States, except among alcoholics, where it results in Wernicke-Korsakoff syndrome, a complex of symptoms that includes memory loss, mental deterioration, abnormal perception, and loss of eye control, leading ultimately to heart failure. Thiamine deficiency also may occur in pregnant women who

experience excessive vomiting, as well as in persons on long-term kidney dialysis. The 1980 Recommended Dietary Allowance for thiamine can be obtained readily from the foods in our diet.

Oral Vitamin B_1 is essentially nontoxic, probably because it is not absorbed into the blood in quantities substantially in excess of 5 mg. Thus, it is probably worthless to consume additional vitamin B_1 supplements.

■ *Vitamin B₂, Riboflavin*

Riboflavin likewise is essential for human functioning. It is required for maintaining the skin, mucous membranes, corneal tissue, and nervous-system structures. Deficiency of riboflavin may result in inflammation of the eyes, lips, mouth, and tongue as well as scaling of the skin. In the United States, riboflavin deficiency is rare, except in alcoholics.

Foods such as milk and milk products, the organ meats, and yeast are rich in riboflavin. Moderate amounts are found also in fruits, grains, vegetables, lean meats, and poultry. Milk and enriched breads and cereals supply substantial amounts of riboflavin in the diet. Amounts above the RDA are excreted in the urine, giving it a bright yellow color.

This vitamin is considered nontoxic.

■ *Vitamin B₃, Niacin*

Sufficient amounts of niacin are necessary to prevent pellagra, a deficiency disease characterized in the early stage by malaise, loss of appetite, and indigestion, and progressing to the "three Ds": dermatitis, diarrhea, and dementia. Ultimately, psychosis, stupor, coma, and death can result. Pellagra was common in the southern states during the early 1900s, due to the high consumption of corn, which contains little tryptophan (converted within the body to niacin). Today, however, pellagra is uncommon except in alcoholics and in persons with debilitating diseases like diabetes, cancer, and cirrhosis.

Niacin is a term for both nicotinic acid, which is found in plant foods, and niacinamide, which is associated with animal foods. Within the body, niacin can be formed from the essential amino acid tryptophan if vitamins B_1, B_2, and B_6 are present. Tryptophan is an important dietary source of niacin, which explains why milk (which

* Linus Pauling, *Vitamin C, the Common Cold, and the Flu* (New York: W. H. Freeman, 1976).

is rich in amino acids) can alleviate deficiency in infants.

Meat and milk products are good sources of tryptophan. Ready-made niacin (nicotinic acid and niacinamide) is high in organ meats, beef, pork, chicken, turkey, halibut, and tuna. Moderate amounts are found in grains, fruits, and vegetables. Sufficient amounts of niacin can be obtained from a varied, balanced diet.

One medical use for nicotinic acid is in the reduction of high blood cholesterol levels. At present, however, nicotinic acid is indicated only for patients with very high blood cholesterol levels that are considered to merit drug therapy. Dietary therapy should be the first choice for combatting high blood cholesterol levels.

Although water-soluble vitamins like niacin are commonly believed to be nontoxic, large quantities of niacin are not innocuous. Megadose niacin may result in headache, itching, and flushing of the face, neck, and chest.

■ *Vitamin B_6, Pyridoxine*

Vitamin B_6 is widely available in nature, and deficiencies are relatively uncommon. Factors that can increase our requirements for the vitamin include: alcoholism, hypothyroidism, a high-protein diet, inadequate intake, malabsorption, stress due to illness, and use of oral contraceptives and medications used to treat arthritis and tuberculosis.

Vitamin B_6 is obtained readily from these foods in our diet:

- meats
- liver
- kidney
- egg yolk
- corn
- whole-grain cereals

Vegetables are good sources also, even though the actual content is often relatively low, because the vitamin is stable during processing. Medical uses of vitamin B_6 include treatment of morning sickness in pregnant women. It has also been used in low doses to reduce the formation of dental caries and kidney stones, and in topical form for dermatitis. There is no proof, however, that it helps arthritis.

Although relatively nontoxic (it is a water-soluble vitamin), extremely high doses of vitamin B_6 may be dangerous. Excessively high doses of vitamin B_6 may cause lethargy, insomnia, brainwave changes, and neurologic symptoms.

■ *Vitamin B_{12}, Cobalamin*

Vitamin B_{12} is essential to a number of body functions: synthesizing genetic material, maintaining nerve tissues, acting to help synthesize an important component of hemoglobin and red blood cells, and, along with folic acid, helping to produce red and white blood cells. Lack of vitamin B_{12} prevents red-cell development and leads to one type of anemia. Deficiency also results in nerve damage, enlargement of the spleen, and ultimately mental disturbances.

Vitamin B_{12} is found primarily in animal foods:
- liver
- kidney
- eggs
- crabs
- clams
- oysters
- salmon
- herring

Lower levels are found in fish, lean meats, cheese, and milk. Minimal vitamin B_{12} is found in fruits, vegetables, and grains. For this reason, strict vegetarians who consume no eggs, milk, or cheese may need supplements. Most Americans, however, get more than ten to twenty times the recommended dietary allowance of vitamin B_{12}.

Vitamin B_{12} absorption requires the presence of *intrinsic factor,* a protein secreted with gastric juice. Some persons are unable to secrete this protein and suffer pernicious anemia as a consequence. These individuals may require B_{12} shots. However, the use of B_{12} shots to treat other problems such as iron-deficiency anemia, fatigue, or emotional problems is useless except as a placebo. Although B_{12} is virtually nontoxic, a few adverse reactions have been reported.

■ *Folic Acid*

Folic acid is essential for production of white and red blood cells, for development of the fetus, for maintaining the nervous system, for maintaining the integrity of the intestinal tract, and in manufacturing the genetic material.
Rich sources of folic acid include:
- liver
- wheat bran
- asparagus
- beans

Moderate amounts are found in grains and in certain vegetables such as corn, beets, turnip greens, and broccoli. Lack of folic acid produces a type of anemia, and the vitamin is clinically useful in treating this deficiency as well as tropical sprue, a disease characterized by weakness, intestinal disorders, and various types of anemia.

Folic acid should not be used to self-treat

fatigue, since self-medication may delay appropriate treatment. Although direct toxicity is uncommon, the Food and Drug Administration requires a doctor's prescription for doses higher than 0.8 mg. Epileptics should not take high doses of folic acid because it can interfere with the protective effects of the commonly used anticonvulsant, Dilantin (diphenylhydantoin).

■ Biotin and Pantothenic Acid

Biotin is essential to the body, but deficiencies are rare, except in individuals who ingest excessive amounts of *raw* egg whites, which contain avidin, a substance that prevents biotin absorption. Loss of appetite, nausea, vomiting, pallor, depression, fatigue, muscle pain are symptoms of deficiency. Most Americans take in up to 100 to 300 micrograms of biotin a day, a more-than-adequate intake. Biotin toxicity has not been reported. Good food sources of biotin include:

- organ meats
- eggyolk
- milk
- yeast
- beans
- nuts
- chocolate
- cauliflower

The term *pantothenic acid* is derived from a Greek word meaning "everywhere," because the substance is so common in foods. Deficiencies are rare because of the ubiquity of the vitamin, but they can occur in combination with other B-vitamin deficiencies in alcoholism, malnutrition, and cancer. Deficiency symptoms are vomiting, fatigue, difficulty sleeping, severe abdominal cramps, tingling in hands and feet. No human toxicity has been reported, but pantothenic acid supplements have no real value. It is unlikely that individuals eating a balanced diet and a variety of foods will develop a deficiency of this nutrient.

Minerals

Minerals, like vitamins, also are required by the body. They are nonliving substances (inorganic) and are often found in rocks and in the soil. Minerals are extracted from the soil by plants: We consume these minerals in the vegetables we eat and also in the meat from animals that have eaten plants.

Some minerals are needed in fairly substantial amounts. These include calcium, phosphorus, magnesium, sodium, potassium, and chloride.

Calcium, which is found in all tissues, helps regulate the heartbeat and keeps muscles and nerves functioning normally. Calcium helps the blood to clot properly and is important for the development of hard bones and strong teeth. Recently calcium has received much attention for its role in the prevention of *osteoporosis*. Especially in women after menopause, a generous intake of calcium (1,200 to 1,400 mg. daily, but no more) helps to maintain bone integrity. The role of calcium is discussed further in the section on aging.

Good food sources of calcium include the following:

- milk (whole milk, skim or low-fat milk, buttermilk evaporated milk)
- cheese
- ice cream
- yogurt

Massive doses (over 2,000 mg.) of calcium, however, have the potential for doing harm. Calcium supplements prepared from bone meal and from dolomite (a type of limestone) can contain significant amounts of lead and may be toxic. Note the source of the calcium in any supplement you buy; oyster shell, for example, is considered a safe, digestible source.

Also important is *phosphorus*, which along with calcium helps maintain bone integrity. Because phosphorus is widely present in foods, however, dietary deficiency is uncommon. High-phosphate diets (where too much meat is consumed) can promote calcium deficiency, creating problems for women past menopause.

Magnesium is essential for nerve-impulse transmission, for utilization of potassium and calcium, and in important body reactions. Although severe dietary deficiency is uncommon, some nutritionists maintain that our intake of magnesium is inadequate, and a recent survey indicated that most Americans consume less than the recommended allowance of magnesium.

Foods high in magnesium include:

- whole grains
- nuts
- green, leafy vegetables

Magnesium deficiency is seen most often in chronic alcoholics and in individuals with intestinal malabsorption. Early signs include nausea, malaise, and appetite loss. Ultimately, neurologic disturbances, mental problems, tremors, convulsions, and death may result. Some reports suggest a role for magnesium deficiency in heart disease (from soft water) and in premenstrual tension. Although there is minimal evidence that large magnesium intakes are harmful in normal individuals, those with poor kidney function, particularly the elderly, may be at risk.

Sodium is discussed in relation to high blood pressure, in the chapter *The Healthy Heart.*

Potassium is used in the body as a regulator of the amount of water in cells, as a buffer for body fluids, as a catalyst in the release of energy from carbohydrates, proteins, and fats; it aids in the transmission of nerve impulses and is important for the proper working of muscles—including the heart. Potassium deficiency occurs only when there is excessive fluid loss resulting from diarrhea, diabetes, laxative use, or diuretic use. Both low and high blood potassium levels can be dangerous, leading to cardiovascular imbalances and potentially fatal arrhythmias (abnormal rhythms). Potassium supplements should be given only under a doctor's supervision: Administration of a potassium supplement along with a diuretic would be a typical instance.

Chloride is important in maintaining fluid balance, in the digestion of foods, and in regulating the function of important body chemicals. Deficiency of chloride is uncommon, however, except in the presence of diarrhea, vomiting, or excessive perspiration.

Sulfur occurs in most of the cells of our body, particularly in two amino acids, methionine and cystine. It performs important body functions, but we have minimal knowledge as yet of its deficiency symptoms and of how much we require.

Iron is a key component of hemoglobin, a critical blood protein. It is found also in a number of other proteins that are important for body functioning. We lose iron through waste excretion, hair growth, nail growth, and, in women, menstruation. The typical American diet gives us 10 to 20 mg. of iron daily, but only about 2 to 10 percent of that is absorbed. Intake must be high of foods rich in this mineral, such as:

- liver (a particularly good source)
- green, leafy vegetables
- potatoes
- raisins
- oysters
- clams
- cocoa

Iron deficiency can result in anemia; even at low levels of deficiency, fatigue and weakness can result. There is some evidence that iron deficiency can adversely affect the learning capacities of children. Iron supplements can be used to treat deficiency, but individuals should not self-treat fatigue, weakness, or anemia without a doctor's advice. If you think you may be suffering from iron deficiency, speak to your physician. He or she can correctly identify the reason for the symptoms, which may arise from a variety of causes.

Iron toxicity can occur accidentally, as in children who ingest iron supplements and adults who take too many supplements. As few as 10 iron tablets can cause signs of poisoning in a child.

Other minerals are found only in trace amounts. They include iodine, zinc, and selenium. *Selenium* deficiency has been implicated in the pathogenesis of cancer. Animal studies suggest that selenium may decrease the frequency of chemically induced cancer. Similarly, individuals living in areas where selenium levels are high are less likely to develop cancer. However, no major health organizations have recommended increasing the daily intake of selenium as yet. In the American diet, typical sources include:

- seafood
- meat
- cereals
- grains

There is no Recommended Dietary Allowance for selenium, but a recommended "safe and adequate intake" (a less strong recommendation by the same organization that sets the RDAs) has been established. Most Americans get about 50 to 150 micrograms a day. There is no evidence on the toxicity of moderate selenium supplements (a few hundred micrograms). On the other hand, there is no evidence for beneficial effects of selenium supplements in humans. Megadoses do have the potential for toxicity, and toxic effects have been reported in animals getting too much selenium in their feed. In short: The verdict is not yet in on selenium.

Zinc is an essential part of enzyme systems controlling major body functions. Sources include:

- meat
- eggs
- liver
- seafood (particularly oysters)

In the early 1960s, zinc deficiency was linked to stunted growth in teenage farm laborers in Egypt. Deficiency of zinc may cause low sperm count, poor appetite, impaired production of white blood cells, dermatitis, diarrhea, loss of hair, and poor wound healing. It has been reported to cause a loss of taste and smell. Until the 1970s, zinc deficiencies were believed to be rare, but today they are believed to occur particularly often in children who eat minimal amounts of meat and dairy products and also in vegetarians.

Analyses of hair samples—a popular but ineffective test for zinc deficiency—do not tell whether an individual is zinc-deficient. An appropriate evaluation tests blood, red cells, and (in men) semen. Zinc supplements may be useful in individuals suffering from certain types of taste and smell alterations, sickle cell anemia, and certain types of growth impairment. Some physicians prescribe zinc for wound healing as well. Its effects on sexual potency and fertility are unproven, unless zinc deficiency has brought on the impotence or infertility.

Surveys have indicated that many Americans get less than the Recommended Dietary Allowance of 15 mg., thus it seems proper to encourage the consumption of zinc-rich foods. However, excessive amounts of zinc, particularly in the form of megadose supplements, are not yet indicated and have the potential for harm. Huge doses result in acute toxicity, and even lower doses may have adverse effects on blood lipoproteins.

Iodine is important for proper thyroid function. A deficiency in the hormones secreted by the thyroid gland leads to goiter, an enlargement of the thyroid. Iodine is now added to table salt, however, and deficiency is uncommon today. Although immediate iodine toxicity is uncommon, steady ingestion of high levels can result in hypothyroidism and goiter. (Both deficiency and excess may cause goiter.) Kelp (dried seaweed) has been promoted as an aid to dieting, but high doses of kelp may induce goiter, which has been reported in Japanese who ingest large quantities of seaweed. Iodine may be useful in treating thyroid disturbances, but only under a doctor's supervision.

Fluorine is essential for strong, decay-resistant teeth. The water supplies of many communities are naturally high in fluoride, and many other communities add it to their drinking water. Although fluorine is toxic in large doses, there is no evidence of any adverse effects at the levels present in fluoridated water systems.

The need for *chromium* in humans has only recently become widely recognized. It is important for maintaining normal metabolism of glucose (blood sugar). Food sources include:

- meats
- cheeses
- whole grains
- eggs
- fruits
- brewer's yeast

The incidence of chromium deficiency in humans is unknown, but may be associated with blood sugar abnormalities in humans. However, high levels of chromium can be toxic. Risks include those from oversupplementation and industrial exposure.

Balance and moderation are the goals of the wellness diet. Consumption of a variety of foods will provide sufficient quantities of vitamins and min-erals for the average individual. Exceptions may include calcium supplements for women past menopause, iron supplements for menstruating women who are deficient, and zinc supplements for vegetarians. Multivitamin (as opposed to megavitamin) supplements are probably not harmful—these contain approximately the Recommended Dietary Allowances of most nutrients—but are probably unnecessary.

The key argument against the use of vitamin and mineral supplements is actually the lack of knowledge of what the vitamins and minerals in our foods really do. For instance, although we know that individuals who consume substantial quantities of foods high in vitamins A and C have a reduced incidence of cancer, we do not know whether the vitamins A and C are responsible or whether some as yet unidentified substances may be responsible for the anticancer properties.

It is for this reason that most medical and scientific experts recommend consuming a *variety of foods* containing enough of the vitamins and minerals we need. And it is here, perhaps, that vitamin and mineral supplements may be the most problematical: The individual may be less apt to consume a varied, balanced, and nutritious diet, reasoning that the vitamin and mineral supplements "make everything OK."

The Nutritional Folklore

Nutritional folklore—the odd assortment of old wives' tales and curious new theories—can neither be accepted without question nor totally dismissed.

■ Herbal Remedies

While advocates preach the benefits of herbs and herbal teas, many physicians dismiss the positive effects of herbal remedies. Although many substances currently used as drugs are derived from herbs and plants, some herbs are potent substances and have potentially toxic and dangerous effects. For example: Ginseng can cause vaginal bleeding, resulting from an estrogen-like effect on the vaginal lining; excessive ingestion of licorice may result in dangerously low serum potassium; sassafras tea contains safrole, a potent carcinogen.

But we cannot entirely dismiss folk remedies. Some studies suggest that garlic may lower blood cholesterol; animal experiments indicate that hot pepper may reduce blood cholesterol; aloe vera may aid in the healing of burns (although this finding is open to question, as the study was uncontrolled and the aloe vera was administered along with aspirin).

Herbal remedies are neither good nor bad, effective nor ineffective, just because they are derived from "natural" sources. They need to be evaluated on the same basis as any other drug—in terms of their benefits as well as their risks.

■ Hair Analysis

A recent addition to the nutritional folklore has been hair analysis. This pseudoscientific technique is poorly regarded in the medical community. Although offered by commercial laboratories to health food stores, beauty shops, nutritionists, and until recently to the general public, the evidence suggests that computerized hair analysis is worthless and—what is more dangerous—likely to be incorrect.

Hair analysis is based on the hypothesis that mineral deficiencies can be determined by assaying the quantities of the mineral in the hair. Although the hypothesis seems logical, often the state of health of the body may be unrelated to the state of one's hair. For instance, hair mineral content may be affected by shampoos and hair dyes used by the individual, and, equally as important, it is unknown to what extent the presence of minerals in the hair reflects the concentration of minerals in the body.

An article appearing in the August 1985 *Journal of the American Medical Association* proves the point. Stephen Barrett, M.D., of Allentown, Pennsylvania, obtained thirteen hair samples from each of two healthy young women. One sample from each woman was sent to thirteen labs, and three weeks later, again twenty-six samples (thirteen from each of the two women) were sent to the labs. The result: fifty-two different reports, each with different findings.

The medical and scientific communities regard hair analysis as unscientific, wasteful, and potentially harmful. The Federal Trade Commission barred one laboratory from advertising to the public, but hair analysis can still be used by licensed as well as unlicensed practitioners.

■ Brain and Food

Can what you eat affect the way you act? It's likely that the answer is yes. The "how," though, is much more mysterious.

From ancient times, foods have been used to induce sleep, cure hangovers, protect against the "evil eye," and enhance libido. The connection between food and behavior has been drawing the interest of behavioral scientists, nutritionists, endocrinologists, pharmacologists, and other scientists, who have been using scientific methodology in their investigations.

Over fifteen years ago, scientists Wurtman and Fernstrom postulated that dietary proteins and carbohydrates influence levels of neurotransmitters, primarily serotonin, in the brain. Evidence also indicates that foods that influence the level of tryptophan (an amino acid) affect how "sleepy" we are. Paradoxically, protein-rich foods lower brain tryptophan, making us sleepier, while carbohydrates raise brain tryptophan, making us less sleepy.

Much of this evidence is essentially preliminary, however, and the scientists involved caution that the results are interesting but not conclusive. Because of the many other factors that may influence behavior, isolating the role of diet is extremely difficult. It's therefore premature to base our dietary choices on these essentially preliminary findings. It's also premature to base any social choices (for example, diets for prison inmates) on such reports. A lot more needs to be done before any firm evidence comes in as to how our meals affect our minds.

■ "Natural Foods"

"All natural" is typical ad copy these days. So-called natural foods are claimed to be "better." Is this really the case?

The term *natural*, applied to food, has no legal definition. When applied to produce, it usually means that the fruits or vegetables being sold are fertilized with natural fertilizers like manure and have not been sprayed with pesticides. However, although certain pesticides have been shown to be harmful, there is no guarantee that water runoff containing pesticides will not leave pesticide residues on the "natural" produce.

Antibiotic and hormone supplementation of animal feed has recently come under attack. The verdict is not yet in, but there is some evidence that antibiotic supplementation favors the development of resistant bacteria that cause harmful infections. Similarly, hormone supplementation may cause problems in susceptible individuals, particularly children. Children in Puerto Rico developed premature sexual characteristics, accounted for by their consumption of chickens whose feed had been supplemented with hormones.

When applied to prepared foods, "natural" is even more nebulous. It usually means that only natural additives like corn sweeteners or honey were used. However, although some additives may be harmful, others are in no way poisonous or carcinogenic and may provide needed protection against contamination.

Even more important, it is critical to recognize that "natural" substances may contain poisons or carcinogens (cancer-causing agents). Aflatoxin, produced by a mold that grows on nuts, grains, and seeds, is a classic example. In 1983, Bruce Ames, writing in the journal *Science*, listed some "natural" toxin-containing foods: the burned material, nitrosamine, produced in frying, cocoa, tea, chocolate, celery, okra, parsnips, mushrooms, rhubarb, potatoes, some herbs and herbal teas, oil of mustard, horseradish, black pepper, fava beans, and figs. As research accumulates, we may be able to minimize our exposure to these "natural" carcinogens.

Essentially, natural substances have to be evaluated in the same way as synthetic substances: for both their benefits and their risks. There is no intrinsic superiority of the "natural" over the "synthetic." Natural substances can have harmful effects; likewise, synthetic substances can be harmful as well. Natural vitamin supplements have not been demonstrated to be in any way preferable to synthetic vitamins. A chemical is a chemical, whether it is extracted from a natural source or whether it is synthesized.

■ Food Additives

Much of the concern over "artificial" substances came from reports on the risks associated with certain food additives. Unquestionably, some food additives have toxic or cancer-causing potential. But food additives also serve important health-related purposes.

Many additives are used to improve the nutritional value of foods: B vitamins in breads and cereals, vitamin C in fruit drinks, vitamin D in milk, iron in infant formulas, iodine in table salt. This type of additive has aided in the eradication of once-prevalent diseases like rickets, pellagra, cretinism, and scurvy.

Other food additives are used to improve flavor or appearance, to preserve freshness, and to help in food processing. Food additives have been regulated since 1960 by the Food and Drug Administration under a provision that makes it the responsibility of the manufacturer to prove an additive is safe. It states (the so-called Delaney clause) that any additive causing cancer in man or animals cannot be used. It was this provision that led to the controversial FDA proposal to ban saccharine.

At the time the law was passed, substances already in use were placed in the GRAS ("generally recognized as safe") category, but even GRAS substances could be removed from this list if new evidence suggested toxicity or cancer-causing potential. In addition, the FDA began a formal review of 450 GRAS substances. The review led to the banning of Red Dye No. 2, then the most widely used coloring agent, because it caused cancer in lab animals. Still under review are BHT and BHA, two of the most widely used preservatives. BHT came under fire because of animal studies suggesting it caused liver enlargement. The FDA has confirmed the safe status of six other additives: benzoic acid, methylparaben, propyl gallate, propylparaben, sodium benzoate, and stannous chloride. Additional additives continue to undergo review.

There is, however, some evidence for the cancer-causing potential of nitrites, which are used to preserve bacon, frankfurters, and other processed meats. Nitrites provide important protection against botulism and other infections, but there is significant evidence relating nitrites to the incidence of cancer. The American Cancer Society, for example, suggests that we limit our intake of nitrite-containing foods. (The National Cancer Institute has made no recommendations.) Meanwhile, the food industry continues to search for substitutes for the nitrites.

Some additives that are safe for most individuals can cause reactions in sensitive persons. Tartrazine, a yellow dye used in foods, beverages, drugs, and cosmetics, may cause hives, swelling, runny nose, and even asthma in sensitive individuals. Similarly, sodium sulfite, a preservative used to maintain the fresh-looking appearance of fruits and vegetables, can cause dangerous asthmatic attacks. And antibiotics used in animal feeds may cause reactions in sensitive persons.

Finally, mention must be made of the so-called Chinese-restaurant syndrome. It was first described as a syndrome consisting of headache and nausea occurring one to two hours after a Chinese meal. Many Chinese restaurants use substantial amounts of monosodium glutamate, or MSG, to enhance flavor, and it is believed that the syndrome is the consequence of eating foods cooked in this way. MSG is also an ingredient of some processed foods, soup cubes, and certain flavor enhancers.

■ *Food Allergy*

Some persons are extremely sensitive to certain foods. Peanuts, for instance, may evoke severe, even fatal reactions in some men and women. One woman died following consumption of chili thickened with peanut butter. In addition, as indicated above, some people are allergic to food additives such as tartrazine or sulfite.

Others suffer classic allergic symptoms: hives, rash, runny nose, and the like. These, for the most part, are readily identified as due to food. Milder reactions are more difficult to attribute to food allergies, however.

Particularly difficult to prove is the role of food allergy in essentially psychiatric or emotional problems. Some evidence does indicate a role for food allergy in the genesis of migraine, but other workers dispute this hypothesis. It has been suggested that food allergies are involved in the irritable bowel syndrome, a complex typified by abdominal pain associated with alternating diarrhea and constipation.

The "proof" that a reaction is allergic is obtained by performing a "double-blind food challenge." An example might be feeding a person who is said to be allergic to a given food both that food and a food that looks like it (a food capsule and a placebo might also be used). This is cumbersome and difficult to accomplish, however. More often used is an elimination diet (an essentially bland diet) followed by the addition, one by one, of foods suspected of causing the allergic reactions. Ideally, the subject should be unaware of the addition. Also commonly used are skin testing and a type of testing known as RAST (radioallergosorbent test).

Like the role of foods in controlling mood, the part played by food allergy in human illness and behavior continues to be "wide open" to question. It is clear that foods may cause adverse and even fatal reactions in certain individuals. Exactly what these reactions are and how many individuals they may affect still needs to be determined.

Dietary Guidelines for Adults

Good nutrition is based on variety and moderation. For healthy eating that helps prevent the major chronic diseases, the 1980 Dietary Guidelines for Americans (U.S. Department of Agriculture and U.S. Department of Health and Human Services) recommend:
• Eat a variety of foods.
• Maintain ideal weight.
• Avoid too much saturated fat and cholesterol.
• Eat foods with adequate starch and fiber.
• Avoid too much sugar.
• Avoid too much sodium.
• If you drink alcohol, do so in moderation.

The old concept of the four major food groups—(1) milk and milk products, (2) meats and equivalents, (3) fruits and vegetables, and (4) bread and cereals—had a certain validity. It ensured a variety of foods as well as the likelihood that individuals would receive the needed amounts of protein, vitamins, and minerals.

Some experts, however, indicate that this concept is to some extent outmoded. An equal amount of attention should be paid to other aspects of the diet—reducing the intake of saturated fats and cholesterol, for instance. Chocolate cake, a food from the bread group, is high in fat, while a baked potato without butter is relatively low in fat. Similarly, skim milk is lower in fat than whole milk, but both are members of the milk group. Still, paying attention to the four food groups will help to ensure that the individual gets sufficient amounts of important vitamins and nutrients.

The American Dietetic Association, in its booklet *Vote for Good Nutrition*, recommends choosing a variety of foods from the four food groups each day:
• *Fruits and vegetables:* 4 or more servings
• *Breads and cereals:* 4 or more servings
• *Milk and dairy products:* 2 or more servings
• *Protein foods (meat and meat substitutes):* 2 servings of about 3 ounces each

Fruits and vegetables. "Servings" vary, depending on the item. For instance, a serving of cooked spinach is equivalent to $\frac{1}{2}$ cup. One medium potato, one medium orange, one half grapefruit are each "one serving." One citrus fruit should be eaten each day, as should other fruits or vegetables high in vitamin C. Fruits and vegetables often are high in vitamins, low in calories, low in fat, and high in fiber. Foods from this group are good sources of vitamin C. Some fruits and vegetables—dark green vegetables, yellow- and orange-colored vegetables, and fruits such as apricots and mangoes—are high in vitamin A. Fruits and vegetables also supply significant amounts of iron. In addition, vegetables from the legume group (beans) are good sources of protein. Note that although many of these foods are not themselves high in calories, they often are consumed with high-calorie garnishes. Broccoli, for example, although low in calories, often is prepared with cheese sauce or butter.

Breads and cereals. One serving of the bread/cereal group is equivalent to one slice of bread; 1 ounce of dry cereal; $\frac{1}{2}$ to $\frac{3}{4}$ cup of cooked cereal; or $\frac{1}{2}$ to $\frac{3}{4}$ cup of macaroni, noodles, rice, or spaghetti. At least four servings from this group should be eaten each day. Foods from this group are good sources of iron, niacin, and vitamins B_1 and B_2. The protein in grains is incomplete; it needs to be combined with legumes (beans), milk, meat products, or other grains.

Meat and meat equivalents. One serving of the meat/meat-equivalent group could be 2–3 ounces of cooked lean meat or fish; $\frac{3}{4}$ can baked beans; 1 cup cooked dried beans, peas, or lentils; two eggs; 2 ounces cheddar cheese; $\frac{1}{2}$ cup cottage cheese; or 4 tablespoons peanut butter. Foods from the meat groups are good sources of vitamins B_1, B_2, and B_3 and of iron and protein. Iron content is highest in the muscle and organ meats; chicken and fish are lower. Muscle meats (steak, roast beef, lamb, veal, pork, for example) also are good sources of zinc and phosphorus. The protein content of meats and meat equivalents varies: 12 percent in pork; 30 percent in fish; 35 percent in dried beans and peas.

Milk and milk products. One serving is equivalent to: 1 cup fluid milk; 2 cups cottage cheese; 1 cup pudding; $1\frac{3}{4}$ cups ice cream; $1\frac{1}{2}$ ounces cheddar cheese; 1 cup yogurt. As lowfat or skim milk can be lower in vitamins A and D, fortified skim or lowfat milks are preferable. Cheeses often are used as substitutes for milk, but some of the vitamins are lost in the processing. Cottage cheese is not the best substitute for whole milk, since the calcium content of cottage cheese is often low. Hard cheeses also tend to have higher fat and calorie contents than whole milk. Ice cream is higher in fat and calories than whole milk. Yogurt, made by fermenting milk, is low in fat, but many commercial yogurts contain substantial amounts of added sugar and fruit.

Eating *only* the recommended number of serv-ings is termed a "foundation diet." Such a diet provides about 90 percent of the vitamin and mineral requirements and about three quarters of the calories most of us need. Normally, however, we eat more than what is included in the foundation diet. Not only do we consume additional servings of foods from the four groups, but we often include supplementary foods like spices, butter, margarine, fat, beverages, sweets, and snacks like cookies and potato chips. Supplementary foods like the fats are often high in calories and may contribute little to important vitamin and mineral needs.

Attention to the four food groups, and to avoiding intake of excessive amounts of saturated fats and cholesterol, will help us maintain a healthy diet. But, although the recommendation of variety applies, this doesn't mean that we have to choose our foods by rote in order to meet the requirements. Nutritional needs can be met by the foods of many cultures, prepared in many different and imaginative ways. Nor is it necessary to choose the most expensive foods in order to obtain a healthy, nutritious diet.

In fact, processed foods are often the most costly and the least desirable. Not only may vitamins be lost in processing, but processed foods often contain excessive amounts of fat and salt. Similarly, expensive cuts of meat are often heavily marbled and high in fat; less expensive cuts or less expensive substitutes like poultry as well as beans (along with a grain) may actually be preferable sources of protein.

To help you plan healthy, nutritious meals, read the food labeling on packaged foods. Although voluntary, the nutrition labeling, usually in terms of percentage of U.S. RDAs, will help you get nutrients in the balanced amounts you need. For some nutrients, the U.S. RDAs may be higher than the actual estimated needs of certain individuals. (U.S. RDAs combine the highest values from the many categories of Recommended Dietary Allowances for males and females of different ages.)

Calorie claims are regulated by the FDA, and the different terms used by manufacturers have different meanings. "Low calorie" means that the food provides 40 calories or fewer per serving (serving size usually is specified on the package or label).

"Reduced calorie" means that the food has at least one third fewer calories per serving (say, 30 instead of 45) than the food normally would have, and that it is not nutritionally inferior.

U.S. RDA

Vitamins, Minerals and Protein	Unit of Measurement	Infants	Adults and Children 4 or More Years of Age	Children Under 4 Years of Age	Pregnant or Lactating Women
Vitamin A	International Units	1,500	5,000	2,500	8,000
Vitamin D	"	400	400[a]	400	400
Vitamin E	"	5.0	30	10	30
Vitamin C	Milligrams	35	60	40	60
Folic Acid	"	0.1	0.4	0.2	0.8
Thiamine	"	0.5	1.5	0.7	1.7
Riboflavin	"	0.6	1.7	0.8	2.0
Niacin	"	8.0	20	9.0	20
Vitamin B_6	"	0.4	2.0	0.7	2.5
Vitamin B_{12}	Micrograms	2.0	6.0	3.0	8.0
Biotin	Milligrams	0.5	0.3	0.15	0.3
Pantothenic Acid	"	3.0	10	5.0	10
Calcium	Grams	0.6	1.0	0.8	1.3
Phosphorus	"	0.5	1.0	0.8	1.3
Iodine	Micrograms	45	150	70	150
Iron	Milligrams	15	18	10	18
Magnesium	"	70	400	200	450
Copper	"	0.6	2.0	1.0	2.0
Zinc	"	5.0	15	8.0	15
Protein	Grams	18[b]	45[b]	20[b]	

[a] Presence optional for adults and children 4 or more years of age in vitamin and mineral supplements.
[b] If protein efficiency ratio of protein is equal to or better than that of casein, U.S. RDA is 45 g. for adults, 18 g. for infants, and 20 g. for children under 4.
Source: U.S. Department of Health and Human Services, Public Health Service, Food and Drug Administration.

Foods can be labeled "for calorie-restricted diets" if the basis for the claim is stated on the label.

Terms such as "dietetic," "diet," and "artificially sweetened" must be reserved for low-calorie, reduced-calorie, or calorie-restricted-diet foods.

Other terms that are likewise regulated are "enriched," "fortified," "restored," and "nutrified." An enriched food has had vitamins and minerals added in compliance with legal regulations. For instance, vitamins B_1, B_2, B_3, and iron can be added to refined grains, which are then termed "enriched." Fortification most often is state-regulated, and includes the addition of vitamins A and D to milk and iodine to table salt. Restoration indicates addition of nutrients lost during processing.

Battling the Bulge

You are "obese"—according to the medical definition of the term—if you weigh more than 20 percent in excess of the "ideal" weight for someone of your sex, height, and build (small-boned to large-boned). Traditionally, the standards for "ideal" weights are those set forth in the Metropolitan Life Insurance Company tables.

Medical evidence continues to accumulate that obesity is undesirable. Obesity is associated with:
- Major risk factors for coronary heart disease, namely, high blood cholesterol and hypertension
- Certain cancers, including those of the breast, colon, and endometrium (lining of the uterus)
- Type II diabetes (maturity-onset)
- Osteoarthritis, especially of the knees and ankles
- Increased incidence of low back pain
- Menstrual disturbances
- Skin disorders
- Increased tendency to accidents

In the mid-1980s two conferences addressed the subject of obesity: A National Institutes of Health Consensus Conference in February 1985, and a conference in mid-1986 at the New York Academy of Sciences.

In the final statement of the NIH Consensus Conference, the panel stressed that weight reduction could be *lifesaving* for extremely obese individuals (twice their desirable weight). The panel also recommended weight reduction for individuals 20 percent or more above desirable weights on the Met Life tables (taking midpoint in the weight range for a medium-build person to figure percentage). Reduction is also desirable, the panel said, for patients with lesser degrees of obesity who have: diabetes or a family history of diabetes; hypertension; or very high blood cholesterol levels. Weight reduction may be helpful also in coronary artery disease and gout as well as in chronic obstructive pulmonary disease and arthritis.

Finally, problems linked to obesity are not limited to the physical. Obese persons often meet with discrimination and prejudice in their work and in social situations, and many respond with feelings of low self-esteem. Their overall mental health, however, is often no different from that of their thinner friends and colleagues.

One distinguished NIH panel member was quoted as saying, "Obesity is a killer. It is a killer as smoking is." Up to 34 million Americans are at least 20 percent or more above ideal weight, and for these persons, treatment and weight reduction are recommended.

■ What Is Overweight?

A number of areas continue to be controversial. What is ideal weight? What about the person who is 5 to 10 pounds overweight? What about the risks of excessive dieting?

News reports after the NIH panel meeting suggested that many people who are as little as 5 to 10 pounds over their desirable weight may be at increased health risk. However, the actual text of the Consensus statement suggests only that weight loss may be desirable for individuals (those less than 20 percent above their ideal weights) who have diabetes, hypertension, and high blood cholesterol. And panel speakers at a New York Academy of Sciences conference indicated that in the absence of other health problems, up to 80 percent of overweight individuals may worry needlessly; many of them may adopt nutritionally unsound diets to lose weight.

Even the experts cannot agree on what is "ideal." The 1959 Metropolitan Life Height and Weight Tables were revised in 1983. Desirable weights are now increased, particularly for people

---

TO MAKE AN APPROXIMATION OF YOUR FRAME SIZE . . .

Extend your arm and bend the forearm upward at a 90 degree angle. Keep fingers straight and turn the inside of your wrist toward your body. If you have a caliper, use it to measure the space between the two prominent bones on *either side* of your elbow. Without a caliper, place thumb and index finger of your other hand on these two bones. Measure the space between your fingers against a ruler or tape measure. Compare it with these tables that list elbow measurements for *medium-framed* men and women. Measurements lower than those listed indicate you have a small frame. Higher measurements indicate a large frame.

Height in 1" heels	Elbow Breadth
Men	
5'2"-5'3"	$2\frac{1}{2}''$-$2\frac{7}{8}''$
5'4"-5'7"	$2\frac{5}{8}''$-$2\frac{7}{8}''$
5'8"-5'11"	$2\frac{3}{4}''$-3"
6'0"-6'3"	$2\frac{3}{4}''$-$3\frac{1}{8}''$
6'4"	$2\frac{7}{8}''$-$3\frac{1}{4}''$
Women	
4'10"-4'11"	$2\frac{1}{4}''$-$2\frac{1}{2}''$
5'0"-5'3"	$2\frac{1}{4}''$-$2\frac{1}{2}''$
5'4"-5'7"	$2\frac{3}{8}''$-$2\frac{5}{8}''$
5'8"-5'11"	$2\frac{3}{8}''$-$2\frac{5}{8}''$
6'0"	$2\frac{1}{2}''$-$2\frac{3}{4}''$

---

of short stature. And, while some experts call for a return to the 1959 tables, others insist that the tables still overestimate the risk, particularly for other individuals. Another point of controversy is the factor of "frame size" in the Met Life tables. What, after all, is frame size? (Elbow width has been suggested as one method of determining frame size.)

The Gerontology Research Center in Baltimore analyzed insurance data (actually, the same data on which Metropolitan Life based its findings) and found that while younger adults should be lighter than the Met Life tables, older individuals could afford to be a few pounds heavier.

The Met Life tables assume that all overweight is alike. Yet evidence suggests that certain individuals are at greater risk from overweight than others. Genetic background is one factor in this. In addition, as indicated by the Baltimore Gerontology Center, younger people may be at more risk from excess weight than their elders. And of course, overweight is a greater risk in persons who are hypertensive or who have adult-onset diabetes.

One measure commonly used by scientists and

1983 METROPOLITAN HEIGHT AND WEIGHT TABLES

| MEN | | | | | WOMEN | | | |
| Height | | Small Frame | Medium Frame | Large Frame | Height | | Small Frame | Medium Frame | Large Frame |
Feet	Inches				Feet	Inches			
5	2	128-134	131-141	138-150	4	10	102-111	109-121	118-131
5	3	130-136	133-143	140-153	4	11	103-113	111-123	120-134
5	4	132-138	135-145	142-156	5	0	104-115	113-126	122-137
5	5	134-140	137-148	144-160	5	1	106-118	115-129	125-140
5	6	136-142	139-151	146-164	5	2	108-121	118-132	128-143
5	7	138-145	142-154	149-168	5	3	111-124	121-135	131-147
5	8	140-148	145-157	152-172	5	4	114-127	124-138	134-151
5	9	142-151	148-160	155-176	5	5	117-130	127-141	137-155
5	10	144-154	151-163	158-180	5	6	120-133	130-144	140-159
5	11	146-157	154-166	161-184	5	7	123-136	133-147	143-163
6	0	149-160	157-170	164-188	5	8	126-139	136-150	146-167
6	1	152-164	160-174	168-192	5	9	129-142	139-153	149-170
6	2	155-168	164-178	172-197	5	10	132-145	142-156	152-173
6	3	158-172	167-182	176-202	5	11	135-148	145-149	155-176
6	4	162-176	171-187	181-207	6	0	138-151	148-162	158-179

Source: Statistical Bulletin, Metropolitan Life Insurance Company.

increasingly used by physicians is the *body mass index*, or BMI. The BMI can be calculated as follows: (1) figure your weight in kilograms (one kilogram = 2.2 pounds); (2) divide this by the square of your height in meters (one meter = 39.37 inches); to get the square, multiply the number by itself).

A body mass index between 23 and 25 is ideal; a BMI between 25 and 30 means that you are overweight; and a BMI over 30 means you are obese.

EXAMPLE:
height: 5 feet 3 inches (63 inches)
weight: 135 pounds

135 lbs ÷ 2.2 = 61 kg.

63 in. ÷ 39.37 in. = 1.6 m.
1.6 × 1.6 = 2.56 m.

61 kg. ÷ 2.56 m. = 23.8 kg.

If you meet the criteria for "obesity," weight loss is highly recommended. But for lesser degrees of overweight, the data are not completely in. In the coming years, additional studies will point the way, as accumulating evidence decides the question.

Another question that has not yet been resolved is this: Why does a given person become obese? Obesity certainly runs in families. Eighty percent of the children of two obese parents are obese, as are 40 percent of the children of one obese parent. A major study compared the weights of adopted persons with the weights of both their natural and their adoptive parents; another study analyzed twins separated at birth. The studies found strong genetic links. Obesity that begins in adult life is fundamentally different from obesity that starts in infancy. People with lifelong obesity have up to five times as many fat cells as those of normal weight, and can achieve a normal body weight only by severe depletion of the fat in these cells. In adult-onset obesity, the number of fat cells does not increase; the existing number simply fill up with lipid oil (which is liquid at body temperature). There is some evidence that people may become obese early in life because of an abnormally low energy expenditure. The studies showed, however, that this is not the only factor. Some of the normal infants had a lower total energy expenditure than some who became overweight. It is highly probable that early-established habits of overeating, derived from obese parents, are a major cause of obesity. If such habits could be shown to lead to an increase in the number of fat cells, much would be explained.

Defining the Diets

The safest and most effective way to reduce weight is to adopt a nutritionally balanced low-calorie diet, to increase levels of physical activity, and to use behavior modification techniques to modify eating behavior.

Sensible dieting is based on including enough foods from the major food groups so as to provide sufficient nutrients. A sensible reducing plan can be implemented in several ways:

• By collecting *meal plans* from nutrition texts, public health clinics, hospital dieticians and nutritionists, state and federal health agencies, and the U.S. Department of Agriculture.

• By following a commercial plan such as Weight Watchers.

• By joining a nonprofit organization such as Overeaters Anonymous or TOPS (Take Off Pounds Sensibly).

• By using the *food exchange systems*, which, although designed for diabetics, can be used effectively by nondiabetic individuals. The food exchange systems were developed by the American Diabetes Association and the American Dietetic Association.

Still, many people are in a hurry for results. Losing pounds sensibly may be time-consuming: Even a loss of just 4 to 8 pounds may take up to two months. What many of us forget is that it may have taken us months to gain the pounds we have put on, and it may take us that much time or more to lose them.

In addition, although planning ahead often makes a diet work, many people say "they just don't have time." The salesman on the road may have trouble finding low-calorie menus. The busy young mother of two may find it a struggle cooking low-calorie meals for herself while her husband and children are calling for more fattening food.

Finally, eating is a major source of pleasure. It provides a social center: How often is "going out to dinner" or "having people over for dinner" a happy event for couples, families, and friends? The temptation to overeat is always there.

One method of "battling the bulge" is to add exercise and physical activity to one's daily routine Modern technology has made everyday tasks like doing the laundry essentially effortless, while more people than ever before do work that is essentially sedentary. With all our "energy-saving devices," we have to make a conscious effort to spend the energy we get in the form of calories from food.

It's quite simple. The more energy we expend, the more weight we can lose. Simple additions to our level of physical activity can be helpful: using the stairs instead of the elevator; walking instead of taking the bus, taking up a new sport.

At the same time, people who are excessively overweight and who have been sedentary all their lives should hesitate before adopting strenuous exercise routines. It is best to consult a physician or other appropriate professional before beginning such a routine. The checkup should evaluate your cardiovascular fitness (by means of a stress test) and your musculoskeletal suitability for the desired activity. And one need not "jump in." An exercise program stands the best chance of working if the individual starts slowly and adopts an exercise that he or she truly likes. (See the discussion of exercise below, under *Fitness.*)

There are tricks to making a diet work. Some methods are borrowed from behavior modification techniques. Under the assumption that "bad" eating behavior is learned through life, behavior modification techniques attempt to alter eating styles and therefore facilitate weight loss. Keeping a food diary can help. Many of us don't really know how much, when, or how we are eating. A food diary provides clues as to whether we are eating in response to hunger or in response to internal cues. Another helpful tactic is to identify and control the stimuli associated with hunger. For instance, you might restrict meals to certain foods or certain times; you might use a small plate and attempt to eat more slowly than usual.

For many persons, group support may be helpful. Commercial programs like Weight Watchers as well as nonprofit groups like Overeaters Anonymous and TOPS base their approach on sensible, nutritionally sound diets and on behavior modification techniques; they may also recommend a moderate program of physical exercise.

There are, however, many "pop" or "fad" diets that most experts in the field regard as nutritionally unsound. Fad diets often bring immediate weight loss, but much of what is lost in the first days of a diet is water weight; we lose fluids when we reduce our food intake. Persons who stay on the diet probably will lose flesh, because they are reducing the number of calories they take in. Over long periods of time, however, these diets provide insufficient amounts of important nutrients.

And their monotony eventually discourages the dieter.

Some fad diets may be potentially harmful. For example, the liquid protein diets of the late 1970s were linked to more than twenty deaths. The company that distributed the Cambridge diet (a liquid, oral formula), popular during the early 1980s, collapsed after the formula was linked to the death of a dieter.

Other "fad" diets may be less hazardous. According to many nutritional professionals, however, many are essentially unsound. Diets criticized in one widely used nutrition textbook* include the Beverly Hills Diet and the Complete Scarsdale Medical Diet. The authors find little justification for the basic premises of the Beverly Hills Diet: that food combinations promote weight loss, and that the enzymes in fresh fruit burn off fat. In addition, the diet provides insufficient amounts of important nutrients. The authors also reject the Scarsdale Diet, which is a high-protein, low-carbohydrate diet that today's knowledge condemns as nutritionally unsound: Not only is it high in fat, but it may result in mineral deficiencies.

There is no "quick fix" for the problem of overweight. There *is* an answer, though: following a sensible reducing plan, increasing one's level of activity, and changing one's eating behavior. *Be patient,* and resolve to make long-term changes in your eating habits.

One caution applies here: Talk to your physician before attempting any weight loss plan. He or she can make sure that the reducing diet is safe for you. A doctor's approval is an *absolute must* for anyone embarking on a diet that provides less than 1,200 calories per day. It is difficult to maintain nutritional adequacy below this level.

Nutrition for Women

Women have certain unique nutritional needs. These needs were codified in September 1986 by the American Dietetic Association. The ADA recommendations for women are these:

1) Eat a variety of foods from each of the major food groups:
- 3 to 4 low-fat servings of diary foods

* T. Randall Lankford and Paula M. Jacobs-Steward, *Foundations of Normal and Therapeutic Nutrition* (New York: Wiley, 1986).

- 2 low-fat servings of meat and/or meat equivalents
- 4 servings of vegetables and/or fruits
- 4 servings of whole-grain breads and/or cereals

2) Maintain healthy body weight:
- Adult women should not not consume less than 10 calories per pound of present body weight. Do not skip meals. Increase exercise activity levels.
- To gain weight, increase caloric intake and exercise in moderation.

3) Exercise regularly:
- 3 days a week

4) Limit total fat to no more than one third of daily calories:
- Select a variety of fat sources: saturated, poly-unsaturated, monounsaturated.
- Limit foods like margarine, butter, cooking oils, salad dressings, cookies, cakes, and creams.
- Choose low-fat selections of meat and milk food groups.

5) Eat at least one half of daily calories as carbohydrates:
- Select complex carbohydrates, such as beans, peas, pasta, vegetables, nuts, and seeds.

6) Eat a variety of fiber-rich foods:
- Make daily selections from fresh fruits with skin, vegetables, legumes (navy, pinto, or kidney beans), whole grains (brown rice, oatmeal, oat, and wheat bran).
- Increase fiber intake gradually.
- Avoid excess fiber intake, especially from one source.

7) Include 3 to 4 daily servings of calcium-rich foods:
- Consume low-fat milk, yogurt, cheese.
- Increase milk in cooking.
- Eat broccoli, sardines with bones, canned salmon with bones, collard greens.

8) Have sufficient amounts of iron-rich foods:
- Selections from lean meats, liver, prunes, pinto and kidney beans, spinach, leafy green vegetables, enriched and whole-grain breads and/or cereals.

9) Limit intake of salt and sodium-containing foods:
- Limit addition of salt in food preparation.
- Limit saltshaker use.
- Watch food labels for sodium-containing additives like monosodium glutamate, sodium bicarbonate, sodium citrate, and other sodium sources.

10) Use vitamin and mineral supplements only when medically prescribed.

11) Limit alcohol intake to one to two drinks daily.

12) Do not smoke.

13) Adjust your diet, exercise, and other health promotional behaviors to correspond with your own identified risk factors.

Eating for Energy

Top performance for the competitive athlete depends not only on training and innate ability but also on nutrition. A diet for the competitive athlete has to provide the needed additional energy (calories) as well as carbohydrates, fats, protein, vitamins, and minerals in sufficient amounts and in the right proportions.

Although there is no "magic recipe" for athletic success, an adequate diet for a competitive athlete might consist of 45 to 55 percent of the calories from carbohydrate; 12 to 15 percent of the calories from protein; and 30 to 40 percent of the calories from fat.

Factors influencing the caloric needs of the athlete include personal characteristics, the type of sport he or she is involved in, and the environment of competition. Depending on the type of competition, an athlete may require from 3,000 to 7,000 calories per day, compared to 2,500 to 3,000 calories for the nonathlete. Protein needs for the athlete also are higher than for the nonathlete: 70 to 90 grams of protein a day. A high-protein diet usually is not necessary, however, since an athlete consuming a high-calorie diet is usually getting enough protein for his or her needs. Younger athletes, though, may need additional protein for developing muscle mass.

Fat may actually be helpful to the athlete, especially in certain sports. For instance, in contact sports like football, fat can provide a cushion against damage. In swimmers, extra fat adds buoyancy and protection against cold.

Athletic activity is fueled by glucose in muscle and by glycogen (a carbohydrate) in liver and muscle. For athletic activity, breakdown of glycogen is an important source of energy. An athlete can plan dietary intake to deposit maximum glycogen in the liver and muscles. This practice—typical of the days before a marathon—is known as *glycogen loading, carbohydrate loading,* or *supersaturation.* To achieve carbohydrate loading, the athlete first exercises intensively about one week before an event. Then, for three or four days, the athlete eats only fats and proteins, while exercising to the extent desired. For the next two days the athlete eats a high-carbohydrate diet and exercises minimally. At the end of the week, the liver and muscles should be loaded with glycogen in preparation for the event; conditioning and training are curtailed 30 to 45 hours prior to the event.

While carbohydrate loading may be beneficial for long-distance marathon events, there is no magic to the actual pregame meal. Performance is based more on what has been eaten days prior to the event. The food preferences and tolerances of the individual are the two main considerations when selecting a pregame meal. The meal should consist of the foods the athlete likes and can digest readily. The last meal should be finished about three hours before the event.

Water is especially crucial to athletes. They need to drink more water than their thirst calls for if they are to perform at their best. If an athlete loses 2 percent or more of his or her body weight due to dehydration, performance worsens. In severe dehydration, pulse rate and body temperature rise, leading to generalized discomfort, fatigue, apathy, and malaise. Water loss can be averted by drinking plenty of fluids before competition.

Extra salt may often be necessary, especially before athletic events in conditions of high temperature and humidity, if heat exhaustion is to be avoided. Salt tablets should be crushed to prevent stomach irritation. Although many "sports beverages" are widely promoted, the athlete's needs are better met by eating a diet that supplies sufficient water and a variety of nutrients.

20

DRUG ABUSE

Drug abuse is a curious term. Usually it refers to the use of any drug that deviates from the approved social norms of a culture. For instance, chronic, disabling intoxication with alcohol may be considered "abuse," but an occasional episode of gross intoxication—getting drunk on New Year's Eve, for instance—is not. Similarly, opiate drugs are used in medical settings for the relief of pain. Sold "on the street," however, heroin (an opiate) is considered a drug of abuse. Similarly, certain hallucinogenic compounds have long been part of the religious rituals of some native American cultures; on the other hand, the widespread experimentation with LSD during the 1960s was considered abuse. And even within a culture the norm may vary: Marijuana was and is considered a drug of abuse by many Americans, but within one subculture—the colleges and universities of the late 1960s and early 1970s—occasional use of marijuana was considered the equivalent of social drinking.

Agents defined as "drugs of abuse," as well as several agents that are essentially accepted within the norms of Western society, have definite health consequences. Among the agents considered socially acceptable are cigarettes and alcohol. Cig-

arette smoking is believed to be responsible for a substantial proportion of the deaths due to cancer and heart disease and is believed to be harmful at whatever level of use. In fact, the addictive potential of cigarette smoking has been compared to that of heroin. Alcohol, while probably harmless in moderate quantities (two drinks a day or less), can be dangerous when it becomes a substance of abuse. Alcohol abuse accounts for about 100,000 deaths annually, due largely to cirrhosis of the liver and other medical consequences, alcohol-related motor vehicle accidents, and alcohol-related murders, and suicides.

The so-called drugs of abuse are generally considered to be illegal substances. Some are illegal under all circumstances, while others are illegal only when used without a doctor's prescription.

Drugs of abuse are regulated by the Controlled Substances Act. Substances (of any kind) are classed under different "schedules":

- Schedule I: High potential for abuse; no accepted medical use and no level of accepted safety.
- Schedule II: High potential for abuse; high potential for dependence of addiction; but drug has accepted medical use.
- Schedule III: Lower potential for abuse than

drugs in Schedules I and II; low to moderate potential for dependence; drug has currently accepted medical use.

- Schedule IV: Drug has low potential for abuse relative to Schedules I, II, and III, drug has accepted medical use; drug has only limited potential for dependence.
- Schedule V: Drug has low potential for abuse relative to Schedule IV; has currently accepted medical use; abuse leads to limited potential for dependence relative to Schedule IV.

Drugs in Schedule I include marijuana, LSD, mescaline, methaqualone, and heroin. Drugs in Schedule II include meperidine (Demerol), cocaine, and phencyclidine ("angel dust"). Drugs in Schedules III and IV include the barbiturates, chloral hydrate, and benzodiazepines like Valium and Librium. Drugs in Schedule I are not available legally. Drugs in the other schedules are regulated. They can be prescribed by a physician only under certain circumstances, and if defined regulations are not followed, sale and distribution, and in some instances possession of these drugs, is subject to certain penalties, including fine and imprisonment.

While the vast majority of individuals "know" that the drugs of abuse are harmful, few have a clear understanding of how these drugs damage the body. It goes without saying that drugs of abuse—heroin, cocaine, sedative/hypnotics, stimulants (unless prescribed for a defined disorder under the direction of a physician), hallucinogens, even marijuana—cannot be part of a healthy life-style. Nor should smoking and alcohol abuse, although legal, be considered healthful.

■ Heroin and Other Opiates

Not only is heroin illegal, it causes both physical and psychological dependence. Many of the health problems relating to heroin abuse are caused by the nature of its use:

- Uncertain dosage levels may result in overdose.
- Contamination with other agents may lead to toxic reactions.
- Lack of sterile equipment may lead to skin abscesses, inflammation, infection of the heart valves, pneumonia, and serum hepatitis as well as AIDS.
- Needle-sharing increases the risk of acquiring HIV, the viral agent responsible for AIDS.

As of this writing, the risk of transmitting AIDS via needles shared by multiple users is of great concern. Intravenous drug abusers now account for about 25 percent of all reported AIDS cases, and the proportion appears to be increasing. It is believed that heroin abuse may also lower the resistance of the immune system—thereby making addicts potentially more vulnerable to the AIDS virus. In some sections of the country, the majority of AIDS cases are seen in intravenous drug users. Moreover, 55 percent of newborns contracting AIDS have a parent who is an intravenous drug user. Partners of those who use intravenous drugs also are at risk for AIDS. Further, prostitutes who are also heroin abusers may transmit AIDS to others via sexual contact.

Overdose of heroin may be fatal. The symptoms of heroin overdose include shallow breathing, clammy skin, convulsions, and coma. Particularly dangerous is the combination of heroin with other agents, such as alcohol or cocaine. As "speedballing" (combining heroin and cocaine) became more common, emergency room admissions due to combined heroin-cocaine dosing increased. Between 1981 and 1985 heroin-related deaths almost doubled; almost 85 percent of these deaths involved other drugs in combination with heroin. The heroin-alcohol combination was responsible for almost 50 percent of the cases.

Because opioids cause physical dependence, cessation of drug use leads to a syndrome of withdrawal, which begins four to six hours after the last dose. Withdrawal symptoms may include uneasiness, cramps, sweating, diarrhea, chills, nausea, and runny nose and eyes. Symptoms are strongest twenty-four to seventy-two hours after they begin; they usually subside within seven to ten days.

Heroin abuse by pregnant women may have tragic consequences, both for themselves and the fetus. Intravenous drug users have more spontaneous abortions, breech deliveries, cesarean deliveries, premature births, and stillbirths. Infants may suffer withdrawal symptoms, and many run the risk of developing AIDS.

Multistage treatment for opioid addiction may involve complete withdrawal in a hospital or as an outpatient; a period of time in a therapeutic community; and outpatient drug-free programs emphasizing counseling. Some treatment programs also involve *methadone maintenance*. Methadone is a synthetic opioid that does not produce a "high" but does prevent withdrawal symptoms. It is often effective because it breaks the cycle of dependence, allowing users to function away from the "street society" of illegal drug use, compulsive drug-seeking, and crime.

While heroin abuse accounts for 90 percent of the opiate drug abuse in the United States, other opiates that have legal medical uses and are available by prescription may be abused as well. They include morphine, meperidine (Demerol), paregoric (which contains opium), and cough syrups containing codeine.

■ Stimulants and Cocaine

The *stimulant drugs* are those agents that tend to increase alertness and physical activity. They include primarily cocaine and the amphetamines.

Cocaine was once considered a rare and relatively harmless drug. Extracted from the leaves of the South American coca plant, it can be used medically as a local anesthetic. Street forms of the drug include:
• powder (usually inhaled, or "snorted")
• injection (under the skin)
• cocaine freebase (smoked in a water pipe; gives a dangerous high)
• coca paste (not yet common in U.S.; smoked as a cigarette)
• "crack" or "rock" cocaine (lends itself to smoking; widely available)

Cocaine often is termed "the champagne of drugs," both because most forms are expensive and because it is considered the drug of the rich and famous: movie stars, sports figures, and the like. Many young, well-paid, "fast-lane" professionals fall into the cocaine habit.

Cocaine is not a harmless drug, and talk of the "hazards" of cocaine use is not just a scare tactic on the part of a conservative, stodgy older generation. The health risks are real.

Health risks linked to cocaine use include the following:
• About 10 percent of those who use the drug recreationally will go on to serious, heavy use. It is difficult for a person to predict the extent to which he or she will become dependent on the drug.
• Regular users of cocaine are often restless, irritable, and anxious. Higher doses and chronic abuse often leads to paranoid attacks. In some cases, there is a total break with reality, with visual, auditory, or tactile hallucinations.
• Daily or binge users often undergo personality changes, becoming confused, depressed, and anxious.
• Occasional use may cause nasal congestion and runny nose. Frequent users who sniff the drug often have a constant runny nose, sores on the nasal membranes, sore throats, and hoarseness.
• There is potential for neural damage, because the drug acts within the brain in the same way as drugs like methamphetamine and MDA (methylenedioxyamphetamine), which are known to cause neural damage.
• Heavy use can cause angina and irregular heartbeat. Even occasional users may be at risk.
• Cocaine may bring on high blood pressure that can cause a blood vessel in the brain to rupture (stroke). Some preliminary evidence indicates that cocaine damages arterial walls.
• Intravenous users risk AIDS, hepatitis, and other infections. Freebase smokers risk lung damage.
• By far the greatest risk is that from overdose, resulting in paralysis of the respiratory muscles, abnormal heart rhythms, and repeated convulsions. Death often comes very quickly. A user with no obvious symptoms may lapse into convulsions, then suffer respiratory collapse. Sudden death, although infrequent, is unpredictable, occurring even among those who have used only small amounts of the drug.
• Suicide and murder is common in the world of the cocaine user. And it is likely that the drug is implicated in substantial numbers of auto accident deaths.

In addition to harming the user, cocaine abuse also affects families, friends, and co-workers. Drug abuse drives up health care costs; it is the most expensive form of drug dependence to treat, costing the nation $25 to $35 billion annually.

Although cocaine does not produce the intense withdrawal syndrome associated with heroin, it can produce a powerful psychological addiction.

Help is available. There are many treatment approaches—on either an inpatient or outpatient basis—and a large number of treatment centers. Telephone hotlines can refer you or someone you care about to treatment. Consult your local telephone directory. There is also a national number: 1-800-662-HELP.

■ Sedative/Hypnotics

Sedatives and hypnotics are drugs that make the body function more slowly. Medically, they may be used for soothing anxiety and achieving sleep. Drugs in this category include the barbiturates and the benzodiazepines. Barbiturates include secobarbital (Seconal) and pentobarbital (Nembutal). Benzodiazepines include diazepam

(Valium), chlordiazepoxide (Librium), and chlorazepate (Tranxene).

Chemically speaking, some sedative/hypnotics are neither benzodiazepines nor barbiturates; these include methaqualone (Sopor, Quaalude), ethchlorvynol (Placidyl), chloral hydrate (Noctec), mebrobamate (Miltown), and glutethemide (Doriden). Originally prescribed for anxiety and as a sleeping aid, methaqualone ("ludes") is today a commonly abused drug causing both mental and physical dependence. No medical uses are currently indicated.

Sedative/hypnotics should not be taken over a long period of time unless under the specific advice of a physician. They can cause physical dependence through increasing tolerance of the drug: The user has to take larger and larger doses to produce the same effects. Physical withdrawal symptoms include restlessness, insomnia, and anxiety and can ultimately progress to convulsions and death.

Combining sedative/hypnotics with alcohol is extremely dangerous, since it multiplies the toxic effects of both the drug and the alcohol. Sedative/hypnotics may also affect the fetus: Babies born to mothers who abuse sedatives during pregnancy may show symptoms of physical dependency, including withdrawal symptoms.

Barbiturate abuse is a factor in nearly one third of all reported drug-related deaths, including suicides and accidental drug poisonings. In addition, barbiturate withdrawal is potentially more serious than heroin withdrawal.

Overdose of the benzodiazepine drugs like chlordiazepoxide (Librium) and diazepam (Valium) is not common. However, users can develop tolerance and dependence if they take high doses over long periods of time.

■ Hallucinogens and PCP

PCP (phencyclidine) is often called "angel dust." Developed as an anesthetic during the 1950s, it was taken off the market because it occasionally produced hallucinations.

The physical effects of PCP are extremely dangerous. Alterations in sensation, mood, and consciousness may occur. Because the consequences of PCP abuse include bizarre behavior and disorientation, there is also a significant risk of accidental injury and death. The alterations of reality sense produced by the drug may lead to violence committed while under its influence. Health risks include not only those of the drug

itself but also those of contaminants mixed with street forms of the drug. PCP can induce a psychotic state exactly like schizophrenia.

LSD, discovered in 1938, is a potent, mood-changing chemical. Popular during the 1960s, its use has since declined. Psychedelic effects are unpredictable and depend on the amount taken, the personality of the user, and the environment of drug use. Feelings and sensations change as well. "Bad trips"—frightening psychological reactions to the hallucinogen—are common; the sensations may last from minutes to several hours and sometimes recur (flashbacks).

Heavy use may alter the mental functioning of LSD users, but such alterations are not present in all cases. Signs of organic brain damage may be present and may include impaired memory, brief attention span, mental confusion, and difficulty with abstract thinking.

■ Look-alike and Act-alike Drugs

These products are often promoted through college newspapers, truckstop handbills, unsolicited literature, and storefront operations. True look-alikes mimic prescription stimulants and sedative/hypnotics in their size, color, shape, and markings. Usually they contain similar substances: Stimulants are mimicked by substances like caffeine or phenylpropanolamine. Act-alikes contain the same ingredients as look-alike drugs but do not physically resemble the stimulants or depressants. Phenylpropanolamine and caffeine can be obtained in legitimately marketed, nonprescription, over-the-counter diet aides.

Look-alikes and act-alikes pose a significant problem in several ways. The legality and availability of these drugs increase the chances that people will develop a pattern of drug use. In addition, users of amphetamines may underestimate the potency of look-alike capsules and take an overdose, with a consequent toxic reaction. Worse yet, those who obtain look-alikes on the street may take real amphetamine, again leading to overdose. Several reports of severe hypertension with cerebral hemorrhage and death have been associated with the ingredients in look-alike drugs.

■ Designer Drugs

MDMA (methylenedioxymethamphetamine) also termed "ecstasy," is one example of a "designer drug," a chemical analog or variation of another psychoactive drug. In 1986 the Controlled Substance Analog Enforcement Act was passed, making it possible to treat designer drugs as controlled substances. Designer drugs—if intended for human use and if used outside the purview of the FDA—are treated as Schedule I controlled substances.

■ *Marijuana*

According to the Surgeon General of the U.S. Public Health Service, "What little we know for certain about the effects of marijuana on human health, and all we have reason to suspect, justifies serious concern."

These health effects have been reported:
- short-term memory impairment
- impaired lung function similar to that found in cigarette smokers
- decreased sperm count and sperm motility
- interference with ovulation
- impaired immune response
- possible adverse effects on heart function
- by-products remaining in body fat for weeks, with unknown consequences

Marijuana is more problematical in the sense that its harmful effects are less obvious than those of cocaine, PCP, and the like, because overdose is not common. It gained a measure of social acceptance in the late 1960s and early 1970s, and was widely believed to be harmless by its users. Today, however, scientific facts are coming available to indicate that this drug is not innocuous.

Summing Up

Drugs of abuse are potent agents whose effects on health range from deleterious to lethal. Important, too, is the fact that most are illegal. There is no reason to use drugs of abuse (except when specifically indicated for medical circumstances): The risk is just not worth it.

Alcoholism

Alcoholism is a chronic and potentially fatal disease typified by physical dependency on alcohol, need for increasing amounts, and organ pathology. It is known to contribute to the development of fatal disorders, including cardiomyopathy (abnormalities of the heart muscle), hypertensive disease, pneumonia, and some cancers. Alcoholism is also responsible for chronic brain damage, and

alcohol-related brain injury is second only to Alzheimer's disease as a known cause of mental deterioration in adults.

Alcohol abuse accounts for about 100,000 deaths annually. Direct causes include cirrhosis of the liver and other medical consequences, alcohol-related motor vehicle accidents and other types of accidents, and alcohol-related homicides and suicides.

The typical alcoholic is not found on skid row. Executives, housewives, construction workers—almost anyone can succumb to alcoholism.

Over 18 million American adults are "heavy drinkers," consuming more than fourteen drinks a week. Some 12 million have one or more symptoms of alcoholism.

The social and economic burdens of alcoholism are enormous. Alcoholism costs the nation over $115 billion annually. And 1 out of 3 American adults says that alcohol abuse has brought trouble to his or her family.

For an individual who is troubled by alcohol abuse, or for the members of his or her family, the basic philosophy of treatment has not changed. Treatment centers teach patients about alcoholism as a disease and furnish counseling. Essentially they try to give alcoholics the skills and support they need for maintaining, complete abstinence, which is seen as the only permanent cure.

The number of treatment centers in the United States has increased substantially over the past few years. It is recognized that many of the personality disorders and behaviors linked to alcoholism—low self-esteem, for example—may be the result, rather than the cause, of the disease. While social, biologic, and genetic factors have all been implicated in the genesis of alcoholism, it is likely to be some years before we know what should be the weight given to each of these factors.

Most treatment centers in the United States are based on the "Minnesota model," a thirty-day, Alcoholics Anonymous–based, strictly abstaining, inpatient program. These programs provide a structured environment, with attending lectures and group and individual counseling sessions all day.

While remaining basically the same over the years, the treatment approaches, have become more subtle. In the past, for instance, most counselors were recovering alcoholics themselves, possessing few if any credentials besides their experience as alcoholics. Today, many are degreed counselors. Many treatment centers have dropped the harsh, confrontational approach once used, which sought to attack and tear down the patient's ego in order to facilitate drastic personal, emotional, and life-style changes; treatment would then restore the patient's ego. Now it is no longer considered necessary to destroy the patient in order to treat him. In another development, the family is being involved to a greater extent in the process of recovery from alcoholism.

Today, too, more alcoholic persons are receiving outpatient treatment. And greater public awareness is bringing in more patients at younger ages. The alcoholic doesn't need to "hit bottom" before seeking a cure. Both inpatient and outpatient treatment centers are having good results with early-stage abusers. For more information about alcoholism:

National Clearinghouse for Alcohol & Drug
  Information
P.O. Box 2345
Rockville, MD 20852
Phone: (301)468-2600

National Council on Alcoholism
12 West 21st Street
New York, NY 10010
Phone: (800)NCA-CALL

Alcoholics Anonymous
General Service Office
P.O. Box 459
Grand Central Station
New York, NY 10163
(or your local AA group)
Phone: (212)686-1100

Al-Anon/Alateen Family Groups
P.O. Box 862
Midtown Station
New York, NY 10018-0862
Phone: (800) 356-9996
or (212) 245-3151 inside New York

21

SAFETY FIRST

To a large extent, accidental death and injury have not received the attention merited by the morbidity and mortality they cause. Accidents are the fourth leading cause of death among people of all ages; they claim more lives than all other causes combined among individuals between 15 and 24 years.

The figures for 1986 give some idea of the kinds of accidents that befall us.

In 1986, some 94,000 Americans lost their lives through accidents. Motor vehicle accidents accounted for 47,900, falls accounted for 11,000, drownings accounted for 5,600, and fires and burns accounted for 4,800. Adding to the toll from accidental injury and death were poisonings, drug reactions, product-related accidents, and recreational accidents. There is much we can do—inside and outside the home—to reduce the chances of falling victim to an accident or injury.

Read the suggestions that follow and rate your home and life-style against the safety guidelines offered. Take steps immediately to remedy anything that may be putting you and your loved ones at risk.

■ Automobiles

Don't drink and drive! Alcohol is a major factor in the thousands of motor vehicle deaths each year. We know that driving and drinking do not mix. Even small amounts of alcohol (or even prescription drugs like Valium) may impair driving performance.

Failure to fasten seat belts is another factor in the rate of injury. Combined lap and shoulder belts almost halve the chances of serious injury and death. And in some localities, driving without seat belts is against the law.

High speeds and poor vehicle design also contribute to vehicular fatalities. Drive at the posted speeds and keep your car in good repair. When your tires become worn, replace them. A bald tire cannot adhere to a wet road.

■ Guns

There are over 30,000 firearms-associated deaths from accidents, suicides, and homicides yearly. This cause of death is continuing to increase. Laws on the control of firearms are a political issue, however. Lacking popular pressure for change, the easy availability of guns is likely to continue—and with it the rising rate of gun-related accidents.

■ Falls

Falls occur primarily at home but also in the workplace. Falls are the most important cause of accidents among seniors. These measures will help prevent falls:

- Wipe up spilled grease and liquids before someone slips and falls.
- Floors are slippery when they are wet or waxed. Do not walk on a wet or waxed floor until it is dry.
- In the tub or shower, use a rubber mat or adhesive decals. A metal grab bar also provides support.
- Install safety railings and handles in the bathroom.
- Be on the lookout for unexpected obstacles.
- Keep traffic lanes free. People should be able to walk through rooms unobstructed.
- Do not carry a load that obscures your vision.
- Use stools to reach things on high shelves. Do not climb on a chair or cabinet, carton, or stack of books.
- Do not let electrical cords hang loose.
- Install window guards for small children.
- Make sure stairways and halls are well lighted.
- If you tend to become dizzy or faint, several measures may help: Sleep with your head raised; use elastic stockings to counteract pooling of blood in your legs; sit on the edge of the bed before trying to stand; and perhaps, too, you may need to see your physician.

■ *Cooking*

Keep pot handles on the range and stove tops turned inward so that youngsters can't reach up and pull hot liquids and food items down. Be sure to follow the manufacturer's instructions regarding operation and safety of microwave ovens. And when cooking, use flat-bottomed utensils that will not tip; do not use utensils that have sharp corners or exposed raw edges; take care with deep fat near open flames.

■ *Electric Appliances*

- Use appliances with the label of the Underwriters Laboratories (UL).
- Dry hands thoroughly before connecting or disconnecting electric equipment.
- Do not overload wall receptacles and plugs.
- Do not handle electric appliances if your hands are sweaty or wet.
- Cords should be plugged into the appliance first, then into the wall outlet.
- Cords should be arranged so that no one can trip over them.

- Disconnect a cord from the wall outlet before removing the cord from the appliance.

■ *Fire*

- Install smoke detectors.
- Store gasoline out of doors in safety cans.
- Store flammable liquids such as oil-base paints in a well-ventilated place.
- Keep oily rags or oily furniture polish cloths in covered containers.
- Never leave paper, fabrics, kindling, paints, turpentine, or other flammable substances near a stove, fireplace, or furnace.
- When disposing of vacuum-cleaner dust, flour, or uncooked cereal, put it securely wrapped in the garbage.
- Never use flammable cleaning fluids.
- Never use kerosene to start an indoor fire.
- Keep grease containers away from the stove or range.

■ *Poisons*

- Keep household products and medicines in a locked cabinet, high up, out of the reach of children. Even everyday products—not just those marked with a skull and crossbones—can be hazardous.

Check the following areas for hazardous products:

Kitchen——

- caustics, drain cleaner, scouring powder, oven cleaner
- furniture polish, floor wax, metal polish, wax remover, wall cleaner, ammonia, floor cleaner, toilet bowl cleaner
- food cupboards: vanilla, almond, and maple extracts (powerful poisons if taken from the bottle, undiluted)

Bathroom——

- medicine cabinets and under-sink cabinets: aspirin, prescriptions, rubbing alcohol, liniment, laxatives, tinctures, boric acid, shampoo, hair spray, hair tonic, after-shave lotion, bowl cleaner

Kids like to climb, and the lavatory provides a platform to reach the medicine cabinet, which probably has no lock. Drugs should be kept in a place that can be locked! Do not make the mistake of telling a child that a medicine is candy. Ask for and use "child-proof" packaging.

Read medicine labels for dosage, and read

again. Take medicine only in prescribed dosages, and not in the dark. Before taking any combination of medicine, ask your physician. Old prescription medicines should be thrown out.

Bedroom——
- hair spray, cologne, nail polish, polish remover, face cream, astringent, depilatory

Utility areas——
- solvents, turpentine, paint, varnish, paint thinner, pesticides, herbicides, auto waxes, polishes, dyes, charcoal starter, drain opener, lye, glues, rat and ant poison, gasoline, kerosene, bleach.

Keep all substances in original containers. Never transfer them to a common container.

What to do if a poisoning occurs:
- Keep calm.
- Call your doctor, the nearest emergency room, or a local poison control center.
- Give all details. Be sure to read the label of the substance swallowed.
- Check the label for an antidote. Follow the instructions carefully.
- If you go to the doctor's office or hospital, take the poison container with you.

Additional information may be obtained from the National Safety Council, P.O. Box 11933, Chicago, Illinois 60611. Telephone: (800) 621-7619 or 1(312)527-4800 inside Illinois.

FITNESS

22

xercise today is more than a trend: It is an integral part of the life-styles of a full 69 percent of all Americans. Individuals who exercise, as well as exercise experts cite many health benefits, which include:

- strengthening the heart and blood vessels
- aiding in control of blood sugar
- improving psychological health
- enhancing immune defenses
- increasing bone and muscle strength

The most important benefits of exercise are those to the heart. Continuing studies of 17,000 Harvard alumni indicate that as little as 2,000 calories expended per week through such activities as walking, jogging, stair-climbing, or sports can reduce the person's risk of heart attack by as much as one third.

Exercise—provided it's carried out prudently and regularly—helps many body mechanisms, but especially blood pressure, blood sugar, metabolism, and reactions to stress. For instance, exercise affects the way the body handles cholesterol: It actually increases the ratio of high-density lipoprotein, the "good cholesterol," to low-density lipoprotein, the dangerous cholesterol. Blood pressure reductions also are achieved by exercise, and, in some individuals, minimal blood pressure elevations can be managed by exercise alone. In addition, a physically fit body distributes oxygen more efficiently to body tissues, in part because the coronary vessels open wider in an active person. The heart pumps more blood with one stroke, thus it works less strenuously. When your heart is fit, the heart rate is lower at any given level of exercise than that of an individual whose heart is not fit.

Exercise also helps in controlling blood sugar. Researchers have found that exercise enhances the sensitivity of an individual to insulin; a physically active diabetic responds more readily to the hormone. In addition, because of its effects on the heart, exercise also aids in controlling the cardiovascular complications of diabetes.

Definite psychological benefits accrue from regular exercise. Depressed people who take up jogging often report a brightening of their mental outlook. In part this is due to the body's endogenous opiates, the endorphins or enkephalins, whose effects, similar to those of morphine, are enhanced through exercise. We've all heard the comments of regular exercisers: "I feel better," "I have more energy," "I work better," and so on.

Exercise is good for the bones too. Sedentary

625

individuals lose calcium from the bones, which makes the bones more fragile. Physical activity, on the other hand, "lays down" calcium in the bones and so helps to protect against osteoporosis and fractures in later years. Exercise, we might say, oils the joints: It increases their mobility and protects against arthritis.

The essential elements of fitness are three: cardiovascular fitness, flexibility, and strength.

Exercises that benefit the *heart* include any activities vigorous enough to raise the pulse rate to 75 percent of maximal (you can estimate your maximal heart rate as equal to 220 minus your age). This takes at least twenty to thirty minutes of continuous exercise, and it should be done three to four times a week, ideally with a day of rest between each exercise session. Good exercises are swimming, cycling, jogging, and brisk walking.

Flexibility is indicative of the amount of mobility in a joint. However, although we have a general impression of what flexibility means, it is essentially an *individualized phenomenon*, not a general phenomenon. We can't say, for example, "Joe is flexible, Mary isn't." Many people who may have limitations in a particular joint may be highly mobile in some other joint.

Strength is the ability to move against force. Like flexibility, it is an individualized phenomenon.

In terms of weight loss, the value of steady, moderate exercise is in its effect on fat metabolism. Steady, moderate exercise burns more fat than intense exercise. And this is why: After ten minutes of moderately strenuous exercise the body is fueling itself as much on fats as on carbohydrates. Later, fatty acids are consumed even more than carbohydrates. Thus if your goal is to lose weight, you can do it best by staying away from programs like fast running, high-energy dance, or rapid cycling; concentrate instead on sustained, more moderate activities like aerobics.

It is a mistake to think that weight loss is the main function of exercise. Its real purpose is increased cardiovascular fitness. Essentially, it's an insurance policy against cardiovascular disease, the premium being a good program of vigorous aerobic activity three to four times a week with a day of rest between each session.

We have emphasized the need to assess your cardiovascular status before embarking on an exercise program. Equally important is your *structure* status. If you have any structural abnormality—for example, flat feet, spinal curvature, or knock-knee—you could exacerbate it by engaging in a high-impact activity like jogging or aerobic dancing.

If you know or suspect that you have a structural problem, it is especially necessary to get professional guidance in setting up an exercise program. And go to knowledgeable sales people for the equipment you need. Something as simple as properly fitted shoes could save you a visit to the foot surgeon.

Preparation for exercise is important to prevent injury. Preparation has two phases. In the first phase you "warm up" to dilate blood vessels in the muscles and become psychologically prepared. In the second phase you stretch the muscles to be used during the activity.

A general exercise, perhaps running in place or walking, will suffice for warming up. The second phase—stretching—is directed to specific muscles. For instance, to counter back pain, exercises for hip flexors, lower back muscles, and weak abdominals are indicated. A swimmer might warm up by doing a few strokes in the pool, then follow with a variety of shoulder stretches. Cyclists and runners need to stretch thigh muscles, calves, and the low back. Some persons are lucky in that they do not even need stretching exercises: They have sufficient flexibility as they are.

It is especially important to adopt an individualized approach. Remember, each body is unique, and different activities use different sets of muscles. Try to tailor your "exercise preps" accordingly.

When performing stretching exercises, comfortable, nonrestricting clothing should be worn. Each stretch should be held at the point of tightness for 15 to 30 seconds. The rest of the body should be relaxed while stretching.

Although exercise is beneficial to most individuals, it is not completely free of risks. In any individual under age 50 with a family history of sudden death, or with a personal history of fainting spells, chest pain, shortness of breath, or cardiac problems, a physician's advice should be sought before beginning an exercise program.

The risks of exercise include injuries to the bony skeleton: sprains, strains, and fractures. *Sprains* are ligament injuries caused by sudden overstretching. *Strains* involve overwork or excessive stretching of a muscle.

Broken bones, or *fractures*, that occur as a result of sports participation require immediate medical attention. If someone complains of severe local pain, it is possible that a break has occurred. Signs to look for include deformity, tenderness, inability to use the extremity, swelling, and bruising.

Emergency splinting of fractures, dislocations, and sprains is necessary before the person can be moved. A splint—a device to prevent movement of the injured part—can be fashioned from any material. All open wounds should be covered with a dry, sterile dressing, with local pressure applied to control bleeding.

Strains, sprains, and any kind of swelling following injury require the attention of a physician. Do not pass off an injury as "just a sprain" or "just a strain." If you do, you may run into problems later.

Ankle injuries are especially frequent and troublesome. A sprained ankle needs to be elevated as soon as possible, and ice should be applied. An elastic bandage can be used for support, and a cane or crutches can be used if pain is severe. When pain subsides and the swelling has gone down, rehabilitation can begin, using exercises to increase the strength and flexibility of the ankle. Time alone will allow the torn ligaments to heal.

In the quest for fitness, minor discomforts are inevitable. One of them is *blisters*. These are small pockets of fluid accumulating just under the skin as a result of heat, friction, or irritation. They occur usually due to unaccustomed exercise or the use of new equipment, such as new shoes. Try to break shoes in gradually, while keeping your comfortable old pair in use.

No treatment, apart from protection, is required for blisters less than an inch across. Larger blisters may need medical attention. They should not be pricked.

Other minor problems include athlete's foot and "jock itch." A good preventive is thorough, daily washing. Keep vulnerable areas dry with talc or cornstarch and wear dry, clean underclothing and socks. Over-the-counter antifungals can be used also; they contain undecylenic acid, tolnaftate, or miconidazole.

"Tennis elbow" is an inflammation of the tendons linking the forearm muscles to the elbow. It results from an overload of pressure on the forearm muscle group and is particularly common in tennis players and other enthusiasts for racket, wall, and net sports. Rest and the use of wide strapping or even steroid injections may be needed.

Whatever type of exercise you do, appropriate exercise preps—warm-ups and stretching exercises—will help prevent injury. And should injury occur, be sure to consult your physician for appropriate treatment.

SENIOR LIVING

23

SENIORS:
A
GROWING
POPULATION

americans living today have a longer life expectancy than ever before in our history. This reflects the combined impact of an ever-expanding pool of medical knowledge, new therapeutic discoveries, and advances in research and clinical technologies. Specifically, today's increased survival is attributed to a decline in maternal, infant, and childhood mortality and to a reduction in deaths occurring later in life from heart disease and stroke. As a consequence of people living longer, the composition of the United States population has undergone striking shifts in age distribution over the twentieth century.

For example, in 1900 the average life expectancy was 47 years, and only 4 percent of the population was over 65 years of age. By 1950 the percentage of the over-65 population had doubled to a little more than 8 percent. Doubtless, this was due at least partly to the ability to control previously fatal infectious diseases though the use of antibiotics and vaccines. The 1960s and 1970s marked an era of major advances in both medical and surgical treatment of various forms of heart disease. In 1984, persons 65 years of age and older

comprised 12 percent of our total population. According to projections by the U.S. Bureau of the Census, the proportion of persons over 65 years of age will increase even more in coming years. It is estimated that by the year 2050 this age group will comprise a little over 20 percent of the total U.S. population.

Today's greater ratio of older to younger persons also stems from an increase that occurred in the annual number of births prior to 1920 and again after World War II. Persons born during the latter period often are referred to as the "baby boom" generation. The aging of the pre-1920s group, together with a dramatic decline in the birth rate after the mid-1960s, has contributed to current age shifts in our population. A significant demographic change was the rise in the median age from 28 in 1970 to 31 in 1984.

Continued life expectancy beyond age 65 is marked by differences between the sexes, with women generally living longer than men. Statistics from the National Institute on Aging show that at 65 years of age a man now has a life expectancy of thirteen additional years, while a woman of 65 can expect to live seventeen more years. In the same way, a man reaching age 75 can expect to live an additional six years, while a woman of the same age has a life expectancy of another twelve years.

Bureau of the Census figures show that the 75- and 85-plus age groups are the fastest-growing age segments in the U.S. population. By the year 2050 these two upper age groups are expected to comprise nearly 50 percent of the total over-65 population. Also, more persons are surviving into their tenth and eleventh decades than ever before. It is not uncommon for older persons to have a surviving parent, and four-generation families are not as unusual as they once were.

Who Are the "Elderly"?

Unlike other stages of life such as adolescence, there is no clear demarcation point for entry to the status of "elderly." The trend toward better health at higher ages has blurred the once appropriate landmarks for the onset of old age. Social trends and changes, too, have reshaped our perception of aging. Consider, for example, the traditional stereotype of the grandmother as a sweet old lady who lives primarily for her grandchildren. Today's grandmother may be no younger chronologically—indeed, she is likely to be older than her ancestor as a result of delayed childbearing—but she could easily be a busy executive who is nevertheless dedicated to her grandchildren.

The selection of 65 as the cutoff point between middle and old age is an arbitrary definition adopted primarily for social purposes. With the passage of the Social Security Act in 1935, 65 came to be accepted as the age at which persons become eligible not only for retirement but for various pensions, discounts, and services reserved for those whom we now call "senior citizens." It does not, however, denote the magic age at which there is a universal decline in individual capabilities, productivity, and potential.

The increase in the number of persons surviving to the upper age brackets has introduced the need for some classification of age groups according to how they differ. Thus, 65 to 74 generally is designated as "young old age," 75 to 84 as "older old age," and 85 and over as "oldest old age."

A major characteristic that has accompanied the increase in absolute numbers of older people in our population is the increasing proportion of women at older ages. Elderly women now out-

number elderly men 3 to 2—a considerable change from 1960 when the ratio of elderly women to elderly men was 5 to 4. In 1984 there were 81 men between 65 and 69 years of age for every 100 women of the same age.

This trend is due partly to mortality rates that favor women at all ages: Mortality from heart disease, lung cancer, and emphysema has traditionally been higher among men than among women—although the rates of heart disease and lung cancer among women rose in the 1980s.

It is believed also that genetic and hormonal differences between the sexes may contribute to women's longevity. For example, estrogen—a naturally occurring female hormone present during a woman's reproductive years—is believed to have a protective effect against heart disease. There is good evidence from clinical studies that estrogen replacement therapy after menopause has beneficial effects upon the cardiovascular system.

■ *Marital Status*

The gap in life expectancy between the sexes creates a situation in which widowhood for women becomes common at older ages. Another contributing factor is that most women are younger than their husbands to begin with. In 1984, half of all older women were widows, and there were over five times as many widows (7.8 million) as widowers (1.5 million) among persons over 65 years of age. Older men, too, were twice as likely to be married as older women.

Older widowers have far greater options for remarriage than do widows. Not only can a man choose from the preponderance of women who are his contemporaries, but he can marry a younger woman without inviting social disapproval. By contrast, an older woman is criticized if she marries someone much younger. And her opportunities for doing so are nowhere near as great as they are for an older man.

For most older women, attracting a partner remains as important as it was in youth, even if the woman is not interested in remarriage. In fact, a woman who has seen a husband through a long and difficult illness may not be at all eager to take on the responsibilities of marriage at a later age. But even widows who are not interested in remarriage usually enjoy having some male companionship. Among members of senior groups and retirement communities it is a source of social status for a woman to have a "boyfriend." And it is not necessarily the former cheerleader or home-coming queen who attracts such companionship, but rather the woman of cheerful and congenial personality.

Still, the merry widow—or widower, for that matter—is probably more the exception than the rule. Both in urban and rural settings, many older persons experience extreme loneliness and isolation. A great many live alone, and their ties to old friends may be altered by illness or severed by death. Children, even when interested and devoted, frequently live far away and are busy with family and career concerns of their own.

■ Geographic Distribution

In recent years the greatest growth in percentage of the older population has been in the "sun belt" states of Arizona, Florida, Hawaii, Nevada, and New Mexico. These regions appeal to older people because of their warm climate and low industrialization.

Indeed, persons 65 years of age and older comprise one of the most mobile segments of the U.S. population. It appears that, aside from factors like cost and urban renewal, relocation among the elderly population is prompted by the desire to find an environment more suitable to the goals and needs of their stage of life.

Studies show that in the younger population mobility rates are highest during the years when families are being formed. After that, there is a decline until retirement age, which represents the second major stage in population mobility: Retirement enables many to move to places where they may have always wanted to live but where there was no work in their profession or industry. The third stage of greatest likelihood for relocation occurs at age 75, when persons may move to a setting that better meets their needs.

■ Housing Status

Approximately two thirds of the over-65 population own their own homes—though this does not necessarily mean they are better off than the rest. Many cannot afford to keep their homes in good repair.

The remainder of the elderly population lives in retirement villages, rented apartments or hotels, low- and middle-income government-subsidized housing, or union-sponsored housing. A few live with relatives or friends.

As a result of urban renewal and the devel-opment of expressways and shopping centers, the metropolitan and suburban communities in which many of the elderly live are under constant threat of demolition. In highly congested urban areas like New York City, the trend toward "bigger and better" has caused the displacement of residents of all ages, as older, affordable buildings make way for expensive high-rise condominiums. Having to relocate can be traumatic for elderly persons. Even if they have the financial means to find satisfactory housing elsewhere, it may be difficult for them to leave a neighborhood where they have lived for many years and where they feel secure.

In 1984, about 30 percent of persons over 65 years of age lived alone or with nonrelatives (41 percent women and 15 percent men). In the two decades from 1964 to 1984, the number of older persons in this category increased by 123 percent, or over 2.5 times the growth rate for the older population in general.

In 1980, only 5 percent of persons over 65 years of age (1.3 million) lived in nursing homes or other institutional facilities. The percentage of institutionalization, however, increases dramatically with age. Data in 1986 showed figures of 2 percent for persons aged 65 to 74, 7 percent for persons 75 to 84 years of age, and 23 percent for persons over the age of 85.

■ Poverty Among the Aged

The elderly rely heavily on Social Security benefits and asset income. Very few persons are able to live on Social Security benefits alone, and Medicare payments cover less than 50 percent of health expenses. A common assumption in policy debates over pension adequacy has been that the financial needs of the elderly are lower than those of nonretired adults. While this may be true to some extent—daily commuting costs to and from work no longer exist—the numbers of older persons living in marginal financial security suggest that most do not have sufficient money from retirement pensions.

Poverty is more prevalent among persons over 65 years of age than in the younger adult population. In 1984, 12.4 percent of persons 65 and older had incomes below the poverty level. An additional 16.7 percent had incomes just above the poverty level. The oldest among the elderly have the lowest money incomes.

Poverty rates are much higher among minority than among white elderly. In 1984 the poverty rate among black elderly was 31.7 percent compared with 21.5 percent among Hispanic elderly and 10.7 percent among white elderly. Poverty rates are highest among minority women living alone. In 1984, nearly 56.6 percent of elderly black women living alone had incomes below the poverty level.

As a general rule, persons who have done well financially during their lifetime can expect to be better off than those who have not. Many people become poor after reaching old age, however, because incomes decline by half or more following retirement. Poverty is a particular problem among women, especially those who are widowed. Many pension plans do not provide widow benefits, and most working women's pensions and Social Security payments are lower than those of men because they are based on a lower income.

The relationship between educational attainment and poverty in old age is not as reliable as one might suppose. While fewer white or black men who attended high school are poor in old age than those who did not, this positive correlation does not hold for black women. Poverty is nearly as prevalent among black women who attended high school as among those with less than six years of schooling. Nor is a college education a sure guarantee against poverty in old age. In 1980, 16.1 percent of black and 5.7 percent of white elderly persons of both sexes who had attended college were poor.

Poverty at any age, but particularly among the elderly, reduces access to adequate housing, health care, and nutrition. These deprivations, in turn, contribute to a greater incidence of illness and higher mortality rates among the elderly poor.

New Outlooks on Aging

Prevailing social values and circumstances affect the quality of life and well-being of older persons living in any given culture. In the United States today, both positive and negative social and environmental forces are shaping our perception and experience of old age.

Over the last few decades, several legislative steps have been taken to ensure a better quality of life for the growing number of elderly persons in our population. The 1965 passage of the Older Americans Act, which established the Administration on Aging, marked an important turning point in our society's policy toward older citizens.

The founding, in 1974, of the National Institute on Aging expressed commitment to continued research on matters relating to human aging. The 1978 amendments to the Age Discrimination and Employment Act raised the minimum age for mandatory retirement to 70 for most types of workers.

Unfortunately, *ageism*—stereotyping and discrimination practiced against people because they are old—has not been eradicated from our society. Ageism still deprives many senior citizens, particularly those from low-income and minority groups, of access to health care, social services, and self-enrichment opportunities.

■ *Health Status*

Perhaps the most common stereotypes about seniors in America today have to do with their health status. Despite findings to the contrary, many persons still believe that older people spend a great deal of time in bed because of illness, have many accidents, or feel tired most of the time. Another prevalent notion is that large portions of the senior population are living in nursing homes, hospitals, homes for the aged, or other institutions.

As mentioned above, only 5 percent of persons over 65 years of age live in such institutions. As for the health status of elderly people living in the community, the majority are relatively healthy and not as limited in activity as is frequently assumed—even if they have a chronic illness.

Contrary to popular opinion, too, the majority of older people view their own health very positively. The 1982 Health Interview Survey conducted by the National Center for Health Statistics showed that 65 percent of elderly persons living in the community described their own health as excellent, very good, or good compared with others of their own age.

■ *Mental Capabilities*

One widespread myth about aging is that old people become "senile." Although not a medical term, the word *senility* has been used by doctors and lay persons to describe forgetfulness or confusion in older persons. There is increasing research evidence that extreme forgetfulness or confusion is not a "normal" sign of growing old, but results from a wide range of medical conditions—many of which respond to prompt treatment. On the other hand, small memory lapses may occur at any age, and may only signify an overload of facts in the brain's storehouse of information.

Another common belief that has long been disproved by a number of studies is that mental faculties—particularly the ability to learn—tend to decline with age. Studies following the same population over a period of years have shown little overall decline in intelligence scores among healthy persons, at least up to the age of 75.

Several studies jointly conclude that persons with advanced education and superior ability show little or no mental deterioration, especially when working without time pressure. There is abundant evidence, both in the arts and sciences, that many people continue to be creative well into their old age.

■ Morale

Another set of stereotypes about the aged is that they are irritable, discontented, and difficult to get along with. Although old age is associated with a considerable incidence of mental depression, this is not a "normal" condition of aging, and it is quite treatable (see "Mental Depression" in Chapter 25).

Life transitions involving major losses can indeed lead to feelings of sadness so overpowering as to progress to clinical depression. Contrary to common belief, however, older persons have fewer mental impairments than other age groups. According to studies by the National Institute of Mental Health (NIMH), persons 65 years of age and older were found to have the lowest rates of all age groups for eight mental disorders. Some years ago, the Minnesota Multiphasic Personality Inventory found a greater degree of satisfaction and happiness in young and older age groups than in middle-aged persons. Similarly, the Duke longitudinal study showed little or no decline in happiness or life satisfaction in their older subjects over a ten-year period.

Other myths include the belief that old people are apathetic, unproductive, and resistant to change. The results of longitudinal studies involving older persons as well as employment statistics refute these generalizations. We now know that a state of apathy depends as much upon personality and life circumstances as on chronologic age. One's ability to adapt to change also does not alter with age, but is a function of lifelong personality traits.

The social value attributed to productivity in the work force—a measure of personal worth in many societies—is perhaps declining in modern America. The recent trend toward early retirement suggests that more people are finding activities other than those related to employment rewarding and worthwhile.

Meanwhile, despite the trend toward early retirement and a declining rate of full-time participation in the labor force with age, part-time employment among persons over 65 years of age is on the rise. Between 1960 and 1984, for example, the proportion of male workers in this age group increased by 16 percentage points.

People's responses to growing older, it is being discovered, are as diverse as the aspects of human personality. Thus, while many older persons may indeed welcome a less hectic life-style with fewer obligations and demands than they had during younger adult years, this is by no means true of all persons as they age.

Progress in Research

Longitudinal studies begun in the 1950s indicate a growing interest in more closely examining the normal process of human aging. The findings from several decades of investigation into various aspects of aging are now available for interpretation. At the same time, research specifically targeted at examining the basic biological processes and social phenomena that occur with aging, such as that being carried out at the National Institute on Aging's Gerontology Research Center (NIA/GRC) in Baltimore, yields interesting new findings each year.

Research evidence constantly confirms that aging is not a disease but a natural part of human development. The study of disease is, therefore, only a part of the work carried out by researchers who study human aging. The ultimate goal of all investigative work is to lengthen the active years of the elderly and to improve the quality of their lives. According to former NIA Scientific Director Dr. Nathan W. Shock—who is often called "the father of aging research"—the objective is "not to increase the number of years of old age and infirmity but rather to allow more people to reach the presently attainable life span with minimum disability."

Over the years NIA/GRC studies have shown quite clearly that chronologic age is not a very good determinant of performance capabilities. Many 80-year-olds are in better physical condition than much younger persons, and their lung function shows relatively little decline. For example, volunteers taking part in the NIA's Baltimore Longitudinal Study of Aging exhibit wide individual differences as they age, with many older persons performing as well as younger persons on some tests. Occasionally, performance is even seen to improve over time, as changes such as daily exercise are incorporated into a person's lifestyle. Research also has laid to rest the theory that there is an adult plateau period when physical functioning is optimal and that this is followed by a steady decline with each passing year. Most changes of aging, it is now established, occur quite gradually.

Gerontology Comes of Age

The two professional disciplines that deal with issues related to aging are *gerontology*, the study of the aging process, and *geriatrics*, the treatment of diseases of the elderly. Until recently, little was known about healthy aging since most investigative efforts focused on diseases associated with aging. As a result of work in gerontology, there is now a growing body of information about the physical and psychological changes that normally occur with age. Gerontology research deals with such issues as the social integration of the aged into society and the ways in which individuals adapt to the changes associated with growing older.

24

THE NATURAL PROCESS OF AGING

The physical evolution of aging is sometimes categorized into primary and secondary types. *Primary aging* refers to those biologic changes that are unrelated to stress, trauma, or disease. When a person first notices that he does not bounce back from strenuous activity as quickly as he once did, he may be experiencing the signs of primary aging—if there is no temporary physical condition to account for the change.

Secondary aging refers to the physical disabilities resulting from trauma and chrônic illness. This chapter deals with the physical and psychological changes associated with primary aging. Those of secondary aging are discussed in chapters 31 and 32.

Some physical changes of primary aging occur during middle age. Graying of the hair—or even baldness in men—is one example. In addition, both men and women may start to notice changes in their general body contour. Often referred to as "middle-age spread," it is due to the redistribution of fat in the body. There is, however, great individual variability with respect to when—and even *if*—these changes occur.

Many people, for example, are able to retain a girlish figure or trim build while others their own age are losing it. Usually, however, it is not because they have been dispensed from nature's rules. In most cases these physical assets are the reward of dedication to a physical fitness program and adherence to a healthy diet. Genetic factors may also play a role. For example, it has been noted that women of Asiatic or northern European extraction have a tendency to "keep their figures" into their later years.

Genetic factors also have much to do with graying and balding. Thus, many people detect their first gray hair in their 20s, whereas others retain their natural hair color well into their 60s. Usually these traits are inherited.

Middle Age and the Transition to Old Age

Middle-age is regarded generally as the period between ages 40 and 65. It is the time when most people are engaged in providing a livelihood for their families and completing the bringing up of children. The middle years of life, too, are a time of transition, when persons of both sexes sometimes experience what is commonly referred to as a "mid-life crisis." At first this can be quite painful and frightening, but studies show that most people adjust remarkably well to the changes and problems of middle life. In fact, for many the middle years are among the most productive and rewarding of their life.

Some time during the mid-life period people become conscious of their own mortality. Seeing children grow up and leave home and parents getting old brings with it an awareness of personal aging. People now develop a new sense of time—they begin to think about how long they have left to live rather than about how long they have lived. Men are aware that the time left to build their careers is dwindling; women undergo personal transition in replacing their diminishing mothering role with outside careers or activities.

Mid-life is a time when people take stock, reassess their lives, and frequently make changes and strike out in new directions. There is the sense that while it may not yet be too late, time also is not limitless, as it seemed during youth. One common response is greater respect for and attention to one's physical health. Action often is taken—perhaps for the first time—to improve the condition of one's body through a commitment to a fitness program. Those who ignored their doctor's admonitions in the past are now more likely to pay attention and take better care of chronic conditions or illnesses as they occur.

The middle-aged person who truly wants to be young again is rare, but most people would like to preserve the good health and energy they enjoyed during youth. At its best, mid-life can be a time of greater sensitivity and self-awareness, a time for putting skills and capabilities to their fullest use and for reassessing values and priorities. These attributes, together with taking better care of one's general health, build an excellent foundation for old age.

Physical Changes of Aging

The changes in physical appearance that come with age are insidious in that they develop slowly over the years. They may go unnoticed in someone we see every day. A middle-aged woman reports of her father, whom she visits frequently, "One day I looked at him and realized that he is old." The physical signs had been there all the time, but something in his stance on a day when his osteoarthritis was particularly troubling caused her to see them for the first time.

Aside from graying and loss of hair, wrinkling of the skin is perhaps the most disturbing physical change associated with growing old. Many women spend a great deal of money on cosmetic products that promise to replace lost moisture, encourage cell turnover, and eliminate wrinkles. But eventually people do develop at least some facial wrinkling as they age, and this change in appearance sometimes remains stubbornly out of keeping with one's self-image. In her book on aging, written at age 86, psychiatrist Olga Knopf notes, "Most old people will tell you that they do not feel old.... looking into the mirror, they expect to see a picture that corresponds to the way they feel—young. What they actually see is the reflection of an old person."* For some, she says, this continues to be a daily shock.

Other physical changes that come with aging include loss of teeth and fading of eyesight and hearing. All these can, of course, be compensated for with the use of dentures, eyeglasses, and hearing aids. They are, nevertheless, disconcerting and can be the source of considerable stress. In addition, there is a redistribution of body fat and a reduction in height. Fat tissue moves away from the face and limbs and settles primarily in the trunk area. Degenerative skeletal changes result in a reduction of height which, by age 80, can amount to as much as 3 inches.

Total body weight decreases gradually with age, primarily as a result of diminished muscle mass. Maximum muscular strength usually is reached by age 25 or 30. Thereafter there is a gradual decrease in both the number and the bulk of active muscle fibers in the body. This reduction in muscle size is referred to as "atrophy" or "wasting" of the muscle. Disuse of muscles at any age very quickly produces atrophy in normal muscles—as anyone who has worn a cast for a long time knows.

Recent research indicates that muscle atrophy is much less pronounced in persons who remain physically active into old age. A survey shows that regular, systematic exercise and proper nutrition are the two most effective ways to offset many of the aches and pains of old age.

The changes in body composition that occur with age are accompanied by a decrease in the basal metabolism rate—the body's process of converting nutrients to energy—as well as an impaired capacity to regulate body temperature. The combination of these changes, in turn, has dietary and life-style implications that will be discussed in chapter 28.

---

* Olga Knopt, *Successful Aging. The Facts and Fallacies of Growing Old* (New York: Viking Press, 1975).

25

THE IMPACT OF LIFE TRANSITIONS

At any age, major life transitions—even happy changes that one anticipates—produce a certain amount of stress. The ability to adapt to change—which varies among persons of all ages—is considered to be at least one of the attributes that makes for successful aging.

One striking aspect of the life transitions that accompany old age has to do with the concept of the "role exit." The number of social roles a person takes on enlarges progressively from infancy to adulthood. Each major role—child, student, employee, parent, boss—is linked closely to one's self-image and social standing. Usually, as a person progresses to adulthood, he or she holds more and more roles simultaneously.

At certain points, however, it becomes necessary to give up, or "exit," old roles in order to take on new ones. Generally, the roles we move on to are at least as valuable or rewarding as the roles we give up—usually more so. For example, the high school graduate may be saddened at the prospect of leaving old friends, but the transition is eased by the prospect of college or a job. In the same way, an executive's promotion may bring heavier personal responsibility and longer hours,

but it is rewarded by an increase in pay and respect in the workplace.

In old age, on the other hand, the number of social roles a person holds usually diminishes—as does the expectation of something better to take the place of a former role. Retirement, for example, represents a major role exit that promises a more rewarding life-style only to those who are ready to relinquish the identity, social position, and financial benefits that accompanied their job.

Ultimately the person reaches a point where there is less hope of achieving something better—at least by the standards that formerly applied. When the sequence of social roles no longer promises greater rewards to come, people must rely on their own resources for a satisfactory adaptation. Those who have gone through life in a well-ordered succession of professional, financial, and social advancements may find it difficult to accept that they have reached the downside of their career.

Some older people respond by using psychological defense mechanisms, for example, denying their need for love or sociability. Others adapt to the loss of former roles by deepening their involvement in those they still hold or by trying to find new roles to take the place of those they have lost.

Common Sources of Stress

Aging frequently brings with it the need to adapt to *a changed physical environment.* As discussed in chapter 23, older people often are forced by urban renewal to leave neighborhoods where they have lived for many years. In other cases, financial considerations make a move necessary. Often, too, it simply becomes impractical for a couple or a single surviving spouse to maintain a large home. Even when a move to a new location, such as a retirement community, is planned and anticipated with pleasure, a certain amount of stress accompanies the adjustment to an unfamiliar environment.

Older people who stay on in an area where they have lived for many years—either because they cannot afford to move or are unwilling to do so— sometimes become trapped in neighborhoods that have become unsafe. This is particularly true of some urban areas today, where the elderly are literally imprisoned in their apartments by their fear of mugging and crime. Even people living in suburban or rural areas are not always safe from these threats. Diminished physical ability to defend themselves makes seniors easy targets for burglary, theft, and other crimes.

Another major stress in the lives of older people is the *sense of loss.* In their human relationships, there may be multiple and simultaneous losses; the deaths of marriage partners, older friends, colleagues, and relatives may occur in rapid succession. For many, the impact of these losses is compounded by loss of their financial security, independence, and familiar social roles.

The loss of a marriage partner has many personal and social implications. The interdependence that develops between two people as a result of living together for many years is considerable, and profound changes in daily living must follow upon the death of a spouse. Usually there is a shift in the relationship between the widowed person and his or her children. While adult children may feel compelled to become more involved with the remaining parent, the extent of this involvement needs to be defined to the satisfaction of both.

It is common for a widowed person to experience a change in social position. Friends and

associates tend to ostracize the widowed man or woman from the social circle to which the couple belonged. There are several reasons for this: pain at being reminded of the death, personal anxiety over one's own aging and impending death, uncertainty and awkwardness in attempting to comfort a grieving person, and uneasiness about accepting a single man or woman into a social setting that is structured around couples. Thus, widows and widowers frequently seek out each other's companionship.

With the narrowing of human contacts, the aging person becomes more aware of the need to lean on a person or a group of peers. As long as the person remains physically healthy, his or her needs are primarily those of sociability and emotional support and understanding. With varying degrees of disability, however, there is also an increased need for the physical support of others.

The sensory changes that occur with age—loss of hearing, vision, smell, and taste—also have an impact on interpersonal relations. It has been observed, for example, that hearing loss causes greater social isolation than blindness. This is because strangers may mistake the hard-of-hearing for being mentally deficient or "senile." In addition, the loud or badly articulated speech that accompanies hearing loss can have a negative effect on others. Having fewer social contacts deepens the sense of isolation from which many older people already suffer. Taking advantage of the technical assistance of a hearing aid, therefore, has more than just practical implications.

Visual loss can hamper one's freedom of movement and prevent visual pastimes such as reading and television viewing. Decreases in the sense of taste and smell affect the enjoyment of meals, and social occasions that involve dining may no longer be as enjoyable as they once were.

Normal Responses to Loss

■ Anxiety

Generalized anxiety tends to increase in elderly people as physical limitations and personal stresses increase their feelings of vulnerability. The need to adapt to changes in one's environment and personal life is a main source of anxiety. The degree of anxiety a person feels is generally proportionate to the amount of adjustment necessary and the resources available for help in adjusting. One source of anxiety is fear of aging.

One sees the consequences of aging in others: sickness, physical helplessness and dependency, poverty. These are major concerns among the elderly.

While some older people are openly anxious and express these feelings, anxiety may manifest itself in different guises. Some people protect themselves by blocking out external stimuli they perceive to be threatening and by adhering to patterns of rigid thinking. Fear of being alone, mistrust of others, and physical illness are other expressions of anxiety.

■ Loneliness

Feelings of loneliness stem less from actually being alone than from a sense that one lacks meaningful contact with others. Thus, many older persons who live alone are not at all lonely, because they have satisfying relationships with others. On the other hand, while social contact has the effect of making one feel less isolated, not all such contacts fulfill inner needs for companionship. Older persons with apparently extensive social contacts can still experience great loneliness if these relationships do not include the sharing of personal feelings and experiences.

Loneliness is perhaps most common among elderly persons who have recently lost a spouse. Efforts to expand one's overall social network are important at this time. While simple social interactions cannot replace the close and intimate relationship enjoyed with a spouse, they are the necessary prelude to the development of friendships. Even one such relationship generally is sufficient to lessen or abolish feelings of intense loneliness.

■ Grief

The death of a marital partner or close friend is a profound source of grief to elderly persons. The actual process of grieving generally does not vary with age. Grief is felt first as a numbness and inability to accept the loss, followed by shock as the reality begins to penetrate. There may be a period of great emotional distress, during which anxiety and longing alternate with depression and despair. The most intense period of grief usually lasts a month or two and then begins to lessen. On the average, the grieving process is largely over in six months to a year, but some reminder of the deceased, new losses, or other stresses can reactivate it.

The importance of mourning as a necessary process for coming to terms with loss must be recognized and supported by others. It has been noted that up to modern times every society in the world had definite rules for mourners to follow, such as the wearing of black clothing for a period of time. While certain rituals still prevail among groups with strong ethnic traditions, the period during which mourning is acceptable in American society has grown shorter and shorter.

Learning to mourn restoratively requires examples in ritual and custom as well as personal experience with others who have mourned. Without such examples to follow, the person may mourn unproductively. Lack of cultural support during mourning can prolong depression and leave grief unresolved. In today's society the social support for mourning ceases after the loved one is buried. After that the mourner is no longer encouraged to express feelings of loss through crying or speaking of the dead person. Yet it is only after the funeral that the survivor's most intense period of mourning begins.

It should be recognized that mourning is an essential part of coping with any loss whether it is a relationship, a major life role, or some other part of one's functioning. Sometimes the apparent withdrawal of an elderly person is part of a mourning process over some personal loss that he or she cannot accept. Take, for example, the older person who has always been a "good provider" throughout life and who, in old age, finds that he can barely make ends meet financially. Younger family members may be puzzled when their offers of financial help do not seem to lift his mood. They do not recognize that he is mourning the loss of his own independence.

The relationship between grief and illness has been the subject of several studies. The findings suggest that bereavement is the single most critical factor in predicting a decline in the physical or emotional functioning of an elderly person. Thus, the death of one spouse sometimes is followed by the physical decline or the actual death of the other within a couple of years. This is particularly likely when other stresses are present and environmental support is weak.

■ The Life Review

The tendency of elderly people to reminisce about the past was once thought to be a way of compensating for loss of recent memory and, therefore, a sign of aging. It is now believed that reminiscence and self-reflection are part of a normal process—the life review—whereby elderly persons come to terms with the prospect of approaching death.

Reviewing the past to better understand one's present life is done at other ages, but the intensity and emphasis on putting one's life in order are more striking in old age. Older people have a particularly vivid memory for the past and can recall early events with remarkable clarity.

The life review offers the opportunity for coming to terms with previously unresolved conflicts and feelings of regret. When this is achieved, it can give new meaning and significance to one's life and lessen fear and anxiety about the present and the future.

■ Guilt and Anger

Reminiscences can bring to the surface feelings of guilt over past mistakes or omissions. Some people deal with guilt by actually trying to make reparations for the past, while others become more active religiously. Guilt feelings in the elderly should not be taken lightly by family or professionals, since their resolution is an essential part of the final acceptance of one's life as worthwhile.

Many older persons also feel anger over the loss of independence, power, and control over their own lives. A sense of helplessness over one's destiny can produce strong feelings of indignation, and some older persons are unable to come to terms with the inevitability of aging and death. It is important that family and caretakers offer as much support and understanding as possible.

Common Adaptive Techniques

All through life people develop individual ways of handling circumstances and emotions that threaten to become overwhelming. These stress-relieving techniques—known as *defense mechanisms*—are internal and unconscious processes whereby the personality attempts to provide psychological stability amid the conflicts and stresses that are part of living.

Defense mechanisms are not totally unique to each individual. Rather, there is a set of well-known defenses—such as rationalization, denial, or selective memory—to which people resort in response to stress. Individuals differ in the type and number of defense mechanisms they use, and

some new defenses may be added and old ones discarded as a person matures. The following are some common defense mechanisms and the characteristics they exhibit in older people.

■ Denial

Denial is a way of eliminating anxiety over something that poses a potential or actual threat to one's welfare. By denial, one refuses to accept that something could, or already does, happen in one's own life. Many older people use a certain amount of denial to help them cope with the stressful realities of their circumstances. In appropriate measures, denial is a necessary and useful technique for maintaining psychological stability and mental equilibrium.

In extreme forms, however, denial may progress to total unacceptance of one's limitations. Denial is no longer healthy when it begins to interfere with the normal developmental processes that take place at any age. The old person who denies that he is sick and refuses to see a doctor or take medication uses denial in a way that no longer serves a protective purpose.

■ Regression

Regression is the return to an adaptive behavior used earlier in life. It occurs not only in the elderly but in people of all ages. Its significance and prevalence in old age are probably very much exaggerated by description of the aged as "childish" or being in their "second childhood." Such designations are disparaging and ignore the accumulation of a lifetime of experience and knowledge that make a true return to childhood coping patterns impossible. Behavior that is labeled "second childhood" may, for example, merely reflect a new-found freedom from responsibility and renewed pleasure in the simple things of life—something younger persons may actually envy!

All adults use the lessons they have learned through past experience to aid them in dealing with present situations. It is only natural that during old age persons would try applying ways of coping that worked for them earlier in life.

■ Selective Memory or Perception

The ability of older people to remember past events with great clarity—coupled with their tendency to reminisce as part of the life review—has been attributed mistakenly to brain changes related to aging. It may, in fact, merely be an attempt to recall happier times. Recent thinking suggests that the recounting of past experiences and achievements can be of psychologic benefit in adjusting to the difficulties or limitations of the present.

Those who are dependent on others for their physical needs may find assistance easier to accept by telling the helping person about their past accomplishments and strengths. This can be an important source of dignity for those who have once been as strong, successful, or courageous.

Selective hearing is most common in older persons who have hearing difficulties, but it is resorted to by others as well. It is believed to be a defense against unwanted information. The person actually hears what is said but registers only as much as he or she can deal with, putting the rest of the information out of mind.

■ *Exploitation of Age and Disability*

The opposite of denial, one might say, occurs when elderly persons exploit their age or disabilities. For example, they may use their seniority to dominate others, or exaggerate a physical disability so as to obtain some secondary gain. An example is the person who insists upon staying in a hospital when he no longer needs medical care. Such persons enjoy the extra attention and sense of importance that come to them as a result of illness. Others may exploit their age and disability as a way of being excused from observing the social amenities and established patterns of behavior.

The Need for Self-Understanding

Despite the comfort found in defense mechanisms, adjustment to life circumstances is not at its best when feelings and behaviors are motivated unconsciously and are thus beyond the person's conscious scrutiny and control. The elderly persons who adjust most easily to life's circumstances share two qualities: an awareness of their own changing needs and capabilities, and a realistic expectation of what the future holds. Understanding of oneself and the realities of life helps the older person decide what to oppose and what to accept, when to struggle and when to give in. Such persons find it easier to accept help with dignity and cooperation.

Self-understanding includes the skill and willingness to use available satisfactions and pleasures to compensate for past losses. Taking advantage of current gains to offset grief over past losses is a widely used and successful method of adaptation observed in healthy older people.

Extreme Reactions in Response to Loss

■ *Mental Depression*

Occasional mood changes are part of the fabric of everyday life. A person who is having "the blues" knows that the feeling of sadness is only temporary and will pass in a matter of hours or days. But when feelings of despondency, hopelessness, and despair persist for weeks or longer, the person may be suffering from depression that requires professional help. In addition to these mood characteristics, depression is accompanied by a sustained lack of interest in one's usual activities or associates, loss of appetite and weight, sleep disturbances (inability to get to sleep, early-morning wakening, or excessive sleeping), and a variety of physical complaints.

Depression can be very frustrating to persons who are close to the sufferer because no amount of encouragement, support, or reassurance appears to have any effect. This is because the depressed person feels totally incapable of looking at the bright side of things or of doing anything about the way he or she feels. Urgings to "cheer up" or "snap out of it" only intensify the depressed person's feeling of exasperation at being unable to respond as expected; the person thus feels all the more powerless and deeply alone. Family and friends who have not experienced depression themselves can easily lose patience when their efforts to help consistently fail.

Although depression can occur at any time in life, the incidence does appear to increase in old age when people experience the loss of many facets of life that once gave joy, pleasure, and satisfaction. Depression also grows out of unresolved feelings of grief, guilt, loneliness, and anger.

As in younger persons, depression in older persons is a very treatable condition. There are a number of effective antidepressant medications, and older patients respond as well as persons in other age groups. Family members and close associates are extremely valuable as intermediaries in detecting a person's need for medical treatment of their depression. It is often necessary to make an appointment with a physician and to accompany the patient there. Depressed persons themselves—no matter how well informed—usually are so despondent that they feel their misery could not possibly be alleviated.

One difficulty physicians face in diagnosing depression in the elderly is that older people are more likely to recognize and report *physical symptoms* of depression rather than *mood changes.* Some patients even strongly deny being depressed and complain only of bodily symptoms. Often a preexisting physical disorder is exaggerated, and the physician finds no signs of a corresponding deterioration to explain the extent of the patient's complaints. Upon direct questioning, however, patients readily admit to symptoms related to depression such as easy fatigability, insomnia, or lack of pleasure in activities that usually bring enjoyment.

The relationship between chronic illness and depression should not be overlooked. It is understandable how the constant physical drain of pain or disability might affect one's mental outlook on life.

■ Suicide in Late Life

Despite the rising rate of suicide among teenagers and young adults reported in the 1980s, persons over 65 still have the highest suicide rate of any age group in the United States. While older persons constitute only 12 percent of the total U.S. population, they commit 17 percent of all reported suicides; suicide ranks among the top ten causes of death in the over-65 age group.

It is difficult to record the exact incidence of suicide in a given group because of underreporting of suicide as a cause of death. This is believed to be particularly true of older persons, who are more likely to have multiple chronic diseases for which they are receiving medications. The elderly are also chronologically closer to death. Consequently they are at greater risk of overdosing on medication without notice, of stopping life-sustaining medications, or of being involved in fatal accidents that are actually disguised suicides. Even where the cause is known, family members may be embarrassed to have the death

of a beloved parent or spouse—who is often a respected member of the community—reported as a suicide; they may find it easier to attribute the death to some existing medical cause.

There are several theories about the causes of suicide in late life. One explanation is the sense of alienation that is often experienced with aging. Support for this view stems from statistical evidence that white men—who, at all ages, commit suicide more often than black men or women—continue to have the highest suicide rate after 65. The prevalence of suicide in this group is believed to reflect a response to the comparatively greater loss of status, power, and influence in society that sets white men apart from other groups.

Control over one's circumstances is believed to be another explanation for late-life suicide. Although death itself is certain, the time and manner in which it will occur are not. Thus, those who commit suicide defy and control death by initiating their own death. Control also extends beyond the grave to survivors, affecting them deeply—often with a legacy of guilt and regret.

As in other age groups, depression is a leading cause of suicide among the elderly. Therefore, aside from alleviating the patient's mental anguish, the treatment of depression can actually prove lifesaving. Yet another cause of suicide—especially prevalent among elderly men—is the rational decision to kill oneself for some practical purpose. For example, an older man with a serious illness may decide to kill himself rather than leave his wife penniless due to long-term medical expenses.

Investigators reviewing epidemiologic trends in late-life suicide note that while thoughts about death and the expressed desire to die are constant over the life cycle, the frequency of suicidal thoughts and attempts is lower in late life. At the same time, the success rate for attempted suicide is much higher among older people (one in 4 succeeds among those 65 and older) than among younger adults (one in 20 among persons under 40). So while older people think about suicide less, they are more likely to be successful if they attempt it. This has the clear implication that family members and mental health personnel should always take the suicide threats of older persons seriously.

26

THE PLEASURES AND PITFALLS OF RETIREMENT

Today's increased life expectancy has led to changes in the way individuals and society view retirement. As a result of living longer, persons now can expect to spend more years in retirement than ever before. Thus, retirement is beginning to be regarded as a natural part of the life cycle rather than another restriction of aging. The increasing trend toward early retirement suggests that a greater number of people are opting for a more leisurely life-style as a result of deliberate planning and choice rather than from necessity.

Past and present trends suggest that early retirement may remain a permanent practice in our society. A 1978 national survey of American attitudes toward pensions and retirement revealed that nearly two thirds of retirees had left work before age 65. According to the results of this survey, people retire at a given age for a variety of reasons including health, availability of private pension benefits, social expectations, and long-held plans.

The results of a 1981 nationwide poll show that almost two third of retirees aged 65 and over report that they left the labor force by choice. Of the remaining one third who reported that they were forced to retire, close to two thirds stated that they retired because of disability or poor health and only one third retired because their employers had a mandatory retirement age.

Unemployment Among the Elderly

Unemployment is a serious problem for elderly persons who need to work for economic reasons or who would like to remain active in the labor force. Older persons who are unemployed usually stay out of work longer than younger people. Moreover, older people are likely to suffer an earnings loss when they do find reemployment. Survey findings show that the wages offered to older workers are frequently so low as to discourage many from seeking work after losing a job. Fringe benefits for older workers are usually inadequate, mainly because most are employed by small firms that offer only limited, if any, benefits for their workers. Thus, prospective workers who have become discouraged in their search for a new job eventually enter the ranks of the retired rather than the unemployed.

Despite findings to the contrary, there is a lingering belief that retirement contributes to health problems and even to premature death. Researchers evaluating overall adjustment to retirement have not confirmed that retirement itself results in either poor physical or mental health. It has been shown, however, that unemployment and failure to find a new job can increase the probability of illness in the elderly. The practical explanation for this is that loss of employment also means loss of health insurance. Lack of health insurance combined with lack of income, in turn, increase the probability of worsened health care during the period of unemployment. Thus, unemployment itself can become the basis for illness which then serves as an obstacle to reemployment.

The Retirement Decision

The decision to retire is one of the most important steps a person takes during life, and many factors affect this decision. Sociologists have identified the personal and environmental determinants that most directly influence the decision to retire.

Social scientists define the retirement decision as a process whereby the older worker weighs the consequences of continuing to work against those of electing retirement. Individual variations in personal goals, preferences, and labor market opportunities explain reported differences in retirement age. On the average, people are motivated to retire if the rewards of retirement appear greater than the rewards of working or seeking employment. The amount of anticipated retirement income is the key determinant.

Retirement income and health are the two most important personal considerations in making the decision to retire. An older worker in poor health is more likely to choose early retirement than one who is in good health. Similarly, persons who expect their retirement income to be adequate to live on are more likely to retire early than those who know they will be needy after retirement.

Conditions in the workplace also play a considerable role in the retirement decision. There is evidence that many older workers would continue to work beyond their planned retirement age if they had more flexible work schedules and opportunities for part-time work.

Public policy regulations have been found to affect the retirement decision somewhat less than might be expected. It has been shown, for example, that the 1978 Amendments to the Age Discrimination in Employment Act barring mandatory retirement before age 70 have had rela-

tively little impact on worker retirement plans. Similarly, the availability of Social Security benefits has been shown to play a relatively negligible role in the retirement decision. Research on the impact of the 1983 Social Security Amendments—which sought to delay retirement age—suggests that a two-year delay in Social Security benefits would raise the average retirement age only by about three months in 2027. The *size* of benefits, however, has been shown to influence the decision to retire, with high benefit levels contributing to early retirement. Thus, factors other than legislated age guidelines and eligibility for benefits appear to influence the decision to retire.

Marital status is another critical factor in the decision to retire, with married men least likely to be early retirees. A man's decision to retire is directly influenced by his wife's working situation: Working spouses generally take retirement at the same time. Thus, whether working or not, wives exert an important influence on their husbands' decision to retire.

Surveys questioning people about what they consider to be the ideal or preferred age for retirement show that opinions change over time. Workers often change their plans in response to changes in pension policies or economic conditions. They are likely to postpone retirement during a recession, in expectation of better times ahead. Also, as workers grow older, the greater their tendency to postpone retirement.

The Retirement Process

A positive psychological adjustment to retirement depends upon many factors, including health, occupation, sex, income, personality, and attitudes toward work and retirement. Most investigators agree that, aside from financial loss, the major problem of retirement is the loss of identification with the work role and separation from the network of social relationships involved in the work role. Although retirement generally is coming to be accepted as a natural part of the life cycle, the step itself nevertheless represents an important status transition. Contemporary American society tends to identify individuals by their occupation, and retirement therefore represents the giving up of a vital role without the acquisition of a new status.

It has also been suggested that adjustment to retirement is a progressive process during which personal adaptation and attitudes change. Thus, retirement often begins as a honeymoon period of enthusiasm which is followed by a period of disenchantment and reorientation. The final adjustment to retirement occurs with the attainment of a level of stability.

Retirement may be accepted as opening up many new possibilities. On the other hand, it can be viewed as a forced change in status reflecting unfavorably on the person's worth. The degree of preparation for retirement often determines whether retirement will be experienced positively or negatively.

Organizing Life in Retirement

In spite of increasing acceptance of retirement as a natural life transition, often there is too little preparation for any but the financial aspects of retirement life. Leaders in business and labor have come to recognize the difficulties many people face as a consequence of abrupt change from regular work schedules to total leisure, and measures have been taken by many employers to ease this transition.

For example, some large companies have begun to offer programs and courses that the soon-to-be-retired worker can take—together with a spouse—on company time prior to retirement. These feature expert speakers on such topics as income planning, Social Security benefits, health insurance and hospitalization, health problems, and family relationships.

In the absence of such aid, however, it appears that those people who would benefit most from preparatory education for retirement are the ones least likely to obtain it. That is, those who are interested and have a positive outlook on retirement will seek out information even if it is not made readily available, while those who dread retirement tend to avoid such information.

On the whole, the more one looks on retirement as a change to a new and desirable way of life rather than the loss of a valued status, the more successful the transition. Occupation is one important determinant of a person's attitude toward and adjustment to retirement. There is evidence that persons in prestigious professions achieve satisfactory adjustment because their professional status generally continues to be a source of personal fulfillment after retirement. In addition, persons who have viewed their work life only as a necessary means to an end, and who have not gained a great deal of personal satisfac-

tion from their work, find the transition to retirement easy because they have not invested much of themselves in the work.

■ *Planning*

Advance planning is the key to satisfactory retirement. Persons who over the years have received most of their gratification from work need to explore ways in which they can achieve the same or similar satisfactions from other activities. It is never too early to begin planning for retirement. It involves identifying one's goals, gathering information, working out a practical and flexible course of action, and developing support systems to replace those that will be lost upon leaving the workforce. Not only does this create a sense of control over one's circumstances, but it usually generates a more enthusiastic view of the future.

Lack of retirement planning, on the other hand, can result in unpleasant surprises. Without satisfactory activities to replace work, time—which is scarce for the working person—may hang heavy during retirement. The result can be boredom and recourse to unsatisfying escapist activities. Some people watch television programs in which they have no real interest merely as a way of filling the time; others indulge in drinking as an escape from boredom.

A good way to begin obtaining information about retirement planning is by writing to the American Association of Retired Persons (AARP) headquarters at 1909 K Street, N.W., Washington, DC 20049. AARP is the largest private, nonprofit, nonpartisan organization in the world. With a membership of over 23 million, AARP is the largest organization of Americans over age 50.

Founded by retired educator Dr. Ethel Percy Andrus in 1958, AARP's stated goals are to enhance the quality of life and promote the sense of independence, dignity, and purpose for older persons. The organization is dedicated also to determining the role and place of older persons in American society and improving the image of aging.

There are 3,300 AARP chapters nationwide, most of which meet monthly. They present programs and conduct community services and educational projects to benefit all ages. Meetings are designed to provide an opportunity for fellowship while also keeping members abreast of legislative issues that concern them.

Many hardcover books and pamphlets—free or at moderate cost—are available through the

AARP. These cover a wide range of subjects of interest to retired persons. Major categories include consumer information, financial planning, health care costs and services, crime and criminal justice, energy-saving tips, housing issues, living alone, safety in the home, tax assistance, driver safety, volunteer work, widowhood, and medical and legal issues of particular concern to older persons.

Community programs sponsored by AARP include driver-improvement programs to help older people update their driving skills and knowledge, as well as programs aimed at lowering the risk of being victimized by crime. Audiovisual programs available to local chapters address street crime, residential burglary, criminal fraud, crime prevention, how to be a witness, how to perform jury duty, rural crime, and Neighborhood Watch programs.

AARP also is educating employers, employees, and the general public about retirement and employment issues affecting older workers through its Worker Equity Initiative program. This program is dedicated to changing those attitudes, policies, and practices that result in unequal treatment of older workers. The major changes AARP is working for on behalf of older workers are:

- increased employment in both public and private sectors
- equal access to promotions and training opportunities
- increased knowledge by older workers about employment protections and retirement options
- increased services for older persons who are entering the work force for the first time, those interested in new careers, and those who become unemployed late in their careers
- elimination of mandatory retirement based on age

Guidelines for Retirement Planning

■ *Strengthening Support Systems*

Long before taking retirement one should identify the existing support systems (colleagues, friends, family, neighbors, clubs, community and religious affiliations) that one relies upon for psychological and emotional well-being. It is important to determine in advance how retirement will affect these supports and how one might find ways to enhance or replace them, if necessary.

■ *Marital Adjustments*

Retirement can place a strain on the best of marriages because of the need for a total change in familiar routines. When a husband retires and spends more time at home, adjustments have to be made in the relationship. Often, this is a time when couples discover that they had drifted apart during their busy working lives. Couples who had stopped communicating with each other must now reestablish their mutual bonds.

Planning *together* for retirement helps couples to make a successful adjustment to their new lifestyle. There are countless stories of the pleasures couples find in retirement. Free time and the lessening of work pressures allow couples to enjoy each other's company and to develop mutual interests and activities. Many husbands begin to share in household chores, thus freeing both partners for the pursuit of mutually enjoyed leisure and social activities. Cooking—one of life's necessities for wives—can turn into an enjoyable new pastime for husbands.

The following are some suggestions from retirees—compiled by the AARP for making a smooth transition into retirement:

- Plan your retirement together and be mutually supportive.
- Encourage friendships and help one another to maintain contact with old friends and develop new friendships.
- Discuss finances candidly so that both partners are aware of the scope and boundaries of the retirement budget.
- Exchange and share household tasks.
- Develop new activities and routines. Allocate time for chores, separate and shared activities, and favorite pastimes. Be flexible. One of the greatest pleasures of retirement is the ability to make spontaneous plans.
- Respect each other's privacy. Too much togetherness can cause friction. Each partner should have a separate place that serves as his or her sanctuary.
- Keep up appearances. Dressing neatly and attractively raises morale and indicates self-respect as well as respect for others.
- Communicate regularly. Talk and listen to one another. Select appropriate times for discussing problems, grievances, or suggestions.

The retirement planning of married couples should also include a realistic acceptance that one partner will outlive the other. Financial planning should include an estimate of income and expenses for each surviving spouse after the death of the other. Each spouse should have a will. If not already specified in the will, there should be a detailed written listing of all assets, their location, and designation for their distribution.

■ *Staying Involved in Life*

Successful retirement begins with a positive and expectant attitude. Getting involved with people and activities outside oneself is a vital part of making life fulfilling during the retirement years. Most people need some level of outside involvement to have a sense of being valued and needed by others.

Many retired people become involved in community and political activities for which they did not have time during their working years. Rewarding outside interests are important at any age, but they become particularly vital as a personal resource when one gets older. Involvement in life and in issues outside one's own realm helps put personal problems into better perspective. Moreover, older people who are actively involved in interesting pursuits are less likely to become preoccupied with, or discouraged over, the infirmities and disabilities that eventually may come with increasing age.

EXPANDING OPPORTUNITIES FOR RETIREMENT

Today's retirees have a greater range of opportunities than ever before for making the retirement years a rich and fulfilling time in life. Retirement now offers many choices for activities, including educational opportunities, volunteer work, second careers, and a wide range of leisure activity programs. The number of available options now, more than ever, makes it possible to re-create one's life according to personal preferences.

Adult Continuing Education

Adult continuing education has gained increasing popularity over the years, and older people today are returning to the classroom in record numbers. A broad selection of subjects is offered in a wide variety of settings including local high schools, colleges, universities, trade schools, correspondence schools, and public libraries. In addition, there are educational programs for older adults sponsored by museums, religious and senior citizen groups, and institutes of specialized learning.

The popularity of continuing education is attributable to several factors. Some people, for example, have had to relinquish educational goals earlier in life because of financial restrictions or family obligations. Thus, adult education programs offer a way to make up for a missed opportunity and to realize a lifelong dream.

Older persons engaged in continuing education programs find the experience of learning personally stimulating. For many, obtaining a degree is not an important objective; just the acquisition of knowledge on subjects of personal interest is rewarding enough. Expanding one's horizons through education promotes a welcome feeling of being in the mainstream of life. Older people engaged in serious academic work often find a new link of communication with younger generations through the shared pursuit of studies.

In recent years, computer know-how has become perhaps the sharpest delineator between the generations. It has become all but mandatory for grade school children to have a home computer for education and play. But older persons who have not learned "computer literacy" feel excluded from this revolutionary development.

Increasingly educational programs for young and old are bringing computers into the classroom, and many older persons find that their learning pursuits quite naturally lead to computer skills. Rather than watching in wonderment as young grandchildren nimbly work out math and word problems on the home computer, grandparents can now comfortably join in the fun. (Doubtless, many a youngster has gained respect for the value of experience by watching grandmother or grandfather solve a third-grade mathematical challenge with just one fleet glance at the screen!)

■ *Public Schools*

The adult education courses available at public schools offer an excellent opportunity for older persons to receive vocational training or retraining, or simply to study for personal enrichment. Some programs allow students to work toward a high school diploma. Most courses are conducted in the evening at special reduced rates for older persons. The Board of Education can provide information about the programs available at local public schools.

■ Community Colleges

The nation's 1,200 community and junior colleges offer two-year programs that correspond to the first two years of a four-year college curriculum, and graduates are awarded the Associate in Arts degree. In many cases older students are permitted to audit a credit course—meaning that they can attend classes but are not required to turn in assignments or take tests. Community colleges generally have lower fees than four-year colleges and universities. Classes are scheduled during convenient daytime or evening hours and are generally held at accessible off-campus locations.

Information about degree programs can be obtained from the admissions office of the local community college. The school's community services office has information about noncredit programs. Information about local community colleges that offer adult continuing education programs may be obtained from the American Association of Community and Junior Colleges, 1 Dupont Circle, Suite 410, Washington, DC 20036.

■ Colleges and Universities

Four-year colleges and universities primarily offer courses for credit toward the bachelor's or graduate degrees, although it is possible to audit credit courses at most schools. Adult education classes may be taken during the daytime or evenings; many are held at extension branches located conveniently throughout the community.

A growing number of colleges and universities offer older persons free or reduced tuition. *The Education Directory*, published annually by the National Center for Education Statistics, lists 3,000 accredited colleges and universities and the programs they provide. The directory is available at local public libraries.

Information about registering as a regular degree student or auditing credit courses may be obtained from the school's admissions office.

The Institute of Lifetime Learning has conducted a national survey of institutions of higher education to determine which schools offer free or reduced tuition benefits and have programs specially designed for older adults. Their listing can be obtained by writing to Institute of Lifetime Learning, AARP, 1909 K Street, N.W., Washington, DC 20049.

Many older persons who are interested in seriously pursuing educational goals may qualify for scholarships and other financial assistance. A school's financial aid office will provide scholarship and grant information. Other sources of information on grants are the *Annual Register of Grant Support* and the *Grants Register*, both usually available at local public libraries.

Another useful publication is *The Student Guide: Five Federal Financial Aid Programs*. A free copy can be obtained by writing to Federal Student Aid Program, P.O. Box 84, Washington, DC 20044.

■ Home Study Courses

Correspondence and home study courses are available for those who prefer to pursue education at home. Colleges, universities, and private organizations offer correspondence courses on a wide range of subjects. Courses offering either high school or college credit are open to all adults, regardless of educational background. Credit students mail in assignments which are reviewed and graded by a specially assigned instructor. In most cases, college credit earned through correspondence can later be applied to a degree program.

Some colleges and universities cooperate with local television stations in presenting televised courses. Viewers earn college credits by completing reading and writing assignments.

The *Guide to Independent Study Through Correspondence Instruction* is available from the National University Continuing Education Association, Peterson's Book Order Department, P.O. Box 2123, Princeton, NJ 08540. The National Home Study Council, representing 109 private correspondence schools, publishes the *Directory of Accredited Home Study Schools*, which may be obtained free by writing to National Home Study Council, 1601 18th Street, N.W., Washington, DC 20009.

Learning Vacations

■ Elderhostel

A particularly popular educational option is the Elderhostel program, which provides an opportunity for persons over 60 years of age to spend a week on a college campus, usually in the summertime. Participants live in the college dormitory during their stay. The cost of the program is restricted to room, board, and transportation; tuition is free.

Elderhostel, established in 1975 by Marty Knowlton, has come to be recognized by educators as a national movement. Participating colleges are encouraged to incorporate the unique qualities of their locale into the educational schedule. The school's regular professors teach the Elderhostel courses, which are abbreviated versions of semester classes—ranging in subject matter from the arts, humanities, and literature to economics, chemistry, and genetic engineering.

Three courses are offered in the usual five-day program, but arrangements can be made for a longer stay. Participants can take one, two, or all three of the courses. With two sessions scheduled in the morning and one in the early afternoon, there is time for field trips and a rest period before the evening's planned activities. Depending upon locale, these may include a night at the opera, a concert, a summer stock theater performance, or a country fair.

Age is the only prerequisite for participation in the Elderhostel program. Its founder specifically ruled out prior education as a requirement. The program thus focuses on education for its own sake, with no set requirements for out-of-class work and no scheduled examinations.

Information about the Elderhostel program may be obtained by writing to Elderhostel, 100 Boylston Street, Boston, MA 02116.

■ Other Vacation Programs

The alumni associations of many colleges and universities conduct organized educational programs during the summer months. *Learning Vacations*, a guide to college seminars, conferences, and educational tours, is available in public libraries. *The National Registration Center for Study Abroad (NRCSA)* lists over 3,000 study programs sponsored by more than 240 foreign countries. Information about these programs can be obtained by writing to NRCSA, 823 N. 2nd Street, Milwaukee, WI 53203.

Volunteer Work

Volunteering can ease the transition from work to retirement by offering many of the same satisfactions that people derive from their jobs. It also provides an opportunity to learn new skills and acquire social contacts.

The opportunities for volunteer work are nu-merous, encompassing a wide range of interests. Several organizations are equipped to provide information about the various types of volunteer activities available. Many communities have volunteer centers that act as clearinghouses for nonprofit and governmental agencies looking for volunteers. These are listed in the local telephone book under "Volunteer Center" or under such listings as "United Way," "Community Chest," or "Council of Social Agencies." In small towns and rural areas the Cooperative Extension Service or the educational branch of the U.S. Department of Agriculture will have information on volunteer jobs.

The Federal Government's ACTION programs offer several volunteer opportunities (some with pay) specifically designed for older persons. These include the Foster Grandparents Program, the Retired Senior Volunteer Program, and the Senior Companion Program. Information about these programs may be obtained by writing to ACTION, 806 Connecticut Avenue, N.W., Washington, DC 20525, or calling the toll-free number: 1-800-424-8580.

The American Association of Retired Persons has a computerized Volunteer Talent Bank that matches the interests and skills of prospective volunteers with the needs of AARP programs and those of other national organizations. The AARP Volunteer Talent Bank is open to AARP members aged 50 and over. A listing of volunteer opportunities and a registration form may be obtained by writing to Volunteer Talent Bank, AARP, 1909 K Street, N.W., Washington, DC 20049.

Second Careers

Some people embark on second careers late in life. These frequently involve the extension of a lifelong interest or hobby to a full-time, paying occupation. Quite often, the second career may be in an area where financial remuneration is not as certain as it was in the original profession or occupation of choice. Thus, the later years—when basic financial security is established—are a good time to launch upon a career that may or may not turn out to be lucrative.

Quite a number of persons have discovered—to their amazement—that the financial rewards of second careers far surpass their expectations. Take, for example, the textile executive who, at age 54, lost his high-paying position due to a corporate merger. As times were bad in the industry, the chances of regaining his former level elsewhere in the corporate structure at his age were not promising. Being a widower with grown children, he decided that he could afford to take a risk. With a little capital he was able to start up a business and, ten years later, is only sorry that he did not have the courage to strike out on his own much sooner.

Second careers are especially common among persons in occupations and professions that have a particularly early retirement age. These include career military personnel, police officers, firemen, and professional dancers. Most such occupations provide a pension upon retirement, which assures basic economic security. This, in turn, makes it possible to enter fields of work that provide personal satisfaction even if they are not very lucrative.

Still other seniors begin *first* careers late in life. For example, many women who have spent earlier years as housewives and mothers go out into the business world in mid-life or later. Some women return to school to complete or obtain vocational or professional education they sacrificed earlier in life for marriage and family. Quite a number of women find satisfaction in occupations such as real estate or catering, for which their years as homemakers have given them excellent preparation.

Popular self-employment options for retired persons include consulting, franchising, and home-based businesses of all kinds. The Service Corps of Retired Executives (SCORE), which is part of the Small Business Administration, offers valuable advice at no cost to persons starting their own business.

Continuing to Work

Retirees may elect to continue work either because of financial necessity or because they wish to retain some involvement with their professional or occupational life after retirement age. The availability of flexible work schedules makes this particularly appealing to retired persons.

One of the most popular work schedules among retirees is the part-time job, the most frequent type of employment among older persons. Other options include flextime programs, which allow individuals to arrange their work time around core work hours. Seasonal work allows older workers to fill in during particularly busy seasons or vacation times. Some employers offer

phased retirement, during which the older employee has a chance to withdraw gradually from the work force. Still another option is job sharing, where two workers split the hours, responsibilities, and benefits of a full-time job. Finally, some older workers do temporary work through an agency which provides work for the time and duration the worker is available. This type of arrangement is particularly suited to private-duty nurses and persons equipped to do temporary office work.

Travel

Whether it be day trips or a month abroad, many retired persons discover the pleasure and stimulation of travel—especially if their busy work schedules and full-time businesses allowed only limited time for vacations earlier in life. During retirement, the ability to plan as long a trip as one wishes, coupled with the eligibility for a variety of senior citizens' cost reductions, makes this time to see the world at one's own pace.

One of the benefits of travel at any age is that it offers the opportunity to get out of one's own world and observe the customs and life-styles of others. Moreover, travel frequently leads to greater involvement in existing interests such as photography, or to the discovery of totally new areas of interest. Thus, a person who has never before seen the Grand Canyon may come back with a resolve to visit all of our country's great national parks—a favorite pastime of retirees.

Planning a trip is in itself a stimulating and pleasurable experience. For those who would rather leave the arrangement of details to others, there are a number organizations that offer special tours and discounts for senior citizens.

Leisure Time Hobbies and Diversions

The availability of free time is the greatest change—and challenge—that comes with retirement. While having no pressure to do things at certain times may at first be a welcome freedom, in time most people find that they develop certain routines. Without some planned activities to fill the day, the retiree's free time begins to weigh heavily and ceases to be the luxury it first appeared.

This is the time of life when people can indulge fully in the leisure activities they have enjoyed all their lives, such as golf, gardening, or stamp collecting—or they can discover new ones. The chosen pursuits depend upon the person's interests, abilities, and possibilities (financial and space considerations, for example). An activity may actually bring a sense of dissatisfaction and frustration if the person lacks the skill or talent to do it well. In time, however, those activities that are fulfilling and rewarding will be discovered and others discarded.

Many retirees find pleasure and a social outlet through regular meetings for bridge games and other group activities. Craft hobbies are quite popular, and include woodworking, ceramic work, quilting, sculpting, needlepoint, and knitting—to name just a few. Crossword puzzles are another favorite pastime; they are stimulating to the mind, distract one from problems or disabilities, and do not depend upon the availability of others.

Senior citizen centers have a great many activities for their members, and offer the opportunity to make new friends and meet people with similar interests. Senior centers also offer information about community cultural and recreational events, which are generally available to seniors at a discount.

To avoid the pitfalls of too much free time, here are some guidelines from other retirees on how to reap the rewards of time well spent:

• Make a daily schedule. It is good to have something to look forward to each day.

• Plan activities around fixed points in the day, such as after breakfast or after lunch. This helps to introduce structure—to which most people are accustomed—into the day.

• Commit yourself to several activities and follow through with them. This will begin the process of discovering those activities that are personally most preferable and fulfilling.

• Involve others in your plans. Both commitment and enthusiasm are contagious.

• Have some occupations that can be enjoyed alone. During the later years companionship is often not so readily available as it once was.

Time for Contemplation

One of the pleasures of increased freedom is that it permits time for contemplation. Throughout adulthood, most people are so immersed in the concerns and problems of daily living that they have little time to step back and "smell the roses." Thus, for many, one of the great satisfactions of retirement is the opportunity it gives them to look anew at themselves and at life.

The process of the life review, discussed in chapter 25, is a natural developmental step whereby the older person reviews his life in order to resolve past conflicts and enhance the sense that his life has meaning. This revised perspective promotes continued personal, emotional, and spiritual growth. For some, the new insights gained through contemplation even lead to creative pursuits such as writing or painting.

ORGANIZATIONS OF INTEREST TO RETIREES

American Association of Retired Persons (AARP)
1909 K Street, N.W.
Washington, DC 20049
Many of AARP's activities are described here.

National Association of Mature People (NAMP)
Box 26792
Oklahoma City, OK 73126
NAMP provides a wide variety of services to persons aged 55 and over. These include information on educational and recreational programs, group discounts on travel, insurance programs, financial counseling, and legislative lobbying.

National Alliance of Senior Citizens (NASC)
101 Park Washington Court
Suite 125
Falls Church, VA 22046
NASC is a membership organization that lobbies state and Federal legislatures and informs the public about the needs of senior citizens and the policies and programs that exist to serve them.

Service Corps of Retired Executives (SCORE)
Small Business Administration
Room 410
1129 20th Street, N.W.
Washington, DC 20416
Established in 1964, SCORE is administered by the Small Business Administration. Its guiding philosophy is that small companies can benefit from the experience of retired business executives. In the more than two decades, of its existence, SCORE executives have counseled over one million small businesses. Advice is given on conducting inventories, ordering stock, keeping records, and cash-flow problems.

Older Women's League (OWL)
1325 G Street, N.W.
Lower Level B
Washington, DC 20005
Founded in 1980, OWL is the only national membership organization that focuses exclusively on women's concerns during mid-life and later. It has over more than eighty chapters nationwide and a membership of 9,000.

27

THE HOME ENVIRONMENT

Human beings of all ages are united by similarities and separated by differences. But no matter how many disparities there are in age, background, or station in life, people share many similar needs. While being old may bring concerns and problems not shared by younger adults, it is important to recognize that fundamental human needs do not change very much with advancing age.

Perhaps the foremost need is the sense of what psychologists call "relatedness," which can be achieved through association with others. The person who feels truly alone or separate suffers personal devastation. This anguish has been expressed in poetry and explored in the writings of philosophers and psychologists. As psychoanalyst Erich Fromm explains it, "The deepest need of man . . . , is the need to overcome his separateness, to leave the prison of his aloneness. The absolute failure to achieve this aim means insanity."*

People who are not poets, philosophers, or psychoanalysts may not be aware of feelings of separateness and the efforts they make to overcome them. Yet at all ages in life we endeavor to create

bonds with others and to establish meaningful relationships that afford an outlet for giving and receiving the love and understanding we all need. As one approaches old age, it is important to become aware of this need so that one can take conscious steps to remain involved with people and create new attachments when old ones are lost.

Friendship with peers is extremely important to older persons, and may be an even more effective alternative to work and marriage roles than relationships with children. Because friendship is based on mutual choice and need and involves a voluntary exchange between equals, it often sustains a person's sense of usefulness and self-esteem better than family relationships. Friendships with peers fulfill the need we all have to give and accept understanding and support. After all, the sharing of common experience is the basis for friendship at all ages.

One concern that may increase with age is the desire to retain as much independence as possible. This is because the interdependencies that exist between persons throughout life—such as those between husband and wife or between parents and children—are characterized by a mutual exchange of needs and gains. Older people, on the other hand, fear dependency because it im-

* Erich Fromm, *The Art of Loving* (New York: Harper & Row, 1956).

653

plies a one-sided relationship in which they are the sole beneficiaries while being able to give little or nothing in return.

Finally, persons of all ages need a sense of security—both financial and personal. This becomes particularly important in old age, however, where incomes generally are fixed and personal security often is threatened by the increasing incidence of burglary and crime committed against elderly persons. Having enough to live on, and living in a safe environment where one has a sense of belonging, are vital factors for the well-being of the elderly.

Staying On in Your Home

■ *The Advantages*

Home holds great significance for many older people. It represents a part of their identity, a place where things are familiar and relatively unchanging, and a setting in which one is accustomed to being in control. For those who have spent many years of their life in one place, home also holds fond memories. The home where one has brought up a family can become a mutually gratifying refuge and provide a sense of place and continuity as grown children return with their own children for holiday visits.

Familiar surroundings are reassuring, and the older person who remains at home avoids separation from a number of valued associations. In addition to remaining close to friends, there are the daily contacts with storekeepers that for many elderly are a source of pleasant and casual daily socializing. By remaining at home, one is not separated from the possessions acquired during a lifetime and which personalize one's surroundings. Pets, too—a significant source of comfort and companionship for the elderly—can remain as part of the household.

It is not surprising then that most older people prefer to remain at home for as long as they possibly can. In fact, many insist upon it, even if it is at great cost to their physical and emotional health or personal security. All too frequently one hears about aged persons who lead reclusive lives in inner city apartments or residential areas where the streets have become unsafe at all times of the day or night. This type of tenacity is often the result of having no other choice.

In many cases, however, the elderly exhibit a fierce determination to remain at home primarily because they view hospitals, nursing homes, and homes for the aged as places where one goes to die. It becomes quite understandable that a person would rather suffer any number of inconveniences rather than give up their sense of freedom and optimism.

■ *When to Consider Moving*

As the years progress, it is necessary to consider how well the home environment will be able to meet the needs and possible limitations of an elderly person. As a person gets older, for example, it may become increasingly difficult for him or her to maintain a large house.

Moreover, the dwelling that housed an entire family may no longer be suited to the needs of a couple or a surviving wife or husband. Thus, many people choose the years after children leave home or after they become widowed as the time to move to smaller and usually less expensive living quarters that are easier to maintain.

In evaluating how appropriate the home environment will be with increasing age, one needs to consider several fundamentals. These include awareness of the basic necessities of daily living, and a knowledge of available services that will provide help when needed.

First, one should make an honest appraisal of the economics of remaining at home. Will it be possible to handle the cost of insurance, taxes, and upkeep on the anticipated retirement income? If so, some other questions need to be answered. For example, will one be able to perform basic household chores and handle the upkeep of the house and yard? Are stores within easy reach? How adequate is public transportation? Is there easy access to physicians and community hospitals? What alternatives exist if, for some reason, one becomes temporarily or permanently unable to drive?

Older couples who have traditionally left the driving to the husband frequently come to regret this pattern in later years. Wives who never learned to drive or who have not driven for many years often wish that they had acquired or maintained driving skills. Consider, for example, the wife who needs to take three buses to visit her husband at the community hospital because there is no direct route. Were she able to drive, she could not only have spared herself this temporary inconvenience, but could serve as a general backup to share the driving with her husband.

Other aspects to consider are the physical characteristics of the house itself. Preferably the layout should have a bedroom and bath on the ground floor. While this may never be needed, it is a feature of the home that will be greatly appreciated during recovery from illness or surgery. Many elderly people, for example, undergo hip operations for osteoarthritis. Following such surgery, it may take a month or longer before the person is able to climb stairs. Similarly, persons recovering from a heart attack generally increase their stair climbing by one step a day. For many, this can mean several weeks before being able to sleep in one's own bed or sit in the downstairs living room.

■ *Home Safety*

Accidents are the third leading cause of death in persons over 65 years of age. The disabilities that result from accidents may end the independence of an older person who lives at home. A hip fracture, for example, is a catastrophic event in old age. This type of fracture is fatal in up to 20 percent of cases and is the cause of long-term nursing-home care in half of those who survive.

Falls are the leading cause of accidental deaths and injuries among the elderly. Loss of muscle strength and coordination, impaired sense of balance, and slowing of reaction time are the primary causes of falls among the elderly. Since most accidents occur in the home, preventive measures can be taken to make the home more accident-proof. Steps should be highly visible and be equipped with good illumination, nonskid treads, and handrails. The most dangerous parts of a staircase are the top and bottom steps, and these areas therefore should be made especially prominent.

Slippery floor coverings, another potential cause of falls, should be removed. Linoleum and small mats and area rugs are especially dangerous. Nonskid floor waxes, wall-to-wall carpeting, rubber-backed rugs, and tacking are wise precautions against falls. Nonskid mats and rails should be used in the bathtub and near toilets and beds. Wearing shoes with corrugated soles helps prevent falls inside and outside of the home.

Burns, cuts, and poisoning are other accidents frequently suffered by the elderly. Especially dangerous habits like smoking in bed should be stopped. The need to revise one's life-style in such small ways may sometimes, however, become a source of conflict within the family. When concerned relatives or friends notice that an older person is somewhat forgetful or has a tendency to nod off to sleep while smoking a cigarette, their cautions are not always well received. The older person may answer that he or she has always smoked in bed or while watching television and doesn't intend to stop now. Usually the person is truly unaware of the changes that others observe. It can often be a delicate matter to bridge such a communication gap before an accident actually does occur.

Care must also be taken with the use of room heaters and heating pads. Fires can start when heating devices tip over, overheat, or burn due to faulty wiring. Another leading cause of fires is the wearing of bedclothes or longsleeved garments while cooking on a gas range. Finally, medication should be handled with care. It is recommended that the label on the medication bottle be read three times—twice before taking the medication and once afterward. The taking of medication on a long-term basis can become so routine that it is easy to forget whether or not one has already taken any given dosage. Dispensing the day's medication dosage in a separate container is a handy way to guard against accidental overmedication.

SUPPORT SERVICES

Home Care

There are many home care facilities available to older persons:

Chore services offer minor household repairs, household, cleaning, and yardwork. Costs average $4 per hour, plus materials.

Home-delivered meals, or "Meals on Wheels," is a service provided by local government or voluntary organizations to deliver nutritious hot meals once or twice a day. Costs per meal vary from $2 to $4.

Friendly visiting volunteers stop by regularly to write letters, run errands, and shop, or simply provide company for older persons who are relatively isolated. There is no charge for the service, which generally is provided through a local religious or voluntary group.

Emergency response systems provide reliable contact with police and medical rescue squads—usually by telephone or electronic device—in the event of home emergencies.

Telephone reassurance is offered by volunteers who make and receive daily phone calls to and from elderly persons living alone.

Other Care Facilities

Senior centers provide older persons with a place to meet and congregate. They provide a wide variety of recreational activities as well as legal, financial, and personal counseling services. Senior centers may be operated independently by volunteers within the community, be affiliated with a senior citizen housing project, or be sponsored by a church or synagogue.

Nutrition sites offer inexpensive, nutritious group meals in settings such as senior centers, housing projects, churches, synagogues, and schools. Transportation sometimes is provided.

Adult day-care centers provide more comprehensive services than do senior centers, ranging from health assessment and care to counseling for social problems. The center may be operated by a hospital, nursing home, local government, or religious or civic group. Transportation sometimes is provided.

Home Health Care

County-run *Home Health Services* comprise a wide range of care performed at home, frequently under a doctor's order and supervision. It can include medical services provided by trained professionals such as nurses or physical therapists, or services performed by homemakers who assist with grooming, dressing, and other health-related services. Typical costs are $9 per hour for a homemaker, $28 for each one- to two-hour visit by a registered nurse, and $50 per visit by a physical therapist.

Medicare is a Federal health insurance program providing benefits to all Americans aged 65 and over. Medicare will pay for home health care only if the patient is confined at home and requires part-time nursing or physical therapy under a set plan prescribed by a physician. There are dollar limits on payments for each type of service, and the consumer must pay the difference between Medicare allowances and actual costs.

In addition, Medicare requires that care be provided by a home health agency that is certified by the state health department. At an added cost to the consumer, Medicare Part B offers optional coverage that provides up to 80 percent reimbursement of the cost for medical equipment such as wheelchairs, hospital beds, and oxygen machines.

Medicaid is a joint Federal and state program originally designed to pay for the medical care of low-income Americans. Today, thousands of formerly middle-income older people who have exhausted their personal financial resources rely on Medicaid to pay nursing-home costs not covered by Medicare. Eligibility for Medicaid is based on personal income and assets.

Medicaid will pay almost all costs of part-time skilled nursing, homemaker services, and medical supplies and equipment. The care must be provided by a home health agency that is certified by the state Department of Health.

Eligibility requirements for services vary from state to state. The local Social Security office, city or county public assistance office, or Area Agency on Aging can provide information about eligibility requirements.

Because they do not provide medical services, home care programs generally are not covered by Medicare, Medicaid, or private health insurers. However, a Federal program under the Older Americans Act funds a comprehensive list of home care and alternative long-term care services. While best known for providing nutritional services, the Act also reimburses home chore and homemaker expenses.

Everyone aged 60 and older is eligible for services provided by the Older Americans Act. There is no charge for these services, but contributions are welcomed. Each state allocates the Federal funds it received under the Act and designates "triple-A agencies"—Area Agencies on Aging (AAAs)—to provide services directly or through local agencies, organizations, or firms. There are more than six hundred AAAs across the country; usually they are listed in the telephone book under "Aging."

Living Alone

Over recent years there has been a sharp increase in the number of older persons living alone (see "Housing Status" in Chapter 23). One out of every 4 mature Americans is either divorced, widowed, or has never been married. Of course, the way individuals adapt to living alone has much to do with their personality and the life-style to which they are accustomed. For many older people living alone is not necessarily synonymous with loneliness. On the other hand, those who have always been part of a large family may find living alone quite dismal and unrewarding.

Widowhood or late-life divorce can be an extremely stressful experience. Today there are more opportunities than ever before for obtaining support during these difficult life transitions. More communities are becoming aware of the needs of divorced or widowed persons and are offering help through education programs, hotlines, and support groups for single adults. The support groups sponsor activities such as fitness programs, breakfast gatherings, trips, and theater attendance. They also provide educational programs that will be of practical help to single adults, such as "Cooking for One," "Traveling on Your Own," or "Developing a Support System."

For those who have never married, living alone is quite commonly a life-long experience, and does not call for any particular readjustment with advancing age—at least while one is healthy. Those who become widowed or divorced, however, necessarily undergo a period of personal adjustment. Both widowed and divorced persons usually need to reexamine their lives and support systems, establish new identities, and make some revisions in their plans for the future.

Being newly widowed or divorced has practical implications. First is the need to take over tasks previously shared with a husband or wife. Women seem to be better equipped than men for living alone because the skills required—such as cooking and homemaking—are those the woman has performed all her life. Certainly, men who have never cooked and taken care of day-to-day household chores may find it difficult to adjust to living alone. Both men and women, however, share the need for companionship. In the absence of a partner at mealtimes, many lose the motivation to cook for themselves.

Elderly persons living alone must be especially careful about matters of home safety and access to emergency services. It is a good idea to have daily telephone contact with a friend or family member, and to have at least a casual relationship with one's neighbors. This will ensure that several people are acquainted with one's habits and schedules. In this way, someone will be sure to notice if anything unusual happens.

The Retirement Community

From relatively simple beginnings in the mid-1930s, retirement communities have become a major part of the real estate industry. Retirement communities are groups of housing units planned specifically to meet the needs of healthy and retired older people. Usually they contain at least one commonly shared nonresidential area, such as a dining room or hall for leisure activities. Some, but not all, retirement communities offer medical services for their residents.

The basic concept of the retirement community as an age-segregated environment has attracted considerable attention among social scientists. Critics have denounced retirement communities as an unnatural way of life, while proponents have hailed them as offering an exciting new concept in meeting the needs of the aged. Residents of such communities have been described variously as bored and disillusioned persons who lead shallow lives in the pursuit of pleasure, and as the fortunate members of a community rich in opportunities for personal growth and fulfillment.

Critics believe that older people prefer to live in age-integrated housing, where the sound of young voices and the presence of children makes them feel part of things. Doubtless, the retirement community is not an ideal setting for some persons. Those who take the view that they would "rather be dead than live in a retirement community" may indeed become demoralized in such a setting. Recent studies, however, have shown that physical proximity alone does not ensure meaningful interaction between the generations. On the other hand, several studies have demonstrated that the social interests of older persons are best served in residential settings in which there is a high concentration of age peers.

To investigate the differences in personal adjustment and life satisfaction of older people in two different environments, a team of investigators compared retired men living in three age-integrated communities with those living in four planned retirement communities in Arizona. The residents of retirement communities were found to have higher morale than those residing in regular age-integrated communities. Although this finding was due partly to different characteristics of these particular populations (the retirement community residents tended to come from higher socioeconomic groups and to be in better health than the others), the structural features of the two community settings were believed to have a significant impact on morale. The retirement community, with its greater opportunities for friendship and interaction with peers, was seen as a supportive environment where residents could adapt more readily to the retirement role.

Time seems to have borne out the alleged benefits of retirement communities—at least for a great many older Americans. More and more seniors are moving into various types of retirement housing, which no longer fit the description of "old age homes." It is estimated that over 1.5 million retirees now live in government- and non-government-sponsored retirement communities throughout the United States. As the characteristics of these communities and their residents amply demonstrate, people do not move to retirement communities to withdraw from active life in their later years. Rather, they select this type of environment because of the positive support and conveniences they provide.

■ Cost Affects Choice of Facility

Retirement communities differ from one another with respect to the emphasis they place on a particular life-style, the extent of health care they provide, and the cost of being a resident. The more luxurious communities offer a country-club style of living, with swimming pools, tennis courts, and golf courses.

Many are actually self-contained communities. A prime example is Leisure World—an activity-oriented retirement community in the Washington, DC, suburbs that has its own twenty-four-hour police force, bank, pharmacy, post office, and library. Residents can choose from a wide range of housing types, including condominiums, apartments in high-rise buildings, and town houses. Purchase prices in 1986 were listed as ranging from $40,000 to $186,000, depending upon the type of accommodation. The main attractions of Leisure World, its residents report, are the high level of security, the low-maintenance life-style, and the emphasis on sports and fitness. Leisure World offers independent living only.

Another option for retirees is to enter a "continuing-care" (or "life-care") retirement community. Continuing-care communities provide the entire spectrum of care—from independent living to twenty-four-hour skilled nursing care for residents whose health needs fall just short of those requiring admission to a hospital. Incoming residents sign a contract assuring them that their daily requirements and health care needs will be met for the rest of their life. Residents pay an entrance fee and monthly fees thereafter, which remain constant (except for inflationary increases) regardless of the extent of care actually utilized. At a lower cost, contracts for specified increments of short-term care are available.

The emphasis at Philadelphia's Cathedral Village is upon continuing one's previous life-style in a continuing-care retirement community. It offers a 146-bed skilled-nursing facility in a country setting of forty acres. Entrance fees for apartments and town houses were listed in 1986 as ranging from $29,500 to $100,000, with monthly fees of $873 to $1,810. According to a current resident and member of the original Cathedral Village Board, the community was developed because "there was a real need for facilities for above-poverty people. There was a need for a controlled environment for people as they grow older." Cathedral Village offers just that: an upper-middle-class setting where gracious living can proceed under conditions of lower maintenance and higher security than would be available in outside communities.

More modest versions of continuing-care retirement communities are financed in part by the Government or by religious or social organizations, making the cost considerably lower for prospective tenants. These generally offer more basic living accommodations without the extra attractions available at more expensive communities. Units usually have features designed to make the residents' lives safer and more comfortable, such as nonslip floors, ramps, low bathtubs, and electrical outlets and shelves at convenient heights.

■ Not All Are Safe Havens

The concept of the life-care community has proved appealing to many thousands of elderly Americans. Today's longer life expectancy, coupled with continuously escalating health care costs, makes the guarantee of lifelong care in pleasant surroundings irresistible. A significant number of older persons have invested in life-care communities, however, only to meet with grave disappointment and broken promises.

In response to increasing popularity and demand, life-care communities have become a big industry. Several have fallen into financial trouble, either because they were unsound enterprises from the start or because they were run by unscrupulous operators who never expected to be able to deliver the promises they held forth. The result is that many older Americans have risked their personal and financial security, with little legal recourse to repair the damages.

The findings of a five-year survey following the financial fortunes of fifty life-care communities show that 10 percent have defaulted on their debts and that another 14 percent are failing to meet the occupancy rates upon which their financial projections were based. For example, in 1985 only seven states required life-care communities to reserve funds for unexpected expenses. Despite the best of intentions, many community operators gravely miscalculate—an error that they then pass on to the consumer in the form of reduced services.

Insurance companies are now experimenting with policies that, together with actuarial reviews, would be used to ensure that life-care contract holders get what they pay for. These include long-term health care insurance—an increasingly popular option today, regardless of the anticipated type of retirement living. Such policies would be sold to individuals or groups—including residents of life-care communities—and would cover all levels of nursing care. In addition, private insurers could assume some of the life-care provider's financial risk in exchange for a portion of the residents' fees. Finally, it is proposed that a rating system—like Moody's in the bond business—could be established to assess the financial strength of life-care communities.

■ Points to Check Before Investing

The substantial entrance and monthly fees of continuing-care retirement communities are likely to take the couple's or the individual's entire assets. For this reason, it is important to obtain good legal counsel before signing any contract. You should know as much as possible about the reputation of a particular retirement community and its financial soundness. You should examine all available financial data concerning the community. And be aware that balance sheet information does not reveal whether a community has sufficient operating funds to cover future health-care costs. Only an actuary can predict that, so it is important to find out if the community has hired an actuary and to examine the actuary's report.

If you find that the community is well recommended and has a sound financial track record and good future projections, there are still some questions to be answered before you sign a contract. It should be established, for example, exactly what premises you will occupy, what services and maintenance you can expect, whether costs are subject to increase, and who pays for the recreational facilities and common areas. In addi-

tion, rights and restrictions regarding visitors, parking, pets, children, and reselling the property should be clarified in advance.

Moving to a Mobile Home

The mobile home is one of the most economical ways of living independently during retirement. It has become increasingly popular with older people who like the simplicity and the sociability that a tightly populated community provides. Originally designed to meet only basic needs, today's mobile homes average 60 to 75 feet in length and incorporate all the amenities of life. (A "mobile home," although it can be trailered, is designed to be semipermanent in its location. A "motor home" is designed for traveling.)

Moving to a mobile home provides a particularly satisfactory solution for retired people on a limited budget. The home usually is anchored in a small lot in a mobile-home park. Many of these parks offer additional facilities such as laundries, food stores, and recreational areas. Lots are rented, not bought, and while this represents a saving in cash outlay, it has the disadvantage of making one a tenant rather than a landowner.

■ Special Considerations for Buyers

An increasing number of mobile-home park owners are operating as developers rather than merely renters of space. This has created the distinction between *closed* and *open* parks. The prime difference is that you cannot move into a closed park with a mobile home you already own; you must buy an already existing or planned unit. The owner of such a home cannot take it with him to another open park. Since it is located in a controlled area, he also cannot sell it on the open market as he would an ordinary home. Instead he must sell the home at the park owner's approval, or sell it back to the park owner—usually at a profit to the developer rather than the individual.

Open parks, too, place certain restrictions on the sale of mobile homes within their confines, so it is necessary to check the rules and regulations before signing a lease.

Another drawback of owning a mobile home is that the resale value is generally low; depreciation rates have been likened to those of an automobile. Although mobile homes were formerly criticized for poor construction and inadequate safety precautions, Congress has passed housing legislation setting new and uniform construction and safety standards for mobile homes.

Finally, mobile home parks usually have many regulations, and it is necessary to learn about these prior to making a permanent commitment.

Urban vs. Rural Living

People who are accustomed to city life may well decide to continue living in the city. As pointed out in chapter 23, however, the escalating costs of housing in urban areas are forcing many elderly and middle-class persons to leave the city for more economical housing in the suburbs.

The advantages of urban living include public transportation, community services, and stimulating cultural activities. The primary drawback of city life is probably the high incidence of crime in urban areas, with elderly persons among its prime victims.

City life, too, is not necessarily proof against loneliness. Unlike small towns or suburban areas, city residents may never make the acquaintance of their neighbors. Nonetheless, while the mere concentration of people in the city does not guarantee companionship, the opportunities for socializing through senior-citizen groups are more numerous than in rural areas.

■ *The Pros and Cons of Rural Life*

The benefits of rural and semirural life are many: fresh air and sunshine, lack of congestion, a leisured life-style, and often friends and neighbors of long acquaintance. The unfavorable features include problems of transportation and more difficult access to medical facilities.

Transportation is a key issue for the rural elderly, who may face driving limitations as a consequence of age. Loss of visual acuity may make driving less enjoyable than it was in the past. Perceptual and motor defects may reduce self-confidence, adding to the hazards of driving. Rural elderly persons therefore often become dependent upon younger friends and neighbors to provide transportation, and this can be a serious limitation in areas where stores and post offices are not within walking distance.

In choosing rural life, one should consider conditions all year round, not just in the summertime when country life is pleasant. The amount of snowfall in the winter, for example, is an important consideration. Shoveling snow is hard work and not recommended for people with potential heart problems.

Medical facilities in rural areas often are inadequate, since most health care and medical services are city-based. However, many rural areas now have sophisticated medical-emergency services and methods of transport to urban medical centers.

Finally, crime—though less common in rural than urban areas—is extending beyond city limits. While most rural residents consider themselves relatively safe, in most parts of the country the unlocked door is a thing of the past.

28

STAYING HEALTHY IN LATER LIFE

Good health in later years, as at all ages in life, is greatly dependent upon an appropriate blend of nutrition, exercise, and rest. Throughout life, foods serve as the building blocks of the body, and, while this does not change with age, some specific dietary requirements for the elderly—differing slightly from the adult Recommended Dietary Allowances (RDAs)—have now been identified. Until recently, the dietary requirements of older people were assumed to resemble those of younger adults, but research aimed at examining the characteristics of normal aging has revealed that older persons have special needs and are prone to certain deficiencies.

Like any machine that gets rusty with lack of use, the body requires regular activity. The benefits of exercise—particularly on the cardiovascular system—are well appreciated by Americans, as reflected by the increased adult participation in running, bicycling, and other sports. Exercise helps to keep the joints in smooth working order and facilitates other bodily processes such as digestion. At all ages, appropriate exercise is generally accompanied by an enhanced sense of well-being.

Finally, sleep and rest restore daily energies, and a good night's sleep is a great rejuvenator.

While individual differences exist, the widely held belief that older people need less sleep than younger adults has been disproved by sleep researchers. Rather, many people may discover that they require more sleep as they grow older, and may find it convenient to take naps to replenish themselves during the day.

Meeting Nutritional Needs

In addition to providing the nutrients that meet basic biological needs, the enjoyment of food is one of life's simple pleasures. At older ages, however, several factors can diminish or altogether eliminate the ability to enjoy food. These include: social isolation and lack of companionship during meals, diminished taste and smell sensation, the limitations imposed by artificial dentures, economic restrictions, disease-related dietary constraints, and lack of mobility and access to convenient shopping facilities.

The likelihood that these factors will result in serious nutritional deficiency—termed "nutritional risk" by scientific workers—increases with the number of these factors present and with advancing age. While surveys indicate that the extent

661

of actual malnutrition among the elderly has been on the decline in recent years, deficient intake of specific nutrients continues. In many cases, dietary deficiencies in the elderly may reflect lack of awareness of needs rather than insufficient resources.

■ Social Factors

The life transitions that accompany aging—particularly the loss of a spouse—exert especially profound effects on nutritional status. It has been shown, for example, that social isolation increases the risk of depression, anxiety, and other mental health problems in the elderly. These, in turn, can strongly influence eating patterns, pointing up the significance of the culturally derived meaning of eating as a social function. In probably all human societies the taking of meals, while fulfilling a very practical need, has also nurtured and symbolized the far more subtle social functions of family intimacy, individual security, and celebration.

For someone who is used to having meals in a social context, solitary eating is a dreary prospect. The elderly widowed person may lack the enthusiasm to prepare a meal for one, so becomes malnourished. Not knowing how to cook causes some widowers to plan their menus for ease of preparation rather than nutritional value. Recognition of the social significance of nutritional habits gave rise to the concept of congregate meals for the elderly. Such meals, now served at community facilities like churches or recreation centers, allow seniors to eat properly in a convivial setting.

■ Diminished Taste and Smell Sensations

Perception of the taste and smell of food is important to nutrition throughout the life cycle. Food preferences, which are formed early in life, based largely on the food's pleasant taste and aroma, are extremely resistant to change later in life. In addition to guiding us in food selection, the sensations of taste and smell serve a protective function in guarding against poisoning from foods that have become spoiled.

Scientific investigations suggest that there are age-related variations in taste and smell sensitivity. The ability to detect and savor particular food substances decreases with age. As a result, older adults may take greater amounts of some substances—such as salt or sugar—in order to achieve the taste sensation they learned to like

earlier in life. And they are less likely to try foods they have not tasted. Thus, older adults often pass up foods that are nutritious because they aren't also tasty.

The sensation of smell in association with food stimulates the appetite and affects the sense of taste. Although there is a normal age-related decline in the sensation of smell, this is particularly pronounced in those who are also in poor health. The enjoyment of food declines with the loss or lessening of this sensation, an effect known to anyone who has had a head cold. Even the most delicious meals taste bland if we are not able to smell the food.

Finally, the way a meal looks and the way it is served have a great deal to do with enjoyment. Attractive place settings and small garnishes using a slice of lemon or a sprig of parsley make food more appealing, as every hostess knows. These small touches should not be overlooked, especially when other appetite enhancers such as taste and smell sensation may be diminished. They are a daily assertion of self-respect rather than a self-indulgence.

■ The Digestive Process

Digestion refers to the processes in the gastrointestinal tract that break food down into simpler components that can be absorbed and used by the body. *Absorption*, in turn, is the process whereby nutrients are removed from the gastrointestinal tract and transferred into the bloodstream, where they become available for use. The gastrointestinal tract includes the mouth, esophagus, stomach, pancreas, liver, and the large and small intestines.

Normally, digestion begins in the mouth, where starch is broken down by the salivary enzyme amylase. On its way to the stomach, food passes through a 10-inch muscular tube called the esophagus (or "gullet"), where it is propelled downward by a special action of the esophageal muscle called peristalsis. The stomach is the site of protein digestion. Its acid environment aids in the breakdown of proteins into their constituent amino acids; it also serves the important function of killing most of the bacteria normally present in food. Most of the important work in digestion and absorption occurs in the small intestine, where enzymes aid in the digestion of fats, proteins, and carbohydrates, and where bile—which enters the small intestine from the gallbladder—makes fat water-soluble.

■ *Prevalent Nutritional Deficiencies of Aging*

Nutritional deficiency is a gradual process to which the body responds by utilizing stored nutrients. Recent clinical research findings have shed new light on age-related nutritional requirements, making it possible to prevent deficiencies before they occur. Since the gastrointestinal tract is the site where dietary nutrients are digested, studies supported by the National Institute on Aging have focused on both nutritional intake and digestive function in the elderly.

These studies show that calcium intake is generally too low in older people, particularly in women. In addition, many older people consume inadequate amounts of protein, iron, vitamin A, the vitamin-B complex, and vitamin C. While the claimed average caloric intake was found to be significantly below the recommended amounts, the prevalence of obesity among the elderly suggests that the caloric recommendation for adults is too high for older persons. These findings indicate that older people should eat more foods rich in vitamins and cut down on fatty foods containing primarily calories. The RDAs for adults are shown vitamin by vitamin in the *Wellness Diet* chapter.

■ *Age-Related Digestive Changes*

Digestive-function studies also show that the protein requirements of the elderly may be higher than those of younger adults because of a decreased absorption of dietary protein. On the basis of this finding, some nutritionists now suggest that the elderly should eat 1 gram of protein per kilogram (2.2 pounds) of body weight, in contrast to the 0.8 gram suggested in the RDAs; this means that 12 percent of the total daily caloric intake should consist of protein. Findings also suggest that nutrients may be absorbed less efficiently in the elderly due to a reduction with age in the total surface area of the small intestine.

Oral glucose tolerance is known to decrease with age, but changes in intestinal glucose absorption are not believed to be responsible. Investigators at the National Institute on Aging Gerontology Research Center in Baltimore have discovered that the standard for defining normal adult glucose levels is inappropriate for older people. By that standard, up to one half of the older population would be diagnosed incorrectly as having diabetes mellitus. Therefore, new classifications for diabetes mellitus and glucose intolerance were established in 1979.

Older people produce less saliva, and this can cause difficulty with very dry foods. Aging also brings about a reduction in the acids secreted by the stomach. The difficulty some older people experience with milk digestion is caused by an age-related reduction in the intestinal enzyme lactase, which breaks down lactose, a principal sugar in dairy products. In addition, intestinal motility—the involuntary folding and unfolding of the intestine that causes food to move through it—decreases with age. Dietary fiber, also referred to as *roughage*, is a particularly vital dietary component of older adults because it facilitates the transit of food through the intestine. Dietary fiber also has a protective function against certain diseases such as colon cancer.

What Do Older People Need?

■ *Food Groups*

A well-balanced diet provides the body with the vitamins, minerals, proteins, fats, and carbohydrates needed for daily energy requirements, continued cell production (which never ceases throughout life), and overall maintenance of good health. The ideal diet has both balance and variety. For seniors, nutritional authorities recommend the following amounts of daily nourishment from each of the four basic food groups:

Bread and cereal: 4 or more servings. These provide proteins, iron, vitamin B, and carbohydrates. Enriched flour and cornmeal offer vitamins B_1, B_2, B_3, B_6 (niacin), and iron. Whole-grain flour, bread, and brown rice contain other B vitamins, minerals, and desirable fiber.

Meat, poultry, fish, and eggs: 2 or more servings. These supply protein, fat, iron, and vitamins.

Fruits and vegetables: 4 or more servings. These supply vitamins, minerals, and fiber. Citrus fruits are an important source of vitamin C, while dark green or yellow vegetables provide vitamin A.

Dairy products: 2 or more cups of milk (or its equivalent). These supply calcium, protein, fat, and vitamins.

A diet that includes foods from each of these four groups daily is well balanced, and sufficient choices exist within each group to provide variety.

Fiber is an important component in a well-balanced diet, because it absorbs water, adding bulk to the food passing through the gastrointestinal tract and facilitating its elimination. Constipation—a common problem in the elderly, and related to a decrease in intestinal muscle tone—can be treated effectively with a high-fiber diet.

■ Vitamins and Minerals

Despite the reduced caloric needs of older people, it is important to maintain ample amounts of vitamins and minerals in the diet. Vitamins are organic substances that have many essential functions in the biochemical processes of the body. Since most vitamins cannot be made in the body and by virtue of their chemical composition are extremely destructible, the availability of sufficient quantities of vitamins depends upon dietary intake.

In 1912, nutritional researchers first isolated fat-soluble and water-soluble substances that prevented disease or death in animals fed a purified diet containing only protein, carbohydrates, fat, and minerals. They had discovered the two distinct classes of vitamins, which they named "fat-soluble A" and "water-soluble B." Today vitamins are still classified into the two major categories of fat-soluble and water-soluble. There are four fat-soluble vitamins: the original vitamin A, plus vitamins D, E, and K. There are eight different water-soluble vitamins: vitamin C and the vitamins of the B complex.

The primary differences in these two classes of minerals are their absorption and storage characteristics. Fat-soluble vitamins are absorbed into the lymphatic system, while water-soluble vitamins are absorbed into the bloodstream. As dietary excess of fat-soluble vitamins is stored by the body for future use, this group is not an absolutely necessary part of daily dietary intake. Excess amounts of water-soluble vitamins, on the other hand, are excreted in the urine and only minimal storage is possible. Thus, water-soluble vitamins must be supplied in the diet every day.

■ Vitamin D and Calcium

Among the fat-soluble vitamins, vitamin D is most frequently seen as deficient in the elderly. Vitamin D is required for the absorption of calcium, and it is believed that insufficient amounts of these two nutrients contribute to loss of bone mass (osteoporosis), which results in brittle bones and fractures in the elderly. Calcium is an important ingredient in the bone mineralization (building) process, and it is now established that prolonged

insufficiency in calcium intake is among the primary factors that predispose to osteoporosis.

Women are at higher risk of osteoporosis than men because they have less initial bone mass, and because the female hormone estrogen plays a vital role in calcium utilization. Menopause—the time during middle age when a woman's body stops producing estrogen—is therefore a period of increased risk for those who do not receive estrogen replacement therapy. The 1984 National Institutes of Health Consensus Conference report recommends a calcium intake of 1,000 to 1,500 milligrams per day for postmenopausal women, depending upon whether or not they are receiving estrogen. Dietary sources of calcium are shown in Table 1, together with their caloric content.

Dietary vitamin D, as well as the form produced in the skin, must be acted upon by the liver and kidney to render it biologically active. A group of investigators at the University of Wisconsin studied the changes that occur with aging in the conversion of vitamin D to its nutritionally active form, a process that diminishes with age. These workers treated a group of patients who had osteoporosis with the active form of vitamin D and observed an improvement in calcium absorption compared to a control group receiving placebo.

■ Water-Soluble Vitamins and Folic Acid

Studies show that the elderly often are deficient in vitamins B_{12} and folic acid. Vitamin B_{12} is essential for cellular function, particularly in the bone marrow, nervous system, and gastrointestinal tract. It is also involved in the metabolism of other nutrients such as protein and carbohydrates.

Vitamin B_{12} is unique among the vitamins in that its absorption requires the presence of a substance called *intrinsic factor*, which is contained in gastric juices. Although low levels of vitamin B_{12} may be caused by low production of intrinsic factor in the stomach, many elderly people do not eat foods sufficiently rich in this vitamin. Milk, eggs, and meat are the best sources of vitamin B_{12}, while fresh fruits and vegetables are high in folic acid.

Folic acid deficiency is a prime cause of anemia in the elderly. Diets low in folic acid are likely also to be low in vitamin C. Bananas, lima beans, liver, and brewer's yeast contain folic acid that is readily available for absorption, while orange juice, romaine lettuce, eggyolk, cabbage, defatted soy bean, and wheat germ contain lower amounts of

Table 1

CALCIUM AND CALORIC CONTENT OF VARIOUS FOODS*

Food	Amount	Ca (mg)	Calories
DAIRY PRODUCTS			
Milk			
Whole, 3.5%	1 cup	288	159
Nonfat (skim)	1 cup	296	88
Butter, stick	½ cup	23	812.5
Buttermilk	1 cup	296	88
Cheese			
Blue or Roquefort	1 cu in	54	64
Camembert	1 wedge	40	114
Cheddar	1 cu in	129	68
Cottage	12 oz	320	360
Parmesan, grated	1 tbsp	68	23
Swiss (natural)	1 cu in	139	56
Swiss (processed)	1 cu in	159	64
American	1 cu in	122	65
Cream			
Half-and-half	1 tbsp	16	20
Light	1 tbsp	15	32
Sour	1 tbsp	12	22
Custard, baked	1 cup	297	305
Ice cream	1 cup	194	257
Ice milk			
Hardened	1 cup	204	199
Soft-serve	1 cup	273	266
Margarine, stick	½ cup	23	816
Pudding			
Chocolate	1 cup	250	385
Vanilla	1 cup	298	283
Yogurt			
made from whole milk	1 cup	272	152
made from partially skimmed milk	1 cup	294	123
MEAT, POULTRY, AND SEAFOOD			
Beef, lean only	2½ oz	10	153
Chicken breast, fried	2½ oz	9	160
Eggs			
Whole	1 egg	27	82
Yolk of egg	1 yolk	24	59
Scrambled with milk and fat	1 egg	51	111
Clams	3 oz	53	65
Crabmeat, canned	3 oz	38	91
Haddock, breaded, fried	3 oz	34	141
Oysters, raw	1 cup	226	158
Salmon, pink, canned	3 oz	167	120
Sardines, canned in oil, drained	3 oz	372	174
Shrimp, canned	3 oz	98	99
Soups			
Canned (prepared with water)			
Clam chowder	1 cup	34	81
Cream of chicken	1 cup	24	94
Cream of mushroom	1 cup	41	134
Minestrone	1 cup	37	105
Tuna, canned in oil, drained	3 oz	7	167
VEGETABLES			
Asparagus, green	1 cup	37	36
Beans			
Lima	1 cup	80	189
Red kidney	1 cup	74	218
Snap (green or yellow)	1 cup	72	31
Beets	1 cup	29	58
Broccoli, cooked	1 stalk	158	47
Brussels sprouts	1 cup	50	56
Cabbage			
Raw	1 cup	39	20
Cooked	1 cup	64	29
Red, raw, coarsely shredded	1 cup	29	22
Carrots	1 cup	45	48
Cashew nuts	1 cup	53	785
Cauliflower, cooked	1 cup	25	28
Celery, pieces	1 cup	39	20
Collards, cooked	1 cup	289	51
Mustard greens, cooked	1 cup	193	32
Onions			
Raw	1 onion	30	44
Cooked	1 cup	50	61
Parsnips, cooked	1 cup	70	102
Peanuts, roasted	1 cup	107	838
Peas, green	1 cup	44	114
Pumpkin, canned	1 cup	57	81
Sauerkraut, canned	1 cup	85	42
Spinach	1 cup	200	41
Squash, cooked	1 cup	55	129
Sweet potatoes	1 med	52	185
Tomatoes	1 med	24	40
Tomato catsup	1 cup	60	289
Turnips, cooked	1 cup	54	36
Turnip greens, cooked	1 cup	252	28
FRUITS AND FRUIT PRODUCTS			
Apricots			
Canned in heavy syrup	1 cup	28	222
Dried, uncooked	1 cup	100	338
Avocados	1 med	26	378
Blackberries, raw	1 cup	46	84
Blueberries, raw	1 cup	21	90
Cantaloupes, raw, medium	½ melon	27	82
Cherries, canned, red	1 cup	37	105
Dates, pitted	1 cup	105	488
Grapefruit, pink	½ med	20	50
Grapefruit juice	1 cup	23	96
Grape juice (canned or bottled)	1 cup	28	167
Lime juice	1 cup	22	64
Oranges	1 med	54	71
Orange juice	1 cup	26	112
Papayas, raw	1 cup	36	73
Peaches, dried	1 cup	77	419
Pineapple, raw	1 cup	27	81
Pineapple juice, canned	1 cup	37	138
Plums, canned	1 cup	36	114
Prunes, cooked	1 cup	60	253
Prune juice, bottled	1 cup	36	197
Raspberries, raw	1 cup	27	70
Rhubarb, cooked	1 cup	212	381
Strawberries, raw	1 cup	31	55
Tangerines	1 med	34	39
Watermelon	4-in wedge	30	111
GRAIN PRODUCTS			
Barley	1 cup	32	698
Biscuits, homemade	1 biscuit	34	103
Bran flakes with raisins	1 cup	28	144
Bread	1 slice	23	74
Cakes (from mixes)	1 piece	55	308
Cupcakes (from mixes)	1 small	43	88
Cornmeal	1 cup	23	433
Farina, cooked	1 cup	147	105
Muffins, enriched white flour	1 muffin	42	118
Oats	1 cup	44	99
Oatmeal	1 cup	22	132
Pancakes			
Wheat flour	1 cake	27	62
Plain or buttermilk	1 cake	58	61
Pie			
Butterscotch	4-in sec	98	344
Custard	4-in sec	125	280
Mince	4-in sec	38	364
Pecan	4-in sec	55	488
Pumpkin	4-in sec	166	272
Pizza, cheese	5½-in sec	107	153
Rice, cooked	1 cup	21	223
Rolls			
Frankfurter or hamburger	1 roll	30	119
Hard	1 roll	24	156
Spaghetti with meatballs			
Home recipe	1 cup	124	332
Canned	1 cup	53	258
Waffles			
Enriched flour	1 waffle	85	209
From mix	1 waffle	179	206
SUGARS AND SWEETS			
Caramels	1 oz	42	113
Chocolate, milk, plain	1 oz	65	147
Fudge, plain	1 oz	22	113
Molasses, blackstrap	1 tbsp	137	43
Sherbet	1 cup	31	259
Sugar, brown	1 cup	187	821
NUTS AND BEANS			
Almonds	½ cup	160	425
Pecans	½ cup	42	406
Tofu (soybean curd)	3½ oz	128	72
Walnuts	½ cup	50	326

* Calcium content derived from M. V. Krause and L. K. Mahan, *Food, Nutrition and Diet Therapy* (Philadelphia: W. B. Saunders Co., 1979). Calorie content derived from *Nutritive Value of American Foods* (U.S. Dept. of Agriculture, 1975).
Table reprinted by courtesy of Marion Laboratories, Kansas City, Mo.

folic acid at lower levels of biologic availability.

Low levels of vitamin C often are found in the elderly, particularly in cigarette smokers, those with digestive disease, and nursing-home residents. Vitamin C deficiency in the elderly usually is not linked to any clinical disease or dysfunction.

While serious deficiencies in water-soluble vitamins are rare in the aged, dietary intake is commonly below recommended levels. The benefits of B-complex and vitamin C supplementation have been promoted by some nutritionists as a source of improved health and vigor in the aged, but there is insufficient scientific evidence to support this. In fact, excess intake of certain water-soluble vitamins has been associated with detrimental effects such as liver damage (niacin) and development of urinary tract stones (vitamin C).

■ *Iron, Zinc, Potassium, and Magnesium*

The primary mineral found lacking in the diets of the elderly is iron. Iron, like vitamin D, requires the presence of a stomach acid (hydrochloric) for conversion to its biological absorbable form. Many older people secrete less hydrochloric acid than normal, and may consequently be absorbing dietary iron poorly. Daily iron-intake recommendations for the elderly range from 10 to 18 milligrams per day. The best way to ensure adequate iron intake without consuming too much red meat is to use iron-fortified foods, particularly cereals.

It is extremely important to remember that older persons should never take iron supplements such as tonics or iron tablets without a doctor's order. This is because one of the most common causes of iron-deficiency anemia in the elderly is slow, unrecognized loss of blood. The most common underlying cause of such blood loss—especially in older age groups—is cancer, and anemia is often the first clue that something is wrong.

The role of zinc in various metabolic processes has been identified relatively recently, and researchers continue to investigate possible links between zinc deficiency and certain ailments. Zinc has been found to hasten wound healing in postoperative patients, while deficiencies in this mineral have been associated with mental changes including memory impairment, confusion, and depression, and impairment of the senses of taste and smell.

The current adult RDA for zinc is 20 milligrams per day. The richest dietary sources of zinc are seafoods, meats, corn, beets, and peas. The zinc contained in whole grains and vegetables is much less readily absorbed than that found in animal products, and foods rich in fiber interfere with the absorption of zinc. Recent recognition of the benefits of zinc and its relative scarcity in foods has resulted in the addition of zinc to fortified foods and vitamin supplements. Zinc overdosage is not believed to cause a problem, unless levels are several times in excess of the RDAs.

Potassium is another mineral in which older people may become deficient, particularly while taking diuretic medications (water pills) for high blood pressure. In the process of promoting the excretion of unwanted salt and fluid from the body, these medications also cause excess loss of potassium—a condition called *hypokalemia*.

Potassium deficiency may cause a feeling of fatigue and listlessness. Common symptoms include muscle weakness, cramps, diarrhea, vomiting, and appetite loss. Potassium is widely distributed in foods, especially meats, milk, vegetables, and fruits. Bananas, oranges, and tomatoes are especially rich sources. As a general rule, potassium supplementation is therefore not necessary, except for persons who are taking diuretic medications.

Another mineral that plays a role in many aspects of body chemistry is magnesium. It is essential for the activation of enzyme systems needed for the proper use of other minerals; it is necessary also for the normal functioning of nerve and muscle cells. While serious magnesium deficiency usually is associated with conditions that cause excessive loss of this mineral (such as alcoholism and prolonged vomiting or diarrhea), marginal deficiencies resulting from inadequate dietary intake are believed to be fairly common. Dietary sources of magnesium include cocoa, nuts, soybeans, whole grains, and molasses.

■ *Protein*

Proteins are found in every cell of the body, and are essential participants in various biochemical processes. Proteins function as structural components of body tissue, as regulators of the body's water balance, and as carriers of oxygen. In reference to nutritional requirements, proteins are categorized generally as either complete or incomplete. *Complete proteins* contain all of the nine essential amino acids the body needs, while *incomplete proteins* do not supply enough of all nine.

The quality of a particular dietary protein is

based roughly on the degree to which its amino-acid pattern is complete. Thus, the higher the quality of the protein food, the less the amount of protein that needs to be included in the diet. Many foods contain significant amounts of protein. All foods of animal origin provide complete proteins, while incomplete proteins come primarily from plant foods such as vegetables, grain products, and nuts. Foods containing incomplete proteins can be rendered complete by combining two different incomplete but complementary proteins that together provide all nine essential amino acids.

As mentioned earlier in this section, recent scientific evidence suggests that the protein requirement for the elderly should be raised to 1 gram of protein per kilogram (2.2 pounds) of body weight per day. This is because the elderly are less able to synthesize dietary proteins. In addition, specific physiological stresses such as surgery, infection, physical injury, burns, and anxiety states impose increased protein needs. However, this issue has not yet been fully resolved, since other believe that protein requirements in the elderly should be lower than the adult RDAs. Some nutritionists believe that reduced ability to synthesize protein should be accompanied by lower protein intake, and that high protein intake may contribute to the development of osteoporosis.

■ Sodium

Studies have shown that most Americans, including the older population, take in more dietary salt (sodium) than the body requires. Through its ability to attract and hold water in the blood vessels, sodium plays a vital role in maintaining blood volume and pressure at normal levels. However, very little sodium intake is required for the performance of these basic functions. Excess salt intake, on the other hand, is one of several factors known to aggravate high blood pressure, and the first step in treating blood-pressure elevations is a reduction in dietary sodium intake.

The National Research Council indicates that a safe and adequate sodium intake for adults is between 1,100 and 3,300 milligrams per day. One teaspoon of salt contains about 2,000mg. of sodium, so the daily requirement is easily fulfilled. In fact, most American diets contain considerably more than the recommended allowance of sodium; estimates place average daily sodium consumption at between 2,300 and 6,900mg.

Thus, the sodium content of foods is usually a concern with respect to avoidance rather than meeting minimal nutritional requirements. As a rule, fresh, frozen, and canned fruits and fruit juices are low in sodium, as are fresh or frozen vegetables and grain products cooked without salt. Milk and dairy products and meat, poultry, and fish contain varying amounts of sodium.

The experienced consumer will soon discover that there are quite dramatic brand-to-brand differences in the sodium content of the same type of food. For example, Arnold's Brick Oven whole-wheat bread contains 69mg. sodium per serving as compared to Wonder brand whole-wheat bread, which contains 375mg. per serving. The careful shopper can cut down considerably on sodium intake simply by taking the time to read the nutritional information labels printed on all food packaging.

■ Carbohydrates

Intake of carbohydrates (sugars and starches) should be limited because these contain primarily calories. Because energy needs generally decrease with age, older people do not require as many calories as younger adults, and excess caloric intake can lead to obesity.

The carbohydrates to choose are those of whole-grain products, fruits, vegetables, and potatoes. These foods also supply B vitamins, vitamin A, iron, various trace minerals, and fiber.

■ Fats

A low-fat diet is recommended for the elderly. There are two major types of dietary fat. Fats made primarily from saturated fatty acids come mainly from animal sources and are called *saturated fats*, while those made from polyunsaturated fatty acids are called *unsaturated fats*. These are mainly vegetable fats. Saturated fats raise the level of blood cholesterol, while unsaturated fats lower it. Excess dietary intake of cholesterol is believed by many to be a major cause of coronary artery disease.

Medical opinion differs about the benefits of cholesterol reduction in older people. While many nutritionists disagree, there is growing evidence that lowering blood cholesterol may be of little value in the prevention of coronary artery disease in persons over 60 or 65 years of age.

To help decrease total dietary fat, skim milk should be substituted for whole milk. Fried foods should be avoided, and all visible fat trimmed off meat prior to cooking. Processed and snack foods are generally quite high in fat, and their intake should be minimized.

Exercise and Aging

Throughout the human life span, the components of body composition—primarily fat distribution and muscle—are modified by both nutritional status and physical activity. While the health-promoting effects of exercise have been demonstrated mostly in younger age groups, gerontologic research has focused recently on exercise response at older ages.

The findings show clearly that exercise improves both overall physical capacity and cardiovascular function in the elderly—particularly when performed with sufficient frequency, intensity, and duration. According to experts, it is possible for healthy aging individuals to delay the physiologic decline and changes in body composition associated with aging by incorporating regular exercise into their daily routine.

Among the many known physiologic benefits of exercise are that it
- improves the circulation and cardiovascular function
- enhances oxygen uptake from the blood
- improves lung function
- increases glucose tolerance
- strengthens bone (weight-bearing exercises)

The gains more directly related to personal satisfaction are that exercise
- alleviates minor aches and pains
- helps improve morale through feeling and looking well
- enhances agility and mobility
- restores elasticity and strength to muscles
- builds endurance
- improves posture

Exercise is also believed to influence both the length and quality of life. It offers a way to attain, or maintain, the physical and mental health necessary for continued enjoyment of a mobile and independent life-style during old age.

Physical activity equips persons of all ages to withstand the stresses of daily life by reducing mental fatigue, tension, strain, and boredom. Older people who engage in daily exercise are less likely to feel chronic fatigue than those who are inactive, since tiredness often results from poor circulation due to lack of exercise. Besides

making one feel better, exercise also helps to keep people looking and acting younger. Studies show that in societies where regular physical activity and a proper diet are part of the life-style, older persons past retirement age continue to be physically vigorous.

A frequently overlooked benefit of exercise is the effect it has upon the general physical agility. This can help reduce the possibility of injury from falls.

Another important benefit of exercise is its ability to aid in weight control. The problem of overweight among older people may be caused as much by inactivity as by overeating. For example, an excess of only 100 calories a day can produce a 10-pound gain in one year; on the other hand, those extra calories can be burned up during a 15- to 20-minute daily walk. According to findings from the Harvard School of Public Health, half hour of proper exercise a day can take off up to 26 pounds a year.

■ Establishing an Exercise Program

Before selecting any exercise—but particularly prior to undertaking strenuous activities such as running—persons over 40 years of age should undergo a physical examination. This is to ensure that there is no underlying health reason, such as undiagnosed heart disease, that would preclude certain exercises. Physicians are prepared to perform exercise stress testing in persons for whom it is indicated, and to advise about appropriate exercise regimens.

The exercise program selected should meet three conditions: 1) Exercise should be commensurate with one's physical capabilities; 2) it should make sufficient demands on the body to be beneficial; 3) perhaps above all, it should be enjoyable. Not all physical activities generally considered under the category of "exercise" offer equal physiologic benefits. Older people should not embark upon regimens that are unrealistically strenuous. Rather, as at any age, one's exercise capacity should be built up gradually through increasing the intensity and/or duration of exercise.

While exercise that benefits the body and makes it stronger and healthier usually requires a certain amount of hard work, exercise does not need to be painful or unpleasant to be good for you. The tendency to equate the degree of pain a fitness activity causes with its level of expected benefit can be downright harmful if overdoing causes damage to tissues or bones.

Finally, exercise should be enjoyable. It is human nature to put off doing what is not pleasant, and exercise that is done purely out of a belief that it is "good for you" is no exception. The type of exercise and the time of day it is done are personal choices that may make a difference between whether or not one adheres to a regular routine. While it is best not to exercise right after a meal (when a greater proportion of the circulating blood should be in the digestive system rather than in the muscles), there is no fast rule that exercises must be performed at a certain time of day. For example, some people, who would abhor the thought of early-morning exercise are quite happy with the same activity performed later in the day.

■ Walking: The Ideal Exercise

Despite the popularity of strenuous endeavors, such as running, and of newer concepts in exercise such as aerobics, walking remains the number one participation sport in the United States. As of 1986, some 55 million Americans were walking for fitness, and almost twice as many are expected to do so by 1990. Thus, walking remains the classic exercise that Hippocrates long ago named "man's best medicine." It benefits the body, eases the mind, and is relaxing and energizing.

Several reasons account for the large numbers of people who walk for fitness. A walking regimen is flexible, it is easy to take up, and it does not require special skills, equipment, or attire. About the only accessory required for walking is a pair of comfortable shoes. Recognizing the popularity of walking, many shoe manufacturers now offer shoes specially designed for walking. These feature a shock-absorbing heel and a flexible, curved sole. However, the primary measure of a good walking shoe remains the comfort it affords the wearer.

Walking is surprisingly beneficial. According to estimates of energy requirements, a brisk walk takes six to seven times the energy required to sit quietly—or about the equivalent of playing singles tennis. Studies have also shown that walking is quite effective for weight reduction. Figure 1 shows the relative amounts of calories burned up

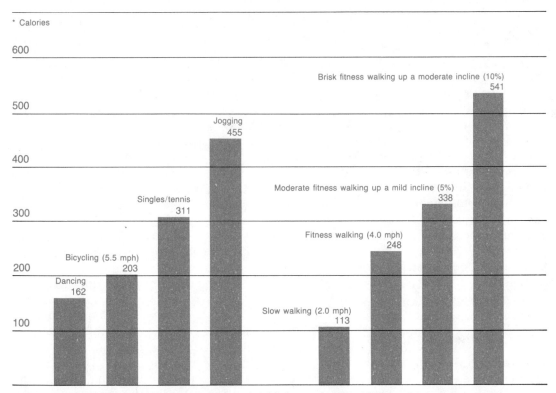

*Calories expended during a typical 45-minute session for each activity for an average-sized (150-pound) male. An average-sized (124-pound) female would burn 20 percent fewer calories.
Source: *Walking*, Jan. 1986, p. 18.

Figure 1 *Fitness Walking for Weight Control*

by walking at various speeds compared with values for other sports or recreational pursuits.

An important recommendation for walking lies in what it does *not* do. Compared to other exercises, walking is a relatively injury-free activity, and this is an important consideration when one is older.

It is reported that fitness can be achieved with daily vigorous walking for regular periods of time, no matter what the person's age or previous level of activity.

■ *Aerobics*

The word *aerobic* means the ability to live, grow, or take place only where free oxygen is present. Aerobic exercises are those that can be persisted in for a sustained period of time, during which the supply of oxygen to the muscles is adequate for their needs. In calisthenics, an oxygen debt is incurred, and after a time, the exercise must stop. The objective is to improve the body's efficiency in processing oxygen for use by various vital organs such as the heart and lungs. Aerobic exercises include fast walking, running, swimming, bicycling—any activity that is continuous rather than stop-and-start.

Several benefits of aerobic exercise have been established in older people. These include:

Heart: The aging heart and the nervous and muscular systems respond well to aerobic training, showing an increase in capacity and enzymatic function.

Bones: Exercised bones do not demineralize (lose density and become brittle) or lose their range of motion as readily as unexercised bones.

Lungs: Exercised lungs still show age-related changes, but lung capacity is far less diminished than that of sedentary older people.

Mental capacity: Studies of the effects of exercise on mental function in persons over 60 show that a sufficiently rigorous regimen lasting ten to twelve weeks improves one's sense of well-being, decision-making ability, and memory function.

Sleep: Exercise promotes sleep.

■ *Some Exercise Pointers for Seniors*

Once an exercise program is begun, here are some pointers to keep in mind:
- Start exercising gradually, for about five to ten minutes at first—especially if you have been inactive.
- Increase the amount of exercise each day.

- Avoid dizziness by pausing briefly before changing direction.
- Breathe deeply and evenly—don't hold your breath.
- Rest whenever necessary.
- Keep a daily written record of your progress.
- Exercise to lively music or TV or with friends to make it more enjoyable.
- Always pay attention to what your body tells you. If you feel much discomfort, you are trying to do too much.
- Consider the benefits as you exercise.

■ *Finding an Exercise Program*

Most communities have centers where older people can join exercise classes and other recreational programs. One can find out about fitness programs at a local church or synagogue, civic center, community college, park or recreation association, senior citizens' center, or service organizations such as an Area Agency on Aging. Community Jewish Centers, YMCAs, and YWCAs usually offer a variety of programs. Organized activities designed for older adults provide many benefits for those who have been inactive or who have specific health considerations.

A list of information sources and free or low-cost publications that describe exercise programs for seniors can be obtained by writing to the National Institute on Aging/Exercise, Building 31, Room 5C35, Bethesda, MD 20892.

Getting Sufficient Rest

The patterns, duration, and quality of sleep change with aging. There is increased difficulty in falling asleep and in sleeping through the night. Up to 15 percent of older people report that they sleep less than five hours a night, and up to 30 percent report frequent nightly wakenings.

Modern sleep research techniques have contributed greatly to better understanding of sleep at all ages. The discovery, in 1953, of rapid-eye-movement (REM) sleep first introduced the concept that not all sleep is alike, but rather that it occurs in stages of varying depth. The REM stage of sleep, characterized by dreaming, takes up only a part of the total sleeping time. Sleep is organized into approximately ninety-minute REM and non-REM cycles.

Non-REM sleep is subdivided into four stages.

Stage 1, the initial stage in falling asleep, is a *transitional sleep* during which the sleeping person can be aroused quite easily. Stage-2 sleep quickly follows and comprises about 50 percent of a normal night's sleep. In stages 3 and 4 the person sleeps deeply and is more difficult to arouse.

Many people notice that they become "lighter" sleepers as they grow older. Sleep researchers have shown that Stage-4 sleep gradually diminishes after age 50, and eventually disappears entirely. Stage 3 sleep either increases slightly, or remains unchanged in the 60s and 70s, and clearly declines after age 80. Thus, the age-related tendency for most sleep to occur in the "lighter" stages accounts for much of the frequent nightly awakenings that older people experience.

Although many older persons believe they need less sleep than they did at younger ages, researchers are finding that this is probably not so. Rather, there is believed to be a redistribution of sleep over the twenty-four-hour period. Because of frequent nightly wakenings or difficulty in sleeping, older people tend to nod off during the day, making up for the sleep they lose at night. Reports of reduced sleep requirements often do not take into account the total daily sleep pattern.

The sleep efficiency—the ratio of total sleep time to time spent in bed—decreases with age. While younger people fall asleep within five to ten minutes of going to bed, it takes longer to get to sleep at later ages. In addition, younger people come to total wakefulness more quickly.

■ Sleep Disturbances

Insomnia is characterized by difficulty in falling asleep and staying asleep, and/or wakening too early in the morning. A common complaint in older people, insomnia stems from a variety of sources. In the elderly, a frequent cause is the psychological stress that accompanies various losses, disappointments, or fears. Depression is linked with insomnia at all ages.

Other causes of insomnia in the elderly include a variety of organic brain syndromes (dementias), including Alzheimer's disease, and several medical conditions; chronic pain from ailments such as osteoarthritis is frequently responsible for sleep disturbances in the elderly.

Treatment of Sleep Disorders in Later Life

Before prescribing sleeping medications, physi-cians usually suggest a number of behavioral adaptations that are frequently effective in overcoming sleep problems. For example, the importance of maintaining a regular sleep-wake cycle is well established. The nine-to-five schedule that most people adhere to from school age onward accustoms the body to expect rest at certain regular periods during the twenty-four-hour cycle, and these periods usually occur at night. Thus, it makes sense to keep to a regular schedule for going to bed and arising.

Some experts suggest that the sleeping area— the bed and bedroom—should be used only for sleeping, and not for reading or television viewing. However, while this practice is helpful for some people, others find that reading or watching TV in bed are pleasant and relaxing ways to prepare for sleep.

Other factors that influence the ability to sleep are room temperature and a comfortable mattress. While mattresses that are too soft are not good for posture and may contribute to orthopedic problems in the elderly, an overly hard sleeping surface makes sleep difficult for many.

Finally, many older people find that they do not sleep well if they eat a large meal or drink caffeine-containing beverages shortly before going to bed.

Sleeping medications may be helpful in overcoming temporary sleep difficulties, but there are several drawbacks associated with their use, especially in the elderly. Increased tolerance with regular use reduces the effectiveness of sedative hypnotic agents, causing some people to increase the dose to obtain the original effect. This poses the risk of accidental overdose or of inducing a state of lethargy in which the person is more likely to stumble and fall.

Because of the incidence of abuse and overdosage, barbiturates are infrequently prescribed today. Instead, most doctors prefer benzodiazepine derivatives such as temazepam or flurazepam. The lower dose of both agents (15mg.) has been found effective in most elderly patients. Patients who have difficulty sleeping because of depression may be treated more appropriately with an antidepressive medication.

Most experts agree that regular use of sleeping medications is not an effective way to treat sleep disorders because of the buildup of tolerance and the likelihood of other adverse effects from long-term use.

Many older people find that they sleep better if they add a little exercise to their daily routine.

29

AGING AND MENTAL HEALTH

A primary concern people express about aging has to do with the fear of losing their mental capabilities. Research into aging has now established that mental deterioration is *not* a normal consequence of aging.

Today's sophisticated medical technologies make it possible to study brain chemistry and function much more precisely than ever before. By these techniques—which include electron microscopy, computerized tomography (CT), and electroencephalography (EEG)—scientists are now able to distinguish between normal and pathologic changes that take place in the aging brain.

The Aging Brain

Many structural changes originally identified in the brains of demented persons (those with irreversible organic brain deterioration) are present also in the normal aging brain. The distinction between normal and pathologic changes lies in the extent, rather than the type, of structural and functional changes that occur.

The normal aging brain loses 5 percent of its total mass by age 70, and this increases to 10 percent by age 80 and to 20 percent by the age of 90. Changes in the protein structure of nerve cells in the cortex (outer layer) of the brain lead to an accumulation of abnormal fibers called *neurofibrillary tangles*. Once considered a unique feature of Alzheimer's disease, this structural alteration has since been identified as part of the normal aging process. In addition, age-related changes have been observed to occur in cerebral neurotransmitter and receptor function.

Senility: Myth or Reality?

Senility is a catch-all term still commonly used to describe a number of mental conditions characterized by forgetfulness or confusion and believed to be directly related to advanced age. While not a medical term, the word *senility* came to be used by professionals and lay persons alike, and was understood to encompass various degrees of age-related mental deterioration. In the past it was believed that almost all people would ultimately get senile if they lived long enough.

Recent scientific evidence indicates that loss of mental capabilities beyond minor lapses in memory is not a normal sign of aging, but rather a manifestation of one of several diseases. The term *dementia* is used now to describe deterioration in mental function from various causes. Dementia is defined as loss of intellectual capabilities of sufficient severity to interfere with social or occupational functioning; it is characterized by impairment in memory and judgment.

Dementias are classified generally into *reversible* and *irreversible* types. *True dementia* occurs with irreversible organic brain changes that exceed those of normal aging, while *pseudodementia* is used to describe transient states of mental deterioration that are generally reversible with appropriate treatment. As in the case of Alzheimer's disease, the term "senile" may be used together with "dementia" to denote conditions that typically appear at older ages.

Alzheimer's Disease

Of the 3 to 4 million older Americans who suffer from some type of dementia, 500,000 have senile dementia of the Alzheimer's type, or SDAT. Senile dementia of the Alzheimer's type accounts for over 50 percent of all dementias that occur in the elderly.

Now regarded as the major form of old-age "senility," SDAT is a disorder that affects the cells of the brain. These changes differ from those associated with normal aging primarily in the extent to which they are present. Although Alzheimer's disease is most prevalent among persons over 65, some individuals are afflicted at much earlier ages.

Like those seen with normal aging, the changes most commonly associated with SDAT occur in nerve cell proteins of the cerebral cortex. The resulting neurofibrillary tangles were first described by the German neurologist Alois Alzheimer in 1906. In addition, groups of nerve endings throughout the cerebral cortex degenerate and disrupt the passage of electrochemical signals between brain cells. These degenerative areas are called plaques, and the greater the number of plaques and tangles, the greater the resulting disturbance in intellectual function and memory. Patients with SDAT have also been found to be particularly deficient in the enzyme choline acetyltransferase.

Until recently, most adult dementia was blamed on poor circulation resulting from "hardening of the arteries." However, studies of brain blood flow demonstrate that circulatory deficits

in patients with SDAT are related to choline-acetyltransferase deficiency and plaque formation rather than to arteriosclerotic changes. Other avenues of research into the possible causes of Alzheimer's disease include examination of toxic, immunologic, and viral factors.

There is evidence, for example, that SDAT is accompanied by excessively high blood levels of aluminum, but it remains to be determined whether the accumulation of trace metals in the brain is an important predisposing factor to the development of SDAT. Other researchers are examining the possibility that SDAT may be transmitted by a slow-acting virus, while still others are investigating the relationship between changes in the immune system and central-nervous-system disease.

The onset of Alzheimer's disease is usually quite imperceptible. At first there are only minor symptoms that can be explained on the basis of an emotional upset or a physical illness. As the disease progresses, however, the afflicted individual becomes increasingly more forgetful, particularly about recent events. Routine tasks such as turning off the oven may be overlooked, and familiar objects like house keys frequently are misplaced.

As time goes on, patients begin to express concern over their forgetfulness and attempt to compensate by making lists and rechecking the performance of routine tasks. Ultimately, the frustrations encountered in day-to-day living lead to increased irritability, restlessness, and agitation. The afflicted person becomes increasingly more confused, and family and friends notice a distinct difference in personality, behavior, and mood. Judgment, concentration, orientation, and even speech become affected, particularly with regard to difficulty in finding the right words. In the most severe cases, the disease eventually renders its victims totally incapable of caring for themselves.

To date, there is no cure for SDAT. The duration of the disease depends upon age of onset, individual health status, available supports, and treatment of concurrent health problems. Although symptoms are progressive, there is great individual variation in the rate at which changes occur. In a few cases, there may be a rapid decline, but more commonly many months go by with little further deterioration.

Even when a loving and caring family is available for support, the victims of Alzheimer's disease usually spend their last days in a nursing home or long-term care facility. Limitations in physical activity during the later stages of the disease may lower resistance to pneumonia and other physical illnesses, which are usually the direct cause of death in patients with Alzheimer's disease. The life span after onset of SDAT ranges from seven to twenty years or longer.

Although there is no treatment for Alzheimer's disease, proper medical care can help reduce many of its symptoms. Several guidelines have been established by medical professionals to assist the victim and the family in coping with the significant impact the disease has on their lives.

Persons suffering from Alzheimer's disease should always be under the care of a physician who will be able to treat the physical ailments that may further complicate the disease. The family general practice physician is an excellent choice because he or she knows the patient and the family and therefore represents continuity of personalized care—an important anchor for those whose lives are losing much of their former stability. All physicians are acquainted with Alzheimer's disease, and it is important to select one who is willing and able to devote the required time and interest to closely monitoring treatment and answering the many questions that will arise.

Judicious use of tranquilizers can lessen agitation, anxiety, and unpredictable behavior. Sleep disturbances—which are a prominent symptom of Alzheimer's disease—may also be improved with medication. Proper nourishment and fluid intake are very important, but specialized diets are not required. Carefully planned exercise is helpful, and physical therapy can assist with the difficulties that may arise in physical functioning.

Family members should aim to maintain activities as close to a normal level as possible. The patient should be encouraged to continue his or her accustomed daily routine. Memory aids can be used to avoid the frustration that stems from inability to remember simple daily routines. These include calendars, lists of daily tasks, and written reminders about routine safety measures.

Although the daily environment should be kept familiar and orderly to avoid the necessity for continuous adaptations, it is important not to prevent the person from trying something new. For example, an individual with Alzheimer's disease may do very well on a trip or social visit when accompanied by a supportive family member or friend.

During the early phase of the disease, Alzheimer's victims can usually be cared for by the family at home. When the condition becomes more advanced, however, a special setting with professional staff and full-time care may become necessary. A great deal of community assistance is now available for victims of Alzheimer's disease and their families.

■ ADRDA Lends a Helping Hand

No matter how loving and motivated the family, care of an Alzheimer's victim is difficult, tiring, frustrating, and seemingly unrewarding. It is painful to witness the progression of a loved one from the preliminary stages of the disease—where only minor memory lapses occur—to a point where the names of immediate family members are forgotten or familiar persons no longer are recognized. The availability of support groups is therefore extremely important to persons caring for an Alzheimer's victim.

The Alzheimer's Disease and Related Disorders Association (ADRDA) is a national organization with headquarters in Chicago. ADRDA chapters offering a wide variety of programs are located in most major cities and rural areas in nearly every state. Each ADRDA chapter sponsors family support groups. Regular meetings provide a forum for caregiving families and friends to share information, get answers to their questions, and listen sympathetically to others who face what has been called "the 36-hour day."

Chapters also provide reliable information about medical, nursing, or respite care in the community. Helpline services assure families of quality advice on the "three A's" of local patient care—availability, accessibility, and affordability.

The Chicago chapter publishes a newsletter sharing information from ADRDA chapters nationwide. Many local ADRDA chapters also publish regular newsletters that inform members about activities and programs in their own vicinities and about research developments in the study of Alzheimer's disease.

Chapter listings appear in the local telephone book under ADRDA. Information can also be obtained by writing to Alzheimer's Disease and Related Disorders Association, Inc., 70 East Lake Street, Chicago, IL 60601.

Other Irreversible Dementias

The other irreversible dementias include multi-infarct dementia and Huntington's disease. The former is more common in men than in women and usually begins in the seventh decade of life.

Multi-infarct dementia is characterized by the presence of multiple areas of infarction (the death of cells resulting from prolonged lack of oxygen supply) throughout the brain.

Cerebral infarction is caused by obstruction of the blood vessels of the brain from any cause, such as thrombosis or embolism. Hypertension is present in most patients with this disorder, but it is not a necessary prerequisite for its development. Multi-infarct dementia accounts for approximately 8 percent of all dementias in the elderly.

Huntington's disease is a hereditary disorder accounting for some 5 percent of all elderly dementias. It is characterized by movement abnormalities stemming from atrophy (wasting away) of brain tissue. Symptoms of the disease usually begin between the ages of 30 and 50, and are characterized most often by increased moodiness, stubbornness, and apathy.

Reversible Dementias

■ Pseudodementia

Pseudodementia is a term used to describe a particular form of depressive illness that causes mental changes similar to those of true dementia. Several clinical factors related to the type of onset and duration of symptoms distinguish pseudodementia from true dementia. Unlike true dementia, the patient with pseudodementia usually shows a relatively well-defined onset and rapid progression of mental dysfunction.

Affected individuals show lack of interest in people and activities around them. They frequently prefer to answer questions with an "I don't know" rather than make the small effort needed to give a thoughtful response. There is a general lack of willingness to perform necessary tasks, and mood changes and memory loss contribute to overall loss of social skills.

Up to 70 percent of patients with pseudodementia respond to tricyclic antidepressant medication, while others benefit from electroconvulsive therapy. Pseudodementia accounts for up to 6 percent of all dementias in the elderly.

■ Normal Pressure Hydrocephalus

In lay language *hydrocephalus* means "water on the brain," a condition that occurs both in infants at birth and in adults at old age. It is caused by a deficiency in the ability to absorb cerebrospinal fluid from the brain into the blood vessels.

The brain contains four reservoirs called *ventricles,* which normally produce about a half quart of cerebrospinal fluid daily. This fluid surrounds the brain, serving as a shock absorber. As new fluid is formed, openings in the brain allow the existing fluid to flow out into the spinal cord. The balance of fluid in the brain is regulated further by large veins in the membranes covering the brain, which also absorb fluid.

Childhood hydrocephalus is a congenital condition in which the head becomes noticeably enlarged, as distention of the cerebral ventricles leads to the spreading apart of still-soft skull bones. Adult hydrocephalus, on the other hand, produces no obvious physical signs, and is suspected in someone who shows mental changes combined with disturbances of gait and urinary incontinence.

The cause of pressure hydrocephalus in the elderly remains unclear, although it may be related to certain central-nervous-system diseases. The usual treatment consists of the surgical creation of an artificial shunt that helps absorption of cerebrospinal fluid. Improvement following this operation is variable, and long-term benefits lasting for years are relatively infrequent. Patients are susceptible to shunt failure as well as to hemorrhagic complications after surgery.

■ Drug-Related Dementia

A variety of drugs can cause dementia—either directly or as a result of the interaction between certain drugs. This is an important cause of dementia among the elderly, many of whom take multiple medications.

The most frequently implicated drugs are antihypertensive agents and drugs that affect central-nervous-system cholinergic activity, such as antiparkinsonian drugs and many antidepressive agents. The reduced central-nervous-system cholinergic activity observed in patients with SDAT suggests that anticholinergic agents may actually unmask some patients with early SDAT. Altering the drug used, or reducing the dose, usually is sufficient to reverse dementias of this type.

■ Other Reversible Dementias

A number of other medical causes account for about 9 percent of the remaining dementias in the elderly. These include diseases such as hyperthyroidism, hypothyroidism, Addison's disease, Cushing's syndrome, and hypopituitarism. In addition, physiologic states such as hypercalcemia (high blood calcium levels) or hypoglycemia (low blood sugar levels) sometimes cause dementia. Certain electrolyte disturbances, characterized by upset of the body's balance of elements such as sodium and potassium, are another potential cause. Certain nutritional deficiencies—particularly those associated with chronic alcoholism—are another leading cause of potentially reversible dementias.

Emotional Well-being in the Elderly

Old age is the period in life when many people are faced with a number of profound personal crises, including widowhood, death of contemporaries, and other major life transitions. During such times, psychological support is extremely important, and may be available from a variety of sources. Often a close contemporary who has undergone some of the same experiences can be an invaluable aid. Friendship with peers is therefore a very positive factor in the emotional well-being of the elderly.

Friendship is distinguished from many other roles in life in that it is optional rather than obligatory. Bonds of friendship generally develop only between people who view one another as equals and have common interests and experiences that they can share freely. For these reasons, friendships most frequently involve persons of the same generation who are at similar stages in life.

Friendships with peers and work associates are often more effective alternatives to marriage than are relationships with adult children. Because friendship is based on mutual choice and need between equals, it often sustains an older person's sense of usefulness and self-esteem more effectively than his family relationships. It has been shown, for example, that the morale of people who are isolated in old age but who have one intimate friendship is as high as that of older persons who have a wider social participation.

■ *Support Groups*

The fundamental concept of support groups is that persons with similar problems can help others through sharing their own experience. This has been demonstrated by programs such as Alcoholics Anonymous, Weight Watchers, and

Mothers Against Drunk Driving (MADD). Support from persons who themselves have confronted and overcome a particular problem appears to be effective because it stems from genuine understanding and empathy. Group members help one another by sharing constructive ways of dealing with similar emotions and life adjustments.

Several such groups are available for senior citizens. The AARP's Widowed Persons' Service offers emotional support to widowed persons through trained volunteers who themselves have been widowed. In addition to group meetings, local services may include volunteer outreach, telephone referral, and public education.

Similarly, the ADRDA sponsors support groups for families of persons with Alzheimer's disease.

One consideration regarding support-group utilization by seniors is acceptance of the group concept. Older generations, brought up with values of self-reliance and stoic perseverance in the face of personal adversities, often are hesitant to reveal their most private problems to a group of total strangers. The conviction that one does not "air one's dirty laundry" in public leaves many seniors facing serious problems alone.

A good example is alcoholism, which can wreak havoc in family relations at all ages. Though less common in older than in younger adults, alcoholism is a recognized problem among the elderly. While some have drunk to excess all their lives, others begin to abuse alcohol only in later years. When the problem becomes sufficiently disruptive in the marital relationship, the nondrinking partner usually turns for sympathy to family members, who generally are not successful in influencing the drinker's behavior. Concerned family members then may recommend a group like Alcoholics Anonymous or Alanon (which helps the families of alcoholics). But all too often no step is taken by the elderly because of shame about disclosing their problem to others.

■ *Psychotherapy*

When many major life transitions and losses occur in close sequence, people may be overcome by their emotional burden. At such times, older people especially need the opportunity to talk and to have a listener. Usually the existing support systems of friends and family help sustain people during difficult times. Occasionally, however, the emotional impact of life transitions may be so great that professional help is needed.

Of all the therapeutic and counseling services, *individual psychotherapy* is the least available to older people. Surveys of mental health clinics and private psychiatric services report a low prevalence of one-to-one therapy sessions between seniors and professionals. While the high cost of private psychiatric care may be a major reason, a certain amount of bias against the aged is believed to exist among professionals. The elderly are often viewed as "poor candidates" for psychotherapy on the basis of an overall pessimism about old age and doubts about the ability of older people to adopt new attitudes and approaches to life problems.

Actual clinical experience shows that the elderly are very receptive to psychotherapy. They often show a particularly strong drive to resolve problems and put their lives in order. The elderly, like the young, can gain from insight, understanding, and an objective evaluation of their circumstances by an empathetic professional. In fact, older people are frequently better prepared for the therapeutic process as a result of already being engaged in a personal life review, which is a part of the natural course of later life.

The potential value of individual psychotherapy in the elderly is most evident in those cases where an older person, during the course of the life review, comes up against feelings of guilt, anger, or conflict that he or she cannot resolve. Frequently, the increased insight into psychologic mechanisms that a professional can provide will help the older person to achieve a satisfactory reconciliation with such unresolved feelings.

■ *Common Themes in Psychotherapy*

Older people often express a wish for a *second chance* of life, to be able to undo some of the patterns of their lives and to give newness to their experience. These people describe the monotony of their daily lives as a kind of "salt losing its savor" feeling. An older woman, for example, who had dedicated herself to home and family may express feelings of depression and uselessness because she no longer has a family to nurture.

The therapist's task then is to guide the patient in relinquishing past roles and exploring new possibilities and new interests that will prove personally rewarding.

Some older people are able to resolve their personal *feelings about death,* while others continue to deny its inevitability without apparent emotional consequences. A number of older persons, however, need help in recognizing their fears and anxieties about death and in coming to terms with the prospect of dying.

Therapists must also be able to recognize disguised fears of death. This may be expressed in a variety of ways, and often dreams are a valuable clue. Once the fear of death has been acknowledged, therapy can be a valuable aid in helping the person come to terms with it. Conscious awareness of the source of generalized anxiety is, in itself, often a source of relief.

People express an obvious *awareness and concern with time* when they realize that the days remaining to them are running short. Younger therapists often have difficulty understanding what it means to someone not to be able to think in terms of the far future.

Adopting a sense of the here-and-now usually leads to simpler enjoyment of life and a feeling of tranquility. This is perhaps the key factor in the outlook of old people who take obvious pleasure in the small satisfactions of day-to-day life.

Many people find that old age affords their first opportunity to enjoy the present free of worries about the future. It is also often the first time they are able to stop long enough to notice the beauties of nature that they never had time to enjoy before. Thus, enhanced quality of life can compensate for decreasing quantity of new experiences.

The value of a sense of presentness is nothing new; it has been recognized throughout history. The Latin phrase "carpe diem"—seize the day— is a dominant theme in ancient and medieval literature. Implicit, too, in the *carpe diem* concept is awareness of the passage of time—at whatever stage in life. Thus, the wise throughout the ages have counseled the importance of seizing the moment.

Psychotherapy in old age also must deal with various types of *grief,* of which the most obvious is grief over loss of loved ones. But people may also grieve over loss of their social roles, physical vitality, or youthful appearance. Grief of this sort can have a profound effect on a person's sense of self-worth, particularly in those who have gone through their lives in occupations where good looks were an important qualification. Loss of physical beauty can be especially devastating for a woman who, unintentionally, may have become accustomed to relying upon her looks and charm to gain desired ends in her interpersonal relationships. Therapy can help such persons explore other areas of personal worth.

While grieving is a normal part of aging, those who are overcome by feelings of sadness and loss may need professional help in regaining perspective in their lives.

Many older people become seriously disturbed over what they perceive to be past *mistakes* or *omissions*. Here, too, the therapist can help by providing insight into human nature and conduct. Often this helps to relieve the older person of the feeling that he or she has behaved in a uniquely evil way.

Atonement and restitution for past mistakes can often be made with spouses, children, or friends. One of the most important goals of therapy is helping the older person find a secure confidant—either a family member or a friend. Sharing one's feelings with an interested and sympathetic listener can in itself be a source of considerable relief.

■ Group Therapy

Group therapy, both in institutional and outpatient settings, can be helpful for elderly persons. It incorporates the therapeutic principles of individual psychotherapy with those of group interaction. It should not be viewed as "second best" to individual therapy. Rather, each type of therapeutic situation has its specific benefits, and—depending on the nature of the problem—some patients may benefit more from one approach than from the other.

For example, older persons who need help in working through their life review process will find that this objective is better accomplished with a therapist on a one-to-one basis. The specific benefits traditionally associated with group therapy include the interchange of a wide range of emotions, which generally results in feelings of empathy and understanding among group members. The group also serves the functions of imparting information, instilling hope, suggesting better ways of adapting to life situations, and generally putting problems into better perspective.

Another form of group therapy that is often beneficial to the elderly is family therapy. The marital problems that frequently arise in later years can often be worked out in a group situation or in counseling sessions. Similarly, the problems of parent-child relationships during the period of the parent's dependency frequently are alleviated by family therapy.

Life Satisfaction in Old Age

A number of characteristics observed in older people signify a healthy understanding of the life cycle as the natural progression from birth to death. Accepting one's own place in the life cycle can bring relief from the fear or denial of death.

■ The "Elder Function"

From middle age onward, people begin to develop a gratifying sense that their years have endowed them with some wisdom about life. Observing the struggles of younger persons serves to remind mature adults of the problems that are now behind them.

The "elder function" refers to the natural propensity of older people to share their accumulated knowledge and experience with the young. The respect that younger people have for such experience creates a satisfying and meaningful tie between the generations.

It is important to a sense of self-esteem to be acknowledged by the young as an *elder*, and to have one's life experience seen as interesting and worthwhile. On the other hand, it can be devastating when one's view are dismissed by the young as irrelevant and old-fashioned. This is less likely to happen, however, if older people express a genuine interest in the lives of the young and keep up to date with current ideas and developments.

■ Leaving a Legacy

Older people tend to develop an emotional investment in physical things that characterize in some way their lives—heirlooms, scrapbooks, antiques, keepsakes, or old letters, for example. Such objects provide a sense of continuity and give comfort and satisfaction.

As people reach old age, they usually become concerned about how their belongings will be distributed and cared for after their death. It is not unusual for people to make lists of persons to whom they would like to leave particular objects—and indeed, it is advisable to do so for valuables not covered under a will. Many of the objects designated for personal distribution have more emotional than monetary worth and therefore are not mentioned in the will.

For legal reasons, it is important to have lists

of such preferences signed by a witness. Many a niece or nephew has seen materially worthless but valued keepsakes, promised to them by word of mouth, disposed of by those who are legally in charge. The relative or friend may feel awkward about coming forward to claim the promised object—especially at a time when the main preoccupation is grief over the death.

In general, old people have a need to "leave something behind" when they die. This legacy may consist of children and grandchildren, professional or artistic accomplishments, personal possessions, or financial wealth. For the older person the legacy is an affirmation that he or she has lived and will continue to live in the memory of others.

■ A Sense of Life Fulfillment

A sense of satisfaction with one's life is more common among the aged than may be recognized, but probably not as common we would hope. It arises from the satisfactory resolution of personal conflicts and the attainment of goals. It is important to note, however, that one's life does not have to be a "success" by social standards to be perceived as fulfilling. Rather, fulfillment comes from the feeling that one has lived one's life according to one's own values, has successfully met challenges and difficulties, and has survived against whatever odds.

Personal accomplishments during life are a source of satisfaction to some who leave a legacy of artistic or professional work. But perhaps equally as many such persons do not derive the full measure of satisfaction from their achievements, because they are aware of the heights that *can* be reached—a quality that, along with talent, sets such persons on the road to unusual accomplishments in the first place.

Thus, the primary prerequisite for a sense of life fulfillment is the personal value one places on what one has achieved and the measure to which life goals and objectives have been attained.

30

SENIORS
AND
THEIR
FAMILIES

As Americans face the end of the twentieth century, the convergence of several social factors is changing the characteristics of family life as it was known earlier in the century. Longer life expectancy has made the four-generation family quite common, and the five-generation family is now on the increase. Thus, it is becoming more and more likely that people over the age of 65 will have living parents. Children of the oldest generations, themselves elderly or nearing old age, may now have obligations not only toward their children and grandchildren but toward their aged parents as well. Both stresses and rewards may result from the multiplication of family demands.

A rise in the divorce and remarriage rate of young adults has dramatically increased the number of children now living in "stepfamilies." Stepfamilies are formed when each of the partners in a new marriage brings children from a previous marriage into the newly formed family unit. The couple may then have one or more children of their own, resulting in half brothers and sisters who are variously related.

Demographic studies predict that by the end of the century one quarter of the elderly will also have been divorced. The trends in divorce and remarriage at all ages may strengthen intergenerational ties in some ways, while weakening them in others. For example, elderly parents who themselves divorce are not likely to be harsh judges of their child's divorce. Theoretically at least, the addition of new family members through remarriage may in part be expected to alleviate the financial and emotional burdens associated with caring for the elderly because responsibilities can be shared by a greater number of individuals. However, as partners in a new marriage will have parents and children of their own, the increase in cross allegiances also carries with it the potential for conflict.

Finally, economic factors have an impact on both the need and the ability of families to care for the elderly. The overall improved finances and health of today's seniors are enabling a segment of the older population to remain independent later into life than ever before. Studies of intergenerational ties suggest that today's relationship between adult children and their elderly parents is based increasingly on cooperation and exchange of emotional support, rather than on dependence for basic needs. In many cases, economic and physical independence later into life affords the time for adult children and their parents to develop a meaningful and affectionate relationship and to resolve the conflicts of the earlier parent-child relationship.

Another social trend expected to affect the caretaking role of adult children is the increased participation of women in the work force. While there has been a distinct rise in career-consciousness, and while professional and executive opportunities for women have expanded, many women still work mainly for the added income. The inflationary economy of 1970s and early 1980s has made the two-income family the rule rather than the exception. Due to the high cost of living, both marriage partners have to contribute financially in order to maintain the standards of middle-class life that their parents were able to achieve on the husband's income alone.

Helping Elderly Parents

On the basis of sociological survey results, there is little evidence that societal changes have lessened the degree of help extended to the elderly not only by their adult children but also—though to a lesser degree—by other family members and friends. According to the results of a 1975 survey, the spouse and children of older persons are the major support in times of illness.

One group of investigators reported that up to 98 percent of elderly persons in their study had someone who could be relied upon in an emergency, and that up to 95 percent of respondents had someone who could come in to give care during an illness. The assistance available to aging parents from their adult children is not limited to times of illness or other crises, but extends to an overall concern about their well-being. The findings of a 1980 survey show that elderly parents received help in a variety of forms from children, including shopping, cooking, housework, financial advice, home maintenance, and repair.

Thus, "taking care of one's own" is still a strong value among younger generations, and help to aging parents is given despite the constraints that social and economic forces may impose.

Several studies have examined the values and characteristics of adult children that influence their helping behavior toward aging parents. Of these, the adult children's feeling of obligation toward their parents, the perceived dependency of elderly parents, and the age and sex of both parents and children were prime factors. The helping functions of adult children tend to be divided up according to gender, with women taking on housekeeping and health-care tasks and men assisting with financial matters and maintenance of a house or car.

Helping elderly parents has also been linked closely to *attachment behavior*, a term used by psychologists to describe the feelings and reactions generally associated with loving someone. Thus, "attachment" is characterized by a desire to maintain closeness, and "attachment behavior" refers to contact and communication with the person to whom one is attached; implicit, too, is a feeling of protectiveness toward that person. Conflict between parents and adult children is another possible factor affecting the willingness and/or ability of grown children to care for aging parents.

■ *Family Conflict: An Age-Old Dilemma*

Conflict—an interpersonal process that occurs whenever the actions of one person interfere with those of another—has been a reality of family life throughout the ages. Conflict can arise also when family members share different values and opinions on issues where a potential for taking only one action exists. For example, family members may quarrel bitterly over political views or religious beliefs.

Typically, conflict is handled in one of three ways. The most positive is finding some resolution through negotiation; this is particularly relevant to issues of behavior, and such conflicts generally are resolved through a form of compromise whereby both sides gain something. Another approach to conflict is for the weaker party simply to back off and pretend to accept the actions or views of the other. Finally, conflict can be ignored by both parties, who tacitly agree to disagree, and further discussion is stopped.

Three types of conflict have been identified as occurring later in life, when parents need support from adult children: continuing conflicts, reactivated conflicts, and new conflicts. *Continuing conflicts* are those that have always been present between parent and child and are still at issue. *Reactivated conflicts* refer to those issues that have been put aside over the years as children and parents lived more independently of each other; these reappear as contact becomes more frequent in the caregiving situation. Finally, *new conflicts* concern issues directly related to the problems of the parent's aging. Unless such conflicts can be resolved, difficulties may be expected to arise in the helping relationship.

In the worst case, severe unresolved conflict can lead to neglect or abuse of aged parents.

A Recent Study of Helping Behavior

The Andrus study was a large-scale investigation of patterns of help to aging parents by their middle-aged children. This study was carried out in Lafayette, Indiana, a city with a population of approximately 50,000.

The study was based on interviews with 164 adult children who had at least one living parent. All the subjects included in the study—both parents and children—were living in the city of Lafayette. The 75 men and 89 women taking part in the study ranged in age from 29 to 71 years. Only 81 of the 164 study participants had a living father, while 148 had living mothers—attesting the greater longevity of women over men. Some fathers, however, had lived to a ripe old age; the age range of fathers was 60 to 95, compared to 55 to 93 for mothers.

Most of the adult children taking part in the study were high school graduates and most had received further education. Fifty-two (32 percent) had some vocational training or college, 22 (13 percent) were college graduates, and 35 (21 percent) had some postgraduate training or an advanced degree. Overall, 75 percent of the study population were employed in either full- or part-time jobs at the time of the interviews, and 58 percent of the households had a woman who worked either full or part time. As to religious preference, 59 percent of the study subjects were Protestant, 29 percent were Catholic, 5 percent were Jewish, 5 percent were of other faiths, and 2 percent had no religious preference.

Participants were asked about their immediate family: the number and ages of children, how many were living at home, and the extent of support they required. The interviews contained sections about each elderly parent individually, their living arrangements, present degree of dependency, and health status. Another set of questions dealt with living siblings and their present or anticipated future role in helping parents. Questions about interpersonal relationships with parents dealt with issues of attachment, conflict, and feelings of obligation.

Finally, a list of sixteen services to elderly parents was given and the participants were asked to respond with respect to perception of present need, which services were currently being provided, and the order of importance of each service. These included homemaking, housing, income, maintenance, personal care, home health care, transportation, psychological support, social and recreational activities, employment, spiritual life, bureaucratic mediation, reading, career education, personality enrichment, and protection.

Respondents also were asked to indicate the services for which they were most likely to receive (or for which it was most appropriate to expect) assistance from siblings and other relatives in the event that increased dependency needs might ultimately surpass the respondents' ability to provide the necessary help.

Although not all were available for this aspect of the study, it was possible at a later date to make comparisons between matched pairs of adult children and their parents in responses to the same questions.

■ Some Surprising Results

There was mutual agreement between older and younger generations about the desirability of separate households. The elderly parents in this study wished to stay in their own houses as long as possible. Adult children, too, preferred this arrangement, believing that conflicts with parents would be most likely to occur when the two generations were living under the same roof.

When faced with the prospect of needing help, elderly parents preferred assistance from adult children above all other potential sources such as relatives, friends, or social agencies. This was in agreement with the expressed feelings of adult children, who perceived themselves as primarily responsible for helping aging parents. However, there was a difference between parents and children in the degree of help expected. Adult children in this study felt obligated to provide elderly parents with much more help than parents expected of them.

While there was general accordance between adult children and parents about the importance of various kinds of help, such as housing, income, homemaking, and house maintenance and repairs, there was disagreement over the importance of other support services. Thus, while adult children tended to rate personal and home health care highly, elderly parents considered these rather unimportant. More important to parents was help with transportation, bureaucratic mediation, obtaining reading materials, and protection—services that were generally rated as relatively low in importance by adult children.

At the time of the study, most elderly parents needed very little help from their adult children, as verified by assessments of both parents and children. The areas in which children actually provided most help were those in which their elderly parents expressed themselves as having the greatest needs: home maintenance, psychological support, transportation, bureaucratic mediation, homemaking, and protection. This implies that some needs which were not seen by children as extremely important (transportation, bureaucratic mediation) were nevertheless met.

Most adult children reported that they felt close or extremely close to their parents and tended to agree with them about most values. They also tended to view parents' personality traits quite positively. Overall, there was not much conflict between adult children and their elderly parents. However, most adult children expected some increase in conflict if the parents were to live with them.

There was slightly more conflict with mothers than with fathers. In particular, mothers tended to be more critical than fathers of children's bad habits, of grandchildren, and of the adult child's life-style. Areas of conflict shared by both parents had to do with the adult children's ideas about what their parents should do and with health matters. Adult children tended to feel that their parents did not take good enough care of themselves or seek sufficient medical attention.

Thus, neither generation welcomed advice on the specifics of how to conduct one's life.

The Stress of Helping

The results of the Andrus study indicate that some degree of personal stress and negative feeling results from adult children's involvement in helping their elderly parents. The degree of stress and negative feelings reported by adult children appeared to be directly related to the degree of the parents' dependency. Older adult children reported more stress and negative feeling than younger adults—probably becauuse the older respondents had older parents requiring more extensive services. This study supports earlier findings that women experience more stress than men, because they play a more prominent role in providing services to elderly parents.

It is interesting that the stresses reported by participants in this study were directly related to the helping relationship rather than to secondary problems with spouses, children, finances, or employment. The most frequently reported complaint was a sense of physical and emotional fatigue and the persistent feeling of being unable to satisfy the parent no matter what one did. More minor stresses involved the feeling of being tied down by a full daily schedule that left little or no time or energy for social or recreational pursuits.

The prospect of the increasing dependence of aging parents is frequently a source of anxiety to adult children. This study explored the attitudes of participants about this aspect.

Present attachment behavior—which includes not only help but general contact with parents through visits or phone calls—is known to be the strongest predictor of an adult child's commitment to provide help in the future. The investigators asked questions about what factors, if any, would limit the study subjects' ability to meet future increasing parental needs.

Twenty-nine percent of study participants anticipated no point at which their help would diminish. Statements like "I'd do whatever it takes," or "I'd take a leave from my job" were common. The remaining 71 percent of respondents gave a variety of situations under which their help would have to become more limited or stop entirely. Most frequently cited were situations that might imperil the respondents' marriage or job, or conflict with the interests of the adult child's own children. Less frequently the respondents cited the additional personal expenditure of time, energy, and emotion. Only 4 percent of the adult children considered financial concerns to be a limitation on future help.

Perhaps because of their own geographical proximity, adult children in this study did not view siblings or other relatives as an important source of present or future help. Nonfamily service providers, such as government agencies, volunteer organizations, friends, and neighbors, also were not strong sources of present help and were not expected to become such in the future. Elderly parents, on the other hand, expected more help from these sources as well as from their adult children if their future needs increased.

Is There a Role Reversal?

There is a general belief that a role reversal often takes place between middle-aged adult children and their elderly parents. That is, while adult children adopt a supportive and protective role toward the aging parent, the parent takes on the child's former dependency role. Such role reversal can be difficult for both sides, since parents often resent the need to be dependent upon children and adult children may react with anger that the parent is no longer the "strong one" in the relationship.

Some gerontologists, however, reject the concept of role reversal and its attendant conflicts, claiming that it happens only when elderly parents and adult children have not continued their normal psychological development in the life cycle. The term "filial maturity" has been proposed as a substitute for role reversal. It implies a responsible attitude on the part of adult children which enables them to adopt a more mature *filial*—rather than a parental—role toward their aging parents.

In a mature filial relationship the adult child is able to see his or her parents as individuals with personal needs and goals, rather than simply as parent figures. The child takes a realistic view of the parents, accepting them as they are rather than as one might wish them to be.

When the adult child reaches filial maturity, he or she assumes a caretaker role toward elderly parents that focuses primarily on willingness to help without placing emphasis on dependency. In such a milieu, feelings of hostility or rejection are less likely to emerge.

Although feelings of affection, respect, and willingness to help improve the quality of the caregiving relationship, one cannot ignore the existence of conflict between adult children and their elderly parents. In most cases the sources of current conflicts date a long way back, and are often well buried in the subconscious. As a result, adult children may either not be aware that they have unresolved conflicted feelings toward their parents or, if they recognize these feelings, they may belittle them as irrelevant and even ridiculous. Nevertheless, it is important to explore one's feelings about the parent-child relationship, otherwise the conflict may prevent both the giving and receiving of help between the generations.

The relationship between parents and their adult children is quite complex. Both carry the "emotional baggage" of whatever happened between them from the birth of the child onward. While many of the exchanges and interactions that once caused pain or conflict may have been long forgotten, they are nevertheless buried in the subconscious. Since no one can completely live up to another's expectations, disappointment and frustration are natural aspects of even the closest and most loving of human relationships.

Making up for the shortcomings of their own childhood is a dominant force in many parents' approach to child-rearing. That is, parents bring up their children in the way they wanted to be brought up when they were young. While this is founded on the best of intentions, often it is accompanied by disappointment when the expected results do not occur. Parents, have to accept their offspring as individual persons whose lives they cannot irrevocably mold to fit their own needs or preferences.

In later years, some parents act out with their children the personal conflicts they were unable to resolve with their own parents. Similarly, some adult children take unconscious revenge on their aged parents for injustices—real or imagined—that they suffered during childhood.

Facing Up to Feelings

It is important for adult children to take stock of their feelings toward their aging parents in order to be able to help them effectively. The more close the attachment to or love for another person, the wider the range of feelings toward that person. There is no strong human relationship that is not a mixture of love and hate—a truth that mature individuals can accept without guilt. This truth was summed up in the "Honeymooners" episode where Ralph, in a moment of pique, says of Norton, "If he weren't my best friend, I'd have nothing to do with him."

In any caring relationship, a whole variety of different—and often conflicting—feelings can be aroused at various times. Not all feelings have the same intensity, and minor annoyances and irritations can easily be overcome. However, when equally strong but opposing emotions exist at the same time, the result can be painful conflict. This is typified by statements like, "If only I didn't love my mother so much, I could really hate her." The most effective way to deal with this type of anguish is to accept conflicting feelings as natural. Once negative feelings are openly acknowledged, they can more easily be put in perspective.

Old feelings from the past are particularly likely to arise when parents get older and are in need of help. While the sense of physical distance—of living in one's own home and having one's own family—may keep unresolved feelings toward parents at bay throughout adult years, the caretaking role can bring about a return to past emotional responses. These are not always unpleasant; old affections and loyalties may become stronger.

There is also the possibility, however, that old wounds will be reopened and forgotten weaknesses reexposed.

Problems That Arise From Unresolved Feelings

■ *Withdrawal*

Many adult children feel guilt over their lack of contact with elderly parents. Some state that despite repeated resolutions to visit or telephone more often, they simply are unable to break a pattern of withdrawal from the relationship with an older parent.

When this happens, the reason may be fear of uncovering feelings—such as anger, resentment, or jealousy—that the child prefers to keep hidden. With the failure to behave differently comes self-condemnation, and the child withdraws still further.

■ *Oversolicitousness*

The opposite of withdrawal, oversolicitousness, is another way to block out feelings of anger or guilt. Expressions of extreme concern over parents' welfare and the spending of unusually large amounts of time with parents may be seen as devotion and an expression of love. Though that is often the case and should not be criticized, oversolicitousness toward aging parents has been recognized by psychologists as one way of dealing with unresolved feelings. In addition, oversolicitous behavior by adult children toward their aging parents may signify fear of losing them. The overly attentive child then feels that as long as he or she is there to take care of things, nothing can happen.

■ *Faultfinding*

When people feel that they are unable or unwilling to meet a responsibility, a common reaction is guilt. Another response is to put the blame elsewhere. Thus, when people are faced with the fact that they are not doing what they feel they should be doing for their parents, there is a tendency to find fault with those who are shouldering the responsibility.

Family members, health care professionals, or other stand-ins then are criticized as being inefficient, inconsiderate, or plainly unqualified to do the job. Whether done consciously or not, faultfinding behavior usually succeeds in distorting matters sufficiently to make the critic feel better temporarily. However, the comfort provided by faultfinding is almost always followed by angry feelings from other family members or caretakers.

■ *Denial*

Some persons cannot confront the increasing helplessness or progressive illness of an aging parent, with its implicit threat of death, and they react by denying reality in the hope that it will go away. Denial of parents' aging by adult children can actually put the parents in danger if the children are the only persons directly responsible for their welfare.

In its most extreme form, this type of denial can cause elderly people to be deprived of medical help until it is too late. Even when doctors are consulted, denial leads many adult children to expect unrealistic miracles from the medical profession.

■ *Scapegoating*

The burdens and problems of adult children's own lives are often taken out on aging parents through the process of *scapegoating*. When people have trouble facing up to problems, they sometimes find release in blaming a totally innocent and uninvolved person for some unrelated thing. Or they may make that person the object of their emotional outbursts. Scapegoating is not usually done deliberately, but it is a very human type of behavior to which anyone may be subjected at one time or another. When carried to extremes, scapegoating can be very destructive to everyone involved, but particularly to its innocent elderly victims.

Common Reactions Toward Aging Parents

■ *Love, Compassion, and Respect*

Love, affection, respect, compassion, and concern generally exist simultaneously in the relationship between adult children and their aging parents. These emotions may all be equal in intensity, or some may be stronger than others. As evidenced in the Andrus study (discussed earlier in this chapter) and by most people's personal experience, the majority of people seem to feel love and affection for their parents. Compassion in the face of need is a natural outcome of affection. The respect felt for one's parents may mature over the years, as adult children learn to appreciate the real strengths and shortcomings of their parents rather than looking up to them as the revered and all-powerful idols of childhood fantasy.

In some cases, however, only one emotion is present, without any of the others. Thus, it is possible to have respect for, and to be concerned about, one's parents without ever having loved or even liked them. A basic lack of affection toward a parent is always a profound source of guilt and remorse, however. It has been pointed out that while love and affection—as expressed in attachment behavior—is the strongest predictor of adult children's helping behavior toward elderly parents, feelings of obligation or a sense of duty are often the only motivators for providing help. It has also been established that family loyalty is in itself an important aspect of intergenerational relationships, and that aging parents' needs are not necessarily neglected even where love is minimal or absent. In this case, helping behavior is motivated by fear of social stigma rather than being the natural outcome of genuine caring.

■ Fear

Many adult children find to their surprise that they still fear their aging parents. Some children live in fear of disappointing their parents' expectations of them, even though their parents may have grown weak and helpless. Aging parents sometimes reinforce such feelings by consciously or unconsciously nourishing childhood dependencies in their adult children. Thus, weak and fragile old men and women may still find the strength to retain command and to continue directing their children's lives, even from a wheelchair or sickbed.

Children's fear of failing to please their parents will dissipate naturally if the parents learn to accept their children as individuals with their own goals and values. But if such acceptance has not developed over the years, adult children need to recognize and assert their right to independence and pursue a life-style that accords with their own values and capabilities.

■ Anger, Hostility, and Contempt

The caretaking role may bring out negative feelings in both adult children and their elderly parents. Anger usually is a passing feeling; when it is present constantly, psychologists usually refer to it as *hostility*. *Contempt* describes the way people feel toward someone they hold in extremely low esteem. At one time or another while they are growing up, children are likely to experience each of these feelings toward their parents. Problems develop only if occasional flare-ups of such feelings evolve into permanent attitudes.

Unfortunately, in many cases such feelings resurface in the caretaking situation. Children may find in it the opportunity to retaliate for perceived parental neglect of their needs. The fact that parents are old and frail may not diminish such responses, especially if parents continue to behave in a way that elicited anger or hostility in the past.

Negative feelings are not the sole domain of adult children, however. Dependent parents may feel a great deal of anger over the loss of their own independence and their present need for help. Their response to helping behavior may be abuse and criticism, rather than expressions of gratitude.

Children can allay their parents' anger in this situation by understanding that it comes from their feelings of impotence. They should assure their aging parents that they are not a burden and encourage them in activities and decision-making that bolster their sense of personal autonomy. Adult children, in turn, must try to identify the source of their own anger toward a parent and attempt to resolve it.

Sometimes the two generations are able to discuss past and present grievances quite openly, and this can lead to better understanding on both sides. If that is impossible, adult children who are caretakers may be helped by talking out their feelings with understanding friends or with a professional counselor.

■ Shame and Guilt

Somewhat intertwined, shame and guilt are

among the prime emotions that mar the parent-child relationship in later years. Adult children suffer shame and guilt over what they believe they are not doing for their aging parents. Usually they deal with these feelings through a number of rationalizations such as "If only I had a bigger house," "If only I didn't have to work," "If only we had more money," and so on.

Guilt and shame are also common consequences of wishing that extremely ill and disabled parents would die. Death wishes directed toward the terminally ill are generally easier to deal with because of the popular attitude that at a certain point death becomes preferable to suffering. A far less acceptable death wish is directed toward a parent who is not terminally ill but is difficult to care for and a drain on the family's physical and emotional resources.

While there are many situations where such feelings are quite understandable, traditionally it has been considered evil to wish anyone dead, and death wishes directed toward aged parents usually carry a heavy burden of guilt.

In addition, the person may feel guilt over the shortcomings of society as a whole in caring for its elderly. In many ways, American society is indeed still ill equipped to help adult children sufficiently in the care of their aging parents. Especially in families where the woman has to work, the care of an elderly parent can be a crushing responsibility. Nursing homes are frequently out of reach financially, and those that are affordable may not offer quality care.

Sometimes adult children feel ashamed of their elderly parents. For example, a professional, self-made person may be ashamed of uneducated, illiterate, unsophisticated, and poor parents and keep them in the background because they do not want the people in their own world—friends, colleagues, neighbors, or in-laws—to know where they came from. If the parent is an alcoholic, the adult child may want to keep that parent out of view in order to avoid embarrassment. Such feelings, in turn, bring about shame over being ashamed of one's parents—which is perhaps the most painful form of shame and the most difficult to resolve.

Viewed in its most positive sense, the feeling of shame over one's parents should provide the person—who presumably has other accomplishments—with a starting point from which to reexamine personal values and feelings of self-esteem and confidence.

Some Other Issues

■ *Can You Accept Your Own Aging?*

The behavior of adult children toward their elderly parents can be profoundly affected by their own perceptions about aging. Many people are reluctant to talk about aging or even to think about it; they make every effort to retain their youthful appearance and demeanor. Such efforts are not negative in themselves, but they become destructive if practiced at the expense of personal growth and a realistic acceptance of one's place in the life cycle.

The visible aging of elderly parents forces adult children to confront the fact of their own aging and mortality—difficult issues for some. If they have, a positive attitude toward their own aging, they will be better equipped to offer concern, compassion, and constructive support to their elderly parents.

In addition, as contact with young children enables adults to relive the gay and carefree times of their own childhood, so witnessing the progression of parents' aging makes some adult children feel that they are being forced to "prelive" their own old age and impending death. Thus, acceptance of the human life cycle is a vital component of healthy adaptation at all ages.

On the more positive side, aged parents set a valuable example of how (and how not) to grow old. Their attitudes and the choices they make in working out age-related adjustments can later serve as guidelines for their children in making their own choices and adaptations.

■ *Can You Accept Your Parents' Aging?*

No one is happy to see signs of aging in his or her parents. Failing hearing or eyesight, a limp, or some other age-related handicap in a parent evokes a variety of emotions in the child, the first of which is often surprise or disbelief. While one consciously knows that parents are aging and will, in fact, be old some day, that day is always somewhere off in "the future." Most adult children find that they are not prepared for the first tangible signs of aging in their parents.

Even though one's parents are no longer depended upon to satisfy basic needs, somewhere in every individual remains the conviction that his or her parents are a source of protection when needed. Thus, when parents themselves come to be in need of help and protection, their potential protective function must be accepted as irrevocably lost.

A parent's mental deterioration—such as forgetfulness or a tendency to repeat a question or statement—can be saddening to adult children, who feel a loss of sharing with their parents. They will find, however, that the typical memory lapses of old age are not a great impediment to meaningful communication; often an aged parent will surprise them by referring back to an item in a conversation that they did not respond to at the time.

When there is sufficient interest and care, adult children and their aging parents can continue to have a rewarding relationship—one that may permit discussion of subjects that previously had been too volatile. Thus it happens that new dimensions in the parent-child relationship sometimes develop at older ages, as the generation gap narrows, due to a more nearly equal experience of life's possibilities and limitations.

■ *Do You Like Your Aging Parents?*

Most people do not answer this question directly, but sidestep it by statements such as, "My mother is pretty ungrateful and critical, but she is still my mother." Persons who do not like one or both of their parents usually find it difficult to admit this even to themselves.

In some cases, children who liked their parents earlier in life begin to dislike many of the traits the parents develop as they become more infirm and dependent. Indeed, some older people do acquire personality traits that are difficult for their adult children to deal with, much less like. It should be remembered that while older people have the right to expect adequate care—with their needs met, their security maintained, their pain diminished, and their loneliness alleviated—they do not have the right to expect to be liked—even by their own children—merely because they are old. An unpleasant manner or mean disposition are not the earned privileges of having lived long.

On the other hand, elderly parents who are healthy and are obviously enjoying their leisure years can be great company. This is a time when the "young old" and their adult children can find mutual enjoyment in many leisure pursuits.

Moreover, the more relaxed attitude of older parents can help put the child's struggle with the "rat race" into perspective. One career woman

says that she feels better about the urgent problems that beset her as soon as she enters her parents' house. Their easy attitude and obvious pleasure in seeing her is somehow contagious, making her feel that the problems she faces have happened to others before and are not as earthshaking as they seem. She is one of many younger adults who find that they benefit from their elderly parents' more serene outlook.

Learning to Help Effectively

■ *Specialized Programs*

Many programs have been developed for the purpose of helping adult children maintain their physical and psychological health while learning how to help aging parents more effectively. Some programs offer instruction in coping with the interpersonal problems of the care taking situation, others teach actual skills needed in caring for the elderly. Some programs offer a combination of theoretical and practical instruction.

These programs also provide information about age-related changes in physical, mental, emotional, and social functioning. They consider common problems of the elderly such as finances, living arrangements, health, widowhood, death of friends and contemporaries, and the usual emotional reactions that occur in response to losses and life transitions. Adult children can thus be better informed about what to expect as their parents get older and not be misled by myths and stereotypes about old age.

Programs aimed at skill training teach adults to deal with the feelings, behaviors, and age-related limitations of older parents. In one program, for example, a caregiver might learn how to communicate with a person who is losing hearing or vision; in another, how to care for a parent who is paralyzed after a stroke.

Other programs are directed primarily toward therapeutic objectives and help adult children in their caregiving role by providing emotional support and maintaining morale. For example, group sessions allow members to share their feelings and frustrations with others. Like all self-help groups, these sessions are a source of mutual support and reinforce the feeling that one's problems are not unique.

Groups further strengthen the helping behavior of their members by considering various approaches to solving the problems they share.

Typical subjects for discussion might include: resolving specific conflicts with parents; becoming more aware of the emotions that arise in the parent-child relationship; learning to modify or accept one's situation.

Information about community programs of this type can be obtained from Area Agencies on Aging or related social service organizations.

■ Family Respite Services

Respite services help families that are caring for a dependent elderly person at home by offering a "respite" from caretaking duties. They provide qualified persons who can come into the home and take over for a weekend or during a vacation, and so allow family members to spend time as they please. The availability of day or night "sitters" enables the family to go out occasionally, or get a good night's rest when an older person requires frequent attention during the night.

Home appliances and aids that alleviate stress on family members, such as wheelchairs, hospital beds, or special handles and bars to assist walking, are readily available through the respite service.

In addition, family respite services smooth the way for short-term hospital admission of elderly persons during times of particular physical decline. Brief stays in the hospital also help to disarm the popular belief that hospitals and institutions are places where one goes to die. The opportunity to "get away from it all" can make even the most physically and mentally draining home-care situations more manageable. The respite helps younger family members renew their energies and dedication to the caretaking role.

Choosing the Caretaker

There is often a question of who will be in charge during the time when aging parents need help. In some families this is answered well in advance, in others it is determined by sheer chance. The caretaker may be chosen by the parents, may volunteer, or may just be the one who lives closest and is in the best position to help.

Experts in family relations have found that middle-aged daughters are more likely than sons to take on the major responsibilities of caretaking. In families where there is only one daughter, she is the one most likely to become the caretaker. Even when aging parents are managing independently and do not need much help, daughters, rather than sons, are generally the ones who keep in closer touch through phone calls and visits.

One particular son or daughter may always have kept in touch regularly and been the one to help when problems arose. Over the years, the parent-child relationship may have been characterized by a mutually gratifying pattern of giving and receiving. Thus, when aging parents need increased help in later years, the son or daughter who has developed strong bonds of affection with parents may also be the one most willing to make personal sacrifices for the sake of his or her aging parents.

The most practical issue in choosing the caretaker is, of course, proximity and availability. The most dedicated child may not be able to care for aging parents as easily as another sibling who lives closer. In cases where there is rivalry between children over who will help parents—and this can occur for a number of reasons—one sibling may officially accept the caretaker role while relegating all its duties to others.

There appears to be no predictable pattern about which child will be selected when parents choose the caretaker in advance. While their preference may always have been known, the child who is singled out by parents as the main source of help may be the oldest, the youngest, the strongest, the weakest, the favorite, or the least favorite. In many cases, however, it is assumed that a child who has no family obligations of her own—such as an oldest daughter who has never married—will become the caretaker.

In some families, the aging parents may place unreasonable demands on their caretaking adult children, while in other families the caretakers themselves insist on shouldering all the responsibility. As their efforts to help are turned down consistently, other family members ultimately stop offering. Then, as burdens increase, the originally overzealous caretaker may find herself alone and in the role of a martyr. Forgetting how the situation came about, this person may complain bitterly about the heavy burden and the selfishness of other family members.

■ Sibling Rivalries

Rivalries between brothers and sisters frequently occur over matters that have to do with gaining their parents' favor. For example, in families where there has always been a "favorite," another child may see the caretaking role as an opportunity to gain missed recognition, if not actual preferment. On the other hand, favoritism may turn into a retaliatory situation: A less favored child feels less obligation, reasoning that the one who was favored over the years should now also take on the caretaking duties.

In many cases, the anticipation of an inheritance plays a role in adult children's rivalry over their parents' care. It may be felt, for example, that those who did the most for parents in their old age are deserving of the greatest reward. Money may be used by adult children both as a substitute and a weapon of power in the caretaking situation. Some adult children feel that they can discharge their obligation by sending money. If parents are indeed in need of financial help, power struggles can occur between siblings over the relative amount of each one's contribution and the degree of authority it confers.

Not infrequently, already fragile relationships between brothers and sisters are permanently broken off as a result of misunderstandings over the care of aging parents. Children whose offers of help were consistently rejected may feel ultimately that the caretaker stood between them and their dying parent, preventing them from making their own final reconciliations with the parent.

Just the opposite may occur, however, when the caretaking function is shared by brothers and sisters who have not been close over the years, and their united effort serves to strengthen the family bond between them.

Games Old People Play

Older people are just as capable as younger persons of using game-playing tactics to gain their ends. In fact, those who have resorted to psychological manipulation of their children over the years are probably better practiced in its techniques than are their less experienced adult children.

One of the more common tactics used by old people is either the denial or the exaggeration of their infirmities. Parents know from experience exactly how their children may be manipulated into certain kinds of behavior and responses. Infirmities frequently are used by older people as a way of controlling their environment. Grandmother's dizzy spells or grandfather's palpitations are effective—though not honest or direct—ways of ending family arguments or getting youngsters to turn down the volume of their music.

Less commonly, older people belittle their in-firmities out of fear of being put into a nursing home. Thus, many older people ignore the efforts of others to further their safety and well-being.

Marriage, Widowhood, Remarriage, and Sex

■ Marital Adjustment in Retirement Years

The retirement years are a time when marriages are challenged by the need to make new adaptations and develop mutually satisfying patterns of living. Couples who have lived together for thirty or forty years may nevertheless find that old differences have not been resolved, that new conflicts appear, or that they do not know each other quite as well as they thought.

Even if there is a strong bond between a husband and wife, periodic quarrels are to be expected, and often these serve to make the relationship even closer. It is unrealistic to expect two people to have resolved all their differences simply by virtue of their long cohabitation. This may be so in some cases—or time may have taken the sting out of some issues—but there is no guarantee that conflict will not occur. In fact, new conflicts related to the stresses and difficulties of aging often arise between spouses in their later years.

As emphasis shifts from career responsibilities to the retirement life-style, people may discover new things about themselves as well as their life-long partners. Some marriage partners find that they easily adopt common interests, while others feel the need to go in different directions.

Adjustment to the retirement life-style does not happen overnight—especially if there has been no advance planning. A wife who over the years wished that she had more time together with her husband may find his constant presence after retirement unsettling. Many wives grow accustomed to having the day to themselves and may resent the duty of providing company—and meals—to a spouse during what previously had been their private time.

A common difficulty in older marriages is the need to adjust to the physical illness of a spouse. One partner then becomes the caretaker of the other, often with little outside support. If the demand for care is sufficiently great, it can drain the energies and emotions of the caregiving spouse, who may not feel as energetic and strong as he or she once was. Such strain can bring about feelings of anger and depression, and it is not unusual for the caregiving spouse to develop physical or emotional symptoms.

While problems are common among elderly married couples—one study reports some degree of deterioration in up to one third of elderly marital relationships—most marriages do not end in late-life divorce. Married couples who reach old age generally have adapted to one another in a way that each finds supportive, or at least more acceptable than the unknown. In addition, children and grandchildren serve as a strong bond between married couples later in life.

In fact, older couples can become extremely dependent upon each other as the sole anchors at a time when many losses are occurring. Marriage often becomes a more valued human relationship during old age because it has turned into the single familiar and comfortable pattern remaining in one's life.

Widowhood

The mutual bond that develops between older married spouses in later years makes loss of the marriage partner through death especially devastating. No matter how troubled the relationship, the very existence of a living spouse implies a continuity of one's total life experience, and widowhood marks the beginning of another period in life.

For both elderly men and women, widowhood almost invariably brings a disruption of established life routines that frequently lasts longer than the actual grief over the death. The surviving marriage partner faces practical as well as emotional demands associated with the loss of a mate. There are financial and insurance matters to be handled (a first-time experience for many widows) as well as adjustments to be made in relationships with friends and family. While adult children may feel compelled to become more involved with the remaining parent, the extent of this involvement needs to be defined to the satisfaction of both generations.

Unless major decisions have been thought out beforehand, it is best to let such questions as whether or not to sell a house or move to a totally new environment wait until the mourning process has run its course. Characterized by stages during which there is a resolution of the loss and a lessening of grief, the mourning process generally is considered to last for six months to one year. (For more on this process, see the discussion in Chapter 25, "Grief.")

Whether due to the loss of a spouse, or the untimely death of an adult child, parental mourning is particularly difficult because of the many reminders that are present in one's home surroundings and the memories that occur at anniversaries, and holidays. Usually at least a one-year cycle of anniversaries, birthdays, Thanksgiving, and the Christmas season must be experienced nostalgically before the survivor is ready again to take the usual pleasure in these events.

■ The Importance of Mourning

As a necessary process for coming to terms with loss, mourning must be recognized and supported by others (see Chapter 25, "Grief"). A common cause of depression in surviving spouses is the feeling that they did not do everything possible for their husband or wife during the last stages of illness. Such persons should be encouraged to discuss these feelings with others who can offer understanding and support.

Contrary to what many people believe, consolation may not be accepted by the mourner. Premature efforts at comforting impose on the survivor the added burden of feeling "comforted." Being pressed to make insincere statements of acceptance may only serve to increase the mourner's feelings of loneliness and isolation. The mourning process is an entirely personal experience, and when bereaved persons are ready to find compensations, they will do it for themselves.

Rather than attempting to reconcile the mourner directly to the loss, it is more helpful to encourage discussion of grief and the feelings of anger that are a common response to the death of a person who is important in one's emotional life. A feeling of envy over the marriage of friends is natural and should not be suppressed. All too often, however, society reinforces such feelings by the exclusion of widowed persons from a social circle of married contemporaries.

Many people find it difficult to communicate with grieving persons, particularly if they have not experienced bereavement themselves. Their comforting words may sound trivial in the face of another person's overwhelming grief. It is not necessary to be profound, however. A simple "I am so sorry" can convey one's recognition of another's pain. The mere presence of friends and family is comforting to the mourner.

■ *Forming New Relationships*

The social isolation of widows can be particularly devastating. If a woman is attractive, married wives may feel threatened by her new availability; if she is dismal and depressed, no one will seek out her company. Self-pity and outrage are futile responses, and constructive action must be encouraged to get the woman back into contact with understanding and nonpatronizing people. Widowers, while experiencing perhaps less social isolation, have unique problems of their own. They may be totally unskilled in cooking, sewing on buttons and all the other tasks for which they have relied upon a wife over the years.

Several self-help groups have been developed in recognition of the specific needs of widowed persons. Groups such as AARP's Widowed Persons' Service offer emotional support to newly widowed persons through trained volunteers who themselves have been widowed. Post-Cana, the Catholic lay association for widows and widowers, assists with the spiritual, psychological, financial, social, and other problems associated with widowhood.

Remarriage

Older men and women who have been widowed sometimes remarry—many in their 70s or 80s. Since widows greatly outnumber widowers, the chances of remarriage are greater for men than women. Even those who during the period of mourning were certain that they would never marry again may surprise themselves and others by doing just that. This is perhaps not so startling, after all: A person who has been happily married is more likely to remarry than one whose experience of marriage was unhappy.

Frequently, widows and widowers who have sought each other's company during the initial period following the death of a spouse share a desire to reenter a marriage relationship. While "May-December marriages"—where an older man marries a much younger woman—do occur, most late-life remarriage take place between persons of approximately the same age.

■ *What Will the Children Say?*

An older widowed parent who contemplates remarriage may worry about how the adult children will react.

There are many reasons why children balk at the prospect of an elderly parent's remarriage. They may refuse to accept that another woman could possibly take the place of their mother in their father's affections (or of their father in their mother's affection). Even the most liberal-minded adults may fear that marriage past a certain age will invite ridicule. Moreover, many children like to ignore the fact that sex plays a role in their parents' lives at any age, let alone during their later years.

Money and health concerns are other factors that can cause an adult child to oppose a parent's remarriage. They may be concerned about the parent's (and their own) potential responsibility in caring for another person who may become ill and disabled. This is a particularly strong factor in cases where the parent who died had a prolonged illness that drained the family's emotional and physical strength. The consequence of remarriage on financial resources is another consideration of adult children, who sometimes feel threatened that their inheritance will decrease because it has to be shared.

Most adult children want what is best for their parents. But they need to feel that the parent is not making a mistake by remarrying. In fact, many adult children actively encourage their widowed parents to find new lives for themselves through remarriage.

What makes a successful late-life marriage? According to researchers in this field, three conditions usually figure: The children encourage it; the partners have known each other for at least eleven years prior to the marriage; and there is sufficient income, with the spouses pooling their resources.

Sex in Later Life: Myths and Realities

The assumption that sexual drives and capabilities vanish with age in both men and women has been, and still is, widely held. Contradicting this are modern studies which confirm that sexual activity among the elderly is far from unusual. The findings of Masters and Johnson show that men and women can, and often do, remain sexually active up to the age of 80 and beyond. It has been shown shown that while sex may be less frequent and perhaps less intense than earlier in life, the sexual experience continues to be important.

Several studies indicate that the "use it or lose it" maxim applies to both men and women, and that a consistent pattern of sexual activity helps maintain one's capabilities. Furthermore, single men and women who have always been sexually active are likely to seek out sexual relationships when they are old. In fact, far from disappearing with age, sexual feelings may be intensified in elderly people. Both men and women undergo some age-related sexual changes, however.

The older man generally takes longer to achieve an erection, but gains increased control over ejaculation. Specifically, men between 50 and 75 years of age are less subject to premature ejaculation than those between the ages of 20 and 40. In addition, after the age of 50 men develop an extended refractory period, meaning that it takes longer—from twelve to twenty-four hours—before sex is again possible. Most men over 60 are satisfied with one or two ejaculations a week, but they can enjoy sex and satisfy a partner more frequently than that because erections are possible.

An important finding from human sexuality studies has been that men do not automatically lose their capacity for erection with age. Rather, when this happens there is a detectable physical or emotional cause. Impotence in older men can often be traced to emotional factors such as depression or fear of failure. Among physical causes of impotence are arteriosclerotic, cardiorespiratory, genitourinary, and neurologic diseases.

The extent to which these diseases affect sexual capacity depends upon the severity of the disease and on other individual variables, thus it should not be concluded that all persons with such diseases are unable to function sexually. Other causes of impotence in men include the use of certain medications (some tranquilizers, antidepressants, and blood-pressure-lowering agents) and alcohol.

Biologically, women experience little sexual impairment as they age. Assuming that a woman is in good health and that her attitude is commensurate, there is no age limit at which a woman must terminate sexual activity. Menopause (also called "change of life") is the time during middle age when a woman's body stops producing the female hormone estrogen. Menopause usually occurs between the ages of 45 and 50, but it may come earlier in some women (premature menopause) and later in others.

The gradual reduction in the body's levels of estrogen results in several physical changes that affect sexual activity. These include a thinning of the vaginal walls, which can result in "senile vaginitis," characterized by localized itching and burning. However, in women receiving estrogen replacement therapy (ERT) at the time of menopause, this problem is not likely to occur. In addition, the bodily secretions that lubricate the vagina may decrease with age. While ERT also minimizes this problem, the use of vaginal lubricants (under the doctor's advice and guidance) is helpful.

In women who are sexually inactive for many years after menopause, there is a tendency for the vaginal cavity to become smaller, making renewed sexual relations difficult at first.

Many people reach older age under the assumption that their sex life will be over after a certain age, only to learn from personal experience that this is not so. Those who are more reticent about speaking of sexual subjects openly with physicians or peers may simply believe that they are an exception to one of nature's laws.

Under such circumstances it is easy to understand how a man who notices that it is beginning to take longer to achieve erection may simply conclude that he is becoming impotent. Concern over sexual potency exacerbates the situation. Men should be aware that many problems, such as excessive drinking, fatigue, worry, or even boredom, can cause temporary periods of impotence *at any age.*

Older women who basically accept the concept of sex in later life but do not fully understand the age-related changes taking place in their bodies may take these changes to mean that sex is over for them. It is a medical fact that the sexual drive of women is not reduced after menopause. Indeed, many women say that sex becomes more enjoyable once the risk of becoming pregnant is past.

Is sex hazardous to the health of people who have conditions such as heart disease or arthritis? The technological data are reassuring. For example, the use of ambulatory monitoring—an electrocardiographic recording made over a twenty-four-hour period and matched to activities recorded in a diary—has shown no differences between the effects of sexual activity and other forms of exertion in patients who have had a heart attack. Furthermore, modern medical opinion holds that sexual activity can actually be therapeutic in reducing tensions and heightening morale.

If you are managing a heart condition, be sure to consult your physician about the advisability of sexual activity. Most doctors tell patients who have had heart attacks that sex—like other activity—should be guided by what the body tells you. That is, if you feel comfortable and have no chest pain during a specific activity, it is usually a sign that it is not causing undue stress on the heart.

Death and the Circumstances of Dying

Facing death—whether it be one's own or that of a loved one—is always difficult. People often avoid talking or even thinking about the subject of dying because of the emotions it evokes. A primary response to the prospect of dying is *fear*. It is quite natural to fear the unknown, and, despite the great strides in our understanding of the process of dying, death is a subject on which no one can speak from first-hand experience. Therefore, no matter how much data medical and scientific scholarship can generate, a certain amount of skepticism will doubtless continue to surround the subject of death.

■ *Where, When, and How Older People Die*

Researchers studying death and dying have emphasized three major concerns: where, when and especially *how* people die. Studies have revealed that in industrial nations older people are more likely to die in a hospital than in their own homes. Opinion varies as to whether it is a setback or an advance that dying, like birth, has been removed from the home to an institutionalized setting. Certainly, many people express the wish to die at home, and often this is made possible by family members and physicians who are able to keep terminally ill patients comfortable and free of suffering. In other cases, the severity of the illness itself precludes home care because of the need for intricate medical equipment and procedures.

Scientific investigations have focused mainly on two aspects of *when* older people die: personal timetables for death, and seasonal influences. The notion that people are more likely to die around the time of their birthdays or on other days with strong emotional associations is not supported by scientific evidence, although dramatic examples have been described. Similarly, personal biorhythms have no apparent effect on when people die. It is generally agreed, however, that more

deaths occur during the winter months than during summer months.

Studies investigating *how* older people die have been more limited and their results are not always consistent or conclusive. It appears, however, that the majority of people in the United States die without severe physical or mental distress. An examination of hospitalized terminally ill patients revealed that 40 percent were unconscious for three hours or more before their death, 15 percent died suddenly (often in their sleep), and the remaining 45 percent died while awake and lucid. Approximately 21 percent of the subjects complained of moderate pain or other discomfort. The most intense suffering occurred among patients with motion-related disorders such as arthritis.

Other research findings about the circumstances of dying show that persons who die under the age of 50 generally undergo greater physical and mental distress than those who are 50 or older. Levels of depression and anxiety have been shown to vary according to the length and discomfort of a terminal illness. People dying at home are more likely than hospitalized persons to be fully alert shortly before death, and are less likely to experience unrelieved physical distress (although this finding may reflect differences in the sickness of patients who are hospitalized and those who die at home). Terminally ill patients share such physical symptoms as pain, difficulty in breathing and swallowing, nausea, vomiting, persistent cough, weakness, and loss of appetite.

Investigations attempting to identify factors that might increase or diminish the fear of death show that persons with strong religious belief show less fear than those with weaker religious convictions. It is interesting that persons with absolutely no religious convictions also show less fear. Study findings indicate too that people are frequently more afraid of pain, physical distress, or chronic disability than of death itself.

■ *The Psychologic Impact of Parental Death*

No matter at what age, the death of a parent always has a major psychologic impact. Even when it is expected because of an incurable illness, or when it is welcomed as an end to suffering, the death of a parent nevertheless represents an irreparable loss. The age at which death occurs appears to have little effect in lightening its impact. Adult children who are in their 60s or 70s will be severely affected by the death of parents who are in their 80s or 90s.

The devastation that parental death poses is understandable. Parents are the most crucial figures in people's lives during early childhood, and a strong bond is established between parents and children over the ensuing years. The death of a mother or father marks the end of the most important chapter in one's own personal history.

While people may try to prepare themselves for the inevitability of a parent's death, it is almost always a source of personal shock when it occurs. Simply knowing that a parent's voice will answer at the ring of a telephone has come to be taken for granted over the years, and the realization that this is no longer possible can be very hard to accept. In addition, death marks the end of any chance for making reconciliations or explanations that may have been put off during the parents' lifetime.

■ Should People Be Told?

There is considerable disagreement about whether people of any age who are dying should be told the truth about their fate. While the law requires that physicians truthfully inform the family, there are no legal dictates regarding the right of patients themselves to know. Traditionally, both medical professionals and family members have leaned toward a "conspiracy of silence" approach, assuring the dying individual that they will get better. It is simply not predictable how an individual will react on hearing that the end is near. Perhaps it is true, as some believe, that people know unconsciously when they are fatally ill.

What is certain is that individuals differ in whether they really do or do not want to know the truth. Some make it plain that they wish to know what to expect, and they insist upon it until they are told. And once informed, such persons usually accept the information well. Only an experienced physician is able to tell whether a person really is ready to hear the truth or whether he is simply looking for confirmation that nothing is seriously wrong.

If the dying person has responsibilities for dependent family members, it is imperative that he know the truth so that he can put his affairs in order. Moreover, once the barrier of silence is broken, both the patient and the family benefit by the opportunity to talk about the wishes and hopes for the future of family members.

■ Death with Dignity

More than they fear actual death, many older people fear that they will be kept alive against their will, though totally incapacitated. The issue of the "right to die" has become extremely complex with the development of technologies that can maintain life.

In addition, the very definition of death has changed as a result of these technologies. Until recently, persons who had lost consciousness, were no longer breathing, and had no heartbeat were pronounced dead as a matter of course. Scientists now suggest that death does not occur until there is an absence of brain electrical activity. These findings have brought about a reevaluation of the methods currently applied for maintaining life through "heroic," artificial means.

There is a growing consensus that people should be allowed to die in peace. Some states have already passed legislation setting forth guidelines for medical intervention to sustain life. They recognize that artificial means, such as the use of respirators and feeding tubes, can cause great emotional pain as well as financial hardship to the family. Because of these considerations, many older people today are making out "living wills" which clearly designate their wishes. A living will differs from an ordinary will in that it stipulates matters regarding one's person rather than one's possessions; it clarifies the maker's wishes in the eventuality that he or she is incompetent to make such decisions when the time comes.

■ Funeral Arrangements

Some knowledge of a person's wishes about where and how they would like to be buried is helpful to family members in making suitable arrangements. For example, it is important to be clear beforehand about such questions as cremation, autopsy, or organ donation. While some religions are strict about such matters—for example, the Orthodox Jewish faith prohibits making one's body available for scientific purposes or donating organs for transplantation—in most cases they are left to the family's discretion. It is extremely difficult to address such issues for the first time during the period of initial bereavement.

Families are extremely vulnerable at this time to the urgings of funeral directors to "do right by the deceased." The fulfillment of this obligation generally translates into an expensive funeral, while little help is offered in dealing with other aspects of the mourning process. Often, the expensive funeral adds to the financial burden of a family whose resources have already been drained by the costs of a prolonged illness.

Nonprofit memorial societies offer simple and dignified funeral arrangements at much lower cost. A memorial society usually is initiated by a church or a ministerial association, sometimes by a labor union. Membership is inexpensive and lightens the burden on survivors because the wishes of the deceased have been clearly defined in advance. There are memorial societies in more than one hundred cities in the United States and Canada.

Memorial, more than funeral, services are believed to have a therapeutic impact upon survivors, since they emphasize the life of the deceased person rather than the ritual of physical burial. An honest appraisal of the deceased helps survivors work through their own complicated feelings. A ceremony of some type is important to the acceptance of the death however. It fills the need of survivors to have some significant homage paid to the passing of a human life.

31

WHEN OUTSIDE HELP IS NEEDED

The longer people live, the greater the likelihood that they will develop disabling conditions requiring skilled care. While such care can sometimes be arranged in the community setting, often the appropriate services are not available and a specialized nursing environment becomes the only solution. While people often prefer to ignore an unpleasant future possibility, in view of the fact that one out of every 4 persons aged 75 and over enters a nursing home, it is prudent to consider how one would handle the situation if it should occur.

Nursing homes vary considerably in quality and in the services that they offer, and the best of them usually have long waiting lists. If a family has acquainted itself with the various facets involved in selecting a nursing home, it may avoid the unfortunate choice forced on so many families when circumstances take them by surprise: that of choosing a facility because it has space, not because it is the one be best suited to the individual concerned.

Categories of Nursing Homes

Nursing homes are classified according to the way they are financed (private or government-funded) and the types of care they offer. Private nursing homes are commercial institutions that have become "big industry" in recent years. While these facilities are designed to operate at a profit to their owners—which are often large chains with publicly owned stock—it should not be assumed that they necessarily stint on the quality of the care they offer. Many of the private institutions offer excellent care. Others, however, do not measure up to standards—another reason why advance investigation is so important. A small number of nursing homes are sponsored by non-profit institutions such as churches and community organizations. Funding by the Medicare and Medicaid programs is largely responsible for the increase in the number of nursing homes over recent decades.

There are two major types of long-term care institutions for the aged that the Federal Government subsidizes through Medicare and Medicaid. These are known as *skilled-nursing facilities* (SNF) and *intermediate-care facilities* (ICF). These categories are referred to also as "levels of care," and complex rules and regulations govern the standards and the reimbursement systems for each.

"Skilled nursing" refers to those services that must be performed by, or under the supervision of, registered professional nurses. "Intermediate care" refers to personal care and simple medical care given under the supervision of a registered professional nurse. Many institutions offer both skilled and intermediate services, allowing for more flexibility as the resident's condition improves or deteriorates.

■ Money Determines Options

Although the financial constraints are no longer as tight as they were prior to the institution of Medicaid, monetary considerations still largely dictate the choice of a nursing home facility. It is essential to determine beforehand which homes are approved for Medicare and Medicaid, and to check on the eligibility of the prospective resident for benefits under either of these programs.

As a rule, Medicare only covers care in an approved skilled nursing facility for one hundred days after hospitalization and for specified conditions. Medicaid, on the other hand, covers the cost of care for eligible persons in approved skilled-nursing facilities for as long as their condition requires it.

Many homes do not accept residents who cannot pay some initial fee, thus they will turn down persons who must be admitted on Medicaid funds from the beginning. Private nursing-home care is very expensive, and without insurance supplementation it can be financially crippling even to a relatively wealthy family. Middle-income families are in a bind: Private nursing-home care is so expensive that it can quickly deplete their financial resources, yet the very existence of these resources makes the parent ineligible for benefits under the Medicaid program.

Under Medicaid regulations, children are not legally responsible for the nursing-home expenses of their aged parents. Husbands and wives, however, are held responsible for one another's nursing-home expenses in every state. The cost of long-term care over and above what is obtained from other sources must be met by the spouse, even if he or she is on a limited income and maintaining a household at the same time. This can cause severe financial difficulties for the relatively well-off and the poor alike.

The financial realities of the cost of nursing-home care are another reason why many older persons refuse to enter a home even at great risk to their well-being. Some older couples divorce so that one will not be financially bankrupted by the nursing-home bills of the other. Only an aged person with no personal resources (including those of the spouse) is eligible for Medicaid.

Thus, careful calculations and projections are essential in appraising the financial consequences of nursing-home placement.

Evaluating Quality

Once questions of eligibility and admission requirements are answered, the family can begin investigating possible choices. Obviously, they will want the home to be within visiting distance. Beyond this, they will need information from reliable sources. The Department of Health, Education and Welfare (HEW) is an excellent source of information on nursing-home selection. Additional sources include local hospital social service departments, county medical societies, Social Security district offices, state and local offices of the aging, and physicians, clergymen, relatives, and friends. Preferably, a favorable recommendation from more than one source should be obtained before the family makes the final decision.

Whenever feasible, the prospective resident should be as much involved as possible in the decision-making process. He or she should certainly be included in the inspection tours of various homes. If this proves too tiring on a repeated basis, the family members can lay the groundwork but they must never make the final decision without the presence and full consent of the prospective resident.

■ What to Look for When Visiting

Actually touring a prospective nursing-home facility is extremely important. Much can be learned from the way you are received, the attitude of the staff, and the general atmosphere that prevails. While it is necessary to be considerate of staff regulations and patients' rights to privacy, you are entitled to see all the areas of a home. Potential residents and their relatives are consumers investing in a way of life, and they have a right to know as much about it as possible. Openness on the part of the staff and willingness to show the facility are good clues to quality, indicating that there is nothing to hide.

■ How Do Residents Look?

Among the obvious things to look for are general cleanliness and the attitude of staff toward patients and visitors. Observing the residents can reveal much about the life-style in a nursing home. Are the residents dressed in nightclothes or streetclothing? Is there an emphasis on active participation, or is there an atmosphere of passivity? The availability of lounges and recreation areas means little if these are not actually used by the residents. A fault of many nursing homes that offer substandard care is their emphasis on ease of patient management; they discourage patients from pursuing activities and may even oversedate them.

Observing the residents also will reveal how much importance is placed on grooming, a part of good morale at any age. Find out whether beauticians and barbers are available. Also check what facilities and arrangements are available for personal laundry and dry cleaning. Access to such services and continued attention to personal appearance do much to enhance the resident's self-esteem and eliminate the feeling that he or she is in a dead-end situation where such things no longer matter.

Is the Atmosphere Cheerful?

The physical environment should be cheerful and homelike. Some things to note are whether patients are allowed to have some of their own possessions and whether they appear to enjoy sufficient privacy. Check whether beds and bedrooms are comfortable and spacious and whether there is enough drawer and closet space. If the building has elevators, are there enough of them, and are they large enough to accommodate wheelchairs? Nice, but not essential, is the availability of pleasant ground facilities, with outdoor gardens and benches. In the absence of these, the neighborhood should be safe for residents to walk through.

One of the major complaints of nursing-home residents is the quality of the food. In this regard you should require whether menus are posted and whether these reflect what is actually served; whether a qualified dietician is in charge of food services; how faithfully specialized diets are provided; whether individual food preferences or dislikes are considered.

The facility should have clean and cheerful dining areas, and patients should be encouraged to eat there rather than at their bedside. The availability of snacks at bedtime or between meals is another consideration, since people living at home may be accustomed to taking a small snack before bedtime. Finally, the scheduling of mealtimes should be at the patients' rather than the staff's convenience.

The availability of group activities, cultural pursuits, and reading materials is another important consideration in evaluating a nursing home. Find out if there is a professionally trained activities director, and whether there is variety in the schedule of activity programs. Are there outings to plays, concerts, and museums for those who are interested? There should be a patients' library and opportunities for adult education courses or participation in discussion groups.

Continued participation in affairs of the outside world is an important factor for the well-being of elderly persons. Nursing homes should make it possible for their residents to take part in local, state, and national elections by providing transportation to the polling places or absentee ballots for those unable to go. Ideally, residents should be able to participate in matters relating to the nursing-home environment itself through resident councils and family organizations. Find out if these exist, and how often they meet.

Safety Conditions

The home should meet Federal and state fire codes. Inquire whether fire drills are held regularly, and ask to see the latest inspection report. The home should be as accident-proof as possible, with adequate lighting and handrails in halls and bathrooms; rooms should not contain scatter rugs.

Medical, Rehabilitation, and Social Services

The availability and quality of medical care are primary considerations. Have it stipulated beforehand whether the home is headed by a medical director qualified in geriatric medicine; whether patients are allowed to have private physicians; whether doctors are available twenty-four hours a day; and how often each patient is seen by a physician. It is also important to know whether the home has a hospital affiliation or a transfer agreement with a hospital. It should be established, too, whether there is provision for dental and eye care as well as other specialized health care services.

The nursing service should be headed by a fully qualified registered professional nurse, and a registered nurse should be on duty at all times. Also, the ratio of nursing staff to residents should be adequate.

Physical therapy may be a current or future concern, and it is necessary to know whether the home has a registered physiotherapist on staff. A professionally trained social worker also should be available to nursing home residents and their families.

■ *Money Matters and Patient Rights*

It is important to be specific about money matters, not only with regard to the basic cost and eligibility for Medicare and Medicaid reimbursement, but regarding any extra charges that might exist. Things to find out include whether the home provides an itemized bill, what provisions are made for residents' spending money, and whether assistance is available with questions about veterans' pensions or union benefits.

Not everyone is aware that nursing homes are subject to standarized legal guidelines defining patients' rights. Thus, while residency in a nursing home does remove a considerable amount of freedom of choice from a person's life, it by no means relegates that person to a state of helpless dependency.

Primary among the rights of nursing-home patients is the right to treatment. Others include the right to receive considerate and respectful care, to be informed periodically of one's current health status by the attending physician, to refuse treatment to the extent permitted by law, and to be informed of the medical consequences of such refusal.

A number of other causes define the patient's right to confidentiality in matters relating to medical care, while others are designed to guard against many other potential pitfalls such as being transferred to another hospital against one's will.

Patients' rights should be posted prominently in a communal area of the nursing home so that everyone can be made aware of them, and family members are entitled to receive a copy.

■ *The Importance of Tact*

As you see, there are many points to cover in making your assessment of a nursing home. Unless you use great tact in pursuing your inquiries, you may easily alienate the staff. Put yourself in their place. Just as you are evaluating the suitability of the nursing home, the staff and current residents are forming impressions about you and

the potential newcomer you represent. It is not necessary—and would be exhausting to all concerned—to find out every item of the suggested guidelines in a single visit to a nursing home. Repeat visits, by appointment, made by different family members, will help to confirm or deny an appealing first impression.

Similarly, social service organizations, hospital social service departments, and the other sources of information mentioned earlier can answer many of the questions by virtue of their experience with a facility. While as much information as possible should be obtained firsthand, professionals who have constant contact with local nursing-home facilities are well informed and reliable.

■ *Families Should Act in Unison*

Nursing homes generally require that all legally concerned relatives—usually spouse and adult children—give written consent for the admission of a resident. Reliable nursing homes, however, will not accept an application from family members alone, but insist that prospective residents themselves—if mentally competent—make the application. These procedures help to avoid the resentment and criticism that often follow when family members feel they have been excluded from the decision-making process.

A family conference over the nursing-home placement of an aging parent can provoke strong discord. But it is better to have disagreements identified before action is taken than afterward. A family conference gives everybody a chance to express their feelings and lessens the likelihood of unpleasant surprises in the future. Often it helps to reinforce the family bond.

Becoming a Nursing-Home Resident

■ *Early Adjustment*

If adequately planned beforehand, the move from the home into the nursing home should take place smoothly. The person who is moving should be allowed to take charge of matters as much as possible, even if this slows things up a little. Family members should not discourage or criticize the person's selection of items to bring along. The temptation may be to replace an old, comfortable robe with a new one for the occasion, but it is best to let this wait for a later time. The familiarity of that well-used garment may offer consolation to the aged person who needs to adjust to a great many new things at once.

Although elderly persons and their families often feel that the worst is over once the decision has been reached and the arrangements made, it is important to be aware that there will be a period of adjustment for everyone involved. The family now has to learn to strike a balance between a hands-off approach and an overly meddlesome one that interferes with the duties and routines of the nursing-home staff. If the new caregivers are trustworthy—and one point of your earlier inquiries was to establish this—they will appreciate your confidence and cooperation. But you should remain vigilant for any change of administration or staffing that could lower the quality of care.

New residents may find the first few days especially stressful; they are making radical adjustments at a time when they are already wearied physically and emotionally by the move. Allow yourself time to linger to help the person get acquainted with the layout of the home, its routines, residents, and staff members.

If the new resident dismisses the family almost at once, he or she may be expressing a need to explore alone or a "let's get it over with" attitude toward saying goodbye. Even if the person seems completely accepting of the nursing-home decision, there is a sense of separation and a fear of losing touch with close family members once the step has been taken. Therefore, you need to be reassuring about your willingness to stay for a while and your intentions to visit often in the future.

As a consequence of the stresses involved, many new nursing-home residents suffer setbacks in their physical condition during the initial adjustment period. These usually are only temporary lapses that reverse themselves with time.

■ Common Mistakes and Misunderstandings

It may take as long as six months for an older person to make a satisfactory adjustment to institutional life. During that time the family will meet with ups and downs in the patient's feelings about his or her new life arrangement. These should not be taken as signs that a mistake has been made and that another facility should be sought. Of course, it is another matter if the adjustment is extremely bad and family members can see good reasons for the patient's dissatisfaction.

Weekend or overnight visits home can be a great pleasure for the nursing-home resident. But if such visits take place too early in the adjustment phase, they only impose an additional strain. Patients who are involved in the step-by-step process of adapting to a new environment usually find it difficult at first to be shuffled back and forth between their old life and the new.

Sometimes, in trying to establish a relationship with staff members, families make excessive demands on their time. Staff members are likely to be more receptive to families who respect routines and abide by rules. Tipping staff members is frowned upon in reputable homes, and some states even prohibit it. The health care team will, however, appreciate a note of thanks for a kindness.

■ Meeting the Needs for Affection

No matter how well an elderly resident adapts to his or her new life and fellow residents, family members remain the primary source of real affection. Although residents come to know one another and the particulars of each others' lives, this familiarity cannot substitute for the shared history and deep affectionate bonds that bind families.

The frequency of visits from family is not nearly as important as their quality. You accomplish much more by setting a particular day on which the family can comfortably visit than by simply dashing in and out at odd times out of a sense of duty. The good feelings that come from a mutually satisfying visit can be enjoyed in retrospect in the days that follow.

■ The Visit Home

Contrary to popular belief, nursing-home residents are not shut-ins unless they are seriously ill or handicapped. While it is usually necessary to be accompanied by a family or staff member, patients can leave the home periodically for a variety of outside activities. These include restaurant meals, movies, concerts, and holidays with family.

By planning such outings well in advance, you show consideration for both the staff and the elderly resident, who is likely to find sudden change disruptive. The rules and regulations governing all outside visits should be carefully checked before residents are taken out. Many nursing homes have specific concerns, and family should be aware and respectful of these.

The most comfortable schedule for visits and outings will become clear with time. Remember, though, that the interest of family members is something of a status symbol among nursing-home residents. It bolsters their self-esteem when people come to see them or invite them out.

■ Continuing Awareness

No matter how activity-oriented and cheerful the nursing home atmosphere may be, residents should not let it limit their sphere of interest. While some older people truly appear to lose interest in community and world affairs, most desire to remain knowledgeable; they welcome newspapers as well as any information the family brings about events and occurrences in the neighborhood and among friends. The telephone is another important means of communication for nursing-home residents.

It is very important to be truthful and honest in all matters pertaining to the nursing-home situation. The elderly person does not need to be protected from information that may be upsetting, such as the death of a contemporary. As a result of long experience in life, older people often accept tragedy better than younger adults.

Family problems should also be discussed openly and advice sought from the elderly nursing-home resident who is mentally lucid and well oriented. While a steady stream of bad news is to be discouraged, the chance to share and contribute to the solution of family problems is vital to dispelling the self-absorption that so often besets persons whose world has become constricted.

Choosing a Nursing Home for the Person with Mental Impairment

An adult with Alzheimer's disease or other irreversible dementia (see Chapter 29) needs increasing help in performing the simple tasks of daily life. Since not all nursing homes are prepared to accept such patients, it may take time to find the right facility.

The family will be asked specifics about the type of care the prospective patient will require: Can the person still perform the routine tasks of self-care, such as dressing, bathing, and eating? To what extent has he or she lost awareness of time, place, and familiar persons and objects?

All the above-mentioned considerations in selecting a nursing home apply to the choice of a facility for patients with intellectual loss. In addition, there are some further aspects that need to be investigated. For example, it is particularly important to observe how staff members speak to and treat patients.

It is a bad sign if staff members use condescension or downright scolding in addressing patients. If they interact as little as possible with patients you may conclude that there is little emphasis on keeping patients active and in touch with reality. Patients should not be isolated in rooms or be left to sit along hallways while the staff congregates at the nursing station or staff lounge.

Reality orientation uses specific means of communication to keep confused patients in touch with what is going on around them. It should be an integral part of the treatment approach rather than something scheduled once a week. The names of personnel should be clearly visible on name tags, and clocks and calendars should be prominently placed to help in the orientation process.

Recreational activities, while necessarily limited by the condition of the patient, are important. Music has been found to be particularly soothing to some patients with Alzheimer's disease, and regular viewing of television programs is often entertaining as well as helpful in reality orientation.

The ideal facility for patients with intellectual loss conveys a positive attitude in helping patients make the most out of their remaining capacities. As family members who have been caring for an Alzheimer's victim are well aware, the job is difficult, frustrating, and often relatively thankless. Nevertheless, this does not entitle professionals who have chosen to work with such patients to take advantage of their limitations by meeting only the most basic of needs.

Homes for the Aging

Homes for the aging—recently renamed "geriatric centers"—represent a much smaller percentage of the institutionalized care available to older persons. These are usually voluntary non-profit institutions, and are sometimes run under the auspices of a religious, benevolent, or fraternal association or by trusts or municipalities.

Religious and fraternal homes are known to be

very selective in their admission standards, and persons without financial means and sustaining family are not likely to be accepted. Such homes also generally do not accept the mentally impaired and the acutely ill. When illness develops during residence, transfer to a hospital is probable if the home is not equipped to offer skilled nursing care.

More recently, however, most geriatric centers have expanded to include facilities for care of the ill. Residents of geriatric centers frequently finance their care by turning over their assets in return for the guarantee of lifetime care. This arrangement—referred to as "life care"—has benefits and drawbacks (see "The Retirement Community" in Chapter 27). The primary factor to check out is the financial soundness of the particular facility chosen.

32

COMMON DISEASES AND DISORDERS OF AGING

The aging process reduces the reserves and resilience of all bodily organs and their functions. The degree to which we experience such reductions depends upon many variables—including our health history, our diet and life-style, and even our attitude. Throughout life, those who dwell on symptoms—real or imagined—seem to suffer more than those who concentrate on health and well-being.

Certain bodily functions decline with age. A familiar example is metabolism, the process whereby nutrients or other substances are converted to forms that the body can use. But such a decline is not the same as disease. For example, an age-related decrease in glucose metabolism has led to a revision of the guidelines for diagnosing diabetes in the elderly: Blood sugar levels that would be considered excessively high in younger adults today are recognized as being within the normal range for older persons.

Geriatricians know that some common diseases may lead to unusual complications in elderly patients. In addition, the typical signs and symptoms that help physicians make a diagnosis are not always present in older persons. The most striking example of this is the painless heart attack.

Older people are known also to have a reduced response to inflammatory conditions. For example, the fever response may be completely absent, allowing infection to go unrecognized. Similarly, the response of the white blood cells (the cells that fight against infecting organisms) may be absent or diminished. Thus, the two clinical markers classically used to detect infection—fever and an elevated white blood cell count—may not be present in the elderly patient. The existence of clinical features unique to elderly patients underscores the importance of geriatrics as a medical specialty.

Throughout life, people are subject to all kinds of diseases. Certain illnesses are more likely to occur with increasing age, however. The most common diseases seen in older persons are discussed in this chapter.

COMMON NUISANCES OF AGING

Constipation

Constipation is a symptom, not a disease. Everyone suffers from constipation now and then, but it seems to become a more prevalent problem as people age. One reason is the age-related decrease in intestinal motility, the process that aids in the passage of food through the intestines.

Older persons are five times as likely as younger persons to complain of constipation to physicians, and some doctors believe that this ailment sometimes is overemphasized by their elderly patients. In some the problem may be fear of colonic dysfunction, as much as dysfunction itself.

In our society much emphasis is placed on bowel regularity, particularly in television commercials depicting the magic effects of laxatives on the way one feels, copes, and enjoys daily living. Such messages lead some persons to worry if they don't have daily bowel movements. The truth is that people vary considerably in the number and timing of bowel movements: What is "regular" for one person may not be regular for another.

Some doctors suggest asking youself the following questions to find out if you are really constipated:

- Do you often have fewer than two bowel movements a week?
- Do you have difficulty passing stools?
- Is bowel movement painful (because of hard stools)?

Although doctors do not know exactly what causes constipation in some persons and not in others, some contributing factors have been identified. Older persons are more likely to suffer from constipation if they eat a poor diet (with insufficient fiber content), drink too little fluid, or misuse laxatives. Additional causes include prolonged bed rest after an accident or during an illness, as well as general lack of physical activity.

Ignoring the natural urge to have a bowel movement can cause constipation at any age. This usually occurs at times when it is inconvenient, or perhaps impossible, to use a bathroom. For example, quite a number of people at all ages find it difficult to use a bathroom when there is insufficient privacy; others prefer to have their bowel movements only at home. The resulting forced holding of the bowel movement can cause constipation if the delay is too long.

It is well known that laxatives and enemas can actually worsen constipation problems if used too often. The body begins to rely on the laxative to bring on bowel movements, and eventually the natural bowel-emptying mechanisms fail to work without the help of these agents. Overuse of mineral oil—the laxative preferred by some people—

may reduce the absorption of vitamins A, D, E, and K.

In the elderly, a common contributing factor to constipation may be the need to use certain medications. Constipating drugs include some medications used to control high blood pressure as well as some of the drugs used to treat depression or sleep disorders. Not all drugs in these categories cause constipation, however, and persons differ in their individual response to various medications.

■ How to Overcome Constipation

While any problem should be brought to the physician's attention to rule out a more serious underlying cause, constipation itself is not a serious medical condition. However, it can certainly be a source of discomfort for those who suffer from it.

Many people are helped by simple changes in their dietary habits and by increasing their exercise. Studies provide strong evidence that foods with a high fiber content result in larger stools, and more frequent bowel movements.

Lack of interest in eating, a common problem in seniors who live alone, may lead to increased use of convenience foods that are generally low in fiber. In addition, loss of teeth may force older people to eat soft, processed foods that also contain little or no fiber. Older people sometimes cut back on their intake of fluids, which add bulk to stools and make bowel movements easier.

Here are some preventive measures to discuss with your doctor:

• Eat more fruits and vegetables—either cooked or raw—and increase your intake of whole-grain cereals and breads. Dried fruits such as prunes, apricots, and figs are especially high in fiber.

• Cut back on highly processed foods and foods with a high fat content. This step is beneficial also for your dietary goals of reducing caloric and sodium intake (see "What Do Older People Need?" in Chapter 28).

• Drink plenty of fluids—1 to 2 quarts daily isn't too much (unless you have heart, circulatory, or kidney problems). You may want to avoid large quantities of milk, however, since this causes digestive problems and increases constipation in some older people.

• Some doctors recommend adding small amounts of unprocessed bran (sold in most health-food stores) to cereals as a way of increasing dietary fiber content. This measure is usually unnecessary if the diet is already well balanced and contains adequate fiber. But it may help if you are constipated.

• Stay active. Taking a brisk walk after meals is a time-honored way of dealing with that heavy feeling that follows a large meal. Furthermore, exercise tones the muscles and stimulates the digestive process.

• Try to develop a regular bowel habit.

• Limit intake of antacids, since some can cause constipation.

Urinary Incontinence

Loss of urine control, or urinary incontinence, is especially common in older women but it also occurs in men. It has been estimated that at least one in 10 persons over the age of 65 has some type of urinary incontinence. The several types of incontinence range from slight loss of urine to severe and frequent wetting.

Persons with this problem often are ashamed to tell their families, friends, or even their doctor. This is unfortunate because several effective treatments are available. Anyone who is having trouble controlling urine should certainly seek medical attention. Even in cases where incontinence cannot be eliminated completely, management methods can greatly lessen its occurrence.

■ Types of Incontinence

When incontinence is persistent, it can usually be diagnosed as one of the following types:

Stress incontinence describes leakage of urine during activities in which contraction of abdominal and pelvic muscles puts pressure on the bladder. Coughing, sneezing, laughing, and some types of exercise have this effect. This type of incontinence can occur in persons of all ages. Usually it is related to poor muscle tone at the bladder outlet.

In *urge incontinence* the person is unable to hold urine long enough to reach a toilet. It is associated with conditions like stroke, senile dementia, Parkinson's disease, and multiple sclerosis, but can occur also in otherwise healthy elderly persons.

Some older people with relatively normal urine control have difficulty reaching a toilet in time because of other disabilities such as arthritis. Such persons can help themselves by responding earlier to bladder signals. It may be possible also

to modify their environment to make reaching the toilet easier.

Overflow incontinence refers to the leakage of small amounts of urine from a constantly filled bladder. A common cause in older men is blockage of outflow by an enlarged prostate gland. Another cause is abnormal contraction of the bladder in some persons with diabetes.

■ Diagnosis and Treatment

The first and most important step in treating urinary incontinence is to see a doctor for a complete physical examination. The clinical history of the problem—its type and duration—will determine whether referral to a urologist, who specializes in urinary tract diseases, is indicated.

Several medications are effective in treating urinary incontinence. Biofeedback and other techniques for behavioral modification have helped some patients in bladder retraining. Exercises to strengthen the muscles that close the bladder outlet frequently are used to treat urinary incontinence.

A number of surgical techniques are available for correcting structural problems that cause incontinence, such as an abnormally positioned bladder or blockage of urinary flow due to prostate enlargement. Prosthetic devices to control urine flow sometimes require surgical implantation.

Specially designed absorbent underclothing is available. Many of these garments are no more bulky than ordinary underwear and can be worn easily under clothing, freeing the person from the embarrassment of incontinence.

It is important to be aware that incontinence can be treated and often cured. Even incurable problems can be managed so as to reduce complications and personal discomfort.

Hearing Loss

A certain degree of hearing loss is a natural consequence of aging, and merely reflects the age-related decline in certain organ functions. Every year after age 50 people lose a little of their hearing ability, and by age 60 or 70 many adults will have some hearing impairment.

Because of fear, misunderstanding, or simple vanity, however, many older people will not admit that they have a hearing problem. About 30 percent of adults aged 65 to 74, and 50 percent of those aged 75 to 79 are believed to suffer some degree of hearing loss. Put another way, more than 10 million older Americans are hearing-impaired.

People with hearing impairment often withdraw socially to avoid the frustration and embarrassment of not being able to hear what others are saying. Their feelings of frustration and powerlessness at being unable to communicate may result in depression. Indeed, it appears that hearing loss is a greater cause of social isolation than blindness.

When ignored and untreated, hearing problems can grow worse, seriously hindering communication, limiting social outlets, and reducing opportunities for leisure activities. In addition, hearing loss or impairment may cause an older person to be wrongly considered "senile," "confused," "unsociable," or just plain "uncooperative," even by close family members who are unaware of the hearing problem.

Fortunately, treatment is available for the various types of hearing loss commonly associated with aging.

■ How Hearing Impairment Is Diagnosed

Since it is a gradual process, hearing loss may become fairly advanced before the person notices it. The following are some common signs of hearing impairment:
- Spoken words are difficult to understand.
- Sounds such as the dripping of a faucet cannot be heard.
- A hissing or ringing background noise is heard continually.
- Another person's speech sounds slurred or mumbled.
- Television programs, concerts, or social gatherings are less enjoyable because much goes unheard.

Persons who fit the above criteria should see a doctor for treatment or for referral to a hearing specialist. They should not ignore the problem, since in some cases it is the sign of a serious medical condition. Hearing impairment can be caused by viral infection, stroke, head injury, a tumor, or by simple buildup of ear wax.

Many times, the diagnosis and treatment of hearing difficulty can be made by the family physician. More complicated problems may require referral to specialists known as *otologists* or *otolaryngologists*. These physicians are doctors of medicine with extensive training in ear problems. They

will conduct a thorough physical examination, take a medical history, and order necessary laboratory tests. They may then refer the patient to an *audiologist*, who performs specialized tests of hearing. This testing is painless, and the combined findings of these specialists then make it possible to determine the most appropriate treatment.

■ Types of Hearing Loss

Contrary to what one might think, there are several types of hearing loss, distinguished by their physiologic causes.

Presbycusis is a common type of hearing loss in older people. It is characterized by changes in the delicate workings of the inner ear that lead to difficulty in understanding speech, and possibly to intolerance for particularly loud sounds, but not to total deafness. Older people with this type of hearing impairment often express their considerable exasperation by saying "Don't shout, I'm not deaf."

Although presbycusis is generally associated with aging, it does not affect everyone (the incidence is about 25 percent in persons between the ages of 60 and 70) and some researchers therefore consider it a disease. It has been shown that prolonged exposure to extremely high noise levels, improper diet, and even one's genetic makeup can determine who does and does not develop this disorder. Although the condition is permanent, there is much a person can do to function well despite this type of hearing deficit.

Conduction deafness is another form of hearing loss sometimes experienced by the elderly. It involves blockage or impairment of mechanical movement in the outer or middle ear, interfering with proper transmission of sound waves through the ear. There are several possible causes, including packed ear wax, retained fluid, abnormal bony growth, infection, and a disease called otosclerosis.

Persons with this problem find that while other people's voices sound muffled, their own voice sounds louder than normal. As a result, they often speak softly. Flushing of the ear, instillation of medication, or surgery are possible treatments, depending upon the cause.

Central deafness is a third type of hearing loss that occurs in the elderly, although it is much rarer than the others. It is caused by damage to the nerve centers within the brain. While sound levels are not affected, understanding of words is generally impaired.

Possible causes include extended illness with high fever, prolonged exposure to extremely loud noises, use of certain drugs, head injury, vascular problems, and tumors. Central deafness cannot be treated medically or surgically, but special speech training can be beneficial.

Physical examination and test results will determine the most effective treatment for a specific hearing disorder. Medical treatment such as flushing of the ear canal may be all that is needed for some persons, while others may require corrective surgery.

In some cases, a hearing aid will be recommended. This is a small device that amplifies sounds. Hearing aids can be purchased only with a written statement from a physician verifying that a hearing impairment has been diagnosed and a hearing aid is recommended.

■ About Hearing Aids

The purchase of a hearing aid should be considered carefully. Many models are available, offering different features for various types of hearing impairment. While one's specific hearing deficit may limit the selection of devices, it is important to choose one that is comfortable and convenient while providing excellent sound quality. These are features only the consumer can judge, and they are important for long-term satisfaction with the device.

Many people do not use their hearing aids once they have them, usually because they find them inconvenient and uncomfortable in day-to-day use. In choosing a hearing aid, one should keep in mind that the most expensive device on the market is not necessarily the best device for every individual. If one that sells for less satisfies more personal criteria, that is the better buy. In addition, one should buy a hearing aid with only the features one needs. Extra features usually add to cost and may be unnecessary. Finally, ease of operation is an important consideration, since many hearing aids have controls that are extremely small and difficult to adjust.

In purchasing a hearing aid, remember that you are buying not only a product but also a set of services. These include adjustments that may be needed after the hearing aid has been worn, counseling on the use and maintenance of the device, and a warranty period during which repair services may be obtained free of charge. Many hearing aid dealers offer a free trial period of up to thirty days before the buyer decides on a specific hearing aid. Take advantage of this if offered, since it may take up to a month to become accustomed to a new hearing device.

■ *Communicating Better with Persons Who Have a Hearing Problem*

Observing the following suggestions helps in better communicating with persons who have a hearing problem:

• Speak slightly louder than normal, but do not shout. Shouting may actually distort the message, rather than making it clearer. Also, do not overarticulate, because this too distorts speech sounds.

• Speak from a distance of 3 to 6 feet, and position yourself in good light so that the person can see your lip movement, facial expression, and any other gestures. All these help to convey your message. Avoid chewing or covering your mouth when speaking to persons with hearing impairment. Many people with hearing loss have learned to read lips as a means of understanding.

• Never speak directly into the person's ear. This prevents the listener from making use of visual clues.

• If the listener does not understand what was said, rephrase the thought in short, simple sentences.

• Arrange seating in living quarters and meeting rooms in such a way that no one is more than 6 feet apart from all persons present, and that all are completely visible.

■ *Organizations That Help*

Several organizations exist that deal specifically with hearing problems. Further information about hearing impairment can be obtained by writing to the following organizations:

• American Academy of Otolaryngologists, Inc., 1101 Vermont Avenue, N.W., Washington, DC 20005. The Academy is a professional society of medical doctors specializing in diseases of the ear and related areas. It can provide information on hearing and balance disorders.

• American Speech-Language-Hearing Association, 10801 Rockville Pike, Dept. AP, Rockville, MD 20852 (or call 1-800-638-8255 for the National Association for Hearing and Speech Action). Either organization can answer questions and mail information on hearing aids, hearing loss, and communication methods. They also can provide a list of certified audiologists in each state.

• The Office of Scientific and Health Reports, National Institute of Neurological and Communicative Disorders and Stroke, Building 31, Room 8A06, Bethesda, MD 20892, is the focal point within the Federal Government for research on hearing loss and other communication disorders. Ask for the Institute's pamphlet, "Hearing Loss: Hope Through Research."

• Self-Help for Hard-of-Hearing People (SHHH) is headquartered at 7800 Wisconsin Avenue, Bethesda, MD 20814. SHHH is a nationwide organization for the hard-of-hearing, and publishes a bimonthly journal reporting the experiences of those with hearing loss as well as new research developments. There are many publications available on request.

Aging and the Eyes

Poor eyesight is not an inevitable consequence of aging, but some physical changes that occur with age can result in vision decline. For example, older people may have difficulty with night driving, and they generally need brighter light for close tasks such as reading. (Incandescent light bulbs—the regular household type—provide better illumination than the fluorescent lights frequently used in offices.)

Certain disorders and diseases of the eyes occur more frequently in old age than earlier in life. Since much can be done to prevent or correct these conditions, it is extremely important to have regular eye checkups. Older people should have a complete eye examination every two or three years. The examination should include a vision evaluation and a check for glaucoma.

Persons with diabetes or a family history of eye disease should have their eyes checked more frequently. Diabetic retinopathy, a condition characterized by the bursting of small blood vessels in the eyeball, is a leading cause of blindness. Some researchers are directing their attention to the vascular effects of diabetes in efforts to find a means of preventing vision loss.

People of all ages should seek medical attention as soon as they notice visual changes such as blurring, dimming or loss of vision, eye pain, excessive discharge from the eye, double vision, or redness or swelling of the eye or eyelid.

■ *Common Eye Complaints*

Presbyopia refers to a gradual decline in the ability to focus on close objects or see small print. This condition is common in persons over the age of 40 and often signals the need for reading glasses. People with this condition hold reading material at arm's length to see it better. An early sign of presbyopia is headache or a feeling of eye strain after prolonged reading or close paperwork.

Floaters are tiny spots or specks that float across the field of vision. Most people notice them in well-lighted rooms or outdoors. While floaters are normal and generally harmless, they may be a warning sign of other eye problems, especially if they are associated with the visual perception of light flashes.

Dry eyes occur when the tear glands produce too little lachrymal fluid. This causes itching or burning, and can even reduce vision. An eye specialist can prescribe special eyedrops called "artificial tears" that correct this problem.

Excessive tears may be a sign of increased sensitivity to light, wind, or temperature changes. Protective measures such as sunglasses usually solve the problem. It is important to check with a doctor, however, since excessive tears sometimes indicate a more serious underlying cause such as eye infection or a blocked tear duct, both of which can be treated.

■ *Eye Diseases Common in the Elderly*

Cataracts are cloudy areas in the lens portion of the eye. A normal lens is clear and allows light to enter the eye. When a cataract forms, it interferes with the passage of light into the eye, thus affecting vision.

Cataracts usually develop gradually, without pain, redness, or tearing of the eyes. While some remain small and do not seriously affect vision, larger cataracts can impair eyesight and need to be surgically removed. Cataract operations are safe in older people and are almost always successful.

Glaucoma occurs when there is too much fluid pressure in the eyeball, causing internal damage and gradually destroying vision. If untreated, glaucoma can lead to blindness, whereas early detection and treatment will prevent vision loss. The treatment of glaucoma consists of the use of special eye drops, medications, and laser therapy or surgery.

Since glaucoma seldom produces early warning signs, it is extremely important to have regular eye examinations that include a check for this condition.

Retinal disorders are a leading cause of blindness in the United States. The retina is a thin lining on the back of the eye. It is made up of nerves whose special function is to receive visual images and pass them on to the brain. Retinal disorders include senile macular degeneration, diabetic retinopathy, and retinal detachment.

Senile macular degeneration is a condition in which the macula, a specialized part of the retina responsible for sharp vision, loses its ability to function efficiently. The first signs may be blurring of reading matter and visual distortion of certain images. Early detection is important, since some cases respond well to laser treatment.

Diabetic retinopathy is one of the possible complications of diabetes, and occurs when the small vessels that bring blood to the retina are damaged. In the early phase of the disease, these blood vessels may leak fluid, causing distorted vision. At later stages, new vessels may grow and release blood, resulting in loss of vision.

Retinal detachment refers to a separation between the inner and outer layers of the retina. A detached retina usually can be reattached surgically, with good—or at least partial—restoration of vision. New surgical techniques are being used with increasing success.

■ *Low-Vision Aids*

Persons who have visual impairment but are not totally blind may be helped by what are called *low-vision aids*. These include various devices that provide more seeing power than regular eyeglasses. Low-vision aids include telescopic glasses, light-filtering lenses, and the age-old magnifying glass. Some are designed to be hand-held, while others rest directly on reading material. Partially sighted persons frequently notice an improvement in their ability to perform daily tasks with the use of low-vision aids.

■ *More Information on Vision*

Additional information on eye care and eye disorders may be obtained from the following sources:

• The National Eye Institute conducts and supports research on eye disease and the visual system. Free brochures on eye disorders may be obtained by writing to the Office of Scientific Reporting, National Eye Institute, Building 31, Room 6A32, Bethesda, MD 20892.

• The National Society to Prevent Blindness is located at 79 Madison Avenue, New York, NY 10016. Upon request, it will send pamphlets containing information on specific diseases affecting the eyes.

• The American Foundation for the Blind, 15 West 16th Street, New York, NY 10011, will mail a list of its free publications upon request.

Diabetes Mellitus

This is a disorder in which the body cannot convert foods properly into energy needs for daily activity.

Normally, dietary sugars and starches are converted into a sugar called glucose. Glucose is a type of fuel that circulates in the bloodstream and is available to meet immediate energy requirements. Glucose exceeding the body's immediate needs is stored in the liver as glycogen for future use.

In diabetes, the mechanism that controls the amount of glucose in the blood does not function normally, and glucose then accumulates in the blood at dangerous levels that may cause damage to body organs. Blood glucose levels that are either too high (hyperglycemia) or too low (hypoglycemia) can lead to serious medical emergencies. In the case of hyperglycemia, diabetic coma is always a danger. Persons who are in diabetic coma should be given insulin, while those in hypoglycemia should be given some source of sugar.

It is important that family members and close associates of persons with diabetes be familiar with the signs and symptoms of these two conditions. Hyperglycemia is characterized by dryness of the skin and flushing, with exaggerated breathing (as if the victim were not receiving sufficient air). Hypoglycemia, on the other hand, is characterized by moist and pale skin, generalized weakness, absence of hunger or thirst, abnormal behavior, and normal or shallow respirations.

In addition to these immediate perils, persons with diabetes are more subject than nondiabetic persons to stroke, blindness, heart disease, kidney failure, gangrene, and nerve damage.

Although diabetes may run in families, causative factors other than heredity have been identified. For example, being overweight can trigger diabetes in susceptible older persons.

There are two main types of diabetes: Type I, or insulin-dependent diabetes, and Type II, or non-insulin-dependent diabetes. The insulin-dependent type is the more severe form of the disease. Although it can appear at any age, insulin-dependent diabetes usually starts at early ages and requires lifelong treatment with insulin.

The far more common form of diabetes is Type II. Previously referred to as "adult onset" diabetes, this type accounts for more than 85 percent of all cases. As its name implies, people with non-insulin-dependent diabetes do not need insulin injections. Usually they can keep their blood glucose levels normal by controlling their weight, exercising, and following a prescribed diet. Often tablets are needed.

■ Detecting Diabetes

Sometimes the first sign of diabetes is detected on routine physical examination through the finding of glucose in the urine. In other cases, the problem is diagnosed through a glucose tolerance test, which measures the level of glucose in the bloodstream before, and at timed intervals after, one drinks a special glucose solution.

As indicated in Chapter 28 (see "Age-Related Digestive Changes"), some increase in blood glucose levels may occur normally with age, and the standards for diagnosing diabetes in older persons have been revised accordingly.

Other symptoms of diabetes include a "rundown" feeling, increased thirst, more frequent need to urinate, unexplained weight loss, blurred vision, infections or itching of the skin, and slow healing of cuts and bruises. Anyone with such problems should report them promptly to a physician.

■ Treatment

While diabetes cannot be cured, it can be controlled. Effective control requires a careful blend of diet, exercise, and, if necessary, the administration of insulin or oral medication.

Diets for diabetics are worked out under the guidance of a physician. In planning a diet, the doctor considers the patient's weight and the amount of physical activity he or she engages in each day. For overweight persons, a weight-reducing diet is essential for achieving adequate blood glucose control. Food exchange lists are helpful in meal-planning, and may be obtained from the doctor or from the American Diabetes Association.

Exercise is important in the management of diabetes because it helps the body burn some of the excess glucose. When a doctor incorporates an exercise regimen into a diabetic's schedule, the patient should adhere to it faithfully.

A person with non-insulin-dependent diabetes may require short-term treatment with insulin during an acute illness. It is necessary, therefore, to alert one's doctor about any changes in health.

Proper foot care is essential for persons with diabetes, since the disease can seriously reduce circulation to the feet. Care includes daily examination for redness, patches, sores, blisters, breaks in the skin, infections, or buildup of calluses. All such changes should be reported to the physician.

Care of the skin on other parts of the body is also important. This should include protection against injury, general cleanliness, and use of skin softeners to treat dryness. To avoid infection, teeth and gums should receive special attention. Persons who have diabetes should tell their dentists that they have this disorder, and consult them promptly about any mouth problems that occur.

Self-care is all-important in the management of diabetes. By adhering to the prescribed diet, a regular exercise plan, and general good health habits, the diabetic should be able to enjoy a normal and productive life. Additional information on diabetes can be obtained by writing to the American Diabetes Association, 2 Park Avenue, Box AP, New York, NY 10016.

Temperature-Related Disorders of Aging

As one ages, the body becomes less able to respond to prolonged exposure to heat or cold. In cold weather, older people may develop hypothermia, a condition characterized by a drop in body temperature which can be fatal if not detected and treated promptly. During hot and humid weather, on the other hand, a buildup of body heat can cause heat stroke or heat exhaustion in the elderly. Persons with heart or circulatory disease, diabetes, or stroke are especially vulnerable to temperature extremes.

■ Hypothermia

Hypothermia is characterized by a body temperature of 95°F (35°C) (normal is 98.6°F [37°C]) or under. It can occur in anyone who is exposed to severe cold, but as persons age they are more easily affected by the cold.

The elderly who are most likely to develop hypothermia are the chronically ill, the poor who are unable to afford adequate heating, and those who are unaware of the danger and therefore do not adequately protect themselves. In a small number of elderly persons, the temperature-regulating mechanisms become impaired to the point that these persons do not feel cold or shiver. They are at great risk, because they cannot produce body heat—the physiologic purpose of the shivering response—when they most need it.

The only way to detect hypothermia is to use a special low-reading thermometer, available in most hospitals. However, a regular thermometer will serve the purpose as long as it is shaken down well below the 98.6°F (37°C) mark. If the body temperature is below 95°F (35°C) or does not register, emergency help is needed. Other signs to look for are an unusual appearance or behavior during cold weather, a slow and sometimes irregular heartbeat, slurred speech, shallow and very slow breathing, a general feeling of sluggishness, and evidence of mental confusion.

■ Heat-Related Illnesses

Heat stroke is a medical emergency requiring immediate treatment by a physician. Symptoms include faintness, dizziness, headache, nausea, and possible loss of consciousness. The body temperature is usually 104°F (40°C) or higher, the pulse is rapid, and the skin is flushed.

Heat exhaustion takes longer to develop than other heat-related illnesses. It results from a prolonged loss of body fluid and salt caused by perspiration. Symptoms include weakness, heavy perspiration, nausea, and a feeling of giddiness. Heat exhaustion is treated by resting in a cool place and drinking plenty of cool liquids.

■ Protective Measures

The ideal room temperature for older persons has not been established scientifically. Most experts agree that 65°F (18.3°C) in living and sleeping areas should be adequate for most people. Measures one can take to prevent accidental hypothermia include:

• Dressing warmly even when indoors, eating enough, and staying as active as possible.

• Keeping warm in bed by wearing enough nightclothes and using plenty of blankets. Hypothermia often starts during the night, when the body's temperature and most biologic functions are at their lowest.

• Asking a doctor's advice on which, if any,

medications taken may predispose to hypothermia.

• Making sure that friends or neighbors look in or call once a day during spells of particularly cold weather. Some communities have a telephone check-in or personal visiting service for elderly persons who are homebound.

In *hot weather*, the best precaution is to remain indoors, preferably in an air-conditioned room, during heat spells. Those who have no air conditioning at home might take a break from the heat by planning to spend the hottest part of the day at air-conditioned places such as libraries, stores, or movie houses.

Other effective ways to cool off include taking cool baths or showers, placing icebags or wet towels on the body, and using electric fans. In addition, it is wise to:

• Stay out of direct sunlight and avoid strenuous activity.

• Wear lightweight, light-colored, and loose-fitting clothing that permits perspiration to evaporate.

• Drink plenty of fluids—especially water, fruit juices, and iced tea—to replace the fluid lost through perspiration. Avoid alcoholic beverages, however, since these do not help in replenishing heat-related fluid loss.

• Seek a doctor's advice before taking salt tablets.

• Pay attention to danger signals such as dizziness, nausea, and general fatigue.

■ How to Get Assistance

Many older people run the risk of hypothermia by trying to save on fuel costs in the winter. They and their families should be aware that there are government-funded programs to help low-income families pay high energy bills, insulate their homes, or even get emergency repairs of heating or cooling devices. The local community-action agency or Area Agency on Aging can refer inquiries to the proper source of assistance.

The brochure, "A Winter Hazard for the Old: Accidental Hypothermia," can be obtained by writing to the National Institute on Aging/Hypo, Building 31, Room 5C35, Bethesda, MD 20892.

Anemia in the Elderly

The incidence of anemia increases with advancing age, and is associated with reduced levels of hemoglobin, a protein present in the red blood cells of circulating blood. Anemia in the elderly generally is believed to stem from dietary deficiencies, particularly of iron, folic acid, and vitamin B_{12}.

There are several types of anemia, the best known of which is iron-deficiency anemia. Anemia can also develop due to chronic inflammatory conditions, such as rheumatoid arthritis, which depress bone-marrow function. This is the type of anemia most frequently seen in the elderly. In some cases, anemia is the first sign of a malignant tumor.

For this reason, older people who learn that they are anemic through a laboratory report should never undertake self-treatment by iron replacement. They should seek a doctor's advice. Proper medical evaluation is extremely important because anemia in the elderly is more likely to have a serious underlying cause than in younger persons.

Anemia is particularly prevalent in the low-income aged population. In one study, about 20 percent of predominantly low-income elderly persons were found to have deficient hemoglobin levels.

Aging Bones and Joints

The two primary diseases of the skeletal system affecting older persons are *rheumatoid arthritis* (RA) and *osteoarthritis* (OA). The term "arthritis" means inflammation of a joint. The disease categories commonly known as arthritis or rheumatism include over a hundred specific conditions which vary in their symptoms and probable cause. Although the underlying pathology of some of these conditions is well understood, the cause of most arthritic conditions remains unclear. In spite of this, many effective treatments are available.

■ *Rheumatoid Arthritis (RA)*

Rheumatoid arthritis is characterized by inflammation of joint membranes—the tissue coverings of joints that facilitate movement and protect against structural damage due to the constant activity of the joint. RA is a condition with a wide range of progression: Some sufferers are only mildly uncomfortable; others are crippled. Approximately three times more women than men are affected, and usually the condition first becomes evident during middle age.

While RA can affect many body systems, the most frequent sites of involvement are the joints of the fingers, wrists, elbows, knees, and ankles. Persistent swelling and pain in affected joints are typical symptoms, and morning stiffness of affected joints is particularly characteristic of RA.

Rheumatoid arthritis should be treated as soon as it is diagnosed, because uncontrolled inflammation of joint membranes can damage joints and worsen the condition.

■ *Osteoarthritis (OA)*

Compared to rheumatoid arthritis, osteoarthritis is often a mild condition that causes no symptoms in many people and only occasional joint pain and stiffness in others. Some people, on the other hand, experience considerable pain and as well as disability from OA.

Osteoarthritis is referred to also as "degenerative joint disease," which many believe to be a more accurate description of its pathology. While wear and tear on the inside surfaces of joints is believed to cause OA in many instances, hereditary factors and overweight are believed to play a role in determining who does and who does not become afflicted.

Although osteoarthritis usually is diagnosed in older people, like RA, it can occur at younger ages, particularly following injury to a joint. The large weight-bearing joints of the knees, hips, and spine are most frequently affected by osteoarthritis.

■ *Treatment Options*

The objectives in treating arthritis are to relieve pain and stiffness, halt further joint destruction, and maintain mobility.

Several medical treatments are used, the most traditional being aspirin. While it is effective is reducing pain and joint inflammation, aspirin should be taken only under medical supervision. This is because quite large doses often are necessary to achieve relief, and a common side effect of aspirin is irritation of the lining of the stomach and even the production of ulcers. "Soluble" aspirin is much safer.

Acetaminophen—an aspirin substitute—does not reduce inflammation but it does relieve pain. So called arthritis-strength aspirin is generally aspirin combined with a small amount of caffeine or antacid.

Newer prescription medications used in place

of aspirin are the nonsteroidal anti-inflammatory drugs (NSAIDs). These include ibuprofen (now also available in over-the-counter preparations), naproxen, fenoprofen, tolmetin, and sulindac. Their painkilling effect is similar to that of aspirin, and they are extremely effective in reducing associated inflammation.

The NSAIDs are a relatively safe class of drugs, and they may have fewer side effects than aspirin. Some may cause fluid retention, which is a drawback in patients with conditions like congestive heart failure. Indomethacin, oxyphenbutazone, and phenylbutazone are older NSAIDs that provide effective pain relief, but they may have more side effects than the newer agents.

Simple physical activity, or a schedule of physical therapy, is vital in the treatment of arthritic conditions. It is natural for persons suffering from painful joints to want to avoid movement, but immobility, while it may reduce inflammation, also causes the joints to stiffen.

Daily exercise like walking or swimming helps maintain joint mobility. Good posture and avoidance of overweight help relieve stress on the large joints of the body.

Surgery may be required in patients with RA or OA who do not obtain sufficient relief from medical therapy. Hip- and knee-joint replacements are now quite common. The purpose of surgery is to relieve pain and restore function when other forms of treatment have been unsuccessful.

■ Arthritis Warning Signs

Any joint symptom lasting longer than six weeks should be checked with a doctor, no matter how mild it appears. A physical examination, X-ray studies, and specific laboratory tests can identify the specific type of arthritis. Important early warning signs are:
- pain, tenderness, or swelling in one or more joints
- pain and stiffness in the morning
- recurring or persistent pain and stiffness in the neck, lower back, or knees
- symptoms such as these that disappear and then return

■ Making Life Easier for Arthritis Sufferers

The American Association of Retired Persons has published "The Gadget Book," which describes the many devices available to help arthritics in the performance of routine daily tasks. It can be obtained by writing to AARP Books, 1900 East Lake Avenue, Glenview, IL 60025.

More information about arthritis treatment and research can be obtained by writing to the Arthritis Foundation, 3400 Peachtree Road, N.E., Room 1101, Atlanta, GA 30326.

Osteoporosis

Osteoporosis, which is characterized by gradual loss of total bone mass with a resulting increase in the risk of fractures, is estimated to affect about 20 million elderly Americans. The condition occurs more often in women than men, and one in every 4 women over 60 years of age suffers fractures of the spine, hip, or wrist.

This disease is a major public health concern, as the consequences can be catastrophic, especially with fracture of the hip. Up to 20 percent of elderly victims of hip fracture die of complications within one year, and half of those who survive require long-term nursing-home care.

Osteoporosis develops silently over a period of many years. Bones maintain themselves throughout life by a process known as remodeling, in which small amounts of old bone are removed and new bone is formed in its place. Beginning at about age 35, more bone is lost than is gained, causing a reduction in total bone mass.

Women are at greater risk of fractures because their total bone mass is less than that of men. In addition, the female hormone estrogen appears to play a preventive role in the disease until menopause, when the body no longer produces estrogen. Calcium is an important factor in bone remodeling, and daily requirements for women change after menopause.

Some physicians recommend that women take 1,000 milligrams of calcium per day prior to menopause, and increase this to 1,500 to 2,000 mg., depending on whether or not they are receiving estrogen replacement therapy (ERT). ERT has been recognized as a major factor in preventing osteoporosis in postmenopausal women. The results of one clinical trial suggest that ERT may be more effective than calcium supplementation in preventing postmenopausal bone loss.

While older men are not exempt from the disease, osteoporosis generally occurs less frequently, and at older ages, in men than in women.

■ Some Risk Factors

Some women are more likely to develop osteoporosis than others because of the presence of several risk factors. These include fair skin, small bone structure, a Northern European extraction, cigarette smoking, heavy drinking, and a family history of osteoporosis. In addition, women who have had their ovaries removed (complete hysterectomy) early are at greater risk than those undergoing natural menopause.

■ Early Signs

Unfortunately, osteoporosis is a disease in which the first symptom often is a traumatic fracture. However, one early sign of the disorder is loss of height that is greater than that which one would normally expect to occur with increasing age. The cause is compression of the spinal column, with eventual fracture and collapse. This is visible as a curving of the spine, and is often referred to as "dowager's hump."

■ Prevention

Certain dietary and exercise habits can help prevent osteoporosis. These include an adequate daily intake of calcium to promote the remodeling of new bone, and weight-bearing exercises to help strengthen existing bone. Older women who exercise should take care not to place undue stress on the spine. Walking, bicycling, and low-impact aerobics are good.

The daily diet should include foods that are high in calcium (see Table 1, Chapter 28). It is also important to get adequate amounts of vitamin D, since this vitamin is needed for the utilization of calcium. Scientists recommend 400 I.U. daily. Fortified milk and cereals, eggyolk, saltwater fish, and liver contain vitamin D.

The treatment of osteoporosis consists primarily of prevention measures to stop further bone loss. Post-menopausal women should discuss with their physicians the important question of estrogen-replacement therapy. For most, this can be very valuable, but for some, risks are involved—especially those with a history of breast cancer.

While calcium and vitamin D will slow the rate of bone loss, they will not stimulate the formation of new bone. Several bone-restoring drugs are under investigation, however, and at least some of them appear promising.

DISEASES OF THE HEART AND BLOOD VESSELS

As people age, their heart and blood vessels become more susceptible to heart attack, congestive heart failure, high blood pressure, and stroke. While some conditions such as high blood pressure can be treated or prevented, the occurrence of a heart attack or stroke is often the consequence of lifelong wear and tear on an organ system.

Hypertension (High Blood Pressure)

Earlier in this guide we discussed the physiology of the heart (see Wellness, "The Healthy Heart"), the meaning of blood pressure (see under The A–Z of Medicine), and the method used to determine blood pressure (see under Tests). Here we will discuss the management of the condition known as "high blood pressure," or hypertension.

Hypertension affects 37 million Americans over the age of 55. It is a potentially dangerous killer, because it does not produce any warning symptoms. Hypertension is a known risk factor for heart attack and stroke—diseases that cause nearly 1 million deaths a year in the United States. As yet, no one knows exactly what causes hypertension, although several theories have been put forth. Body chemistry, emotion, hereditary factors, overweight, and high sodium intake are believed to have causative roles.

■ Hypertension Can Be Controlled

Because hypertension is a risk factor for heart attack and stroke, it is important that the condition be diagnosed and treated promptly. Most hypertension falls into the category called "essential," meaning that there is no known underlying cause. Only a small percentage of persons with high blood pressure have "secondary hypertension" stemming from certain other medical problems.

The good news about hypertension is that in most people it can be controlled with diet and/or medical therapy. The type and severity of high blood pressure, as well as consideration of associated medical conditions, determines whether medical therapy is indicated. A wide variety of medications is available for the treatment of hypertension.

Many people are under the mistaken impression that once their blood pressure is brought down by medical or dietary measures, it is no longer necessary to adhere to the diet or to take medication. On the contrary: If the doctor has prescribed a medication for high blood pressure, it is probably necessary to take it for the rest of one's life, although the dosage may be altered to accommodate changing needs. For example, some medications have the effect of building up tolerance when used over a long period of time, and slight increases in the dosage are needed to overcome this response. Such increases should never be initiated by patients themselves, however. In addition, doctors may prescribe another drug if the one being taken causes side effects.

Persons whose blood pressure elevation is mild may not need to take medication, provided they reduce their sodium intake and their weight. Those with high blood pressure can help control their condition by remembering that:

• A person with hypertension may not feel sick, but hypertension is serious and should be treated by a doctor.

• Blood pressure can be lowered with medications, but it will rise again if medicine is not taken regularly.

• Taking medication at the same time each day helps establish a regular and easily remembered routine.

• Weight reduction, reduced salt intake, and exercise are helpful, but they are not a substitute for medical therapy in many people with high blood pressure.

The long-term presence of untreated hypertension leads to many serious conditions in older people, including stroke, heart disease, and kidney failure. One can reduce the risk of developing these problems by getting, and adhering to, proper treatment.

Further information on hypertension may be obtained by writing to the High Blood Pressure Information Center, 120/80 National Institutes of Health, Bethesda, MD 20892.

Atherosclerosis

Atherosclerosis, formerly referred to as "hardening of the arteries," contributes directly to heart attack and stroke. It is a slow, progressive condition that begins early in life. The development of atherosclerosis may be prevented or slowed, however, when risk factors such as high blood pressure, cigarette smoking, and elevated blood cholesterol are modified.

In atherosclerosis, the inner walls of the arteries become thickened and irregular as a result of the deposition of fatty substances. When the inner diameter of the artery—called the *arterial lumen*—becomes narrowed, the blood cannot flow as efficiently to the various parts of the body. There is an increased risk of clot formation due to "platelet aggregation." This refers to the tendency of blood platelets to congregate at sites of damage or injury (in this case, fatty deposits). In turn, clot formation in the arteries blocks off blood supply to the brain, heart, or other vital organs. The result can be a heart attack or a stroke, depending upon where the circulatory blockage occurs.

Coronary Artery Disease

Coronary artery disease is caused by atherosclerosis involving the three major coronary arteries that supply the heart with the blood it needs to function. This is the most common form of serious heart disease in the United States, and it is the major cause of chest pain (angina pectoris) and heart attack (myocardial infarction).

■ Angina Pectoris

Angina pectoris is not a heart attack. Rather, it refers to the chest pain felt when the supply of blood to the heart muscle is insufficient to meet energy needs. The coronary arteries are the source of the heart's own blood supply. Angina occurs during intense physical activity when the demand for oxygen increases; it occurs also in cold temperature, when normal vascular constriction in response to cold causes a decrease in blood supply. Thus, angina is known to stem from two primary causes: an increase in the demand for, or a decrease in the supply of, oxygenated blood.

Episodes of angina usually are brief, lasting for a few minutes. Patients describe anginal pain as a feeling of heaviness, tightness, burning, pressure, or squeezing around the breastbone. Other symptoms include a feeling of tightness in the jaw and pain in the arms or the back. Some persons experience discomfort at the level of the upper abdomen, just below the breastbone. This type of angina can easily be mistaken for indigestion.

Angina pectoris is brought on by physical exertion or emotional stress, and is relieved by rest and by taking nitroglycerin. While attacks of angina are uncomfortable—and may be disabling if they produce severe pain and occur frequently—they do not permanently damage the heart. Permanent damage as a result of cell death due to a prolonged inadequate supply of oxygen to the heart muscle is the feature that distinguishes heart attack from angina. Angina is viewed as a warning signal that heart attack may occur however.

In patients with angina pectoris, indications for seeing a doctor include:

• *First occurrence of angina.* While a chronic pattern of recurrent attacks is not necessarily dangerous, at the time of the first angina attack the seriousness of the underlying atherosclerosis has not yet been established. Atherosclerotic obstruction of the coronary arteries may not produce symptoms until it is far advanced, thus it is important to establish the status of these vessels. This is best done by *coronary angiography*, also called *cardiac catheterization.*

• *Change in the pattern of angina.* A sudden change in the pattern of angina may signal an impending heart attack. Similarly, an increase in the frequency of attacks, or a lessening of the amount of activity necessary to provoke chest pain, must be reported to the physician at once.

• *Rest pain.* In persons who usually had angina only on physical or emotional exertion, the development of chest pain while at rest must be reported to the physician, since this may signify a worsening of the underlying coronary artery disease.

• *Prolonged pain that persists longer than usual* and is not promptly relieved by nitroglycerin may signify a developing heart attack. This constitutes a medical emergency.

■ *Coronary-Artery Bypass Surgery*

When angiography reveals a certain type or severity of coronary arterial obstruction for which surgical intervention is appropriate, the patient usually is encouraged to undergo coronary bypass surgery. This operation is frequently performed, and the techniques are sufficiently advanced to allow surgery regardless of age in those who are otherwise healthy candidates.

Coronary bypass surgery involves implanting grafts to bypass obstructed areas in the coronary arteries. Usually the grafts are taken from the saphenous vein of the thigh. It is now possible to bypass more than one coronary artery, and each such bypass increases the oxygen supply to the heart muscle.

Much educational help is available today about the coronary-artery bypass operation, its aftermath, and what it will and will not accomplish. Reading materials on the subject are available at bookstores and libraries.

Those who are hesitant to undergo this operation, on the basis of age or other reasons, should know about the group called "Mended Hearts." This is a voluntary association of persons who have had bypass operations and are willing to share their experience with those considering such surgery.

Heart Attack

Heart attack, or *myocardial infarction*, refers to the occurrence of a prolonged reduction of oxygen supply to an area of the heart, resulting in the death of cells in that region. A heart attack produces irreversible damage, and functioning of necrotic (dead) muscle cannot be restored by coronary-artery bypass surgery. Thus, no benefit would be obtained from surgical bypass of coronary arteries leading to such an area. Benefit might be derived, however, from bypass to undamaged areas of heart muscle when the coronary artery supplying those areas is found to be obstructed. Thus, a heart attack does not automatically rule out the potential for benefit from bypass surgery.

In all persons who have had a heart attack, an area of the heart muscle is no longer able to participate in the total work of contraction. If the damaged area is large enough, this can contribute ultimately to the development of complications such as congestive heart failure.

■ *Heart Rhythm Disturbances*

Several serious complications are associated with heart attack. These include life-threatening disturbances of heart rhythm (arrhythmias) and heart failure. The likelihood of arrhythmic complications is greatest during the immediate period after the heart attack when patients are in the hospital and under constant monitoring. Medical treatment consists of the use of several drugs, including propranolol and nitroglycerin (either sublingually to prevent angina, or in a long-acting slow-release form). In addition, patients usually are given an antiarrhythmic agent such as quinidine.

The majority of heart rhythm disturbances are not life-threatening, though many require some type of treatment.

A condition that may develop in older people is *heart block*—interference with the functioning of the heart's conduction system. Normally, the heartbeat is regulated by the conduction of electric impulses from one chamber to the other. Together these result in a uniform contraction of the heart, which is felt as the pulse rate.

Some forms of heart block require treatment by implantation of a pacemaker, a device that establishes a more reliable rhythm by regulating the heartbeat electronically.

Modern pacemaker technology is quite advanced; pacemakers now include such features as external programming and telephone monitoring. The former means that the physician can readjust the device according to changing demands without the need to remove and reimplant it, as was necessary in the past. Telephone monitoring enables patients with a pacemaker to transmit a recording of their heart rhythm to a central medical facility where it is received and interpreted.

The actual implantation of a pacemaker device is considered a minor operation, requiring only a day or two of hospitalization. Patients with pacemakers often report great relief of symptoms like dizziness or feelings of faintness.

Stroke (Cerebral Vascular Accident)

The word *stroke* originally was used to describe any sudden catastrophic illness. Today it is used almost exclusively to describe sudden paralysis caused by brain damage.

There are two major types of stroke. Most common are strokes caused by interruption or blockage of the circulation to a part of the brain—much like the obstruction that causes angina or a heart attack. The second type of stroke is caused by sudden bleeding into the brain substance, caused by the rupture of blood vessels.

Brain tissue that is deprived of oxygen for even a few seconds stops functioning. When blood circulation to the brain stops for a few minutes, brain tissue cells die. The resulting loss of voluntary motion is called *paralysis*. Paralysis usually is confined to the side of the body where function is regulated by the affected portion of the brain.

Risk Factors

There are a number of identifiable risk factors known to increase the risk of stroke. These include hypertension, atherosclerosis, heart disease, diabetes, and a family history of heart disease and/or stroke.

Other conditions, less certainly identified as risk factors but also believed to contribute to the likelihood of stroke, include high blood levels of cholesterol, obesity, and cigarette smoking. Individuals who have one or more of these conditions or habits are considered to be at greater risk than persons in whom they are fewer or absent.

Statistics indicate that although stroke can occur at any age, it is more common in people over 60. Men have more strokes than women, and blacks have more strokes than whites.

Transient Ischemic Attack (TIA)

A stroke can develop gradually or occur suddenly. An example of a gradual pattern of stroke onset is the occurrence of transient ischemic attacks (TIAs). *Ischemia* is a medical term meaning that the oxygen supply to a particular part of the body is insufficient to meet its cellular demands for sustaining life.

The occurrence of TIAs warrants immediate medical attention, since they may be a warning sign of impending stroke. Symptoms consist of a brief period of weakness and loss of speech or sensation, usually lasting for minutes to hours. TIAs are believed to be caused by a sudden, but temporary, decrease in blood flow to a portion of the brain.

Usually a person with TIAs reports one or more of the following: sudden onset of numbness, a sensation of tingling or weakness on one side of the body, temporary blindness in one or both eyes, difficulty in understanding words and using them correctly, dizziness, nausea, vomiting, staggering, and fuzzy speech. Consciousness is not lost during an attack, and victims quickly recover with no after effects.

When any of these symptoms is noted, it is extremely important to notify a physician immediately, even though the episode may pass as quickly as it came. Knowing and heeding such symptoms can help prevent the occurrence of a complete stroke with permanent damage.

The medical evaluation of TIAs includes a complete neurologic examination to determine whether the cause of the condition can be corrected. Most TIAs are caused by the buildup of atherosclerotic deposits on the interior surfaces of arterial walls.

Most commonly, the site of arterial obstruction is in the carotid artery, which is accessible to surgical removal of the atherosclerotic material. Such debridement of the carotid artery is one of the treatments of TIA. In addition, medications such as aspirin that reduce blood clotting or prevent blood platelets from clumping together can help stop TIAs and reduce the chance of stroke.

■ Cerebral Infarction

Stroke may be caused by cerebral infarction or hemorrhage. The *cerebrum* is the medical term for the brain, and *infarction* describes the condition in which a portion of the brain dies as a result of inadequate blood supply. The blockage is caused either by atherosclerotic obstruction of blood vessels supplying the brain or by a blood clot in one or more of these vessels.

The consequences of a stroke are weakness, paralysis, and loss of sensation. These symptoms usually become evident in those parts of the body controlled by the affected portion of the brain. The primary distinguishing feature of stroke from TIA is that the effects do not disappear quickly.

Stroke victims need to be hospitalized to make certain that there is no further progression. There is no actual medical treatment for stroke, but improvements in nerve functioning may occur spontaneously. In addition, physical therapy helps restore persons with stroke to optimal physical function.

■ Intracerebral Hemorrhage

Sometimes a major vessel in the brain ruptures, causing bleeding into the brain which permanently destroys or temporarily disrupts brain-cell function. Normally, blood flows to the brain through arteries that are under extremely high pressure. Thus, vessels weakened at their walls are especially susceptible to rupture in the brain. Because the extent of the hemorrhage can be severe—with accompanying damage to large portions of brain tissue—strokes caused by intracranial hemorrhage are more likely to be fatal than those caused by cerebral infarction.

■ Rehabilitation After Stroke

The treatment of paralysis following a stroke is aimed at restoring as much function as possible. This is accomplished by physical therapy, which should be started as soon after a stroke as possible.

At first, rehabilitation is a passive process whereby the therapist moves paralyzed limbs to maintain their potential for motion. Gradually it becomes more action-directed, with the objective of preparing the person for life in the home environment. Physical therapists aim to teach the person to walk alone or with the support of a walker, and to become reasonably independent in the performance of the activities of daily living. In addition to physical therapy, the rehabilitation process may include speech and occupational therapy, nutritional and psychological counseling, and family education programs.

The family is often a key factor in the success of the total rehabilitation effort, since they usually are involved in the long-term care of the stroke victim. With patience and determination, most stroke patients can get better—though they may not recover to the full range of activity they had prior to suffering a stroke.

URINARY TRACT AND RELATED PROBLEMS

Urinary Tract Infection (UTI)

Urinary tract infection (UTI) occurs much more frequently in elderly persons than in the general adult population. In fact, UTI is the second most common cause of febrile illness in those over 65, and the tenth leading cause of death in that population. The fatalities reported with urinary tract infection are related to the development of bacteremia, or infection of the bloodstream. More often, UTI is a chronic and recurrent condition requiring repeated medical treatment.

The incidence of UTI in elderly persons is influenced by environmental factors, with persons living at home having the lowest incidence. The prevalence of UTI in nursing-home patients is considerably greater, but is exceeded by that of the hospitalized elderly. One reason for this is that hospitalization often necessitates urinary catheterization, a procedure that, despite preventive measures, is still associated with a high risk of infection.

Several age-related factors contribute to the development of UTI in the elderly. Both men and women have poorer emptying of the bladder with increasing age, and this results in the retention of residual urine. Incomplete voiding is a problem mainly because it creates an environment that encourages the growth and multiplication of organisms. In addition, many older people drink insufficient fluids and this results in a drop in urinary acidity that favors bacterial growth.

Some anatomic changes that commonly occur in older persons may exacerbate the problem of residual urine retention. These include urinary obstruction caused by prostate enlargement and problems associated with muscle control. Compromise of normal bladder defense mechanisms also contributes to the development of UTI in the elderly.

Despite its prevalence, UTI is often difficult to diagnose in elderly patients and exemplifies how some diseases have unusual presentations at older ages. In younger persons, UTI is easily detectable on the basis of complaints like pain and burning on urination and urgency or frequency of urination. These symptoms may be entirely absent in older patients. On the other hand, many older people who exhibit the typical symptoms do not have UTI.

The primary objectives of treatment are to eradicate the infection and prevent its recurrence. It is extremely important to take medications for the length of time they are prescribed, even if symptoms have disappeared. In this, like many other infections, taking a full course of antibiotic therapy is essential to ensure that organisms do not gain a permanent foothold.

Prostate Problems

The prostate is a male organ about the size of a walnut; it lies under the urinary bladder, around the urethra. During sexual activity, it secretes a fluid that enhances the motility of sperm.

Several prostate problems can occur in men over 50. These include acute and chronic prostatitis (infection of the prostate gland), prostate enlargement, and cancer of the prostate. Most of these problems can be effectively treated without affecting sexual function.

Acute prostatitis is a bacterial infection of the prostate gland that can occur at any age. Symptoms include fever, chills, painful or difficult urination, and pain in the lower back and between the legs. Acute prostatitis can be treated successfully with antibiotics.

Chronic prostatitis is, as the term suggests, a recurring prostate infection. The symptoms are similar to those of acute prostatitis, but are generally milder. Fever is uncommon.

Chronic prostatitis can be difficult to treat, since sometimes no disease-causing bacteria can be identified. Often the condition clears up spontaneously, but symptoms may last a long time.

Benign prostatic hypertrophy (BPH) is, in lay terms, enlargement of the prostate. It is caused by small, noncancerous tumors that grow inside the gland. The cause is uncertain but may be related to hormone changes that occur with aging.

An enlarged prostate gland may eventually obstruct the urethra (the passageway for urine), causing difficulty in urination. Dribbling after urination and the urge to urinate are common symptoms of BPH. In rare cases, the patient is unable to urinate.

Doctors can diagnose prostate enlargement at physical examination. This requires a rectal exam, as well as a measure of how much urine is left in the bladder following urination. This is determined by injecting a dye into a vein. (The dye is safe, and soon disappears from the body.) After injection, the dye serves as an X-ray marker for outlining the urine in the bladder. The physician may also examine the prostate and bladder by inserting an instrument called a cystoscope through the penis.

No drugs are available for the treatment of BPH, and surgery to remove the overgrown portion of the prostate gland may be indicated in severe cases.

Prostate Cancer

Prostate cancer is one of the types of tumors that older persons are particularly prone to develop. In the early stages, the disease remains localized within the prostate gland and does not endanger life. Without treatment, the cancer can spread to surrounding tissues and eventually become fatal through involvement of other body organs.

Prostate cancer generally progresses very slowly, and regular physical checkups (including a rectal exam) usually ensure early detection. While prostate cancer may produce no symptoms, when symptoms do appear they are usually similar to those of BPH.

A *urologist* (a specialist in diseases of the urinary system) is best qualified to diagnose and treat prostate cancer. If a suspicious area is found in the bladder, the urologist may recommend a biopsy, a simple surgical procedure in which a tiny piece of tissue is removed for microscopic examination.

When the cancer is confined to the prostate gland, the cure rate is high. Even cancers that have spread beyond the gland often are controlled for long periods.

■ Prostate Surgery

Prostate surgery is performed either to treat BPH or prostate cancer. Such surgery is quite safe, and patients recover rapidly.

For the treatment of BPH, it is common to remove only the portion of the prostate gland directly obstructing the flow of urine through the urethra. This is referred to sometimes as a *simple prostatectomy*. This procedure does not damage the nerves that cause erection of the penis, and resumption of normal sexual activity is possible soon after the operation. Transurethral resection of the prostate (TURP) is another surgical procedure commonly used to correct slight or moderate prostate enlargement.

Sexual problems following prostate surgery are usually psychological rather than physiological in origin. Reassurance from one's physician about this aspect of the operation may be all that is necessary to alleviate the problem. If impotence continues, psychological counseling may be indicated.

Aging and Cancer

The ability of certain immune cells to kill human tumor cells diminishes markedly after the age of 50. As a result, many cancers occur more often in people over 50 than in younger persons. When cancers are detected early, the likelihood of successful treatment is greater. The chances of surviving cancer are better today than ever before. It is important to be aware of the early warning signs of cancer, however, and to have regular physical examinations.

■ Common Cancers in Persons Over 50

Lung cancer should be suspected if a cough is persistent, if one is coughing up blood, or if one is short of breath.

Breast cancer should be suspected if lumps appear in the breast, if there is a change in the shape of a breast, or if there is discharge from a nipple.

Colon or rectal cancer should be suspected if there is a change in bowel habits or bleeding from the rectum, or if the stool is black in appearance. Black stool may come from other causes—such as taking certain iron supplements—but it also can indicate bleeding—the blood being responsible for the dark color.

Prostate cancer should be suspected if there is difficulty or pain while urinating or if there is a need to urinate often, especially at night.

Uterine, ovarian, or cervical cancer should be suspected if vaginal bleeding occurs after menopause, if there is an unusual vaginal discharge, or if there is abdominal enlargement or pain during intercourse.

Skin cancer should be suspected if sores do not heal, or if there is a change in the shape, size, or color of an existing wart or mole or the sudden appearance of a new mole.

Persons suspecting a cancer on the basis of the above symptoms should see their doctor at once. Early detection is vitally important in the treatment of all types of cancers. It is not unusual for elderly persons to ignore legitimate medical symptoms on the basis that they are simply part of the aging process. This can lead to the underreporting of significant complaints.

Recommended Medical Tests

Certain medical or laboratory tests are recommended on a regular basis in persons over 50 to facilitate the early detection of some kinds of cancers. Some well-known tests are rectal examination for colon cancer and pelvic examination and Pap smear for cervical cancer. More recently, mammography has come to be considered a vital part of the examination for the prevention of breast cancer.

On the basis of one's medical history and the generally accepted guidelines, the family physician is able to advise how often specific tests should be performed. In persons with a prior history of cancer, tests will be required more frequently than in those who do not have a personal or family history of cancer.

In addition to rectal examination for colon cancer, doctors may request a stool specimen for examination for traces of blood. Simple kits are available for collecting the sample at home.

Pelvic examinations and Pap smears, familiar routine examinations for most adult women, should be continued despite the cessation of reproductive function at the menopause. In fact, this is an important time to see the gynecologist regularly in order to monitor the changes that are taking place in the body.

Breast examination by mammography, a special type of breast X ray, is recommended for all women over 50. Mammography is designed so as to produce the least possible exposure to radiation.

More information about cancer can be obtained from the Cancer Information Service (CIS). The toll-free number is 1-800-422-6237—which is more easily remembered as 1-800-4-CANCER.

Older People and Medications

Although many factors—such as body size and gender—contribute to how an individual responds to medications, one of the most important variables is age. Specifically, scientists are now learning that for many drugs the dosage levels appropriate for middle-aged adults are often too high for the elderly.

This is accounted for partly by age-related changes in the efficiency of some organs such as the kidneys. In addition, changes in the water, fat, and lean-tissue contents of the body that accompany aging may influence the way the body handles drugs. Moreover, older people often receive several medications at once for the treatment of different diseases, and it is well known that some drug interactions can cause undesirable effects.

For these reasons, it is recommended that older patients and their doctors attempt to work together to achieve the simplest possible medical regimen. All too often, older people receive prescriptions from several different physicians who may be unaware of the other medications that person is taking. This can happen, for example, if a patient with a cardiac condition forgets to tell his rheumatologist what heart medications he is taking.

Older people with multiple diseases that require the use of several medications each day may need help in keeping track of their drug schedule. It is helpful to make out simple charts outlining each medication according to how many pills should be taken and at what times to take them. In addition, it is a good idea for patients and physicians to review periodically the existing drug regimen to eliminate those that may no longer be necessary or useful.

Adverse drug reactions are more likely to occur in patients who are taking many drugs. Some of the drug categories most often responsible are:

■ Digitalis Preparations

Several reports have shown that doses of digitalis can be reduced in older patients to lessen the possibility of developing digitalis toxicity. This condition develops gradually as a consequence of long-term buildup of drug levels in the body.

Symptoms of digitalis toxicity include fatigue, loss of appetite, vision problems, nausea, and psychological disturbances. It is common for older people to be given digitalis for longer periods and in larger doses than necessary.

■ Antihypertensive Agents

Many older people receive some type of medication to lower blood pressure. The diuretic type of antihypertensive agents (often called "water pills") cause loss of potassium from the body which in turn can cause fatigue. Potassium in this case should be replenished (see "Minerals," Chapter 19).

In addition, blood-pressure-lowering agents may sometimes lower the pressure suddenly, causing a feeling of faintness. This is especially likely to occur when the person stands up from a lying position.

Other possible side effects of antihypertensive agents in older patients include depression and drowsiness.

■ Sedatives and Tranquilizers

The elderly are more likely than younger adults to experience adverse effects from this widely prescribed class of drugs. Barbiturates are particularly dangerous and may cause reactions ranging from mild restlessness to psychosis (a mental derangement characterized by loss of contact with reality).

Many of the drugs called "minor tranquilizers" belong to a group known as benzodiazepines. It is believed that older people are more likely to have unwanted side effects—which include drowsiness, confusion, and loss of muscular coordination—from this class of drugs than are younger persons.

Some commonly prescribed tranquilizers include diazepam and chlordiazepoxide. Although these drugs are preferable to more powerful tranquilizing agents, it is recommended that each of these agents be used at a lower dosage in elderly persons.

The study of the movement of drugs in the body, called *pharmacokinetics,* is a relatively recent medical discipline. Thus, much more is known today than ever before about the intricate inter- actions that determine specific drug effects and the individual variations that occur.

Physicians are aware of the findings of recent pharmacokinetic studies, and will appreciate their patients' understanding of issues concerning the role of medications in their general health care.

33

ISSUES OF SPECIAL CONCERN TO OLDER PEOPLE

Crime and the Elderly

Crime is a social problem that affects people of all ages and occurs—to a greater or lesser extent—in most regions of the United States. The subject of the elderly as crime victims has received considerable media coverage for some time, and resulting public awareness has led to measures for protecting persons from becoming crime victims.

Increasing emphasis is now placed on crime prevention techniques through such programs as "Neighborhood Watch" (where residents are urged to report to the police any suspicious person or unusual event) and classroom education programs on practical ways to avoid becoming a crime victim. Despite increased public awareness, however, many older people still live in great fear of crime.

In some large urban areas, neighborhoods exist where the elderly are prisoners of their home because of the prevalence of crime. These are generally people who have lived in a particular apartment for many years, and who are reluctant to move because of rent control and the general shortage of housing.

■ *The Elderly as Crime Victims*

Old people are more likely to be victims of crime than younger persons, and they are victimized in a number of ways. In addition to robbery, assault, and murder, old people suffer beating and rape. Their Social Security or Public Assistance pension checks often are stolen from mailboxes, and many are sought out by fortune hunters seeking to make money by a number of schemes ranging from the sale of useless hearing aids to investment fraud.

Addressing the issue of whether stronger police protection and tougher laws are enough to win the battle against crime, a Public Interest Report published in *Aging and Human Development* suggests that cooperation between law enforcement and social service agencies may be a promising future approach to crime prevention. The report concludes that "continuing efforts must be made to deepen our culture's sensibility toward older people and to inaugurate fundamental reforms in income security and social services." It also proposes that "growing political awareness and organization of older people will help in these respects, for they have a massive vote." In other words, older people have considerable political power to help bring about desired changes on their own behalf.

The same report cites the 1970 demonstration study called "Project Assist," which established a network of police-community relations to benefit the old, as a useful model for the development of similar programs in other communities. In the study, conducted in the Washington, DC, metropolitan area, some 220 older persons received direct help such as emergency money, replacement of food stamps, medical assistance, and shelter through social service efforts initiated by police contact with the elderly.

Seventy was the mean age of the Project Assist study population, and robbery was the number one crime. Women were victimized more frequently than men, and blacks more frequently than whites. Many participants in the study were physically and/or mentally impaired in some serious way, adding to their vulnerability to crime. The majority of the study population were poor, and more were on Old Age Assistance than in the city's population as a whole. Widows and single persons were also disproportionately represented in the sample. These findings indicate that to be old, poor, widowed, and a woman increases the chances of crime victimization and/or police contact.

■ Patterns of Crime Against the Elderly

The majority of crimes committed against the elderly population are recorded as "larceny with contact" and include such things as purse-snatching and wallet-stealing. Robberies of all kinds outnumber actual murders of older persons. The incidence of robberies—including the stealing of benefit checks from mailboxes—is greatest in communities where there is a high concentration of older residents. There is also an increasing likelihood of crimes of larceny in areas where older people congregate, such as public housing projects and public transportation facilities. Purse-snatchings are particularly common in supermarkets and shopping malls where people are likely to be carrying money.

The rural community, once considered a haven from the ills of urban life, is no longer safe against crime. The following are some of the research findings from studies conducted by the National Rural Crime Prevention Center at Ohio State University:

- 20 percent of the rural residences and farms occupied by persons aged 60 and over are victimized each year by at least one property crime incident
- vandalism is the leading crime in the countryside
- larceny near the house or on the premises, residential burglary, trespassing, and criminal fraud are also major crime problems for the rural elderly
- less than 40 percent of the crimes committed against older persons are reported to the police or sheriff
- older rural crime victims believe that reporting is useless or that nothing can be done

Since the most frequently committed crimes in rural areas are crimes of opportunity, crime prevention is best furthered by reducing opportunity.

The American Association of Retired Persons (AARP) publishes several pamphlets on specific issues concerning crime and the elderly. These include such topics as how to spot the con artist, how to protect one's rural home, how to conduct a security survey, and how to protect one's car from theft. These may be obtained through any regional AARP branch.

Elder Abuse

Increasing interest in the study of normal aging uncovered an unexpected problem—abuse of the elderly. According to a 1980 report in the *Journal of the American Medical Association*, "Abuse of the elderly is at a stage that child abuse was at 20 years ago. People are horrified at this notion." In 1981, the nationwide occurrence of elder abuse was estimated at 500,000 to 1 million cases per year.

■ Types of Abuse

One issue that social scientists now face is exactly how to define abuse. While several complex definitions have been put forth, they tend to agree on certain common features. It is recognized generally that abuse can be either passive—consisting of general neglect as well as failure to take action in the face of a known need—or active. Active abuse includes the categories of physical, verbal, psychological, financial, and material abuse. (Material abuse refers to measure such as the withholding of food, which, of course, also has psychological effects.)

In fact, the types and patterns of abuse comprise a rather complex problem, involving reporting and identification of the abused. For example, because abuse generally takes place in a family setting, there is a tendency for it to be underreported. Elderly victims of abuse may fear family reprisal and thus not admit to the problem. In addition, medical detection of elder abuse— even when it is physical—is not as certain as with other abused groups.

While abused children and battered wives can generally be identified readily on physical examination, the greater prevalence of bruising injuries among the elderly often makes it hard to distinguish signs of abuse from normal injuries. Since visual, hearing, and circulatory impairments and changes in the skin, soft tissue, blood vessels, and bones that occur with age can result in bruises and pathologic fractures in the course of everyday life, even medical professionals may find it difficult to prove that an elderly patient has been slapped, pushed, or hit.

■ Some Profiles of the Abused and Their Abusers

Despite the potential for all elderly to become victims of abuse, certain characteristics have been identified that give a potential profile of the elderly abused. Based on limited data, abused older people have been identified as predominantly low- or middle-class Protestant women with an average age of 84, who live with relatives. In fact, the term "granny-battering" has been coined to emphasize the frequency of ill treatment of older women—not only in the home but in hospital environments.

However, evidence from more recent research somewhat changes the stereotype of the elderly abuse victim. The results of a recent controlled study assessing risk factors for elder abuse show that the concept of the frail elderly parent as the victim of overburdened or downright cruel family members is not as valid as was commonly believed. The study was more revealing about the abusers and their personality problems.

The notion that physical abuse arises from the strain of caring for a dependent old person found little support in this study. Nor did the study cite prior exposure to family violence as a contributing factor. Instead, the abuser emerged in profile as a psychologically troubled person who resorts to violence as a means of gaining money or goods to compensate for the absence of power in his or her relationship with the victim. Thus,

the trouble often stemmed from dependency of the caretaker on the older family member, rather than the other way around.

The problems surrounding family-violence intervention are well known. Families are reluctant to call for help. When they do, police have little jurisdiction over domestic conflicts occurring in the home. Social service providers and other professionals need to be educated about the potential for spouse abuse among the elderly, and about elder abuse in general.

SUMMARY

As Americans face the twenty-first century, several factors affect the lives of older persons. For one, people are living longer today, and both men and women have a greater life expectancy. The elderly population, therefore, is continuing to increase; it will reach record numbers in the early decades of the next century.

Although the characteristics of family life have changed as a result of divorce, remarriage, and the formation of more and more "step families," the basic functioning of family units remains intact. In general, the relationships between aging parents and their adult children are gratifying, and the ties between the generations usually remain strong.

While economic and social changes have altered the patterns of family life, such factors as the greater participation of women in the work force do not appear to affect the ability of adult children to meet the needs of their aging parents. The younger generation's commitment to act as primary caretakers of aged parents remains strong. And with most aging parents, their children are the preferred source for such help.

Recognition of the often unique clinical needs of older persons has led to greater overall acceptance of geriatrics as a separate branch of medicine. Continued study of the normal aging process by gerontologic researchers can be expected to generate much valuable information about this lengthening stage of the human life cycle.

The insights gained into the medical and social issues of aging are enabling older Americans to lead enjoyable, productive lives long after retirement. No longer looked upon as the end of the most interesting and vital years of one's life, retirement is now viewed as the beginning of an era during which new objectives and goals can be reached.

Increased visibility of seniors, due to their ex-panding ranks, will lead, it is hoped, to increasing efforts to find solutions to problems such as poverty, the high cost of health care, and crime and abuse against the elderly.

THE
FAMILY
HEALTH
RECORDKEEPER

The following charts will help you keep your medical records up to date and readily accessible. By maintaining a comprehensive history, you can enhance communication between yourself and your physician as well as between different specialists caring for you. If you change doctors or move, this record will help ensure the continuity of your care as well as your children's.

The charts are designed to help you start your own record. The medical problems listed will give you an idea of the kind of information that may be called for.

To fill in the charts as fully and correctly as possible, you may need to inquire about the medical histories of relatives, but the effort is worth making. And be sure to keep the charts up to date.

By photocopying these charts, you can keep a record of the medical history of each family member.

FAMILY MEDICAL HISTORY

The purpose of the family medical history is to provide information about family predispositions to particular illnesses. It is an aid to correct diagnosis and thereby to effective treatment. And most important, it can serve as a tool for the prevention of illness. Note all medical problems that have occurred in the members of your immediate family—your mother, father, siblings, maternal and paternal aunts, uncles, and grandparents. If members are deceased, list the cause of death and age at death. The list might include hereditary diseases such as:

ankylosing spondylitis
cystic fibrosis
Down's syndrome
Ehlers-Danlos syndrome
Fabry's disease
galactosemia
glucose-6-phosphate
   dehydrogenase deficiency

hemophilia
Huntington's chorea
Klinefelter's syndrome
Marfan's syndrome
osteogenesis imperfecta
phenylketonuria

retinoblastoma
sickle cell anemia
Tay-Sachs disease
thalassemia
Turner's syndrome
von Willebrand's disease

You should also track those medical problems that are not strictly hereditary but do have a tendency to run in families. These might include:

alcoholism
Alzheimer's disease
anemia
arthritis
asthma
bleeding disorders
cancer
colitis
congenital heart disease
depression
diabetes

hay fever
heart attack
high blood pressure
hypercholesterolemia
kidney disease
leukemia
migraine headache
multiple sclerosis
nervous breakdown
obesity
schizophrenia

seizure disorder (epilepsy)
stroke
suicide
syphilis
thyroid disease
tuberculosis
ulcers
urticaria

FAMILY MEMBER	MEDICAL PROBLEM	AGE AT DEATH	CAUSE OF DEATH

PERSONAL MEDICAL HISTORY

Record your medical problems, both past and present. Include treatments, operations and diagnostic procedures, screening tests, and immunizations.

Name _____

Date of Birth _____ Place of Birth _____ Blood Type _____

CONDITIONS

List conditions such as heart disease, blood vessel disorders, high blood pressure, cancer, adult chest disorders, intestinal diseases (including liver), blood diseases, genito-urinary diseases, ear, nose and throat problems, eye disorders, psychiatric problems, sexually related diseases, infertility, etc.

CONDITION	AGE	DATE	REMARKS

INFECTIONS AND CHILDHOOD ILLNESSES

This list might include cases of botulism, bronchitis, chicken pox, chorea, convulsions, diphtheria, German measles (rubella), gonorrhea, hepatitis, influenza, malaria, measles (rubeola), mononucleosis, mumps, pneumonia, rabies, rheumatic fever, scarlet fever, syphilis, tetanus, tonsillitis, toxoplasmosis, TB, typhoid fever, whooping cough, etc.

ILLNESS	AGE	DATE	REMARKS

CHECKUPS

It's a good idea to keep a list of your visits to the doctor, dentist, etc. This will help you remember when you should make another appointment. In the Remarks column under "Medical Exam," you may want to note blood pressure and weight to give you a long-term perspective on how you are doing.

MEDICAL EXAM	DATE	REMARKS

DENTAL CHECKUP	DATE	REMARKS

EYE EXAM	DATE	REMARKS

HEARING EXAM	DATE	REMARKS

GYNECOLOGIC AND OBSTETRIC RECORDS

	DATE	REMARKS
Start of Menstruation		
Pregnancies		
Miscarriages/Abortions		
Start of Menopause		
Other		

HOSPITALIZATIONS AND SURGICAL PROCEDURES

	AGE	DATE	REMARKS

IMMUNIZATIONS AND SCREENING TESTS

	DATE(S)	REMARKS
DPT (diphtheria, pertussis, tetanus) vaccine		
Hepatitis B vaccine		
Pneumococcal vaccine (pneumonia)		
Polio vaccine		
Rubella vaccine (German measles)		
Influenza vaccine (flu shot)		
Foreign travel protection (malaria, yellow fever, polio, typhoid, etc.)		
TB skin test		
Breast exam/mammogram		
Pap smear		
Blood in stool test		
Cholesterol level/lipid profile		
Osteoporosis test		
Electrocardiogram		
Other		

ALLERGIES AND ALLERGIC REACTIONS

These include hay fever, asthma, hives, insect bites, eczema, plants (ivy, oak, sumac, etc.), foods, chemicals and household products, antibiotics, other medications, and blood transfusions.

ALLERGY	AGE	DATE	REMARKS

ADDITIONAL FACTORS

HISTORY OF (CHECK IF PERTINENT):	REMARKS
Smoking	
Alcohol use	
Caffeine	
Foreign travel (outside North America and Europe)	
Military service	
Exotic pets	
Environmental or toxic exposure (describe):	

MEDICATIONS

It is important to know the names of the medications you are taking, the dosages and the reasons for taking them. When a medication is eliminated from your regimen, make sure to throw out the bottle; otherwise you run the risk of taking more medicine than you need, and increase the chance of side effects, unwanted reactions, and using medicines that have expired. Whenever you visit your physician or the hospital, always bring all your bottles of medication; one of the first questions your doctor will ask you is to name all the medications you are taking. This list also should include vitamins and sedatives.

MEDICINE	DOSAGE AND FREQUENCY	REASON FOR TAKING	DATE

YOUR CHILD'S MEDICAL RECORDS

With this chart you can keep track of your child's development and medical history. Your accurate notations and observations can help a pediatrician better evaluate your child, and will allow you to have a permanent record of your child's growth and milestones.

Child's Name _____

Date of Birth _____ Place of Birth _____ Blood Type _____

AGE	HEIGHT	WEIGHT	AGE	HEIGHT	WEIGHT
At birth					
3 months					
9 months					
1 year					
18 months					
2 years					
3 years					

IMMUNIZATIONS

Parents should ask the pediatrician for a schedule of their child's vaccines in order to know when each booster is due.

IMMUNIZATION	DATE	BOOSTER	BOOSTER
DPT (diphtheria, pertussis, tetanus)			
TOPV (trivalent oral polio vaccine)			
PPD (purified protein derivative — for TB)			
MMR (measles, mumps, rubella)			
DT (diphtheria, tetanus)			
HIB (hemophilus influenza — type B vaccine)			
Other			

TESTS AND ASSESSMENTS

	AGE	DATE	REMARKS
Scoliosis check			
Eye exam			
Hearing test			
Dental checkup			
Other			

ILLNESSES

Childhood illnesses may include chicken pox, German measles (rubella), measles, mumps, whooping cough, diphtheria, roseola, croup, ear infections, convulsions (specify), gastroenteritis, urinary infections, skin disorders (specify), influenza, infectious mononucleosis, etc.

ILLNESS	DATE	REMARKS

OBSERVATIONS AND MILESTONES

Fill in what you would like to record about your child's development. At what age did she first smile? How many months old was he when he began to walk?

ACTIVITY	AGE	REMARKS

OBSERVATIONS AND MILESTONES

ACTIVITY	AGE	REMARKS

INDEX